PRECIS V

An Update in Obstetrics and Gynecology

acog
The American College
of Obstetricians
and Gynecologists
409 12th Street, SW
Washington, DC 20024-2188

Precis V: An Update in Obstetrics and Gynecology represents the knowledge and experience of experts in the field and does not necessarily reflect College policy. Methods and techniques of clinical practice that are currently acceptable and used by recognized authorities are described in this publication. The recommendations do not dictate an exclusive course of treatment or procedure to be followed and should not be construed as excluding other acceptable methods of practice. Variations taking into account the needs of the individual patient, resources, and limitations unique to the institution or type of practice may be appropriate.

Medicine is an ever-changing field. As new research and clinical experience emerge, changes in treatment and drug therapy are required. Every effort has been made to ensure that the drug dosage schedules contained herein are accurate and in accordance with standards accepted at the time of publication. Readers are advised, however, to check the product information literature of each drug they plan to administer in order to be certain that there have been no changes in the dosage recommended or in the contraindications for administration. This is of particular importance for new or infrequently used drugs.

Copyright © 1994 by the American College of Obstetricians and Gynecologists. All rights reserved. Printed in the United States of America. No part of this publication may be reproduced, stored in a retrieval system, or transmitted in any form or by any means, electronic, mechanical, photocopying, recording, or otherwise, without the prior written permission of the publisher. Requests for photocopies should be directed to the Copyright Clearance Center, 222 Rosewood Drive, Danvers, MA 01923.

1234/87654

ISBN 0-915473-22-4

Design
Christine Draughn

Managing Editor
Mary F. Mitchell

CONTENTS

Contributors iv
Preface v

1 Primary and Preventive Care 1
Screening, Counseling, and Immunizations 2
Health Maintenance 8
Management of Medical Disorders 15

2 Office Practice 55
Fertility Control 56
Preconceptional Care 64
Low Abdominal and Pelvic Pain 66
Premenstrual Syndrome 71
Breast Disorders 75
Vaginitis 77
Sexually Transmitted Diseases 82
Pelvic Infections 94
Sexuality and Sexual Dysfunction 97
Crisis Intervention 103
Ethical Issues in Obstetrics and
    Gynecology 111
Epidemiology and Statistical
    Interpretation 116

3 Obstetrics 123
Antepartum Care 124
Physiology of Pregnancy 143
Complications of Pregnancy 152
Medical Complications 163
Intrapartum Management 189
The Newborn 200
The Puerperium 202

4 Gynecology 209
Diagnostic and Surgical Procedures 210
Preoperative Care 224
Nonmalignant Disorders of the Vulva 227
Anatomic Support Defects and
    Dysfunction 230
Urogynecology 234
Disorders of the Uterus 245

Tubal and Peritoneal Factors 250
Disorders of the Ovaries 255
Wound Healing: Techniques and Materials ... 260
Postoperative Care 266
Surgical Complications 270
Sterilization 287
Pregnancy Termination 290

5 Oncology 297
Genetics and Gynecologic Cancer 298
Cancer of the Breast 301
Cancer of the Vulva 307
Cancer of the Vagina 314
Cervical Neoplasia 317
Cancer of the Uterine Corpus 321
Cancer of the Ovary and Uterine Tube 326
Gestational Trophoblastic Disease 337
Cancer and Pregnancy 342
Quality of Life Considerations 354

6 Reproductive Endocrinology
and Fertility 359
Receptor Physiology 360
Neuroendocrinology 361
The Menstrual Cycle 368
Prostaglandins 376
Genetics 379
Pediatric and Adolescent Gynecology 384
Disorders of Menstruation 391
Menopause 401
The Thyroid Gland 407
The Adrenal Gland 409
Infertility 417
Recurrent Spontaneous Abortion 433
Assisted Reproductive Technologies 439
Endocrine Assays 443

Appendix A. Reference Values 447
Appendix B. ACOG Resources 451
Index 457

CONTRIBUTORS

Editor
Harrison C. Visscher, MD

Associate Editor
Rebecca D. Rinehart

Primary and Preventive Care
Leon Speroff, MD,
   Section Editor
Ellen L. Brock, MD
Thomas A. Buchanan, MD
Ronald A. Chez, MD
David S. Cooper, MD
Leo J. Dunn, MD
Sebastian Faro, MD, PhD
J. Leonard Goldner, MD
Ralph W. Hale, MD
Susan Hellerstein, MD, MPH
William H. Hindle, MD
Siri L. Kjos, MD
Paul W. Ladenson, MD
Stephen B. Levine, MD
Michael McClung, MD
Thomas E. Nolan, MD
Miriam B. Rosenthal, MD
Benjamin P. Sachs, MBBS, DPH
Stephen Silberstein, MD
Richard Wernick, MD
James R. Woods, Jr, MD

Office Practice
William Droegemueller, MD,
   Section Editor
Joanna Cain, MD
Robert C. Cefalo, MD, PhD
Stanley A. Gall, MD
Phillip Heine, MD
Paula J. A. Hillard, MD
Susan R. Johnson, MD
David G. Kleinbaum, PhD
Douglas J. Marchant, MD
Merry-K. Moos, FNP, MPH
Herbert B. Peterson, MD
Donna Shoupe, MD
David E. Soper, MD

John F. Steege, MD
Diane H. Stenchever, MSW
Morton A. Stenchever, MD
Pamela Van Hine, MSLS
Alan J. Wabrek, MD

Obstetrics
Larry C. Gilstrap III, MD,
   Section Editor
Thomas Albert, MD
Charles E. L. Brown, MD
Bruce R. Carr, MD
Susan M. Cox, MD
Patrick Duff, MD
Jay D. Iams, MD
Mark B. Landon, MD
Bert B. Little, MD
Jeffrey M. Perlman, MD
Jeffrey P. Phelan, MD
Philip Samuels, MD
Andrew J. Satin, MD
Isabelle Wilkins, MD
Edward R. Yeomans, MD

Gynecology
Henry A. Thiede, MD,
   Section Editor
Jacques S. Abramowicz, MD
J. Thomas Benson, MD
Daniel L. Clarke-Pearson, MD
Sebastian Faro, MD, PhD
Andrew J. Friedman, MD
Kenneth D. Hatch, MD
Nicolette S. Horbach, MD
Jaroslav Hulka, MD
Robert Israel, MD
Raymond H. Kaufman, MD
Charles M. March, MD
Byron J. Masterson, MD
Ana Alvarez Murphy, MD
David H. Nichols, MD
Kenneth L. Noller, MD
Steven J. Ory, MD
Lisa M. Peacock, MD
P. G. Stubblefield, MD
John D. Thompson, MD

Oncology
Philip J. DiSaia, MD,
   Section Editor
Vicki V. Baker, MD
Patricia J. DiSaia, RN, MSW
Donald George Gallup, MD
Howard D. Homesley, MD
William J. Hoskins, MD
Howard W. Jones III, MD
John R. Lurain, MD
Douglas J. Marchant, MD
James W. Orr, Jr, MD
Pamela Jo Orr, RN, OCN
C. Robert Stanhope, MD

Reproductive Endocrinology and Fertility
Kamran S. Moghissi, MD,
   Section Editor
Eli Y. Adashi, MD
Charla M. Blacker, MD
Richard A. Bronson, MD
Richard E. Blackwell, MD, PhD
Sandra A. Carson, MD
M. Yusoff Dawood, MD
Barry W. Donesky, MD
Sherman Elias, MD
Marc A. Fritz, MD
Kenneth A. Ginsburg, MD
Mary G. Hammond, MD
Ray V. Haning, Jr, MD
Joseph P. Holt, Jr, MD, PhD
Rogerio A. Lobo, MD
Paul G. McDonough, MD
David R. Meldrum, MD
Morris Notelovitz, MD, PhD
Robert W. Rebar, MD
John A. Rock, MD
Joseph S. Sanfilippo, MD
Luther M. Talbert, MD
Michelle P. Warren, MD

Editorial Consultant
Albert B. Gerbie, MD

PREFACE

Precis V: An Update in Obstetrics and Gynecology is a broad, yet concise, overview of information relevant to the specialty. As with earlier editions, the emphasis is on innovations in clinical practice, presented within the context of traditional approaches that retain their applicability to patient care. It is a compendium of the field written by over 100 of its leading authorities especially for practicing obstetricians and gynecologists.

Precis is an educational resource for preparation of the cognitive assessment of clinical knowledge, regardless of the form of the assessment—formal or informal, structured or independent. It takes on renewed emphasis in today's medical environment, which dictates the need for a measurable knowledge base. *Precis* is one of the recognized vehicles on which the recertification and recredentialing processes are based, and it is designed to complement those evaluations. It can also serve as a review for those physicians who are self-motivated to excellence.

One of the most timely changes in *Precis V* is the addition of a completely new section on primary and preventive care. Primary and preventive care has emerged as a means of confronting and controlling spiraling health care costs. As obstetricians and gynecologists have always recognized, it is also a means of promoting better health. The role of the obstetrician–gynecologist in providing total women's health care, which has long been practiced, has now been defined. The information contained here serves as a primer to primary and preventive care. It offers guidelines for screening and assessment, counseling about high-risk behaviors, and promoting early detection and initial management of high-prevalence medical disorders.

Each of the sections in *Precis V* includes exciting new information—updated management guidelines for sexually transmitted diseases, strategies for the active management of labor, advances in urogynecology and management of problems encountered in older women, cancer screening and prevention, and rapidly evolving areas in reproductive endocrinology. New and emerging techniques are presented from a balanced perspective that takes into consideration their practical, beneficial, and economic incorporation in practice.

Although some repetition is unavoidable and, at times, even desirable in a work of this magnitude, the information has been organized to unify coverage of a topic into a single section, even though that topic may be relevant to several sections. Some information from the previous edition continues to be of value and thus has been retained and woven into the new structure. The efforts of authors contributing to previous editions, as well as those providing new material, must be recognized with gratitude. Collectively, they represent the expertise of the specialty. With such a breadth of representation, differences of opinion are inevitable and have been respected.

The format of *Precis V* also reflects innovations aimed at making this edition more practical to use. The bibliographies have been moved in proximity to the relevant text to promote ease of reference. Two appendixes have been added, one presenting conversions of common reference values and one listing current ACOG Committee Opinions and Technical Bulletins, educational publications that complement *Precis*.

Precis V is an educational vehicle for review, reference, and evaluation. It encompasses a broad scientific basis that establishes a current educational and practice objective for the delivery of quality health care for women. It serves as an intellectual approach to education, rather than a statement of ACOG policy. An effort has been made, however, to ensure consistency with ACOG recommendations. Variations in patient care, adapted to individual patient, community, and physician circumstances, must always be anticipated.

The Editors

Primary and Preventive Care

In the past 30 years, mortality from stroke has declined by 60% and from coronary heart disease by 30% in the United States. Advances in medical and surgical care can account for some of this decline, but 60–70% of the improvement is the result of preventive measures. Data from epidemiologic studies and clinical trials demonstrate a decline in morbidity and mortality as a result of smoking cessation, blood pressure reduction, and lowering of cholesterol. There is a strong and growing scientific basis for preventive medicine and health promotion efforts in clinical practice. These efforts focus on routine assessments, identification of risk factors, and counseling regarding life style modification and disease prevention.

Life style influences health and the acquisition of risk factors for chronic disease or premature mortality and disability. The best health strategy is to postpone the illness and, if it is postponed long enough, effectively prevent it. The methods for postponing illness are obvious: exercising, eliminating cigarette smoking and excessive alcohol consumption, controlling obesity, preventing heart disease and osteoporosis, maintaining mental well-being (including sexuality), screening for cancer, and practicing family planning and safe sex.

The physician is in an ideal position to influence behavioral change and health promotion by identifying risks and with authority pointing out potential consequences. Routine periodic assessments provide opportunities to screen for certain diseases, to counsel patients about behavior modification and risk factors, and to detect early signs of problems. Early detection of problems can lead to early intervention, thus enabling the obstetrician–gynecologist to function as a primary care physician in providing continuity of care.

Physicians should develop individualized preventive health programs for asymptomatic patients and initiate modification of unhealthy life styles. Predisposing factors, including values and perceptions of the patient, or enabling factors—peer pressure, family, health education in the community, and work site pressures—may have resulted in the behavior. All of these factors can affect the motivation for behavioral change and should be explored in doctor–patient interaction. This is a never-ending effort, and physicians who practice this approach have a great deal to offer their patients.

Leon Speroff, MD

Screening, Counseling, and Immunizations

Screening can identify individuals who are free of evidence of or at low risk for the development of a disease or a condition. It also identifies individuals who are susceptible to the development of a disease or a condition or who have a precursor of a disease or condition. Finally, screening may identify an individual who has a disease or condition before it becomes clinically manifest, when it is more susceptible to cure, or who has a disease or a condition that poses risk to others.

Tests for screening need to be evaluated in terms of accuracy, risks, and cost. These factors are usually expressed in terms of *sensitivity*, which is the number of persons correctly identified by the test as having the disease divided by the number of persons actually having the disease. Also of importance is *specificity*, which is the number of persons correctly identified as not having the disease divided by the number of persons who do not have the disease. The value of a test used in a population is affected by how many persons in that population have the disease or condition.

Screening is generally considered as testing a person who does not have signs or symptoms of the disease or condition under consideration. This is in contrast to the use of the same test for diagnosing a disease based on symptoms or findings. However, screening also applies to the use of tests in individuals or populations who do not have manifestations of the disease but are identified as being at high risk for the disorder because of a distinctive characteristic. Therefore, the presence of a high-risk factor may be the primary indication for screening, or it may determine the age at which screening is started or influence the frequency with which it is done.

Identification of high-risk factors by means of a medical, social, and behavioral history is becoming of increasing importance, as is the physician's responsibility for detecting them. Self-administered histories offer one method by which more complete data can be obtained with an economy of physician time. A system by which risk factors are identified and displayed in the record for easy review at subsequent visits will enhance the quality of an office practice.

The American College of Obstetricians and Gynecologists has outlined a broad role in health maintenance for women, which includes health screening and disease prevention. Patients should be made aware of services available and whether the obstetrician–gynecologist is serving as a specialist or a primary care physician. Following are guidelines for providing such primary and preventive care for physicians who practice in this role.

The initial evaluation is a complete assessment of a patient with whom a primary care relationship is established, regardless of the patient's age. Subsequent periodic evaluations as part of continuing care, represented by age group, include an interval history and focused physical examination, screening, counseling, and immunizations appropriate for the patient's age and needs. The periodic evaluations are planned as scheduled appointments for the asymptomatic patient. The specific schedule is yearly or as appropriate, based on the patient's needs and the physician's discretion. Additional services may also be provided; in some cases, it may be necessary for the obstetrician–gynecologist to make referrals for certain screening procedures (eg, colonoscopy, tonometry) or counseling. If the patient is being seen for specific signs or symptoms, an additional appointment may be necessary for the periodic evaluation.

High-risk categories are provided to focus further specific assessment and intervention where necessary (Table 1-1). During evaluation the patient should be made aware of high-risk conditions that require targeted screening or treatment.

In addition to high-risk factors related to each age group, the physician should be aware of the leading causes of death and leading causes of morbidity of women by age group.

AGES 12 YEARS AND UNDER

Most patients in this age category will be under the care of a specialist in pediatrics or a specialist in family medicine. Therefore, the screening necessary for all children should be done by that physician. The obstetrician–gynecologist usually serves in the capacity of a consultant, and any tests or evaluation performed would most likely be directed toward diagnosis, not screening.

AGES 13–18

Screening

Periodic History
Reason for visit
Health status: medical, surgical, family
Dietary/nutritional assessment
Physical activity
Tobacco, alcohol, other drugs
Abuse/neglect
Sexual practices

Periodic Physical
Height
Weight
Blood pressure
Secondary sexual characteristics (Tanner staging)
Pelvic examination
Yearly when sexually active or by age 18
Skin (HR1)

Laboratory Tests
Periodic
Pap test
Yearly when sexually active or by age 18

High-Risk Groups
Hemoglobin (HR2)
Bacteriuria testing (HR3)
Sexually transmitted disease testing (HR4)
Human immunodeficiency virus testing (HR5)
Genetic testing/counseling (HR6)
Rubella titer (HR7)
Tuberculosis skin test (HR8)
Lipid profile (HR9)

Evaluation and Counseling

Sexuality
Development
High-risk behaviors
Contraceptive options
 • Genetic counseling
 • Prevention of unwanted pregnancy
Sexually transmitted diseases
 • Partner selection
 • Barrier protection

Fitness
Hygiene (including dental)
Dietary/nutritional assessment
Exercise: discussion of program

Psychosocial Evaluation
Interpersonal/family relationships
Sexual identity
Personal goal development
Behavioral/learning disorders
Abuse/neglect

Cardiovascular Risk Factors
Family history
Hypertension
Hyperlipidemia
Obesity/diabetes mellitus

Health/Risk Behaviors
Injury prevention
 • Safety belts and helmets
 • Recreational hazards
 • Firearms
 • Hearing
Skin exposure to ultraviolet rays
Suicide: depressive symptoms
Tobacco, alcohol, other drugs

Immunizations

Periodic
Tetanus–diphtheria booster
Once between ages 14–16

High-Risk Groups
Measles, mumps, rubella (MMR) (HR7)
Hepatitis B vaccine (HR10)
Fluoride supplement (HR11)

Leading Causes of Death
Motor vehicle accidents
Homicide
Suicide
Leukemia

Leading Causes of Morbidity
Nose, throat, and upper respiratory conditions
Viral, bacterial, and parasitic infections
Sexual abuse
Injuries (musculoskeletal and soft tissue)
Acute ear infections
Digestive system conditions
Acute urinary conditions

AGES 19–39

Screening

Periodic History
Reason for visit
Health status: medical, surgical, family
Dietary/nutritional assessment
Physical activity
Tobacco, alcohol, other drugs
Abuse/neglect
Sexual practices

Periodic Physical
Height
Weight
Blood pressure
Neck: adenopathy, thyroid
Breasts
Abdomen
Pelvic examination
Skin (HR1)

Laboratory Tests
Periodic
Pap test
  Physician and patient discretion after 3 consecutive normal tests
Cholesterol
  Every 5 years

High-Risk Groups
Hemoglobin (HR2)
Bacteriuria testing (HR3)
Mammography (HR12)
Fasting glucose test (HR13)
Sexually transmitted disease testing (HR4)
Human immunodeficiency virus testing (HR5)
Genetic testing/counseling (HR6)
Rubella titer (HR7)
Tuberculosis skin test (HR8)
Lipid profile (HR9)
Thyroid-stimulating hormone (HR14)

Evaluation and Counseling

Sexuality
High-risk behaviors
Contraceptive options
  • Genetic counseling
  • Prevention of unwanted pregnancy
Sexually transmitted disease
  • Partner selection
  • Barrier protection
Sexual functioning

Fitness
Hygiene (including dental)
Dietary/nutritional assessment
Exercise: discussion of program

Psychosocial Evaluation
Interpersonal/family relationships
Domestic violence
Job satisfaction
Life style/stress
Sleep disorders

Cardiovascular Risk Factors
Family history
Hypertension
Hyperlipidemia
Obesity/diabetes mellitus
Life style

Health/Risk Behaviors
Injury prevention
  • Safety belts and helmets
  • Occupational hazards
  • Recreational hazards
  • Firearms
  • Hearing
Breast self-examination
Skin exposure to ultraviolet rays
Suicide: depressive symptoms
Tobacco, alcohol, other drugs

Immunizations

Periodic
Tetanus–diphtheria booster
  Every 10 years

High-Risk Groups
Measles, mumps, rubella (MMR) (HR7)
Hepatitis B vaccine (HR10)
Influenza vaccine (HR15)
Pneumococcal vaccine (HR16)

Leading Causes of Death
Motor vehicle accidents
Cardiovascular disease
Homicide
Coronary artery disease
Acquired immunodeficiency syndrome (AIDS)
Breast cancer
Cerebrovascular disease
Uterine cancer

Leading Causes of Morbidity
Nose, throat, and upper respiratory conditions
Injuries (musculoskeletal and soft tissue, including back and upper and lower extremities)
Viral, bacterial, and parasitic infections
Acute urinary conditions

AGES 40–64

Screening

Periodic History
Reason for visit
Health status: medical, surgical, family
Dietary/nutritional assessment
Physical activity
Tobacco, alcohol, other drugs
Abuse/neglect
Sexual practices

Periodic Physical
Height
Weight
Blood pressure
Oral cavity
Neck: adenopathy, thyroid
Breasts, axillae
Abdomen
Pelvic and rectovaginal examination
Skin (HR1)

Laboratory Tests
Periodic
Pap test
   Physician and patient discretion after 3 consecutive normal tests
Mammography
   Every 1–2 years until age 50, yearly beginning at 50
Cholesterol
   Every 5 years
Fecal occult blood test
Sigmoidoscopy
   Every 3–5 years after age 50

High-Risk Groups
Hemoglobin (HR2)
Bacteriuria testing (HR3)
Mammography (HR12)
Fasting glucose test (HR13)
Sexually transmitted disease testing (HR4)
Human immunodeficiency virus testing (HR5)
Tuberculosis skin test (HR8)
Lipid profile (HR9)
Thyroid-stimulating hormone (HR14)
Colonoscopy (HR17)

Evaluation and Counseling

Sexuality
High-risk behaviors
Contraceptive options
  • Genetic counseling
  • Prevention of unwanted pregnancy
Sexually transmitted disease
  • Partner selection
  • Barrier protection
Sexual functioning

Fitness
Hygiene (including dental)
Dietary/nutritional assessment
Exercise: discussion of program

Psychosocial Evaluation
Family relationships
Domestic violence
Job/work satisfaction
Retirement planning
Life style/stress
Sleep disorders

Cardiovascular Risk Factors
Family history
Hypertension
Hyperlipidemia
Obesity/diabetes mellitus
Life style

Health/Risk Behaviors
Hormone replacement therapy
Injury prevention
  • Safety belts and helmets
  • Occupational hazards
  • Recreational hazards
  • Sports involvement
  • Firearms
  • Hearing
Breast self-examination
Skin exposure to ultraviolet rays
Suicide: depressive symptoms
Tobacco, alcohol, other drugs

Immunizations

Periodic
Tetanus–diphtheria booster
   Every 10 years
Influenza vaccine
   Annually beginning at age 55

High-Risk Groups
Mumps, measles, rubella (MMR) (HR7)
Hepatitis B vaccine (HR10)
Influenza vaccine (HR15)
Pneumococcal vaccine (HR16)

Leading Causes of Death
Cardiovascular disease
Coronary artery disease
Breast cancer
Lung cancer
Cerebrovascular disease
Colorectal cancer
Obstructive pulmonary disease
Ovarian cancer

Leading Causes of Morbidity
Nose, throat, and upper respiratory conditions
Osteoporosis/arthritis
Hypertension
Orthopedic deformities and impairments (including back and upper and lower extremities)
Heart disease
Hearing and vision impairments

65 YEARS AND OLDER

Screening

Periodic History
Reason for visit
Health status: medical, surgical, family
Dietary/nutritional assessment
Physical activity
Tobacco, alcohol, other drugs, polypharmacy
Abuse/neglect
Sexual practices

Periodic Physical
Height
Weight
Blood pressure
Oral cavity
Neck: adenopathy, thyroid
Breasts, axillae
Abdomen
Pelvic and rectovaginal examination
Skin (HR1)

Laboratory Tests
Periodic
Pap test
 Physician and patient discretion after 3 consecutive normal tests
Urinalysis/dipstick
Mammography
Cholesterol
 Every 3–5 years
Fecal occult blood test
Sigmoidoscopy
 Every 3–5 years
Thyroid-stimulating hormone test
 Every 3–5 years
High-Risk Groups
Hemoglobin (HR2)
Fasting glucose test (HR13)
Sexually transmitted disease testing (HR4)
Human immunodeficiency virus testing (HR5)
Tuberculosis skin test (HR8)
Lipid profile (HR9)
Colonoscopy (HR17)

Evaluation and Counseling

Sexuality
Sexual functioning
Sexual behaviors
Sexually transmitted diseases

Fitness
Hygiene (general and dental)
Dietary/nutritional assessment
Exercise: discussion of program

Psychosocial Evaluation
Neglect/abuse
Life style/stress
Depression/sleep disorders
Family relationships
Job/work/retirement satisfaction

Cardiovascular Risk Factors
Hypertension
Hypercholesterolemia
Obesity/diabetes mellitus
Sedentary life style

Health/Risk Behaviors
Hormone replacement therapy
Injury prevention
 • Safety belts and helmets
 • Occupational hazards
 • Recreational hazards
 • Hearing
 • Firearms
Visual acuity/glaucoma
Hearing
Breast self-examination
Skin exposure to ultraviolet rays
Suicide: depressive symptoms
Tobacco, alcohol, other drugs

Immunizations

Periodic
Tetanus–diphtheria booster
 Every 10 years
Influenza vaccine
 Annually
Pneumococcal vaccine
 Once
High-Risk Groups
Hepatitis B vaccine (HR10)

Leading Causes of Death
Cardiovascular disease
Coronary artery disease
Cerebrovascular disease
Pneumonia/influenza
Obstructive lung disease
Colorectal cancer
Breast cancer
Lung cancer
Accidents

Leading Causes of Morbidity
Nose, throat, and upper respiratory conditions
Osteoporosis/arthritis
Hypertension
Urinary incontinence
Heart disease
Injuries (musculoskeletal and soft tissue)
Hearing and vision impairments

TABLE 1-1. HIGH-RISK FACTORS

Factor	Description	Groups at Risk
HR1	Skin	Persons with increased recreational or occupational exposure to sunlight, family or personal history of skin cancer, or clinical evidence of precursor lesions (eg, dysplastic nevi, certain congenital nevi)
HR2	Hemoglobin	Persons of Caribbean, Latin American, Asian, Mediterranean, or African descent or with a history of excessive menstrual flow
HR3	Bacteriuria Testing	Persons with diabetes mellitus
HR4	Sexually Transmitted Disease (STD) Testing	Persons with a history of multiple sexual partners or a sexual partner with multiple contacts, sexual contacts of persons with culture-proven STD, persons with a history of repeated episodes of STD, and persons who attend clinics for STDs
HR5	Human Immunodeficiency Virus (HIV) Testing	Persons seeking treatment for STDs; past or present drug use by injection; persons with a history of prostitution; women whose past or present sexual partners are HIV positive or bisexual or who inject drugs; persons with long-term residence or birth in an area with high prevalence of HIV infection; and persons with a history of transfusion between 1978 and 1985
HR6	Genetic Testing/Counseling	Women of reproductive age who are exposed to teratogens or who contemplate pregnancy at age 35 or beyond; patient, partner, or family member with history of a genetic disorder or birth defect; and persons of African–American, Eastern European Jewish, Mediterranean, or Southeast Asian ancestry
HR7	Rubella Titer/Vaccine	Women of childbearing age lacking evidence of immunity. A second measles immunization, preferably as MMR (measles, mumps, and rubella vaccine), for all women unable to show proof of immunity.
HR8	Tuberculosis (TB) Skin Test	Patients infected with HIV; close contacts (sharing the same household or other enclosed environments) of persons known or suspected to have TB; persons with medical risk factors known to increase the risk of disease if infection has occurred; foreign-born persons from countries with high TB prevalence; medically underserved, low-income populations; alcoholics and intravenous drug users; residents of long-term care facilities, correctional institutions, mental institutions, nursing homes and facilities, and other long-term residential facilities; and health professionals working in high-risk health care facilities
HR9	Lipid Profile	Persons with an elevated cholesterol level; history of parent or sibling with a blood cholesterol level of 240 mg/dl or higher; history of a sibling, parent, or grandparent with documented premature (aged less than 55 years) coronary artery disease; presence of diabetes mellitus or smoking habit
HR10	Hepatitis B Vaccine	Intravenous drug users; current recipients of blood products; persons in health-related jobs with exposure to blood or blood products; household and sexual contacts of hepatitis B virus carriers; prostitutes; and persons with a history of sexual activity with multiple partners in the previous 6 months
HR11	Fluoride Supplement	Persons living in areas with inadequate water fluoridation (less than 0.7 parts/million)
HR12	Mammography	Women aged 35 and older with a family history of premenopausally diagnosed breast cancer in a first-degree relative
HR13	Fasting Glucose Test	Every 3–5 years for persons with a family history of diabetes mellitus (one first- or two second-degree relatives), who are markedly obese, or who have a personal history of gestational diabetes mellitus
HR14	Thyroid-Stimulating Hormone (TSH)	Individuals with a strong family history of thyroid disease and patients with autoimmune diseases (there is some evidence that subclinical hypothyroidism may be related to unfavorable lipid profiles)
HR15	Influenza Vaccine	Residents of chronic care facilities; persons with chronic cardiopulmonary disorders; and persons with metabolic diseases, including diabetes mellitus, hemoglobinopathies, immunosuppression, or renal dysfunction
HR16	Pneumococcal Vaccine	Persons with medical conditions that increase the risk of pneumococcal infection (eg, chronic cardiac or pulmonary disease, sickle cell disease, nephrotic syndrome, Hodgkin disease, asplenia, diabetes mellitus, alcoholism, cirrhosis, multiple myeloma, renal disease, or other immunosuppression)
HR17	Colonoscopy	Persons with a personal history of inflammatory bowel disease or colonic polyps or a family history of familial polyposis coli, colorectal cancer, or cancer family syndrome

BIBLIOGRAPHY

American College of Obstetricians and Gynecologists. The adolescent obstetric–gynecologic patient. ACOG Technical Bulletin 145. Washington, DC: ACOG, 1990

American College of Obstetricians and Gynecologists. The obstetrician–gynecologist and primary–preventive health care. ACOG Task Force Report. Washington, DC: ACOG, 1993

National Cancer Institute. 1987 Annual cancer statistics review, including cancer trends: 1950–1985. Bethesda, Maryland: NCI, 1988

National Center for Health Statistics. Vital statistics of the United States, 1988. Vol II: mortality, part A. Washington, DC: Public Health Service, 1991

Health Maintenance

Changing unhealthy behavior can make a difference in a patient's health and well-being. Once any risk factors have been identified, most patients will benefit from guidance on how their life style can be modified to promote their health and prevent disease. Such counseling should be an integral component of routine care.

Routine periodic assessments also provide opportunities for physicians to counsel patients about family planning and prevention of sexually transmitted diseases, including human immunodeficiency virus (HIV). These topics are integral components of office practice. The benefits of hormone replacement therapy should also be discussed with appropriate patients.

SMOKING CESSATION

Cigarette smoking is the single greatest cause of preventable morbidity and mortality in American women. It is responsible for 55% of cardiovascular deaths in women aged less than 65 years, and women smokers are 12 times more likely to die of lung cancer than women who have never smoked. Lung cancer has now surpassed breast cancer as the number one cause of cancer deaths in women. Smoking increases the risk of oral cancer, laryngeal cancer, bladder cancer, pancreatic cancer, and probably cervical cancer, as well as chronic obstructive pulmonary disease.

Approximately 30% of American women smoke cigarettes, and 19–30% continue to smoke during pregnancy. The prevalence is higher among older, less educated, and African-American women. Women are more likely than men to have never tried to quit smoking. Physicians and other health care professionals can have a dramatic effect on influencing smokers to reduce or quit smoking with counseling and smoking cessation guidance.

In addition to learning about the general ill health effects of smoking, patients can be informed of the effects of smoking on childbearing:

- Decreased fertility
- Twice the rate of ectopic pregnancy
- Increased rate of spontaneous abortions (1.2–1.8 times higher)
- Greater likelihood (39%) of aborting a chromosomally normal fetus
- Increased rates of abruptio placentae, placenta previa, and premature rupture of membranes
- Increased relative risk of preterm births compared with nonsmokers (1.2–1.5 times higher)
- Decreased mean birth weight of infants

Women smokers have other risks in addition to those effects of smoking in the childbearing years:

- Early menopause (an average of 1.7 years earlier than non-smokers)
- Higher risk of osteoporosis
- Greater risk of myocardial infarction and stroke if over age 35 years and oral contraceptives are used

Smoking cessation can reverse many of the risks associated with smoking. By 10 years after smoking cessation, a former smoker's risk of lung cancer returns to that of a nonsmoker. Smoking reduction in pregnancy improves the birth weight of the infant, especially if cessation occurs before 16 weeks of gestation. It is estimated that if all pregnant women stopped smoking a 10% reduction in fetal and infant deaths would be observed.

Smoking Cessation Strategies

The obstetrician–gynecologist should take an active role in promoting smoking cessation. The high motivation of the pregnant patient may provide a window of opportunity to achieve smoking cessation. Thirty percent of women are smokers at the time they conceive. Approximately 20% of smokers quit by their first prenatal visit but only 6% give up smoking later in pregnancy despite regular obstetric visits and antismoking advice. In the general population 65% of those who stop smoking relapse within 3 months of quitting, 10% relapse after 3–6 months, whereas only 3% relapse after 6–12 months.

Many approaches are used to promote smoking cessation. The American Cancer Society suggests the following five-step approach:

1. Begin by obtaining a patient history of smoking habits and assessing the patient's motivation to stop smoking.
2. Give clear advice to stop smoking, emphasizing the benefits of cessation.
3. Set a specific goal (eg, a realistic date to stop smoking).
4. Suggest cessation strategies.
5. Arrange a visit or phone call to monitor progress.

Patient education about the benefits of smoking cessation, clear advice to quit smoking, and physician support improve smoking cessation rates, although 95% of smokers who successfully quit do so on their own without formal smoking cessation programs. However, during pregnancy, the most successful efforts in smoking cessation involve interventions that emphasize a pragmatic approach to smoking cessation, rather than merely providing antismoking advice. Prospective, randomized, controlled clinical trials of intensive smoking reduction programs with frequent patient contact and supervision have been shown to aid in smoking cessation and result in increased infant birth weights.

It can be helpful to discuss nicotine withdrawal symptoms with patients. These generally last less than 1 week and may include tobacco craving, irritability, anxiety, insomnia, fatigue, difficulty with concentration, dizziness, drowsiness, depression, gastrointestinal disturbance, and headache. There is a wide range of severity and duration of these symptoms. Many patients are concerned about weight gain with smoking cessation, which averages 2.3–4.5 kg (5–10 lb) over the first few months because of changes in metabolism and eating behaviors.

There are many behavioral modification approaches to smoking cessation. The health care practitioner may use smoking cessation charts to track a patient's contacts and to reinforce positive behavior. Many free self-help manuals are available from the National Cancer Institute, the Office of Smoking and Health, and the Health Promotion Group. Additionally, there are community-based support groups, organized by local chapters of the American Cancer Society and the American Lung Association, that may be of interest to some smokers.

Nicotine Replacement Therapy

Nicotine replacement therapy as chewing gum or a transdermal patch has been demonstrated to increase the effectiveness of smoking cessation programs by approximately 50% when evaluated 6 months after the intervention. For patients who are highly nicotine dependent (greater than 20–25 cigarettes per day) and unable to stop on their own, physicians may consider nicotine replacement therapy combined with a structured cessation program or professional counseling.

A pack-a-day smoker (20 cigarettes per day) systemically absorbs approximately 20 mg of nicotine, 200–300 mg of carbon monoxide, and many other of the 2,500 chemicals identified in tobacco smoke. Blood concentrations of nicotine build up at an average of 20–35 ng/ml in a pack-a-day smoker. To help alleviate the symptoms of nicotine withdrawal, nicotine chewing gum is recommended for heavy smokers; it is prescribed for use of one piece when the patient feels the urge to smoke, with an average consumption of 10–12 pieces per day and not more than 30 pieces per day. It is contraindicated in patients with a recent myocardial infarction, severe angina, or life-threatening arrhythmias and in pregnant and nursing women. With use of 12 pieces of chewing gum, about 12 mg of nicotine is absorbed, resulting in a peak plasma level of 10–15 ng/ml, which is much lower than the level of a pack-a-day smoker. Transdermal nicotine systems also result in a peak plasma nicotine level of 10–15 ng/ml. Patients should begin to self-wean from nicotine replacement by 3 months of use. Patients should be warned that while on nicotine therapy they should never smoke.

The package inserts of nicotine replacement therapies suggest that pregnant women not use these therapies because nicotine is considered an important cause of the adverse effects of smoking on the mother and the fetus. However, nicotine is only one of the toxins absorbed from tobacco smoke, and cessation of smoking and nicotine replacement would certainly reduce fetal exposure to carbon monoxide and other toxins. For women who smoke more than 20 cigarettes per day and who are otherwise unable to decrease smoking it may be reasonable to advise nicotine replacement as an adjunct to counseling during pregnancy. In the absence of sufficient data concerning nicotine replacement this must be an individualized therapeutic decision, and the patient should be informed about the presumed risks and benefits.

EXERCISE

Exercise has become an important aspect of the life style of many women. From recreational participants to elite athletes, women are using exercise to control weight, to feel better, and to compete. Therefore, obstetrician–gynecologists should be able to answer patients' questions and counsel them about exercise.

Exercise can alter lipid profiles by increasing high-density lipoprotein (HDL) and reducing low-density lipoprotein (LDL), helping to prevent heart disease. Exercise is a major component of "fitness," a broad term that encompasses cardiovascular fitness, endurance, and weight control. Cardiovascular fitness occurs when the body increases its aerobic capacity by increasing oxygen storage capacity at the cellular level. A major byproduct of the increase in aerobic capacity is the ability to prolong the capacity for physical activity, resulting in more energy. An exercise program is helpful for women who wish to lose or maintain weight. A weight-control program that combines diet and exercise is more effective and longer lasting than either program alone. Once a desired weight has been achieved, exercise can help to maintain it. In addition, exercise can increase muscle strength, flexibility, and coordination. An active fitness program that includes weight-bearing exercise can also increase bone density, an important factor in preventing osteoporosis.

As part of a physician's overall program for the patient, questions should be asked about the amount of exercise the patient has on a weekly basis. For those patients who have a sedentary life, an active exercise program should be recommended. For the average patient, the main goals of an exercise program are cardiovascular fitness or weight control, or both.

Cardiovascular Fitness

Oxygen storage capacity increases with the duration of exercise. This response is usually referred to by the patient as "conditioning." In the laboratory, this response is called aerobic capacity and is measured by determining maximum oxygen uptake ($\dot{V}O_2$ max). Measurement of the heart rate during exercise is an excellent method by which to evaluate cardiovascular fitness and estimate the $\dot{V}O_2$ max. As conditioning (ie, cardiovascular fitness) improves, the heart rate will stabilize at a fixed rate of exercise. It is possible to establish the heart rate at which conditioning will develop by using the following formula to determine the target range: (220 − age) × 60–80% = target range. For example, a 45-year-old patient would have a target range of 105–140 (220 − 45 = 175 × 0.6–0.8). During her exercise program, she would need to maintain her heart rate within these parameters to achieve fitness levels.

To attain cardiovascular fitness, a woman must exercise at a level that elevates the heart rate into a target range, based on her age, for 20 or more minutes, at least three times a week. A gradual "warm-up period" of approximately 5 minutes should precede exercise at the target heart rate. By slowly increasing activity, there is a more uniform supply of blood to large muscle groups, which helps prevent muscle injury. Likewise, slowly decreasing activity in a "cool-down period" allows the large quantity of blood in the skin and muscles to return to the central vasculature, thus helping to prevent dizziness, nausea, and fainting as the heart rate returns to normal.

Weight Control

Weight loss from exercise is based on the premise that more calories are used than ingested, and the resulting deficit is met by modifying fat stores. Thus, for any exercise program designed for weight control to be effective, a negative caloric balance must be achieved (ie, caloric intake must be less than calories expended).

Since each pound of body fat contains 3,500 kcal, if a woman uses 500 kcal/d exercising and does not increase her caloric intake, she will lose 1 lb/week. Thus, weight loss will take time, and the patient should be encouraged in her efforts. Furthermore, as a woman exercises she will gain muscle, and muscle per unit volume is approximately twice as heavy as fat. Therefore, a woman may be losing fat without losing weight. The patient needs to be aware of these facts when entering a weight-loss program so that she does not soon become discouraged and quit. The physician can help by evaluating the patient's weight on a regular basis, which also provides an opportunity to review the level of activity of her exercise program.

Developing a Program

Any exercise program must be designed to fit the needs of the woman. Initially, the physician should determine the woman's goals. With that information, specific encouragement and recommendations can be offered. If the patient is under age 45 and has no history of chronic illness or injury, it is probably not necessary for a physical examination or special laboratory tests to be performed. After age 45, a lipid profile and electrocardiography are usually recommended as a base line. Regardless of the type of program the patient undertakes, she should be cautioned about the warning signs of overexertion. The patient should stop exercising and contact her physician for further follow-up if any of the following signs occur: sudden sharp pain, excessive fatigue, difficulty breathing, persistent lethargy, nausea, vomiting, faintness, dizziness, excessive muscle soreness or pain, or any irregularity of the heartbeat.

Activities that are commonly recommended as exercise are those that promote aerobic endurance. The most common are jogging or running, bicycling, brisk walking, cross-country skiing, swimming, and aerobic dancing. Other sports such as racquetball, tennis, and volleyball are also good if they require continuous activity for 20 minutes or more and do not have intermittent rest periods.

Exercise programs and aerobic dance classes should be of the low-impact type, especially for perimenopausal and postmenopausal women, to avoid muscle, ligament, and bone injury. Indoor exercise machines also are good sources of physical activity. They have the advantage of a secure, protected environment and the ability to exercise at any time of day. To avoid boredom, many women watch television, listen to a radio, or even read at this time, depending on the exercise machine used.

For the occasional patient who wants to develop strength as well as cardiovascular fitness, one of the newer innovations is circuit training. Many city parks and recreation areas offer these programs, which consist of running, climbing, pulling, pushing, and jumping. If strength alone is the patient's goal, then a specific weight-training program should be developed. This program is best developed with and supervised by an instructor who is specifically trained to use this program.

Exercise should be an integral part of a healthy life style. A specific exercise program should be based on the patient's ability and interests. At each visit, regardless of the reason, the patient should be questioned about her exercise program and how she is progressing. This takes very little time but gives her positive reinforcement and encouragement.

NUTRITION AND WEIGHT CONTROL

Patient motivation to seek medical care related to nutrition and weight control usually reflects a wish to improve appearance. In contrast, medically based motivations to assess and treat in these areas include the avoidance of chronic deficiency and disease states and the amelioration of existing diseases. Both viewpoints relate to the individual perception of quality of life. Although seemingly disparate, both perspectives can be melded effectively via an efficient process of screening, counseling, diagnosis, and management implemented in the office.

All evidence indicates that diet influences the risk of several major chronic diseases, especially atherosclerotic cardiovascular diseases and hypertension. The evidence is highly suggestive for many forms of cancer. Other health problems influenced by diet include dental caries, chronic liver disease, diabetes mellitus, and, of course, obesity.

A high fat intake is associated with atherosclerotic cardiovascular disease and certain cancers. Saturated fatty acid intake is the major determinant of the serum total cholesterol and LDL cholesterol levels. The substitution of polyunsaturated and monounsaturated fatty acids results in lowering of total cholesterol and LDL cholesterol. Diets high in plant foods (fruits, vegetables, legumes, and whole-grain cereals) are associated with a lower occurrence of coronary heart disease (CHD) and cancers of the lung, colon, esophagus, and stomach. There is no evidence that daily multiple vitamin–mineral supplements are either beneficial or harmful for the general population.

Screening

The purposes of screening questions related to current dietary practices are to reinforce appropriate eating practices, to identify inappropriate practices, to correct misinformation, and to identify overt disease states. The answers allow the physician to determine which patient needs additional in-depth assessment.

Opening questions can be asked about the patient's attitude toward her present weight, its distribution, and her body image. A 24-hour diet recall history will provide information about food intake and meals taken and skipped. Further questions can relate to food avoidance, eating habits, special diets, and mineral and vitamin supplements used.

Diagnosis

History is the most important assessment tool for the diagnosis of illness related to inadequate or inappropriate diet. Clues derived from the patient's answers may be reinforced by findings on physical examination.

Weight related to height will provide body mass index (kilograms per square meter). This number, coupled with a clinical judgment about the distribution of fat and muscle mass, is the most practical way to evaluate for normal weight, overweight, and underweight categories. Although obesity and anorexia can be recognized, the bulimic patient may have a normal body habitus.

It is unusual to find signs of hypovitaminosis. Furthermore, dermatitis and changes in skin texture, hair texture, and mucous membranes are not specific for the diagnosis of deficiency states.

Blood chemistry levels are not helpful in the evaluation of malnutrition, but the presence of both macrocytic and microcytic anemia may be. Lipid profiles are pertinent in patients with a family history of cardiovascular disease. Laboratory tests to rule out endocrine disorders should be ordered only if there is a specific clinical suspicion derived from both history and physical examination.

Counseling

There is great diversity in the diets and eating habits of Americans. Cultural, ethnic, and religious backgrounds, among others, are important influences that are difficult to modify. However, there are tenets of healthful nutrition that are applicable to all diets. Most people in the United States, regardless of race, education, or income, do not follow these tenets. Therefore, all patients will benefit from current information about nutrition, healthful diet composition, and weight control. The following recommendations represent the conclusions of the Committee on Diet and Health of the National Research Council:

- Total fat intake should be reduced to 30% of calories or less. Saturated fatty acid intake should be less than 10% of calories, and the intake of cholesterol should be less than 300 mg daily.
- Every day, five or more servings should be eaten of a combination of vegetables and fruits, especially green and yellow vegetables and citrus fruit. The daily intake of starches and other complex carbohydrates should be increased by eating six or more servings of a combination of breads, cereals, and legumes.
- Protein intake should be maintained at moderate levels (less than 1.6 g/kg of body weight).
- Alcoholic beverages should be limited to less than 1 oz of alcohol per day (equivalent to two cans of beer, two glasses of wine, or two average cocktails).
- Total daily intake of salt should be limited to 6 g or less.
- Vitamin–mineral supplement intake should not exceed the recommended dietary intake per day.

Individual patients with abnormal findings, including food faddism, malnutrition, medical disease with special diet requirements, and low and high body mass index, all require more intense and knowledgeable counseling to effect change. To do this, the physician needs more detailed information from the patient. Core data include an assessment to understand the patient's present goals, previous attempts at change, motivation for change, and daily activities. Who determines what food is purchased and the manner in which it is cooked and when it is eaten are additional areas of inquiry.

Management

In most instances, remedial actions related to abnormal findings in nutrition and weight control involve a combination of changes in amount and type of food eaten, implementation of a fitness program, and behavior modification therapy. Success in effecting permanent change is enhanced when there is mutual agreement by patient and provider as to realistic goals for outcome, realistic time frames for change, and realistic commitment to long-term maintenance once change is achieved.

Throughout this frequently extended process, the physician is challenged not to make negative value judgments, to offer positive feedback and reinforcement, and to assess for barriers and patient constraints that need to be overcome. Frequently, referral both to other health care professionals and to self-help peer groups is required. The challenge for the physician is to maintain a supportive role during the time of change and then during the time of maintenance once change has occurred.

STRESS MANAGEMENT

Dynamic physiologic, psychologic, and social balance—historically referred to as homeostasis—is usually maintained by inapparent, minor adjustments at biochemical, cellular, organ system, psychologic, interpersonal, and social levels of a person's functioning. Homeostasis is routinely threatened by external and intrinsic forces called "stressors." The resultant state of disharmony is "stress," which typically manifests itself at each of these levels.

The physiologic processes of homeostasis are often nonspecific and involve central and peripheral cortisol and adrenergically mediated responses. These dependably increase arousal, vigilance, and attention, and prepare the individual for aggression whether facing a new demand at work, a family member's chronic illness, or a tiger in the jungle.

The forces that begin the psychologic homeostatic process involve mechanisms of defense. These largely automatic mental maneuvers dampen emotional intensity and enable behavioral responses that are often judged as either good or poor coping. What is perceived as stressful varies greatly from one person to another according to the meaning that the stressor has to the individual. Individuals use highly specific defenses and coping behaviors. It is widely assumed that the frequent use of "immature" defenses—projection and denial—is associated with less effective coping. Poor coping may lead to social changes that are referred to as a maladjustment and sometimes may lead to a psychologic disorder, as well.

Invocation of the term *stress* implies that the person's threshold for a comfortable life as usual has been exceeded and her emotional life has become unpleasant. The presence of stress predicts that a demand for an accommodation to some change exists. Although these demands traditionally have been viewed as stimuli to emotional and intellectual growth, more recently the culture has come to regard stress as largely negative. Remedies for stress are sought in general approaches that are widely applicable to the public's health. Many techniques are now widely available for stress management of these educational, vocational, relationship, health, and environmental stressors (see box). Wellness programs consist of one or more of these techniques.

Stress Management Techniques

Relaxation Techniques
  Progressive muscle relaxation
  Stretching
  Guided visual imagery
  Self-hypnosis
  Meditation or prayer
  Yoga
  Biofeedback
  Massage
  Music
  Self-help, problem-focused groups

General Health Maintenance
  Exercise programs
  Regular and adequate sleep patterns
  Nutritional programs
  Discontinuation of poor habits
   Smoking
   Alcohol and other substances of abuse

Counseling
  Clergy
  Mental health professional
  Other health professional

Prescription Medication

SUBSTANCE ABUSE

Substance abuse is a chronic, relapsing disease. Drug abuse often is associated with medical risks such as hepatitis and heart disease and therefore may not seem to be an integral component of women's reproductive health care. As primary care providers, however, obstetrician–gynecologists are positioned uniquely to identify and initiate counseling for substance abuse. The obstetric or gynecologic needs of substance-abusing women often bring them into medical care systems for the first time. The obstetrician–gynecologist should seize the opportunity to address their presenting health complaints and their nonverbalized health problems. Because of the effects that substance abuse may have on pregnancy, preconceptional counseling may be warranted.

Recent Trends in Substance Abuse

Although alcohol consumption among women of all ages has increased only slightly in the past three decades, abuse by women of childbearing age has increased dramatically. Caucasian women are more prone to drinking than are African–American or Hispanic women and are apt to be heavier drinkers. Overall, alcohol consumption appears to be highest among unmarried Caucasian women of middle to upper socioeconomic status. For African–American women, alcohol consumption appears to be correlated inversely with socioeconomic status.

Alcohol abuse frequently is tied to illicit drug use, deteriorating mental health, and suicide. Despite educational efforts, fetal alcohol syndrome remains one of the leading causes of mental retardation. Continued alcohol abuse throughout pregnancy is seen more frequently among women who are younger, who are abusing illicit drugs, and who previously were subjected to sexual or physical abuse—as evidence of dysfunctional family settings.

Marijuana

Marijuana remains the leading illicit drug of abuse in the United States, and women aged 18–25 years represent the largest marijuana-using population. Marijuana smoking has been associated with tachycardia, exercise intolerance, bronchitis, sinusitis, and pharyngitis. Chronic consumption leads to anovulation and decreased sperm count and motility.

Cocaine

Cocaine use in the past decade declined until approximately 1988, when crack cocaine—a cheap, highly addictive, smokable form of cocaine—surfaced in U.S. urban regions. Crack abuse appears to be more prevalent among the African–American population, particularly among young, unmarried women of low education and socioeconomic status. These women are more prone to abuse alcohol and other illicit drugs; and, through prostitution to purchase drugs, they are exposed frequently to sexually transmitted diseases such as chlamydia, gonorrhea, syphilis, and HIV. During pregnancy, most women decrease their cocaine use. Those who continue their addictions are more likely to be older, unmarried, African–American women with low education and socioeconomic status but with higher gravidity and parity and with a history of multiple abortions.

Heroin

Heroin abuse, although frequently overlooked because of media attention to cocaine, is making a comeback. Characteristics of the heroin-abusing woman resemble those of cocaine users. In the 1980s, fear of needles and acquired immunodeficiency syndrome (AIDS) contributed to the decline of heroin use, as smokable cocaine became readily available. The popularity of snorted heroin portends a new cycle of heroin abuse during the 1990s.

Barriers to Care

Women with substance addiction freely acknowledge a love–hate relationship with the medical community. Commonly dwelling in communities where "everyone does drugs," these women lose their children to foster care, and their partners often sell drugs to subsist and support their drug habits. These women's own childhoods frequently have been affected by sexual abuse, rape, or physical violence. In such an environment, these women understandably suffer low self-esteem. They may use sex and pregnancy as a means to hold onto a male partner, sex as a way to pay for drugs, and drugs as the social glue in an otherwise friendless community. Isolation, depression, and denial may dominate their days. Is it surprising, then, when during a hurried visit to an obstetrician-gynecologist they are asked, "Do you take drugs?" that they would mistrust the examiner and respond negatively to the question?

Interviewing Techniques

Questions about substance abuse must be asked in an empathetic and sensitive manner. Despite their many problems, substance abusers are quick to recognize insincerity. But even the empathetic questioner may wish to structure his or her questions:

- Sequence the questions from least to most threatening (ie, medication, smoking, alcohol, licit drugs, illicit drugs).
- Be specific about the type of drug. A woman may deny alcohol abuse but admit to consuming wine coolers.
- Be specific about the period of time in question. The question, "How much wine did you drink in the month prior to your pregnancy?" might be followed by, "Has that pattern changed since you found out that you were pregnant?"
- Be aware that most women addicts *do* worry about their unborn babies. A reasonable question might be, "Do you worry that drugs you used early in your pregnancy might have harmed your baby?"
- A number of systems have been developed to question for alcohol abuse. One of the more popular methods is known as the CAGE technique:
  — C: Have you ever felt that you ought to Cut down on your drinking?
  — A: Have people Annoyed you by criticizing your drinking?
  — G: Have you ever felt bad or Guilty about your drinking?
  — E: Have you ever had a drink first thing in the morning to steady your nerves or to get rid of a hangover (Eye opener)?

A woman's affirmative response to substance abuse questions should be considered a call for help and a unique opportunity for intervention. The scope of the problem should be defined in a nonjudgmental way, such as, "Drug X is known to have harmful effects that you may wish to avoid." This approach may clarify how the woman herself assesses the risks of the drug. Some type of plan should be mutually agreed upon. Does the woman want to become drug free? What is her motivation to do so, and how will that affect her family (children)? What are her greatest fears if she so chooses? Does she require hospitalization to avoid withdrawal? Will she require residential treatment, or can she be treated in an outpatient facility?

This type of discussion requires that the obstetrician–gynecologist inquire about drug, alcohol, and mental health treatment programs in his or her community. This information will provide the care provider with the knowledge that he or she is not acting in isolation. It also will diminish anxiety that if he or she identifies a woman with substance abuse, the obstetrician–gynecologist will have little to offer the woman. Addiction medicine is a critical part of primary care.

BIBLIOGRAPHY

Smoking Cessation

American College of Obstetricians and Gynecologists. Smoking and reproductive health. ACOG Technical Bulletin 180. Washington, DC: ACOG, 1993

Centers for Disease Control. Cigarette smoking among reproductive-aged women: behavioral risk factor surveillance system, 1989. MMWR 1991;40:719–723

Centers for Disease Control. Cigarette smoking among adults—United States, 1988. MMWR 1991;40:757–759, 765

Lumley J, Astbury J. Advice for pregnancy. In: Chalmers I, Enkin M, Keirse MJNC, eds. Effective care in pregancy and childbirth. Oxford, England: Oxford University Press, 1989:237–254

Petersen L, Handel J, Kotch J, Podedworny T, Rosen A. Smoking reduction during pregnancy by a program of self-help and clinical support. Obstet Gynecol 1992;79:924–930

U.S. Department of Health and Human Services. The health benefits of smoking cessation: a report of the Surgeon General. Washington, DC: U.S. Department of Health and Human Services, 1990: v–vi, 245; publication no. (CDC) 90-8416

U.S. Department of Health and Human Services. Female: pregnancy and pregnancy outcome. In: The health benefits of smoking cessation: a report of the Surgeon General. Washington, DC: U.S. Department of Health and Human Services, 1990:371–423; publication no. (CDC) 90-8416

Exercise

American College of Obstetricians and Gynecologists. Women and exercise. ACOG Technical Bulletin 173. Washington, DC: ACOG, 1992

Nutrition and Weight Control

Institute of Medicine. Improving America's diet and health: from recommendations to action. Washington, DC: National Academy Press, 1991

Institute of Medicine. Nutrition during pregnancy and lactation: an implementation guide. Washington, DC: National Academy Press, 1992

Kant AK, Block G, Schatzkin A, Ziegler RG, Nestle M. Dietary diversity in the US population, NHANES II, 1976–1980. J Am Diet Assoc 1991;91:1526–1531

U.S. Department of Agriculture. Cross-cultural counseling, a guide for nutrition and health counselors. 1986. Washington, DC: U.S. Government Printing Office, 1987

Stress Management

American College of Obstetricians and Gynecologists. Stress in the practice of obstetrics and gynecology. ACOG Technical Bulletin 149. Washington, DC: ACOG, 1990

American Psychiatric Association. Diagnostic and statistical manual of mental disorders. 3rd revised ed. Washington, DC: APA, 1987

American Psychiatric Association. Stress management by behavioral methods. In: Treatments of psychiatric disorders. Vol 3. Washington, DC: APA, 1989:2532–2548

Chrousos GP, Gold PW. The concepts of stress and stress systems disorders: overview of physical and behavioral homeostasis. JAMA 1992;267:1244–1252

Girdano DA, Everly GS, Dusek DE. Controlling stress and tension: a holistic approach. 4th ed. Englewood Cliffs, New Jersey: Prentice-Hall, 1993

Ivancevich JM, Matteson MT, Freedman SM, Phillips JS. Worksite stress management interventions. Am Psychol 1990;45:252–261

Substance Abuse

Allen PM, Sandler M. Critical components of obstetric management of chemically dependent women. Clin Obstet Gynecol 1993;36: 347–360

American College of Obstetricians and Gynecologists. Substance abuse. ACOG Technical Bulletin 194. Washington, DC: ACOG, 1994

Blume SB. Women and alcohol: a review. JAMA 1986;256:1467–1470

Chasnoff IJ, Landress HJ, Barrett ME. The prevalence of illicit drug or alcohol use during pregnancy and discrepancies in mandatory reporting in Pinellas County, Florida. N Engl J Med 1990;322:1202–1206

Day NL, Cottreau CM, Richardson GA. The epidemiology of alcohol, marijuana and cocaine use among women of childbearing age and pregnant women. Clin Obstet Gynecol 1993;36:232–245

Ewing JA. Detecting alcoholism: the CAGE questionnaire. JAMA 1984;252:1905–1907

Klein RF, Friedman-Campbell M, Tocco RV. History taking and substance abuse counseling with the pregnant patient. Clin Obstet Gynecol 1993;36:338–346

Management of Medical Disorders

By routinely assessing a woman's health, obstetrician–gynecologists have an opportunity to detect medical problems and ensure that they receive attention. Periodic screening, evaluation of risk factors, and observation of physical signs and symptoms can disclose a medical disorder in early stages of development, when treatment is often most effective. Most of these initial interventions are within the scope of the obstetrician–gynecologist who is providing primary care. That physician can monitor the patient's care and suggest referral as needed to ensure continuity. Management of these disorders in pregnancy may require specialized care, which will not be covered here.

PULMONARY AND UPPER RESPIRATORY PROBLEMS

Acute diseases of the respiratory system are the most common reasons that patients will seek medical attention in a primary care practice. Cough, sputum production, chest and head pain, and dyspnea are the major manifestations of this group of diseases. Sinusitis is usually secondary to an upper respiratory infection or allergic rhinitis. Bronchitis in many cases is related to viral infection, but the bronchi may become secondarily infected by bacteria or fungi. Asthma is common among young patients, and afflicts 5% of the population. Pneumonia may be community acquired or may be secondary to surgery. Early recognition of these disorders, treatment, and occasionally referrals are important in daily practice.

Sinusitis

One of the most common problems encountered by physicians is posed by the patient who presents with "sinus problems." Multiple other medical problems are blamed on the sinuses, such as headaches, postnasal drainage, halitosis, and dyspepsia. The sinuses are one part of the respiratory system and may be affected by other anatomic areas such as the nose, bronchial tree, or lung. Even though the entire respiratory system may be infected by a particular virus or pathogen (the sinobronchial syndrome), one anatomic area will produce the most symptoms. In evaluating the patient with sinusitis, the focus should be broadened to consider other systemic infections.

Multiple chemical, infectious, nervous, physical, emotional, and hormonal stimuli will influence the mucosa of the nose and sinus. Poor health, systemic diseases, and nutritional deficiencies also contribute to chronic sinusitis. Work and geographic environment, especially if cold, wet, and humid, are factors in the development of sinusitis. Other contributory factors that predispose to sinus disease include infections, atmospheric pollutants, tobacco smoke, dental conditions, skeletal deformities, and neoplasms.

Infectious agents are viral, bacterial, and fungal. Viral infections of the contiguous nose and nasopharynx are the usual mode of spread. Viral infections affect the ciliary function of the sinus, and with the edema of inflammation, predispose to superinfection with bacteria. The most common bacterial agents are *Streptococcus pneumoniae, Haemophilus influenzae, Staphylococcus aureus, Streptococcus pyogenes,* and alpha streptococcus species. In chronic sinusitis, complicated by inadequate drainage and compromised local defense mechanisms, opportunistic anaerobic bacteria predominate. Mixed infections with both aerobic and anaerobic organisms are frequently identified.

Acute infection can affect any of the sinuses, with the maxillary and frontal sinuses most commonly affected in the adult. The prototypical infection is in the maxillary sinus. Fever, malaise, and vague headache are early symptoms. There is a feeling of "fullness" in the face, and on sudden motion, pain in the underlying teeth. On physical examination there is pain to pressure and percussion over the cheeks. Inspection of the nose will reveal purulent exudates in the middle meatus or in the nasopharynx. Radiologically, early infections will reveal thickened mucosa followed by opacification of the sinus by fluid. The final stage will demonstrate the classic air fluid levels that require both supine and upright views. Cultures, unless obtained by direct needle drainage, should be viewed with suspicion.

Antibiotic coverage should be broad to cover the common aerobes and anaerobes. Appropriate choices include ampicillin, amoxicillin, erythromycin with sulfonamide, and cefaclor. Decongestant drops such as phenylephrine and systemic medications such as pseudoephedrine should be used only in the first few days of therapy. Hot packs over the affected areas and analgesics can be helpful. Improvement should be noted in 2 days and complete resolution of symptoms by 10 days. Radiologic improvement may lag by up to 3 weeks. In patients who do not rapidly improve, resistance to the antibiotics may be present or there may be abscess formation due to lack of drainage. Referral for irrigation of the affected sinus is recommended.

Chronic sinusitis is the result of repeated infections with inadequate ventilation and drainage. In the preantibiotic era, chronic sinusitis was the result of repeated acute sinusitis with incomplete resolution. Incomplete regeneration of surface ciliated epithelium results in impaired mucus removal. This results in an environment that enhances growth of opportunistic organisms, creating a vicious cycle. Allergies increase edematous mucosa and hypersecretion, which result in ductal obstruction and infection. Chronic sinusitis causes a vague feeling of fullness of the face and may be associated with chronic cough and laryngitis. Acute infections are more common because of the altered environment.

Treatment is directed at the underlying etiology, such as allergies and infection. Occasionally surgical drainage with formation of nasoantral windows is necessary. Computed tomography in conjunction with endoscopic surgery has increased the success of sinus surgery, especially in cases involving polyps.

Complications of untreated infections may lead to orbital cellulitis, subperiosteal abscess formation, orbital abscess, and cavernous sinus thrombosis. Hospital admission, parenteral antibiotics, and surgical drainage are the mainstays of therapy. Acute meningitis may result from bacterial spread either through venous channels or by local spread. Dural abscess and brain abscess are usually due to direct spread and may present as a dull headache with systemic findings of fatigue, weight loss, and vomiting. Recognition by computed tomography scan with appropriate surgical intervention is mandatory. Neoplasms of the sinus are unusual and malignant tumors rare.

Bronchitis

Acute bronchitis is an inflammatory condition of the tracheobronchial tree. It occurs most commonly in the winter during the peak of viral infections. The common cold viruses (rhinovirus and coronavirus), adenovirus, influenza virus, and a nonviral pathogen, *Mycoplasma pneumoniae*, are the most common infectious agents. Cough, hoarseness, and fever are the most common symptoms and are found in all age groups. After 3–4 days, the symptoms of rhinitis and sore throat resolve, but the cough persists and may last as long as 3 weeks. Sputum production is present in one half of cases, and may be prolonged in cigarette smokers.

Physical examination will demonstrate rhonchi and coarse rales, but without consolidation and alveolar involvement. Auscultation of the chest should be performed carefully for signs of pneumonia. If questions of parenchymal disease still exist, chest radiographs should be obtained. As the syndrome subsides, the sputum may become more purulent. Cultures of sputum tend to grow multiple organisms and are of limited value. Treatment is directed at symptomatic relief. The use of cough suppressants with either dextromethorphan or codeine may afford some degree of relief. Expectorants are of limited value and their efficacy has not been proven beneficial. Treatment with antibiotics is not indicated unless infection with *M. pneumoniae* is suspected or the chest radiograph is suggestive of pneumonia. Erythromycin is the drug of choice in patients with *M. pneumoniae*.

Chronic bronchitis is defined as a productive cough for at least 3 months of the year for 2 consecutive years. Prevalence has been estimated to be between 10% and 25% of the adult population. It is strongly associated with cigarette abuse and usually classified as a form of chronic obstructive lung disease. Other etiologies include chronic infections and the inhalation of environmental pathogens in dust. Incessant cough is the cardinal manifestation of disease. Expectoration of sputum occurs during the day, but it is most prominent on arising. Most of these patients have other associated pulmonary diseases and require follow-up frequently. Because of the chronic nature of these patients' diseases, specialized care is recommended.

Asthma

Asthma is a clinical syndrome of recurrent airway obstruction that resolves either spontaneously or with bronchodilator therapy. Asthma is associated with hyperresponsiveness of the airways to various chemical and physical stimuli resulting in bronchoconstriction. Common stimuli that may initiate an attack include viral infections, oxidant air pollutants (such as nitrogen dioxide or sulfur dioxide), allergens in susceptible individuals, pharmacologic stimuli (such as aspirin), exercise, occupational factors, and emotional stress. The clinical hallmarks of the disease are wheezing and dyspnea. During periods of quiescence, spirometry will be normal. The etiology remains unknown and may represent multiple distinct disease entities that defy classification schemes. The male–female ratio is 2:1 in childhood but is 1:1 by age 30. Initial attacks occur before age 25, but may appear at any age. The symptoms are variable and range from a chronic cough to life-threatening episodes of hypoxia.

The pathophysiology of an asthma attack consists of 1) constriction of smooth muscle in the airway, 2) thickening of the airway epithelium, and 3) liquids in the airway lumen. Constriction of the airway is considered the most important event in an asthma attack and may be due to bioactive mediators and neurotransmitters. Histamine, acetylcholine, kinins, adenosine, leukotrienes, and other mediators are felt to have some role in bronchoconstriction. During acute airway obstruction, airway resistance increases while flow rates of gases decrease. The decrease in flow is most noticeable during the expiratory phase rather than during the inspiratory phase. During resolution of the obstruction, the large airways return to normal, followed by the peripheral airways.

The presenting symptom is usually shortness of breath that may be associated with cough, wheezing, and anxiety. Physical examination is significant for tachypnea, with a rate to 25–40 breaths per minute. The chest will be hyperinflated, with a prolonged expiratory phase. Accessory neck muscle usage is common. Auscultation will reveal wheezing and rhonchi in all lung fields. Decreasing wheezing may be a sign of impending respiratory arrest.

Laboratory findings will reveal a decrease in vital capacity. Multiple spirometric variations have been described. The most useful test is the peak expiratory forced rate, which can be performed with a simple device in the emergency department. During the resolution of the attack, the peak expiratory forced rate will begin to approach normal. Chest radiographs should not be routinely obtained unless there is a strong suggestion of pneumonia. Determination of arterial blood gases may be helpful in assessing the severity of an attack. In early stages of asthma, respiratory alkalosis is found, and the partial pressure of carbon dioxide, arterial (Pa_{CO_2}), is 25–35 mm Hg. The Pa_{O_2} is usually 55–75 mm Hg on room air. As the attack worsens, pH will normalize because of metabolic acidosis, and a "normal Paco$_2$," signals impending pulmonary failure. In the final stages of "status asthmatica," just before respiratory arrest, there will be a sharp rise in Paco$_2$ with a profound drop in pH due to physical tiring of the patient. Intubation and intensive care transfer are mandatory.

Inhalation agents have become the mainstay of therapy for the patient with asthma. These drugs are topically and locally absorbed, which lessens many systemic side effects. Because of the increased safety of the more specific beta-2 medications, many older therapies, such as the use of subcutaneous epinephrine, have been replaced. Most emergency department and pulmonary physicians now use inhalation agents for primary therapy. Bronchial dilatation in the constricted airways is caused by stimulating beta-2 receptors in the pulmonary tree. Older inhalation agents such as epinephrine and isoproterenol stimulate both beta-1 and beta-2 receptors. An uncomfortable side effect of beta-1 stimulation is tachycardia. Beta-2–selective drugs common in clinical use are metaproterenol and albuterol. Patients tolerate these newer medications better, and they have the additional benefit of longer half-lives (approximately 5–6 hours, compared with 2–3 hours). A third medication available is an aerosolized atropinelike compound, ipratropium bromide. Ipratropium blocks the parasympathetic stimulation that alters the balance toward the sympathetic system and therefore bronchodilation. This drug's usefulness is limited to a very select subset of patients and should not be considered to be primary therapy.

Theophylline was the mainstay of therapy for many years. The mechanism of action continues to be debated. Significant problems with theophylline have included toxicity and a wide variation of metabolism that is affected by age, concurrent medications, and cigarette smoking. Laboratory expenses for frequent monitoring of levels increase total cost. In more severe cases of asthma, corticosteroids are used. The mechanism of action is debated, but it is probably secondary to decreasing the effects of inflammatory cells in the tracheobronchial tree. Patients who do not respond quickly to outpatient maneuvers should be started on intravenous dosages of corticosteroids. There is no consensus on interval and dosage schedules, but 20–80 mg of methylprednisolone is commonly used. Once the patient responds, 40–60 mg of prednisone per day is begun. Prednisone is decreased by 5 mg daily until finished or baseline daily dosage is reached.

Pneumonia

Pneumonia is defined as inflammation of the distal lung that includes terminal airways, alveolar spaces, and the interstitium. Additional information is added to better characterize the etiology or location, such as aspiration pneumonia, acute bacterial or viral pneumonia, lobar pneumonia, and bronchopneumonia. Pneumonia is generally classified as either community acquired or nosocomial. This distinction is important in determining the prognosis and therapy. Mortality increases with age, with a 30% mortality rate in patients older than age 65. Other risk factors in mortality are chronic cardiopulmonary diseases, alcoholism, diabetes, renal failure, malignancy, and poor nutrition. Clinical features associated with poor outcome include the following: more than two-lobe involvement, respiratory rate greater than 30 breaths per minute on presentation, severe hypoxemia, hypoalbuminemia, and septicemia. Pneumonia that progresses to adult respiratory distress syndrome has a 70% mortality rate.

Signs and symptoms of pneumonia are variable and depend on the organism and the patient's underlying immune status. Typical pneumonia syndrome presentation is characterized by high fever, productive cough, chills, and pleuritic chest pain; the patient appears to be in a toxic condition. Chest roentgenogram often will show infiltrates. The most common agents are bacterial in two thirds of cases, including *Streptococcus pneumoniae* ("pneumococcal pneumonia"), *H. influenzae, Klebsiella pneumoniae*, and gram-negative and anaerobic bacteria. Atypical pneumonia is more insidious in onset with moderate fever but without chills, nonproductive cough, headache, myalgias, and mild leukocytosis. Chest roentgenogram will show a more diffuse interstitial pattern, or bronchopneumonia. The patient will not appear as clinically ill as the radiograph would suggest. Common etiologic agents include viruses, *M. pneumoniae, Legionella pneumophila, Chlamydia pneumoniae* (also called the TWAR agent), and other rare agents.

A strong index of suspicion is required in diagnosis, especially in elderly patients and immune-impaired patients. These groups may have a more elusive presentation, despite infection with "typical agents." Confusion in the elderly or exacerbation of other illnesses may be the only clue. Fever, while prominent in younger patients, may be absent in the elderly. An increased respiratory rate of greater than 25 breaths per minute is the most reliable sign of pneumonia. Mortality in these groups of patients is correlated with the ability of the patient to mount normal host defenses such as fever, chills, and tachycardia. Tests helpful in the diagnosis of community-acquired pneumonia are sputum Gram stain with culture and blood cultures. Adequate sputum is defined as having more than 25 neutrophils and fewer than 10 epithelial cells per low-power field on microscopic examination. *L. pneumophila* may be demonstrated by direct fluorescent antibody staining of sputum or by serologic tests using enzyme-linked immunosorbent assays. *Mycoplasma pneumoniae* is suspected when cold agglutinins are positive with the appropriate clinical syndrome.

Therapy should be directed at the responsible pathogen, if it can be identified. Streptococcal pneumonia classically presents with a sudden onset of fever and chills with gram-positive cocci (so-called coffee bean cocci) on Gram stain. Bacteremia may be present in up to 25% cases, and occasionally the diagnosis is made on results of blood culture prior to sputum culture. Procaine penicillin G, 600,000 U, is given intramuscularly every 12 hours until clinical resolution, when penicillin V potassium, 500 mg four times daily, may be substituted. Most patients respond within 48 hours of initiation of therapy. Alternative therapy is 2.4–4.8 million U daily of penicillin G given intravenously every 4 hours. Penicillin-allergic patients may receive intravenous erythromycin 500 mg every 6 hours, and after improvement may be switched to oral preparations. Penicillin-resistant strains have been identified in the past 15 years and are associated with nosocomial infections or with treatment with β-lactam antibiotics.

Mycoplasma pneumoniae infections may be treated with erythromycin, 2 g daily, in divided doses. Clinical severity will determine the need for hospitalization and intravenous antibiotics versus outpatient therapy with oral preparations. *Legionella pneumophila* requires doses of 2–4 g intravenously per day. After the patient has been afebrile for 2 days, oral erythromycin, 500 mg four times daily, is begun and given for a total of 3 weeks of therapy. In severe infections, rifampin, 600 mg every 12 hours, is added. In many cases, exact identification of the organism cannot be determined, and therapy is directed at the most likely organism. Erythromycin is active against the three most likely organisms, *Streptococcus*, *Mycoplasma*, and *Legionella*, and should be used in immunecompetent patients. In elderly or immune-compromised patients, a second- or third-generation cephalosporin should be added. Hospitalization is necessary for patients who are elderly, in a toxic condition, or immunocompromised. Hydration and oxygen therapy are important in all patients, and chest physiotherapy should be used when copious sputum and ineffective cough are present.

Tuberculosis

Tuberculosis is caused by *Mycobacterium tuberculosis*, which is part of a complex of five species: *M. tuberculosis*, *M. bovis*, *M. africanum*, *M. ulcerans*, and *M. microti*. *M. tuberculosis* is responsible for most human disease. Most individuals who contract *M. tuberculosis* do not develop the disease, with only 5–15% developing active tuberculosis.

Transmission occurs when aerosolized droplets containing the tubercle bacillus are inhaled and carried to the deep alveolar spaces. Chest X-rays of patients with primary tuberculosis reveal dense infiltrates in the lower or middle lung. Marked hilar or mediastinal lymphadenopathy will also be noted. The patient may develop fever, lassitude, and a brassy cough. Patients with chronic tuberculosis have disease in the posterior regions of the lungs' apices due to increased oxygen tension and low lymphatic drainage.

Individuals with primary tuberculosis are more likely to have disseminated disease. Tubercle bacilli can enter the lymphatics draining the lungs and establish foci of infection in the ipsilateral hilar lymph node. The bacilli can enter the thoracic duct and the circulation, thereby infecting various organs. Dissemination can also result in infection of the posterior regions of the apices of the upper lobes of the lung and the superior segments of the lower lobes, resulting in chronic pulmonary tuberculosis.

Within 2–6 weeks after infection, the host develops hypersensitivity to tubercle bacilli and a granulomatous inflammatory reaction at sites of infection. Calcification of granulomas results in formation of a Ghon complex typically found in the lungs and hilar nodes.

Tuberculosis is often diagnosed by detection of cutaneous hypersensitivity to tuberculin through the intracutaneous injection of purified protein derivative (PPD) of tuberculin, 5 tuberculin U (intermediate-strength PPD). A positive reaction is defined as a wheal of induration of at least 10 mm at the injection site within 72 hours of administering the PPD. Individuals who have a negative-to-intermediate reaction can be administered a second-strength PPD, which is equivalent to 250 tuberculin U. False-positive tests are due to injection of nontuberculous mycobacteria (eg, *M. kansasii*). False-negative reactions (anergy) can occur in patients with active tuberculosis and pregnant patients.

Therapy for tuberculosis is based on the following considerations:

- Within a population of tubercle bacilli, spontaneous resistant forms exist, although the given population has not been previously exposed to antituberculous agents.
- The bacteria exist in three different populations: extracellularly in cavitary lesions, in closed caseous lesions, and within macrophages.

Multiple antimicrobial therapy is necessary to prevent a resistant organism from becoming dominant. A bactericidal combination is frequently used to achieve effectiveness against the rapidly proliferating organisms found extracellularly and the more slowly growing bacilli found in caseous lesions and macrophages.

Isoniazid and rifampin are commonly used as initial agents for the treatment of tuberculosis. A third agent, such as streptomycin, pyrazinamide, or ethambutol, is often given along with isoniazid and rifampin. Streptomycin is active against extracellular organisms. Pyrazinamide is bactericidal against intracellular bacteria. Although ethambutol is not bactericidal, it is effective against extracellular and intracellular bacteria, reducing the risk of selection of resistant forms.

Patients who convert from a negative PPD test to a positive one with no evidence of active disease should receive isoniazid for 1 year. Individuals older than age 35 years with a positive skin test, no evidence of conversion, and no known contact with an individual with active disease should not be given isoniazid. Although older individuals are more susceptible to developing isoniazid hepatotoxicity, isoniazid therapy should be considered for the older patient with a positive skin test who has HIV infection or fibrotic pulmonary lesions.

COMMON INFECTIOUS PROBLEMS

Influenza

There are three types of influenza viruses—A, B, and C. Types A and B are responsible for febrile respiratory disease. These viruses tend to spread by aerosolization, being easily spread from one person to the next by coughing, sneezing, or talking. Once the virus has been inhaled, the incubation period is 1–3 days. After this short incubation period, the patient develops acute onset of fever, chills, headache, myalgia, lumbosacral pain, and fatigue. The patient tends to have headache and myalgia that increase in intensity with exacerbation of the fever. Resolution of the fever is associated with a cough, rhinorrhea, and pharyngitis.

A diagnosis can be made by isolating and cultivating the virus in tissue culture. In the absence of tissue culture facilities, serologic detection of antibodies can be performed. Influenza A and B stimulate the production of specific immunoglobulin M (IgM), IgG, and IgA antibodies. Immunoglobulin M antibodies appear within 1–2 weeks after the onset of infection and remain elevated for 2–3 months. Immunoglobulin G antibodies remain elevated for several years, whereas IgA antibodies remain elevated in nasal secretions for 3–6 months. Although only 1% of cases of influenza result in pneumonia, mortality rates of 30% have been reported. Influenza pneumonia is more likely to occur in patients with chronic illness, such as rheumatic mitral stenosis, and in healthy pregnant women. Elderly patients who develop influenza pneumonia are likely to develop secondary bacterial pneumonia.

The best prevention for influenza is vaccination with a trivalent vaccine. Patients who are exposed but have not been vaccinated can be administered amantadine. The basic treatment for viral pneumonia is supportive.

Urinary Tract Infections

Urinary tract infections are among the most common medical problems encountered by obstetrician–gynecologists. It is estimated that 10–20% of women will, during their lifetime, experience a symptomatic urinary tract infection. Urinary tract infections can be divided into three types: urethritis, bladder infections (asymptomatic bacteriuria and acute cystitis), and pyelonephritis. In addition to being one of the causes of urethritis, coliform organisms, particularly *Escherichia coli*, are the most common causes of asymptomatic bacteriuria, cystitis, and pyelonephritis.

Urethritis

Although it is sometimes found in sexually active women, urethritis is relatively uncommon. Such patients are more likely to have cervicitis than urethritis. They are often mistakenly treated for cystitis. Symptoms often persist if the patient is treated with urinary antiseptic or nitrofurantoin, a cephalosporin, or ampicillin. The diagnosis should, therefore, be established in any patient who presents with dysuria. A urinalysis usually shows pyuria but yields no bacteria. However, a Gram stain and cultures can guide the clinician in treatment. A swab inserted into the urethra can be used to obtain a specimen for Gram staining and cultures for *Neisseria gonorrhoeae*, *Chlamydia trachomatis*, *Mycoplasma*, and *Ureaplasma*. If *N. gonorrhoeae* is present, the Gram stain will usually reveal intracellular gram-negative diplococci. A stained specimen revealing polymorphonuclear leukocytes but no bacteria suggests the presence of *C. trachomatis*, *Mycoplasma*, or *Ureaplasma*.

Urethritis caused by *N. gonorrhoeae*, *C. trachomatis*, *Mycoplasma*, or *Ureaplasma* can be treated with several agents. Nonpregnant patients who are not treated with ofloxacin (300 mg twice daily for 7 days) or ciprofloxacin (250 mg twice daily for 7 days) should receive doxycycline (100 mg twice daily for 7 days) plus ceftriaxone (250 mg intramuscularly). If the patient is pregnant, erythromycin (500 mg four times daily for 7 days) should be substituted for doxycycline. Norfloxacin is effective against *N. gonorrhoeae* but has no activity against *C. trachomatis*. Other organisms which may cause urethritis are *Mycoplasma*, *Ureaplasma*, and *Trichomonas vaginalis*. Tetracycline is effective against *Mycoplasma*. Erythromycin is not effective against *Mycoplasma*, but may be used in pregnant patients for treatment of *C. trachomatis* or *Ureaplasma*.

Lower urinary tract infections should be differentiated from vaginitis. Information regarding the patient's symptoms will aid in the diagnosis; that is, do her symptoms or dysuria originate inside the body with the onset of micturition or are they experienced on the vulva or perineum after voiding? The acute onset of dysuria is characteristic of bacterial urethrocystitis associated with *E. coli* or *Staphylococcus saprophyticus*. The patient with a new sexual partner should be suspected of having *N. gonorrhoeae* or *C. trachomatis*. *N. gonorrhoeae* usually has an abrupt onset, in contrast to the gradual development of symptoms seen with *C. trachomatis*. It is important to determine whether *N. gonorrhoeae* or *C. trachomatis* is present in the urethra because, if present, the organism will probably be found in the endocervix as well.

Bladder Infections

The diagnosis of cystitis can usually be made on the basis of physical findings and laboratory tests. A bimanual pelvic examination can be helpful by eliciting pain on compression of the empty bladder between the intravaginal examining fingers and the hand on the abdomen. Urine should be examined for the presence of leukocytes. Microscopic hematuria, uncommon in other dysuric syndromes, is indicative of acute cystitis. If bacteria are seen, then a Gram stain should be performed to help in selecting antibiotic therapy. If the specimen is gram negative, a member of the Enterobacteriaceae family should be suspected; if it is gram positive, *Streptococcus agalactiae*, *Staphylococcus*, or *Enterococcus* should be suspected. The number of bacteria per oil immersion field of uncentrifuged urine suggesting a concentration of $\geq 10^5$ colony-forming units (CFU) per milliliter of urine is also diagnostic. Biochemical tests (eg, leukocyte esterase and leukocyte esterase/nitrate strip) as well as other commercially available tests can be helpful. A routine culture is not necessary unless the patient fails therapy, experiences recurrent infections, has a debilitating disease, or receives antibiotic therapy for another condition.

The standard measure of infected urine has been $\geq 10^5$ uropathogens per milliliter of voided urine. This standard was originally established because voided specimens of women were easily contaminated. However, it has subsequently been learned that many women with cystitis due to *E. coli*, *S. saprophyticus*, *Proteus*, or other uropathogens have counts between 10^2 and 10^4 CFU per milliliter of urine, which makes acceptable a count of a known uropathogen of $\geq 10^2$ CFU per milliliter of urine. Antibiotics used for treatment of acute cystitis are listed in Table 1-2.

Bacteriuria is common in the geriatric female population. During the perimenopausal and postmenopausal periods, bacteriuria is uncommon, occurring in <5% of the women in this age group. Among women aged 65 years and older, bacteriuria occurs in 3–50%; among women aged 80 years and older, in 20–50%. Nonhospitalized ambulatory patients with asymptomatic bacteriuria should not be treated because it is a transient condition. However, debilitated or hospitalized patients with bacteriuria should be treated because they are likely to experience dissemination of bacteria, resulting in significant illness. If the patient is to undergo an operative procedure involving the genitourinary tract, the presence or absence of bacteriuria should be determined and, if present, treated appropriately. If such a patient is not treated for her asymptomatic bacteriuria and she undergoes gynecologic surgery, the bacteria are likely to be disseminated.

Asymptomatic bacteriuria is a condition of importance in pregnant patients. Roughly 98% of pregnant patients with asymptomatic bacteriuria will have bacteriuria at the first prenatal visit. If untreated, approximately 25% will develop pyelonephritis during the pregnancy or in the postpartum period.

Pyelonephritis

Women who have acute pyelonephritis should be hospitalized for treatment with intravenous antibiotics. Potential serious complications of pyelonephritis include bacteremia, septic shock, adult respiratory distress syndrome, and preterm labor in pregnant women.

Vaccines

Influenza

Influenza vaccine is made from killed influenza types A and B viruses. The vaccine is trivalent because it represents a variety of subtypes. The vaccine should be administered to adults and children with chronic pulmonary or cardiac disease or metabolic disease. Nursing home patients and patients older than age 55 years should be vaccinated annually. In addition, pregnant women with underlying illnesses should receive the vaccine. Health care workers should also be vaccinated because they can transmit the virus. Family members of high-risk patients should receive the vaccine as well.

Pneumococcal

Pneumococcal vaccine is a 23-valent polysaccharide obtained from multiple serotypes. The vaccine is recommended for children younger than age 2 years who have had a splenectomy or who have sickle cell disease, HIV infection, or nephrosis. Patients aged 65 years and older and adults with medical conditions that increase the risk of pneumococcal infection (eg, chronic cardiac or pulmonary disease, sickle cell disease, nephrotic syndrome, Hodgkin disease, asplenia, diabetes mellitus, alcoholism, cirrhosis, multiple myeloma, renal disease, or other immunosuppression) should receive the vaccine. Repeat vaccination is suggested every 6 years secondary to poor antibody response in elderly patients.

Hepatitis B

Infection with hepatitis B virus (HBV) is not uncommon. In the United States, serologic evidence is found in 4.8% of the total population, in 3.2% of the white population, and in 14% of the African–American population. Although there does not appear to be any difference with regard to sex, positive serology does correlate with increasing age. A higher prevalence of HBV-positive serology is seen among individuals from Southeast Asia. Transmission is primarily by parenteral, sexual, or vertical routes. Therefore, this disease is particularly important to the obstetrician–gynecologist because he or she is exposed to 1) multiple bodily fluids and 2) congenital infection. The following groups should receive HBV vaccine: intravenous drug users; current recipients of blood products; persons in health-related jobs with exposure to blood or blood products; household and sexual contacts of HBV carriers; prostitutes; and persons with a history of sexual activity with multiple partners in the previous 6 months.

TABLE 1-2. ANTIBIOTICS FOR TREATMENT OF ACUTE CYSTITIS

Regimen	Dosage
Pregnant patients	
7-Day	
Nitrofurantoin	100 mg q 12 h × 7 d
First-generation cephalosporin	500 mg q 6 h × 7 d
Amoxicillin	500 mg q 8 h × 7 d
Nonpregnant patients	
1 Dose	
Nitrofurantoin	200 mg
Trimethoprim (TMP)	400 mg
TMP/sulfamethoxazole	300 (1,600) mg
Amoxicillin	3 g
Ampicillin	3.5 g
First-generation cephalosporin	2 g
Sulfisoxazole	2 g
7-Day	
TMP	100 (200) mg q 12 (24) h
TMP/sulfamethoxazole	160/800 mg q 12 h
Nitrofurantoin	100 mg q 12 h
Amoxicillin	500 mg q 8 h
First-generation cephalosporin	500 mg q 9 h
Norfloxacin	400 mg q 12 h
Ofloxacin	200 mg q 12 h
Ciprofloxacin	250 mg q 12 h
Sulfisoxazole	500 mg q 6 h
Tetracycline	500 mg q 6 h

Passive immunization can be accomplished by administering hepatitis B immune globulin (HBIG). Before administering HBIG to an exposed individual, blood should be drawn for determination of hepatitis B surface antigen (HBsAg) antibody status. If the serology is negative, HBV vaccine should be administered. Pregnancy is not a contraindication to the administration of HBV vaccine or HBIG.

Infants born to mothers who are HBsAg positive should receive HBIG and HBV vaccine, particularly if the mother had acute hepatitis B in the third trimester or is HBsAg and HBeAg (hepatitis B envelope antigen) positive. Individuals who are HBeAg positive are more likely to infect their infants. The presence of anti-HBe (antibody to e antigen) reduces the potential for infectivity. However, the presence of anti-HBe in the mother should not deter the physician from administering HBIG and HBV vaccine to the newborn.

CARDIOVASCULAR DISORDERS

Coronary artery disease is one of the most common causes of death in women in the United States. Lowering cholesterol levels and controlling hypertension, in addition to using hormone replacement therapy, can help prevent coronary disease and reduce the death rate from it. Patients should be counseled about these factors as well as other risks, such as smoking, that they can control through a combination of life style modification and treatment.

Hypertension

Although hypertension contributes less to subsequent cardiovascular morbidity and mortality in women than it does in men, it is still the most common chronic disease in older women and a significant risk factor for stroke, congestive heart disease, and renal disease. Beginning at age 50, hypertension is more common in women than in men, and more common in African–American patients. A sustained blood pressure greater than 140/90 mm Hg requires treatment.

Measuring Blood Pressure

"White coat" or office hypertension is a real phenomenon. For this reason office measurement of blood pressure should be standardized, and ambulatory monitoring is worthwhile. In the office, the patient should be allowed to rest for 5 minutes in a seated position. There should be no use of cigarettes or caffeine for at least 30 minutes before measurement. Because higher readings are found inexplicably in the right arm, the cuff should be applied to the right arm, 20 mm above the bend of the elbow. The cuff size should be matched with arm size, using the adult size for most patients and the obese cuff for large arms (greater than 32-cm circumference).

Readings are made with the arm raised and parallel to the floor. The cuff is rapidly inflated until the brachial pulse cannot be palpated. After deflation, the cuff is reinflated after a pause of 30–45 seconds, to a systolic pressure 30 mm Hg greater than the pressure at which the pulse disappeared. The cuff should be deflated no faster than a rate of 2 mm Hg/s.

The phase V Korotkoff sound is used to measure diastolic pressure, the pressure at which all sound disappears. Measurements should be repeated with at least 2 minutes of rest between readings, if blood pressure readings are inconsistent. Automated sphygmomanometer readings should be correlated with the standard method of blood pressure measurement.

Diagnosis

Key information to be obtained from the history and physical examination is as follows:

- Previous history of hypertension
- Previous history of antihypertensive treatment
- Medical information of specific interest: headaches, coronary artery disease, chest pain, prior stroke, renal disease
- Family history of cardiovascular disease, especially early age of onset
- Dietary history, especially excessive sodium or alcohol intake
- Relevant medications, such as glucocorticosteroids, sympathomimetic amines, nasal decongestants
- Other cardiovascular risk factors: smoking, cholesterol–lipid profile, obesity, diabetes mellitus, stress

The blood pressure classification established in 1988 is shown in Table 1-3. A single elevated diastolic pressure less than 105 mm Hg should not be treated but should be rechecked within 2 months. When the diastolic pressure is greater than 105 mm Hg, the patient should be treated. A diastolic pressure greater than 115 mm Hg requires immediate attention. Malignant hypertension is a diastolic pressure greater than 140 mm Hg with papilledema. Patients with a systolic blood pressure greater than 160 mm Hg will benefit from treatment.

Patients with hypertension require the following minimal laboratory evaluation:

- Urinalysis
- Hemoglobin or hematocrit

TABLE 1-3. BLOOD PRESSURE CLASSIFICATION

Blood pressure (in mm Hg)	Result
Diastolic pressure	
< 85	Normal
85–89	High normal
90–104	Mild hypertension
105–114	Moderate hypertension
> 115	Severe hypertension
Systolic pressure	
< 140	Normal
140–149	Borderline systolic hypertension
150–159	Moderate systolic hypertension
> 160	Isolated systolic hypertension

- Creatinine
- Potassium
- Fasting glucose
- Cholesterol–lipid profile
- Electrocardiography

The common causes of secondary hypertension are as follows:

- Renal: renal vascular disease, polycystic kidney disease, collagen vascular disease, and renin-secreting tumors
- Endocrine: adrenal problems (aldosteronism, adrenal hyperplasia, Cushing disease, pheochromocytoma), hyperparathyroidism, acromegaly
- Cardiac: coarctation of the aorta
- Drugs and chemicals: glucocorticoids, mineralocorticoids, sympathomimetics

Treatment

The first line of defense is dietary and life style changes rather than pharmacologic interventions. Weight loss, control of sodium intake, exercise, elimination of excess alcohol intake, calcium supplementation, stress management, and cessation of smoking are all important treatment interventions for hypertension. Only after these efforts have failed should pharmacologic therapy be considered. Patients who respond to nonpharmacologic treatment require close monitoring, because a significant percentage will progress to higher levels of blood pressure and will require drug therapy.

Women with diastolic blood pressures greater than 100 mm Hg should be treated with drugs if blood pressure levels cannot be lowered with nonpharmacologic methods. Women with diastolic blood pressures of 90–100 mm Hg should be treated with drugs if they are African–American, have a systolic blood pressure greater than 160 mm Hg, or have other cardiovascular risk factors.

Drug therapy (Table 1-4) should be individualized, and consideration must always be given to the effect of a given drug on another health problem or medication. The first line of therapy is a drug from one of the following classes: diuretic, beta blocker, calcium antagonist, or angiotensin-converting enzyme (ACE) inhibitor. Potassium-sparing diuretics are preferred (spironolactone, triamterene, or amiloride). Patients with hyperlipidemias should avoid beta blockers, as should patients with pulmonary disease or congestive heart failure. Alpha-adrenergic drugs have the advantage of having a positive impact on the cholesterol–lipid profile and are often used as first-line therapy. Angiotensin-converting enzyme inhibitors are relatively safe with few side effects. Calcium channel blockers are especially effective in elderly and African–American patients. Schemes for primary and secondary combinations are given in Table 1-5.

TABLE 1-4. SELECTED MEDICATIONS AND DOSAGE FOR CONTROL OF ESSENTIAL HYPERTENSION

Class and Medication	Normal Daily Dosage in mg/d (Interval*)	Dispensing Unit (mg)
Angiotensin-converting enzyme (ACE) inhibitors		
Captopril	75–450 (tid)	12.5, 25, 50, 100
Enalapril	5–40 (qd, bid)	2.5, 5, 10, 20
Calcium channel blockers		
Nifedipine (sustained release)	30–90 (qd)	30, 60, 90
Diltiazem (sustained release)	120–240 (bid)	60, 90, 120
Verapamil (sustained release)	120–480 (qd, bid)	120, 180, 240
Alpha blockers		
Prazosin	2–20 (bid, tid, qid)	1, 2, 5
Terazosin	1–20 (qd)	1, 2, 5, 10
Mixed alpha and beta blockers		
Labetalol	200–800 (bid)	100, 200, 300
Diuretics		
Hydrochlorothiazide	12.5–50 (qd)	25, 50
Furosemide (loop diuretic)	20–1,000 (qd–bid)	20, 40, 80
Triamterene (potassium sparing)	50–100 (bid)	50, 100
Beta blockers		
Propranolol (lipid soluble)	60–160 (qd)	60, 80, 120, 160
Atenolol (water soluble)	50–100 (qd)	50, 100
Central agents		
Methyldopa	250–2,000 (bid)	125, 250, 500
Clonidine	0.2–0.6 (bid)	0.1, 0.2, 0.3

*Intervals are defined as follows: qd, daily; bid, twice daily; tid, three times daily; qid, four times daily.

TABLE 1-5. SCHEMES FOR CONTROL OF ESSENTIAL HYPERTENSION*

Primary Medications	Secondary Combination†
ACE inhibitor‡	Beta blockers, diuretics, central agents
Calcium channel blockers	Diuretics, beta blockers, central agents
Alpha blockers	Diuretics, beta blockers

* Monotherapy and long-acting agents are recommended for compliance. Fixed combinations are discouraged because of the inability to modify doses selectively; however, they have the advantage of compliance. If hypertension remains uncontrolled despite use of a secondary drug, referral to an internist is suggested for further work-up and management.
† Secondary combinations are added to primary medications if adequate control is not achieved.
‡ ACE indicates angiotensin-converting enzyme.

Monitoring Therapy

Patients on drug therapy should monitor their blood pressures at home at least one or two times per week, at the same time during the day. A record of these measurements should be reviewed with the physician 2–4 weeks after beginning therapy. If side effects are encountered, treatment should be shifted to another class of the first-line drugs. An interval of 1–3 months should be allowed to evaluate the response to initial therapy. Patients not responding to first-line drugs require referral.

The doses of estrogen and progestin used for postmenopausal hormone therapy do not cause hypertension (except for the very rare idiosyncratic reaction). Because of the protective effect of appropriate estrogen therapy on the risk of cardiovascular disease, women with controlled hypertension are in need of that specific benefit of estrogen.

Cholesterol

High blood pressure and high blood cholesterol frequently coexist in adults in the United States. Both are risk factors for CHD. Classification of total cholesterol, LDL, and HDL levels is shown in Table 1-6. A patient's risk for CHD is assessed by evaluating cholesterol levels as well as additional risk factors:

- Age
  —Men ≥ age 45 years
  —Women ≥ age 55 years or premature menopause without estrogen replacement therapy
- Family history of premature coronary heart disease (definite myocardial infarction or sudden death before age 55 years in father or other male first-degree relative, or before age 65 years in mother or other female first-degree relative)
- Current cigarette smoking
- Hypertension
- Low HDL cholesterol levels
- Diabetes mellitus

High risk is defined as the presence of two or more risk factors other than high levels of LDL cholesterol. An HDL level of ≥60 mg/dl is considered a negative risk factor; if present, one risk factor should be subtracted (because high levels decrease the risk of CHD).

There are important differences in lipoprotein risk factors between women and men. Low-density lipoprotein cholesterol is more important in men than in women, whereas in women, HDL cholesterol and triglycerides are more important. Diabetes is a more important risk factor in women, perhaps because of effects on the lipoproteins. Life style-induced changes in lipoprotein levels may be more difficult in women. Nevertheless, the major risk factors for CHD have predictive value in both men and women, and the overall treatment strategy is the same.

For primary prevention of CHD (ie, prevention in patients without established CHD), the total blood cholesterol and HDL cholesterol levels in the nonfasting state should be measured for all patients aged 19 years and older at least once every 5 years. Those determined to be at low risk should be given general educational materials about dietary modification, physical activity, and risk-reduction activities. Patients with borderline high or high levels of LDL should be evaluated clinically to determine whether secondary causes, relevant familial disorders, or other risk factors exist for CHD.

Initial therapy for those at risk primarily consists of dietary modification and physical activity. Diet should be modified to include only 8–10% of total calories from saturated fat, 30% or less calories from total fat, and less than 300 mg of cholesterol per day. Weight reduction in overweight patients and increased physical activity are extremely important elements of therapy because they not only reduce cholesterol levels but also reduce triglycerides, raise HDL levels, reduce blood pressure, and decrease the risk for diabetes mellitus. Total cholesterol should be reevaluated at 4–6 weeks and at 3

TABLE 1-6. CLASSIFICATION OF CHOLESTEROL LEVELS IN INDIVIDUALS WITHOUT CORONARY HEART DISEASE*

Cholesterol Level (mg/dl)	Classification
Total	
<200	Desirable
200–239	Borderline high
≥240	High
HDL cholesterol	
<35	Low
35–59	Normal
≥60	High
LDL cholesterol	
<130	Desirable
130–159	Borderline high risk
≥160	High risk

* HDL is high-density lipoprotein; LDL, low-density lipoprotein.
Expert Panel on Detection, Evaluation, and Treatment of High Blood Cholesterol in Adults. Summary of the second report of the National Cholesterol Education Program (NCEP) Expert Panel on Detection, Evaluation, and Treatment of High Blood Cholesterol in Adults (Adult Treatment Panel II). JAMA 1993;269:3015–3023

months. Further dietary modification may be necessary if patients have not reduced cholesterol to appropriate levels. A minimum of 6 months of intensive dietary therapy and counseling generally should be carried out before initiating drug therapy as an adjunct to, not a substitute for, dietary therapy.

Drug treatment may be considered for patients with high levels of LDL despite dietary therapy. Because drug therapy is likely to continue for many years and may have side effects, and because premenopausal women generally have a low risk for CHD, maximal efforts should be made to achieve lower cholesterol levels by diet, exercise, and reduction of other risk factors in such women before drug therapy is initiated. For postmenopausal women, estrogen replacement therapy is a possible alternative or adjunct to drug therapy. The major drugs used for treatment are bile acid sequestrants, nicotinic acid, and hydroxymethylglutaryl coenzyme A reductase inhibitors (statins).

DIABETES

Diabetes mellitus denotes a group of diseases that are identified on the basis of hyperglycemia and that are associated with acute metabolic complications (ketoacidosis and hyperosmolar coma), as well as long-term complications involving capillaries (retinopathy and nephropathy, "microvascular" complications), arteries (atherosclerosis, "macrovascular" complications), and nerves (several forms of peripheral neuropathy).

Classification and Diagnosis

Diabetes mellitus occurs in two general forms in nonpregnant adults. Type I diabetes (insulin-dependent diabetes; IDDM) is an autoimmune disorder directed at the pancreatic B cells. The disease generally occurs in children and young adults, and the autoimmune B cell destruction leads to a complete lack of endogenous insulin production. Thus, patients are "dependent" on exogenous insulin for day-to-day survival; they will develop ketoacidosis if they are not treated with insulin.

Type II diabetes (non–insulin-dependent diabetes; NIDDM) encompasses all other forms of chronic hyperglycemia severe enough to meet current diagnostic criteria for diabetes. Patients with NIDDM have some degree of endogenous insulin production, so that they rarely develop ketoacidosis. They develop hyperglycemia because of an imbalance between the amount of insulin that the pancreas can produce and the amount of insulin that is required to keep blood glucose levels normal. The relative contribution of decreased insulin supply and increased insulin demands varies widely among patients, consistent with the concept that NIDDM is not one disease with a single pathogenesis, but a group of disorders that share hyperglycemia as a common feature. Patients with NIDDM may require insulin treatment to attain good glycemic control, but they are not insulin "dependent" for day-to-day survival in the way that patients with IDDM are. Both IDDM and NIDDM have important genetic components (eg, specific human leukocyte antigen [HLA] associations with IDDM), although the two disorders appear to be genetically distinct.

The diagnosis of diabetes is based on the demonstration of hyperglycemia in the absence of an acute intercurrent illness. Diagnostic criteria currently in use in the United States require 1) unequivocal hyperglycemia (≥200 mg/dl) in association with typical symptoms of diabetes (polydipsia, polyuria, weight loss); or 2) fasting glycemia ≥140 mg/dl on two or more occasions; or 3) results of a 2-hour, oral glucose (75 g) tolerance test in which the 120-minute glucose value *and* at least one other of the 30-, 60-, and 90-minute values are ≥200 mg/dl. The diagnosis of diabetes should be based on venous serum or plasma glucose concentrations measured by a certified clinical laboratory. Diabetes should not be diagnosed by reflectance meters.

Some distinction between IDDM and NIDDM can be made on the basis of clinical characteristics (Table 1-7), but the distinction can be made with certainty only by demonstrating in patients with IDDM either 1) serum markers of autoimmunity (antibodies directed against pancreatic islet cells or against insulin itself) before or soon after the onset of hyperglycemia or 2) the absence of endogenous insulin production (no C peptide response to a mixed meal) several years after the onset of hyperglycemia. At present, neither of these tests is important for routine patient care. However, as methods to preserve residual B cell function early in the course of IDDM are developed, the tests for autoimmunity may become indicated in young patients who present with diabetes.

The vast majority (>90%) of adults with diabetes have NIDDM, a disease of insidious onset and subtle progression. Screening studies suggest that approximately 50% of persons with NIDDM in the United States are undiagnosed. Those persons may have subtle or no symptoms of diabetes, but they are at risk for long-term diabetic complications and their diabetes should be detected and treated. The American Diabetes Association (ADA) recommends that people with one or more of the following risk factors be screened for diabetes: 1) family history of diabetes in parents or siblings; 2) obesity (body weight >120% of ideal); 3) high-risk ethnicity (Native American, Hispanic, African–American); 4) history of glucose intolerance; 5) hypertension or hyperlipidemia (total cholesterol >240 mg/dl or total triglyceride >250 mg/dl); or 6) history of gestational diabetes or a baby weighing >4 kg (9 lb) at birth.

TABLE 1-7. CLINICAL CHARACTERISTICS OF IDDM AND NIDDM*

Characteristic	IDDM	NIDDM
Ketoacidosis	Frequent	Rare
Age at onset[†]	<30 years	>40 years
Body habitus[‡]	Lean	Obese
Family history of diabetes	Occasional	Frequent

* IDDM indicates insulin-dependent diabetes melitus; NIDDM, non–insulin-dependent diabetes mellitus.
† Age shown is usual age; both types can occur at any age.
‡ Habitus shown is usual habitus; patients may be lean or obese with either disease.

Screening should consist of a fasting serum or plasma glucose measurement. Concentrations of <115 mg/dl are normal and warrant nothing more than repeated measurements at 3-year intervals. Concentrations of ≥140 mg/dl are consistent with diabetes and should be repeated once to confirm the diagnosis. Concentrations of 115–139 mg/dl are abnormal but not diagnostic of diabetes.

The ADA recommends "diagnostic testing" (presumably an oral glucose tolerance test) for individuals with such nondiagnostic fasting glucose levels. However, since the therapeutic implications of an abnormal oral glucose tolerance test in the absence of fasting hyperglycemia of >140 mg/dl are unclear, it seems reasonable to advise such patients regarding measures that may reduce their risk of overt diabetes (eg, weight loss, exercise, and avoidance of medications that can worsen hyperglycemia) and to monitor their fasting glucose levels at 3–6-month intervals.

Management

Routine care should be delivered with two goals in mind: minimization of the risk of long-term diabetic complications and maintenance of a good quality of life for patients. In general, the risks of diabetic retinopathy, nephropathy, and neuropathy parallel the severity and duration of hyperglycemia. Thus, those three types of complications are thought to result from the impact of chronic metabolic decompensation on microvascular and nervous tissues in susceptible individuals. Atherosclerosis is less closely correlated with glycemic control.

One of the major advances in the care of diabetic patients was the recent demonstration by two long-term, controlled trials in patients with IDDM that intensive diabetes management to lower ambient glycemia reduced the rates of development and progression of diabetic eye, kidney, and nerve disease without worsening atherosclerosis. That finding mandates that the care of patients with IDDM, and probably of patients with NIDDM as well, be directed toward maintaining circulating glucose levels as close to normal as possible, since the studies revealed no threshold of glycemia above which diabetic complications began to occur. Ideally, a multidisciplinary approach (at a minimum a physician, diabetes educator, and nutritionist) should be used in the management of diabetes.

Insulin-Dependent Diabetes

Initial Evaluation. The medical history should include specific queries regarding 1) current and previous insulin and glucose self-monitoring programs and education; 2) dietary habits and nutritional education; 3) acute metabolic complications (ketoacidosis and coma); 4) symptoms, evaluations, and treatment of chronic complications (retinopathy, nephropathy, neuropathy, atherosclerosis); 5) other cardiovascular risk factors (smoking, hypertension, family history, obesity, lipids); 6) hypoglycemic episodes and symptoms; and 7) exercise and activity patterns.

The physical examination should focus on 1) height and weight, 2) blood pressure, 3) retinal examination, 4) periodontal examination, 5) cardiovascular examination (including examination for peripheral pulses and bruits), 6) foot and skin examination, and 7) neurologic examination.

Initial laboratory determinations should include 1) serum or plasma glucose (preferably fasting); 2) fasting serum lipids (total and HDL cholesterol and total triglycerides); 3) glycohemoglobin (eg, hemoglobin A_1 or A_{1c}); 4) serum potassium, urea nitrogen, and creatinine; and 5) urinalysis. Quantitation of urinary albumin excretion by a sensitive method (eg, immunoassay) is indicated in postpubertal patients who do not have proteinuria on routine urinalysis, since the excretion of small quantities of albumin (30–300 mg/24 hours) is indicative of early diabetic nephropathy.

Initial Care. It is beneficial for patients to meet with a nutritionist who is experienced in nutrition for patients with diabetes. Patients with IDDM are generally not obese, so that a weight-maintaining diet (30–32 kcal/kg) providing <30% of calories as fat and <20% as protein may be recommended for most patients. Timing of meals should be consistent with activity schedules and insulin regimens.

Patients need to learn diabetes self-management skills, including insulin administration, glucose self-monitoring, recognition and treatment of hypoglycemia, and foot and skin care. Ideally, these skills should be taught by a certified diabetes educator or a similarly qualified individual. Presentation of a large body of information at the onset of IDDM may overwhelm some patients, so that basic management skills (eg, insulin injection) should be taught first, followed by additional skills (eg, self-adjustment of insulin doses) as patients become familiar with basic management skills. Likewise, therapeutic goals may be less rigid at the outset of therapy than they will be once patients have mastered their self-management skills.

Insulin therapy is required for all patients with IDDM. Some patients experience a "honeymoon" for up to 12 months after diagnosis, during which they require little or no exogenous insulin to maintain good glycemic control. However, all patients require insulin therapy eventually. Initial doses can be based on the patient's weight (eg, approximately 0.3–0.4 U of insulin per kilogram of body weight per day), and at least two doses of short-, intermediate-, or long-acting insulin should be given daily. All patients should perform capillary glucose monitoring, preferably several times each day. The complexity of the insulin- and capillary-monitoring regimens often need to be increased in order to improve glycemic control as patients become more skilled at diabetes management.

Continuing Care. Follow-up examinations should take place at 1-week–3-month intervals to review the status of the patient's metabolic management and any long-term complications. Blood glucose levels should be kept as close to normal as possible to minimize the risk of long-term diabetic complications. Most patients will need three or four injections of insulin per day or continuous insulin infusion therapy

(Table 1-8) to achieve their optimal glycemia level, and most will need to learn to adjust their own insulin doses on the basis of premeal capillary glucose results. The process of learning these self-management skills initially requires frequent, sometimes daily, contact with the management team. Glycohemoglobin levels measured every 2–3 months are useful to assess overall glycemic control in the face of varied daily blood glucose measurements.

Detection and early treatment of incipient complications should be a major focus of continuing care. With regard to retinopathy, visual symptoms are a very late finding, so that all patients should see an ophthalmologist annually beginning within the first 5 years of IDDM. Laser photocoagulation therapy can reduce greatly the risk of blindness in patients who develop diabetic retinopathy.

Incipient diabetic nephropathy is also asymptomatic, but it can be detected by the urinary excretion of >30 mg of albumin per 24 hours in the absence of proteinuria detected by dipstick. Patients with such "microalbuminuria" have been shown to benefit from relatively low-dose ACE inhibitor therapy (eg, enalapril, 10 mg/d) even in the absence of arterial hypertension. Patients who develop more marked proteinuria (>300 mg/24 hours; usually detectable on routine dipstick urinalysis) have more severe nephropathy and they frequently have some degree of hypertension. Those patients benefit from maintenance of arterial pressure well within in the normal range.

No specific therapies currently are available for the prevention of diabetic neuropathy except for maintenance of good metabolic control. However, patient education and routine examination of the feet for calluses, blisters, and skin breakdown are critical in the prevention of limb loss related to diabetic neuropathy and peripheral vascular disease. Serum lipid concentrations should be assessed annually and treated in accordance with the recommendations of the National Cholesterol Education Program.

Hypoglycemia is a frequent complication of intensive insulin therapy. Patients with IDDM may have a limited ability to sense and to recover from such hypoglycemia. Thus, all patients should receive education about the symptoms and treatment of hypoglycemia. It is important to note that "tight" blood glucose control lowers the blood glucose threshold for epinephrine release. Thus, initial symptoms of hypoglycemia may change from adrenergic (tremor and sweating) to neuroglycopenic (confusion and lethargy) during intensive diabetes management. Patients and families should be aware of these changes, and family members should be instructed in the use of subcutaneous glucagon to treat severe hypoglycemia.

Pancreas transplantation is a viable therapeutic option for patients with IDDM. Centers experienced in pancreas transplantation report 3-year cure rates (patients normoglycemic without exogenous insulin) in the range of 60–70%. However, chronic immunosuppression is necessary to prevent graft rejection, so that many centers limit pancreas transplantation to patients who have had or will soon have a renal transplantation for diabetic nephropathy. Transplantation of isolated pancreatic islets and immunotherapy to retard B cell destruction early in the course of IDDM remain experimental at present.

All diabetic women of reproductive age should receive education about the risk of birth defects when periconceptional glycemic control is poor. Those women should use effective contraception when they are not planning to become pregnant, and they should be encouraged to participate in special preconceptional care programs, where they exist, when they want to have a baby.

Non–Insulin-Dependent Diabetes

The basic goal of management for patients with NIDDM is similar to that for patients with IDDM: the prevention of morbidity and mortality through careful metabolic regulation to prevent long-term complications and through early detection and treatment of complications that develop. Because patients with NIDDM are often obese and because they possess some capability for endogenous insulin release, several therapeutic options are available. As is true for IDDM, NIDDM is best managed by a multidisciplinary team with expertise in diabetes in order to ensure optimal metabolic control and the prevention of complications. The remaining discussion focuses on the management of NIDDM as it differs from the management of IDDM.

Initial Evaluation. The initial evaluation is similar to that for IDDM except that patients with NIDDM often have had diabetes for a considerable period of time before the diagnosis is made. Thus, the initial history, physical examination, and laboratory evaluations should focus more carefully on signs and symptoms of atherosclerosis, peripheral neuropathy,

TABLE 1-8. INSULIN REGIMENS FOR INTENSIVE THERAPY OF PATIENTS WITH IDDM*

Regimen	Before Breakfast	Before Lunch	Before Dinner	At Bedtime
1	Short + intermediate	—	Short + intermediate	—
2	Short	Short	Short + intermediate or long	—
3	Short	Short	Short	Intermediate or long
4	←——————————— Constant infusion pump ———————————→

* "Short" (eg, regular or semi-Lente), "intermediate" (eg, neutral protamine Hagedorn [NPH] or Lente), and "long" (eg, ultra-Lente) refer to the duration of action of the insulin preparation. Regimen 1 may be useful soon after the diagnosis of IDDM, when many patients have some residual endogenous insulin secretion. Regimens 2–4 are generally required to achieve good glycemic control during long-term treatment.

retinopathy, and nephropathy, any of which may be present at the time NIDDM is first diagnosed. All patients should be examined by an ophthalmologist, and all should have 24-hour urine collection for determination of albumin excretion if they do not already have dipstick proteinuria. Assessment of cardiovascular risk factors is particularly important in patients with NIDDM, since they frequently have hypertension and hyperlipidemia.

Initial and Subsequent Care. In general, therapies for NIDDM are designed to reestablish a normal balance between the body's insulin demands and supply by improving insulin action or by improving insulin secretion. Weight loss, exercise, and ingestion of diets high in complex carbohydrates are examples of therapies that improve insulin action. Sulfonylurea drugs enhance insulin secretion from the pancreas, and insulin injections provide additional insulin directly.

The choice of initial therapy is based on each patient's body habitus and degree of hyperglycemia. Lean patients (≥120% of ideal weight) generally derive only small benefit from dietary therapy alone, since weight loss is not indicated in such patients.

On the other hand, lean patients with mild-to-moderate fasting hyperglycemia (≥250 mg/dl) often achieve a therapeutic benefit from sulfonylurea drugs. Second-generation sulfonylurea drugs such as glipizide and glyburide are not systematically more efficacious than older preparations such as chlorpropamide and tolbutamide, but the second-generation drugs cause fewer side effects and are preferred. Lean patients with fasting glycemia in the range of 250–300 mg/dl and above frequently fail to respond to sulfonylurea therapy, and insulin is recommended as the primary therapy for such patients.

Recent data indicate that lowering of fasting glucose levels by administering intermediate insulin (neutral protamine Hagedorn [NPH] or insulin–zinc suspension [Lente]) with dinner or at bedtime can greatly improve overall glycemia in NIDDM while causing a minimum degree of hyperinsulinemia. Thus, a stepped-care approach that starts with evening NPH or Lente insulin (approximately 0.2–0.3 U/kg of body weight) to normalize fasting glycemia, followed by addition of an oral hypoglycemic agent or insulin in the morning if daytime hyperglycemia persists, appears to be a rational approach. However, many physicians initiate therapy with twice-daily injections of regular and intermediate insulin (Table 1-8), using total daily doses of approximately 0.5 U/kg to compensate for the insulin resistance present even in lean patients with NIDDM. In either case, capillary glucose monitoring should be employed to assess day-to-day glycemic control, and glycohemoglobin levels should be measured at 2–3-month intervals to assess overall glycemia.

As in IDDM, glycemia should be kept as close to normal as possible to minimize the risk of long-term complications. However, glycemic goals may be modified in response to advancing age or medical illnesses that minimize the relevance of a risk of long-term diabetic complications.

Therapy for obese patients should begin with a hypocaloric diet. The degree of caloric restriction must be individualized according to patient compliance, but greater caloric restriction generally results in greater and more rapid declines in blood glucose levels. Even obese patients with marked hyperglycemia may experience a significant lowering of blood glucose in response to caloric restriction. Patients who show no signs of improvement within 8–12 weeks of initiating diet therapy and those who stabilize at glycemic levels that are less than ideal should receive sulfonylurea treatment, then insulin if needed to achieve the desired glycemia. Rational combination therapy with insulin and oral hypoglycemia agents is limited to the use of overnight insulin to normalize fasting glycemia plus an oral agent to minimize daytime hyperglycemia. Patients should be seen at 1–3-month intervals, and renal, retinal, neuropathic, and vascular complications should be assessed and managed as described for IDDM.

Goals of Management

It has now been shown convincingly that intensive diabetes management can prevent or delay the development of retinopathy, nephropathy, and neuropathy in patients with IDDM. It is likely that careful blood glucose control will have a similar beneficial effect on patients with NIDDM. Thus, for diabetic patients who do not already have end-stage diabetic complications, their care should include measures to maintain blood glucose levels as close to normal as possible.

For patients with IDDM, a disease in which insulin deficiency is the predominant metabolic defect, care should be directed at intensive insulin replacement therapy delivered by a multispecialty team in a setting of patient education and self-management. For patients with NIDDM, who generally have defects in insulin action and secretion, diet and exercise therapies should be used to improve insulin action. Oral hypoglycemic agents and exogenous insulin may be needed to correct the insulin deficiency in patients who present with severe hyperglycemia and in patients who fail to maintain optimal glycemic control with diet and exercise. In both types of diabetes, routine assessments for retinal, renal, neural, and atherosclerotic disease are required to detect at an early and treatable stage any long-term complications that develop.

Future directions for therapy of IDDM include transplantation of isolated pancreatic islets, closed-loop insulin delivery systems, and immunologic interventions to arrest the B cell destruction early in the course of the disease. Future treatments for NIDDM include new pharmacologic agents that improve insulin action directly.

BREAST CANCER

Breast cancer is the most common invasive cancer occurring in women. Its incidence and mortality are more than twice that of all the female pelvic cancers combined, and it is the cancer most often encountered in women by their primary care physicians. Furthermore, it is the fear of breast cancer that motivates women with breast symptoms and concerns to consult their physicians. Obstetrician–gynecologists should respond by offering their patients regular breast examinations, instructing them in breast self-examination (BSE), ordering screening mammography, and evaluating breast signs and symptoms. The diagnosis of breast disease and the treatment of benign breast conditions often can be performed in the office setting.

Although numerous risk factors for breast cancer have been identified, the epidemiologic association is weak and only a woman's advancing age can be strongly correlated with increasing incidence of breast cancer. A personal history of breast cancer and breast cancer in a first-degree relative increase a woman's relative risk of breast cancer. There is conflicting evidence whether maintaining body weight within the normal range for age and height and limiting alcohol intake to moderation or less decrease the risk of breast cancer.

Breast Cancer Screening

While mammography is the most effective screening method for detecting nonpalpable breast cancers, clinical breast examination (CBE) and BSE are still important. Screening for breast cancer should include CBE, as the Breast Cancer Detection Demonstration Project has revealed that about 10% of palpable breast cancers will not be detected by mammography. Although BSE has not yet been shown to improve the overall survival of treated breast cancer patients, regular BSE promotes awareness of anatomic variations and encourages women to consult their physicians about breast changes, signs, and symptoms.

Clinical Breast Examination

Clinical breast examination is most effectively performed by using the systematic methods developed by the California division of the American Cancer Society. (This is the same technique taught to the patient for her own BSE.) Annual routine examinations should include CBE. Precise recording of the performance of CBE and any clinically significant findings is essential. If an indistinct lesion is palpated in a menstruating woman, another examination should be performed after the next menstruation.

Breast Self-Examination

Women should be instructed in BSE beginning at age 18. Effective instruction consists of describing the BSE technique while doing the CBE and then having the patient demonstrate her interpretation of what has been taught. Alternately, BSE education and demonstration can be performed by properly trained allied health care personnel. The optimum time for BSE is a few days after the cessation of menstruation or on a monthly calendar day for women who are not menstruating. Breast self-examination instruction and the patient's feedback demonstration should be a part of each annual gynecologic evaluation.

Screening Mammography

Current ACOG guidelines recommend that women age 40–49 have mammography every 1–2 years and yearly beginning at age 50. The mammography report should be obtained by the ordering physician and the patient informed of the result. Women aged 35 and older with a family history of premenopausally diagnosed breast cancer in a first-degree relative should have an annual mammogram. Screening mammography is the keystone to decreasing the mortality from breast cancer. Only mammography can detect small nonpalpable cancers which, when treated, have an excellent 90% 10-year disease-free survival prognosis.

Diagnosis

The diagnostic evaluation of the patient with breast symptoms begins with a careful history including the date of examination and the chief complaint. The age of the patient, the menstrual and family history, and the age of the patient at the time of her first child should be noted. For specific symptoms such as nipple discharge, it is important to note the date of onset, the character of the discharge, and whether it is bilateral, spontaneous, or provoked. The history should be recorded in a legible and logical sequence, and the diagnostic plan should be outlined, including the disposition of the case and recommendations for follow-up.

Physical Examination

Careful physical examination is essential to a correct diagnosis and appropriate treatment. Obvious findings represent late signs of malignancy, for which current treatment methods are ineffective. Thus, the examiner should look for subtle changes and, in order to detect these changes, the patient should be examined in both the sitting and supine positions. These changes may be exaggerated by asking the patient to elevate her arms or place her hands on the hips to contract the pectoral muscles. The axillae should be palpated with the patient in the sitting or the standing position.

The physical findings represent a judgment call. The patient's chief concern may be a lump. This may or may not be confirmed by careful evaluation. The usual finding is thickening, particularly in the upper outer quadrant of the breast. The physical findings may vary depending on the amount of adipose tissue. In a woman who has recently lost a considerable amount of weight, the breasts feel lumpy. The cushion of fatty tissue is absent, and palpation reveals the normal, lumpy breast tissue. On the other hand, in very obese patients, it is unlikely that anything but the most obvious lesion will be observed by routine breast examination, and a large breast is an indication for mammography to enhance what in most cases will be an inadequate physical examination.

The physical findings should be carefully documented in a narrative form with a diagram. The diagram is helpful because it clearly indicates which breast is involved and the location and size of the lesion and associated conditions, such as skin dimpling or regional involvement.

Once a lesion has been characterized as a mass or a lump and measured or drawn, it must be resolved. This may require additional examination, for example, at another time during the patient's menstrual cycle, an attempt at aspiration, or referral for open biopsy. At the completion of the physical examination it is important to reinforce the practice of BSE. Most breast cancers continue to be self-detected. Women who practice monthly BSE may have a more favorable pathologic stage, and if it is true that early detection is possible through breast examination, this examination could affect mortality. The true impact of BSE will remain unanswered, however, until a well-designed prospective study is available.

Diagnostic Studies

If a dominant mass is discovered, it may be cystic or solid, benign or malignant. If the mass appears to be cystic, an attempt should be made to aspirate the lesion. It is a mistake to assume that a very firm mass represents a solid lesion. A cyst under considerable pressure feels very firm, and an attempt should be made at aspiration. This can be done with an ordinary syringe and a 23–25-gauge needle without local anesthesia.

If the fluid is clear or cloudy and no residual mass is palpated, follow-up examination 1 month later with reassurance and reinforcement of monthly BSE is recommended. The mass must completely disappear at the time of initial aspiration and should not return on follow-up examination in 1 month. Since the incidence of breast cancer is extremely low in patients under 20 years of age, solid masses in this age group that appear to be benign by ultrasonography can be monitored without biopsy at the discretion of the physician.

The deliberate aspiration of multiple macrocysts, noted on either breast examination or by other diagnostic aids such as mammography and confirmed by ultrasonography, is not necessary. On the other hand, a tender macrocyst should be aspirated. Cytologic evaluation of cyst fluid is seldom rewarding and is not recommended as a routine procedure.

Fine needle aspiration is quite accurate when applied correctly. A standard disposable syringe can be used with a 23–25-gauge needle. It is not necessary to use special syringes, and large needles should be avoided. Local anesthesia is preferred because several "passes" may be required to obtain an adequate sample. The technique in essence provides an evaluation of "tissue juice." It is therefore important that sufficient material be withdrawn into the needle and placed on the slide for appropriate evaluation. This technique is most useful for the obvious dominant mass with signs suggesting carcinoma, either on physical examination or confirmed by a mammographic finding. A positive fine needle aspiration permits immediate treatment planning and a discussion of alterative treatments with the therapeutic team. Except in unusual instances, this finding must be confirmed by open biopsy at the time of definitive treatment. Some radiologists prefer that mammography be performed prior to fine needle aspiration because of the potential of distorted anatomy by hematoma formation.

Additional studies include mammography and ultrasonography. Although ultrasonography is not useful as a diagnostic screening method, it may be valuable as an imaging technique in distinguishing cystic lesions from solid lesions, especially with an occult lesion. Mammography is the most accurate technique for detecting early-stage breast cancers and for defining certain benign conditions. Although mammography is sensitive, it does not detect all cancers, and a negative mammogram should not obviate further investigation, particularly open biopsy. Mammography is the only method capable of detecting microcalcifications or asymmetric densities that may be associated with malignant lesions. In these cases, a decision must be made to repeat the films to clarify the diagnosis, to repeat the films in several months to assess stability, or to recommend localization and biopsy. This requires considerable judgment on the part of the radiologist. Most of these lesions are benign; however, approximately 15–20% may represent early carcinoma. Consultation with the radiologist is essential.

COMMON GASTROINTESTINAL SYNDROMES AND DISEASES

The most important aspect of care for the patient with gastrointestinal disease is the distinction between acute and chronic disease. Acute problems such as hematemesis, rectal bleeding, and appendicitis require early and accurate intervention. Many diseases, however, such as gastroesophageal reflux and irritable bowel syndrome, are chronic and require long-term therapy. Additionally, many diseases are more prevalent in women, such as gallbladder disease, and may be first seen by the gynecologist. Recognition and initial workup will facilitate care and timely referral, when indicated.

Gastroesophageal Reflux

The reflux of gastric acid to the sensitive esophagus causes heartburn, the cardinal manifestation of gastroesophageal reflux disease. The most common etiology is the decrease in tone of the lower esophageal sphincter pressure. Symptoms are most common after consuming large meals, after consuming certain foods, and upon assuming the recumbent position. Prolonged exposure of acid to the esophagus may lead to stricture formation and dysphagia. Nocturnal aspiration may occur and be mistaken for asthma. Erosive esophagitis from chronic reflux can lead to subclinical chronic bleeding and eventually to iron deficiency anemia.

Empirical therapy has been advocated in patients with uncomplicated gastroesophageal reflux disease. Before initiation of therapy, medications that contribute to reducing lower esophageal sphincter pressure, such as diazepam and calcium channel blockers, should be eliminated. Nonsteroidal anti-inflammatory drugs (NSAIDs) are common medications in gynecologic practice and contribute to direct damage to the esophageal mucosa. Patients with anemia, excessive weight loss, symptoms consistent with pulmonary aspiration (sudden awakening with cough, choking, wheezing, or laryngospasm), and dysphagia should undergo further evaluation. Initial studies may be either an air-contrast barium swallow (less sensitive) or upper gastrointestinal endoscopy. Information from these studies will eliminate other potential causes of gastroesophageal reflux disease that include esophageal motility disorders, erosive esophagitis, and peptic ulcer disease (gastric or duodenal).

Therapy requires life style adjustments as well as medication. Cigarette smoking contributes to lowering lower esophageal sphincter pressure, delays esophageal acid clearance, and therefore subjects the esophagus to prolonged acid exposure. Patients should not lie down for 2–3 hours after consuming large meals. Postural changes contribute to lower esophageal sphincter relaxation and reflux. Postural therapies, by either placing the bed on 6–8-in blocks or using a bed wedge, have been shown to decrease acid exposure time and are as effective as medication in healing reflux esophagitis. Diet should be modified by eliminating liquids with high acid content (eg, orange juice), which may evoke symptoms. Fatty foods and chocolate decrease lower esophageal sphincter pressure and delay gastric emptying, which contribute to symptoms. Carminatives are natural substances found in onions, garlic, peppermint, and certain after-dinner liqueurs that increase gas, induce belching, and reduce lower esophageal sphincter pressure. Foods that contain carminatives should be eliminated from the diet.

Initiation of pharmacologic therapy should begin with life style adjustments. Prior to the widespread availability of H_2 antagonists, antacids were prescribed. Because of the dosage interval of 1–3 hours after meals and at bedtime, compliance is a problem. Antacids contain inorganic salts, and depending on the type used, result in diarrhea, bloating, and constipation. A trial of antacids in mild disease may be helpful to some individuals. In the mid-1970s, H_2 antagonists were introduced and dramatically changed the treatment of gastroesophageal reflux disease and peptic ulcer disease. Cimetidine, ranitidine, and famotidine are common medications in this class and are prescribed for use twice daily. A new medication, omeprazole, has been approved for use in resistant gastroesophageal reflux disease. The mechanism of action is the inhibition of the hydrogen–potassium pump in gastric acid-producing cells. Because of a lack of long-term follow-up, this drug may be taken for 8–12 weeks. Referral of patients with this degree of disease severity is prudent. Additionally, if a chest pain component is present and is consistent with cardiac distribution or symptoms, then appropriate referral is indicated.

Peptic Ulcer Disease

Peptic ulcer disease is the result of disruption of host factors in the stomach or duodenum in the presence of acid and pepsin. Peptic acid secretion is controlled by three endogenous chemicals: 1) acetylcholine, which is released by the vagus nerve; 2) gastrin, which is released by protein in food; and 3) histamine, which is secreted by mastlike cells via a paracrine mechanism. Three levels of defense are postulated to protect sensitive gastric and duodenal mucosa. Surface epithelial cells secrete mucus and bicarbonate, which creates a neutral pH at the mucosal level while maintaining an acid environment in the lumen. Blood flow to the mucosa is extensive, and it removes acid quickly from the mucosal epithelium. Cell renewal is ongoing and rapidly replaces sloughed cells. Endogenous prostaglandins stimulate mucus and bicarbonate production, increase blood flow, and enhance cellular renewal. The disruption of prostaglandin production may be important in the genesis of peptic ulcer disease.

Patients may have multiple abnormalities that lead to ulcer formation. A hereditary link has been described in patients with multiple endocrine neoplasia syndrome and other rare syndromes. Little evidence supports a strong genetic basis for the disease in the majority of patients. Up to 40% of patients have an increased secretion rate of acid; however, the larger group of patients have normal rates of secretion. Breakdown of the mucosal barrier is probably the most important factor in peptic ulcer disease. Definite factors that contribute to disruption of the mucosa include 1) infection with *Helicobacter pylori*, 2) cigarette smoking, and 3) NSAIDs. Many etiologies, such as alcohol use, stress, and adrenocorticosteroids, are now thought to be less important.

H. pylori infection has been isolated in 95% of patients with duodenal ulcers and 70% of patients with gastric ulcers. Normal volunteers accidentally exposed to *H. pylori* became ill with acute symptomatic gastritis. *H. pylori* is associated with inflammation that disrupts the mucosal barrier and allows for the disruptive action of acid and pepsin. Cigarette smoking is associated with increased acid formation, alteration in blood flow, and interference with prostaglandin production. Nonsteroidal antiinflammatory drugs have a direct effect on disruption of the mucosal barrier and range from superficial lesions to deep ulceration.

Symptoms of peptic ulcer disease are referred to as dyspepsia, which represents a constellation of disorders. Nausea, vomiting, anorexia, fullness, and bloating, in addition to pain in the upper abdomen, are common. Pain is described anywhere in the upper abdomen and may consist of cramping, gnawing, or burning. Pain may last only a few minutes, and response to meals is variable. A correlation between symptoms and demonstrated ulcers is poor, and a high degree of suspicion is necessary in the diagnosis. Physical examination is rarely helpful, unless a more serious complication such as perforation or obstruction is present. Diagnosis is made either by radiographic studies (which may miss as many as 20% of cases) or more commonly by endoscopy.

Several therapies have been shown to be efficacious in treating ulcers. Ulcers usually require 12 weeks of therapy to heal. Antisecretory agents include H_2 receptor antagonists (cimetidine, ranitidine, and famotidine), antimuscarinic drugs (rarely used because of side effects of blurred vision and dry mouth), and prostaglandins (misoprostol). Antacids, once a mainstay of therapy, are rarely used because of frequent dosage changes and side effects of diarrhea or constipation, depending on the agent. Sucralfate is an aluminum hydroxide salt of sucrose octasulfate, which is effective in duodenal ulcers. Omeprazole, a substituted benzimidazole, inhibits the hydrogen–potassium pump. The use of this drug is limited to 8–12 weeks of therapy because of a lack of long-term follow-up. Finally, in patients with *H. pylori* infection, a combination of bismuth emulsion and an antibiotic (metronidazole, 250 mg every 6 hours; tetracycline, 500 mg every 6 hours; or amoxicillin, 500 mg every 8 hours) has been recommended for 2 weeks. Side effects of dark or black stools from bismuth and complications of antibiotic therapy such as pseudomembranous diarrhea may limit the usefulness of this regimen. The influence of *H. pylori* in peptic ulcer disease is still controversial, and prospective studies may help to better characterize its role in disease evolution and treatment.

Gallbladder Disease

Gallbladder disease affects three times more women than men. The reason for sexual predilection is unknown; however, hormonal influences are noted to increase the incidence. Gallbladder disease occurs at any age, with 70% of patients over age 40 years. Obesity is a commonly recognized risk factor. A patient who is 6.8–9 kg (15–20 lb) overweight has a twofold increase in the risk of cholelithiasis, whereas an increase of 27.7–34 kg (50–75 lb) above ideal body weight increases the risk sixfold. Paradoxically, extreme weight loss increases the risk of cholelithiasis. Medical conditions such as cirrhosis, diabetes, and Crohn disease also increase the risk of cholelithiasis. Native Americans, Mexican–Americans, pregnant women, oral contraceptive users, and estrogen replacement users have an increased risk of gallstones.

Cholesterol gallstones form as a result of abnormal liver metabolism, rather than problems in the gallbladder or biliary tree. Gallstones are formed when there is a precipitation of bile salts (cholesterol) on a nidus. Roughly 80% of stones are of the cholesterol type. The remaining 20% of stones are pigmented stones and are classified as either brown or black. An altered cholesterol–bile acid ratio increases the risk of precipitation and therefore gallstone formation. Biliary stasis occurs for many reasons: mechanical or structural alterations in the biliary tree, and diet or hormonal factors, such as pregnancy or estrogen replacement. Stasis further increases the risk of cholesterol precipitation, causing stone formation. Once a small stone is formed, it may acquire further layers of cholesterol, mucin, and bilirubin salts, growing until it is detected and creates symptoms.

Common symptoms include dyspepsia, fatty food intolerance, biliary colic, and jaundice. Biliary colic occurs as a result of intermittent obstruction of the biliary tree and presents as right upper quadrant or scapula pain, fever, nausea, or vomiting. Jaundice, which may be confused with hepatitis, fortunately is rare and occurs with common duct obstruction. The most common complication of gallbladder disease is acute cholecystitis. Untreated cases may progress to ischemia and gangrene of the gallbladder. Vomiting is present in 75% of patients and may spontaneously resolve within 12–18 hours if the obstruction is transient. Acute cholecystitis may lead to chronic cholecystitis with varying degrees of repeated clinical attacks. Cholangitis, or inflammation in the bile-collecting system, is associated with colicky pain, fever, and jaundice. If untreated, the infected gallbladder is associated with significant morbidity. Pancreatitis is a serious complication of gallstone passage. Approximately 50% of pancreatitis is considered to be secondary to biliary tract disease.

The diagnosis of cholelithiasis is based on history, physical examination, and laboratory investigation. Classically, patients with cholelithiasis complain of fatty food intolerance, variable right upper quadrant pain with radiation to the back or scapula, nausea, or vomiting. Symptoms are often mistaken for "indigestion." Determination of serum alkaline phosphatase may indicate obstruction. Alkaline phosphatase is often elevated during pregnancy, compromising the utility of this test in pregnant patients. An elevated serum bilirubin may be useful in diagnosing obstruction, and serum amylase may indicate the presence of pancreatitis. Elevated serum levels of aspartate or alanine aminotransferase can indicate altered metabolic function of liver cells in cases where obstruction causes damage. The standard diagnostic tool is abdominal ultrasonography and is 96% accurate in making the diagnosis of sludge or stone in the gallbladder.

Management of cholelithiasis depends on a number of factors, including patient and physician preference. Variables considered in therapeutic options include the severity and character of symptoms, stone composition and size, and availability of various treatment modalities. For years, surgical therapy was the definitive therapy for gallstones. Surgical complications are common, with a 0.7–1.2% mortality rate in asymptomatic patients, which rises to almost 5% in patients with acute cholangitis or pancreatitis. Risks of complications triple when associated with common duct exploration. The risk of surgery also increases with age. Fortunately, complications are less common in women than they are in men.

Laparoscopy is rapidly becoming an alternative to "open" cholecystectomy. Complications occur in about 5% of cases and include bleeding from the cystic artery or liver bed, bile leakage, or damage to the common duct. Recent studies have cited a 5% conversion from laparoscopy to conventional surgery because of unexpected findings or problems.

Lithotripsy, first made popular in the treatment of ureteral lithiasis, is now being applied to gallstone dissolution. Obesity, a common etiologic factor, is a contraindication to this therapy.

Depending on the size and character of the stones, oral therapy may be an option. Chenodeoxycholic acid has been used to shrink cholesterol stones by decreasing cholesterol secretion and promoting the reabsorption of cholesterol stones. Ursodeoxycholic acid is used to increase the solubility of cholesterol in bile by promoting the formation of a lecithin–cholesterol liquid layer on the stone surface. Ursodeoxycholic acid therapy also causes a decrease in the secretion and reabsorption of cholesterol. The rate of stone dissolution (approximately 1 mm/mo) limits its applicability to stones larger than 1.5–2 cm. Unfortunately, 50% of patients experience a recurrence of stones after cessation of therapy, which limits the drug's usefulness.

Irritable Bowel Syndrome

Functional gastrointestinal symptoms are found in up to 30% of patients, two thirds of whom are women. The irritable bowel syndrome (IBS) is the most common clinical entity seen in clinical practice and has a 2:1 female–male ratio. Patients with IBS have altered motor reactivity to different stimuli, including meals, psychologic stress, and balloon distention of the rectosigmoid. Most affected patients are young to middle aged. Irritable bowel syndrome is a common etiology for chronic pelvic pain in the younger patient, and a history of bowel irregularity should be sought in this group. There are three common clinical variants: 1) "spastic colitis," characterized by chronic abdominal pain and constipation; 2) intermittent diarrhea, which is usually painless; and 3) a combination of both clinical entities with alternating diarrhea and constipation. Colonic wall motility is altered in these patients, and evidence suggests altered colonic sensitivity to cholinergic drugs. Transit time in the gut is modified and results in pain, constipation, and diarrhea.

The diagnosis of IBS is made by careful history and exclusion of underlying pathologic lesions. A travel history, looking for exposure to possible bacterial or parasitic infections, should be obtained. Lactase deficiency, which may masquerade as a diarrhea variant of IBS, responds to the elimination of dairy products from the diet. A rectal examination should be performed on physical examination. A history of bloody stools requires a barium enema and sigmoidoscopy. If the history is suggestive of ulcerative colitis or inflammatory bowel disease (by the intensity of symptoms or the presence of bloody stools), the patient should be referred for colonoscopy.

Treatment of IBS is difficult because of the chronicity of the condition. Many of these patients have hysterical, depressive, and bipolar personality disorders that complicate treatment. Psychologic support, after organic abnormalities have been ruled out, is important. If the patient's symptoms change significantly, further diagnostic studies are indicated. Bulk agents and increased dietary fiber in association with patient education may be helpful. Mild sedation with phenobarbital and tranquilizers may afford some relief.

Colon Cancer and Screening

Colorectal cancer is the second most common cause of cancer in the United States. The mortality rate for women has decreased slightly over the past 40 years, whereas the rate for men has not changed. Most cases develop in patients aged 50 years or older; however, up to 8% are discovered before age 40. In the past several decades, the predominant site of origin has changed from the rectum to the proximal descending colon. A genetic predisposition, a deletion on chromosome 5, is reported to be associated with the development of colorectal cancer. Multiple correlations exist among high dietary fats, meat protein, and caloric intake, in addition to hypercholesterolemia and coronary artery disease. High-fiber diets are thought to decrease stool transit time and therefore limit bowel wall contact with potential carcinogens (such as anaerobic bacteria) in fecal material.

Symptoms of bowel cancer are nonspecific and do not correlate with disease stage or prognosis. Rectal bleeding may be the first sign of bowel cancer; however, it is not necessarily associated with early lesions. Classic symptoms of bowel cancer result from partial obstructions and include abdominal pain, bloating, constipation, and diarrhea. Bright red bleeding may be associated with left-sided colonic lesions; right-sided lesions are usually associated with occult bleeding due to the mixing of stool with the blood. Dark or clotted blood has no clinical significance to location or prognosis. Low rectal carcinomas are associated with hematochezia, tenesmus, and narrowing of stool.

Patients may present with symptoms of anemia, including new-onset angina, increasing frequency of angina, heart failure, or general malaise. Any patient with iron deficiency anemia should be considered at high risk for or highly suspicious for carcinoma of the gastrointestinal tract until proven otherwise. An upper gastrointestinal series (to investigate possible esophageal and gastric lesions), in addition to a lower tract workup, is indicated. Prognosis is directly related to size and penetration of lesions into underlying mucosa and tissues. Blood in the stool is the primary sign for large bowel cancers. Initial screening is done in two steps: 1) the rectal or rectovaginal examination and 2) a modified guaiac test.

Before age 40, the occurrence of false-positive results is high, which makes routine guaiac testing difficult to justify. The false-positive rate for guaiac testing in a normal population is approximately 6%. False-negative results in patients with cancer may reach as high as 50% because of the intermittent nature of bleeding in most lesions. Prospective studies on the usefulness of guaiac testing are ongoing; however, at present, it is the best available method and women over age 40 should have an occult blood sampling annually or as appropriate. Heme-positive stools may be secondary to many conditions, including hemorrhoids, red meat in the diet, inflammatory and infectious diseases of the colon, and carcinoma.

If no mass is felt, multiple stool sampling should be done. The patient should be instructed to consume a red meat–free diet for several days before initiation of testing. A sample of the next six stools should be placed on guaiac test cards and brought to the office for development. If any of these samples is positive, more invasive diagnostic testing should be ordered.

Two radiographic techniques are available: 1) a single stream of barium, which is the easiest test to perform and the most comfortable for the patient; and 2) the air contrast technique, which has greater sensitivity, but is time consuming for the radiologist and uncomfortable for the patient. Flexible sigmoidoscopy is performed after the barium enema to examine the first 25 cm of the rectum and sigmoid, which are poorly visualized because of the catheter placed for dye instillation. If a lesion is found, colonoscopy is performed to inspect the entire colon and to biopsy abnormal lesions. Patients who are at risk of colorectal cancer (ie, those with a personal history of inflammatory bowel disease or colonic polyps or a family history of familial polyposis coli, colorrectal cancer, or cancer family syndrome) should undergo colonoscopy at 3–5-year intervals after age 50. In general, all women aged 50 and older should undergo sigmoidoscopy every 3–5 years.

JOINT AND BONE DISEASE

Approximately 50% of people aged 65 or older have arthritis or rheumatism (pain and stiffness in some portion of the musculoskeletal system). Osteoarthritis is present in 85% of people who become elderly. Musculoskeletal symptoms are therefore common daily problems for older people. Because of their prevalence, these conditions commonly will be encountered in the primary care of patients.

Rheumatoid Arthritis

Rheumatoid arthritis (RA) is the most common inflammatory disease of joints, affecting 1% of adults. Seventy percent of patients are women, and the peak incidence is in the fourth to sixth decades. Although etiology remains unknown, the characteristic chronic inflammation of synovium is immunologically driven, and T-cell immunity plays a central role. In addition, RA is associated with particular inherited HLA alleles involved in the binding and presentation of antigen to T-lymphocytes.

Clinical Features

The diagnosis of RA should be considered in patients with polyarthritis for 6 or more weeks. Pain and stiffness are accentuated in the morning or after prolonged inactivity (gelling), as occurs for inflammatory arthritis of other causes. Joints commonly involved in early RA are proximal interphalangeal, metacarpal–phalangeal, wrist, knee, and metatarsal–phalangeal, but virtually any joint except those in the lumbar area may be affected. Most patients with RA experience constitutional symptoms of fatigue and malaise, and subcutaneous rheumatoid nodules can be found over pressure points such as the proximal ulna in 25% of these patients. The diagnosis of RA is a clinical one that can be supported by characteristic joint space narrowing or juxtaarticular erosions on hand radiographs or by the presence of rheumatoid factor in serum. Test results for rheumatoid factor are positive in 75% of patients with RA by 1 year, but the sensitivity of this test may be lower early in the disease course. Rheumatoid factor also is present in 15% of healthy elderly women, in 35% of patients with lupus, and in other chronic inflammatory and rheumatic diseases. A diagnosis of RA should never be based on this test alone, however.

In younger patients with chronic polyarthritis, the differential diagnosis revolves around psoriatic arthritis, in which there is concurrent or a history of typical psoriatic skin or nail involvement in 90% of cases, and systemic lupus erythematosus (SLE). The multisystem involvement of female-predominant SLE should be sought by a targeted history and physical examination, and laboratory testing for hematocytopenia and proteinuria. In older patients, osteoarthritis (OA) can be differentiated easily in most cases by its differing joint distribution and lack of inflammation. Arthritis caused by viral infections—such as hepatitis B, parvovirus infection, and rubella—is characterized by a symmetric joint distribution similar to that in RA but usually resolves within 2 months.

Treatment

The goals of therapy are to reduce discomfort, maintain or restore function, and prevent joint destruction. Optimal management usually requires early consultation with physical therapy, occupational therapy, and rheumatology; orthopedic surgery is often needed during the course of the disease.

Rheumatoid patients should perform daily exercises to maintain joint motion and muscle strength, and an aerobic conditioning program—walking, swimming, or stationary bicycling—may result in diminished discomfort. Assistant devices may help make certain activities easier to accomplish or less stressful on inflamed joints. Orthotics may cushion the impact of subluxed metatarsal heads. Patients must be educated about the chronic nature of RA and its often-fluctuating course. Sexual and vocational counseling may be required.

Pharmacologic therapy is directed at decreasing inflammation within the joint. In general, therapy is begun with an NSAID. Approximately 20 such drugs are available in the United States; with the exception of the nonacetylated salicylates, NSAIDs inhibit prostaglandin production. All are effective within a few weeks and share antipyretic and analgesic activity. None is consistently more effective than any other for RA. However, responses are idiosyncratic and vary greatly from patient to patient; thus, three or four sequential trials of different NSAIDs are often needed. For any single NSAID, a rheumatoid cohort derives approximately 30% benefit for pain and stiffness.

Some patients (25–40%) develop nonspecific abdominal symptoms while taking NSAIDs. Of greater concern, clinically significant gastric or duodenal ulcers develop in 2–4% of patients treated with a prostaglandin inhibitor for 1 year. The correlation between abdominal symptoms and peptic ulcer is poor, and ulcers often present with hemorrhage or perforation. Investigators have estimated a mortality from ulcer complications of 1/1,000 patients given 1 year of prostaglandin inhibitor therapy. Risk factors include a history of peptic ulcer disease, older age, debility, glucocorticoid therapy, and higher doses of NSAID. Risk appears to be lower with use of enteric coated aspirin and nabumetone.

Acute renal insufficiency, generally mild and reversible, may occur as a result of inhibition of production of renal prostaglandins, which normally autoregulate renal blood flow. Patients at risk usually are elderly or have renal insufficiency or decreased renal blood flow. For patients at risk, serum creatinine should be measured at base line and repeated after five half-lives of the administered NSAID. Hyperkalemia may develop in patients with sodium or volume depletion, diabetes mellitus, or renal insufficiency, or in those receiving medications that raise serum potassium levels. Potassium should be measured at base line and repeated after five half-lives of the NSAID. Other adverse effects include bronchospasm in 10–20% of asthmatics and mild cognitive defects or headaches in 5–10%.

Choice of NSAID can be dictated by consideration of cost, convenience, and risk. The least expensive options include plain aspirin, ibuprofen, and indomethacin. Patients may prefer NSAIDs with longer dosing intervals for the sake of compliance. Nonacetylated salicylates have the best toxicity profile but may have somewhat less efficacy than prostaglandin inhibitors.

After rheumatologic consultation, virtually all patients with rheumatoid disease should be started within the first few months of the disease on a disease-modifying antirheumatoid drug (eg, parenteral gold, methotrexate, sulfasalazine, hydroxycholoroquine) in conjunction with an NSAID. In contrast to NSAIDs, disease-modifying antirheumatoid drugs may slow progression of RA. The disease-modifying antirheumatoid drugs are slower acting than NSAIDs—benefit from methotrexate requires 4–8 weeks and from injectable gold or hydroxychloroquine up to 6 months. Many patients (50–75%) derive benefit from any single agent; however, with the exception of methotrexate and perhaps sulfasalazine, efficacy usually wanes after several years.

Glucocorticoids may be added as an adjunct in the form of prednisone, 7.5 mg or less per day, while awaiting a response to a disease-modifying antirheumatoid drug. Intraarticular steroid may benefit inflamed joints, but injections should not be repeated frequently.

At present there is much debate over the appropriate intensity of treatment for RA; nevertheless, there is a distinct trend toward earlier and more aggressive therapy, at least partially fueled by recent evidence demonstrating that patients have not only diminished quality of life, but also decreased life expectancy as a result of RA.

Osteoarthritis

Osteoarthritis, also known as degenerative joint disease, is the most prevalent form of arthritis. Over 50 million people in the United States have at least radiographic evidence of disease, and almost 200,000 patients are severely disabled; prevalence increases with age. Osteoarthritis is characterized by erosion of cartilage and bony proliferation at joint margins, and its pathogenesis involves biomechanical, biochemical, genetic, and immunologic factors. Obesity is a risk factor for OA of the knee, particularly for women. Although recent studies suggest that running does not lead to OA, definitive longitudinal data do not exist.

Clinical Features

Patients with OA typically have an insidious onset of pain and stiffness that is worse after use and better with rest. Morning stiffness may occur, but it lasts for only 30 minutes or less. Most commonly involved joints include distal interphalangeals (Heberden nodes), proximal interphalangeals (Bouchard nodes), basal joints of the thumb, cervical and lumbar spine, hips, knees, and first metatarsal–phalangeals. Physical examination may reveal painful or limited range of motion, firm bony enlargement or effusion, and crepitus. Typical signs of inflammation are minimal. Although a single joint may be involved initially, OA becomes polyarticular in over 90% of cases. Radiographs may demonstrate nonuniform joint space narrowing, subchondral bony sclerosis, or marginal osteophyte formation. In general, radiographic changes correlate poorly with symptoms. Differential diagnosis of distal interphalangeal arthritis, particularly for postmenopausal women with erosive inflammatory OA, includes psoriatic arthritis and gout. Patients with generalized symmetric disease may be misdiagnosed as having RA, particularly if the rheumatoid factor test result is positive. Medial knee pain from a torn medial meniscus or anserine bursitis may mimic that of OA.

Treatment

Osteoarthritis is a slowly progressive arthropathy that causes minimal disability if limited to small joints. Knee or hip involvement often leads to total joint replacement, and more than 100,000 total hip replacements are performed each year for this indication. Treatment modalities include physical measures, adaptive devices, medications, and orthopedic surgery. Three to five times body weight is loaded across the joint surface with weight bearing; thus, patients with lower extremity OA may benefit from a cane, crutch or walker, and weight loss. Range-of-motion exercises may help to maintain motion. Heat or ice may provide symptomatic benefit.

Pharmacologic therapy is driven by patient discomfort, and in some cases none is indicated. However, for symptomatic patients, acetaminophen in a dosage up to 4 g daily is the preferred initial therapy. It is inexpensive and well-tolerated, and has efficacy comparable to that of NSAIDs for this relatively noninflammatory arthropathy. Should it fail, a nonacetylated salicylate such as salsalate, 3–4 g daily, should be tried for 3–4 weeks. For patients who derive no benefit, analgesic dosages of a prostaglandin inhibitor such as enteric coated aspirin, 2–3 g daily; ibuprofen, 1,200 mg daily; or nabumetone, 1,000 mg daily may be tried. Patients with more severe symptoms may require higher dosages or the addition of a mild opioid preparation. Of great concern in this older cohort is NSAID-induced gastrointestinal or renal toxicity (see "Rheumatoid Arthritis"). If, despite maximal medical therapy, pain remains severe and function remains compromised, total joint arthroplasty may be indicated for the involved knee or hip.

Polymyalgia Rheumatica

Polymyalgia rheumatica (PMR) is a clinically defined syndrome of patients over age 50, two thirds of whom are female, and characterized by severe proximal pain and stiffness that are worse in the morning. Although patients may note subjective muscle weakness, muscle strength and serum creatine kinase are normal in this condition. When the diagnosis is suspected, the erythrocyte sedimentation rate should be determined; it is greater than 30 mm/h in 99% of cases. The diagnosis of PMR hinges on a dramatic response within 1 week to 15–20 mg of prednisone per day. A slow taper may be instituted after 2–4 weeks toward a maintenance dosage of 5–7.5 mg/d, guided by PMR symptoms. Although the median duration of PMR is 1–2 years, many patients require long-term therapy and may experience relapse.

The major differential diagnosis is RA, which may begin proximally in the older patient. Often differentiation can only be made with observation over time. The clinician should monitor for and educate the patient about signs of concomitant giant cell arteritis, which occurs in a small minority of patients presenting with PMR. The presence of this vasculitis would mandate higher doses of prednisone.

Giant Cell Arteritis

Giant cell arteritis is an idiopathic granulomatous vasculitis of large arteries, particularly cranial, which occurs in the same demographic group as PMR. It affects 0.1% of persons over age 50, a prevalence one fourth that of PMR. Giant cell arteritis is associated with the presence of a subtype of HLA-DR4, but its pathogenesis is poorly understood.

Clinical manifestations can be divided into arteritic and nonarteritic; the former include headache (75%), temporal artery tenderness (69%), diminished temporal artery pulse (40%), and sudden loss of vision (40%). Sixty percent of patients relate jaw claudication—discomfort with mastication—which improves with rest. Nonarteritic manifestations include weight loss (55%), PMR (40%), fever (20%), and peripheral arthritis (20%). Permanent visual loss secondary to optic nerve ischemia is the most feared complication and occurs in 10–15% of untreated patients. In most cases it is preceded by other symptoms of giant cell arteritis by weeks to months.

The diagnosis of giant cell arteritis should be considered in any patient over age 50 with new headaches, amaurosis fugax, jaw claudication, fever of undetermined origin, or unexplained weight loss. The erythrocyte sedimentation rate is usually markedly elevated. Definitive diagnosis requires cranial artery biopsy, usually of the temporal artery. Because the vasculitic pathology occurs in a patchy distribution, it is mandatory to obtain a specimen at least 4 cm in length. The sensitivity of this test is probably no greater than 75%, and thus the diagnosis cannot be excluded by negative biopsy results from a patient with a compatible clinical picture.

Treatment consists of prednisone, 40–60 mg/d, which should be started as soon as the diagnosis is seriously considered. Biopsy performed within 5 days of initiation of prednisone should not be affected by therapy. After 1 month, a slow taper should be instituted with a goal of 5–10 mg daily after 5 months. The dosage should be titrated to symptoms and not to level of erythrocyte sedimentation rate. In this older cohort of patients, steroid toxicities of vertebral fracture, myopathy, and cataracts may occur.

Gout

Gout is characterized by recurrent attacks of inflammatory arthritis caused by the presence of monosodium urate crystals in synovial fluid. Usually caused by hyperuricemia, supersaturation of monosodium urate within the joint leads to deposition in synovial tissue. When monosodium urate crystals are autoinjected into synovial fluid, they are phagocytosed by neutrophils, which release proinflammatory lysosomal enzymes. Hyperuricemia is usually a result of decreased renal excretion of uric acid, which may be caused by chronic renal disease; lactic acidemia produced by alcohol ingestion; ketosis; dehydration; or drugs, such as low-dose salicylate or diuretics. Many patients have an idiopathic defect in uric acid excretion. In 15% of cases, gout is associated with uric acid overproduction, usually of unknown cause.

Approximately 1.9% of men and 0.8% of women have gout, which presents predominantly in middle-aged men and postmenopausal women. In men, uric acid levels rise during puberty, but in women this rise is delayed until menopause. This discrepancy explains the later onset of the disease in women.

Clinical Features

Gout is divided into three clinical stages, beginning with acute gouty arthritis, which is characterized by the rapid onset of severe inflammation of the first metatarsal–phalangeal, ankle, and knee joints in descending order of frequency. Most attacks involve only one or two joints. Physical examination usually reveals marked tenderness and florid inflammation that may mimic soft tissue infection. Attacks may be precipitated by medical illness, surgery, trauma, or alcohol binge. Untreated attacks usually resolve within a few weeks, and involved joints return to their baseline state without permanent damage. Definitive diagnosis of gout and the exclusion of sepsis and pseudogout require synovial fluid analysis and the finding of negatively birefringent, needle-shaped monosodium urate crystals. Crystals may be missed in 10–20% of cases. Serum uric acid plays no role in diagnosis.

The intercritical stage is asymptomatic, but 80% of patients have a recurrence within 1–2 years. Over time, attack frequency, duration, and extent generally increase. After 10 years of inadequate treatment, 50% of patients develop the final chronic tophaceous stage, in which collections of monosodium urate—tophi—develop over the olecranon, extensor proximal forearm, or joints. Intraarticular tophi may insidiously erode subchondral bone and cartilage, leading to permanent joint damage. With modern therapy, such cases have become uncommon.

For the minority of gouty patients who are overproducers of uric acid, there is a risk of uric acid nephrolithiasis, particularly with excretion of 1,100 mg/d or more. However, chronic renal insufficiency—"gouty nephropathy"—is caused by coincidental conditions and not by gout itself.

Women with gout may diverge from the classic picture described. Disease in postmenopausal women taking long-term diuretics may develop more insidiously, with a polyarticular distribution that includes hands and accompanying tophi over fingers. Such patients may be misdiagnosed as having RA with accompanying rheumatoid nodules.

Treatment

For acute gout, treatment choices include nonsalicylate NSAIDs, intravenous colchicine, corticosteroid, and corticotropin. Any single agent is efficacious in 75–90% of cases, and treatment works best if begun early in the attack. An NSAID such as ibuprofen, naproxen, or indomethacin in antiinflammatory dosage is prescribed, unless contraindicated, for 10–14 days or until the attack has completely resolved. Colchicine by the oral route produces gastrointestinal toxicity too frequently to be recommended. Intravenous colchicine may be used for selected patients; however, relatively small dosing errors may be fatal. Corticosteroids may be given intraarticularly or by mouth in the form of 20–30 mg of prednisone daily. Corticotropin may be given intramuscularly or subcutaneously at a dosage of 40–80 IU with little risk of toxicity. Patients should be instructed to avoid salicylates, which may alter the serum level of uric acid and precipitate an acute attack, and to use moderation in their intake of alcohol.

After a gouty attack has resolved fully, prophylaxis is indicated for patients with frequent recurrences. Colchicine, 0.6 mg twice daily, is moderately effective in preventing recurrent attacks and produces minimal toxicity. However, antihyperuricemic therapy has greater efficacy. For underexcretors (less than 600 mg of uric acid in a 24-hour urine), the uricosuric agent probenecid may be prescribed, but it is contraindicated with renal insufficiency or history of kidney stone. In such cases the xanthine oxidase-inhibitor allopurinol, which decreases uric acid production, can be administered. Allopurinol is also indicated for prophylaxis in overproducers of uric acid and for all patients with tophaceous gout. The appropriate dosage of either antihyperuricemic agent is that dosage at which serum uric acid falls below 6 mg/dl, at which level intraarticular microtophi will begin to dissolve. During the first 6–12 months of antihyperuricemic therapy, colchicine, 0.6 mg twice daily, should be given concomitantly to prevent recurrent attacks.

Pseudogout

Pseudogout is the most common clinical form of calcium pyrophosphate dihydrate deposition disease, which is often asymptomatic and manifest only by radiographic calcification of cartilage (chondrocalcinosis). Named because of its propensity to mimic gouty attacks with rapidly developing inflammation of one or a few joints, pseudogout occurs when calcium pyrophosphate dihydrate crystals are shed from cartilage and phagocytosed by polymorphonuclear leukocytes, resulting in release of lysosomal enzymes. Pseudogout is half as common as gout, and its prevalence increases with age. Knee involvement is most common, but attacks may involve the great toe or wrist. Diagnosis requires the identification of weakly positively birefringent calcium pyrophosphate dihydrate crystals under polarized light. Calcium pyrophosphate dihydrate crystals are easily missed, and thus their absence does not exclude the diagnosis. Rarely, hyperparathyroidism or hemochromatosis will be found in patients with pseudogout. Treatment of acute attacks is similar to that of gout; NSAIDs, intravenous colchicine, and corticosteroids have comparable efficacy. Prophylaxis can be achieved with low-dose colchicine.

Osteoporosis

Osteoporosis is a multifactorial disorder of skeletal fragility due to low bone mass and altered bony architecture. Fractures are the complications of osteoporosis and most commonly occur in the spine, hip, and distal radius, but fractures of other skeletal sites (pelvis, ribs, humerus, metatarsals) can also occur.

Low bone mass may be the consequence of inadequate peak bone mass or of increased bone loss. Peak bone mass is achieved in early adulthood and is strongly influenced by genetic factors. Lack of exercise and low calcium intake or absorption during growth years limit the attainment of peak bone mass. Estrogen is necessary for the increase in bone density associated with puberty. Low peak bone mass is observed in patients with hypogonadal states such as Turner syndrome and exercise-induced amenorrhea.

Bone mass is usually stable in women until menopause. Estrogen deficiency results in increased osteoclastic bone resorption, particularly in trabecular bone, causing accelerated bone loss for a few years after menopause. The loss of bone mass, particularly evident in the spine, is prevented by the administration of estrogen in most women. A relatively short phase of accelerated bone loss is a major component in the increased risk of osteoporosis in women compared with men. As a woman continues to age, the rate of bone loss diminishes but continues at a slower rate for the remainder of life. This age-associated loss of both cortical and trabecular bone is similar to that seen in men and appears to be the result of an age-related impairment in osteoblastic or bone-forming activity, coupled with inefficiencies in calcium balance that lead to increased bone resorption. Increased calcium intake, estrogen, and other antiresorptive drugs (ie, calcitonin, biphosphonates) are variably effective in suppressing age-related bone loss and in decreasing the incidence of osteoporotic fractures of the spine and hip.

Other medical and metabolic disorders may augment the rate of postmenopausal and age-related loss of bone mass. Alcohol intake suppresses bone formation. Endogenous or iatrogenic hyperthyroidism, hyperparathyroidism, anticonvulsant therapy, vitamin D deficiency, intestinal malabsorption of calcium and vitamin D, chronic renal or liver disease, and generalized skeletal disorder such as multiple myeloma can contribute to the loss of bone mass. Glucocorticoid therapy impairs bone formation and leads to accentuated bone resorption, often causing rapid loss of bone in the first several months of therapy.

Skeletal radiography is useful for the detection of fractures and severe bone loss but is not sensitive enough to detect the early loss of bone or to monitor the skeletal response to therapy. Bone mass can be assessed accurately by several techniques, including single-photon absorptiometry of the radius or calcaneus, dual-energy X-ray absorptiometry of the spine and proximal femur, and quantitative computed tomography of the spine. Bone density can be used effectively to assess the skeletal status of a patient, to predict the risk of future osteoporotic fractures, and to monitor skeletal response to therapy. Measurement of spinal bone density is the most sensitive indicator of bone loss in the early postmenopausal years. Direct measurement of the proximal femur is the best indicator of the risk of hip fracture. For monitoring therapy, bone density methods and laboratories that provide very precise measurements must be employed.

The management of symptomatic osteoporosis begins with identifying and correcting factors that contribute to bone loss, including vitamin D deficiency, excess alcohol intake, and hormone therapy. Total calcium intake (dietary and supplements) should be 1,000–1,500 mg daily. Vitamin D, 400–800 U daily, is appropriate, particularly in older individuals, but large doses should be reserved for patients with documented vitamin D deficiency.

Estrogen and salmon calcitonin are the antiresorptive agents currently approved by the U.S. Food and Drug Administration (FDA) for the treatment of osteoporosis. Both drugs suppress osteoclastic bone resorption. Estrogen is effective even in women beyond menopause and will decrease the risk of subsequent fractures in patients with osteoporosis.

Etidronate is a bisphosphonate drug that also inhibits bone loss and vertebral fracture frequency in postmenopausal osteoporosis. While approved for the treatment of Paget disease, etidronate has not yet been approved by the FDA for the indication of osteoporosis. When etidronate is used, it is given cyclically, because prolonged continuous therapy impairs mineralization of newly formed bone. New bisphosphonates will be effective alternatives to estrogen for the treatment of osteoporosis.

Adjunctive therapeutic measures include exercises to strengthen the legs, hips, and extensor muscles of the back, both to diminish back discomfort and to decrease the frequency of falls. Other measures to prevent falls and injuries, including proper body mechanics, avoidance of sedatives and alcohol, correction of orthostatic hypotension, and improving the home environment, are appropriate for patients with osteoporosis.

Prevention of osteoporosis can be achieved by maximizing peak bone mass during adolescence. Maintaining adequate calcium intake and correcting estrogen deficiency when it occurs are important steps in this goal. Estrogen replacement therapy is very effective for the prevention of postmenopausal bone loss. Exercise and high calcium intake are insufficient in blunting skeletal loss in early postmenopausal women but are important components of preventing bone loss in older women.

Paget Disease of Bone

Paget disease is a patchy disorder of the skeleton usually occurring in adults over age 40. Increased osteoclastic activity, thought to be caused by paramyxoviral infection of the cells, causes localized bone resorption followed by haphazard production of new bone with enlargement and frequent distortion of the affected bone. Any skeletal site may be involved, although the spine, pelvis, skull, and large bones of the extremities are most often affected. Pagetic activity may progress to involve an entire bone, but spread from one bone to another or the occurrence of pagetic activity of a new skeletal site has not been reported. Pagetic disease is associated with pain of involved bones; bowing of affected weight-bearing bones in the lower extremity; degenerative arthritis of the hip, spine, and ankle; pathologic fractures of pagetic bone in the spine or extremities; and compression of nerves or spinal cord by the bony enlargement. Headache and deafness may be complications of cranial involvement. However, many patients, even some with extensive Paget disease, are asymptomatic.

Paget disease is usually suspected because of symptoms or incidental discovery of elevated alkaline phosphatase concentrations or radiographic abnormalities. The radiographic features of mixed lytic and sclerotic areas with enlargement of the bone are generally sufficient to confirm the diagnosis. Biopsy of bone may be necessary when isolated, predominately lytic lesions are found. Bone scan is useful to identify the distribution of pagetic activity in the patient. Serum alkaline phosphatase and urinary hydroxyproline levels reflect total pagetic activity and generally correlate well with each other.

Therapy to decrease osteoclastic bone resorption is indicated in patients with symptoms, with involvement of the skull or weight-bearing long bones, and with widespread distribution of skeletal lesions, and before orthopedic surgery involving pagetic bone. Increased calcium intake and postmenopausal estrogen replacement therapy may be of benefit. Suppression of osteoclastic activity with salmon or human calcitonin or with etidronate (a bisphosphonate drug) is a current mainstay of therapy. These drugs are moderately effective, usually causing a 50–60% reduction in alkaline phosphatase activity in most patients. Several new bisphosphonate drugs appear to be very effective inhibitors of bone resorption. These drugs are currently undergoing clinical trial in the United States and are not available or approved for treatment of Paget disease. Pamidronate is available in intravenous form for the management of hypercalcemia of malignancy and has been shown to be a useful therapeutic approach in patients unresponsive to conventional therapy.

BACK PAIN

Back pain covers a wide spectrum and may be categorized by specific syndromes. Low back pain affects the area between the last rib and the upper pelvis. Muscular–ligamentous strain is a common cause of low back pain. Sciatica, low back pain with radiation to the extremities, results from lesions involving the intervertebral disc and the lumbar nerve roots and is occasionally accompanied by sensory and motor defects. Facet joint syndrome causes back and buttock pain and may cause deep aching of the thighs. It may be due to synovitis, injury, or degeneration of the facet joints. Secondary muscle tension ("spasm") of the lumbosacral muscles may occur.

Spondylolysis or spondylolisthesis, although relatively rare, occurs often enough to warrant additional studies in certain patients who have recurrent or persistent back and thigh pain. Many patients with these conditions or with disc pathology are managed by limited physical activity, controlled exercise, and awareness of the cause of their intermittent back pain. Surgery is usually not required. Patients who have more persistent or severe nerve root irritation may require surgery.

Causes

A frequent cause of low back pain is degeneration of the intervertebral disc complex. If the annulus fibrosis, the fibrocartilaginous unit that surrounds the nucleus pulposus, is damaged by physical activity or by a familial cartilaginous defect, the nucleus can bulge out against the intact annulus; alternatively, the annulus may stretch and the nucleus may bulge and cause direct or indirect nerve root irritation.

Individuals who participate in stressful physical activity, particularly in repetitive bending and twisting, may have a higher incidence of injury to the disc complex if they lift or exercise incorrectly. Individuals with or without back pain should know how to lift by bending the knees and maintaining a straight back, how to avoid sudden jerking twisting motions, and how to shorten the length of the lever arm from the back to the object being lifted. Obesity, fluid retention, smoking, and excessive alcohol intake can affect the strength of both osseous tissue and the intervertebral disc complex. Other factors that cause or accentuate pain are related to mental health, such as job dissatisfaction, anxiety, or depression. Many patients have multiple physical and emotional complaints, and backache may be either the result of specific pathology or a depressive equivalent.

The exact cause of low back pain cannot always be determined immediately. The age of the patient is important, as specific lesions occur in particular decades. The younger patient is typically affected by muscular and ligamentous factors and the older by degenerative arthrosis and osteopenia. Malignant changes are rare in the young, but more common in the geriatric group.

Diagnosis

History

A detailed history and a diary of daily activities can help the physician classify back pain of recent origin. The duration, quality, location, and severity of the pain should be determined. The patient's age and occupation and a description of daily activities and incidents that coincided with the onset of pain are very helpful in determining whether the pathologic lesion is muscular–ligamentous or related to the intervertebral disc or osseous structures.

Physical Examination

The detailed physical examination includes observation of the gait, digital palpation of the spinous processes and the paravertebral muscles, and an estimate of leg length (done by comparing the level of the iliac crest while the patient is standing). Flexibility of the spine is determined by flexion, extension, right and left lateral bending, and rotation. Maneuvers that might give pain relief may be noted during the examination. The patient should be examined in the standing, sitting, and supine positions.

Standing Position. The spine is examined for lateral curvature, a round back, unequal height of the shoulders, or an unequal pelvis. Evaluation of the posture includes assessment of the abdominal muscles, the degree of lumbar lordosis, and the patient's ability to perform a pelvic tilt. Irregular or prominent spinous processes detected through palpation suggest a local lesion such as spondylosis, spondylolisthesis, or trauma. If the pain is acute and severe, digital palpation may cause discomfort over inflamed areas such as an intervertebral disc infection. If the problem is of longer duration and associated with systemic disease, back pain may indicate a metastatic lesion.

Mobility of the spine is assessed by having the patient bend forward and attempt to reach the floor with her fingertips. Pain on flexion, lateral bending, or extension may be related to the primary pathology. For an acute or chronic pain problem, increased muscle tension, commonly referred to as "spasm," should be observed and palpated.

A quick way to survey strength in the lower extremities is to have the patient walk on tiptoe, walk on her heels, and do a half knee bend with her hands on her hips. Obvious weakness of dorsiflexion of the foot or weakness in attempting to push up on the forefoot suggests muscle weakness due to nerve root irritation.

Chest expansion should also be measured. The average expansion varies with age, but 4–6 cm is adequate. Expansion of 2.5 cm or less requires additional diagnostic studies, because ankylosing spondylitis should be suspected.

Sitting Position. Deep tendon reflexes in the upper and the lower extremities should be tested. Absent knee or ankle reflex in a patient under age 50 suggests nerve root compression or a peripheral neuropathy. Symmetrical diminished or absent reflexes are not unusual in geriatric patients; if asymmetrical, however, a more proximal lesion should be suspected.

In straight leg raising, the patient places her hands on the table to support her trunk, so that she does not flex her back. Also, the lower extremity is adducted during the test because the abducted position relaxes the sciatic nerve. The left knee is straightened, the examiner places the left hand under the patient's left heel and the right hand on the patient's shoulder, and then flexes the entire left lower extremity. Pain during the test indicates either muscle-tendon stretch, if the hamstrings are tight, or possible nerve root irritation. The occurrence and the location of pain when the extremity is at an angle of 45° or 60° to the hip indicates a positive straight leg raising test. If the extremity can be flexed to 70° or 80° with the knee extended, the test is considered negative. These findings are confirmed by repeating flexion of the hip to a point where pain occurs and the complaint is determined to be either nerve irritation or hamstring tightness. The extremity is then lowered to a point where pain disappears. This maneuver is repeated three times.

Supplementary tests include passive dorsiflexion of the foot after a positive straight leg raising test. There is a correlation between the degree of straight leg raising and the onset of pain with foot dorsiflexion. Foot dorsiflexion will aggravate the sciatic radiation if the irritation is below the nerve root, but will tend to relieve it if the irritation is above the root. Furthermore, head flexion done after the flexed position of the extremity causes pain will reinforce the nerve root irritation. If the nerve root compression is above the root, head flexion will aggravate the pain; if it is below the root, head flexion will lessen the pain. The pain should be characterized as feeling like an electrical shock; shooting into the thigh, back, or foot; or localized to the back.

Popliteal nerve compression is done by rolling the peroneal or the tibial nerve in the popliteal region. This isolated compression may cause back pain and localize the site of the lesion to the neural structures rather than the hamstring muscles.

Supine Position. Straight leg raising is performed by adducting the extremity, straightening the knee, and slowly flexing the hip with the examiner's hand under the patient's heel. Back pain or shooting pain to the thigh, calf, or foot suggests nerve root irritation. As the angle at which pain occurs is determined, passive foot dorsiflexion is performed to aggravate the pain. Also, at the point where pain is most noticeable, head flexion is done to increase or decrease the intensity of pain. Popliteal compression is repeated. The physical findings observed in the sitting and the supine position should coincide.

With the patient in the supine position with her hips and knees flexed, the abdomen is palpated for masses, localized tenderness, rebound pain, or a possible source of referred pain to the back. A rectal examination may give information about the uterus, rectal masses, and referral of pain to the coccyx or the sacrum. A pelvic examination is also necessary. In endometriosis, for example, aberrant endometrial implants may cause back pain, pain in the pelvis, or even sciatica.

Tests

Findings of the history and physical examination may assist the physician in determining the need for radiographic studies. Radiographs are taken if the back pain is chronic, if there has been acute trauma, or if there has been a known systemic disease. Radiographs are not necessary at the first visit if the history and physical findings suggest a muscular or ligamentous problem, if the complaints have been of short duration, and if the patient is otherwise in good health. Radiographs are necessary when a patient has a distant known primary tumor, persistent rest pain and severe unexplained weight loss, or fever, malaise, and chills suggesting a bacterial infection.

Other tests that may be useful include:

- Glucose
- Thyroid-stimulating hormone
- Complete blood count
- Sedimentation rate
- Urinalysis
- Serum calcium and phosphorus levels
- Alkaline phosphatase
- Bone density
- Bone scan

Management

Most patients with acute or sub-acute low back pain require only short-term treatment. Limitation of activity is recommended, but absolute bed rest is usually unnecessary. Two days of rest are optimal, and longer periods are unnecessary. The patient should be advised to initiate mild back stretching and limited muscle strengthening and to avoid unbalanced lifting, twisting, and turning. Analgesics in conjunction with limited activity will usually reduce or eliminate back pain within 1–2 weeks in most patients with pain caused by a nonspecific condition. Other aspects of treatment include a limited physical therapy program, local heat in a bath tub or shower, or ice application for temporary improvement. Patient education includes daily postural exercise and elimination of activities that are likely to induce back complaints. Proper car, office, and home seating and lifting techniques should be reviewed. Group instruction is advisable in certain industries in which back complaints are common and movements of the spine during daily lifting, bending, twisting, and turning may result in misuse rather than overuse of the back.

Medications referred to as "muscle relaxants" are frequently prescribed for back pain, but such medications do not actually act as relaxants. Most of their benefit lies in their central effect on pain, not their antiinflammatory response at the site of the injury. Certain NSAIDs such as aspirin or other medications help some patients, but not others.

Manipulative therapy includes soft tissue massage, point pressure techniques, manual traction, and ultrasonography. This therapy is usually offered by physical therapists, chiropractors, or osteopathic physicians. Certain patients respond well to "hands-on therapy" while others obtain the same result at less expense and time through a graduated home exercise program and by changing their daily physical routine. The effectiveness of manipulative therapies is controversial. Limited trials with some comparative control studies have shown short-term improvement after manipulative therapy, but no long-term preventive or curative benefits. For a compliant patient who is compulsive about following directions, a home exercise program will usually manage infrequent but recurrent episodes of mild back pain.

If back pain persists and if there is evidence of nerve root irritation that causes sciatica, limited activity and a short course of oral steroids may abort the root irritation. If the complaint does not respond, an epidural steroid injection which provides a greater concentration of the medication in the area of nerve root irritation may be beneficial. Epidural steroid treatment may be helpful in determining whether the pain is caused by nerve root irritation or by some other condition.

Patients with persistent sciatica, reflex alteration, a discrete sensory dermatome, and motor weakness who do not respond to limited activity and antiinflammatory medication over a 4–6-week period may require discectomy. This operation is preceded by magnetic resonance imaging and electromyography to document nerve root irritation and muscle denervation.

Chemonucleolysis requires the injection of chymopain or collagenase into the intervertebral disc to decrease the water content, diminish the swelling, and cause the disc complex to recede from the nerve root. This procedure may be helpful in patients who have sciatica and an unruptured annulus. A small percentage of patients may develop a neurologic complication due to the mixture of the chymopain and blood; although this risk is low, the severity of the maloccurrence may be high and the risk–benefit ratio is too high when safer options exist.

For the patient who has spondylolisthesis, spondylolysis, or severe degenerative intervertebral disc disease with nerve root irritation, nerve root decompression and spinal fusion should be considered. If the major problem is a ruptured disc or a bone spur pressing on a nerve root, and if the disc bond is otherwise stable, nerve root decompression alone is the initial treatment of choice. Spine fusion is used after failed discectomy or in those patients who have persistent chronic back pain associated with degenerative arthrosis. The indications are clear and the results are usually predictable if the patient is emotionally stable, if secondary gain is not a major factor in recovery, and if union of the bone segments occurs.

DEPRESSION

Most mental health disorders are first recognized, diagnosed, and sometimes treated in primary care settings. Recent epidemiologic data suggest that 30% of persons using general medical services, including those of obstetricians and gynecologists, have a psychiatric disorder. However, the recognition of these illnesses in primary care is less than 50%; even when they are recognized, there is often inadequate treatment and no referral to a mental health professional. The problem is further compounded by the frequent presentation of psychologic distress as physical symptoms in patients, referred to as somatization.

The most common psychiatric illnesses seen in obstetric and gynecologic practice are depression and anxiety. The term *depression* is used imprecisely. It may refer to a symptom (ie, a sad mood in response to loss or disappointment) or to a syndrome with a very specific set of symptoms. Affective disorders are synonymous with depressive ones. The term *mood* refers to internal emotional states, whereas *affect* is the external expression of emotional states.

Types of Disorders

Depressive disorders can be unipolar or bipolar (manic–depressive). In obstetric and gynecologic settings, these disorders are often seen early accompanied by anxiety symptoms and vague somatic complaints. Patients often fear that if they express any psychologic distress their physical complaints will be discounted.

Specific criteria are diagnostic of depression (see box). When these symptoms are accompanied by periods of elation and grandiosity, a bipolar condition should be considered. A psychotic form of depression is accompanied by hallucinations and delusions. A melancholic form more often seen in older patients features more psychomotor retardation, a lack of reactivity to usually pleasant stimuli, a worsening of mood in the early morning, and considerable dysphoria. Two types of atypical depressions have been described, one a vegetative type with more overeating, hypersomnia, weight gain, and symptoms of oversensitivity to interpersonal rejection. The anxious type of atypical depression is characterized by excessive anxiety, difficulty in falling asleep, phobic symptoms, and symptoms of sympathetic arousal. A seasonal mood disorder has been described, with episodes occurring during a particular time of the year, generally when there is less sunlight. Treatments for these varying types of depressive disorders differ, hence the need for careful history taking.

Etiology and Risk Factors

The etiology of depressive disorders is complex, with biologic, psychologic, and social theories interacting in vulnerable individuals. Neurotransmitters implicated in depression are serotonin, norepinephrine, dopamine acetylcholine, and γ-aminobutyric acid. Neurohormonal theories are based on the observations that the major vegetative signs of depressions show alterations in the hypothalamus in the centers regulating feeding, sexual behaviors, circadian rhythms, and the synthesis and release of hypothalamic releasing hormones. Hypercortisolism is the most consistent neuroendocrine finding in depression. Thyroid function may be disturbed. Circadian rhythm hypotheses note the disruption of biologic rhythms.

Depressive disorders may develop at any age, but usually start in the mid-20s and 30s. More than half of those who develop a single episode will have a recurrence. The course is

---

Diagnostic Criteria for Major Depressive Episode

At least five of the following symptoms have been present during the same two week period and represent a change from previous functioning; at least one of the symptoms is either 1) depressed mood, or 2) loss of interest or pleasure. (Do not include symptoms that are clearly due to a physical condition, mood-incongruent delusions or hallucinations, incoherence, or marked loosening of associations.)

1. Depressed mood (or can be irritable mood in children or adolescents) most of the day, nearly every day, as indicated either by subjective account or observation by others
2. Markedly diminished interest or pleasure in all, or almost all, activities most of the day, nearly every day (as indicated either by subjective account or observation by others of apathy most of the time)
3. Significant weight loss or weight gain when not dieting (eg, more than 5% of body weight in a month), or decrease or increase in appetite nearly every day (in children, consider failure to make expected weight gains)
4. Insomnia or hypersomnia nearly every day
5. Psychomotor agitation or retardation nearly every day (observable by others, not merely subjective feelings of restlessness or being slowed down)
6. Fatigue or loss of energy nearly every day
7. Feelings of worthlessness or excessive or inappropriate guilt (which may be delusional) nearly every day (not merely self-reproach or guilt about being sick)
8. Diminished ability to think or concentrate, or indecisiveness, nearly every day (either by subjective account or as observed by others)
9. Recurrent thoughts of death (not just fear of dying), recurrent suicidal ideation without a specific plan, or a suicide attempt or a specific plan for committing suicide.

American Psychiatric Association: *Diagnostic and Statistical Manual of Mental Disorders. Third Edition, Revised.* Washington, DC, American Psychiatric Association, 1987

very variable, and generally there is a return to usual functioning with recovery. Most untreated cases last 6–24 months, with considerable morbidity.

Major episodes of depression occur in 4–8% of medical outpatients and minor depression occurs in 6–14%. Depression may coexist with other medical illness and with other psychiatric disorders, such as bulimia, anxiety disorder, and organic brain syndromes. Primary risk factors for major depressive disorders are as follows:

- History of depression
- Family history of depression
- Prior suicide attempts
- Female gender
- Age of onset under 40 years
- Postpartum state
- Medical comorbidity
- Lack of social supports
- Stressful life events
- Current alcohol or substance abuse

Women have twice the risk for depressive disorders as men. The prevalence for major depressive disorders in Western industrial nations is 2.3–3.2% for men and 4.5–9.3% for women. The lifetime risk for developing a major depression is 20–25% in women and 7–12% in men. Rates of depression increase during adolescence more for girls than for boys. A number of factors are thought to predispose women to depression, including early childhood losses, physical and sexual abuse, poverty, genetic predisposition, role stress (combining home, career, family), perinatal loss, and reproductive events.

Depression and Reproductive Events

Obstetricians and gynecologists often recognize that relationships exist between depressive disorders and reproductive events such as menses, pregnancy and the puerperium, infertility, and menopause.

Premenstrual depression has been found to have a prevalence rate of 65% in patients with current or past histories of depressive illnesses. Patients with premenstrual depression often later develop a depressive syndrome.

While many women during pregnancy and the postpartum period may appear more emotionally distressed and anxious, they may not meet the criteria for any specific psychiatric illness. Mental illnesses can occur during pregnancy, but they occur more frequently in the postpartum period. Mood disorders are the most common, but schizophrenia, organic brain syndromes, and anxiety disorders are also seen. Postpartum blues and the relatively rare sequela of postpartum psychosis may occur as well.

Diagnosis

Information about psychologic problems can be elicited from patients in a relatively brief time. There needs to be a high degree of awareness of signs of depression. Some clues may be complaints of low energy, anhedonia, irritability, anxiety, and sexual complaints. Recent stressful life events and lack of social supports may precipitate psychologic distress. Patients should be asked about changes in mood, behavior, and cognition that have occurred recently. The medical history should include questions about the patient's psychiatric history; family psychiatric illness; alterations in sleep, eating, concentration, and libido; obsessional thoughts; suicidal ideas; and alcohol or substance abuse. Asking questions about suicide does not cause patients to have such thoughts and often comes as a relief. Patients need to know that their physicians do not consider them to be "crazy" if they have concerns about mental health and that if they have psychiatric disorders their physical complaints will still be taken seriously. An introductory statement about the mind–body connection is often very reassuring.

Hospitalized patients should be asked about orientation to time, place, and person, to determine the state of cognitive functioning in order to obtain informed consent for procedures. Patients who are hearing voices, seeing visions, or receiving messages from radio or TV, or who feel that their thoughts are being controlled, or who are violent or agitated should receive mental health care immediately even though their condition may be a medical one.

Treatment

A treatment plan should be developed in three phases: 1) acute (0–12 weeks), aimed at improvement of mood and vegetative signs; 2) continuation of treatment (4–9 months), aimed at prevention of relapse; and 3) maintenance treatment, aimed at prevention of recurrence in patients with prior episodes. Essential to any plan is patient education, regular monitoring of side effects of any medications used, monitoring regularly of psychiatric symptoms and change in treatment plan if no improvement, and assessment of compliance. Commonly used therapeutic regimens and side effects are shown in Tables 1-9 and 1-10.

The treatment for major depression includes antidepressant medication and psychotherapy. The varying types of psychotherapy include short-term therapy—interpersonal, cognitive, or behavioral. This may be the therapy of choice for patients with mild or moderate depression and may be as effective as the use of antidepressant medications. Patients who are good candidates for psychotherapy alone are those who have less severe depression, less recurrent chronic or disabling disease, absence of psychotic symptoms, and a positive response to the psychotherapy; those who refuse medication or for whom it is contraindicated; and those who prefer psychotherapy alone. For many patients, the most helpful treatment is a combination of psychotherapy and medication given in adequate dosage.

If primary intervention is ineffective, referral to a mental health professional may be considered. Knowing a number of psychiatrists or psychologists and their special interests and skills will make the referral more smooth and less stressful for both the patient and the physician.

TABLE 1-9. PHARMACOLOGY OF ANTIDEPRESSANT MEDICATIONS

Drug	Therapeutic Dosage Range (mg/d)	Average (Range) of Elimination Half-Lives (h)*	Potentially Fatal Drug Interactions
Tricyclics			
Amitriptyline (Elavil, Endep)	75–300	24 (16–46)	Antiarrhythmics, MAO inhibitors
Clomipramine (Anafranil)	75–300	24 (20–40)	Antiarrhythmics, MAO inhibitors
Desipramine (Norpramin, Pertofrane)	75–300	18 (12–50)	Antiarrhythmics, MAO inhibitors
Doxepin (Adapin, Sinequan)	75–300	17 (10–47)	Antiarrhythmics, MAO inhibitors
Imipramine (Janimine, Tofranil)	75–300	22 (12–34)	Antiarrhythmics, MAO inhibitors
Nortriptyline (Aventyl, Pamelor)	40–200	26 (18–88)	Antiarrhythmics, MAO inhibitors
Protriptyline (Vivactil)	20–60	76 (54–124)	Antiarrhythmics, MAO inhibitors
Trimipramine (Surmontil)	75–300	12 (8–30)	Antiarrhythmics, MAO inhibitors
Heterocyclics			
Amoxapine (Asendin)	100–600	10 (8–14)	MAO inhibitors
Bupropion (Wellbutrin)	225–450	14 (8–24)	MAO inhibitors (possibly)
Maprotiline (Ludiomil)	100–225	43 (27–58)	MAO inhibitors
Trazodone (Desyrel)	150–600	8 (4–14)	—
Selective Serotonin Reuptake Inhibitors			
Fluoxetine (Prozac)	10–40	168 (72–360)[†]	MAO inhibitors
Paroxetine (Paxil)	20–50	24 (3–65)	MAO inhibitors[‡]
Sertraline (Zoloft)	50–150	24 (10–30)	MAO inhibitors[‡]
Monoamine Oxidase Inhibitors (MAO Inhibitors)[§]			
Isocarboxazid (Marplan)	30–50	Unknown	For all 3 MAO inhibitors: vasoconstrictors,[‖] decongestants,[‖] meperidine, and possibly other narcotics
Phenelzine (Nardil)	45–90	2 (1.5–4.0)	
Tranylcypromine (Parnate)	20–60	2 (1.5–3.0)	

* Half-lives are affected by age, sex, race, concurrent medications, and length of drug exposure.
[†] Includes both fluoxetine and norfluoxetine.
[‡] By extrapolation from fluoxetine data.
[§] MAO inhibition lasts longer (7 days) than drug half-life.
[‖] Including pseudoephedrine, phenylephrine, phenylpropanolamine, epinephrine, norepinephrine, and others.

Depression Guideline Panel. Depression in primary care: detection, diagnosis, and treatment. Quick reference guide for clinicians, No. 5. Rockville, Maryland: U.S. Department of Health and Human Services, Public Health Service, Agency for Health Care Policy and Research, 1993:15; AHCPR publication no. 93-0552

TABLE 1-10. SIDE EFFECT PROFILES OF ANTIDEPRESSANT MEDICATIONS

Drug	Anticholi-nergic[†]	Central Nervous System Drowsiness	Insomnia/ Agitation	Orthostatic Hypotension	Cardiac Arrhythmia	Gastrointestinal Distress	Weight Gain (over 6 kg)
Amitriptyline	4+	4+	0	4+	3+	0	4+
Desipramine	1+	1+	1+	2+	2+	0	1+
Doxepin	3+	4+	0	2+	2+	0	3+
Imipramine	3+	3+	1+	4+	3+	1+	3+
Nortriptyline	1+	1+	0	2+	2+	0	1+
Protriptyline	2+	1+	1+	2+	2+	0	0
Trimipramine	1+	4+	0	2+	2+	0	3+
Amoxapine	2+	2+	2+	2+	3+	0	1+
Maprotiline	2+	4+	0	0	1+	0	2+
Trazodone	0	4+	0	1+	1+	1+	1+
Bupropion	0	0	2+	0	1+	1+	0
Fluoxetine	0	0	2+	0	0	3+	0
Paroxetine	0	0	2+	0	0	3+	0
Sertraline	0	0	2+	0	0	3+	0
Monoamine Oxidase Inhibitors	1	1+	2+	2+	0	1+	2+

* Numerals indicate the likelihood of side effect occuring ranging from 0 for absent or rare to 4+ for relatively common.
† Dry mouth, blurred vision, urinary hesitancy, constipation
Depression Guideline Panel. Depression in primary care: detection, diagnosis, and treatment. Quick reference guide for clinicians, No. 5. Rockville, Maryland: U.S. Department of Health and Human Services, Public Health Service, Agency for Health Care Policy and Research, 1993:14; AHCPR publication no. 93-0553

HEADACHE

Headache affects almost 93% of men and 99% of women during their lives. Headache is usually part of a primary headache disorder (migraine, tension-type headache, or cluster headache), but it may be a symptom of another illness, such as a brain tumor, cerebral hemorrhage, or meningitis.

Classification

The International Headache Society has published criteria for classification and diagnosis of a broad range of headache disorders. Migraine and tension-type headache are among the most common (see box).

Migraine Headache

Migraine is an episodic headache disorder usually lasting 4–24 hours, which may be initiated by a prodrome and preceded by an aura. The headache, of moderate to severe intensity, may be unilateral or bilateral. It typically, but not always, is throbbing. Patients with migraine usually are photophobic and phonophobic and have nausea and sensitivity to movement. Vomiting and diarrhea are less common.

Common migraine is now called "migraine without aura," and classic migraine is called "migraine with aura." Types of aurae (the complex of focal neurologic symptoms preceding an attack) include the following: 1) homonymous visual disturbance (most common, includes fortification spectra [bright scintillating lights in a zigzag pattern moving across the field of vision], photopsia [sparks or flashing lights], and visual obscurations [visual illusions or distortions]); 2) unilateral paresthesias or numbness; 3) unilateral weakness; and 4) aphasia or unclassifiable speech difficulty. *Status migrainosus* refers to bouts of migraine that last longer than 72 hours. It may be associated with nausea, vomiting, and dehydration.

Tension-Type Headache

The most common headache type, tension-type headache, is the new International Headache Society term for tension headache. The pain is typically bilateral; dull, deep, or bandlike; mild to moderate in severity; not aggravated by exertion; and lasts from 30 minutes to 7 days. Associated symptoms may include anorexia, photophobia, phonophobia (fear of noise), and pericranial muscle tenderness. Patients with episodic tension-type headache (occurs <15 days per month) should be distinguished from those with chronic tension-type headache (formerly chronic daily headache). Most patients with chronic tension-type headache have almost daily head pain (present >15 days per month) that is similar to that of episodic tension-type headache. These patients frequently overuse medications and are depressed.

Tension-type headache is present for at least 15 days per month for at least 6 months. Many patients have chronic tension-type headache and acute exacerbations of headache that fit the criteria for migraine. Tension-type headache was previously called mixed tension–vascular headache.

Tension-type headache may be difficult to differentiate from migraine; both can be episodic, bilateral, nonthrobbing, and

> **Migraine and Tension-Type Headache**
>
> **Migraine Without Aura (Common Migraine)**
> A. At least 5 attacks
> B. Headache lasting 4–72 hours
> C. Headache has at least two of the following characteristics:
>   1. Unilateral location
>   2. Pulsating quality
>   3. Moderate or severe intensity
>   4. Aggravation by routine physical activity
> D. During headache at least one of the following:
>   1. Nausea and/or vomiting
>   2. Photophobia and phonophobia
>
> **Migraine with Aura (Classic Migraine)**
> A. At least 2 attacks
> B. At least 3 of the following 4 characteristics:
>   1. One or more fully reversible aura symptoms indicating focal cerebral cortical or brain stem dysfunction
>   2. At least one aura symptom develops gradually over more than 4 minutes or 2 or more symptoms occur in succession
>   3. No aura symptom lasts more than 60 minutes
>   4. Headache follows aura with a free interval of less than 60 minutes (It may also begin before or simultaneously with the aura)
>
> **Episodic Tension-Type Headache**
> A. At least 10 previous headache episodes
>   Headache days <180/year (<15/month)
> B. Headache lasting from 30 minutes to 7 days
> C. At least 2 of the following pain characteristics:
>   1. Pressing/tightening (nonpulsating) quality
>   2. Mild or moderate intensity (may inhibit, but does not prohibit activities)
>   3. Bilateral location
>   4. No aggravation by routine physical activity
> D. Both of the following:
>   1. No nausea or vomiting (anorexia may occur)
>   2. Photophobia and phonophobia are absent, or one but not the other is present

of moderate severity, and both can have associated anorexia, photophobia, and phonophobia. The aura, if present, allows an easy diagnosis. Nausea, vomiting, and diarrhea may be associated with migraine; these symptoms are not seen with tension-type headache. Migraine and tension-type headache may be part of a spectrum of benign headache differing only in pain severity.

Cluster Headache

Cluster headache is a nonfamilial disorder predominantly affecting men. The attacks are brief (30–90 minutes), frequent, strictly unilateral, and usually occur in clusters lasting weeks. The pain is excruciatingly severe and frequently associated with unilateral autonomic signs, such as nasal stuffiness and lacrimation. There is no prodrome, aura, or postdrome, and usually no associated gastrointestinal symptoms. Whereas the migraineur is passive during the attack, the cluster patient is active.

Diagnosis

Since most headache patients have normal results of neurologic and physical examinations, headache diagnosis depends almost exclusively on the history:

- Present illness: new, progressive, or recurrent headache
- Age at onset
- Location
- Frequency
- Onset, duration, character, and severity: migraine is throbbing; cluster is deep and boring; tension-type headache is dull, bandlike
- Course: a progressively worsening headache is worrisome
- Prodromes and aura
- Associated signs and symptoms: nasal congestion, tearing (cluster); nausea and vomiting (migraine); teeth grinding and neck tenderness (tension-type headache)
- Signs of depression and cognitive dysfunction
- Signs of neurologic dysfunction: weakness, paresthesia, aphasia, diplopia, visual loss, vertigo, faintness
- Precipitating factors: bright lights; fatigue; loss of sleep; hypoglycemia; stress; certain drugs, alcohol, food additives; menstruation
- Family history
- Multiplicity: patients frequently have different headache types

The physical and neurologic examinations can rule out systemic and neurologic causes of headache. Laboratory testing can exclude secondary causes of headache, provide a base line for potential side effects, monitor drug levels, and confirm or rule out medication overuse. Some patients will require neurodiagnostic testing or a lumbar puncture to rule out an organic central nervous system cause of headache.

Patients may present with a headache that is worrisome. Causes for concern include the following:

- The first or worst headache of the patient's life (particularly if it is of acute onset)
- Progressively worsening headache
- A headache associated with fever, nausea, and vomiting that cannot be explained by a systemic illness
- A headache associated with focal neurologic findings, papilledema, a stiff neck, or changes in consciousness or in cognition (such as difficulty in reading, writing, or thinking)
- No obvious identifiable headache etiology
- Medication overuse
- Failure to respond to therapy

If any of these conditions exist, medical or neurologic consultation, neuroimaging studies (magnetic resonance imaging or computed tomography), or a lumbar puncture may be indicated.

The first or worst headache of a patient's life should be assumed to be an acute neurologic disorder. If the current headache is similar to multiple prior headaches, one can be less concerned about a new problem.

Acute recurrent headaches are usually tension-type headache or migraine. Less common causes include subarachnoid hemorrhage, cerebrovascular insufficiency, intermittent hydrocephalus, pheochromocytoma, trigeminal neuralgia, cluster headache, and pseudotumor cerebri.

Subacute headache, present for days or weeks, may be the beginning of chronic tension-type headache but usually signifies a primary neurologic disorder and demands a complete neurologic evaluation.

Chronic daily headache may be related to analgesic overuse, pseudotumor cerebri, or an underlying psychologic problem. Patients may present to the emergency department with the "last straw" syndrome. The patients typically have chronic tension-type headache with superimposed, more severe, migraine headaches.

Headache should be evaluated with the same intensity and completeness as any other clinical condition. The diagnosis of migraine should not be made without excluding condi-

TABLE 1-11. MEDICATIONS FOR TREATMENT OF HEADACHE

Drug	Route of Administration*	Dosage Range
Simple analgesics ± caffeine		
Acetaminophen, 250 mg, and/or aspirin, 250 mg; caffeine, 65 mg	PO	Limit dose to 1 g stat, 4 g/d; avoid daily use
Combination analgesics ± butalbital		
Aspirin, 325 mg, or acetaminophen, 325 mg; butalbital, 50 mg; caffeine, 40 mg	PO	Limit dose to 1 or 2 stat, 6/attack, 24/mo
Aspirin, 650 mg, or acetaminophen, 325 mg; butalbital, 50 mg	PO	
Combination analgesics with narcotics		
Aspirin, 325 mg; butalbital, 50 mg; caffeine, 40 mg; codeine phosphate, 30 mg	PO	Limit dose to 1 or 2 stat, 6/attack, and 16/mo
Aspirin, 325 mg; codeine, 30 mg	PO	
Acetaminophen, 125, 300, or 325 mg; codeine, 7.5, 15, 30, or 60 mg	PO	
NSAIDs commonly used		
Naproxen sodium, 275 mg	PO	Maximum initial dose, 825 mg[†]
Ibuprofen, 200, 300, 400, 600, or 800 mg	PO	Maximum initial dose, 800 mg[†]
Meclofenamate sodium, 50 or 100 mg	PO	Maximum initial dose, 100 mg[†]
Indomethacin, 25, 50, or 75 mg	PO	Maximum initial dose, 50 mg[†]
Ketoprofen, 25, 50, or 75 mg	PO	Maximum initial dose, 75 mg[†]
Diclofenac sodium, 25, 50, or 75 mg	PO	Maximum initial dose, 75 mg[†]
Sympathomimetic agents		
Isometheptene, acetaminophen, dichloralphenazone	PO	Dose: 2 stat, can repeat in 1 h (limit: 3 times/wk)
Ergotamine tartrate[‡]		
Caffeine, 100 mg; ergotamine tartrate, 1 mg	PO/PR	Dose: up to 6 mg (oral) or 2 suppositories stat Limit monthly use to 8 events or 24 mg (oral) or to 12 suppositories
Dihydroergotamine mesylate[‡]		
Dihydroergotamine mesylate, 1 mg/ml ampule	IM/IV	Dose: up to 1 mg stat, 3 mg/d. Limit monthly use to 12 events or 18 ampules
Serotonin agonists[§]		
Sumatriptan	SC	6 mg; can be repeated after 1 h (limit: 2 injections/24 h)

* Route: PO, per os; PR, per rectum; IM, intramuscular; IV, intravenous; SC, subcutaneous.
[†] Up to maximum dose may be taken stat.
[‡] Keep 3 days between dosing with ergotamine in patients with frequent or daily headache.
[§] For protracted migraines, serotonin agonists may be used.

tions that can mimic it. Diagnostic testing cannot replace, but should be an adjunct to, a comprehensive history and physical examination.

Treatment

Prophylaxis is designed to reduce the frequency and severity of headache attacks. Treatment is aimed at stopping individual attacks, reducing the severity and duration of head pain, and alleviating associated symptoms, including nausea and vomiting. Patients can use medication for the treatment of headache even if they are using prophylactic agents. Medications for treatment include analgesics, anxiolytics, NSAIDs, ergots, steroids, major tranquilizers, narcotics, and, most recently, sumatriptan, a direct-acting serotonin agonist (Table 1-11).

Prophylactic medication use should be considered when 1) a patient has at least two or three attacks per month; 2) the attacks are incapacitating, associated with focal neurologic signs, or of prolonged duration; 3) the patient is unable to cope with his or her headache; and 4) there are contraindications or adverse reactions to medications used for treatment.

Following are guidelines for the use of prophylactic medication:

1. Start with a low dose and increase it slowly.
2. Give a full trial of the medication (1–2 months).
3. Ensure that the patient is not taking interfering medications and is not overusing medications for treatment.
4. Be sure that a female patient is not pregnant and is using effective contraception.
5. Attempt to taper and discontinue the prophylactic medication once headaches are well controlled.

The major drugs used for migraine headache prophylaxis, recommended dosages, contraindications, and side effects are given in Table 1-12. Patients with frequent headaches may overuse analgesics or ergotamine. Overuse consists of using simple analgesics daily, combination analgesics containing barbiturates or sedatives more often than three times a week, or ergotamine tartrate more often than twice a week. Overuse can produce chronic tension-type headache with growing dependence on symptomatic medication and refrac-

TABLE 1-12. MEDICATIONS FOR PREVENTION OF MIGRAINES

Drug	Daily Oral Dosage Range	Comments
Beta blockers		
Propranolol	40–320 mg/d	Effective. Side effects: drowsiness, nightmares, insomnia, depression, memory disturbances, decreased exercise tolerance
Atenolol	50–150 mg/d	
Nadolol	40–240 mg/d	
Timolol maleate	10–30 mg/d	
Calcium channel blockers		
Verapamil	240–720 mg/d	Benefit may lag 3–4 weeks. Side effects: hypotension, edema, headache, constipation
Nifedipine	30–180 mg/d	
Diltiazem	120–360 mg/d	
Antidepressants		
Nortriptyline hydrochloride	10–125 mg/d	Effective independent of antidepressant effect
Amitriptyline hydrochloride	10–300 mg/d	
Doxepin hydrochloride	10–150 mg/d	
Fluoxetine hydrochloride	20–80 mg/d	Fewer anticholinergic effects than tricyclics
Monoamine oxidase inhibitors		
Phenelzine	30–90 mg	Side effects: hypotension, weight gain, edema. Requires close medical supervision and tyramine-free diet
Anticonvulsant		
Divalproex sodium	250–1,500 mg	Gastrointestinal disturbances, sedation, tremor, hepatotoxicity, transient hair loss
Serotonin antagonists		
Methylergonovine maleate	0.2–0.4 mg qid*	Lacks significant peripheral vasoconstrictive effect
Methysergide maleate	2–8 mg	Idiosyncratic fibrotic reaction (1/5,000)

*qid indicates four times daily.

toriness to prophylactic medications. Stopping the overused medication frequently results in headache improvement following a period of increased headache (analgesic washout period).

THYROID DISEASES

Thyroid disorders are common in women, as are potentially misleading clinical and laboratory findings that can falsely suggest thyroid diseases. There are important interrelationships between thyroid dysfunction and female reproductive disorders and pregnancy.

Clinical Physiology

Thyroid hormones act in target tissues by binding to nuclear receptors, which ultimately induce changes in gene expression. Triiodothyronine (T_3) binds the receptor with higher affinity and is the more biologically active thyroid hormone; thyroxine (T_4), the main product of the thyroid gland, provides a stable hormonal reservoir for extrathyroidal conversion to T_3. Pituitary thyroid-stimulating hormone (TSH) is the principal regulator of thyroid growth and hormone production. In turn, TSH is regulated by hypothalamic thyrotropin-releasing hormone (TRH) and thyroid hormone negative feedback. Thyroid-stimulating immunoglobulins that bind to the TSH receptor are the cause of hyperthyroid Graves disease.

Over 99% of circulating T_4 and T_3 are bound by plasma proteins, predominantly thyroxine-binding globulin (TBG). Changes in levels of these plasma proteins alter the serum total, but not the free, thyroid hormone levels and therefore do not affect patients' clinical status. In women, TBG excess is common because estrogens increase the TBG plasma concentration by decreasing its TBG clearance.

Thyroid function tests may be misleading in women with systemic illnesses or those taking certain drugs. Conversion of T_4 to T_3 is decreased in a variety of illnesses (eg, sepsis, malignancy, and hyperemesis gravidarum) and with propranolol and amiodarone administration. Severe nonthyroidal illnesses can also cause low serum T_4 and TSH concentrations. In heathy women, puberty, menopause, and aging do not alter free thyroid hormone concentrations.

Fetal thyroid development begins late in the first trimester and is independent of the mother. There is minimal transplacental passage of maternal thyroid hormones, but their role in normal fetal development remains unclear. Maternal immunoglobulins causing autoimmune thyroid diseases cross the placenta and can cause transient thyroid dysfunction in the fetus and neonate. The fetus is also exposed to the drugs commonly used to treat hyperthyroidism.

Hypothyroidism

Overt hypothyroidism occurs in 2% of women, and at least an additional 5% develop subclinical hypothyroidism. Transient hypothyroidism affects approximately 5% of postpartum women.

Causes

The principal cause of hypothyroidism is autoimmune (Hashimoto) thyroiditis. Although there is a familial predisposition, the specific genetic and environmental factors that trigger this condition are unknown. Autoimmune thyroiditis is increasingly prevalent with age, affecting 15% of women over age 65. Most have mild thyroid failure, termed subclinical hypothyroidism, defined by an elevated serum TSH concentration with a normal serum free T_4 level. Some patients with subclinical hypothyroidism, in fact, experience symptom reversal by thyroid hormone.

Patients with underlying autoimmune thyroiditis usually have a diffuse, firm, and painless goiter, although the gland may be nonpalpable in the atrophic variant of the disease. Autoimmune thyroiditis may be associated with other endocrine (eg, IDDM, primary ovarian failure, adrenal insufficiency, and hypoparathyroidism) and nonendocrine disorders (eg, vitiligo and pernicious anemia).

Hypothyroidism also occurs frequently after surgical or radioactive iodine therapy for hyperthyroidism. Thyroid gland irradiation in the course of treatment for head and neck tumors can also cause hypothyroidism. All patients who have received these therapies should be monitored yearly for the possible development of hypothyroidism. Thyroid gland inflammation causes spontaneously resolving hypothyroidism in postpartum thyroiditis and subacute thyroiditis (see below). Hypothyroidism is rarely the result of pituitary or hypothalamic diseases causing TSH deficiency.

Clinical Features

Manifestations of hypothyroidism include fatigue, lethargy, cold intolerance, dry skin, hair loss, constipation, myalgia, carpal tunnel syndrome, and weight gain, which typically is less than 5–10 kg (11–22 lb). Common neuropsychiatric symptoms include impaired memory, depression, irritability, and dementia. Menstrual dysfunction is common: menorrhagia is most frequent, but amenorrhea also occurs. Anovulation may cause infertility, but thyroid hormone is not useful therapy for anovulatory euthyroid women. Hypothyroidism does not cause premenstrual syndrome, and thyroid hormone therapy for premenstrual syndrome is no more effective than placebo. Hypothyroidism can cause precocious or delayed puberty. Hyperprolactinemia and galactorrhea are unusual manifestations of hypothyroidism. In patients with amenorrhea, galactorrhea, and modest hyperprolactinemia, it is vital to distinguish primary hypothyroidism from a prolactin-secreting pituitary adenoma by measuring the serum TSH level.

Diagnosis

Clinical diagnosis of hypothyroidism requires laboratory confirmation. Overt primary hypothyroidism is characterized by a low serum free T_4 or free T_4 index and an elevated serum TSH level. In hypothyroid women, during pregnancy the serum total T_4 level may remain normal because of the increased TBG level; accurate diagnosis can be ensured by serum TSH measurement. Autoimmune thyroiditis can be confirmed by the presence of serum antithyroid peroxidase (formerly antimicrosomal) antibodies. Central hypothyroidism is characterized by a low or low-normal serum free T_4 with a low or inappropriately normal serum TSH concentration.

Therapy
The treatment of choice for hypothyroidism is L-thyroxine (T_4). Its conversion to T_3 restores a physiologic milieu. Thyroxine is well absorbed, unless there is co-administration of cholestyramine, ferrous sulfate, aluminum hydroxide, or sucralfate. The T_4 dose requirement is weight related (approximately 1.6 µg/kg), decreases in elderly women, and should be adjusted to maintain the serum TSH level within the normal range. In approximately one half of pregnant women, the T_4 dose requirement is increased by 25–100%. Consequently, serum TSH should be reassessed during pregnancy. Postpartum, the prepregnancy T_4 dose can usually be resumed.

Treatment of subclinical hypothyroidism may be justified under three circumstances: 1) the presence of antithyroid antibodies, which predict progression to overt hypothyroidism; 2) symptoms consistent with mild hypothyroidism; and 3) an elevated serum LDL cholesterol concentration, which may improve with T_4 therapy.

Administration of excessive T_4 doses should be avoided. Even mild T_4 excess, which is recognizable solely by a suppressed serum TSH, has been associated with cortical bone loss and atrial fibrillation, particularly in older women. A low initial T_4 dose should be used in women with known or suspected ischemic heart disease, which can be exacerbated by T_4 therapy.

Hyperthyroidism

Hyperthyroidism affects 2% of women during their lifetime. It occurs most often during the childbearing years.

Causes
Graves disease, by far the most common underlying disorder, is caused by immunoglobulins that bind to and activate the TSH receptor. In addition to hyperthyroidism, Graves disease is associated with orbital inflammation and a characteristic dermopathy, pretibial myxedema. The environmental factors that trigger the onset of Graves disease in genetically susceptible women are, as yet, unidentified, but stress and cigarette smoking may be risk factors.

Less often, hyperthyroidism may be due to autonomously functioning benign thyroid neoplasia—toxic adenoma and toxic multinodular goiter. Transient thyrotoxicosis also results from the unregulated glandular release of thyroid hormone in subacute (painful) thyroiditis and in postpartum (painless, silent, or lymphocytic) thyroiditis. Rarely, thyroid gland overactivity is caused by a human chorionic gonadotropin-secreting choriocarcinoma or a TSH-secreting pituitary adenoma. Ovarian teratomas (struma ovarii) can produce thyroid hormones ectopically. Thyrotoxicosis is also caused by iatrogenic prescription or factitious ingestion of T_4 or T_3, the latter often occurring in patients with eating disorders.

Clinical Features
Classically, thyrotoxic patients complain of fatigue, heat intolerance, palpitations, dyspnea, nervousness, and weight loss, although one fourth of younger women actually gain weight because of increased appetite. Thyrotoxicosis may present with vomiting, particularly in pregnant women, in whom it may be confused with hyperemesis gravidarum. Tachycardia, lid lag, tremor, proximal muscle weakness, and warm, moist skin are often present on examination. Elderly women may lack these typical symptoms and signs and often present with unexplained weight loss, atrial fibrillation, or angina pectoris. Hyperthyroidism may cause or exacerbate osteoporosis. Most thyrotoxic patients have regular menses with lighter flow, although amenorrhea occurs in 10% of patients. Anovulatory menses and associated infertility are common. Goiter is present in most younger women with Graves disease but is absent in 50% of affected older patients.

Ophthalmologic signs of Graves disease, including lid retraction, periorbital edema, and proptosis, occur in less than one third of women, whereas more severe ophthalmologic complications (eg, corneal ulceration, extraocular muscle dysfunction, and vision loss) occur in less than 5%. Rarely, orbital inflammation can occur in patients without hyperthyroidism, so-called euthyroid Graves disease.

Toxic nodular goiter is associated with homogeneous gland enlargement. In subacute thyroiditis, the gland is tender, hard, and enlarged; in postpartum thyroiditis it is minimally enlarged and nontender.

Diagnosis
Most thyrotoxic patients have elevated total and free T_4 and T_3 concentrations. However, as discussed above, high serum total T_4 or T_3 levels are not pathognomonic of hyperthyroidism. In euthyroid individuals, elevations of thyroid hormone concentrations can be due to increased protein binding, decreased peripheral conversion of T_4 to T_3, or (rarely) congenital tissue resistance to thyroid hormones.

In all of the common forms of thyrotoxicosis, the serum TSH concentration is undetectable or very low in sensitive assays (ie, ones with detection limits ≤0.1 mU/L). Consequently, serum TSH measurement is an extremely accurate way to exclude the diagnosis of hyperthyroidism. Patients with a low TSH concentration despite normal free T_4 and T_3 concentrations are said to have subclinical hyperthyroidism, which is associated with increased risk of osteoporosis and atrial tachyarrhythmias.

It is essential to differentiate accurately among the causes of hyperthyroidism, since distinct forms of treatment are often indicated. The radioiodine uptake and scan are useful in the differential diagnosis of chemically established hyperthyroidism. There is homogeneously increased uptake in Graves disease, heterogeneous tracer concentration in toxic nodular goiter, and diminished gland radioisotope concentration in thyroiditis and medication-induced thyrotoxicosis. In patients with Graves disease, serum immunoglobulins that mimic TSH-mediated adenylate cyclase activation (TSI) or compete with TSH for receptor binding (TBII) can be detected, but are seldom required for diagnosis. High maternal TSI levels do predict a greater likelihood of neonatal hyperthyroidism in pregnant women with Graves disease, including those who may themselves be euthyroid after previous thyroid ablation therapy. The erythrocyte sedimentation rate is increased in patients with subacute thyroiditis. The serum TSH level is appropriately elevated or normal in rare patients with TSH-secreting pituitary adenomas.

Therapy
The antithyroid medications, methimazole (10–30 mg/d) and propylthiouracil (50–150 mg every 6–8 hours), or radioiodine, are widely considered to be the treatments of choice for women with hyperthyroid Graves disease. The antithyroid drugs block thyroid hormone biosynthesis and may have additional immunosuppressive effects. Although propylthiouracil also partially inhibits extrathyroidal T_4 to T_3 conversion, this benefit is outweighed in most patients by the longer half-life of methimazole, which can be administered in a single daily dose. Euthyroidism is typically restored in 3–10 weeks, and treatment is usually continued for 6–24 months. Although continued antithyroid medication is effective in controlling hyperthyroidism, sustained remissions after a course of drug therapy occur in less than one half of patients. All patients should be cautioned about the drugs' minor side effects (eg, fever, rash, and arthralgias, which are infrequent [5%]) and particularly about major drug toxicities (eg, hepatitis, vasculitis, and agranulocytosis, which are rare [0.2–0.5%]). If a remission is achieved, lifelong follow-up is warranted. Relapses are particularly common in the postpartum period.

Iodine 131 therapy leads to permanent cure of hyperthyroidism in 70–80% of patients within 2 to 6 months. The principal drawback to radioactive iodine therapy is the high rate of postablative hypothyroidism, which occurs in at least 50% of patients within 1 year and continues to develop at a rate of 2–3% per year. Large retrospective surveys have failed to demonstrate any increased carcinogenic or teratogenic risk for women treated with radioactive iodine, regardless of age at treatment. The estimated ovarian radiation in the course of radioactive iodine therapy for hyperthyroidism is 0.2 rad/mCi administered, or approximately 1–2 rads total, a dose that is similar to widely used diagnostic procedures (eg, barium enema with fluoroscopy and hysterosalpingography). Since hyperthyroidism may be temporarily exacerbated by radioactive iodine therapy, pretreatment with antithyroid medication is advisable in severely thyrotoxic individuals, older patients, and those with intrinsic cardiopulmonary disease.

Beta-adrenergic blocking drugs represent useful adjunctive therapy for control of sympathomimetic symptoms in hyperthyroid patients. Beta blockers are usually the sole treatment for patients with spontaneously resolving hyperthyroidism caused by thyroiditis. Patients with subacute thyroiditis are also treated with aspirin or other nonsteroidal antiinflammatory agents for relief of thyroid pain. In 20% of patients, a 2–8-week course of glucocorticoids is required. In the rare woman with thyrotoxicosis due to primary trophoblastic, ovarian, or pituitary diseases, surgical excision of the responsible tumor is obviously indicated.

Thyroid Nodules and Cancer

Thyroid nodules are extremely common, being detectable on examination in 5% of women and demonstrable by ultrasonography in as many as 30%. Although more than 90% of thyroid nodules are benign, malignancy and hyperthyroidism must be excluded. Most thyroid nodules are symptomatic and are discovered on routine examination. A history of childhood therapeutic head or neck irradiation implies a higher risk of malignancy.

Virtually all nodules require evaluation; routine surgical excision of all nodules is inappropriate. Thyroid function testing by serum TSH measurement is indicated, since an elevated serum TSH level may reveal benign autoimmune thyroiditis, whereas a suppressed or low TSH level suggests an autonomous nodule or toxic multinodular goiter. Since the vast majority of nodules are "cold" on radionuclide thyroid scan and hence require a tissue diagnosis, routine thyroid scanning is not cost-effective. Neither is ultrasonography generally definitive, since benign lesions cannot be distinguished from malignancies with certainty.

Fine needle aspiration biopsy is the diagnostic procedure of choice. In several large series, the positive predictive value of fine needle aspiration biopsy was 95–100%, with low false-negative rates (1–5%). Approximately 20% of nodules will be classified as "indeterminate" or "suspicious" by fine needle biopsy. At surgery, only 20% of these will actually prove to be malignant. Thus, surgery is usually indicated if a suggestive biopsy result is obtained, although a 3–6-month trial of T_4 suppression is an acceptable alternative. Should the nodule fail to decrease in size, surgical excision should be performed.

Papillary thyroid carcinoma, which accounts for 70% of thyroid cancers, generally has a favorable prognosis. Patients less than age 50 years, with small (<4 cm) tumors and no evidence of extraglandular spread have a life expectancy similar to that of the general population. The presence of cervical node metastases does not alter the prognosis. Discussion of the controversies related to the extent of surgery, radioiodine ablation of thyroid remnants, and follow-up of patients with thyroid cancer with serum thyroglobulin measurement and radioiodine scanning are beyond the scope of this review. However, lifelong T_4 suppression therapy is mandatory.

In the pregnant woman discovered to have a thyroid nodule, fine needle aspiration biopsy is the test of choice; radionuclide thyroid scanning is contraindicated. If the results of the biopsy are benign or suggestive, T_4 suppression therapy should be initiated. In the case of a suggestive nodule, surgery could be performed after delivery, should the nodule fail to shrink. If the patient clearly has thyroid carcinoma, two options can be considered: thyroid surgery in the second trimester or T_4 suppression therapy and close observation for tumor growth with postpartum surgery. The latter option would be particularly reasonable for papillary tumors, which typically have an indolent growth pattern.

DERMATOLOGIC CONDITIONS

Common dermatologic conditions include contact dermatitis, atopic dermatitis, fungal infections, bacterial infections, viral infections, scaling disorders, infestations, and acne. These conditions are diagnosed by history, physical examination, and, in some cases, some simple laboratory techniques. Pharmacologic treatment most often consists of antihistamines or corticosteroids. Nonpharmacologic therapies include the use of wet dressings and soaks, ointments or lotions, and mild soaps.

Diagnosis

The history should allow the physician to assess the nature and duration of the condition. The following questions may be helpful:

- How long has the rash or itching been present?
- How has the appearance changed?
- Is it constant or recurrent?
- Are there factors that seem to make it better or worse?
- Has a similar problem occurred in a family member?
- Has it been treated at home or by another physician?
- Are any drugs being taken, either prescription or nonprescription?

In addition, the patient's age, occupation, habits, and physiologic state (eg, menses or pregnancy) may be helpful in determining the diagnosis.

During the physical examination, the appearance and distribution of lesions should be noted. Primary lesions include:

- Macules and patches: flat areas that differ in color from surrounding skin
- Papules, nodules, and tumors: solid, elevated lesions of increasing size
- Vesicles, bullae, and pustules: raised, fluid-filled lesions of varying size and fluid composition
- Wheals: elevated, edematous, transitory lesions
- Petechiae and purpura: circumscribed deposits of blood or blood pigments

Secondary lesions evolve from a visible lesion and include scales, crusts, ulcers, fissures, and excoriations.

The use of a filtered ultraviolet light is helpful in diagnosis because it makes some lesions fluoresce. In addition, microscopic examination of samples can aid in identifying unusual lesions. The addition of potassium hydroxide to the sample may aid in the diagnosis of fungal infections.

Common Conditions

Contact dermatitis can be caused by a weak irritant, a strong irritant, or an allergic reaction. In each case, eliminating or preventing further exposure is an important part of treatment.

Contact dermatitis caused by a weak irritant such as soap or detergent typically appears as a poorly demarcated patch of erythema with pruritus. Scratching may cause excoriation and crusting. The patient should be instructed to keep the affected area dry. Topical corticosteroids may be prescribed.

Strong irritants, such as acids, alkalis, or other caustic materials can also cause dermatitis. In such cases, exposure is often related to the patient's occupation, and prevention requires protective clothing and frequent washing. Irrigation has been effective.

An allergic reaction to poison oak, poison ivy, or poison sumac results in dermatitis that is papulovesicular, often occurring in a linear formation, and is extremely pruritic. An allergic reaction to a variety of other substances, including fabrics, cosmetics, and foods, may also cause dermatitis. Allergic dermatitis appears as a sharply demarcated, red, pruritic area of inflammation. Nondrug treatment consists of cool compresses, tub soaks, and colloidal oatmeal. Calamine lotion and topical corticosteroids may help.

Atopic dermatitis is another form of dermatitis that is often associated with a personal or family history of allergic disorders, including hay fever and asthma. In adults, it appears on flexor surfaces, neck, scalp, and chest as scaly, lichenified, erythematous lesions. Atopic dermatitis may be affected by psychologic or physical stress or dietary factors (ie, avoidance of eggs, peanuts, milk, and fish may reduce cutaneous reactions). Patients should use a mild soap or a soap substitute and emollients. Cool baths and wet dressings are recommended. Antihistamines and topical corticosteroids may also be helpful.

Fungal infections include candidiasis and tineas (also known as dermatophytoses). Candidiasis produces moist, red, and scaly lesions. In addition to the vulva, candidiasis may also affect the skin under the breasts; in the axillae, umbilicus, and groin; between the fingers and toes; and in the gluteal folds as well as the oral cavity. Tineas are typically discrete, well-defined, scaly, elevated patches with distinct red borders and a fading center. Tineas are contagious. Tinea capitis is usually seen in children and appears as scattered patches of inflammation and scaling on the scalp; an immunologic reaction can cause a kerion (an inflamed lesion on the scalp) which can scar. Other tineas affect the inner thighs and pubic areas or the foot. Because treatment of tineas can involve systemic griseofulvin, which has potential adverse side effects, the diagnosis should be confirmed by culture or positive potassium hydroxide preparation before beginning therapy. Tinea capitis must be treated with griseofulvin; other fungal infections may be treated either topically or systemically.

A common viral infection is molluscum contagiosum. It is characterized by flesh-colored, translucent papules that are dome shaped with central umbilication. It is contagious and is frequently seen in people with AIDS. It can be transmitted sexually or by contact (such as that which occurs during contact sports). Scratching causes the virus to spread. Treatment involves cryosurgery with liquid nitrogen. Curettage and topical vesicants such as those used for warts are also effective in removing molluscum contagiosum. If left untreated, lesions will spontaneously subside in 6–9 months as immunity to the virus develops. However, treatment is recommended in adults to prevent transmission. Other common viral infections are herpes simplex and herpes zoster.

Most bacterial infections are caused by group A beta-hemolytic streptococci and *Staphylococcus aureus*. Some of the most common are impetigo, cellulitis, folliculitis, erysipelas, and superficial lymphadenitis. Impetigo appears in two forms, bullous or crusted. It occurs more frequently in hot, humid climates; it is associated with crowded conditions and poor hygiene and is highly contagious. Cellulitis appears as elevated, warm, red, tender patches of inflammation with poorly demarcated borders. It may be accompanied by fever and constitutional symptoms and may be potentially life-threatening. A history of a puncture or scrape wound may suggest cellulitis. In individuals who have diabetes or are immunocompromised, cellulitis can be induced by *E. coli*, *Pseudomonas*, *Enterobacter*, *Proteus*, and other infections. Folliculitis is pustules of the hair follicles. It is characterized by erythema and crusting at the openings of hair follicles in a patchy distribution, often in areas injured during shaving. Diabetes and occupational exposure to tars and oils predispose to folliculitis. Superficial lymphadenitis is an isolated swollen lymph node with no apparent source of infection. Impetigo can be treated topically or with cleansing plus systemic antibiotics. Other bacterial infections must be treated with systemic antibiotics.

Some other common dermatologic conditions are scaling disorders, such as seborrheic dermatitis and psoriasis, and infestations, such as scabies and lice. In addition, acne is a well-known condition that is frequently seen in adolescents.

Seborrheic dermatitis usually appears in adults as dandruff on the scalp. It may also occur on the chest, eyebrows, cheeks, ears, and nasolabial folds. It responds well to 1% hydrocortisone solution, 2% ketaconazole cream applied twice daily, or 2% ketaconazole shampoo. Shampooing with commercial products that contain tar, zinc pyrithione, selenium sulfide, or sulfur and salicylic acid is also effective. Fluorinated corticosteroids rubbed into the scalp twice daily may also be used, but facial areas should be avoided because of the potential for atrophy and permanent telangiectasia.

Psoriasis is a lifelong hereditary condition that produces scaling and often symmetrically distributed lesions on the hairline, scalp, eyebrows, eyelashes, elbows, lower back, and knees. Plaques may be thick, hyperkeratotic, erythematous, and have a silvery scale with clearly defined margins. Pruritus occurs in about half of patients. Treatment of psoriasis requires an understanding of the various clinical manifestations of the disease and consists of corticosteroids, keratolytic agents, tars, phototherapy with or without psoralens, and use of antimetabolites. Mild psoriasis can be managed with emollients and steroids and, possibly, topical tars. Severe psoriasis should be managed by a dermatologist

Scabies can be transmitted sexually and by household contact. Lesions appear as excoriated papules; the primary lesion is the burrow, about 2 mm in length, caused by the female mite burrowing into the skin to lay eggs. Affected areas are usually the flexural surfaces of the elbows, wrists, finger webs, external genitalia, belt line, and areola. Secondary lesions may be seen on the trunk, legs, and arms. Pruritus develops about 2–3 weeks after infestation and is most pronounced at night; it may persist for 2 weeks after successful treatment. Calamine lotion may relieve this symptom. The diagnosis is established by identifying a burrow and, through microscopic examination of a skin scraping, revealing a mite or eggs. Scabies tends to be overdiagnosed in patients with dry skin or viral exanthems. Lindane or the synthetic pyrethroid 5% permethrin is used for treatment. Lotion is applied to the entire body and left on for 8–12 hours, then washed off. Retreatment within 1 week is often recommended. Clothes and bedding should be washed in hot water and dried with heat.

Lice infestation is a highly contagious condition spread through both sexual and casual contact that can affect the head, body, or genitals. It can be diagnosed by the presence of nits, tiny pearl-colored ova, attached to hair shafts or by intensely pruritic macules and papules. Lice can be treated topically with lindane or permethrin. As with scabies, clothes and bedding should be washed in hot water and dried with heat.

Finally, acne consists of a variety of lesions. It is a self-limited condition but can have long-term effects. Acne or similar lesions can occur with use of certain drugs (eg, corticosteroids, iodides, bromides), occupational exposure to coal tar derivatives and some oils, or from exposure to some cosmetics or detergents. Many patients do not require medical therapy for acne. Estrogen therapy is not appropriate for routine acne. Patients already taking an oral contraceptive will have improvement of acne with a more estrogenic pill, but the side effects of higher estrogen doses should be considered. Retinoic acid is an effective therapy; however, the patient may need to take some precautions to avoid skin irritation, such as reducing exposure to sunlight. Benzoyl peroxide is available in various strengths and mediums. Combined therapy with retinoic acid and benzoyl peroxide is effective but carries the same precautions as use of retinoic acid alone. Systemic antibiotics such as tetracycline, minocycline, or erythromycin may be needed. However, tetracycline should not be prescribed for pregnant women. Topical antibiotics include tetracycline, erythromycin, and clindamycin.

BIBLIOGRAPHY

Pulmonary and Upper Respiratory Problems

Barnes PJ. A new approach to the treatment of asthma. N Engl J Med 1989;321:1517–1527

Burrows B. The natural history of asthma. J Allergy Clin Immunol 1987;80:373–377

Daley CL, Sande M. The runny nose: infection of the paranasal sinuses. Infect Dis Clin North Am 1988;2:131–147

Eddy NB. Codeine and its alternates for pain and cough relief. Ann Intern Med 1969;71:1209–1212

Evans FO, Sydnor JB, Moore WE, Moore GR, Manwaring JL, Brill AH, et al. Sinusitis of maxillary antrum. N Engl J Med 1975;293:735–739

Farr BM, Kaiser DL, Harrison BD, Connolly CK. Prediction of microbial aetiology at admission to hospital for pneumonia from the presenting clinical features. Thorax 1989;44:1031–1035

Gwaltney JM Jr. Acute bronchitis. In: Mandell GL, Douglas RG Jr, Bennett JE, eds. Principles and practice of infectious diseases. 3rd ed. New York: Churchill-Livingstone, 1990:529–531

Hamory BH, Sande MA, Sydnor A Jr, Seale DL, Gwaltney JM Jr. Etiology and antimicrobial therapy of acute maxillary sinusitis. J Infect Dis 1979;139:197–202

Hilger PA. Diseases of the paranasal sinuses. In: Adams GL, Boies LR Jr, Hilger PA, eds. Boies fundamentals of otolaryngology. 6th ed. Philadelphia: WB Saunders, 1989:249–270

Nolan PE, Bass JB. New drugs for treating lung infection. Chest 1988; 94:1076–1079

Stott NC, West RR. Randomized controlled trial of antibiotics in patients with cough and purulent sputum. BMJ 1976;2:556–559

Woodhead MA, MacFarlane JT, McCracken JS, Rose DH, Finch RG. Prospective study of the aetiology and outcome of pneumonia in the community. Lancet 1987;1:671–674

Common Infectious Problems

Beasley RP, Hwang LY, Lee GC, Lan CC, Roan CH, Huang FY, et al. Prevention of perinatally transmitted hepatitis B virus infections with hepatitis B immune globulin and hepatitis B vaccine. Lancet 1983;2:1099–1102

Bloom HG, Bloom JS, Krasnoff L, Frank AD. Increased utilization of influenza and pneumonococcal vaccines in an elderly hospitalized population. J Am Geriatr Soc 1988;36:897–901

Boscia JA, Kobasa WD, Knight RA, Abrutyn E, Levison ME, Kaye D. Therapy vs no therapy for bacteriuria in elderly ambulatory non-hospitalized women. JAMA 1987;257:1067–1071

Carlson KJ, Mulley AG. Management of acute dysuria: a decision-analysis model of alternative strategies. Ann Intern Med 1985;102:244–249

Douglas RG Jr. Prophylaxis and treatment of influenza. N Engl J Med 1990;322:443–450

Filice GA. Pneumococcal vaccines and public health policy: consequences of missed opportunities. Arch Intern Med 1990;150:1373–1375

Fowler JE Jr. Urinary tract infections in women. Urol Clin North Am 1986;13:673–683

Glezen WP. Serious morbidity and mortality associated with influenza epidemics. Epidemiol Rev 1982;4:25–44

Grayston JT, Campbell LA, Kuo CC, Mordhorst CH, Saikku P, Thom DH, et al. A new respiratory tract pathogen: *Chlamydia pneumoniae* strain TWAR. J Infect Dis 1990;161:618–625

Iravani A, Richard GA. Amoxicillin-clavulanic acid versus cefaclor in the treatment of urinary tract infections and their effects on the urogenital and rectal flora. Antimicrob Agents Chemother 1986;29:107–111

Jenkins RD, Fenn JP, Matsen JM. Review of urine microscopy for bacteriuria. JAMA 1986;255:3397–3403

Kim JH, Langston AA, Gallis HA. Miliary tuberculosis: epidemiology, clinical manifestations, diagnosis, and outcome. Rev Infect Dis 1990;12:583–590

Ruben FL. Prevention and control of influenza: role of vaccine. Am J Med 1987;82(suppl 6A):31–34

Sobel JD, Kaye D. The role of bacterial adherence in urinary tract infections in elderly adults. J Gerontol 1987;42:29–32

Stamey TA. The role of introital enterobacteria in recurrent urinary infections. J Urol 1973;109:467–472

Stamey TA. Recurrent urinary tract infections in female patients: an overview of management and treatment. Rev Infect Dis 1987;9(2 suppl):195s–210s

Stamm WE, Wagner KF, Amsel R, Alexander ER, Turck M, Counts GW. Causes of the acute urethral syndrome in women. N Engl J Med 1980;303:409–415

Cardiovascular Disorders

Byyny RL, Speroff L. A clinical guide for the care of older women. Baltimore: Williams and Wilkins, 1990

Nolan TE. Evaluation and treatment of uncomplicated hypertension in the gynecologic patient. Female Patient 1992;17(10):13–21

1988 Report of the Joint National Committee on Detection, Evaluation, and Treatment of High Blood Pressure. Arch Intern Med 1988;148:1023–1038

Summary of the second report of the National Cholesterol Education Program (NCEP) Expert Panel on Detection, Evaluation, and Treatment of High Blood Cholesterol in Adults (Adult Treatment Panel II). JAMA 1993;269:3015–3023

Diabetes

American Diabetes Association. Clinical practice recommendations: 1992–1993. Diabetes Care 1993;16(5 suppl 2):1–118

American Diabetes Association. Role of cardiovascular risk factors in the prevention and treatment of macrovascular disease in diabetes. Diabetes Care 1989;12:573–579

American Diabetes Association. Pancreas transplantation for patients with diabetes mellitus. Diabetes Care 1992;15:1668–1672

Cryer PE, Binder C, Bolli GB, Cherrington AD, Gale EA, Gerich JE, et al. Hypoglycemia in IDDM. Diabetes 1989;38:1193–1199

Diabetes Control and Complications Trial Research Group. The effect of intensive treatment of diabetes on the development and progression on long-term complications in insulin-dependent diabetes mellitus. N Engl J Med 1993;329:977–986

National Diabetes Data Group. Classification and diagnosis of diabetes mellitus and other categories of glucose intolerance. Diabetes 1979;28:1039–1057

Ravid M, Savin H, Jutrin I, Bental T, Katz B, Lishner M. Long-term stabilizing effect of angiotensin-converting enzyme inhibition on plasma creatinine and proteinuria in normotensive type II diabetic patients. Ann Intern Med 1993;118:577–582

Reichard P, Nilsson BY, Rosenqvist U. The effect of long-term intensified insulin treatment on the development of microvascular complications of diabetes mellitus. N Engl J Med 1993;329:304–309

Yki-Jarvinen H, Kauppila M, Kujansuu E, Lahti J, Marjanen T, Niskanen L, et al. Comparison of insulin regimens in patients with non-insulin-dependent diabetes mellitus. N Engl J Med 1992; 327:1426–1433

Breast Cancer

Bender HG, Schnurch HG, Beck L. Breast cancer detection: age-related significance of findings on physical exam and mammography. Gynecol Oncol 1988;31:166–175

Boring CC, Squires TS, Tong T. Cancer statistics, 1993. CA Cancer J Clin 1993;43:7–26

Duffy SW, Tabar L, Fagerberg G, Gad JL, Grontoff O, South MC, et al. Breast screening, prognostic factors and survival: results from the Swedish two county study. Br J Cancer 1991;64:1133–1138

Edmiston CE Jr, Walker AP, Krepel CJ, Gohr C. The nonpuerperal breast infection: aerobic and anaerobic microbial recovery from acute and chronic disease. J Infect Dis 1990;162:695–699

Fletcher SW, O'Malley MS, Earp JL, Morgan TM, Lin S, Degnan D. How best to teach women breast self-examination: a randomized controlled trial. Ann Intern Med 1990;112:772–779

Gateley CA, Miers M, Mansel RE, Hughes LE. Drug treatments for mastalgia: 17 years experience in the Cardiff Mastalgia Clinic. J R Soc Med 1992;85:12–15

Henderson IC. What can a woman do about her risk of dying of breast cancer? Curr Probl Cancer 1990;14:161–230

Hindle WH. Breast masses: in-office evaluation with diagnostic triad. Postgrad Med 1990;88:85–87, 90–94

Hindle WH, ed. Breast disease for gynecologists. Norwalk, Connecticut: Appleton & Lange, 1990

Miller BA, Feuer EJ, Hankey BF. The increasing incidence of breast cancer since 1982: relevance of early detection. Cancer Causes Control 1991;2:67–74

National Cancer Institute. Division of Cancer Prevention and Control. Cancer statistics review: 1973–1989. Bethesda, Maryland: NCI, 1992; NIH publication no. 92-2789

National Cancer Institute. Division of Cancer Prevention and Control. 1987 Annual cancer statistical review, including cancer trends: 1950–1985. Bethesda, Maryland: NCI, 1988; NIH publication no. 88-2789, III-36

Saunders KJ, Pilgrim CA, Pennypacker HS. Increased proficiency of search in breast self-examination. Cancer 1986;58:2531–2537

Sterns EE. The natural history of macroscopic cysts in the breast. Surg Gynecol Obstet 1992;174:36–40

Common Gastrointestinal Syndromes and Diseases

Drossman DA, Thompson WG. The irritable bowel syndrome: review and a graduated multicomponent treatment approach. Ann Intern Med 1992;116:1009–1016

Everson GT, McKinley C, Kern F Jr. Mechanisms of gallstone formation in women: effects of exogenous estrogen (Premarin) and dietary cholesterol on hepatic metabolism. J Clin Invest 1991;87:237–246

Feldman M, Burton ME. Drug therapy: histamine$_2$-receptor antagonists: standard therapy for acid-peptic disease: 1. N Engl J Med 1990;323:1672–1680

Feldman M, Burton ME. Drug therapy: histamine$_2$-receptor antagonists: standard therapy for acid-peptic disease: 2. N Engl J Med 1990;323:1749–1755

Harvey RF, Gordon PC, Hadley N, Long DE, Gill TR, Macpherson RI, et al. Effects of sleeping with the bed-head raised and of ranitidine in patients with severe peptic oesophagitis. Lancet 1987;2:1200–1203

McSherry CK, Ferstenberg H, Calhoun WF, Lahman E, Virshup M. The natural history of diagnosed gallstone disease in symptomatic and asymptomatic patients. Ann Surg 1985;202:59–63

Michelassi F, Block GE, Vannucci L, Montag A, Chappell R. A 5- to 21-year follow-up and analysis of 250 patients with rectal adenocarcinoma. Ann Surg 1988;208:379–389

Mitchell CM, Drossman DA. The irritable bowel syndrome: understanding and treating a biopsychosocial illness disorder. Ann Behav Med 1987;9:13–18

Peterson WL. *Helicobacter pylori* and peptic ulcer disease. N Engl J Med 1991;324:1043–1048

Sastic JW, Glassman CI. Gallbladder disease in young women. Surg Gynecol Obstet 1982;155:209–211

Simon JB. Occult blood screening for colorectal carcinoma: a critical review. Gastroenterology 1985;88:820–837

Soll AH. Pathogenesis of peptic ulcer and implications for therapy. N Engl J Med 1990;322:909–916

Southern Surgeons Club. A prospective analysis of 1518 laparoscopic cholecystectomies. N Engl J Med 1991;324:1073–1078

Joint and Bone Disease

Arnett FC, Edworthy SM, Bloch DA, McShane DJ, Fries JF, Cooper NS, et al. The American Rheumatism Association 1987 revised criteria for the classification of rheumatoid arthritis. Arthritis Rheum 1988;31:315–324

Brooks PM, Day RO. Nonsteroidal anti-inflammatory drugs: differences and similarities. N Engl J Med 1991;324:1716–1725

Chuang T-Y, Hunder GG, Ilstrup DM, Kurland LT. Polymyalgia rheumatica: a 10-year epidemiologic and clinical study. Ann Intern Med 1982;97:672–680

Connolly JF, Jardon OM. Orthopedics. In: Rakel RE, ed. Textbook of family practice. 4th ed. Philadelphia: WB Saunders, 1990:1005–1090

Frymoyer JW. Back pain and sciatica. N Engl J Med 1988;318:291–300

Goldner JL, Nitka J, Howson P, Tobey B. Painful arthropathies. In: Tollison CD, Satterthaite JR, Tollison JW, eds. Handbook of pain management, 2nd ed. Baltimore: Williams and Wilkins, 1994:369–373

Huston KA, Hunder GG, Lie JT, Kennedy RH, Elveback LR. Temporal arteritis: a 25-year epidemiologic, clinical, and pathologic study. Ann Intern Med 1978;88:162–167

Liang MH, Fortin P. Management of osteoarthritis of the hip and knee. N Engl J Med 1991;325:125–127

Meyers OL, Monteagudo FS. A comparison of gout in men and women: a 10-year experience. S Afr Med J 1986;70:721–723

Prince RL, Smith M, Dick IM, Prince RI, Webb PG, Henderson NK, et al. Prevention of postmenopausal osteoporosis: a comparative study of exercise, calcium supplementation and hormone-replacement therapy. N Engl J Med 1991;325:1189–1195

Riggs BL, Melton LT 3d. The prevention and treatment of osteoporosis. N Engl J Med 1992;327:620–627

Shmerling RH, Delbanco TL. The rheumatoid factor: an analysis of clinical utility. Am J Med 1991;91:528–534

Depression

Blume SB, Russell M. Alcohol and substance abuse in the practice of obstetrics and gynecology. In: Stewart D, Stotland N, eds. Psychological aspects of women's health care. Washington, DC: American Psychiatric Press, 1993:391–409

Depression Guideline Panel. Depression in primary care: Vol 1. Detection and diagnosis. Clinical practice guideline, no. 5. Rockville, Maryland: U.S. Department of Health and Human Services, Public Health Service, Agency for Health Care Policy and Research, 1993; AHCPR publication no. 93-0550

Feldman E, Mayou R, Hawton K, Ardern M, Smith EB. Psychiatric disorder in medical in-patients. Q J Med 1987;63:405–412

Gitlin MJ, Pasnau RO. Psychiatric syndromes linked to reproductive function in women: a review of current knowledge. Am J Psychiatry 1989;146:1413–1422

Gold PW, Goodwin FK, Chrousos GP. Clinical and biochemical manifestations of depression: relation to the neurobiology of stress (1). N Engl J Med 1988;319:348–353

Gold PW, Goodwin FK, Chrousos GP. Clinical and biochemical manifestations of depression: relation to the neurobiology of stress (2). N Engl J Med 1988;319:413–420

Goldberg D, Huxley P. Common mental disorders: a biosocial model. London, Tavistock, Routledge, 1992

Groves JE, Kucharski A. Brief psychotherapy. In: Cassen NH, ed. Massachusetts General Hospital handbook of general hospital psychiatry. St Louis: CV Mosby, 1991:321–341

Jensvold MF. Psychiatric aspects of the menstrual cycle. In: Stewart DE, Stotland NL, eds. Psychological aspects of women's health care. Washington, DC: American Psychiatric Press, 1993:165–192

McGrath E, Ketia GP, Strickland BR, Russo NF. Women and depression: risk factors and treatment issues. Washington, DC: American Psychological Association, 1990

O'Hara MW, Schlechte JA, Lewis DA, Wright EJ. Prospective study of postpartum blues: biologic and psychosocial factors. Arch Gen Psychiatry 1991;48:801–806

Phillips KA, Gunderson JG, Hirschfeld RM, Smith LE. Review of the depressive personality. Am J Psychiatry 1990;147:830–837

Russell M, Bigler LR. Screening for alcohol-related problems in outpatient ob/gyn clinic. Am J Obstet Gynecol 1979;34:4–12

Russell M, Skinner JB. Early measures of maternal alcohol misuse as predictors of adverse pregnancy outcomes. Alcohol Clin Exp Res 1988;12:824–830

Sichel DA, Cohen LS, Rosenbaum JF, Driscoll J. Postpartum onset of obsessive-compulsive disorder. Psychosomatics 1993;34:277–279

Ylikorkala O, Stenman UH, Halmesmaki E. gamma-Glutamyltransferase and mean cell volume reveal maternal alcohol abuse and fetal alcohol effects. Am J Obstet Gynecol 1987;157:344–348

Headache

Linet MS, Stewart WF, Celentano DD, Ziegler D, Sprecher M. An epidemiologic study of headache among adolescents and young adults. JAMA 1989;261:2211–2216

Raskin NH. Headache. 2nd ed. New York: Churchill-Livingstone, 1988

Silberstein SD. Office management of benign headache: the science and the art. Postgrad Med 1993;93:223–240

Silberstein SD, Merriam GR. Sex hormones and headache. J Pain Symptom Manage 1993;8:98–114

Silberstein SD, Saper JR. Migraine: diagnosis and treatment. In: Dalessio DJ, Silberstein SD, eds. Wolff's headache and other head pain. 6th ed. New York: Oxford University Press, 1993:96–170

Thyroid Diseases

Emerson CH. Thyroid disease during and after pregnancy. In: Braverman LE, Utiger RD, eds. The thyroid: a fundamental and clinical text. 6th ed. Philadelphia: JB Lippincott, 1991:1263–1279

Hayslip CC, Fein HG, O'Donnell VM, Friedman DS, Klein TA, Smallridge RC. The value of serum antimicrosomal antibody testing in screening for symptomatic postpartum thyroid dysfunction. Am J Obstet Gynecol 1988;159:203–209

Nelson M, Wickus GG, Caplan RH, Beguin EA. Thyroid gland size in pregnancy: an ultrasound and clinical study. J Reprod Med 1987;32:888–890

Nikolai TF, Turney SL, Roberts RC. Postpartum lymphocytic thyroiditis: prevalence, clinical course, and long-term follow-up. Arch Intern Med 1987;147:221–224

Roti E, Gnudi A, Braverman LE. The placental transport, synthesis, and metabolism of hormones and drugs which affect thyroid function. Endocr Rev 1983;4:131–149

Dermatologic Conditions

Roaten S Jr, Lea WA Jr. Dermatology. In: Rakel RE, ed. Textbook of family practice. 4th ed. Philadelphia: WB Saunders, 1990:1111–1148

Schwartz RA, Fox MD. Office dermatology. American family physician monograph. Kansas City, Missouri: American Academy of Family Physicians, 1992

Office Practice

Every practitioner appreciates that we spend most of our time in office practice. Five years ago in the introduction to this section I wrote: "Emphasis on cost containment and preventive medicine is bound to increase...over the next 5 years. Similarly, increasing emphasis on primary care for women by obstetrician–gynecologists is an important priority of most practitioners."

To keep pace with these changes, this edition of *Precis* includes a separate section on primary and preventive care. Obviously, to the editors and the readers there is not a clear delineation of subjects included in these respective sections. However, the Office Practice section provides an appropriate bridge from the section on Primary and Preventive Care to the section on Gynecology, which focuses on an in-depth approach to the medical and surgical management of gynecologic disorders.

Each author has revised and updated his or her contribution to present the reader with the latest information in the field. The subsections on sexually transmitted diseases, viral infections, and pelvic infections include the latest recommendations in therapy from the Centers for Disease Control and Prevention. Many topics have been expanded, especially the discussions of premenstrual syndrome, crisis intervention, and ethical issues in obstetrics and gynecology. With more couples actively planning the timing of their pregnancies, the section on preconceptional counseling is a topical and important subject to patients and physicians alike.

The goal of the Office Practice section is to provide the reader with an update of a wide range of relevant topics. Since this book is a condensed update, readers are encouraged to explore the bibliographies and other forms of postgraduate education as well.

William Droegemueller, MD

Fertility Control

CONTRACEPTIVES: USE IN THE UNITED STATES AND EFFECTIVENESS

Overall, 56% of the 6.4 million pregnancies in the United States each year are unplanned. Of the 39 million women in the United States who are at risk for unintended pregnancy (ie, they are currently sexually active, fertile, and not pregnant or seeking pregnancy), 90% use some form of contraception. The 10% of women who do not use contraception account for 53% of unintended pregnancies, half of which end in abortion.

The choice of a contraceptive method is heavily dependent on whether the couple intends to have any more children. Women who intend to have children in the future are most likely to choose oral contraceptives (OCs) (48.8%), while those who do not intend to have any children in the future most often choose sterilization (61%). The estimated percentage of all women using no method is 9.9%; periodic abstinence, 2.1%; withdrawal, 2%; condom, 13.1%; spermicides, 1.7%; sponge, 1%; intrauterine device (IUD), 1.8%; OCs, 27.7%; tubal sterilization, 24.8%; and vasectomy, 10.5%.

The contraceptive choices presently available vary widely in effectiveness. Tubal sterilization, vasectomy, and injectable and implantable contraceptives are the most effective contraceptive methods. Oral contraceptives and IUDs also have low failure rates. Couples who rely on periodic abstinence from or interruption of intercourse have a 14–27% chance of having a contraceptive failure. Failure rates of condoms range from a low of 12% to a high of 18.5%; those of sponges run from 16% to 52%, and of spermicides from 22% to 26%. The low rates refer to low rates of pregnancy among groups of women who are more likely than average to use the method correctly and consistently. The higher rates refer to high rates of pregnancy among women who are more likely to use the method incorrectly or less consistently.

There are often large differences associated with methods in which coitus-related activities are required, such as use of a diaphragm (12–39%). There are very small differences between the high and low failure rates with female sterilization (0.4% for both high and low), injectables (0.4% for both high and low), and implants (0.05–0.5%). There are slightly higher differences with OCs (3.8–8.7%) and IUDs (2.5–4.5%).

One of the most important factors influencing contraceptive failure rates is user motivation. Contraceptive failure is more common in couples seeking to delay a birth, compared with those who want no more births. Age of the woman, socioeconomic class, and level of education have a strong correlation to contraceptive failure rates. Younger women are usually less experienced users, may become pregnant more easily than older women, and—especially those aged 20–24 years—may have intercourse more frequently.

VAGINAL FOAM, CREAM, SUPPOSITORIES, JELLY, AND SPONGE

Vaginal foam, cream, suppositories, jelly, and sponges contain a spermicide, usually nonoxynol-9, that kills or immobilizes spermatozoa on contact. Women often report that these methods are difficult to use and messy. Couples often do not use these methods correctly and consistently, and relatively high failure rates are often associated with them. The effectiveness of vaginal spermicides increases greatly with increasing age, approaching the effectiveness of the IUD in women over age 30. The 1-year failure rate for the sponge is about 15%, which is slightly higher than that for the diaphragm. For highest effectiveness, when a spermicide is used without a device to hold it in place, it needs to be inserted shortly before intercourse. Spermicides are most effective when used with barrier devices such as a diaphragm, cervical cap, or condom.

Sponge users have a slightly greater risk of toxic shock syndrome (TSS), especially if it is used during menses or the puerperium or is left in the vagina for more than 24 hours. The overall incidence is estimated to be about one infection per 2 million sponge users. Spermicides may inhibit certain sexually transmitted diseases of bacterial and viral origin and the development of cervical cancer.

DIAPHRAGM AND CERVICAL CAP

The diaphragm and cervical cap are barrier methods of contraception that have similar effectiveness rates. The largest diaphragm that is comfortable to the user should be fitted. The cervical cap comes in four sizes. It is smaller than a diaphragm, fits closely over the cervix, and relies on suction to stay in place.

Users should place spermicide inside the cup and may place the device in the vagina several hours before intercourse. Spermicide should be inserted in the vagina with repeated intercourse. The device should be left in place for at least 8 hours after the last coital act and no longer than 24 hours.

Use of the diaphragm lowers the risk for developing clinical gonorrheal infection. Former diaphragm users have lower incidences of tubal disease, infertility, and cervical neoplasia. Users have a significantly higher rate of urinary tract infections than do nonusers, probably because of compression and irritation of the urethra.

MALE AND FEMALE CONDOMS

The condom is highly effective in couples with high motivation. Latex condoms can reduce the transmission rate of sexually transmitted diseases, including chlamydial infection, gonorrhea, herpes, and human immunodeficiency virus (HIV) infection. The incidence of cervical neoplasia is also reduced.

Most male condoms are made of latex rubber, although about 1% of those sold in the United States are made from lamb intestines. These are used by men allergic to rubber or those who desire greater sensitivity. Condoms made from lamb intestines, however, do not provide protection against HIV.

The female condom is a sheath worn by women that is approved by the U.S. Food and Drug Administration (FDA) to prevent sexually transmitted diseases, including acquired immunodeficiency syndrome (AIDS), and unintended pregnancy. While the 1-year failure rate is reported to be as high as 25%, this rate is primarily the result of improper use. The female condom is available without prescription, and the cost is approximately $2.50.

The female condom is made of polyurethane, a thin but strong material that resists tears during use. It consists of two flexible rings within a loose-fitting sheath. One of the rings is used to insert the condom and hold it inside the vagina. The other ring remains outside and covers the woman's labia and the base of the penis during intercourse. The female condom is prelubricated and lines the vagina after insertion. It is disposable and designed for a single sexual act. One advantage of the female condom over the male condom is that it can be inserted several hours before sexual intercourse. It can be used during menses and by postpartum women.

PERIODIC ABSTINENCE: NATURAL FAMILY PLANNING

Abstaining from sexual intercourse during the "fertile interval" of the menstrual cycle is the method of choice of couples who desire a method that involves no drugs, devices, or surgery. The effectiveness of this method is highly dependent on accurately predicting when the fertile interval will occur. There are several methods for determining this interval, including the calendar rhythm method, the basal body temperature method, the cervical mucus (Billings) method, and the symptothermal method. Women who have irregular menses are poor candidates for these methods.

With the calendar rhythm method, the fertile interval is determined by subtracting 18 days from the length of the woman's previous shortest cycle and 11 days from her previous longest cycle. With the basal body temperature method, the fertile interval starts with the first day of menses and continues until the third consecutive day of an elevated basal body temperature. With the cervical mucus method, abstinence is required until 4 days following the last day of wet, slippery mucus (peak mucus day). The symptothermal method uses calendar calculations, basal body temperature, and cervical mucus changes to estimate the fertile period.

The necessity to abstain from sexual intercourse for many days of each menstrual cycle is a major reason for the lack of a general acceptance of the method and the relatively high failure rates. Enzyme immunoassays for urinary estrogen and pregnanediol that can be performed at home may help to define the fertile interval more accurately. Such assays could lead to a reduction in the number of days of abstinence and may improve the effectiveness and acceptance of this method.

ORAL CONTRACEPTIVES

Formulations

Combination OCs contain both a synthetic estrogen and progestin and are taken continuously for 3 weeks, followed by a 1-week steroid-free period. The only estrogen used in current formulations is ethinyl estradiol. Five long-standing progestins are used: norethindrone, norethindrone acetate, ethynodiol diacetate, norethynodrel, and norgestrel and its active isomer levonorgestrel; and three new progestins, desogestrel, norgestimate, and gestodene. A second type of OC contains only a progestin.

The multiphasic combination OCs were developed to lower the total dose of steroid, primarily the progestin, while maintaining bleeding control. The dose of the progestin, or of both the progestin and estrogen components, is changed two or three times during the cycle.

Combination OCs that contain 30–35 µg of synthetic estrogen are associated with pregnancy rates similar to those with the 50-µg and higher formulations. However, these lower-dose OCs have significantly lower incidences of both serious adverse events and minor side effects.

Effects

Many of the most frequent symptoms produced by combination OCs are due to the estrogenic component and include nausea, breast tenderness, and fluid retention. The incidence of these side effects is much lower today because the current formulations contain less estrogen than earlier formulations.

Cardiovascular Disease

During the 1960s and 1970s, studies suggested that women using high-dose OCs were at increased risk for thromboembolism, myocardial infarction, and stroke. The relevance of these observations to current clinical practice has been questioned for three reasons. First, current OC formulations have a threefold to fourfold lower dose of estrogen and a 10-fold lower dose of progestin than older formulations. Second, early studies failed to take into account the effects of independent risk factors for vascular disease, including smoking and hypertension. Finally, physicians are now less likely to prescribe OCs to women at high risk for vascular disease, including older women who smoke.

Past use of OCs does not increase the risk of cardiovascular disease. Furthermore, limited evidence suggests that OC use may even reduce the risk of atherosclerosis. These findings led to the conclusions that OC use does not cause coronary atherosclerosis, the leading cause of death of U.S. women, and that, in those rare cases in which myocardial infarctions occur in current OC users, they have a thrombotic rather than an atherosclerotic etiology.

Nonsmoking OC users, regardless of age, do not appear to be at increased risk for myocardial infarction. Women over age 35 who smoke, however, have an increased risk of cardiovascular disease. Such women should not be prescribed OCs. Otherwise, women over age 35 may continue to use OCs provided that no other risk factors are present.

The increased risk of thromboembolism noted in women using OCs appears to be related to the estrogenic component. Use of low-estrogen OCs is associated with less risk of thromboembolism than higher-estrogen OCs. Whether the risk of thromboembolism is higher in women using low-dose OCs than in nonusers is not known. If women using low-dose OCs are at any increased risk, however, such risk is of low magnitude. There is no evidence that combination OCs increase the risk of postoperative thrombosis in women without other risk factors. The risk of pregnancy must be weighed against any theoretic risk in women using low-dose preparations in deciding whether to discontinue OCs prior to surgery.

Reproductive Tract

The absence of withdrawal bleeding while using OCs does not indicate less contraceptive effectiveness. However, bleeding is an important marker signaling that probably the user is not pregnant, and switching to a more estrogen-dominant OC is advised.

Users of OCs are a high-risk group for the development of cervical neoplasia. Unlike earlier studies that linked OCs to cervical cancer, recent studies have accounted for many factors known to influence the incidence of invasive cervical cancer, such as age at first coital experience, use of barrier contraceptives, number of sexual partners, smoking, and exposure to human papillomavirus (HPV). Although several of these studies have shown no higher incidences in OC users, the complete effect of OCs on cervical cancer is unknown. Use of barrier methods (with or without OCs) in high-risk women and yearly Pap tests in OC users is recommended.

Breasts

The relationship between OCs and breast cancer is not clear. Through age 54, breast cancer is equally common among women who have and have never used OCs. Additionally, women who first used OCs at age 25 or later have the same incidence of breast cancer as women who never used OCs, regardless of duration of OC use. However, some studies report that women who use OCs for prolonged periods during their teens and early 20s are more likely than those who did not to develop breast cancer in their 30s and early 40s. After this age, these women are then less likely to develop breast cancer. The largest American study failed to find any increases in breast cancer in this high-risk group and also reported no increased risk among users with benign breast disease or with a first-degree relative with breast cancer.

Liver and Bile Ducts

Oral contraceptive users have about twice the risk of developing cholelithiasis in the first few years of use, compared with nonusers, but the incidence declines below that of controls after a few years of OC use. The estrogen component appears to accelerate the appearance of clinical symptoms but does not increase the incidence of the disease.

Although active liver disease is a contraindication to OC use, women with a history of hepatitis who currently have normal liver function test results are candidates. Benign liver cell adenoma is a rare complication attributed to OCs that has been linked to long-term use. These tumors can rupture and cause pain and have led to death from intraperitoneal bleeding. The annual incidence of these tumors is less than 1/50,000 users of OCs. Routine palpation of the liver is recommended in all users.

Two British studies reported increased incidences of liver cancer among OC users. However, during the three decades of use of OCs by American women, the rate of death from this disease has remained unchanged.

Central Nervous System

Nausea and emesis is increased in OC users, especially during the first months of use. Nausea is linked with the estrogen component.

Depression also is believed to be an estrogen-mediated metabolic effect, due to alterations in tryptophan metabolism that lead to increased levels of serotonin in the brain. Treatment with vitamin B_6 may reverse this effect, but discontinuation of OCs is the recommended treatment.

The incidence of migraine headaches is increased in women taking OCs. Women who develop severe migraines, visual loss, or any peripheral neurologic changes should stop OC use.

Skin

Chloasma, similar to that seen in pregnancy, may develop in some OC users. Exposure to sunlight tends to exacerbate this problem.

The progestins used in current OCs are structurally related to testosterone and may produce certain androgenic side effects, including acne. Additionally, progestins increase sebum production, and although OCs are generally useful in treating acne, they may actually cause acne to develop in some women. Recently two new progestins, desogestrel and norgestimate, have been added to the U.S. market and reportedly are associated with low incidences of androgenic side effects.

Some studies show an increased incidence of malignant melanoma in OC users, whereas others show no effect or a decrease. If there is any increased risk, it is small.

Subsequent Fertility

The incidence of amenorrhea lasting more than 6 months after stopping OCs is 0.2–0.8%. This incidence is similar to the incidence of secondary amenorrhea in nonusers. During the time of use, OCs will mask an otherwise amenorrheic state that will be noticed clinically only after OCs are stopped.

After stopping OCs, there may be a delay in the return of fertility because of a delay of several months in the return of ovulation. After 2–3 years, fertility rates are the same for former OC users as for users of other methods of contraception, including barrier methods.

Several studies of large numbers of babies born to women who stopped taking OCs have reported no greater chance that these infants will be born with any type of birth defect. Rates of congenital anomalies, chromosomal abnormalities in abortuses, and spontaneous abortion are not increased in women who conceive shortly after stopping OCs.

Contraindications

With few exceptions, OCs can be prescribed to most healthy women of reproductive age. There are only a few absolute contraindications for their use. The most common contraindication is cigarette smoking by a woman over age 35 years. Other strong contraindications include a present or past history of vascular disease, including stroke, thromboembolism, or systemic vascular disease such as hemoglobin SS disease or lupus erythematosus. Additionally, uncontrolled hypertension, diabetes mellitus with vascular disease, and hyperlipidemia are contraindications of OC use.

A contraindication listed by the FDA is cancer of the breast or endometrium. Patients with active liver disease should not receive OCs, since steroids are metabolized in the liver. Women with a history of liver disease whose liver function test results are normal may take OCs.

Relative contraindications to OC use include heavy cigarette smoking (more than 15 cigarettes per day) in younger patients, depression, and migraine headaches. Oral contraceptive users who develop frequent or severe headaches, fainting, paresthesias, or loss of speech or vision should stop taking OCs immediately.

Noncontraceptive Health Benefits

Oral contraceptives offer women a substantial number of noncontraceptive health benefits, in addition to protecting them from unwanted pregnancy. Because of the antiestrogenic action of the progestins, the endometrium is thinner than that in a normal cycle. This change results in less blood loss and a 50% reduced risk of iron deficiency anemia. Users are less likely to develop menorrhagia or irregular menstruation and about half as likely to develop endometrial cancer.

By inhibiting ovulation, OCs decrease dysmenorrhea and premenstrual tension and protect against functional ovarian cysts. In one study, the incidence of benign ovarian neoplasms was reduced by 64% in OC users, and another study showed that only 2% of women discharged from the hospital with the diagnosis of functional ovarian cysts were taking OCs, in contrast to 20% of the control subjects.

Oral contraceptive users have a 40% reduced risk of developing ovarian cancer. The relative risk of developing ovarian cancer in a user is 0.6. The longer the use, the better the protection. As little as 6 months of OC use provides definite protection that lasts for at least a decade after stopping OCs.

The progestin component of combination OCs decreases the synthesis of estrogen and progesterone receptors by the endometrial cells, resulting in less endometrial proliferation and less menstrual bleeding. Oral contraceptive users have lighter menstrual flow, with a total monthly blood loss of 20 ml compared with 35 ml in an average menstrual cycle. This mechanism is also responsible for the protective effect of OCs against endometrial cancer. Women who use OCs for 1 year or longer have a relative risk of 0.5 of endometrial cancer, compared with nonusers. This protective effect increases with longer use and persists for at least a decade after OCs are stopped.

The incidence of developing clinical salpingitis among OC users is one half that of a control group using no method of contraception. There are two studies showing a 50% reduced risk of developing rheumatoid arthritis. There appears to be increased bone density of the lumbar spine associated with long-term use, which may decrease the risk of postmenopausal osteoporosis. Additional benefits include less hirsutism, acne, and benign breast disease. Another possible benefit is less risk of developing uterine leiomyomas.

Prescribing Guidelines

After an initial history and physical examination, including a breast and pelvic examination with a Pap test, the potential user should be told about the risks and benefits of OC use, and this should be noted on the patient's chart. Blood pressure and weight should also be recorded.

Oral contraceptives have not been shown to interfere with the action of other drugs. However, some drugs can interfere clinically with the action of OCs by inducing liver enzymes that convert steroids to less active metabolites. These include barbiturates, cyclophosphamide, sulfonamides, and rifampin.

Adolescents

Oral contraceptives are a good choice for the sexually active adolescent provided that she has normal adolescent development and has had two or three spontaneous menses. Advantages of OC use include less dysmenorrhea, acne, and irregular bleeding, which are common problems in this age group. Compliance is a particular problem in this age group, and adequate counseling on OC use and potential side effects is necessary. Because high rates of sexually transmitted diseases are a concern in this age group, the use of condoms should be encouraged.

Following Abortion

The first bleeding episode in postabortal women is generally preceded by ovulation, which can occur as early as 2 weeks after the pregnancy loss. Oral contraceptives should be started immediately after a spontaneous or induced abortion to prevent conception.

During Breast-feeding

After a term delivery, OCs may be taken once the milk flow has become established. Use of combination OCs can reduce the quantity and duration of lactation. Progestin-only OCs do not impair lactation and in fact may increase the quality and duration of lactation. Thus, progestin-only OCs are an alternative. When initiated within 1 week postpartum, progestin-only OCs have not been shown to adversely affect lactation or infant development.

INTRAUTERINE DEVICES

Intrauterine devices are a highly effective method of birth control with a lack of systemic metabolic effects. A single act of motivation is required for use, with no coitally related responsibility. Since a visit to the health care facility is necessary for discontinuing this method, IUDs have one of the highest continuation rates of all reversible methods of contraception.

Types

There are two types of IUDs, each with a monofilament tail string, approved for use by the FDA that are currently marketed in the United States. These are the Copper T380A (Paragard) and a progesterone-releasing device (Progestasert). The Copper T380A was approved in 1988. It has 380 mm^2 of surface copper, 300 mm^2 on the vertical arm and 40 mm^2 on each of the horizontal arms. The FDA has approved continuous use of the Copper T380A for 8 years and of the Progestasert for 1 year.

Adverse Effects

Expulsion

Generally, during the first year of IUD use, the expulsion rate is about 10%. Up to one fifth of all expulsions are unnoticed by the user, and one third of all accidental pregnancies are due to unnoticed expulsions. The rate of expulsion diminishes with increasing duration of use.

Uterine Bleeding

The presence of a copper-bearing IUD significantly increases the amount of blood loss in each menstrual cycle, whereas a progesterone-releasing IUD significantly reduces the blood loss. In a woman with normal cycles, about 35 ml of blood is lost per month. In women with a copper IUD, 50–60 ml is lost each cycle, and in women wearing a progesterone-releasing device about 25 ml of blood is lost.

If women develop heavy menses while using an IUD, the hemoglobin and hematocrit should be checked and possibly the serum ferritin should be measured. Serum ferritin concentrations are a more sensitive marker for iron deficiency. If any of these parameters is low, iron supplementation should be initiated.

An IUD user with excessive bleeding should be carefully evaluated for the presence of concurrent abnormalities. In the months after IUD insertion, mild to moderate increases in cyclic bleeding may be treated with supplemental iron therapy and reassurance. Bleeding frequently diminishes with time as the uterus adjusts to the presence of a foreign body. Continued heavy cyclic bleeding may be treated with prostaglandin synthetase inhibitors.

If heavy, bothersome bleeding continues, removal of the device should be considered. After a 1-month wait, another IUD may be inserted, preferably a progesterone-releasing device, as it is associated with less blood loss.

Perforation

Although uncommon, one of the serious adverse events associated with IUD use is perforation of the uterine fundus. Perforation most often occurs at the time of insertion; it is best prevented by careful, gentle insertion, with careful determination of the size and position of the uterus by palpation and use of a uterine sound. Fundal perforation rates are reported to be about 1/1,000 to 1/2,000 insertions. Perforation should be suspected if the tail string is not visualized and the patient did not notice expulsion.

Intrauterine devices that have moved outside the uterus should be removed on an elective basis. Rarely, complications such as bowel perforation, bowel obstruction, adhesions, or peritoneal reaction have been reported. Copper-containing devices are especially irritating, and they should be removed. Removal through a laparoscope is usually possible unless severe adhesions have developed.

Perforation of the uterine cervix is reported to occur in about 1/600 to 1/1,000 insertions. On follow-up visits of users of T-shaped devices, the cervix should be carefully inspected and palpated for perforation. Cervical perforations may be difficult to detect, since perforations often do not extend completely through the cervical epithelium. An IUD that has perforated the cervix should be removed. Displacement of the IUD is associated with decreased contraceptive effectiveness.

Missing Strings

The cervix should be carefully palpated, and the cervical canal should be gently probed. If the strings are not located, a pregnancy test should be done prior to any probing of the endometrial cavity.

There are three possibilities for the location of the IUD: there has been an unnoticed expulsion of the IUD, the IUD is located within the endometrial cavity, or the IUD is in an extrauterine location. The uterine cavity should be probed with a sound or biopsy instrument in an attempt to locate the lost IUD. If the IUD is not found within the cavity, an ultrasound examination of the pelvis and abdomen should be performed. Roentgenography may be necessary to determine the location of the missing IUD. Roentgenographic studies should include a lateral and an anteroposterior view with either contrast material or a sound within the endometrial cavity.

Pregnancy-Related Complications

There is no evidence for any increased incidence of fetal anomalies in infants born to women with any type of IUD in situ. If a patient becomes pregnant with an IUD in place and the IUD is not removed, the incidence of spontaneous abortion is about 55%, or about three times higher than the incidence of spontaneous abortion in women without IUDs. If the woman wants to continue the pregnancy and the tail strings are visible, the IUD should be removed by traction. This will reduce the chance of spontaneous abortion. If the tail strings are not visible, an attempt to remove the IUD may be preformed under ultrasound guidance.

The risk of a septic abortion is increased if an IUD remains in place in a pregnant patient. If removal of the IUD is not possible, the patient should be informed of the increased risk of sepsis and the importance of reporting any symptoms of infection or bleeding promptly. If an intrauterine infection does develop, antibiotics should be given and uterine evacuation should be performed.

Intrauterine devices prevent intrauterine pregnancies better than they prevent ectopic pregnancies. The IUD reduces endometrial implantation by 99.5–97% but reduces tubal implantation by only 90–95% and ovarian implantation not at all. For this reason, if pregnancy does occur, the chance that it will be ectopic is about fivefold to 10-fold greater than that when an IUD is not used. Thus, if conception occurs in an IUD user, it is important to document the location of the pregnancy by ultrasonography.

Several studies suggest an increased incidence of preterm labor in pregnancies with an IUD in situ. If removal of the IUD is not possible and the patient wishes to continue the pregnancy, she should be warned of this possible complication in addition to the increased risk of spontaneous and septic abortion. There is no evidence that there are any other obstetric complications. Additionally, previous IUD use does not increase complication rates of future pregnancies.

Infection-Related Complications

The use of a copper-releasing IUD increases the risk of developing pelvic inflammatory disease (PID). In a multicenter, case–control study, the increased risk of salpingitis in IUD acceptors was limited to the first 4 months of use after insertion. This suggests that use of an aseptic insertion technique, thereby decreasing the number of bacteria introduced into the endometrial cavity during insertion, is important. Use of an IUD without tail strings does not reduce the overall risk of pelvic infection.

Case–control studies have examined the association of infertility with IUD use in nulliparous women. The relative risks of infertility due to tubal factor for women who had used copper-bearing IUDs were 1.3 and 1.6 in the two studies. In one study, women with only one sexual partner and an IUD did not have an increased risk of tubal infertility, and parous women who had previously used the copper-bearing IUDs did not have an increased risk of tubal infertility. Use of an IUD by married women with one sexual partner did not increase their risk of pelvic infection.

In women who have clinical evidence of PID, the IUD should be removed after therapeutic levels of appropriate antibiotics are achieved. There are reports that IUD users have an increased risk for colonies of *Actinomyces israelii* in the upper genital tract. At present the recommendation is to screen for these organisms on the routine cytologic test. If actinomycosis is detected, antibiotic therapy should be given and another cytologic test done. Persistent cases necessitate removal of the IUD until the organisms disappear.

Populations at risk for developing PID include those with multiple sexual partners, women with a history of PID, and nulliparous women under age 25 years. Women in these high-risk groups are not good candidates for an IUD and should be advised regarding methods that reduce pelvic infections, such as barrier methods.

The best candidates for an IUD are parous women with stable, monogamous sexual relationships. For those women who have completed their families but do not opt for tubal sterilization, or women who cannot take OCs, this may be the method of choice.

LONG-ACTING PROGESTINS

Implants

Contraceptive implants are a highly effective, estrogen-free, reversible, and long-term method of contraception. The implant system approved for use in the United States consists of six capsules made of polymeric silicone tubing that contain levonorgestrel. The amount of steroid released is related to the surface area of the delivery system. The daily release rates of levonorgestrel are 80 µg initially, 50 µg at the end of the first year of use, and 30 µg from the second through the fifth years.

The implant capsules are placed just under the skin of the arm in the upper inner area. This site allows for easy insertion and removal. Six capsules are placed in a fanlike pattern through a 3-mm incision. Local anesthesia is needed for the procedure.

The mechanisms of action of the subdermal implants are probably due to several factors. The major mechanism of action during the first year of use is suppression of ovulation. In successive years, the incidence of ovulatory cycles increases, and other mechanisms involving the cervical mucus and endometrial cavity maintain the contraceptive effectiveness. Estrogen levels fluctuate within early proliferative phase levels of a normal cycle.

The pregnancy rate during the first year is approximately 0.2/100 users, and the 5-year cumulative pregnancy rate is 1.1/100 users. There has been concern that women who weigh more than 70 kg (154 lb) may have diminished efficacy during the fourth and fifth years of use. However, the capsules now available are composed of soft polymeric silicone tubing, which allows for therapeutic levels of levonorgestrel throughout the 5 years of use. When the implant system is removed, ovulation usually occurs within 2–4 weeks. Fertility is restored promptly.

The major side effect of the implants is an increase in the number of bleeding and spotting days per month. The total blood loss is reduced, however, and increases in hemoglobin and hematocrit often are reported, even in users with bothersome bleeding patterns. Usually with each successive year of use, the number of bleeding and spotting days decreases. However, this continues to be the greatest inconvenience of the method. Appropriate patient education before initiation as well as supportive follow-up measures help promote patient acceptance. Other nuisance side effects include headache, weight gain, acne, depression, hirsutism, and anxiety. The subdermal capsules require both surgical insertion and surgical removal. If the capsules are not placed subdermally, removal may be difficult. Other disadvantages are the initial upfront expense and the visibility and elevation of the skin over the implants.

The sustained delivery system allows for low levels of steroid. This reduced steroid level has minimal impact on carbohydrate metabolism and lipid metabolism. The few changes reported result in values within the normal range and appear to have no clinical significance.

The best candidates for implants are women who are seeking long-term birth control. Women who have completed their families but do not desire permanent sterilization are excellent candidates. Women who have had problems with other methods or those demonstrating poor compliance should consider implants. Teenaged mothers, women who are postpartum and are breast-feeding, and women who need to avoid estrogen are excellent candidates.

Depot-Medroxyprogesterone Acetate

Depot-medroxyprogesterone acetate (DMPA) provides a highly effective, long-acting, reversible method of family planning. This method is widely used throughout the world, with more than 50 million users of DMPA since 1960. There are more than 90 countries in which DMPA is used, and more than 1,000 scientific articles on the method have been published.

Depot-medroxyprogesterone acetate is an aqueous suspension of microcrystals that is given by intramuscular injection every 12 weeks. The injection site should not be massaged after injection because massaging increases the absorption and may decrease the effectiveness. The first injection is generally given within the first 5 days after menses. Contraceptive protection is immediate. Women with IUDs may have the injection at any time but should not have the IUD removed until the onset of the next menses.

Depot-medroxyprogesterone acetate has not been demonstrated to be effective against sexually transmitted diseases. It probably offers some protection similar to that of OCs but less than that of barrier methods.

Postpartum women may receive DMPA. Nonlactating mothers may start the progestin within 5 days after delivery. Breast-feeding mothers should delay an injection until lactation is established. Depot-medroxyprogesterone acetate does not decrease the volume of breast milk or adversely affect its composition. Patients who have spontaneous or induced abortions should receive their first injection immediately after the pregnancy termination.

The most important mechanism of action of DMPA is suppression of ovulation by prevention of the midcycle luteinizing hormone surge. Estrogen levels are similar to those in subdermal implant users and are within the early follicular phase levels. Other antifertility effects include the formation of thick, viscous, cervical mucus that impedes sperm motility and the formation of an atrophic endometrial lining that is unfavorable for implantation.

Suppression of ovulation lasts for at least 14 weeks after each injection of 150 mg of DMPA. The general clinical approach is to repeat the injections every 12 weeks. If a woman delays her visit to more than 14 weeks, pregnancy should be excluded before another injection is given. Following an injection, serum levels peak in 10 hours, then decline gradually. Depot-medroxyprogesterone acetate has been detected in serum for more than 200 days after a single injection.

The failure rate in clinical practice is 0.4/100 woman-years and is similar to the rate for the contraceptive implant system. Women who have been using DMPA may experience a delay in the return of fertility. Recovery of the reproductive axis is variable but may occur as early as 4 months and as late as 31 months or longer after stopping the progestin. The median time to conception is 10 months.

The most common reasons for discontinuing the method are disruption of cycle control and menstrual irregularities. About one third of new starters will have increased numbers of episodes of bleeding and spotting. With continued use of the method, however, 50% of users will have amenorrhea by 1 year.

Benefits of DMPA include less dysmenorrhea, less blood loss, and possibly improvements in premenstrual syndrome (PMS). Side effects include headache (17%), abdominal discomfort (13%), nervousness (11%), dizziness (5.4%), decreased libido (5.4%), depression (1.7%), and acne (1.3%). The average weight gain during the first year of use is 2.3 kg (5 lb), with 1.4 kg (3 lb) more by the end of the second year.

The effects of DMPA on lipid metabolism vary from one study to another. Low-density lipoprotein cholesterol values are reported as unchanged, increased, or decreased. Most studies demonstrate a decrease in high-density lipoprotein cholesterol values. There are mild changes in glucose metabolism and almost no changes in coagulation factors. One study reports a 7% reduction in bone mineral density.

Depot-medroxyprogesterone acetate was approved in 1960 for endometriosis and habitual spontaneous abortion. Approval of DMPA as a contraceptive was delayed in the United States because of concerns about mammary tumors in beagle dogs. The World Health Organization Collaborative Study was conducted to determine cancer risks in DMPA acceptors. The study concluded that the method does not increase the risk of breast, cervical, or ovarian cancer. Depot-medroxyprogesterone acetate has no neoplastic effects, except in reducing the risk of endometrial cancer.

Depot-medroxyprogesterone acetate does not increase the risk for congenital anomalies, spontaneous abortion, ectopic pregnancy, stillborn infants, or premature births. In utero exposure to DMPA does not appear to be detrimental to pregnancy outcome.

Depot-medroxyprogesterone acetate injection is a good method for women who need a long-acting, coitus-independent, highly effective, and convenient method of family planning. For women with sickle cell disease, the method is an excellent choice. Other candidates are those who cannot take estrogen or those who dislike taking a pill daily.

Depot-medroxyprogesterone acetate is highly effective and minimizes patient responsibility. The major disadvantages are menstrual bleeding changes, weight gain, and delay in the return of fertility.

BIBLIOGRAPHY

Brache V, Alvarez-Sanchez F, Faundes A, Tejada AS, Cochon L. Ovarian endocrine function through five years of continuous treatment with Norplant subdermal contraceptive implants. Contraception 1990;41:169–177

Cramer DW, Schiff I, Schoenbaum SC, Gibson M, Belisle S, Albrecht B, et al. Tubal infertility and the intrauterine device. N Engl J Med 1985;312:941–947

Croft P, Hannaford PC. Risk factors for acute myocardial infarction in women: evidence from the Royal College of General Practitioners' oral contraception study. BMJ 1989;298:165–168

Daling JR, Weiss NS, Metch BJ, Chow WH, Soderstrom RM, Moore DE, et al. Primary tubal infertility in relation to use of an intrauterine device. N Engl J Med 1985;312:937–941

Garza-Flores J, De la Cruz DL, Valles de Bourges V, Sanchez-Nuncio R, Martinez M, Fuziwara JL, et al. Long-term effects of depot-medroxyprogesterone acetate on lipoprotein metabolism. Contraception 1991;44:61–71

Godsland IF, Crook D, Simpson R, Proudler T, Felton C, Lees B, et al. The effects of different formulations of oral contraceptive agents on lipid and carbohydrate metabolism. N Engl J Med 1990;323:1375–1381

Hardy E, Goodson P. Association between contraceptive method accepted and perception of information received: a comparison of Norplant and IUD acceptors. Contraception 1991;43:121-128

Harlap S, Kost K, Forrest JD. Preventing pregnancy, protecting health. New York: Alan Guttmacher Institute, 1991

Huovinen K, Tikkanen MJ, Autio S, Harkonen T, Lommi L, Varonen S, et al. Serum lipids and lipoproteins during therapeutic amenorrhea induced by lynestrenol and depot-medroxyprogesterone acetate. Acta Obstet Gynecol Scand 1991;70:349–354

Konje JC, Otolorin EO, Ladipo OA. Changes in carbohydrate metabolism during 30 months on Norplant. Contraception 1991;44:163–172

Lee NC, Rubin GL, Borucki R. The intrauterine device and pelvic inflammatory disease revisited: new results from the Women's Health Study. Obstet Gynecol 1988;72:1–6

Liew DF, Ng CS, Yong YM, Ratnam SS. Long-term effects of Depo-Provera on carbohydrate and lipid metabolism. Contraception 1985;31:51–64

Mishell DR Jr, Shoupe D. Oral contraceptives for women over the age of 35. In: Shoupe ED, Haseltine FP, eds. Contraception. New York: Springer-Verlag 1993:85–92

Porter JB, Hunter JR, Jick H, Stergachis A. Oral contraceptives and nonfatal vascular disease. Obstet Gynecol 1985;66:1–4

Powell MG, Mears BJ, Deber RB, Ferguson D. Contraception with the cervical cap: effectiveness, safety, continuity of use, and user satisfaction. Contraception 1986;33:215–232

Prentice RL, Thomas DB. On the epidemiology of oral contraceptives and disease. Adv Cancer Res 1987;49:285–401

Rekers H. Multicenter trial of a monophasic oral contraceptive containing ethinyl estradiol and desogestrel. Acta Obstet Gynecol Scand 1988;67:171–174

Rothman KJ, Louik C. Oral contraceptives and birth defects. N Engl J Med 1978;299:522–524

Rubeck-Peterson KR, Skouby SO, Dreisler A, Kuhl C, Svenstrup B. Comparative trial of the effects of glucose tolerance and lipoprotein metabolism of two new oral contraceptives containing gestoden and desogestrel. Acta Obstet Gynecol Scand 1988;67:37–41

Schlesselman JJ. Cancer of the breast and reproductive tract in relation to use of oral contraceptives. Contraception 1989;40:1–38

Shoupe D. Effects of desogestrel on carbohydrate metabolism. Am J Obstet Gynecol 1993;168:1041–1047

Singh K, Viegas OA, Loke DF, Ratnam SS. Effect of Norplant implants on liver, lipid and carbohydrate metabolism. Contraception 1992;45:141–153

Sivin I. International experience with Norplant and Norplant-2 contraceptives. Stud Fam Plann 1988;19:81–94

Stadel BV. Oral contraceptives and cardiovascular disease (first of two parts). N Engl J Med 1981;305:612–618

Stadel BV. Oral contraceptives and cardiovascular disease (second of two parts). N Engl J Med 1981;305:672–677

Stampfer MF, Willett WC, Colditz GA, Speizer FE, Hennekens CH. A prospective study of past use of oral contraceptive agents and risk of cardiovascular disease. N Engl J Med 1988;319:1313–1317

Stolley PD, Strom BL, Sartwell PE. Oral contraceptives and vascular disease. Epidemiol Rev 1989;11:241–243

Vessey MP, Lawless M, Yeates D. Efficacy of different contraceptive methods. Lancet 1982;1:841–842

Vessey M, Mant D, Smith A, Yeates D. Oral contraceptives and venous thromboembolism: findings in a large prospective study. BMJ [Clin Res] 1986;292:526

Vessey MP, Meisler L, Flavel R, Yeates D. Outcome of pregnancy in women using different methods of contraception. Br J Obstet Gynaecol 1979;86:548–556

Vessey MP, Wright NH, McPherson K, Wiggins P. Fertility after stopping different methods of contraception. BMJ 1978;1:265–267

World Health Organization. Breast cancer and depot-medroxyprogesterone acetate: a multinational study. WHO Collaborative Study of Neoplasia and Steroid Contraceptives. Lancet 1991;338:833–838

Zacharias S, Aguilera E, Assenzo JR, Zanartu J. Effects of hormonal and nonhormonal contraceptives on lactation and incidence of pregnancy. Contraception 1986;33:203–213

Preconceptional Care

Over the last several years, preconceptional care has received increasing attention as an appropriate primary prevention strategy for obstetricians and gynecologists. In part, the emphasis has evolved because of changing patterns in infant mortality. In the past decades, congenital anomalies have replaced low birth weight as the leading cause of infant death. The traditional access point for information relative to the prevention of poor reproductive outcomes is the first prenatal visit. In many cases, this is too late. Because organogenesis occurs between day 17 and day 56 after fertilization, many compromised pregnancy outcomes are determined before women have had opportunity to initiate prenatal care.

Preconceptional health promotion should be thorough and systematic. Basic components include identification and evaluation of risks, education individualized to patient need, and the initiation of interventions desired by the woman. Recommended components for prepregnancy care are as follows:

- Systematic identification of preconceptional risks through assessment of medical, reproductive, and family histories; nutritional status; drug exposures; and social concerns of all fertile women
- Provision of education based on risks
- Discussion of possible effects of pregnancy on existing medical conditions for both the prospective mother and the fetus and introduction of interventions, if appropriate and desired
- Discussion of genetic concerns and referral, if appropriate and desired
- Determination of immunity to rubella and immunization, if indicated
- Determination of hepatitis status and immunization, if indicated
- Laboratory tests, including hemoglobin or hematocrit; D (Rh) status (unless already recorded), gonorrhea testing, syphilis testing, chlamydia culture, Pap test, and urine dipstick for protein, sugar, and leukocytes (risk status may suggest other testing, such as for tuberculosis and HIV)
- Nutritional counseling on appropriate weight for height, sources of folic acid, and avoidance of oversupplementation; referral for in-depth counseling, if appropriate and desired
- Discussion of social, financial, and psychologic issues in preparation for pregnancy
- Discussion regarding desired birth spacing and real and perceived barriers to achieving desires, including problems with contraceptive use
- Emphasis on importance of early and continuous prenatal care and discussion of how care may be structured based on the woman's risks and concerns

Risk identification involves investigation of reproductive, medical, and family histories; nutritional habits; drug exposures; and social issues. The assessment elicits information about issues and risks that may affect future childbearing and includes a strong health promotion and disease prevention emphasis.

MEDICAL CONDITIONS

Many of the data supporting the benefits of preconceptional care come from experiences of women with medical conditions that exist prior to pregnancy. Women with insulin-dependent diabetes represent the best example. The offspring of diabetic women have major congenital anomalies at a rate two or three times that of the general population. The likelihood that the offspring of diabetic women will be born healthy can be increased by achieving strict glucose control in the preconceptional period and by maintaining control throughout organogenesis and pregnancy. Ideally, the patient's hemoglobin A_{1C} level should be within normal limits for the specific reference laboratory; this level is generally achieved by maintaining the fasting blood plasma glucose levels at 60–100 mg/dl and the 2-hour postprandial plasma glucose levels at 120–140 mg/dl.

Diabetes illustrates other benefits of preconceptional care: women or couples should gain information about the potential risks to the woman should pregnancy occur; they should be aware of the likely course of prenatal care, and they should be able to place their risks in perspective. This information will allow informed decision-making about future reproduction. Informed couples or women can decide to accept the risks that pregnancy may pose to the health of the woman or to the health of future children, to modify their risks, or to forgo childbearing.

In the case of diabetic women, laboratory and diagnostic studies, including analysis of a 24-hour urine specimen for creatinine clearance and total protein concentration, ophthalmologic examination, and electrocardiography, should be performed to assess the prospective mother's risks. Although pregnancy does not accelerate the natural course of diabetic nephropathy, the complications of pregnancy in the presence of renal disease and hypertension are serious and potentially life threatening. The risks of pregnancy to the life of the mother should be carefully reviewed, preconceptionally, with diabetic patients who have a reduced creatinine clearance and hypertension.

Patients should be aware that diabetic retinopathy may either progress or regress during pregnancy but that no controlled, prospective studies suggest that pregnancy permanently alters the natural course of the disease. Patients should also be aware that many of the preconceptional tests will be repeated during pregnancy and that serial ultrasound examinations and fetal evaluation tests will also be needed.

Because of the increased incidence of neural tube defects (NTDs) in the offspring of diabetic mothers, patients should be made aware preconceptionally of maternal serum alpha-fetoprotein screening. Finally, the diabetic patient and her partner should understand that it is not possible to reduce the incidence of congenital malformations to zero, as there is a 2–3% incidence of severe congenital anomalies in the offspring of the general, nondiabetic, population.

The same steps of evaluation, counseling (including anticipatory guidance), and initiation of desired interventions should be basic to the preconceptional care of all women with preexisting medical conditions. Other diseases of potential importance include phenylketonuria, asthma, heart disease, chronic hypertension, deep vein thrombosis, kidney disease, systemic lupus erythematosus, epilepsy, and cancer.

Prescribed treatments for medical conditions should also be evaluated for safety in the preconceptional period so that, if possible, timely alterations can be made. For instance, coumarin and its derivatives readily cross the placenta and have been associated with warfarin embryopathy. Because heparin does not cross the placenta and is not teratogenic, appropriate prevention includes counseling women about changing to heparin therapy before conception. In general, the best choice is to eliminate unnecessary medications and, for essential therapies, to choose drugs that have the best and longest track record during pregnancy.

REPRODUCTIVE HISTORY

Some obstetric events tend to repeat themselves. A preconceptional reproductive history offers an important opportunity for identifying factors that may have contributed to a previous outcome and that may be amenable to intervention. It is important to categorize poor outcomes as early or late spontaneous abortions, second- or third-trimester fetal deaths, preterm births, or neonatal deaths, because each category suggests different areas for preconceptional exploration.

Potential contributors to early pregnancy loss are:

- Chromosome defect
- Immunologic disorder
- Corpus luteum defect
- Uterine anatomic abnormality (eg, intrauterine adhesions, septate uterus)
- Infections
- Ectopic pregnancy
- Cigarette smoking

Some contributors to second- and third-trimester losses are:

- Immunologic disorder (eg, lupus anticoagulant or anticardiolipin antibodies)
- Infections (eg, group B streptococci, *Mycoplasma hominis, Listeria, Haemophilus influenzae*)
- Uterine or cervical anatomic abnormality (eg, cervical incompetence, septate uterus, uterine anomaly caused by exposure to diethylstilbestrol)
- Placental abruption
- Placenta previa
- Maternal disease
- Chromosome defect
- Cigarette smoking
- Regular or occasional use of illicit substances (eg, heroin, cocaine)
- Alcohol ingestion

Some contributors to neonatal loss are:

- Premature delivery/premature rupture of membranes (contributors may include genital tract infection, uterine anomalies, polyhydramnios, maternal cigarette smoking, use of alcohol or other mood-altering drugs)
- Congenital malformation
- Perinatal infection (eg, group B streptococci, *Neisseria gonorrhoeae*, herpes, TORCH [toxoplasmosis, other viruses, rubella, cytomegalovirus, herpes simplex viruses (HSVs)] organisms)

Factors such as uterine malformations, maternal autoimmune disease, endocrine abnormalities, and genital infection lend themselves to diagnosis and therapies that may decrease the risk for recurrent fetal and neonatal losses. Cigarette smoking, alcohol ingestion, and their reproductive complications should be addressed prior to conception, with encouragement and support for preconceptional cessation.

GENETIC ASSESSMENT

Preconceptional assessment of genetic risks offers a number of advantages over making inquiries at the first prenatal visit. Associated counseling may be prospective if an affected child has not yet been born or retrospective if the parents have had a child with a genetic defect and desire information on the likelihood of a recurrence.

Carrier screening for autosomal recessive inheritance risks is of special preconceptional significance because it allows for relevant counseling before the first affected pregnancy. Prospective carrier screening can be offered based on the ethnic or racial background of the couple: Tay–Sachs disease testing for the Ashkenazic Jewish population; β-thalassemia for Greeks and Italians; α-thalassemia for Southeast Asians and natives of the Philippines; and sickle cell anemia for African–Americans.

The family and personal histories may reveal other risks for genetic diseases, such as fragile X and Down syndromes or constellations of birth defects. Genetic counseling should be offered to couples with identifiable risks so that they may understand the risks to their future children as well as the opportunities and limitations of prenatal testing in their given circumstances.

NUTRITIONAL CARE

In recent years, research findings have accumulated that support the wisdom of women's achieving optimal nutritional status prior to conception. The protective effects of folic acid on the occurrence of NTDs have resulted in the following recommendation by the U.S. Public Health Service: "All women of childbearing age in the United States who are capable of becoming pregnant should consume 0.4 mg of folic acid per day for the purpose of reducing their risk of having a pregnancy affected with spina bifida or other NTDs." This level of consumption can be realized through dietary choices or through supplementation, although supplementation can pose problems, considering the large number of unplanned pregnancies, the difficulties associated with taking a pill daily throughout the reproductive years, and the variability of folate in foods.

Good sources of folic acid in the diet include leafy, dark-green vegetables; citrus fruits and juices; yeast; bread; beans; and fortified breakfast cereals. Folic acid supplements and daily multivitamin preparations containing 0.4 mg of folic acid are also widely available. However, the latter choices require cautions that women do not suppose that supplements will meet all of their nutritional needs around conception and during pregnancy. The preconceptional visit offers an excellent opportunity to counsel about the needs for increased protein, calcium, and calories during pregnancy and to prepare women for the weight gain recommendations that will accompany a gestation.

BIBLIOGRAPHY

Cefalo RC, Moos MK. Preconceptional health promotion: a practical guide. Rockville, Maryland: Aspen Publishers, 1988

Jack BW, Culpepper L. Preconception care: risk reduction and health promotion in preparation for pregnancy. JAMA 1990;264:1147–1149

Kitzmiller JL, Gavin AL, Gin GD, Jovanovic-Peterson L, Main EK, Zigrang WD. Preconception care of diabetes: glycemic control prevents congenital anomalies. JAMA 1991;265:731–736

Moos MK. Preconceptional health promotion: a health education opportunity for all women. Women Health 1989;15:55–68

Scheffler RM, Feuchtbaum LB, Phibbs CS. Prevention: the cost-effectiveness of the California diabetes and pregnancy program. Am J Public Health 1992;82:168–175

Low Abdominal and Pelvic Pain

Low abdominal pain is one of the most common symptoms encountered in gynecologic practices and continues to present important diagnostic challenges, despite recent technologic advances in pregnancy testing, diagnostic imaging, and gynecologic endoscopy. Detailed and thorough history-taking, selective use of diagnostic tests, and a well-considered differential diagnosis usually lead to an accurate diagnosis and appropriate therapy. Diagnostic laparoscopy may be necessary for establishing a pathologic diagnosis or, equally important, for excluding a visible pathologic condition.

HISTORY

The history of any patient with abdominal pain must include descriptions of the onset, character, location, and radiation pattern of the pain, in addition to modifiers of the pain pattern, such as urination, bowel movements, intercourse, activity, and stress. Menstrual, sexual, and contraceptive histories must be recorded meticulously; gastrointestinal, urinary tract, medical, and orthopedic screening questions should be included. A direct inquiry regarding the patient's impression of the cause of the pain may be revealing, especially if her fears are mainly focused on cancer, infertility, or sexual function.

Diagnosis, treatment, and therapeutic response in previous episodes may add important historic information, but one should not assume that the previous diagnosis was necessarily correct, especially if it was not confirmed by a laparoscopic or tissue diagnosis. This point is important in women with a poorly substantiated diagnosis of pelvic infection or endometriosis.

Correspondingly, if the patient states that the present attack of pain is the same as or similar to that of previous episodes, it is most likely that there is a single underlying etiology, but this cannot be assumed. Early evaluation of records from previous hospitalizations, surgical procedures, or radiologic or pathologic consultations can be a critical step in instituting the appropriate therapy and avoiding the repetition of costly, uncomfortable, or dangerous procedures.

PHYSICAL EXAMINATION

Complete physical examinations, including systematic abdominal and pelvic examinations, are done routinely, with attention focused on the location and intensity of the pain. Voluntary vaginal contraction and relaxation should be requested at the start of digital vaginal examination in order to detect vaginismus. A rectovaginal examination is a necessity for complete evaluation. An effort should be made to re-create the pain with separate motions of the hands on the abdomen and in the vagina, thus completing palpation of the abdominal wall, vulva, vaginal walls, uterus, adnexa, and uterosacral ligaments. The examiner should note whether the pain is similar to that described during the history.

The position and extent of the pain should be mapped on a diagram to document whether there have been changes from visit to visit. Pain that is of a pelvic origin may be noted ventrally or both dorsally and ventrally but almost never as back pain alone. This dorsal zone of pelvic pain typically is caudal to the posterior iliac spine and is less likely to be of pelvic origin when the pain moves progressively cephalad. Pain from the cervix, bladder base, and upper vagina may be centered deep in the pelvis but may be also experienced in the buttocks and sacral area and may radiate down the backs of the thighs.

The initial classification scheme in the diagnosis of pelvic pain differentiates acute and subacute pelvic pain from chronic pelvic pain that has been present for 6 months or more. Chronic pelvic pain is further classified as episodic chronic pelvic pain, such as dysmenorrhea or dyspareunia, or as continuous chronic pelvic pain that waxes and wanes but is rarely or never completely absent. In each category, causes are further subdivided by gynecologic or nongynecologic origin. A few conditions, such as endometriosis, may be acute, episodic, or continuous and must be considered in the differential diagnosis of each pattern.

ACUTE PELVIC PAIN

Office or emergency room evaluation of acute abdominal pain hinges on the severity of the patient's symptoms and the urgency of prompt diagnosis and treatment. If the initial evaluation reveals that there is no need for immediate surgery or hospitalization, a stepwise approach to diagnosis is acceptable as long as contact with the patient can be maintained and an acute exacerbation of the patient's symptoms can be evaluated expeditiously.

The first stage of evaluation usually begins with screening tests, including complete blood count, sedimentation rate, and routine urinalysis. A pregnancy test is virtually always indicated when a woman of reproductive age has acute abdominal pain.

Culdocentesis is performed sometimes when there is suspicion of a hemoperitoneum secondary to a ruptured ectopic pregnancy or extracapsular ovarian hemorrhage. It can also be used to help confirm a diagnosis of acute salpingitis and to obtain a sample of peritoneal fluid for culture.

The use of ultrasonography in evaluating acute abdominal pain is confined primarily to pregnancy diagnosis. Ultrasound evaluation of the adnexa in patients with a suspected ectopic pregnancy is helpful if a gestational sac or fetus is localized; otherwise, an adnexal examination does not exclude the possibility of an ectopic gestation, nor does the finding of an adnexal cyst support the possibility of an ectopic pregnancy.

Other applications of ultrasonography in the diagnosis of acute abdominal pain include the demonstration of adnexal masses or cul-de-sac fluid in patients who cannot be examined otherwise because of pain, obesity, vaginal stenosis, or other conditions. Serial ultrasound examinations may be the best way to follow a medically treated tuboovarian abscess or pyosalpinx, since examination is usually difficult early in the course of treatment. Ultrasonography may also be helpful in localizing an IUD in a user with acute abdominal pain when no string is visible. Conversely, the patient with a clearly negative pelvic examination should not be subjected to an ultrasound procedure, as the likelihood of positive ultrasound findings is quite low.

Diagnostic laparoscopy has developed as an important advance in the ability to diagnose acute abdominal pain, which is the indication for more than 50% of diagnostic laparoscopic procedures. Two criteria should be met in deciding to use diagnostic laparoscopy in the diagnosis of acute abdominal pain: first, laparoscopy should be able to provide an accurate, definitive diagnosis, which is necessary to determine appropriate therapy; second, there must exist a possibility that laparoscopic findings may preclude the need for laparotomy.

Studies that compare preoperative diagnoses with laparoscopic findings confirm that there is a high rate of clinical misdiagnoses for both salpingitis and ectopic pregnancy that are corrected only by laparoscopic visualization. Laparoscopy can be used to exclude certain diagnoses such as acute appendicitis or tubal pregnancy, thereby avoiding the need for laparotomy. Conversely, when there is a high likelihood or certainty that laparotomy is necessary, laparoscopy needlessly adds anesthetic and operative time before the laparotomy is performed.

The gynecologic causes of acute pelvic pain include pelvic infection, early pregnancy complications, adnexal problems, endometriosis, and acute degeneration or torsion of a leiomyoma. Pelvic pain can also stem from nongynecologic causes, which should be considered in the diagnosis.

Pelvic Infection

Pelvic infections include acute salpingitis and its complications of tuboovarian abscess, pyosalpingitis, and perihepatitis. The diagnosis should be suspected in women with bilateral lower-quadrant pain and tenderness when the pelvic examination reveals a purulent cervical discharge, corpus tenderness, cervical motion tenderness, and bilateral adnexal tenderness.

Classic gonococcal salpingitis occurs near the time of the menses, is more likely to be associated with fever or peritoneal signs, and responds rapidly to therapy. Nongonococcal salpingitis, in which upper-tract *Chlamydia trachomatis* has been implicated as an etiologic agent, is less likely to be associated with acute peritonitis or fever and is slower to respond to therapy. Cervical culture for gonorrhea and tests for *C. trachomatis* may identify the infecting organisms, although most upper-tract infections are presumed to be polymicrobial and should be treated as such. Because early, aggressive treatment may minimize the risks of sequelae such as infertility, chronic pelvic pain, and ectopic pregnancy, a trend has developed toward the more liberal use of hospitalization for parenteral antibiotic therapy, as opposed to outpatient therapy.

Early Pregnancy Complications

Complications of pregnancy that may produce pelvic pain include spontaneous abortion, septic abortion, and ectopic pregnancy. Pregnancy-related complications should be highly suspected in any woman of reproductive age with acute or subacute pelvic pain; for this reason, a sensitive pregnancy test is a mandatory component of the evaluation. If ectopic pregnancy is part of the differential diagnosis, a qualitative or quantitative determination of the beta subunit of human chorionic gonadotropin with a high sensitivity should be performed.

If a pregnancy test is positive, a diagnostic vaginal ultrasound examination may be valuable for diagnosing intrauterine pregnancy (after 5 weeks from the last menstrual period) and, therefore, for ruling out ectopic pregnancy, except for rare heterotopic (combined) gestations. In cases in which the pregnancy test result is positive but the gestation is too early for ultrasound visualization, serial quantitative human chorionic gonadotropin determinations at 48-hour intervals have been used to differentiate normal intrauterine pregnancies from abnormal pregnancies. In this case, a 66% rise over the baseline suggests a normal pregnancy, although 13% of abnormal pregnancies also exhibit this pattern.

Adnexal Problems

Pelvic pain may arise from ovarian torsion, intracapsular or extracapsular ovarian hemorrhage, or rupture of an ovarian cyst. The pain is either acute or hyperacute at the time of onset. Colicky unilateral pain is associated with ovarian torsion, and bilateral pain localized to a predominant side is associated with ovarian rupture or extracapsular hemorrhage. An associated history of intercourse, intense physical activity, or abdominal trauma is commonly noted with these types of adnexal problems. A history of anticoagulant treatment makes ovarian hemorrhage more likely.

If a pelvic examination does not reveal the needed information because of pain or abdominal guarding, a pelvic ultrasound examination may be helpful in outlining an adnexal mass or fluid in the cul-de-sac. If extracapsular hemorrhage or a ruptured ovarian cyst is suspected, culdocentesis may provide important information, although the procedure is relatively contraindicated if there is a fixed mass in the cul-de-sac. Low-grade fever, leukocytosis, and an increased sedimentation rate are characteristic of torsion; these findings are usually absent in patients with ovarian hemorrhage or rupture. Diagnostic laparoscopy has replaced both laparotomy and observation in patients for whom the diagnosis is unclear.

Nongynecologic Causes

Other causes of acute pelvic pain are most commonly gastrointestinal in origin and include acute appendicitis, diverticulitis, viral gastroenteritis, acute bacterial ileitis, and acute mesenteric (viral) lymphadenitis. Inflammatory bowel disease, which includes regional enteritis and ulcerative colitis, more commonly presents as episodic subacute or chronic pelvic pain but on occasion may cause acute abdominal pain and, in some cases, mimics a tuboovarian abscess. Sigmoidoscopy and imaging studies of the gastrointestinal tract—as well as stool examination for the presence of blood, leukocytes, bacteria (culture and sensitivity), and ova and parasites—may provide important information.

Renal colic secondary to a renal or ureteral stone may be a cause of lower abdominal and flank pain that is very intense and may radiate to the groin, labia, or vagina. Passage of a stone or gravel and a history of hematuria confirm the diagnosis. Intravenous pyelography remains the mainstay of diagnosis, although ultrasonography can also be used to demonstrate hydroureter, hydronephrosis, or a stone. Acute cystitis may be accompanied by midline lower abdominal pain, in addition to dysuria, urgency or frequency of urination, or hematuria.

Numerous medical conditions may be associated with recurrent acute lower abdominal pain, but this is rarely an isolated or presenting symptom. These problems include sickle cell crisis, acute intermittent porphyria, and connective tissue diseases such as familial Mediterranean fever, Henoch–Schönlein purpura, systemic lupus erythematosus, and hereditary angioneurotic edema. Untreated endocrine conditions such as hyperthyroidism, addisonian crisis, and hyperparathyroidism occasionally may be associated with lower abdominal pain that is vague and poorly localized. Herpes zoster virus infection may present with unilateral lower abdominal pain located in the T-10–T-12 dermatomes and is characterized as burning in nature, progressively severe, and associated with cutaneous hyperesthesia. The pain is followed by the outbreak of vesicles in the same dermatomal pattern.

CHRONIC PELVIC PAIN

Communication between the physician and the patient is a critical component of management, and the patient should be provided with a realistic assessment of outcome; however, the physician should neither promise a cure nor predict failure. Physical examination not only should serve to establish or exclude pathologic findings but also should be used for evocative testing, such as cervical traction to evaluate pain caused by the loss of pelvic support, or nerve blocks to aid in the diagnosis of adenomyosis.

Ultrasonography, barium enema, intravenous pyelography,

and other noninvasive procedures should be used, but they should not be indiscriminately ordered as screening tests when there is a low likelihood of positive findings. Diagnostic laparoscopy should be used in women with chronic pelvic pain to either confirm a presumptive diagnosis or exclude an undetected pathologic state. If chronic pelvic pain syndrome is confirmed, pain amelioration, rather than rejection of the problem as irremediable, must be considered as the therapeutic goal.

Episodic Chronic Pelvic Pain

Cyclic recurrent episodes of pain that have been present for longer than 6 months and are associated with pain-free intervals are described as episodic chronic pelvic pain. Such pain can be related to sexual intercourse or stages of the menstrual cycle.

Dyspareunia

Dyspareunia is traditionally described by location: superficial, vaginal, or deep. Superficial dyspareunia is commonly related to an irritative lesion, such as vulvitis or bartholinitis, or an anatomic lesion, such as atrophic dystrophy with introital shrinkage, infected urethral diverticulum, constrictive hymenal remnant, tender episiotomy scar, or overcorrected posterior colporrhaphy. Introital dyspareunia caused by a posterior fourchette ulcer or vulvar vestibulitis can be treated by chemical or thermal destruction or surgical excision.

Involuntary vaginal introital muscle spasm, or vaginismus, may be diagnosed by history or physical examination and often responds to behavioral management with vaginal relaxation exercises. Vaginal dyspareunia may be irritative secondary to chronic infection or may be related to inadequate lubrication or vaginismus.

Deep dyspareunia is commonly associated with an underlying pelvic abnormality, such as endometriosis, chronic salpingitis, or severe pelvic adhesions with encasement and fixation of the ovaries; it may also be a component of the pelvic pain syndrome. Deep dyspareunia after hysterectomy without salpingo-oophorectomy may be due to prolapse of a fallopian tube through the vaginal cuff, chronically infected cuff granulation tissue, or the residual ovary syndrome with adhesion of one or both ovaries to the vaginal apex. Medical treatment for the latter condition can be attempted with ovarian suppression, but usually reoperation is indicated for either ovarian suspension or oophorectomy.

Midcycle Pelvic Pain

Midcycle pelvic pain is usually a manifestation of peritoneal irritation caused by the release of blood or follicular fluid from the ovary at the time of ovulation. The pain is generally unilateral and dissipates within a few hours, but in some women it is quite intense and prolonged. Treatment is not usually required; when necessary, systemic analgesics, nonsteroidal antiinflammatory agents, or ovarian suppression with OCs can be used. Less commonly, endometriosis or other organic conditions may be associated with isolated midcycle pain or midcycle exacerbation of continuous chronic pelvic pain.

Dysmenorrhea

Dysmenorrhea may be primary, with no associated organic pathology, or secondary, with demonstrable organic pathology. Primary dysmenorrhea is caused by prostaglandin-induced uterine contractions and ischemia and is currently managed with prostaglandin synthetase inhibitors or OC therapy. Secondary dysmenorrhea is usually due to endometriosis or adenomyosis but may also be due to chronic salpingitis, an IUD, or congenital or acquired outflow tract obstruction, including cervical stenosis.

Symptom profiles of primary and secondary dysmenorrhea are helpful in triage and may avoid prolonged therapy with prostaglandin synthetase inhibitors when other treatment is needed. Primary dysmenorrhea has a tendency to occur with the onset of ovulatory cycles and usually improves with time, coincides with the onset of menstrual bleeding, and frequently is associated with other prostaglandin-mediated symptoms such as nausea, vomiting, diarrhea, and dizziness. Dyspareunia is generally absent, although mild dyspareunia may be present during menses. The pain is sharp and crampy and is located in the midline without a lower-quadrant or adnexal component. Pelvic examination in a nonmenstruating patient with primary dysmenorrhea should not demonstrate tenderness or other pathologic changes.

In contrast, secondary dysmenorrhea most commonly begins in women who are in their 20s and progressively worsens, although it may improve temporarily after childbirth. The pain may begin long before menses and continue during and even after it. Dyspareunia is commonly present throughout the month and is worse with menses. Menorrhagia and secondary dysmenorrhea suggest the possibility of adenomyosis, an endometrial polyp, or a pedunculated submucous myoma. Menstrual pain in a patient with secondary dysmenorrhea involves not only midline structures but, in some cases, one or both lower quadrants. Pelvic examination will demonstrate uterine or adnexal tenderness and, possibly, fixed uterine retroflexion, uterosacral nodularity, or a palpable pelvic mass.

When the history or physical examination is suggestive of primary dysmenorrhea, medical treatment with prostaglandin inhibitors or OCs should be prescribed before proceeding with other diagnostic procedures. If the patient fails a trial of either or both therapies, diagnostic laparoscopy is indicated for further evaluation of causes. Alternatively, if the initial evaluation reveals the likelihood of secondary dysmenorrhea, further diagnostic steps should be continued without delay, so that any secondary condition can be treated expeditiously. Fifteen percent of patients with early-onset dysmenorrhea have secondary (organic) causes; therefore, a definitive diagnosis should not be postponed simply because of a patient's young age.

Continuous Chronic Pelvic Pain

Noncyclic recurrent pelvic pain that has been present for 6 months or longer is defined as continuous chronic pelvic pain. The gynecologic causes of continuous chronic pelvic pain are endometriosis, adenomyosis, chronic salpingitis, and pelvic congestion syndrome.

Other, less well-defined and more controversial, causes of chronic pelvic pain are loss of pelvic support and the presence of dense pelvic adhesions. Uterine descensus and prolapse are associated with pelvic pain or pressure in one quarter of women with this condition, although it is rarely severe enough to be a primary complaint. Pelvic adhesions are the only finding in 10–25% of laparoscopies for chronic pelvic pain, but it is still unclear whether such adhesions are the cause of the pain or an incidental finding. Doubt exists because of the large percentage of women with adhesions who have no complaint of pelvic pain. Adhesions that are located between the bowel and the pelvic organs and that could put traction on either structure are a possible cause of chronic or episodic pain. Operative laparoscopy, including laser use, deserves extensive study to determine its appropriate role in the treatment of adhesions.

Endometriosis

Endometriosis classically presents with dysmenorrhea, deep dyspareunia, and infertility as chief complaints; 50% of women who have symptomatic endometriosis, however, have continuous pelvic pain that may or may not worsen with menses. Other, less common, symptoms include dyschezia, dysuria, and tender nodules on the vagina or other pelvic surfaces. Physical examination may reveal a tender uterus and adnexal structures, an adnexal mass caused by an endometrioma, fixed uterine retroflexion, or nodularity of the uterosacral ligaments or posterior corpus. Therapy is medical or surgical, depending on the severity of the disease and the patient's reproductive plans.

In a young woman with endometriosis, every effort should be made to achieve prompt diagnosis and therapy to maximize future fertility and to minimize subsequent pelvic pain. Surgery for pain control, such as presacral neurectomy and division of the uterosacral and ligaments, remains controversial and is appropriate for only a very limited number of patients who also desire to preserve their fertility.

Adenomyosis

Adenomyosis is another important cause of continuous chronic pelvic pain, although, like endometriosis, it may be associated only with dysmenorrhea and dyspareunia. Adenomyosis should be suspected in women of late reproductive age who have the aforementioned symptoms associated with a mildly enlarged, boggy, and tender uterus—especially during menses. Adnexal findings should be negative unless there is concomitant peritoneal endometriosis. Temporary relief of pelvic pain with a uterosacral paracervical block has been proposed as a helpful diagnostic aid.

Chronic Salpingitis

Chronic salpingitis is a sequel to acute infection and may be associated with continuous or intermittent chronic pelvic pain, dyspareunia, or dysmenorrhea. The mechanism of the pain in patients with chronic salpingitis is unknown. It may be that repeated infection; a chronic, smoldering infection; neurovascular damage; or anatomic distortion secondary to adhesion formation contributes to the pain pattern.

Pelvic examination reveals varying degrees of adnexal tenderness that is commonly associated with adnexal matting and, occasionally, fixed retroflexion of the uterine corpus. An elevated sedimentation rate is consistent with the disease but is not necessary for diagnosis.

Long courses of oral or parenteral antibiotics and perimenstrual antibiotic prophylaxis have been suggested, but neither is a proven therapy. Conservative surgery, such as unilateral adnexectomy, should be limited to unilateral disease. Operative laparoscopy is a promising but unproven approach to treating pain associated with adnexal adhesions. For patients who have become physically or socially debilitated secondary to pelvic pain from chronic pelvic infection, extirpative surgery may be the only effective therapy when the laparoscopic approaches fail.

Pelvic Congestion Syndrome

A syndrome of chronic pelvic pain was described as "pelvic congestion syndrome" by Taylor in 1949. A patient with pelvic congestion syndrome typically complains of bilateral lower abdominal pain, usually with low back pain in the sacral area and radiation to the backs of the legs or the inner aspects of the thighs. The pain is most commonly continuous but is worse at day's end, premenstrually or menstrually, and may be accompanied by deep dyspareunia and increased intensity of pain while standing or jumping.

A pelvic examination reveals tenderness of both the adnexa and the posterior fornix without induration or masses. Laparoscopy may show a normal pelvis or perhaps prominent, enlarged, broad ligament veins. The true importance of these veins in the pathophysiology of the syndrome is uncertain.

Chronic Pain Syndrome

Many women with pain continue to function surprisingly well, even though they may have extensive organic abnormalities. A substantial number, however, will, with time, develop chronic pain syndrome demonstrating the following symptoms:

- Incomplete relief by most surgical or medical treatments
- Significantly impaired function at home or at work
- Signs of depression (early-morning awakening, weight loss, anorexia)
- Pain that bears little relation to the amount of organic pathology
- Altered family roles

The traditional model of physiologic versus psychogenic origin of disease is of limited usefulness in the case of chronic pelvic pain; instead, the picture is one of an intricate interaction of physiologic and psychologic factors that are ultimately manifest as pain. Management of such patients should involve simultaneous attention to physical and psychologic factors.

The history should be expanded to include evidence of past or present physical or sexual abuse, alcohol- or drug-related problems, medication habituation, and domestic discord. Because it is usually impossible to assign the relative degrees of contribution of these factors to the total pain problem, a more productive approach is to devote balanced diagnostic and therapeutic attention to all important factors.

Once the hallmarks of a chronic pain syndrome are evident, psychologic assessment is indicated, either by the gynecologist or a consulting mental health professional. Management may include development of specific skills for coping with the pain, relaxation training, biofeedback, individual psychotherapy, marital therapy, and sexual counseling. Narcotic medication should be prescribed cautiously; antidepressants, together with continuous nonnarcotic analgesics, often suffice, especially when they are combined with behavioral and psychotherapeutic measures. When multiple therapeutic approaches seem to be indicated, these may be handled best by a multidisciplinary pain center.

Nongynecologic Causes

Other causes of chronic pelvic pain include gastrointestinal problems such as inflammatory bowel disease, diverticulitis, and functional bowel syndromes exemplified by spastic colon syndrome. Chronic or interstitial cystitis may be associated with recurrent or chronic midline lower abdominal pain in addition to other urinary tract symptoms such as urgency or frequency of urination.

Orthopedic etiologies are distinctly uncommon causes of chronic pelvic pain, although chronic low-back pain caused by disk disease or other musculoskeletal conditions may be confused with gynecologic problems that cause a combination of abdominal and sublumbar pain.

BIBLIOGRAPHY

Cunanan RG Jr, Courey NG, Lippes J. Laparoscopic findings in patients with pelvic pain. Am J Obstet Gynecol 1983;146:589–591

Goodkin K, Gullion CM. Antidepressants for the relief of chronic pain: do they work? Ann Behav Med 1989;11:83–101

Kresch AJ, Seifer DB, Sachs LB, Barrese I. Laparoscopy in 100 women with chronic pelvic pain. Obstet Gynecol 1984;64:672–674

Reiter RC, Gambone JC. Demographic and historic variables in women with idiopathic chronic pelvic pain. Obstet Gynecol 1990;75:428–432

Steege JF, Stout AL. Resolution of chronic pelvic pain following laparoscopic adhesiolysis. Am J Obstet Gynecol 1991;165:278–281

Steege JF, Stout AL, Somkuti S. Chronic pelvic pain in women: toward an integrative model. Obstet Gynecol Surv 1993;48(2):95–110

Stout AL, Steege JF, Dodson WC, Hughes CL. Relationship of laparoscopic findings to self-report of pelvic pain. Am J Obstet Gynecol 1991;164:73–79

Walker E, Katon W, Harrop-Griffiths J, Holm L, Russo J, Hickoc LR. Relationship of chronic pelvic pain to psychiatric diagnoses and childhood sexual abuse. Am J Psychiatry 1988;145:75–80

Premenstrual Syndrome

Premenstrual symptoms, including physical and emotional changes, occur in a large majority of women between menarche and menopause. A number of surveys of widely varying populations suggest that 85–90% of all women report having experienced premenstrual symptoms at some point during their reproductive lives.

The term *PMS* is commonly used by gynecologists to describe the occurrence of premenstrual physical or emotional changes that are of sufficient severity to disrupt daily activities of work or life style. Depending on how strictly these changes are defined, the prevalence of PMS is much less than the overall prevalence of premenstrual symptoms. A number of studies suggest that approximately 20% of women of reproductive age experience clinically significant symptoms but that fewer than 5% report symptoms severe enough to meet a stricter diagnosis of PMS.

The cause of PMS is unclear, although now there is more clarity of definition, thus facilitating the differentiation of PMS from other psychiatric disorders and aiding an assessment of various therapies. In 1985, the term *late luteal phase dysphoric disorder* was proposed to the American Psychiatric Association as a new diagnostic category needing further study. This term is used in the psychiatric literature, whereas the term *PMS* is found in the gynecologic literature and may refer to a wider range of symptoms. *Diagnostic and Statistical Manual of Mental Disorders* suggests the inclusion of yet another term, *premenstrual dysphoric disorder*, although the issues of definition and placement as a psychiatric diagnosis have been controversial. Progress has been made in defining the diagnosis for research purposes, and well-designed clinical studies are ongoing.

HISTORY

Women presenting with a self-diagnosis of PMS require careful evaluation and sensitive history-taking. Most of them have read something about the subject, and many have attempted to deal with their symptoms through a variety of self-help manipulations of diet or exercise. The way in which a clinician is willing to listen to a description of symptoms and to respond in an empathetic and understanding manner to validate the degree of emotional distress is critical in the formation of a therapeutic alliance. It is important for the clinician to discuss what is and is not known about premenstrual symptoms, to describe what will be necessary to confirm a diagnosis of PMS and rule out other problems, and to formulate as a realistic goal of therapy an increase in an ability to cope with symptoms, not a "magic cure."

An open-ended interview question, such as "Tell me what is troublesome to you about your PMS," can be helpful at the initial visit. After allowing the patient to describe her problems, more specific information can be elicited, including the relationship of symptoms to the menstrual cycle. As with any medical symptoms, the onset, duration, alleviating or exacerbating factors, and previous therapies should be determined. The patient can be asked to describe which symptoms are most bothersome to her. She can be asked about the impact of PMS on her family, friends, and colleagues. She should be asked questions about her social situation and social support.

Specific screening for a history of physical or sexual abuse should be a part of the general history-taking, as with all gynecologic patients. The general medical and gynecologic history should not be neglected, nor should a review of systems and a family history.

The woman can be asked about any complicating psychologic factors that she feels may be contributing to her problems. If any aspect of the screening history suggests vegetative symptoms of major depression, it is essential that the patient be questioned about suicidal ideation, intent, and plans. Formal psychologic testing or referral may be appropriate after the initial visit, particularly if the symptoms are severe or suggest major psychiatric illness.

DIAGNOSIS

From the clinician's perspective, the key diagnostic criteria include 1) the presence of characteristic symptoms, 2) occurrence with a luteal phase pattern, and 3) disruptive severity.

More than 150 symptoms have been described as occurring with PMS. Mood disturbances, somatic symptoms, cognitive symptoms, and behavioral changes have all been described (see box). These symptoms are not unique to PMS or even to women, and a key issue is the differentiation of PMS from other clinical entities (see box). Disorders that should be distinguished include psychiatric diagnoses such as depression and anxiety, which may be noncyclic or have a premenstrual exacerbation.

The diagnosis of PMS is generally reserved for situations in which an underlying psychiatric disorder has been excluded. Psychiatric diagnoses may also be classified as a primary diagnosis, such as major depression, with a premenstrual exacerbation. Medical disorders such as vascular headaches ("menstrual migraines"), irritable bowel syndrome, hypothyroidism, perimenopause, and medication-induced side effects (such as those occurring with combination OCs and implantable or injectable contraceptives) should be differentiated from PMS.

Symptoms of Premenstrual Syndrome

Mood Disturbances
Anxiety
Irritability
Tension
Mood swings/lability
Depression
Anger
Hostility

Cognitive Symptoms
Confusion
Difficulty concentrating
Oversensitivity
Forgetfulness

Somatic Symptoms
Fatigue
Bloating
Breast tenderness
Acne
Swelling
Gastrointestinal symptoms
Increased appetite
Headache
Hot flashes
Insomnia
Joint pain
Constipation

Behavioral Changes
Food cravings
Social withdrawal
Argumentative behavior
Social isolation
Crying spells

Differential Diagnosis of Premenstrual Syndrome

Psychiatric Illness
Major depressive disorder
Bipolar disorder
Panic disorder
Posttraumatic stress disorder
Somatization disorder
Personality disorders
Substance abuse
Eating disorders

Medical Illness
Vascular headaches
Cardiovascular disease with edema
Renal disease
Hepatic disease
Hypothyroidism
Irritable bowel syndrome

The differentiation of PMS from other medical disorders is facilitated by the pattern of symptoms occurring in the luteal phase. Prospective charting of symptoms with a rating of their severity is essential, and a variety of charts have been formulated to facilitate an overview of symptoms. Charting for several cycles should be reviewed. More than one half of women presenting to PMS clinics do not have a diagnosis of PMS confirmed by prospective charting. Prospective charting should reveal an interval, from approximately cycle day 4 through cycle day 12, that is relatively symptom free. An additional research criterion for diagnosis is an increase of at least 30% in symptom scoring in the late luteal phase (last 7 days of the cycle) over the midfollicular phase (cycle days 3–9). Even women who describe symptoms that are only mildly troublesome should be asked to confirm the premenstrual timing of their symptoms by prospective charting, because sometimes the exercise itself can be therapeutic.

The criterion for the diagnosis of PMS that symptoms be severe is difficult to standardize or measure. Self-assessment of marital and relationship problems, problems of parenting, legal difficulties, problems with work or school performance, suicidal ideation, or medical treatment can sometimes be identified and confirmed by a partner or family member.

ETIOLOGY

Although the symptoms of PMS are closely associated with the luteal phase of the menstrual cycle, most studies have not shown any consistent differences in levels of estrogen or progesterone or estrogen–progesterone ratios between women with PMS and those without. Therefore, it appears that ovarian steroid hormones do not provide a biochemical marker for the diagnosis of PMS. It has been demonstrated, however, that temporary reduction of estrogen and progesterone to postmenopausal levels with gonadotropin-releasing hormone agonists or permanent reduction with oophorectomy results in a marked reduction of PMS symptoms. The administration of mifepristone (RU 486), with its antiprogesterone activity, to induce early menses was shown not to result in the earlier disappearance of PMS symptoms. Thus, it is not believed that fluctuations in estrogen or progesterone levels are causative of PMS symptoms, but they may be mediators or inducers of central nervous system neuroendocrine changes.

Studies have not shown consistent links of PMS to abnormal levels of thyroid hormone or an abnormal thyroid-stimulating hormone response to thyrotropin-releasing hormone. Nor are prolactin levels consistently different between women with PMS and normal controls. Other attempts to find differences in the hypothalamic–pituitary–adrenal axis through sampling of urinary or plasma cortisol levels or responses to serial dexamethasone suppression tests have found no significant differences between the follicular and luteal phases in women with PMS and controls.

The role of endogenous opioids in PMS has been investigated, with some studies noting differences in plasma β-endorphin premenstrually between PMS patients and controls. Other studies have suggested a relationship between PMS symptoms and endogenous opioids by showing a correlation between the degree of placebo response and plasma endorphin levels.

Neurotransmitters have been widely studied and are known to play a mediating role in disorders of mood and behavior. The role of serotonin, in particular, has been investigated in PMS and other affective disorders. A premenstrual deficit in the serotonin system has been suggested in PMS.

The relationship between ovarian steroid hormones and brain activities is not yet well understood. Although the serotoninergic system may be involved, it alone or any other single system is unlikely to be solely causative of symptoms. The "cause" of PMS symptoms has not been demonstrated. Thus, treatment for PMS is not specifically focused toward a single cause. The most promising recent treatments have been aimed not toward correcting an underlying abnormality but toward providing relief of the symptoms.

MANAGEMENT

After the initial visit in which the history of PMS symptoms is reviewed and a differential diagnosis is developed, the patient is asked to keep a prospective symptom chart for two or three cycles. At the initial visit, additional testing may be helpful to exclude underlying medical conditions. At the next visit, the symptom charting is reviewed for symptom patterns that suggest PMS, based on the absence of symptoms during the postmenstrual phase. The presence of an underlying condition, such as depression, as a primary diagnosis is suggested by the presence of symptoms throughout the month with little or no consistent symptom-free interval. Symptoms suggesting an underlying depression with a premenstrual exacerbation or with the superimposition of additional premenstrual symptoms should prompt a more detailed evaluation.

If it is determined that the symptoms suggest PMS and are of sufficient severity to be disruptive, therapy should be individualized; it may consist of a variety of medical and nonmedical approaches.

Nonmedical Treatment

A variety of nonmedical treatments have been proposed, including vitamin and mineral supplementation, dietary modifications, exercise, and stress reduction. Most of these therapies are inexpensive and safe, and thus deserving of some focus. Anecdotally, but without a great deal of scientific evidence to support their efficacy, many women report a reduction of symptoms with a dietary program. Such regimens usually involve reducing sodium, simple sugar, caffeine, and alcohol consumption; increasing complex carbohydrates; and having more frequent meals. These recommendations are generally health promoting and thus deserving of a trial.

Dietary supplementation of both calcium and magnesium has been reported to reduce PMS symptoms. Other supplements, such as pyridoxine, may have some benefit, although the therapeutic window between a safe dose and a toxic one is relatively narrow. Doses of as little as 200 mg/d have been reported to be associated with symptoms of peripheral neuropathy.

Exercise has been shown to decrease symptoms in depression and theoretically may be beneficial in PMS through an alteration of endorphins. Moderate regular exercise and likely dietary modifications are generally good recommendations for health maintenance, and women who adopt such a regimen will be addressing the most prevalent cardiovascular risk factor: physical inactivity.

Other therapies, such as efforts to reduce stress by meditation or relaxation exercise, may also be helpful. Preliminary studies suggest some possible relief from PMS symptoms by altering circadian rhythms through sleep deprivation or phototherapy.

These nonmedical therapies may be most beneficial for women who have mild-to-moderate symptoms, some of whom may not qualify for a strict diagnosis of PMS or late luteal phase dysphoric disorder. Patients with significant psychosocial stressors, while not qualifying for a psychiatric diagnosis, may nonetheless benefit from counseling to address their own personal issues, including marital discord or past sexual or physical abuse.

Medical Treatment

The goal of medical treatment of PMS is the alleviation or reduction of symptoms. Since the etiology of PMS has not been well established, pharmacologic therapy cannot be targeted specifically to an underlying pathophysiology. Treatment with medication is usually considered after self-help therapies, including dietary modification, supplementation, and exercise, have provided insufficient relief.

Initial therapy can target isolated symptoms. Nonsteroidal antiinflammatory drugs, such as 250 mg of mefenamic acid three or four times daily, can be used to treat dysmenorrhea, headaches, or joint pain. Spironolactone, 25 mg four times daily, can relieve bloating and fluid retention. Low-dose danazol, 200 mg once or twice daily, or bromocriptine, 2.5 mg daily, is effective for breast symptoms or tenderness. Oral contraceptives are helpful for women requiring contraception who have symptoms such as dysmenorrhea.

Progesterone vaginal suppositories, although widely prescribed for PMS, have been shown to be no more effective than placebo. There is some evidence for the benefit of oral micronized progesterone; however, its lack of easy availability in the oral form makes other, more effective, alternatives a preferable choice for therapy.

Two psychotropic medications have been shown to result in a marked decrease in symptoms in double-blind, placebo-controlled studies. The serotonin uptake inhibitor fluoxetine has been used in a dosage of 20 mg daily. Alprazolam, a benzodiazepine, has also been shown in some studies to be effective, although the studies are less consistent in showing a benefit. Alprazolam has an addictive potential. It is best used during the second half of the cycle, at an initial dosage of 0.25 mg three times daily, increasing to a total daily dosage of 4 mg. At the onset of menses, the dose should be decreased by 25% each day. Other antidepressants, including clomipramine or tricyclics, have also been used with some success.

Additional therapies that have been shown to be of benefit include those that produce anovulation. Although gonadotropin-releasing hormone agonists are effective in relieving symptoms, their long-term use is precluded by their hypoestrogenic effects, including development of osteoporosis. Danazol has also been used, although its expense (like that of gonadotropin-releasing hormone agonists), metabolic effects (on lipids), and side effects compromise its long-term use. Medroxyprogesterone acetate, 10–20 mg daily, orally, or DMPA has also been used and is relatively inexpensive. The therapies of ovulation suppression are generally considered as second- or third-line therapies, to be used after nonmedical and other medical therapies have failed.

The goals of therapy include an improvement in functioning and a reduction or control of severe symptoms. The treatment of PMS, more than the treatment of most other gynecologic conditions, requires attention to the biologic, psychologic, and social factors of the illness. It requires that the clinician practice the art of medicine while awaiting the science to provide further explanation of the causes and elucidation of effective therapies.

BIBLIOGRAPHY

Demers LM. Premenstrual, postpartum, and menopausal mood disorders. Baltimore: Urban & Schwar-zenberg, 1989

Harrison WM, Endicott J, Nee J. Treatment of premenstrual dysphoria with alprazolam: a controlled study. Arch Gen Psychiatry 1990; 47:270–275

Jensvold MF. Psychiatric aspects of the menstrual cycle. In: Steward DE, Stotland NL, eds. Psychological aspects of women's health care: the interface between psychiatry and obstetrics and gynecology. Washington, DC: American Psychiatric Press, 1993:1–11

Johnson SR. Premenstrual syndrome. Clin Obstet Gynecol 1987;30: 365–480

Rapkin AJ. Premenstrual syndrome. Clin Obstet Gynecol 1992; 35:585–701

Rubinow DR. The premenstrual syndrome: new views. JAMA 1992; 268:1908–1912

Schmidt PJ, Nieman LK, Grover GN, Muller KL, Merriam GR, Rubinow DR. Lack of effect of induced menses on symptoms in women with premenstrual syndrome. N Engl J Med 1991;324:1174–1179

Sheftell FD, Silberstein SD, Rapoport AM, Rossum RW. Migraine and women: diagnosis, pathophysiology, and treatment. J Womens Health 1992;1:5–19

Strickler RC. Premenstrual syndrome. In: Sciarra JJ, ed. Gynecology and obstetrics. Vol 1. Philadelphia: JB Lippincott, 1992:1–13

Wood SH, Mortola JF, Chan YF, Moossazadeh F, Yen SS. Treatment of premenstrual syndrome with fluoxetine: a double-blind, placebo-controlled, crossover study. Obstet Gynecol 1992;80:339–344

Breast Disorders

It has been estimated that one of every four women in the United States will require medical attention for breast problems, most of which are benign. More than half of all women have some degree of symptomatic fibrocystic changes during their lifetimes.

DEVELOPMENTAL ANOMALIES

Congenital absence of the breast usually is associated with a deformity of the muscles and bones of the chest wall. The defect is quite obvious, and treatment consists of appropriate plastic surgery to reconstruct the absent breast. Premature breast development may present as a unilateral breast mass. Results of hormone studies are normal, and there are no other manifestations of sexual maturation. This is a benign, self-limiting condition and does not require treatment. Surgical removal of the mass in the belief that this is a tumor must be avoided, as removal will result in complete absence of the breast on the affected side.

Asymmetric breast development is not uncommon. Minor breast asymmetry is common in adult women and occasionally represents excessive development of the pectoral muscles on the affected side. The finding is of no clinical significance and requires no treatment. Significant asymmetry, on the other hand, may require augmentation mammoplasty for cosmetic purposes.

Breast hypertrophy is a rather rare situation that occurs in young patients and is characterized by the rapid growth of one breast. Endocrine studies are normal. The process continues over a period of years, and both the patient and the parents must be counseled to wait for full development of the hypertrophy. A reduction mammoplasty performed prematurely will result in continued hypertrophy requiring additional reduction surgery.

Occasionally, particularly during pregnancy, massive breast overdevelopment may occur, resulting in local areas of ulceration. The cause is unknown, and treatment is bilateral mastectomy.

FIBROCYSTIC CHANGES

Fibrocystic changes represent an exaggerated physiologic response to a changing hormonal environment and include painful breasts (mastalgia), macrocysts, and nipple discharge. The epidemiology of fibrocystic changes is poorly understood. The peak incidence occurs between ages 30–50 years. The fact that breast tenderness often occurs premenstrually suggests that progesterone may play some role in the development of the symptomatology of cystic "disease." The proportional effect of estrogen and progesterone and the etiology of benign breast conditions need further clarification. Most, if not all, women experience these changes, and to label this condition as a disease is inappropriate. Typically, the patient complains of discomfort, and examination often discloses a generalized lumpiness or granular feeling located in the upper, outer quadrant and beneath the nipple–areola complex.

Often a careful family history reveals similar findings in several daughters, the mother, and possibly even the grandmother. In some patients, the findings and the symptoms may be related to an end-organ defect that is as yet incompletely understood. The use of medication, particularly OCs and certain tranquilizers, should be documented; knowledge of the patient's physical activity also is important.

The symptoms of fibrocystic changes are difficult to treat. The treatment usually is based on the patient's symptoms and physical findings rather than a definitive diagnosis obtained by open biopsy. These clinical impressions often are inaccurate and do not reflect the pathophysiology of the condition. Mastodynia, or painful breasts, is best managed with simple analgesics, a well-fitting bra, and restriction of fluids, particularly premenstrually. Almost every form of medical treatment has been recommended, including vitamins, hormonal therapy, tamoxifen, bromocriptine, androgens, progesterone, and most recently danazol. None of these treatment modalities is entirely successful and many have significant side effects, especially bromocriptine and androgens.

Caffeine restriction, in particular, has been recommended in women with fibrocystic changes. Recent studies have indicated that initial information did not provide unequivocal scientific evidence that methylxanthines are related to the development of fibrocystic changes. Additional dietary recommendations, including the use of various vitamins, have not proved helpful. In short, none of the treatment regimens proposed for the symptomatic relief of fibrocystic changes has been totally effective.

NIPPLE DISCHARGE

Nipple discharge may be spontaneous or provoked. Inappropriate lactation with or without amenorrhea may be due to excessive prolactin secretion, resulting in lactation. The higher the prolactin level the greater the likelihood of an underlying pituitary tumor. Appropriate diagnostic studies should be carried out not only to confirm the diagnosis but to plan the appropriate therapy. In the office setting, galactorrhea can be distinguished from ductal disease by the use of an appropriate stain for fat. A positive fat stain indicates a physiologic secretion because of either inappropriate lactation or possibly the use of tranquilizers.

The patient should be questioned concerning the nature of the discharge to determine whether it is bilateral, unilateral, clear, yellow, greenish, watery, serosanguineous, or bloody. Spontaneous discharge may be associated with ovulation or the use of tranquilizers or contraceptives. Most physiologic discharges are white or green. Occasionally the discharge may be clear or yellow.

Unilateral discharge raises the possibility of an underlying malignancy, and serosanguineous or bloody discharge must be investigated. The most common lesion is a benign, intraductal papilloma. Breast cancer occurs in 5–15% of these patients. Therefore, the diagnosis must be confirmed by histologic evaluation. Usually the involved quadrant can be located by firm pressure, and exploration of this area is performed under local anesthesia. The involved duct is located and excised for pathologic evaluation.

Two additional causes of spontaneous discharge should be included in the differential diagnosis. Patients who jog several miles per day, particularly those not using a support bra, may have a spontaneous nipple discharge; aerobic exercise, when associated with weight lifting, stimulates the pectoral muscles and produces nipple discharge. Discharge from a nonlactating nipple is seen in approximately 5% of women. It is most frequent in premenopausal patients, and galactorrhea is the most common cause. Reported rates of malignancy in patients with serosanguineous or frankly bloody discharge range from 7% to 17%. The risk increases with the finding of a palpable mass. Cytologic study of the discharge may be helpful, but false-negative results often are obtained.

MASTITIS

With the usual form of puerperal mastitis, there is a localized area of inflammation and tenderness and a slight elevation of temperature. Treatment includes continuation of breastfeeding or emptying the breast with a pump and the use of appropriate antibiotics. If the treatment is ineffective and the tenderness and fever persist, a breast abscess should be suspected. Because of the unique anatomy of the breast, there is far more destruction of breast tissue than a superficial physical examination would suggest. Treatment requires adequate drainage under general anesthesia in an operating room setting. Antibiotics must be continued and given in full therapeutic doses for 7–10 days after adequate drainage.

Squamous metaplasia or nonpuerperal mastitis is not uncommon. Whether infection occurs first, followed by squamous metaplasia, or whether the squamous metaplasia initiates the obstruction and subsequent infection is not known. The usual history reveals the presence of a multicolored discharge, either through the nipple or near a Montgomery follicle. A palpable swelling may be noted. The patient usually states that several attempts at drainage have not resulted in cure. As the process continues, there is thickening of the wall of the duct and occasional retraction of the nipple. Successful treatment requires complete excision of the involved duct system, usually under general anesthesia. The location of the sinus tract is noted, cultures are taken, and the involved duct system is removed. It is important to excise the sinus tract completely. The duct system is submitted to the pathologist in a fresh condition so that a frozen section can be obtained to rule out carcinoma.

Women who have recently lactated may develop a galactocele. A mass usually is palpable and generally located in the central area of the breast. Aspiration produces a thick, creamy secretion. The diagnosis can be confirmed by ultrasonography, and no additional treatment is required. The mass or masses usually subside within a few weeks.

BENIGN NEOPLASMS

The most common benign neoplasm is the fibroadenoma. This appears predominantly in young women and presents as a firm, painless, and mobile mass. The lesions tend to be multiple but may be bilateral in 10–20% of patients. Usually they are discovered by accident. Unlike fibrocystic changes, the fibroadenoma does not change during the menstrual cycle. It may grow rapidly during adolescence, pregnancy, or menopause associated with exogenous estrogen administration. If the size of the mass increases dramatically, the possibility of a cystosarcoma phylloides or a sarcoma must be considered.

Surgical removal may be considered. The lesions do not disappear and, over a period of years, may increase in size, making removal more difficult. It may be difficult to provide medical follow-up over an extended time.

A more difficult problem occurs when multiple fibroadenomas are discovered. One solution is to perform an ultrasound examination to determine exactly how many lesions are present in each breast. Once the number of lesions has been determined, a decision can be made concerning elective removal. Nonpalpable lesions should not be removed, at least in young patients. They can be considered asymmetric densities and followed later by mammography to assess their stability. Obvious and symptomatic lesions should be removed through cosmetic incisions. However, judgment and tact are required in young patients with multiple lesions.

Lipomas usually are superficial and easily documented by mammography. They may be seen in young as well as elderly patients and can be removed with ambulatory surgery under local anesthesia.

Occasionally, patients complain of discomfort immediately beneath the nipple. A small mass is palpated, and this may represent an adenoma of the nipple, including epithelial changes in the nipple itself. Excision biopsy is required to confirm the diagnosis.

Some patients present with an irregular, tender mass. This may be related to trauma, with fat necrosis. Most patients do not recall the actual traumatic incident. The mammogram is nonspecific, as is the ultrasound scan. If there is a clear-cut history and obvious ecchymoses, a period of watchful waiting is in order. Otherwise, an open biopsy under local anesthesia should be performed.

Mondor disease or superficial angiitis may present as a distinct cord or dimpling with erythematous margins. It is a self-limited condition; however, it should be confirmed by appropriate diagnostic studies, including mammography and reexamination. If there is any uncertainty, a biopsy should be performed.

Rarely, patients present with marked breast tenderness with no antecedent history of trauma. Physical examination reveals erythema and tenderness but no edema or dominant mass. This symptomatology occasionally is associated with ipsilateral lymphadenopathy, and the mammogram is negative. The lesions resolve within a few days and probably are the result of the rupture of a large, previously undetected macrocyst that has spilled its contents throughout the breast stroma, causing chemical irritation. If there is any question and if the areas are associated with significant edema, a biopsy, including the skin, should be performed to rule out inflammatory carcinoma.

BIBLIOGRAPHY

American College of Obstetricians and Gynecologists. The role of the obstetrician–gynecologist in the diagnosis of breast disease. ACOG Committee Opinion 67. Washington, DC: ACOG, 1989

Battersby S, Anderson TJ, King RJB, Going JJ. Influence of oral contraceptives on normal breast epithelial proliferation. In: Bresciani F, Lippman ME, King RJB, Raynaud J, eds. Progress in cancer research and therapy. Vol 35: hormones and cancer, III. New York: Raven Press, 1988

Fletcher SW, O'Malley MS, Bunce LA. Physicians' abilities to detect lumps in silicone breast models. JAMA 1985;253:2224–2228

Going JJ, Anderson TJ, Battersby S, MacIntyre CC. Proliferative and secretory activity in human breast during natural and artificial menstrual cycles. Am J Pathol 1988;130:193–204

Huguley CM Jr, Brown RL, Greenberg RS, Clark WS. Breast self-examination and survival from breast cancer. Cancer 1988;62:1389–1396

Marchant DJ. Breast disease and the gynecologist. Curr Probl Obstet Gynecol Fertil 1992;15:5–37

Vaginitis

Symptoms of vulvovaginal inflammation or infection are among the most common problems encountered in gynecologic practice. Understanding of the causes of these symptoms has improved in the last decade, so that accurate diagnosis and effective treatment are usually possible.

When evaluating vaginal discharge or vulvar irritative symptoms, the clinician should consider sites other than the vagina as the source. Not all symptoms are caused by infection. For example, cervicitis often leads to an increase in discharge without irritative symptoms. Vulvovaginal infections, urethritis, and cystitis may be accompanied by the same voiding symptoms, and various dermatologic conditions may be confused with either vulvar or vaginal infections.

Normal vaginal discharge is white, nonhomogeneous, and odorless, and pools in the posterior fornix. The normal pH during the reproductive years is 3.5–4.2. The pH becomes more alkaline on exposure to semen or menstrual blood. With estrogen deficiency, the pH is usually in excess of 6. Microscopically, a normal discharge is characterized by superficial epithelial cells, flora composed of lactobacilli (long, stringlike bacteria), and occasional leukocytes. The addition of 10% potassium hydroxide to the discharge does not change the odor (the amine test).

The microbiology of the normal vaginal flora is complex. Briefly stated, it is composed of a mixture of aerobic and anaerobic organisms. Organisms that are pathogens under some circumstances, such as *Escherichia coli*, *Bacteroides fragilis*, *Staphylococcus aureus*, group B streptococci, and *Candida* species, can be found in the normal flora.

EVALUATION

In most cases, a diagnosis is based on the history, the physical examination, and the performance of simple office tests. This process is facilitated by proper timing of the office visit. Women should not use tampons or diaphragms for at least 2 days and avoid intravaginal medications for at least 5 days. In acute cases these guidelines may not be necessary. However, when the initial examination is not diagnostic, the symptoms are mild, or the problem is a chronic one that has defied previous evaluations, following this advice will improve the likelihood of establishing a diagnosis.

The principal complaints that may signal an infection are an increase in the amount of discharge, irritative symptoms (itching, burning, or dysuria), and abnormal odor. Although individual infections have characteristic symptoms, these signals are an inaccurate way to establish a diagnosis. The history should include the chronology of the current infection, associated symptoms, current and recent medications (especially antibiotics), recent medical or self-treatment, and comparison with any previous episodes. Inquiry about sexual partners is usually necessary, because they may be at risk of acquiring infection or of being part of the reinfection cycle. The review of symptoms should focus on questions relating to PID (eg, pelvic pain, fever, and exposure to sexually transmitted diseases) and urinary tract infection (eg, urinary frequency, urgency, and hematuria).

Physical examination should include careful inspection of the vulva and perirectal area, looking for nonspecific signs such as erythema, ulceration, or excoriation and for more specific lesions such as pigmentation suggesting intraepithelial neoplasia, satellite lesions (cutaneous candidiasis), condyloma acuminatum, pediculosis pubis, genital herpes, or molluscum contagiosum. No lubricant, other than warm water, should be used for the speculum examination. The color, quantity, and consistency of the vaginal discharge should be noted. Does it pool in the fornix, or does it cling to the vaginal walls? Are there signs of inflammation or discrete lesions (eg, ulceration or condyloma)? The endocervical mucus should be examined separately from the vaginal discharge. This can be accomplished by wiping the vaginal discharge from the cervix with a large swab, inserting a small cotton swab into the endocervical canal, and examining the discharge obtained on that swab. Normal endocervical mucus is either clear or white. Signs of cervicitis include easily induced contact bleeding (friability), purulent or yellow cervical mucus (mucopus), and inflammation. Tenderness of the cervix, uterus, and adnexa should be assessed by bimanual examination.

DIAGNOSIS AND MANAGEMENT

Certain diagnostic tests should be routine, while the use of others depends on the clinical presentation. Routine tests include determination of vaginal pH, microscopic examination of the vaginal discharge (the wet preparation), and the amine (whiff) test.

The vaginal pH can be determined easily by using pH indicator paper that makes distinctions of at least 0.5 U between pH 3.5–6.0. The indicator paper can be touched directly to the vaginal wall (while care is taken to avoid cervical mucus), or, after the speculum is removed, it can be dipped into the discharge collected in the lower blade.

The wet preparation can be prepared by collecting a sample of vaginal discharge on a cotton-tipped swab and then placing it in a test tube containing a small amount of room-temperature normal saline. This specimen is best examined immediately. The cotton swab can be used to transfer several drops of the saline mixture onto a glass microscope slide. A coverslip should be placed on the slide, and the slide should be examined under both low and high powers. Several high-power fields should be systematically examined to characterize the epithelial calls, the predominant flora, the number of leucocytes, and the presence of any pathogens.

A 10–20% potassium hydroxide preparation should also be examined. A drop of potassium hydroxide can be added to the edge of the original coverslip, or a second slide can be made and potassium hydroxide added directly to the discharge before placing the coverslip on the slide. As the potassium hydroxide is added, the examiner should note whether a "fishy" odor is released (the amine test).

Other tests that should be performed selectively include cultures or rapid tests for gonorrhea, chlamydia, or herpes; urinalysis and culture; culture for *Candida* species; and Gram stain of the vaginal or cervical discharge. Occasionally, a colposcopic examination or a vulvar, vaginal, or cervical biopsy specimen may be indicated. Aerobic or anaerobic cultures of the vagina are virtually never indicated.

Excessive Discharge

Some women report a chronic vaginal discharge that has been treated on several occasions for a diagnosis of nonspecific vaginitis, yet they have a normal vaginal discharge according to all the aforementioned criteria. This condition has been referred to as normal but excessive physiologic vaginal discharge.

The diagnostic approach to excessive discharge should include careful clinical examination of the vulva and vagina, assessment of vaginal pH, and microscopic examination of the discharge. A culture for *Candida* species is helpful if the patient complains of irritation or itching, since the wet preparation is relatively insensitive with mild symptoms. Cervical cultures for chlamydia and gonorrhea should be performed, as cervicitis is associated with increased secretions. If these tests are negative, it is helpful to reexamine the patient during a different part of her menstrual cycle or when the symptoms intensify. There is no specific therapy for this problem, but most women feel reassured by the knowledge that infection is not present.

Bacterial Vaginosis

In the past, bacterial vaginosis has been known as nonspecific vaginitis and *Gardnerella* vaginitis. The latter name reflects Gardner's pioneering work in describing the infection and identifying the organism. The current name reflects the growing recognition that bacteria in addition to *Gardnerella* species are involved. Current information suggests that the flora, which is usually predominately aerobic lactobacilli, is dominated by anaerobic lactobacilli and various obligate anaerobic species (including *Bacteroides* species, *Mobiluncus* species, and anaerobic cocci), along with *Gardnerella vaginalis*. Overall, the concentration of total bacteria in the vagina increases at least 100-fold. Despite these dramatic alterations in the flora, there is little inflammatory response. One of the metabolic byproducts of the new flora is an increase in the metabolic production of certain amines. These chemicals can cause mucosal irritation and, when alkalinized, release the characteristic fishy odor.

Depending on the population characteristics, 5–30% of women of reproductive age have asymptomatic bacterial vaginosis. It is found more often in women who are sexually active, who use an IUD or barrier method, and who have multiple sexual partners. It can occur in women of all ages, and after hysterectomy.

Although bacterial vaginosis is seen more often in women who are sexually active, the role of sexual transmission has not been clearly defined. Treatment of male sexual partners has not been shown to improve the cure rate or to reduce the risk of recurrence. Bacterial vaginosis occurs in women who have never had sexual relations or who are in stable, monogamous relationships.

Symptomatic bacterial vaginosis is characterized by a malodorous vaginal discharge that is sometimes accompanied by mild itching or burning. Symptoms may worsen after menses or intercourse. The vaginal discharge is homogeneous, gray-green, and often frothy.

In addition to the appearance of the discharge, the following criteria are used to establish the diagnosis: 20% or more clue cells, background flora consisting of small rods and cocci (and, as a corollary, reduced or absent lactobacilli), pH 5–5.5, and a positive amine test. Clue cells are defined as epithelial cells with bacteria attached so that the border of the cell is obscured. Culture for *G. vaginalis* is not useful and, in fact, will lead to overdiagnosis, since as few as half of the women with a positive culture meet the diagnostic criteria for the infection.

The symptomatic, nonpregnant woman should be treated. There is no consensus on the advisability of treating the asymptomatic woman. Because there appears to be an increased risk of upper genital tract infection in women with bacterial vaginosis who undergo surgical procedures, therapy should be considered in the asymptomatic woman prior to an invasive procedure such as endometrial biopsy, hysteroscopy, IUD insertion, or hysterectomy.

An association between bacterial vaginosis and several pregnancy-related complications, including premature labor, premature rupture of membranes, chorioamnionitis, and postpartum endometritis, has been found. However, there is no consensus on the need to treat symptomatic bacterial vaginosis during pregnancy. Also, there are insufficient data to recommend routine treatment of male sexual partners, although this may be considered in cases of frequently recurring infection.

Metronidazole and clindamycin are superior to topical sulfa cream, ampicillin, erythromycin, and tetracycline for treatment of this disorder. For metronidazole, the usual treatment is 500 mg twice daily for 7 days. A recent metaanalysis of published treatment trials found no difference in short-term cure rates for a single 2-g dose or for 2 g/d for 2 days, 5 days, or 7 days of therapy. Long-term differences between these regimens have not been studied. There are fewer data on oral clindamycin, but a dosage of 300 mg twice daily for 7 days has been shown to have a short-term cure rate in excess of 90%. Effective intravaginal therapy with these two agents is now available. Metronidazole gel is administered in a dosage of 400 mg twice daily for 7 days, and 2% clindamycin cream is given as a 5-g dosage once daily for 7 days.

Recurrence is common and poses a difficult management problem. Because it is not always desirable to administer antibiotics repeatedly, other sources of symptomatic relief may be considered. An acidifying agent may help to reduce the odor associated with the infection. A douche with 1.5% hydrogen peroxide has been recommended. Povidine–iodine vaginal pessaries, used twice daily for 14 days, may be useful. If semen appears to be an exacerbating factor, use of a condom may be helpful.

Trichomoniasis

Trichomoniasis makes up 5–10% of all vaginal infections. Although management of this problem is usually straightforward, both diagnostic and therapeutic dilemmas occasionally arise. The infectious agent is *Trichomonas vaginalis,* a motile unicellular protozoan. The pathophysiology of this infection is incompletely understood. It appears that the organism releases toxins that, in part, disrupt the epithelial lining of the vagina, resulting in a host inflammatory response. There may be differences in toxin production among various strains that account for the wide range of symptom severity seen in clinical practice.

Trichomoniasis is usually sexually transmitted, although it has been reported in women who have never had sexual relations. The female-to-male transmission risk is estimated to be 80%. The spectrum of disease includes both acute and chronic infection. The latter is difficult to diagnose because the *Trichomonas* organism is difficult to identify on a wet preparation. Recently, *T. vaginalis* has been associated with preterm rupture of membranes, preterm labor, and postsurgical infections. There is also an ill-defined relationship between *T. vaginalis* and HPV, such that some women have both condyloma and vaginal trichomoniasis. In these women, the condyloma may resolve after metronidazole therapy for the trichomoniasis.

The acute onset of intense, irritative symptoms and an increase in vaginal discharge signal acute trichomoniasis. Clinical examination reveals an abundant, sometimes frothy, gray–green, and homogeneous discharge. Clinical signs are similar to those of bacterial vaginosis except that there is commonly evidence of inflammation. The classic finding is the "strawberry" cervix, which is seen in only a small number of cases with the naked eye but in almost all cases with the colposcope.

The pH of the vaginal discharge exceeds 4.5. The wet preparation shows parabasal and basal epithelial cells from the deep layers of the disrupted squamous epithelium. The background flora is replaced by rods and cocci, and more leukocytes are present than epithelial cells. In contrast to bacterial vaginosis, there are few if any clue cells. These changes are all reflective of the underlying inflammatory process. The *Trichomonas* organism (which is slightly larger than a leukocyte and has four flagella) is usually obvious. In chronic cases, however, the organism may be round and relatively immotile, thus resembling a leukocyte.

Studies in which wet preparation identification of the trichomonad has been compared with culture diagnosis suggest that the wet preparation is 60–97% sensitive. Asymptomatic and minimally symptomatic cases are more likely to have a negative result on the wet preparation. The organism becomes nonmotile below room temperature and is very sensitive to ionic concentration, so it is critical that room-temperature physiologic saline be used for dilution of the wet preparation. Cultures are not commonly performed, in part because the medium required (eg, Diamond or Feinberg–Whittington medium) is not widely available, and up to 1 week is needed for final results. Monoclonal antibody tests are being developed that may be more practical and that may allow for a more accurate diagnosis in women with a suspected *Trichomonas* infection who have negative results on wet preparations.

Cytologic findings consistent with the *Trichomonas* organism may be found with a Pap test. Because the sensitivity of Pap test diagnosis is only 50%, cytology alone is not sufficient for the diagnosis of symptomatic infections. However, the more common clinical dilemma is deciding what action to take when the Pap test analysis of an asymptomatic woman returns showing a possible *Trichomonas* infection. The positive predictive value of the Pap test (the percentage of cases in which the cytologic findings correctly predict an infection) in a patient population with an average prevalence of infection is low (approximately 40%). Therefore, when this finding is reported, a clinical examination should be performed to determine whether treatment is necessary.

The *Trichomonas* organism is usually highly sensitive to metronidazole. Either a short course (250 mg three times daily for 7 days or 500 mg twice daily for 5 days) or a single dose of 2 g can be used. Patients should be warned about the disulfiramlike effect that can lead to nausea and vomiting if alcohol is taken concomitantly. Ideally, the patient should be reexamined to be sure that the infection has cleared. Although 80% of male partners acquire the organism during sexual contact with an infected women, 60% spontaneously revert to negative within 2 weeks of exposure. Sexual transmission between women has not been studied but theoretically can occur. Currently, the usual clinical practice is to treat sexual partners with one of the same regimens used for the patient.

The management of *Trichomonas* infection during pregnancy is essentially the same as that described previously. The safety of metronidazole in the first trimester has not been established. Even though no specific teratogenic risk has been established, treatment should be postponed until the second trimester if the patient's symptoms are mild. If the symptoms in the first trimester are severe, intravaginal clotrimazole given for 1 week may be helpful.

A strain of *T. vaginalis* that is relatively resistant to metronidazole has been reported. It is still rare, but it should be suspected in a woman who has taken the 7-day course of metronidazole, has not been reinfected, and yet has a persistent infection. The initial approach should be to retreat the woman with the usual dose, but if there is still no improvement, culture with sensitivity testing should be considered. So far, all of the women infected with the resistant species have eventually responded to metronidazole, although they sometimes require high doses given intravenously (IV).

Candidiasis

Candida vulvovaginitis is the second most common vaginal infection, and the lifetime risk of at least one episode has been estimated to be 75%. Most cases are caused by *Candida albicans*; the remainder, about 20%, are caused by *Candida glabrata* (formerly *Torulopsis glabrata*) and *Candida tropicalis*. These latter two strains may be relatively resistant to the commonly used imidazole antifungal agents, and therefore they must be considered in cases of persistent and recurrent infections.

Risk factors include pregnancy, antibiotic use, systemic antibiotic or corticosteroid use, diabetes, and immunosuppressive disorders (including AIDS), although most women with sporadic infections do not have any of these risk factors. There is controversy over the effect of OC use. While OC users may be more likely to be colonized with *Candida* species, it is not clear that they are more likely to develop acute infections. Because estrogen appears to encourage the growth of *Candida* species, low-dose OCs may be less likely to be a cofactor than high-dose ones. There is no reason to discontinue the use of OCs simply for a single acute infection. For women with recurrent infections, the contraceptive needs of the woman must be considered before recommending discontinuation of the drug. Although in most cases this infection is not acquired via sexual transmission, male partners may acquire the organism and may be a source of reinfection.

Vaginal candidiasis presents with the acute onset of itching and burning but with minimal vaginal discharge. Dysuria is common and is characteristically described as burning of the vulva during urination (vulvar dysuria). Clinical examination may reveal erythema and adherent patches of white discharge on the vulva and the vaginal walls (thrush patches), although these signs appear in less than one half of patients with the infection. Candidiasis should be suspected if the appropriate symptoms are present, even if the findings of the examination are normal. Conversely, candidiasis is often mistakenly suspected in women who have a heavy "curdlike" discharge and no other symptoms; if pruritus is absent, candidiasis is unlikely.

The vaginal pH is most often 4.5 or less, although *Candida* species can grow at a higher pH and may be present with either bacterial vaginosis or trichomoniasis. The wet preparation shows normal superficial epithelial cells, normal background lactobacilli, and few leukocytes. *C. albicans* typically appears in its mycelial form, although spores may be present as well. *C. tropicalis* also forms hyphae and is indistinguishable from *C. albicans* by microscopic examination. However, *C. glabrata* forms spores that are about half the size of erythrocytes, and on wet preparation they are often seen in clusters. The addition of 10–20% potassium hydroxide to the wet preparation will dissolve epithelial cells and blood cells, making the *Candida* organisms easier to identify.

The wet preparation has a sensitivity of only 80%, and so it may be negative when an infection is present. Therefore, if *Candida* organisms are not demonstrated but the patient is symptomatic, a culture should be obtained. The Pap test is relatively insensitive as a diagnostic test. Because *Candida* organisms commonly colonize the vagina without causing symptoms, however, treatment should not be recommended merely on the basis of a positive culture in the absence of symptoms.

C. albicans can be treated with 1% gentian violet, nystatin, or one of the newer antifungal agents. Because the topically applied imidazole or triazole agents (miconazole, clotrimazole, butoconazole, and terconazole) are superior to nystatin and are easier to administer than is gentian violet, these agents are the usual treatment of choice. The effectiveness rates of the three drugs are similar; both creams and suppositories are available, and it appears to make little difference which form is chosen. The duration of treatment depends on the specific drug. Women should be encouraged to finish the complete course of treatment to reduce the risk of relapse. When there is vulvar inflammation, the addition of a cream combined with a corticosteroid will reduce symptoms more rapidly.

Systemic therapy with ketoconazole is not recommended for uncomplicated acute vaginal infections because there is the potential for hepatotoxicity, the cure rates are similar to those with topical therapy, and the therapy is more expensive. This drug may be useful for the occasional patient who is unable to use a vaginal therapy. Routine treatment of asymptomatic sexual partners is not indicated. There is no evidence of teratogenicity, and these topical agents are commonly prescribed during pregnancy. Common sense suggests that their use should be minimized during the first trimester; care should be taken with the use of the vaginal applicator during the later stages of pregnancy. This infection may require a longer course of therapy during pregnancy.

Frequently recurring candidiasis is a difficult management problem. Each of the following five factors has a potential role:

1. Relapse from incomplete treatment of the primary infection—This may occur when treatment is stopped prematurely.
2. Infection with a strain resistant to the treatment used—Some strains of *C. tropicalis* are resistant, and *C. glabrata* may require a dose several times higher than that required for *C. albicans*. A culture will help to identify these species.
3. A defect in host defense—Most women with recurrent candidiasis do not have any of the classic risk factors but instead have subtle immunologic defects that reduce the host defenses specifically against *Candida* species.
4. Autoinoculation from an extravaginal reservoir—The gastrointestinal tract may be the primary site. Support for this concept comes from a multicenter European study in which improved cure rates in patients with acute infections were obtained with a combination of topical imidazole and oral nystatin. Other studies have not confirmed benefits of treating the gastrointestinal tract.
5. Reinfection from a sexual partner—Sources of *Candida* can be the mouth, rectum, and ejaculate. However, treatment of the male partner has not resulted in improved cure rates in women with recurrent infections in most clinical trials.

While a permanent cure may prove elusive, control can be achieved by using one of several approaches. These include the use of a longer course of treatment for acute infections; the use of a prophylactic topical imidazole premenstrually, if that is a time of recurrence, and during periods of antibiotic use; discontinuation of OCs; and treatment of the sexual partner if the partner's culture is positive. If these methods do not result in a long-term improvement, the patient may need to use a topical imidazole twice weekly for several months or years. Alternatively, low-dose daily ketoconazole (eg, 100 mg for 6 months) may be effective. Patients must be aware of the potential for a rare (1/100,000) idiosyncratic hepatotoxicity. Unfortunately, although these regimens control infection while the drug is taken, they do not usually result in long-term elimination of the problem.

Atrophic Vaginitis

Postmenopausal women may suffer from any of the aforementioned infections; they may also have a specific estrogen deficiency-related vaginitis. Symptoms are primarily irritative and are often accompanied by vaginal dryness and dyspareunia. The vaginal epithelium appears thin, with a watery yellow discharge. The pH exceeds 6 (as it does in all estrogen-deficient women whether or not they have symptoms). The wet preparation shows numerous leukocytes, along with basal epithelial cells and a background flora of rods and cocci. The most effective treatment is either topical or oral estrogen. After several weeks of daily topical therapy, the frequency can be reduced to two or three times weekly.

Desquamative Vaginitis

The uncommon disorder of desquamative vaginitis, which appears to be a variation of lichen planus, presents with chronic vaginal discharge and dyspareunia. Examination shows ulceration, usually at the apex of the vagina, and sometimes there is partial coaptation. Wet preparation shows numerous leukocytes and decreased lactobacilli. A herpes culture and vaginal biopsy may be needed to rule out other disorders. Characteristic lichen planus lesions are often seen in the mouth. Intravaginal steroid cream for at least 2 weeks may be effective. Recurrence rates are high, and retreatment may be necessary.

Foreign-Body Vaginitis

The most common foreign body is a forgotten tampon. Once other infections are ruled out, no treatment, other than removal of the object, is usually necessary. Washing of the vagina with povidone–iodine during the office visit may reduce the odor more quickly, but antibiotic treatment is not usually needed. Ulceration is uncommon, but biopsy is not needed unless there are persistent ulcers.

BIBLIOGRAPHY

Biswas MK. Bacterial vaginosis. Clin Obstet Gynecol 1993;36:166–176

Ernest JM. Topical antifungal agents. Obstet Gynecol Clin North Am 1992;19:587–607

Graves A, Gardner WA Jr. Pathogenicity of Trichomonas vaginalis. Clin Obstet Gynecol 1993;36:145–152

Grossman JH 3d, Galask RP. Persistent vaginitis caused by metronidazole-resistant trichomonas. Obstet Gynecol 1990;76:521–522

Kurki T, Sivonen A, Renkonen OV, Savia E, Ylikorkala O. Bacterial vaginosis in early pregnancy and pregnancy outcome. Obstet Gynecol 1992;80:173–177

Larsson PG, Platz-Christensen JJ, Thejls H, Forsum U, Pahlson C. Incidence of pelvic inflammatory disease after first-trimester legal abortion in women with bacterial vaginosis after treatment with metronidazole: a double-blind, randomized study. Am J Obstet Gynecol 1992;166:100–103

Lugo-Miro VI, Green M, Mazur L. Comparison of different metronidazole therapeutic regimens for bacterial vaginosis: a meta-analysis. JAMA 1992;268:92–95

Reed BD. Risk factors for Candida vulvovaginitis. Obstet Gynecol Surv 1992;47:551–560

Schmitt C, Sobel JD, Meriwether C. Bacterial vaginosis: treatment with clindamycin cream versus oral metronidazole. Obstet Gynecol 1992;79:1020–1023

Thomason JL, Gelbart SM, Scaglione NJ. Bacterial vaginosis: current review with indications for asymptomatic therapy. Am J Obstet Gynecol 1991;165:1210–1217

Sexually Transmitted Diseases

BACTERIAL DISEASES

Chlamydia trachomatis is the most prevalent bacterial sexually transmitted infection in the United States today. Many sexually active women have been exposed to this organism; 20–40% have chlamydial antibodies. The prevalence of *C. trachomatis* in the endocervix of asymptomatic women ranges from 3% to 26%, and its prevalence among symptomatic women is higher than that of *Neisseria gonorrhoeae*. *C. trachomatis* is especially prevalent in teenaged patients in urban adolescent medical clinics. The high prevalence of *C. trachomatis* is due to several factors: most infected women have minimal or no symptoms, the incubation period is long (mean, 10 days), a persistent carrier state exists, and women are unlikely to be treated unless a male sexual partner develops a symptomatic infection.

In many respects, the epidemiologies of *C. trachomatis* and *N. gonorrhoeae* are similar; indeed, about 25–40% of women with gonococcal infections have a concomitant chlamydial infection, which has important implications for treatment.

Since 1975, the number of reported cases of gonorrhea in the United States has stabilized, with a total of about 1 million cases reported annually. The highest age-specific rates of gonorrhea in women occur among those aged 20–24; women who are members of minority groups have higher reported rates than do Caucasian women.

In 1983, the first U.S. outbreak of penicillin-resistant *N. gonorrhoeae* that did not produce penicillinase was reported; this resistance is presumably chromosomally mediated. Penicillinase-negative isolates from patients in whom recommended therapy has failed should be screened by laboratories for penicillin susceptibility, preferably by the disk diffusion method.

There has been a recent increase in the incidence of syphilis. Between 1985 and 1990, new cases of syphilis totaled 50,223, representing a 75% increase in the incidence of disease. These rates, however, were not geographically or racially uniform. Rates are highest in the southeastern United States and in Texas, although changes have been reported nationwide. The rates for African–Americans have increased dramatically, while rates for other subgroups have remained relatively stable.

The AIDS epidemic and the concomitant epidemic of illegal drug usage, particularly crack cocaine, have coincided with the recent surge in syphilis. Behavioral changes in the mid-1980s among homosexual men, mainly in response to AIDS, have led to a decline in the incidence of syphilis in this population with a resultant decrease in the male–female ratio of cases. Exchange of sex for drugs or money contributes greatly to risk of syphilis, and the association between syphilis and drug use makes partners difficult to trace and adequately treat.

Chlamydial Infection

The most common manifestations of chlamydial infections in women are mucopurulent cervicitis and salpingitis. The endocervix is the most frequent site of infection, which results in a hypertrophic appearance of the cervix and a mucopurulent discharge. *C. trachomatis* infection appears to be common in women with ectropion of the cervix; since OCs induce ectropion of the cervix, this may account for the association between OCs and lower-tract *C. trachomatis* infection.

The second principal chlamydial infection is salpingitis. Both culture results and serologic evidence implicate *C. trachomatis* as an etiologic agent in acute salpingitis. The microbiology of salpingitis is complex, however; the contribution of *C. trachomatis* to acute salpingitis has not been accurately measured.

A less common manifestation is the acute urethral syndrome, which is defined as the acute onset of dysuria and frequency of urination in women whose urine is either sterile or contains fewer than 10^5 bacteria per milliliter. *C. trachomatis* is an important cause of this syndrome. In addition to these infections, *C. trachomatis* is also associated with the Fitz–Hugh–Curtis syndrome, postpartum endometritis, and infertility.

Diagnosis

The lack of an inexpensive and rapid diagnostic test for *C. trachomatis* has been a major obstacle in the diagnosis and treatment of chlamydial infections. Serologic tests cannot be used reliably to diagnose *C. trachomatis* infections, since many women have antibodies from previous infections. Culturing of *C. trachomatis* on cycloheximide-treated McCoy cells is the most sensitive means of diagnosis; this procedure is expensive and laborious, and the delay of diagnosis is not optimal.

Two alternatives to cell culture are available for standard use. One approach is an enzyme-linked immunoassay. The second test is a direct antigen-detection system in which monoclonal antibodies are used. Refinement of antigen-detection systems and enzyme immunoassays over the last several years has improved their sensitivity and specificity such that their use in populations with high prevalence rates is justified. In low-prevalence populations, however, predictive values of positive results will be unacceptably low. Other diagnostic techniques recently used include nucleic acid probes specific for chlamydia and gene amplification using the polymerase chain reaction. Many clinicians feel that the polymerase chain reaction will ultimately become the modality of choice for diagnosing chlamydial infections.

Treatment

The recommended regimen for treatment of uncomplicated urethral, endocervical, and rectal infections is as follows:

- Doxycycline, 100 mg orally twice daily for 7 days, or
- Azithromycin, 1 g orally in a single dose

Alternative treatments for uncomplicated infections include:

- Ofloxacin, 300 mg orally twice daily for 7 days, or
- Erythromycin base, 500 mg orally four times daily for 7 days, or
- Erythromycin ethylsuccinate, 800 mg orally four times daily for 7 days, or
- Sulfisoxazole, 500 mg orally four times daily for 10 days

Ofloxacin is not recommended for treating adolescents aged 17 years or younger nor for pregnant women. The efficacy of sulfisoxazole is inferior to that of other regimens.

Because the antimicrobial resistance of *C. trachomatis* to the recommended regimens has not been observed, test-of-cure evaluation is not necessary when treatment has been completed. Exceptions would include inadequate treatment of sexual partners and patients with persistent symptoms.

Sexual partners of patients with *C. trachomatis* infection within the previous 30 days should be tested for *C. trachomatis*. If testing is not available, they should be treated with the appropriate antimicrobial regimen.

Infections During Pregnancy

Diagnostic testing for *C. trachomatis* should be considered during pregnancy, based on risk factors. Women who are at high risk (age less than 25 years, a history or presence of another sexually transmitted disease, a new sexual partner within the past 3 months, or multiple sexual partners) should be tested during the third trimester. Ideally, pregnant women with gonorrhea should be treated for *C. trachomatis* on the basis of diagnostic studies, but if chlamydial testing is not available, then treatment should be given because of the high likelihood of coinfection.

The recommended regimen is erythromycin base, 500 mg four times daily for 7 days. If this is not tolerated, the following regimens are recommended:

- Erythromycin base, 250 mg four times daily for 14 days, or
- Erythromycin ethylsuccinate, 800 mg four times daily for 7 days, or
- Erythromycin ethylsuccinate, 400 mg four times daily for 14 days

Azithromycin has not yet been tested in pregnancy but likely will become a drug of choice. The alternative therapy if erythromycin cannot be tolerated is amoxicillin, 500 mg orally three times daily for 7–10 days. Erythromycin estolate is contraindicated during pregnancy, as drug-related hepatotoxicity, although rare, can occur when the drug is administered during pregnancy. Ofloxacin and other quinolone antibiotics are contraindicated during pregnancy.

Gonorrhea

Gonorrhea can lead to a complex spectrum of diseases. In women, the primary infection usually occurs in the cervix, although sites such as the urethra, rectum, and pharynx can be infected. Gonorrhea can remain localized, can ascend to the upper genital tract (salpingitis or PID), or can spread through the circulation (disseminated gonococcal infection).

Because 40–60% of young women with gonorrhea have symptoms, gonorrhea may be less "silent" than previously thought. The infection can lead to increased vaginal discharge from a purulent cervicitis, and it can also cause dysuria and frequent urination.

Diagnosis

The presumptive diagnosis of a cervical gonococcal infection may be based on an endocervical culture, Gram stain, or identification of gonococcal enzymes, antigens, fragments, or nucleic acids in genital secretions. The endocervical culture with selective culture media remains the cornerstone of diagnosis. The sensitivity of a single endocervical culture is usually about 80–90%; this yield is improved only slightly by a simultaneous second endocervical culture or a rectal culture. Cultures from extragenital sites, especially the pharynx, should be confirmed by a biochemical or immunologic test.

Gram stain evaluation of endocervical bacteria provides the only immediate laboratory information on which to base clinical decisions. This simple diagnostic test is probably underused. When carefully prepared and examined for gram-negative intracellular diplococci by an experienced microscopist, this test has a moderate sensitivity (50–70%) but a high specificity (97%). Use of the Gram stain enables a larger proportion of patients to be treated at the time of the initial visit.

Treatment of gonococcal infections in the United States is influenced by the following trends: 1) the spread of infection caused by antibiotic-resistant *N. gonorrhoeae*, including penicillinase-producing *N. gonorrhoeae*, tetracycline-resistant *N. gonorrhoeae*, and strains with chromosomally mediated resistance to multiple antibiotics; 2) the high frequency of chlamydial infections in persons with gonorrhea; and 3) recognition of the serious complications of chlamydial and gonococcal infections. All cases of gonorrhea should be diagnosed or confirmed by culture to facilitate antimicrobial susceptibility testing. The susceptibility of *N. gonorrhoeae* to antibiotics is likely to change over time in any locality. Therefore, gonorrhea control programs should develop a procedure of regular antibiotic sensitivity testing of a surveillance sample of *N. gonorrhoeae* isolates, as well as samples of all isolates associated with treatment failures. Because of the wide spectrum of antimicrobial therapies that are effective against *N. gonorrhoeae*, the following guidelines are not intended to be a comprehensive list of all possible treatment regimens.

Treatment

Single-dose efficacy is a major consideration in choosing an antibiotic regimen to treat uncomplicated urethral, endocervical, and rectal *N. gonorrhoeae* infections. Another important concern is coexisting chlamydial infection, which has been documented in up to 45% of patients with gonorrhea. In some populations if chlamydial testing is not readily available it is generally more cost-effective to treat presumptive chlamydial infections in all persons with gonorrhea. Simultaneous treatment of all gonorrhea infections with antibiotics that are effective against both *C. trachomatis* and *N. gonorrhoeae* may lessen the possibility of gonorrhea treatment failure because of antibiotic resistance.

The recommended regimen is ceftriaxone, 125 mg intramuscularly (IM) once, plus doxycycline, 100 mg orally twice daily for 7 days. Some authorities prefer a dose of 250 mg of ceftriaxone IM because theoretically it may delay the emergence of ceftriaxone-resistant strains, but the Centers for Disease Control and Prevention (CDC) now recommends the 125-mg dose. At this time, both doses appear to be highly effective for mucosal gonorrhea at all sites. Some practitioners mix 1% lidocaine (without epinephrine) with ceftriaxone to reduce the discomfort associated with the injection. No adverse reactions have been associated with the use of lidocaine diluent.

Other recommended treatments include ciprofloxacin, 500 mg orally once; cefixime, 400 mg orally once; and ofloxacin, 400 mg orally once. Oral therapy may be optimal in that needle-stick exposure is avoided. All of these regimens are followed by azithromycin, 1 g orally once, or doxycycline, 100 mg orally twice daily for 7 days. If infection was acquired from a source that was proven not to have penicillin-resistant gonorrhea, a penicillin such as amoxicillin, 3 g orally, with probenecid, 1 g, followed by oral azithromycin or doxycycline, may be used for treatment. Doxycycline and azithromycin are not considered adequate therapy for gonococcal infections, but they are added for the treatment of coexisting chlamydial infections.

Tetracycline may be substituted for doxycycline; however, compliance may decrease, since tetracycline must be taken in a dosage of 500 mg four times daily between meals, while doxycycline is taken in a dosage of 100 mg twice daily without regard to meals. Moreover, at current prices, tetracycline is not significantly less expensive than generic doxycycline.

For patients who cannot take a tetracycline (eg, pregnant women), erythromycin may be substituted (erythromycin base or stearate, 500 mg orally four times daily for 7 days, or erythromycin ethylsuccinate, 800 mg orally four times daily for 7 days).

Patients with an uncomplicated pharyngeal gonococcal infection should be treated with ceftriaxone, 125 mg IM once. Patients who cannot be treated with ceftriaxone should be treated with ciprofloxacin, 500 mg orally as a single dose. Since experience with this regimen is limited, such patients should be evaluated with a repeated culture 3–7 days after treatment.

All patients diagnosed with gonorrhea should have a serologic test for syphilis and should be offered confidential testing for HIV infection. Most patients with incubating syphilis (those who are seronegative and have no clinical signs of syphilis) may be cured by any of the regimens containing β-lactams (ceftriaxone) or tetracyclines. Spectinomycin and the quinolones (ciprofloxacin and norfloxacin) have not been shown to be active against incubating syphilis. Patients who are treated with these drugs should be monitored with a serologic test for syphilis in 1 month.

Persons exposed to gonorrhea within the preceding 30 days should be examined, and a sample should be obtained for culture; they should be treated presumptively.

Follow-up

Treatment failure following combined ceftriaxone–doxycycline therapy is likely to be rare; therefore, a follow-up culture (test of cure) is not essential. In many instances, a more cost-effective strategy may be to reexamine the patient by the culture method 1–2 months after treatment (rescreening); this strategy detects both treatment failures and reinfections. Patients should be advised to return for an examination if any symptoms persist at the completion of treatment.

Symptoms that persist after treatment should be evaluated by obtaining cultures for *N. gonorrhoeae*, and any gonococcal isolate should be tested for antibiotic susceptibility. Symptoms of urethritis may also be caused by *C. trachomatis* and other organisms associated with nongonococcal urethritis. Additional treatment for gonorrhea should be ceftriaxone, 250 mg, followed by doxycycline. Infections that occur after treatment with one of the recommended regimens are commonly due to reinfection rather than treatment failure and indicate a need for improved sexual partner referral and patient education.

Infections During Pregnancy

Samples for culture for *N. gonorrhoeae* may be obtained from pregnant women at the first prenatal visit based on their risk factors. A second culture for gonorrhea (as well as tests for chlamydia and syphilis) should be obtained late in the third trimester in women at high risk for these sexually transmitted diseases..

Ideally, pregnant women with gonorrhea should be treated for chlamydia on the basis of chlamydial diagnostic study results. If chlamydial diagnostic testing is not available, then treatment for chlamydia should be given. Tetracyclines (including doxycycline) and the quinolones are contraindicated during pregnancy because of the possibility of adverse effects on the fetus.

The recommended treatment regimen is ceftriaxone, 125 mg IM once. Erythromycin, in the dosage listed in "Treatment," is the recognized treatment for presumptive or diagnosed chlamydia in pregnancy.

Pregnant women who are allergic to β-lactam antibiotics should be treated with spectinomycin, 2.0 g IM once (followed by erythromycin). Follow-up cervical and rectal cultures for *N. gonorrhoeae* should be obtained 3–7 days after the completion of treatment

Syphilis

It is thought that approximately one third of patients exposed to early syphilis will acquire the disease. Primary, usually painless, lesions (chancres) will develop about 21 days after exposure (range, 10–90 days). Within a few weeks to several months after the primary lesion, secondary syphilis resulting from widespread hematogenous and lymphatic dissemination develops. This is characterized by low-grade fever, malaise, sore throat, headache, adenopathy, and the cutaneous or mucosal rash. This is the stage in which the classic rash on the soles of the feet or palms of the hands is present. If untreated, patients enter a variable period of latency followed by development of tertiary syphilis in 15–40% of patients. The most common manifestation of tertiary syphilis is benign latent syphilis (gumma) affecting mostly skin, bone, and mucosa. The more serious cardiovascular and neurologic manifestations of tertiary syphilis occur in approximately 5–20% of patients.

The rise of infection in female patients has led to an increased incidence of congenital syphilis. Untreated patients with primary or secondary disease have a vertical transmission risk of approximately 50%. Half of these patients will deliver preterm or have a stillbirth. Early latent syphilis transmission rates are approximately 40%, but only 20% of these pregnancies result in preterm delivery or perinatal mortality. Late syphilis has a frequency of transmission of 10%, and there is no increase in preterm delivery or perinatal mortality.

Diagnosis

Serologic testing is the technique most widely used for the diagnosis of syphilis. For screening, the quantitative nontreponemal reaginic tests, such as the Venereal Disease Research Laboratory test or the rapid plasma reagin test, are used. These tests become positive shortly after patients enter the primary stage and climb to their highest levels during the secondary or early latent stages. Importantly, as many as 25% of Venereal Disease Research Laboratory tests may become nonreactive in patients with late syphilis.

As numerous conditions cause false-positive reaginic and nontreponemal tests, confirmation is required with specific treponemal testing. These include the fluorescent treponemal antibody absorption test, and the microhemagglutination assay for *Treponema pallidum*. Although these tests are slightly more sensitive and considerably more specific, they are more expensive and technically more demanding and therefore are not used for screening. One circumstance under which they can be especially useful is when early primary syphilis is suspected and the reaginic tests are negative. This is because the treponemal tests are positive before the screening tests.

Treatment

The goals of therapy in syphilis are to prevent transmission and avoid the late complications. Penicillins are the best studied and are considered the treatment of choice for syphilis. Depot preparations are preferred because of ease of administration, decreased expense, and the fact that in early stages they do not require readministration. Primary, secondary, and early latent disease are treated with benzathine penicillin, 2.4 million U IM one time. This regimen is also used for sexual contacts of persons with infectious syphilis. Late latent syphilis or syphilis of unknown duration is treated with the same dose of benzathine penicillin, but it is repeated for 2 successive weeks for a total of three doses. As benzathine penicillin may fail to produce treponemicidal concentration in cerebrospinal fluid, neurosyphilis is treated with aqueous crystalline penicillin G, 12 million–24 million U/d IV (2 million–4 million U every 4 hours) for 10–14 days. Alternatively, penicillin G procaine, 2 million–4 million U/d IM, plus probenecid, 500 mg orally four times daily, for 10–14 days may be used.

Treatment of patients allergic to penicillin involves use of other antibiotics that may require administration of multiple doses. Efficacy will depend on compliance. If taken appropriately, doxycycline is as efficacious while erythromycin has higher failure rates. Use of first-generation cephalosporins, ceftriaxone, and amoxicillin has been encouraging, but more information is needed before routine use can be recommended.

All pregnant women should be tested for syphilis during their first prenatal visit. Penicillin is the drug of choice for treatment during pregnancy. Treatment guidelines are the same as for nonpregnant patients. As tetracyclines are contraindicated during pregnancy and erythromycin provides inadequate treatment for the fetus, a patient who is allergic to penicillin should be hospitalized and desensitization should be attempted.

After adequate treatment, serial Venereal Disease Research Laboratory or rapid plasma reagin titers should be followed. Titers will decline more rapidly in patients at earlier stages of infection, in those with low titers at initiation of therapy, and in patients without a previous history of syphilis. A decline of two or more serial dilutions after appropriate therapy has classically been used to define therapeutic efficacy. Recent data, however, suggest that a fourfold titer decrease at 6 months and an eightfold decrease at 12 months may better define treatment success.

VIRAL DISEASES

Herpes Simplex Virus Infection

There are two major types of HSV: HSV type 1 (HSV-1) and HSV-2. Multiple strains of each virus type exist. About 50% of the DNA sequences of HSV-1 and HSV-2 are the same. Herpes simplex virus type 2 is thought to be the major etiologic agent in 80% of patients with genital herpes, with HSV-1 being the agent for the other 20%. The virus is widespread, and greater than 70% of women have serologic evidence of prior exposure to one or both HSV types. Exposure to HSV-1 occurs in early childhood, and exposure to HSV-2 occurs after sexual activity has begun, with peak incidence occurring at ages 14–30.

Humans are the sole natural host for HSV. Transmission of the virus occurs by the genital–genital, genital–oral, and oral–oral routes. On rare occasions, transmission may occur by contact with fomites that have been freshly contaminated with infected body fluids.

Of the 150 million people in the United States who are thought to harbor antibodies to HSV, 20 million have as many as four recurrences per year. The CDC projects that there are approximately 300,000 new cases per year—an increase. However, many practicing physicians have seen a decrease in the number of patients with genital HSV infections in the last 5 years. Herpes simplex virus infection is present in members of all socioeconomic groups. In recent years, however, the highest incidence has been reported in middle-class Caucasian women.

Herpes simplex virus infections have been associated with genital cancers in a number of studies published over the past 20 years. Women with HSV-2 antibodies have a higher incidence of cervical intraepithelial neoplasia and invasive cancer than women without antibodies. Because an epidemiologic association exists between HSV-2 and genital cancers, it may be proved in the future that HSV-2 is a cocarcinogen along with HPV in the development of squamous genital cancer. These epidemiologic associations indicate that women with genital HSV infections should have Pap test screening yearly.

Clinical Manifestations
The initial infection with HSV can be symptomatic or asymptomatic. If it is symptomatic it may be primary or nonprimary. A primary infection occurs in a patient without a history of prior HSV infection as evidenced by a lack of antibodies to either HSV-2 or HSV-1. A nonprimary first genital infection is caused by reactivation of latent virus and occurs in a patient with HSV antibodies. Recurrent infections are characterized by the presence of active lesions in a patient who has had previous ulceration at specific anatomic sites.

Herpes simplex virus enters the skin and replicates in parabasal and intermediate cells. The virus passes from cell to cell, and because it is neurotropic, it seeks out nerve cell endings in the epithelium, thereby gaining access to local ganglia.

Productively infected cells develop intranuclear inclusions and undergo ballooning, which is followed by degeneration and death. Polymorphonuclear leukocytes and monocytes are found at the periphery of the developing infection. As a result of this process, typical fluid-filled vesicles on an erythematous base develop within the superficial epithelium. After local invasion and replication, dissemination of the infection is possible by local spread; by hematogenous routes that include viremia, infected leukocytes, and mononuclear cells; and by ascension along local peripheral nerves to regional ganglia. The sacral root ganglia are the reservoirs that are involved in genital HSV infections. Additional replication can occur at the sites of dissemination or in the nerve cell ganglia. Initially, there is a polymorphonuclear, followed by a lymphocytic, immune response. As viral replication becomes restricted, lesions reepithelialize and a state of viral latency is established. The actual mechanism of latency development is unknown, but when latency has been established, no detectable viral antigens are expressed by the nerve cells.

The clinical manifestations of HSV-2 genital infections vary, depending on the presence of serologic evidence of prior experience with HSV-2. First episodes of genital herpes infections often are associated with systemic symptoms, involve multiple genital and nongenital sites, and have a prolonged duration of viral shedding. The incubation period from the time of exposure is 3–9 days. Prodromal paresthesia, tingling, burning, and pruritus may occur for 1–2 days prior to vesicle formation. The patient is infectious during this period, as virus can be cultured from the involved vulvar areas. Systemic symptoms include fever, malaise, and myalgia in 70% of women. The systemic symptoms usually reach their peak within 7 days after the appearance of the first vesicle and resolve gradually.

Pain, pruritus, dysuria, vaginal and urethral discharges, and tender, painful, inguinal adenopathy are the predominant local symptoms of the disease. Painful lesions are reported in virtually 100% of women, with a mean duration of 12.2 days for primary HSV infection. Subsequently, the vesicles crust over on cutaneous surfaces or reepithelialize on mucosal surfaces. In most instances healing is complete. Secondary bacterial infection may complicate recovery in an occasional patient. Lesions in various stages of development are common. Herpes simplex virus can be cultured from 1–2 days before lesion formation to after crusting has developed. During primary HSV infection, virus can be isolated from the urethra, vagina, and cervix in 80% of women. Extensive ulceration and necrosis of the cervix can occur to the extent that it mimics cervical carcinoma. Under those circumstances a profuse watery discharge is common. The clinical symptoms of pain and irritation from lesions gradually increase during the first 6–7 days after the onset of infection, reaching a maximum intensity between days 7–11 of the disease, and then gradually recede. The tender inguinal adenopathy usually appears during the second and third weeks and is the last symptom to resolve. The inguinal and femoral lymph nodes are tender to palpation, firm, and nonfluctuant. Suppurative lymphadenopathy is uncommon.

The median duration of viral shedding in patients with primary HSV infection is 14 days, when the first day of shedding is calculated to occur with the onset of genital paresthesia and to last until crusting has occurred. Since mucosal lesions do not crust, patients should be considered infectious until the lesions have completely reepithelialized.

Complications of primary genital HSV infections include urinary retention, aseptic meningitis, transverse myelitis and autonomic nervous system dysfunction (hyperesthesia or anesthesia of the lower back, sacral regions, and perineum), difficulty in urinating, and constipation. Additional complications are extragenital lesions in 16% of patients (buttocks, thighs, groin, fingers, and eyes). On rare occasions in non-immunocompromised hosts, severe systemic disease and death result from hematogenous disseminated infection.

The recurrence rate from reactivation of a latent genital herpes infection is 90%. In the natural history of recurrent infections a decreasing number of clinical infections occur over time. In contrast to the primary infections, the signs, symptoms, and anatomic sites of recurrent genital HSV infections are localized to the same areas within the genital region. The symptoms of itching and paresthesia are less intense, the duration of the episode usually ranges from 8–12 days, and the duration of viral shedding is decreased by 50% compared with that of the primary infection.

Asymptomatic reactivation of HSV after a primary HSV-2 infection is two or three times more frequent in the first 3 months after resolution of the primary first-episode HSV-2 infection than later in the time course. In contrast, the frequency of symptomatic reactivation during early time points is similar to that during later time points of infection. Newer data would also suggest a protective effect of prior HSV-1 antibody for asymptomatic vulvar but not cervical shedding of HSV-2. Prior infection with HSV-1 reduces the risk of acquiring genital HSV-2 infection.

There is substantial risk of HSV transmission during periods of asymptomatic shedding. A recent report indicated that in 70% of patients transmission appeared to result from sexual contact during periods of asymptomatic viral shedding. The risk for acquisition was higher in women than in men. Public health and private consultative strategies for the prevention of genital herpes must take into consideration the important role of subclinical reactivation in horizontal transmission.

Diagnosis

The diagnosis of HSV infection is suspected from the typical history of genital paresthesia, itching, and painful vesicular lesions, especially if there is a history of recurrence. In general, painful vesicular genital lesions should be considered to be symptoms of HSV infection until this diagnosis is ruled out. The differential diagnosis includes syphilis, chancroid, lymphogranuloma venereum, granuloma inguinale, herpes zoster virus, Behçet disease, Crohn disease, local excoriation, ulcerative vulvitis, and carcinoma of the vulva or cervix.

The clinical diagnosis should be confirmed by laboratory studies. Viral cultures are the most sensitive and specific means of establishing HSV as the etiologic agent. Vesicular fluid should be obtained, placed in appropriate transport media, and cultured. Herpes simplex virus grows in a wide variety of human and animal cell lines, and a diagnosis can be made in 90–95% of patients within 48–72 hours. Cytology is useful in establishing a diagnosis. This technique suffers from a low sensitivity, 65% at best. When cytology is used, the vesicle must be unroofed and the margins scraped. When present, multinucleated giant cells and cells with typical intranuclear inclusions confirm the diagnosis. Culture backup is strongly recommended.

The rapid diagnostic HSV kits are not advised for routine use, as they lack specificity and sensitivity when used in routine diagnostic laboratories. The presence of HSV-specific immunoglobulin M (IgM) is useful in making the diagnosis. Routine IgG serology is usually of little use unless prior knowledge of a negative antibody screen is known. Current tests to detect HSV are approved to detect the large amounts of HSV present in clinical lesions. The use of routine testing for detection of the asymptomatic shedding patient is not reliable.

Treatment

The goals of therapy for genital herpes include 1) shortening the clinical course of disease, 2) preventing complications, 3) preventing recurrences, and 4) decreasing the transmission of disease. Chemotherapy of genital HSV infections has been revolutionized by the introduction of acyclovir. Acyclovir is a synthetic acyclic purine nucleoside. It is highly specific for HSV-infected cells, causes minimal toxicity, and at the recommended doses has minimal carcinogenic and teratogenic potential.

The most common method of administration of acyclovir is the oral route, 200 mg five times daily for 10–14 days. Topical acyclovir, a 5% cream, can be placed directly on the lesions every 3–4 hours but is less acceptable to patients. It is the preferred route of administration in pregnant patients. For serious systemic disease, intravenous acyclovir can be administered at a dosage of 5 mg/kg of body weight over 45–60 minutes every 8 hours. The major benefit from acyclovir is to reduce the length of time of viral shedding, shorten the healing time, and decrease the severity of symptoms. It is most effective if treatment is started early in the course of disease. Acyclovir can be used for the prevention of recurrent disease at a dosage of 200 mg three times daily.

Human Papillomavirus Infection

Human papillomavirus infections of the genital tract are the most common sexually transmitted viral infection in the United States. It has been recognized for centuries as a sexually transmitted disease; however, there has been a dramatic increase in the number of patients seen in physicians' offices and in hospitals for the management of HPV disease. There was a 6.7-fold increase in physician–patient consultation for genital warts from 1966 to 1984. The data are difficult to interpret, but gynecologists in active practice are inundated with patients with HPV disease. Manifestation of HPV disease includes overt condylomata acuminata, subclinical papillomavirus infection, Bowen disease of the vulva, and cervical, vulvar, and vaginal intraepithelial neoplasia.

The information regarding the prevalence of HPV in the general population is constantly expanding. It is known that 1–3% of Pap tests will show cytologically detectable HPV disease (active, productive infection). When the same material is tested for HPV DNA types 6, 11, 16, 18, 31, 33, and 35, approximately 10% will be positive. When tested by polymerase chain reaction, approximately 50–60% will be positive for HPV DNA. A recent study of asymptomatic university women showed 42% positive for HPV DNA when the polymerase chain reaction technology was used. Most of these patients never had manifestations of HPV disease. But clinicians must be aware of the possibility of reactivation from latency of the HPV disease to manifest itself as overt condylomata acuminata; subclinical HPV infection; cervical, vulvar, and vaginal intraepithelial neoplasia; Bowen disease; or invasive squamous malignancies of the genital tract.

Clinical Manifestations

The biology of HPV infection is not completely understood. Most genital warts are seen in young adults, with mean age of onset being 16–25 years. Other manifestations of HPV disease, such as abnormal genital cytology, intraepithelial neoplasia, and invasive neoplasia, usually occur later.

It is generally agreed that the initial infection occurs through inoculation of HPV in areas of microtrauma of the genital tract at the time of coitus. Since HPV is a hardy virus and resists drying, fomite transmission as well as autoinoculation can occur. Human papillomavirus enters the basal and parabasal cells and induces stimulation of these cells. At this point, there is episomal DNA replication, and the virus is not incorporated into the host genome at this time. Usually an incubation period of 2 months is present, at which time a condyloma will be noted. The incubation period is variable (1–6 months), or the infection can go directly to latency without ever manifesting itself either as a condyloma acuminatum or abnormal cytology. Those patients who develop a condyloma usually have a period of active viral replication (6–9 months).

Eventually, when enough cells have become clustered, the lesion is called a genital wart. Mature virus can be found in the superficial layers of the wart; when the virus is shed, other epithelial cells are infected, and the cycle continues. The number of HPV virions needed to cause an infection is unknown. Cellular proliferation occurs mainly in the acanthotic stratum spinosum, which constitutes most of the bulk of the wart. Many mitotic figures are seen, but the epithelial cells show an orderly arrangement and the border with the dermis is sharp.

Within several months there is activation of the immune system, at which time HPV usually enters latency. The immunology of HPV disease is poorly defined and has not been helpful in the diagnosis or management of HPV infections.

It seems to be clear that HPV disease is sensitive to the competency of the immune system. The most difficult problems with condylomata acuminata occur in transplant patients who are receiving exogenous immunosuppressive agents or patients with HIV infection who are endogenously immunosuppressed. Other immunosuppressive agents are exogenous steroids, cigarette smoking, other viruses such as HSV-2, and metabolic deficiencies. Patients who are immunosuppressed will respond to therapeutic modalities at a much slower rate and will manifest more recurrences or progression of the disease.

The entire lower genital tract may be involved, starting from the perianal area to the perineal body, the vulva, the vagina, and the cervix. Two thirds of women with overt condylomata acuminata or subclinical HPV infection (abnormal genital cytology) of the cervix have evidence of HPV elsewhere in the genital tract. Similarly, more than 33% of women with HPV disease of the vulva have HPV disease elsewhere in the genital tract as well.

Relation to Malignancy

It is now recognized that HPV may have neoplastic potential in the genital tract and is considered a cocarcinogen by most investigators. This consideration has resulted from the finding of HPV DNA in more than 90% of patients with intraepithelial and invasive squamous cell carcinoma of the genital tract. Evaluation of the relationship of HIV to genital malignancies is still evolving, but several facets are becoming clear.

Certain HPV DNA types are associated with infection at specific anatomic sites. Human papillomavirus DNA types 6 and 11 are generally thought to be present in condylomata acuminata of the lower third of the vagina, vulva, and perianal area. Human papillomavirus DNA types 6 and 11 are thought to have little or no oncologic potential, as these types cannot become integrated into the host genome. In contrast, HPV DNA types 16, 18, 31, 33, 35, and others are usually present in lesions in the upper third of the vagina and the cervix. These types are able to be integrated into the host genome and are associated with advanced grades of intraepithelial neoplasia and squamous cell carcinomas. It appears that integration of HPV DNA into the host genome is necessary for malignant transformation of the host cells. Apparently, HPV DNA types 6, 11, and 42 are unable to be transformed, whereas HPV DNA types 16, 18, 31, 33, 35, and others can be integrated into the host genome and cause malignant transformation. The process of integration usually disrupts the region of the viral genome involved with early transcription. This is reflected clinically by the disappearance of HPV antigens as the lesion advances to carcinoma in situ and invasive cancer. Additional cocarcinogens or factors must be present for malignancy to occur. Candidates for cocarcinogens include cigarette smoking, HSV-2 or other viruses, and nutritional factors.

Diagnosis

The overt condylomata acuminata that are found in 30% of all patients with HPV disease usually appear as a soft pink or white vascular, sessile tumor with multiple fine, fingerlike projections. Clinicians are encouraged to confirm the clinical impression with a biopsy of the vulva, vagina, or cervix. Frequently, management becomes lengthy and complicated, and a correct diagnosis is mandatory.

Vulva. Overt condylomata acuminata may be seen on the vulva. The most common sites are the posterior fourchette and adjacent labia minora, labia majora, clitoris, and urethra. In nonmucosal areas, the condylomata become keratotic. Human papillomavirus infection of the vulva can also produce small (3–7 mm), smooth, flat papules. These 'esions may be pigmented or nonpigmented. These papules may coalesce to produce a larger area of disease. The vulva should be examined by colposcopy or with a magnifying lens after application of 5% acetic acid. Samples from abnormal areas should be obtained for biopsy.

Subclinical HPV infection can be detected only after application of 5% acetic acid and colposcopic examination. This permits identification of three distinct types of lesions in patients with subclinical HPV infections:

1. **Vestibular papillae**—Vestibular papillae are multiple, small, villous projections that are largely confined to mucous membranes. Each microscopic projection resembles an individual exophytic frond of a condyloma acuminatum. These papillae are most commonly found on the posterior fourchette, labia minora, introitus, and external urethral meatus. It is important to differentiate these vestibular papillae from normal anatomic variants around the labia minora and introitus.
2. **Fused papillae**—When individual papillae fuse, they give the vulvar skin a granular rather than a villous appearance. Fused papillae are associated with burning vulvar discomfort, which may be erroneously attributed to chronic yeast infection.
3. **Acetowhite epithelium**—Acetowhite epithelium is normal-appearing vulvar skin that turns white after application of 5% acetic acid. This abnormality is frequently associated with productive HPV infection, 5–10% being associated with vulvar intraepithelial neoplasia grades 2–3.

Vagina. The presence of HPV infection in the vagina has not aroused great interest because the lesions are usually asymptomatic and the malignant potential is significantly less than that for lesions of the cervix and vulva. It is now recognized that vaginal involvement is very common and may represent a significant reservoir for sexually transmitted HPV infections. Vaginal condylomata acuminata can be detected in as many as one third of women who have vulvar condylomata acuminata and in nearly 50% of women who have cervical condylomata acuminata. The distribution is usually in the upper and lower third of the vagina in a patchy manner. The lesions appear as raised, dense, white elevations that are made up of microcondylomata. The course over time is variable, but in some patients spontaneous regression occurs. Patients with immunosuppressive diseases tend to have intractable and persistent disease.

Subclinical vaginal HPV infections are largely undiagnosed, therefore making the use of 5% acetic acid and colposcopy necessary to determine the extent of disease. Three patterns of subclinical HPV infection have been described:

1. **Elongated vaginal papillae**—Elongated vaginal papillae are elongated, single clusters of projections that appear to be similar to the individual fronds of vulvar condylomata acuminata.
2. **Acetowhite epithelium**—Acetowhite epithelium is a sharply defined area of flat vaginal epithelium that becomes white. It occurs more frequently in the upper third of the vagina, and punctation and mosaicism may be found. Colposcopic findings resemble those of vaginal intraepithelial neoplasia, and a biopsy is required.
3. **Reverse punctation**—Reverse punctation is the finding of a few to many tiny acetowhite dots against a pink mucosa. These dots represent the parakeratotic epithelium. This change can be made more prominent by staining the mucosa and the dots with one-quarter-strength Lugol solution. The mucosa stains the expected mahogany brown, and the parakeratotic dots turn yellow. This finding is best interpreted as minimal HPV expression within latently infected tissues.

Cervix. Condylomata acuminata are readily recognizable as papillary projections in a single, multiple, or scattered pattern or a confluent pattern. The lesions are usually found within the transformation zone but may also involve the original squamous epithelium of the portio.

Subclinical cervical HPV infection makes up the bulk of infections and manifests itself after the application of 5% acetic acid. This is one of the most common sexually transmitted diseases with cytopathic effects, specifically koilocytotic atypia, dyskeratosis, and multinucleation, and is found in 2–3% of routine cervical cytologic smears. During colposcopy, the lesion margin, color, vascular pattern, and iodine staining should be used as a guide to directing a biopsy of the most severe area of disease.

Subclinical HPV infection is characterized colposcopically by indistinct acetowhitening or snowy-white lesions, an irregular outline with jagged margins, and the presence of satellite lesions. The capillary patterns may be pronounced and confused with mosaicism and punctation of characteristic cervical intraepithelial neoplasia grades 2–3. The vascular patterns of subclinical HPV infection are more ordered, with a fine meshwork of uniform-caliber vessels arranged horizontally. Capillary loops may run to the surface but maintain a uniform vessel caliber throughout their course. Staining with one-quarter-strength Lugol solution denotes glycogenesis, whereas negative staining is seen in areas of transformed cervical intraepithelial neoplasia.

Subclinical HPV infection represents the earliest lesion in the cervical intraepithelial neoplasia hierarchy that is capable of progressing to invasive squamous cell carcinoma. Patients with subclinical HPV infection can progress to advanced-stage cervical intraepithelial neoplasia within a 12–24-month period. This departs from traditional teaching, which states that the transit time to malignancy is long. Clinicians must be aware of the changing pattern of transit time and the more aggressive nature of HPV infections.

Patients must be approached with the view that the entire lower genital tract may harbor evidence of overt or subclinical HPV infection. Therefore, the lower genital tract should be examined with a colposcope if disease is detected in any area. Liberal biopsy of suspected lesions is indicated to determine the extent of disease. Since these patients are considered to be at high risk for malignant disease, they should be evaluated every 6 months by at least a Pap test but also, more importantly, by colposcopy.

At present, the availability of HPV DNA typing does not alter the clinical management of HPV disease and should therefore be considered a research tool. Peroxidase–antiperoxidase techniques for the detection of HPV antigens are useful and are available in many areas.

Management

Clinical management of overt condylomata acuminata, and particularly of subclinical HPV infection of the vulva, varies greatly. This has resulted because of the lack of basic knowledge concerning the biology of HPV and the absence of convenient modalities of therapy. The persistence or recurrence of HPV disease is very common after all therapies, and this leads to physician and patient frustration.

The most important part of clinical management is to help the patient understand her disease. It is important for the patient to understand that she has acquired an infection that is lifelong and that it may recur at any time at any anatomic site within the lower genital tract. The patient should be told that the goal is control and not cure of her HPV infection.

After a histologic diagnosis is made and the extent of disease is known, a variety of modalities and agents are available for management. These therapeutic modalities include keratolytic agents (podophyllin, trichloroacetic acid, and 5-fluorouracil cream), physical agents (cryotherapy, laser therapy, and electrocautery), surgical resection, and immunotherapy (autologous vaccine, dinitrochlorobenzene, and interferon). At present, there is no standard approach to treat overt or subclinical HPV infection. The agents have been used singly and in combination.

Keratolytic Agents. Podophyllin (podophyllum resin) acts by poisoning the mitotic spindle and causing intense vasospasm. It is applied directly to the lesion and is allowed to dry. The patient is instructed to wash off the podophyllin in 6 hours. It can be applied weekly until the wart disappears. The side effects are unpredictable and include a severe local reaction at the time of application and systemic toxicity from excessive absorption. This agent should be applied with caution to nonkeratinized epithelial surfaces because of the danger of excessive absorption. It is contraindicated during pregnancy. Many physicians have abandoned the use of podophyllin. Its use should be restricted to patients with minimal vulvar or anal disease (lesions up to 1 cm). Results have shown clearing of overt warts in up to 75% of patients, with a relapse rate of 65–78%.

Trichloroacetic acid (85%) acts by precipitation of surface proteins. Application should be via a cotton-tipped swab. The application may be done under colposcopic direction for vulvar and anal subclinical HPV infections. It is not necessary to apply paraffin to the adjacent skin, as this is cumbersome and counterproductive. The trichloroacetic acid produces a white slough that peels off in several days. Therapy may be repeated in 2–3 weeks. It is indicated for vulvar, anal, and vaginal lesions and can be used for cervical lesions.

5-Fluorouracil is a pyrimidine antimetabolite that causes necrosis and sloughing of growing tissue. The 1% or 5% cream can be used. It may be used intravaginally or for vulvar, anal, or urethral lesions. Condylomata acuminata that are located on nonkeratinized surfaces respond better than do lesions that are located on keratinized surfaces. 5-Fluorouracil may be applied in one of several protocols. The first method is for use in vulvar or anal lesions. The 5-fluorouracil is applied directly to the lesion on a daily basis until erythema or vesiculation occurs, usually on days 7–10 of therapy. The course may be repeated. This protocol leads to marked erythema and discomfort in patients. The alternative protocol calls for the administration of 5-fluorouracil on a weekly basis for 10–12 weeks. This protocol is better tolerated by patients. For vaginal lesions, 5-fluorouracil may be applied nightly for 7 nights; however, a better-tolerated approach is to use 3 g (two thirds of a vaginal applicator) of 5-fluorouracil weekly for 12 weeks. Control rates of 80% have been reported. Persistent vaginal ulceration has been reported with the use of 5-fluorouracil cream in higher doses. The patient's vagina should be examined for ulceration after four to six applications.

Physical Agents. Cryotherapy of anogenital warts uses either single or repetitive 1–2-minute freeze–thaw cycles to destroy wart tissue. Cryotherapy may be performed by probe or with liquid nitrogen. Most patients need three to six treatments to control the warts. In comparative studies, cryotherapy is more effective than podophyllin and is as effective as laser therapy. Success in controlling overt warts varies from 62% to 79%.

Laser therapy offers the theoretic advantages of precise control of depth, margins, and hemostasis. Recurrence occurs in 25–100% of patients. Some clinicians have extended their field of treatment to account for latent HPV at the margins. Recent information suggests that control rates are not improved and morbidity is excessive. Patients must be given an anesthetic for most laser applications.

The use of electrocautery destruction of warts has been found to be effective. It is a useful technique for the destruction of small lesions in the office setting.

Immunotherapy. Autologous vaccines are made from the host's own condylomata acuminata. Results in blinded trials have shown no benefit when compared with that of a placebo.

The use of dinitrochlorobenzene is unique in that the host's cell-mediated immunity is used to destroy the warts. Dinitrochlorobenzene is used to sensitize the patient and, when accomplished, the dinitrochlorobenzene is placed on the wart. A delayed-type hypersensitivity reaction occurs, destroying the wart. This therapy has problems because of an inability to sensitize patients with warts to dinitrochlorobenzene; varying patient sensitivities to dinitrochlorobenzene, with the potential for a severe reaction; and the hesitancy of some patients to have a hypersensitivity reaction in the perineal area.

Interferons are a family of proteins with antiviral, antiproliferative, and immunomodular properties. Two interferons, interferon alfa 2-b (Intron-A) and interferon alfa-n3 (Alferon N Injection), are currently approved for condyloma acuminatum therapy. Interferons are administered by the parenteral route. The potential advantages of therapy with interferon are that 1) multiple HPV-infected areas can be treated concomitantly, 2) there is no local discomfort from destructive procedures, 3) general anesthesia is not needed, and 4) it can be used as a primary agent, as well as for adjuvant therapy.

The exact dosing and scheduling for administration of interferon has not been standardized. Interferon can be administered intralesionally, subcutaneously, or IM. The dosing recommended in the package insert advises using 250,000 U per wart for up to five warts two or three times weekly for 3–8 weeks. An alternative dosage is 2.5–3.0 million units two or three times per week injected subcutaneously into the anterior thigh by self-administration. The length of administration should be at least 6 weeks to attain the best effect.

Interferon can be used to treat small or large lesions. It lends itself particularly well to the treatment of intravaginal HPV disease. Systemic therapy is also successful in patients with recurrent disease or in patients who have extensive genital tract HPV disease.

A special circumstance may warrant the use of interferon in children. Interferon has been used successfully in children for the therapy of anogenital condylomata acuminata. The interferon is administered at the dosage of 3.0 million units per square meter three times per week. It is well tolerated, and this therapy minimizes the additional physical and psychologic trauma of surgical procedures.

Administration of interferon can be carried as an adjuvant therapy with the laser. Data suggest that use of interferon, 1.0 million units three times per week for 10 weeks, started at the same time as the laser ablation was performed, gave superior results to laser alone.

Administration of interferon causes side effects that are dose related and usually minimal at a dosage of 3 million units per square meter three times weekly. The most frequent side effect is fever, which is associated with the first injection. Other common side effects include malaise, fatigue, and headache. Transient decreases in leukocyte count and increases in hepatic aminotransferase levels may occur in less than 15% of patients.

In general, topical therapy is best used when the lesions are external and few in number; intralesional interferon therapy may be used for patients with few lesions. Systemic interferon therapy, laser therapy, or cryotherapy, or combinations of these therapies seem to be most effective for large wart volumes. Newer agents or combinations of agents are being sought to improve management options.

Human Immunodeficiency Virus Infection

Adult AIDS was first recognized in the early 1980s, and the etiologic agent HIV type 1 (HIV-1) was isolated in 1984. As of December 31, 1993, approximately 361,000 cases of AIDS in the United States were reported to the CDC. The number of deaths was approximately 220,000, with the number of deaths being approximately half of the number of reported cases. The U.S. Public Health Service has estimated that 2.0 million Americans are infected with HIV-1. This indicates that approximately 0.7% of the total population is assumed to be infected. Acquired immunodeficiency syndrome is the fifth leading cause of death in women of reproductive age in the United States.

It was estimated that women made up 13% of the AIDS cases diagnosed in 1992. There has been a gradual increase in the percentage of women diagnosed with AIDS. It is estimated that the sex ratio of new cases of AIDS will be 1:1 by the year 2000. This dramatic change from an initial sex ratio of 15:1 to 1:1 is caused by the dramatic increase in heterosexual transmission.

Human immunodeficiency virus infection is considered a sexually transmitted disease. Among women and men from high endemic areas who entered the U.S. Armed Forces, the rates of HIV infection were similar for both sexes (males, 10.6/1,000, and females, 8.3/1,000). Human immunodeficiency virus seropositivity affects minority populations more than it does white populations. When adjusted for population size, the rates of AIDS are much higher in African–American and Hispanic women than in white women (13 and 11 times, respectively).

Acquired immunodeficiency syndrome is also increasing as a cause of childhood mortality. An estimated 1.5/1,000 U.S. women giving birth in 1989 were infected with HIV-1. The available data regarding perinatal transmission has varied from a low of 12% to a high of 65%. Most recent data suggest an overall perinatal transmission rate of 15–40%.

Pathogenesis

The transmission of HIV occurs by three primary routes: intimate contact with bodily secretions of infected individuals, exposure to blood or blood products infected with HIV, and perinatally from an infected mother to her fetus or infant. Epidemiologic data indicate that HIV is not transmitted through casual contact, immune globulin preparations, the hepatitis B vaccine, or contact with insects.

Acquired immunodeficiency syndrome is now known to be the result of immunosuppressive phenomena caused by the retrovirus HIV. The characteristic feature of retroviruses is the possession of an enzyme called reverse transcriptase that enables these RNA viruses to make a DNA copy that can be inserted into the host genome, leading to latent infection. The characteristics of this family of viruses include their long genome (9.7 kilobases), highly variable envelope antigens, induction of slow disease, cytopathic properties in cell cultures, and infectivity of brain tissue.

Human immunodeficiency virus may infect a number of cell types. It has been generally accepted that cells that possess the CD4 antigen complex on the cell membrane become targets for HIV. The frequency of expression of the CD4 antigen complex on cells varies with the type of cell, and this frequency is directly proportional to the ease with which the cells become infected. In addition, a direct interaction between the protein gp120 on the virus and the CD4 antigen receptor has been demonstrated by showing that both proteins are required for infection. The types of cells that have become infected include T and B lymphocytes, macrophages, promyelocytes, astrocytes, oligodendrocytes, Langerhans cells of the skin, and bowel epithelia.

Following the interaction of the viral gp120 and the CD4 antigen–receptor complex, the virus enters the cell; its RNA is released from the central core; and, by the mechanism of reverse transcriptase, double-stranded DNA, which circularizes, goes into the nucleus. The complementary DNA integrates with the host genome and exists as proviral DNA. At this stage it can remain latent for an indefinite time period, with little or no viral RNA or protein being made.

Alternatively, the infected cell may enter an active virus production phase in which the proviral DNA makes viral RNA and proteins, leading to infectious virus release. The factors, cofactors, and conditions that initiate active viral production or activation from latency are not well defined. Based on observations in patients with AIDS, however, coinfection with other viruses (ie, cytomegalovirus, hepatitis B virus, or HSV) or allogeneic stimulation (by exposure to proteins found in blood, semen, or allografts) provides some stimulus for viral genomic transcription. Once transcription begins, viral proteins are synthesized and posttranscriptional processing is performed.

The amount of time involved from initial infection of the cell to its death is variable. The infected cell may circulate with continuing internal viral production until a cell-to-cell fusion or syncytium is formed, with ballooning of the cell and death. The relative density of CD4 antigen complexes influences the cell's ability to escape syncytium molecules (ie, macrophages and monocytes) that have fewer receptors, which are more resistant than those with a higher density (ie, T4 cells). The existence of cells that are relatively resistant to cell death creates an important viral reservoir, which may account for the persistence of infection and infectivity of the host.

As each cell becomes infected or dies, its function either is altered or ceases. This leads to the malfunction of the immune system. This diminution of immune system function allows opportunistic infections and malignancies to develop, leading to death of the host.

Clinical Manifestations

The CDC clinically defines primary HIV infection as a syndrome similar to mononucleosis, with or without aseptic meningitis, with seroconversion for HIV antibody. The initial exposure to HIV results in this acute syndrome in approximately 90% of patients. Febrile pharyngitis is the main sign of infection, with fever, sweats, lethargy, arthralgia, myalgia, headache, photophobia, and lymphadenopathy starting acutely and lasting 3–14 days. The lymphadenopathy usually begins in the second week and is usually generalized. The incubation period from the time of HIV exposure to the onset of acute clinical illness has ranged from 5 days to 3 months, with most investigators reporting an incubation period of 2–4 weeks.

The clinical manifestations of disease after recovery from the primary HIV infection are usually absent, during which time patients are either asymptomatic carriers or are undergoing a prolonged incubation period. Studies indicate that HIV infection is persistent. The virus is usually shed into many body fluids, including semen, saliva, cervical secretions, amniotic fluid, breast milk, and urine, in addition to blood. The titer of virus is low during asymptomatic periods.

At some point, as the immune system decreases in efficiency, opportunistic infections will occur and the seropositive individual will develop symptoms. Very few infected persons (< 5%) develop AIDS within 3 years, and the mean time from infection to AIDS is over 10 years. Five years after infection 35% will have progressed to AIDS. Evidence of immune dysfunction may be observed in a deteriorating clinical condition manifested by persistent generalized lymphadenopathy, fever, night sweats, diarrhea, weight loss, fatigue, and central nervous system dysfunction. Infections such as herpes zoster or oral candidiasis may occur.

The final stage of HIV infection is AIDS. This is a clinical condition characterized by certain malignancies or opportunistic infections resulting from immune dysfunction. In addition, individuals who are HIV positive and have CD4 counts of less than 200 mm^3 or a CD4 percentage of less than 14 should be considered as having AIDS. Infections such as *Pneumocystis carinii* pneumonia are the most prevalent opportunistic infections in the United States, but tuberculosis, cryptococcal meningitis, HSV, toxoplasmosis, cryptosporidiosis, and other infections are not uncommon. Several otherwise rare malignancies occur in patients with AIDS; they include Kaposi sarcoma, non-Hodgkin lymphoma of the high-grade or B-cell type, and Burkitt lymphoma.

Diagnosis

Following primary infection, seroconversion occurs, with the development of specific antibodies directed against three main gene products of HIV: *gag* (p55, p24, p18), *pol* (p31, p51, p68), and *env* (gp160, gp120, gp41). Within 2 weeks of the acute illness, IgM antibody, followed by IgG antibody, is detected by immunofluorescence assay. Enzyme-linked immunosorbent assay detects antibodies at 1–2 months. Western blot analysis first detects antibodies to p24 and gp41 gene products. Recent studies have shown that, in rare cases, seroconversion may not be documented until 15 months after exposure.

The standard method to screen for the presence of HIV antibodies is by the enzyme-linked immunosorbent assay technique. These kits vary in their sensitivities and specificities, which are from 93% to 99%. This creates some false-positive and some false-negative results. The predictive value of the enzyme-linked immunosorbent assay screening test is dependent on the prevalence of HIV in the population to be tested. In a low-prevalence population, an estimated 1/200 persons is infected; a specificity of 99% yields about 100 false-positive results per 10,000 individuals tested, for every 25 infected individuals identified as HIV antibody positive. Therefore, a confirmatory test is necessary.

The Western blot test is used as a confirmatory test. In this test, the patient's antibodies can be separated and precisely identified by their ability to migrate in an electrophoretic gel.

The newest technique for the diagnosis of HIV-infected individuals is the polymerase chain reaction. This is currently a research tool but is coming into increasing clinical use. The polymerase chain reaction technique was developed for in vitro gene amplification of RNA or DNA, and as such can amplify extremely small amounts of RNA or DNA to recognizable levels. It is currently being used to assess neonatal diagnosis or to determine seroconversion.

Management

The dysfunction of the patient's immune system can be monitored with CD4 lymphocyte counts. As the CD4 count decreases, the risk for opportunistic infection increases. Although there is no curative therapy for HIV infections, two drugs have been released for palliative therapy. The initial drug released for treatment of AIDS was azidothymidine (now known as zidovudine), and dideoxyinosine was released more recently. Zidovudine has been recommended to be started when the CD4 count is less than 500/mm³; *P. carinii* pneumonia prophylaxis is initiated when the CD4 count drops to 200/mm³. The various opportunistic infections and malignancies are treated by standard therapies.

Numerous drug trials with zidovudine, dideoxyinosine, inteferons, and newer experimental drugs are occurring. Preliminary studies show that zidovudine therapy can reduce by two thirds the risk of transmission of the virus from pregnant women to their infants. Evaluation of the neonates suggests minimal toxicity, with infants showing macrocytosis in their bone marrow. Side effects of zidovudine include hematologic toxicity with granulocytopenia, severe anemia, severe headaches, and (rarely) neurologic changes.

In the absence of an effective therapy, efforts must be directed to the prevention of the spread of HIV. The greatest number of women who become infected with HIV today are infected through heterosexual transmission. Education continues to be the most important preventive measure at this time.

BIBLIOGRAPHY

Bacterial Diseases

Berry MC, Dajani AS. Resurgence of congenital syphilis. Infect Dis Clin North Am 1992;6:19–29

Centers for Disease Control. Antibiotic-resistant strains of *Neisseria gonorrhoeae*: policy guidelines for detection, management, and control. MMWR 1987;36(5 suppl):1s–18s

Centers for Disease Control and Prevention. Recommendations for the prevention and management of *Chlamydia trachomatis* infections, 1993. MMWR 1993;42(RR-12):1–39

Centers for Disease Control and Prevention. 1993 Sexually transmitted diseases treatment guidelines. MMWR 1993;42(RR-14):50–61

Chapin-Robertson K. Use of molecular diagnostics in sexually transmitted diseases. Diagn Microbiol Infect Dis 1993;16:173–184

Hook EW 3d, Marra CM. Acquired syphilis in adults. N Engl J Med 1992;326:1060–1069

Martin DH, Mroczkowski TF, Dalu ZA, McCarty J, Jones RB, Hopkins SJ, et al. A controlled trial of a single dose of azithromycin for the treatment of chlamydial urethritis and cervicitis: the Azithromycin for Chlamydial Infections Study Group. N Engl J Med 1992;327:921–925

Pearlman MD, McNeeley SG. A review of the microbiology, immunology and clinical implications of *Chlamydia trachomatis* infections. Obstet Gynecol Surv 1992;47:448–461

Phillips RS, Hanff PA, Wertheimer A, Aronson MD. Gonorrhea in women seen for routine gynecologic care: criteria for testing. Am J Med 1988;85:177–182

Trachtenberg AI, Washington AE, Halldorson S. A cost-based decision analysis for chlamydia screening in California family planning clinics. Obstet Gynecol 1988;71:101–108

Viral Diseases

Campion MJ, McCance DJ, Cuzick J, Singer A. Progressive potential of mild cervical atypia: prospective cytological, colposcopic, and virological study. Lancet 1986;2:237–240

Douglas GC, King BF. Maternal-fetal transmission of human immunodeficiency virus: a review of possible routes and cellular mechanisms of infection. Clin Infect Dis 1992;15:678–691

Gall SA, Hughes CE, Mounts P, Segriti A, Weck PK, Whisnant JK. Efficacy of human lymphoblastoid interferon in the therapy of resistant condyloma acuminata. Obstet Gynecol 1986;67:643–651

Gibbs RS, Amstey MS, Sweet RL, Mead PB, Sever JL. Management of genital herpes infection in pregnancy. Obstet Gynecol 1988;71:779–780

Jha PK, Beral V, Peto J, Hack S, Hermon C, Deacon J, et al. Antibodies to human papillomavirus and to other genital infectious agents and invasive cervical cancer risk. Lancet 1993;341:1116–1118

Koutsky LA, Stevens CE, Holmes KK, Ashley RL, Kiviat NB, Critchlow CW, et al. Underdiagnosis of genital herpes by current clinical and viral-isolation procedures. N Engl J Med 1992;326:1533–1539

Kulhamjian JA, Soroush V, Au DS, Bronzan RN, Yasukawa LL, Weylan LE, et al. Identification of women at unsuspected risk of primary infection with herpes simplex virus type 2 during pregnancy. N Engl J Med 1992;326:916–920

Levy JA, Kaminsky LS, Morrow WJ, Steimer K, Luciw P, Dina D, et al. Infection by the retrovirus associated with the acquired immunodeficiency syndrome: clinical, biological, and molecular features. Ann Intern Med 1985;103:694–699

National Institute of Allergy and Infectious Diseases. Clinical alert: important therapeutic information on the benefit of zidovudine (AZT) for the prevention of the transmission of HIV from mother to infant. Bethesda, Maryland: NIAID, 1994

Selwyn PA, Schoenbaum EE, Davenny K, Robertson VJ, Feingold AR, Shulman JF, et al. Prospective study of human immunodeficiency virus infection and pregnancy outcomes in intravenous drug users. JAMA 1989;261:1289–1294

Pelvic Infections

PELVIC INFLAMMATORY DISEASE

Pelvic inflammatory disease is the result of an ascending infection by bacteria that have colonized the endocervix. The most commonly incriminated microorganisms are the sexually transmitted pathogens, *Neisseria gonorrhoeae* and *Chlamydia trachomatis*. Infection of the endocervix with these pathogens causes inflammation (endocervicitis). With ascending spread, these pathogens produce inflammation throughout the upper genital tract (endometritis, salpingitis, peritonitis). Respiratory pathogens, such as *Haemophilus influenzae, Streptococcus pneumoniae*, and *Streptococcus pyogenes*, are found in approximately 5% of cases. These microorganisms appear to reach the upper genital tract through canalicular spread. Other cases are caused by endogenous vaginal microorganisms such as *Streptococcus agalactiae* (group B streptococcus), *Escherichia coli*, and bacterial vaginosis microorganisms (*Gardnerella vaginalis, Bacteroides* [*Prevotella*] species, and *Peptostreptococcus* species). Retrograde menstruation may also play a role in contaminating the fallopian tubes and peritoneum with microorganisms. A polymicrobial infection with aerobic and anaerobic bacteria has been identified in up to 40% of patients with laparoscopically proven acute salpingitis. Many of the bacteria recovered from the upper genital tracts of patients with PID are those present in high numbers in the vaginas of women with bacterial vaginosis. Anaerobic bacteria are commonly present in patients with tuboovarian abscesses.

Diagnosis

Lower abdominal pain is the most frequent symptom noted in patients with PID. The pain is usually bilateral and is not necessarily severe. Associated symptoms generally represent infection of other anatomic structures with *N. gonorrhoeae* or *C. trachomatis*. For example, endocervicitis may be manifest by the complaint of an abnormal vaginal discharge. Urethritis symptoms, such as dysuria, may be due to concomitant infection of the urethra. Breakthrough bleeding while the patient is taking OCs or persistent vaginal spotting after elective termination of pregnancy may be indicative of endometritis. More systemic symptoms, such as fever and the association of nausea with or without vomiting, reflect peritoneal inflammation and more severe clinical disease.

Physical findings consistent with the diagnosis of PID include a saline preparation of the cervical secretions demonstrating a marked increase in the number of inflammatory cells (leukorrhea) or endocervical mucopus. This simple test can be used to exclude a genital infection and, consequently, PID in a woman with abdominal pain. Adnexal tenderness, usually associated with uterine and cervical motion, is also present in women with PID. It is usually associated with uterine and cervical motion. Additional clinical findings supportive of infection and inflammation improve the specificity of the clinical diagnosis of PID. Elevated temperature, palpation of an adnexal complex, leukocytosis, elevated erythrocyte sedimentation rate or C-reactive protein, and positive tests for a lower genital tract infection with *N. gonorrhoeae* or *C. trachomatis* are considered adjunctive criteria for the diagnosis of PID. The presence of a palpable adnexal mass suggests the presence of a tuboovarian abscess.

Although laparoscopy can play a role in the diagnosis of PID (acute salpingitis), its applications are limited. Laparoscopic examination may not detect endometritis or subtle, chronic inflammation of the fallopian tubes. Laparoscopy should be considered in patients for whom the diagnosis is in question, especially if ectopic pregnancy is a possibility. Also, patients with a history of multiple treatments for PID as outpatients should undergo laparoscopy to rule out an alternative, treatable diagnosis such as endometriosis. Endometrial biopsy revealing either acute or chronic inflammation offers an alternative, objective method of documenting upper genital tract inflammation.

Treatment

Most women with PID are treated as outpatients. In its 1993 guidelines the CDC recommends the following two regimens for ambulatory management of PID. The first is either cefoxitin (2 g IM) plus probenecid (1 g orally) combined with a 14-day course of doxycycline (100 mg orally, twice daily), or a combination of ceftriaxone (250 mg IM) plus the 14-day course of doxycycline. This regimen maximizes coverage against the gonococcus and chlamydia but provides little in the way of coverage for significant facultative and anaerobic soft tissue infections. An alternative regimen uses ofloxacin (400 mg orally, twice daily for 14 days), a quinolone antibiotic with excellent activity against *N. gonorrhoeae* and *C. trachomatis*. Because of concern related to ofloxacin's lack of anaerobic coverage, a 14-day course of oral clindamycin (450 mg, four times daily) or oral metronidazole (500 mg, twice daily) is added.

Patients with suspected anaerobic infections, as associated with tuboovarian abscess or IUD use, should be hospitalized. Generally, patients with severe clinical disease, those unable to tolerate oral therapy, and HIV-positive patients should be admitted. Recommended inpatient antibiotic regimens cover *N. gonorrhoeae* and *C. trachomatis* as well as anaerobes and facultative bacteria. The combination of cefoxitin (2 g IV every 6 hours) or cefotetan (2 g IV every 12 hours) and doxycycline (100 mg every 12 hours orally or IV) is recommended when sexually transmitted microorganisms are thought to play a role in the etiology of PID. The combination of clindamycin (900 mg IV every 8 hours) plus an aminoglycoside such as gentamicin, loading dose (2 mg/kg) IV, followed by a maintenance dose (1.5 mg/kg) every 8 hours, provides excellent coverage for mixed anaerobic and aerobic infections. Both regimens have been studied extensively and are associated with clinical cure rates in the 90% range. After the patient has been discharged, regimens should be followed by a 14-day course of either doxycycline, 100 mg orally two times daily, or clindamycin, 450 mg four times daily. Most failures are associated with tuboovarian abscess formation and the need for surgical drainage.

The therapy for PID should also include the epidemiologic treatment of all male sexual partners with an antibiotic regimen for gonococcal and chlamydial infection. In addition, patient education concerning the sexually transmitted nature of PID may lead to the practice of safer sex and prevent recurrence.

Sequelae/Prevention

Pelvic inflammatory disease leads to tubal factor infertility, ectopic pregnancy, and chronic abdominal pain. The risk of tubal factor infertility roughly doubles for each episode of PID. Overall, after one, two, and three or more episodes the infertility rates are 8.0%, 19.5%, and 40%, respectively. In addition, the rate of ectopic pregnancy is increased fourfold in women with documented salpingitis. The key to the prevention of these sequelae is the detection of uncomplicated lower genital tract infection with chlamydia and *N. gonorrhoeae*. Targeted screening for these sexually transmitted diseases is recommended for high-prevalence groups (ie, age <25 years and a new sexual partner within the last year). Diagnosis and treatment of mucopurulent endocervicitis can likewise prevent ascending infection. Encouraging the use of barrier contraceptives may reduce the likelihood of acquiring sexually transmitted diseases.

Atypical Disease, or "Silent Salpingitis"

Most women with tubal factor infertility have no history of PID. However, antibodies to the sexually transmitted pathogens, *C. trachomatis* or *N. gonorrhoeae*, are noted in most of these patients, suggesting that prior infection has occurred. In addition, both morphologic and physiologic examination of the fallopian tubes of women with tubal factor infertility fail to show a difference between those patients with or without a history of PID. These data suggest that women may develop salpingitis and subsequent tubal damage without manifesting the typical clinical symptoms, primarily lower abdominal pain and fever, associated with the traditional diagnosis of PID. Atypical PID may be defined as pelvic inflammation of the endocervix, endometrium, or fallopian tubes in the absence of a chief complaint of abdominal pain. Patients may present with the clinical manifestations discussed above (vaginal discharge, dysuria, breakthrough vaginal bleeding) or in some cases with no symptoms whatsoever ("silent salpingitis"). The diagnosis is based on the concurrent findings of leukorrhea and pelvic organ tenderness, suggesting pelvic organ inflammation.

TOXIC SHOCK SYNDROME

More than 20 years after the highly publicized epidemic of staphylococcal TSS, fewer than 300 cases are reported annually to the CDC. However, recently two additional microorganisms, *S. pyogenes* (group A streptococcus) and *Clostridium sordellii*, have been associated with TSS in obstetric and gynecologic patients. These rare but commonly fatal infections challenge clinicians both diagnostically and therapeutically (Table 2-1).

Staphylococcal Toxic Shock Syndrome

The TSS associated with *Staphylococcus aureus* is commonly associated with fever (>102°F), a diffuse or palmar erythroderma progressing to subsequent peripheral desquamation, and mucous membrane hyperemia. Vomiting and diarrhea are common, and multiple organ system dysfunction with rapid progression to hypotension and shock can be seen in severe cases. Menstrually related TSS occurs in young (ages 16–30) women using tampons with high absorbency for water. These tampons promote the production of toxic shock toxin 1, an exotoxin unique to *S. aureus*, which is responsible for the clinical manifestations of this disease. Nonmenstrually related cases have been associated with surgical wound infections, postpartum infections, and nonsurgical focal infections such as mastitis.

Streptococcal Toxic Shock Syndrome

The pathogenesis of streptococcal TSS involves the acquisition of *S. pyogenes*. Mucous membranes serve as the source of this microorganism without manifesting signs of a symptomatic infection. Tissue invasion occurs, and if pyrogenic exotoxin A or B is expressed, shock, multiorgan failure, and tissue destruction ensue. Streptococcal TSS has been reported in cases of septic abortion, postpartum endomyometritis, necrotizing fasciitis, and postoperative infection. The case definition requires the isolation of the group A streptococcus, hypotension, and evidence of multisystem dysfunction.

TABLE 2-1. CLINICAL MANIFESTATIONS OF TOXIC SHOCK SYNDROMES

Characteristic	Staphylococcus aureus	Streptococcus pyogenes	Clostridium sordellii
Menstrually related	+	–	–
Not related to menses	+	+	+
Fever	+	+	–
Rash	+	–	–
Hypotension	+	+	+
Spreading edema	–	–	+
Multiorgan dysfunction	+	+	+
Hemoconcentration	–	–	+

A rash is not a prominent presenting sign in patients with streptococcal TSS.

Clostridium sordellii–associated Toxic Shock Syndrome

The TSS associated with *C. sordellii* is characterized by the sudden onset of weakness, nausea, and vomiting, followed by progressive refractory hypotension associated with local and spreading edema. It is distinguished from staphylococcal TSS by the absence of *S. aureus*, fever, and rash. The classic *C. sordellii*-associated TSS has been described in patients with episiotomy infection, but it has also been associated with postpartum infections, wound infections, a vaginal foreign body, and a degenerating cervical myoma. The pathogenesis involves the production by *C. sordellii* of toxins similar to those produced by *Clostridium difficile*.

Management

All patients with TSS present with an evolving clinical picture resulting in shock. Initial management includes clinically supporting the patient, beginning broad-spectrum antimicrobial therapy, and in selected cases, surgical intervention. Once the diagnosis is clarified, more specific antimicrobial treatment (such as penicillin for streptococcal TSS or a β-lactamase–resistant antibiotic for *S. aureus* TSS) can be initiated. Initial considerations during the physical examination involve the removal of tampons, sponges, or other foreign bodies from the vagina. Cultures of the mucous membranes (oropharynx, vagina), blood, focal lesions (ie, endometrium), and urine should be performed to detect one of the potential pathogens. Fluid replacement to correct hypotension and monitoring in an intensive care setting are required. Recent reports suggest that intravenous immune globulin therapy may play an important role in the treatment of these syndromes.

PELVIC TUBERCULOSIS

Although pelvic tuberculosis is rare in the United States, continued consideration of the diagnosis is important, particularly in HIV-positive and immigrant populations. Although it is usually asymptomatic, common complaints associated with this disease include infertility, abdominal or pelvic pain, and abnormal uterine bleeding. Pelvic pain may be manifest by dysmenorrhea or deep dyspareunia. Pelvic examination is abnormal in only half of cases, and the findings, such as a pelvic mass, are nonspecific. Menstrual fluid collection and culture appear to be the most reliable diagnostic test, but granulomas are present in a premenstrual endometrial biopsy in up to 75% of women with this infection. Endometrial involvement occurs from seeding by organisms draining from the fallopian tubes directly. Infection in the fallopian tubes is acquired hematogenously or, rarely, by lymphatic spread from a primary focus in the lung or gastrointestinal tract.

Because of the increasing prevalence of drug-resistant tuberculosis, a four-drug regimen (isoniazid, rifampin, pyrazinamide, and ethambutol or streptomycin) is preferred for the initial, empirical treatment of tuberculosis. Susceptibility testing should be performed on isolates of *Mycobacterium tuberculosis* from all patients. If the isolate is susceptible, two-drug therapy (usually isoniazid and rifampin) is adequate. If treatment fails or pain persists, total abdominal hysterectomy and bilateral salpingo-oophorectomy are indicated.

BIBLIOGRAPHY

Barry W, Hudgins L, Donta ST, Pesanti EL. Intravenous immunoglobulin therapy for toxic shock syndrome. JAMA 1992;267:3315–3316

Brunham RC, Binns B, Guijon F, Danforth D, Kossein ML, Rand F, et al. Etiology and outcome of acute pelvic inflammatory disease. J Infect Dis 1988;158:510–517

Centers for Disease Control and Prevention. Initial therapy for tuberculosis in the era of multidrug resistance: recommendations of the Advisory Council for the Elimination of Tuberculosis. MMWR 1993;42(RR-7):1–8

Centers for Disease Control and Prevention. 1993 Sexually transmitted diseases treatment guidelines. MMWR 1993;42:75–83

Centers for Disease Control. Pelvic inflammatory disease: guidelines for prevention and management. MMWR 1991;40(RR-5):1–25

Centers for Disease Control and Prevention. Recommendations for the prevention and management of *Chlamydia trachomatis* infections, 1993. MMWR 1993;42(RR-12):1–29

Kahn JG, Walker CK, Washington AE, Landers DV, Sweet RL. Diagnosing pelvic inflammatory disease: a comprehensive analysis and considerations for developing a new model. JAMA 1991;266:2594–2604

Margolis K, Wranz PA, Kruger TF, Joubert JJ, Odendaal HJ. Genital tuberculosis at Tygerberg Hospital—prevalence, clinical presentation and diagnosis. S Afr Med J 1992;81:12–15

McGregor JA, Soper DE, Lovell G, Todd JK. Maternal deaths associated with Clostridium sordellii infection. Am J Obstet Gynecol 1989;161:987–995

Peterson HB, Walker CK, Kahn JG, Washington AE, Eschenbach DA, Faro S. Pelvic inflammatory disease: key treatment issues and options. JAMA 1991;266:2605–2611

Soper DE, Brockwell NJ, Dalton HP. Microbial etiology of urban emergency room acute salpingitis: treatment with ofloxacin. Am J Obstet Gynecol 1992;167:653–660

Wager GP. Toxic shock syndrome: a review. Am J Obstet Gynecol 1983;146:93–102

Wasserheit JN, Bell TA, Kiviat NB, Wolner-Hanssen P, Zabriskie V, Kirby BD, et al. Microbial causes of proven pelvic inflammatory disease and efficacy of clindamycin and tobramycin. Ann Intern Med 1986;104:187–193

Westrom L. Clinical manifestations and diagnosis of pelvic inflammatory disease. J Reprod Med 1983;28(10 Suppl):703–708

Wolner-Hanssen P, Kiviat NB, Holmes KK. Atypical pelvic inflammatory disease: subacute, chronic, or subclinical upper genital tract infection in women. In: Holmes KK, Mårdh P, Sparlin PF, Wiesner PJ, eds. Sexually transmitted diseases. New York: McGraw-Hill, 1990:615–620

Working Group on Severe Streptococcal Infections. Defining the group A streptococcal toxic shock syndrome: rationale and consensus definition. JAMA 1993;269:390–391

Sexuality and Sexual Dysfunction

Many women perceive their obstetrician–gynecologist as the initial contact for exploring all aspects of their health, including their sexual health. If physicians do not respond to these concerns, patients may become discouraged about discussing their sexuality and may have their fears and doubts reinforced.

Both the patient and the physician share some of the difficulties inherent in talking about sexual issues. A physician's casual answer to even the most innocent question of a sexual nature may reinforce a patient's concerns or contribute to her feelings of inadequacy or inferiority. If the physician is particularly busy at the moment, it is better to listen to the woman for a few minutes, then tell her of the time dilemma, and schedule a 20–30-minute visit, preferably at the end of an office day, within the next week. A physician who only half listens and is distracted by other concerns may leave the woman feeling that her concerns are not important for discussion.

Predictably, certain events in a woman's life may produce sufficient changes to cause her to be concerned about her sexual health. These include development or absence of secondary sexual characteristics, onset or absence of menarche, sexual activity and intercourse, the use of contraception, pregnancy, menopause, surgical procedures that affect future childbearing, menstruation or sexual function, and change in the status of marriage or an intimate relationship. As long as physicians perceive their patients' sexual health as an integral part of these life changes, sexuality can be discussed as part of overall health care.

THE SEXUAL RESPONSE CYCLE

The first stage of sexual response is desire. This is comparable to the energy that either permits or allows an individual to initiate or respond to sexual stimulation. The second stage of sexual response is arousal. Both physical and emotional excitement may lead to breast and genital vasodilatation. Dilatation and engorgement of the blood vessels in the labia and tissue surrounding the vagina produce the orgasmic platform, the area at the distal third of the vagina where blood becomes sequestered. Localized perivaginal swelling and vaginal lubrication constitute the early changes in this stage of sexual response. Subsequently, ballooning of the proximal portion of the vagina and elevation of the uterus into the false pelvis occur.

The third stage of the cycle—orgasm—occurs as one or both individuals maximize the physical and emotional excitement that has been generated. It requires that individuals relinquish their sense of control and experience the feelings of the moment. Physiologically, in the female a series of involuntary 0.8-second contractions of the ischiocavernous and pubococcygeal muscles occur during orgasm. In the male, reflex contractions of the vas deferens, prostate gland, and seminal vesicles propel ejaculate to the posterior urethra. This is followed by 0.8-second contractions of the bulbocavernous and ischiocavernous muscles that propel the ejaculate out of the urethra.

In the psychology of sexual response, an individual may review and evaluate a sexual experience and may also interpret it in terms of success or failure. This interpretation contributes to greater or lesser desire for future sexual experiences. If the experiences are pleasant and enjoyable, desire will be enhanced; experiences that are painful, uncomfortable, or psychologically threatening will contribute to decreased desire.

A recurrent barrier or interruption during any of the stages of the sexual response cycle can result in sexual dysfunction. Lack of desire, lack of arousal, and lack of orgasm are examples of such barriers. Performance anxiety, misconceptions about human sexual response, a generally discordant relationship, a reaction to illness, and some medical or surgical treatments are some of the causes of these barriers that may lead to the sexual difficulties.

SOURCES OF SEXUAL DYSFUNCTION

There are many real and potential causes of sexual difficulties, but the most common ones may be grouped under relationship difficulties, intrapsychic factors, or medical and biologic factors. Sexual problems may be either primary (onset when the individual became sexually active) or secondary (situational).

Relationship Factors

In some instances when a woman complains of sexual difficulty, the cause is an interpersonal problem with her partner. If relationship problems begin and are chronic or progressive, it is probably only a matter of time before the difficulty includes sexual problems. In other cases, the difficulty is sexually based, in which the partner may not know what appropriate sex play is or the woman may be unable or unwilling to respond. Blame may be assigned to the partner. The woman needs to assume some responsibility for her own sexual pleasure and be able to communicate her needs effectively to her partner. If her partner rejects explicit requests, the difficulty is a relationship problem and not strictly a sexual one.

In dealing with sexual and interpersonal health, the obstetrician–gynecologist should offer education, counseling, and techniques that are appropriate for brief evaluation and treatment. Basic information about the variety of interpersonal, family, and sexual patterns is helpful. Physicians should understand the importance of prevention and learn the appropriate procedures and skills to help resolve conflicts in the earliest stages. By developing a clinical awareness of the interplay between family stresses and illness and having resources for referrals when they are indicated, obstetrician–gynecologists can be helpful to their patients.

Intrapsychic Factors

Individual or intrapsychic problems that may affect sexual functioning sometimes stem from faulty learning or conditioning in childhood or adolescence. Inhibitions may be due to specific traumatic events and their emotional sequelae, such as sexual abuse as a child. Some women who have been abused as children believe that their sense of trust has been violated and may have extraordinary difficulties relating in an intimate and sensual way to their partners. Other women respond by totally losing their sexual desire or their ability to experience orgasm. Usually, if an intrapsychic factor is responsible, there will be other manifestations of the intrapsychic process.

Medical and Biologic Factors

Patients may perceive any illness, problem, or changes in the reproductive tract as a threat to sexual functioning. These feelings may revolve around reproductive events or be related to a medical condition or resultant surgery.

Pregnancy

Masters and Johnson reported on sexual changes during pregnancy by using two study groups. In the first group of six pregnant women, sexual functioning was directly observed and measured in the research laboratory. In the second group of 111 pregnant women, regular verbal reports on sexual functioning were obtained as their pregnancies progressed. Accordingly, they found that sexual frequency decreased in the first trimester (mostly because of psychologic factors), increased in the second trimester (allegedly because of increased pelvic congestion), and decreased in the third trimester (because of physical discomfort). In the 1970s, interviews of 260 women just after childbirth revealed that intercourse decreased in a linear fashion once pregnancy was discovered; orgasmic ability and sexual interest also decreased. In a study of women's desire to be held during pregnancy, more than one half of the women noted a change in their wish to be held, and of those who did, approximately three of four reported an increased desire.

Menopause

From a sexual perspective, postmenopausal women with no hormone replacement typically have more difficulty with vaginal lubrication and find insertion and penetration painful at times. Because the vaginal epithelium is thinner and more atrophic, it is more susceptible to trauma and abrasions. A vicious cycle can result, with decreased lubrication, painful penetration resulting in muscular spasm, more pain at penetration, a further decrease in lubrication, and, possibly, a secondary vaginismus. Estrogen replacement therapy—assuming that there are no contraindications—and the use of a vaginal dilator for a short period of time may be extraordinarily helpful in alleviating these sexual difficulties.

For many elderly women, the frequency of sexual intercourse decreases somewhat but not dramatically. If there is a significant decrease in sexual frequency, an important reason is the partner's inability to obtain or maintain an erection of sufficient rigidity to have intercourse. This may occur because of medication, vascular disease, or some other illness.

For those couples who are attitudinally and behaviorally comfortable with sexual stimulation to orgasm without intercourse, sexual frequency is much more likely to be maintained. These behaviors may include manual stimulation of the partner's genitals, oral–genital stimulation, or simply rubbing the partially erect penis against the vaginal opening or clitoris. For these couples the frequency of their lovemaking may not change; only the form that it takes may change.

For other couples who simply are not comfortable with sexual stimulation outside of intercourse, sexual frequency may decrease dramatically. For some couples, a life of celibacy may be well tolerated and accepted, but for others significant marital strife may result.

Cancer

One study found that only 4 of 60 women reported having discussions with their physicians on how mastectomy might affect their sexuality, in contrast to almost 50% of the women who indicated a desire for such a discussion but thought that this would be an inappropriate topic because no health care professional brought it up. Important findings from that study included the following:

- Forty-nine percent of women resumed intercourse within 1 month of discharge from the hospital, but one third of the women did not resume intercourse by 6 months.
- The number of women who never used the female superior position for intercourse increased threefold after mastectomy, suggesting that looking directly at the mastectomy site was discomforting for the woman, her partner, or both.
- The frequency of breast stimulation decreased substantially, indicating both avoidance of the remaining breast by the partner and a definite avoidance of single-breast stimulation by some women.
- Thirty-eight percent of men had not viewed the mastectomy scar in the first 3 months postoperatively.

Virtually all diagnoses may have—in the woman's mind—some influence on her sexual functioning. For the woman, her assumption is her reality, and that is why it is important that a dialogue about the sexual implications of disease take place between the physician and the patient.

Acute or Immediate Sources

Whatever the past or remote causes, there are always immediate factors that contribute to the lack of sexual pleasure and satisfaction. These include performance anxiety, spectatoring, communication difficulties, avoidance of sex, or ineffective arousal.

Almost everyone who has problems with sexual performance develops anxiety. An anxious individual approaches sex with a foreboding of failure that is sufficient to inhibit arousal or orgasm. As a consequence of this attitude, a woman may begin to monitor her own responses, a process called spectatoring. She wonders whether she will respond or experience orgasm. She worries about her partner's possible reaction and whether her failure will produce anger and rejection on her partner's part. Monitoring of her own performance effectively interferes with her appropriate participation with her partner and decreases her capacity to receive signals from her own body.

In the presence of performance anxiety and spectatoring, the partner may feel tension that makes it difficult to talk openly and freely about their sexual difficulties. This common communication disorder frequently takes the form of not talking about the problem at all, having discussions that lead to angry exchanges, blaming each other, or rationalizing one's own difficulty in responding. This communication difficulty may be nonverbal, with the partners indicating to each other in various ways their unhappiness in the sexual relationship. Sexual encounters may become demanding or selfish or may result in a stereotyped pattern, none of which can produce effective arousal. This situation may deteriorate to the point of almost precluding sex altogether; months may elapse between sexual encounters. There may be a conspiracy of silence about the situation, with neither partner actively complaining. The woman may bring this trouble to her gynecologist after it has been present for a number of years.

MANAGEMENT

Treatment of patients with sexual dysfunction involves a series of steps in behavior modification aimed at reducing the demand for performance, eliminating the emotions that inhibit appropriate responses, or teaching the woman and her partner what types of external physical and internal psychologic behaviors are needed to augment their responsiveness. In addition to assuming the role of educator, the physician can relieve much anxiety and guilt by showing a nonjudgmental attitude. The physician's immediate task is to reduce the patient's immediate anxiety and gather enough information to make a proper diagnosis; the physician can than treat the patient or provide a proper referral.

The interview should be conducted in a comfortable and private setting. It is best not to conduct the interview in an examination room, and it is definitely best not to conduct the interview with the patient in a hospital gown, on an examination table. If there is insufficient time for a relaxed discussion, the interview should be rescheduled appropriately. Before treatment starts, the physician needs to be honest with himself or herself about the capabilities and interests he or she has for providing this type of therapy. If the physician is too busy or does not feel sufficiently confident to undertake this treatment, referral is the best choice.

Lack of Desire

The lack of sexual desire is the most common female sexual dysfunction for which women seek advice from physicians. More research is needed to help increase physicians' understanding of this important aspect of sexual functioning. It is already known that some disturbances of sexual desire are dyadic, or interpersonal, in origin, often as a consequence of anger or resentment. These feelings may be secondary to the relationship interaction or the result of previous sexual failures. Conditioning may also inhibit the sexual response cycle at this level. For example, a woman who has had difficulty experiencing orgasm over a number of years may develop a defeatist attitude about her ability to be orgasmic, and over time she may find that her ability to be aroused is also decreased. As sexual interaction continues, the process may erode further so that by the time she sees a gynecologist her chief complaint will be the lack of desire.

Some women with low levels of desire are able to be aroused and are able to be orgasmic with relative ease, but they simply have relatively little interest in starting the process or in having the process started by their partner. Most women who present with a low sexual desire have some difficulty with arousal or orgasm. Occasionally, a woman's desire is inhibited because she has repressed sexual fantasies or homosexual impulses and worries that these impulses might be put into action if she were to become sexually interested.

When a woman is reacting to angry feelings toward her partner, and if this is secondary to repeated sexual failures in the past, a qualified sex therapist can intervene effectively. If the problem is primarily due to difficulties in the relationship, referral to an appropriate marriage or relationship counselor is indicated. Treatment of patients with low sexual desire or desire-phase dysfunctions can be trying and difficult for the woman and possibly for her partner and her gynecologist. If, after taking a history of the patient's psychologic relationship and sexual history, the gynecologist does not see an obvious cause, and particularly if the problem is of long duration, the best choice is referral.

Lack of Arousal

Difficulty with becoming sexually aroused may occur if there is insufficient holding, touching, kissing, or caressing or if the woman is experiencing fear, anger, or guilt. Any of these factors may be either self-generated or interpersonally generated. Whatever the cause, the woman with this type of arousal-phase dysfunction fails to achieve the necessary degree of arousal. This may be manifest either physiologically by insufficient vasocongestion or psychologically. Both psychologic and physiologic factors are important for high levels of arousal both to occur and to be appreciated.

If a woman is unable to become aroused with appropriate stimulation, other causes for the arousal-phase dysfunction must be explored. These may include attitudinal concepts whereby sexual arousal is not part of her self-image. It is also possible that she is not comfortable communicating to her partner her specific likes or dislikes or that if she does communicate them, the partner may have trouble doing what she likes.

To clarify these issues, the use of the sensate focus exercises as originally described by Masters and Johnson can be helpful. In these exercises both the man and the woman are nude in a warm room, and they decide in advance who will be the giver and who will be the receiver. If the man is to be the receiver, he lies on his abdomen on the bed and the woman sits beside him. During the next 15 minutes there should be no conversation—except to say that something is painful. The woman uses a warm lotion and gently caresses his entire body. She starts at the back of his neck, caresses first one arm and then the other arm, and then continues caressing down his back. This is followed by the buttocks, one leg, the other leg, and both feet. After the man rolls over, she caresses one leg and then the other leg, skips the genital area, and caresses the lower abdomen, chest, and neck. After that the couple changes roles. The man becomes the giver, the woman becomes the receiver, and he caresses her in a similar fashion.

One purpose of the exercise is to help teach a couple that they can successfully relate to each other physically and do not need to experience performance pressure or performance anxiety. As the couple is able to do sensate focus and have it be a pleasurable experience for each partner, the couple goes on to breast and genital touching or stimulation. In the classic position, the man is sitting on the bed leaning with his back against some pillows, while the woman is leaning with her back to his chest. He reaches his arms around her body and she puts her hands on each of his hands and guides and directs him on how she would like her breasts, lower abdomen, inner thighs, and genital area to be touched and stimulated. By nonverbally communicating her desires about where and how she would like to be touched and when, an effective learning process for the man takes place. As the man learns how to stimulate her to orgasm—under the tactile direction of her hand on top of his—the couple is ready to proceed to additional sexual activity.

Lack of Orgasm

At one time, women who were unable to have an orgasm during intercourse were considered to be dysfunctional or frigid. This is no longer the case. More than 90% of women are able to experience orgasm. For some of these women, orgasms occur with self-stimulation or with partner stimulation manually, orally, or with a vibrator. Accurate statistics are difficult to obtain, but in most studies only approximately 30–40% of women are able to experience orgasm during intercourse, and a number of these women require simultaneous stimulation of the clitoral area for an orgasm to occur.

It is still questionable whether coital orgasmic dysfunction is pathologic or a normal variation, but most authorities consider it normal. Orgasmic dysfunction is categorized as either primary (existing from the beginning of sexual activity) or secondary (situational), either with one or the other partner or under one set of circumstances and not another. In some cases the woman may complain of having difficulty experiencing orgasm, and on specific questioning the physician may learn that she also has an arousal-phase dysfunction. Orgasms can occur only from high levels of arousal, but if the woman has never experienced an orgasm she may have trouble differentiating high from low levels of arousal.

If a woman has a primary orgasmic dysfunction and has never had experience with self-stimulation, an effective, behaviorally oriented, time-limited treatment program has been broken down into the following nine steps:

1. The woman is gently told that she needs to get in touch with her own body and increase her self-awareness. She is instructed to stand nude in front of a full-length mirror in her home and gently run her hands over her body. The woman is instructed to use a hand mirror to examine her genitals, closely identifying the various areas with the aid of diagrams. Many women find the genital exploration to be somewhat more acceptable if done shortly after bathing.

2. The woman is instructed to explore her genitals with her fingertips as well as visually. Over time, by actually touching and feeling the entire vulva and labia, the woman usually will become somewhat desensitized to the sight and feel of her genitals.

3. Next, the woman is instructed to locate those sensitive areas of her genitals that produce pleasurable feelings. She is instructed to explore the entire genital region, including the clitoral shaft and hood, the labia majora and minora, the vaginal opening, and the perineum. Many woman find the clitoris and clitoral area to be the most pleasurable.

4. After the pleasure-producing areas are located, the woman is told to concentrate on manual stimulation of these areas, again in the privacy of her home. A lubricating jelly may help to prevent irritation.

5. As sexual arousal continues, the woman is instructed to increase the intensity and duration of the self-stimulation. It is helpful to introduce the concept of a sexual or erotic fantasy to increase sexual arousal. The concept of fantasizing during self-stimulation does not seem to occur spontaneously in many women.

6. If an orgasm has not been reached in the previous step, the woman is instructed to purchase a vibrator that either straps onto her hand, causing her fingers to vibrate, or can be applied directly to the genital area. For some women, fears about the loss of control during an orgasm may be so important that it is necessary to role-play an orgasm.

7. Once a woman has achieved orgasm through masturbation, the focus shifts to enabling her to experience orgasm through stimulation from her husband or partner. As a first step in the process, the woman is instructed to stimulate herself with her husband lying beside her in bed. This helps desensitize her to visibly displaying arousal and orgasm in his presence and also functions as an excellent learning experience for the husband. He learns what techniques of genital stimulation are effective and pleasurable for her.

8. This step involves having the husband or partner manually stimulate the woman's genital area. On some occasions it may be helpful if her hand rests on top of his, guiding him nonverbally. Nonverbal instruction tends to work better for many couples. Ultimately, he needs to learn what to do; simply learning what not to do by exclusion does not teach him what he should do.

9. Once high levels of arousal and, possibly, orgasm have occurred in step 8, the couple is instructed to engage in intercourse. For some women it is extremely important to have an orgasm during intercourse. Therapeutically, use of the so-called bridge technique, in which the clitoris or clitoral area is manually stimulated simultaneously with intercourse, can be helpful. Either her hand or her partner's hand can be used, depending on the one that is psychologically most acceptable, most physically accessible, and most effective. If the couple prefers the woman in the supine position during intercourse, manual clitoral stimulation is technically best achieved with her hand.

Various group treatments, the so-called preorgasmic groups, have become quite popular for women who want and need the group support of other women dealing with a similar problem.

Vaginismus and Dyspareunia

Vaginismus is a spasm of the levator ani muscle, making penile penetration into the vagina difficult and painful. The diagnosis covers a spectrum from the point in which the woman is unable to be examined gynecologically to one in which she is quite comfortable in the gynecologist's office but is extremely fearful of penile vaginal penetration. In some cases of vaginismus, the onset may be related to a previous painful episode, either psychologic or physiologic. Most cases of vaginismus are primary in nature, with the problem being present during the first coital attempt. The appropriate treatment consists of behavior-modifying muscle-awareness (Kegel) exercises and vaginal-dilation exercises in combination with counseling.

In muscle-awareness exercise, one of the examiner's fingers is placed inside the vaginal introitus, and the woman is instructed to contract the same muscles that she uses to stop the flow of urine. Once these have been identified, the woman inserts her own finger into the vagina. The next step is to have the woman transfer her conscious attention from her finger that is being squeezed to the vaginal muscles that are doing the squeezing. Most women are able to identify the sensation of their finger being squeezed before they can identify the sensation of the vaginal muscles doing the squeezing.

With a relatively normal pubococcygeal muscle, the primary sexual effect of the Kegel exercises is probably to help the woman develop a cognitive awareness of the feelings and sensations coming from the lower vagina. This includes recognition of the distinction between a contracted and a relaxed pubococcygeal muscle. The process is continued at home, and once a woman can identify the appropriate muscles, isometric vaginal contractions can be done without placing a finger in the vagina.

The psychophysiologic process of vaginal-dilation exercises enables a woman to learn that something put into her vagina under her control does not cause pain. Although plastic syringe covers can be used, vaginal dilators are preferred by a number of women.

The small dilator is approximately the size of the fifth finger and is initially placed in the vagina by the woman. As each dilator is replaced by the next larger size without pain, a change from muscle spasm to muscle relaxation occurs. In the absence of scars or stenosis, dilators do not cause mechanical dilation or relaxation of the introitus. Symptom resolution is highest when the woman inserts the dilators into her vagina.

Erectile Dysfunction

Erectile dysfunction or impotence is difficulty obtaining or maintaining a penile erection of sufficient rigidity to allow for vaginal penetration. Unfortunately, lack of scientific knowledge about the pathophysiology of erectile dysfunction, lack of precise objective examinations to document the erectile dysfunction, and lack of communication between physician and patient have all contributed to the common belief that erectile dysfunction is mostly of psychogenic etiology.

Most investigators have found that a sudden onset of erectile dysfunction that occurs intermittently is mostly associated with a psychogenic etiology, whereas erectile dysfunction that has a gradual onset and is persistent or progressive is mostly associated with an organic cause. The significant pathophysiologic factors in erectile dysfunction are vascular, pharmacologic, neurologic, endocrine, surgical, and miscellaneous.

The diagnosis is based on nocturnal penile tumescence monitoring and a vascular assessment, which may include the direct injection of vasoactive drugs into the corpora cavernosa, infusion pharmacocavernosometry, pharmacocavernosography, duplex ultrasonography, and arteriography. These assessments may be used singly or in combination.

Following are six characteristics of nocturnal penile tumescence:

1. Nocturnal penile tumescence occurs consistently in healthy males between the ages of 3 and 79.
2. Most (80–90%) periods of rapid eye movement are accompanied by erections.
3. Nocturnal penile tumescence occurs every 90–100 minutes during a normal night's sleep and lasts an average of 20–40 minutes per episode.
4. The quantity of nocturnal penile tumescence is related to age. In adolescence, nocturnal penile tumescence constitutes 32% of total sleep. It remains at this level until approximately age 40, then declines to about 20% for a man in his 60s.
5. The quality of nocturnal penile tumescence is also age related. During adolescence there are approximately 90 minutes of full erections during a night's sleep, in middle age about 45 minutes, and in the 70s about 20 minutes.
6. Both rapid eye movement and nocturnal penile tumescence are more prominent in the latter portion of a normal night's sleep than in the earlier portion.

The usual working assumption for the clinical use of nocturnal penile tumescence in the differential diagnosis of erectile dysfunction is that a nondepressed man with a normal nocturnal penile tumescence for age has a psychogenic etiology for the dysfunction. Either no nocturnal penile tumescence or partial nocturnal penile tumescence or insufficient penile rigidity in the presence of a normal night's sleep indicates an organic etiology. For reasons not well understood, significant psychologic repression in selected cases may cause abnormal nocturnal penile tumescence patterns.

The direct injection of vasoactive pharmacologic agents into the corpora cavernosa for both diagnostic and therapeutic purposes has become quite popular since the mid-1980s. The drugs most commonly used are papaverine hydrochloride (a smooth muscle relaxant) and phentolamine mesylate (a sympathetic antagonist). Some urologists prefer prostaglandin E_1 instead. These pharmacologic agents help a man obtain and maintain an erection by increasing blood flow through the penile arteries and by helping to close the corporal–venous occlusive mechanism. In approximately 80% of the cases the men with erectile dysfunction will—with the injection of these vasoactive drugs—be able to achieve an erection that is sufficiently rigid for intercourse. A 27-gauge, 0.5-in needle attached to a 1-ml syringe is used. These medications do not interfere with either ejaculation or orgasm. Test dosing should be done in the morning; if an erection lasts longer than 4 hours, pharmacologic detumescence must be considered. Scarring inside the corpora may be a troublesome complication.

The treatment of erectile dysfunction will depend in part on the diagnosis. For men with an erectile dysfunction secondary to a well-defined organic etiology, the treatment options include 1) giving up sex; 2) a sexual relationship that includes holding, touching, kissing, caressing, and stimulation to orgasm even though the couple is unable to have intercourse; 3) pharmacologic erections; 4) a vacuum constriction device; 5) a penile implant; or, in selected cases, 6) penile vascular surgery.

The concept that a couple would accept an option of a celibate relationship may seem quite foreign to most physicians, but there are some couples who will opt for that choice. If one member of the couple decides that is what he or she would like to do, and the couple is in a marital relationship, it is obviously important that the choice be acceptable to the partner. One factor that couples should be warned about is that, behaviorally, when couples stop having a sexual relationship it becomes easy to stop all physical interaction, so there may be no touching in the living room or hugging in the kitchen or kissing in the dining room. For many couples this lack of physical contact outside of the bedroom may be more burdensome than the lack of sexual contact in the bedroom. The concept of sex without intercourse can be frightening for some, unnatural for others, and making the best out of an awkward situation for others.

Couples who have previously enjoyed noncoital stimulation, perhaps to orgasm, are more likely to maintain their sexual activity without intercourse. If the physician does not believe that sex without intercourse is an acceptable option, that attitude may be inadvertently conveyed nonverbally to the couple. A book that illustrates different sexual techniques may be helpful. Some couples will want and need specific information on what sex without intercourse means. A number of men do not know that they can ejaculate without an erection.

Stimulation of the flaccid, or partially erect, penis against the clitoris or vaginal opening may provide a considerable amount of sexual enjoyment, perhaps orgasm, for many couples. For others, "heavy petting" to high levels of arousal or orgasm is a possibility, and for still others oral–genital stimulation may be preferred. An emphasis on good hygiene and sexual involvement after taking a shower may need to be emphasized. If a couple seems interested and willing to experiment, it may be helpful to prescribe some reading material and see them in several months to discuss what their experiences have been like.

For many couples intercourse is the only acceptable sexual behavior, and sexual frequency typically decreases because of the erectile dysfunction. For some of these couples the resumption of intercourse by whatever means will be the goal. The insertion by a urologist of a penile implant inside the corpora cavernosa is a possibility. Implants come in a variety of sizes and shapes and commonly are made of silicone. The two basic types are solid and inflatable. The precise measurement both in length and width is determined at the time of surgery. All implants produce a penis that is at its erect length all of the time, although it is flexible enough to bend and go down the pant leg.

A penis cannot be made larger by implantation. One inflatable penile implant consists of two hydraulic cylinders, one inside each corpus cavernosum, and an inflate–deflate pump is placed in the right hemiscrotum above the testis. To make the penis sufficiently rigid for intercourse, the man or his partner squeezes on the pump through the wall of the scrotum, transferring several ounces of fluid from the reservoir into the hydraulic cylinders. This makes the penis thicker and more rigid. The increased girth will be maintained even after ejaculation until the deflate portion of the pump is squeezed, thereby returning the fluid back to the reservoir.

For some women the thought that their husband or partner has a penile implant may create fear and anxiety, particularly if the device is inserted at a time in life when their own interest and desire are decreasing. If the husband's expectation is that sexual activity will be increasing, maybe dramatically, while the wife's concern is that her desire is decreasing, a future marital problem could develop. Prescribing physicians need to be sensitive to these issues.

For men in whom the cause of the erectile dysfunction appears to be primarily psychogenic, it is important to identify as clearly as possible the source of stress. If marital dysfunction is present, particularly if it is progressive and chronic, referral to a competent marriage counselor is the best treatment choice. If the marriage is intact, and particularly if the wife is interested and cooperative, it is always helpful to have her included. Sexual counseling entails teaching the couple how to enjoy a "nondemand" sexual interaction. Sensate focus exercises and genital stimulation exercises, as detailed by Masters and Johnson, are helpful.

The man's "performance anxiety," whereby he becomes so concerned about the outcome of the sexual interaction that he fails to attend to the erotic stimulation and other aspects of the sexual experience, needs to be addressed. This fear must be reversed and can be best taught by a sexual interaction pattern that is nondemanding and does not include intercourse. If couples make progress, they should be encouraged to continue. If the psychologic and behavioral treatment is getting bogged down, referral may be the best option. With some time and patience, many couples will be helped by the intervention of the practicing physician.

BIBLIOGRAPHY

Ekelund L, Forsberg L, Olsson AM. Pharmacoangiographic assessment of penile arteries in patients with erectile failure. Urology 1988; 31:271–274

Frank D, Dornbush RL, Webster SK, Kolodny RC. Mastectomy and sexual behavior: a pilot study. Sex Disabil 1978;1:16–26

Fuchs AM, Mehringer CM, Rajfer J. Anatomy of penile venous drainage in potent and impotent men during cavernosography. J Urol 1989;141:1353–1356

Hollender MH, McGehee JB. The wish to be held during pregnancy. J Psychosom Res 1974;18:193–197

Kinsey AC, Pomeroy WB, Martin CE, Gebhard PH. Sexual behavior in human females. Philadelphia: WB Saunders, 1953

LoPiccolo J, Lobitz WC. The role of masturbation in the treatment of orgasmic dysfunction. In: LoPiccolo J, LoPiccolo L, eds. Handbook of sex therapy. New York: Plenum Press, 1978:187–195

Masters WH, Johnson VE. Human sexual inadequacy. Boston: Little, Brown, 1970

Masters WH, Johnson VE. Human sexual response. Boston: Little, Brown, 1966:141–144

Rollin B. First you cry. New York: New American Library, 1976

Schover LR. Sex after cancer: help your patient avoid dysfunction. Female Patient 1988;13(1):34–40

Solberg DA, Butler J, Wagner NN. Sexual behavior in pregnancy. N Engl J Med 1973;288:1098–1103

Stief CG, Benard F, Diederichs W, Bosch R, Lue TF, Tanagho EA. The rationale for pharmacologic cavernosography. J Urol 1988;140: 1564–1566

Stief CG, Diederichs W, Benard F, Bosch R, Lue TF, Tanagho EA. The diagnosis of venogenic impotence: dynamic or pharmacologic cavernosometry? J Urol 1988;140:1561–1563

Vincent CE, Vincent B, Greiss FC, Linton EB. Some marital-sexual concomitants of carcinoma of the cervix. South Med J 1975;68:552–558

Wabrek AJ. Nocturnal penile tumescence (NPT). Conn Med 1981; 45:559–562

Crisis Intervention

Obstetricians and gynecologists have the opportunity to identify and modify acute and chronic social problems involving their patients and their patients' families. During the evaluation of a new patient or a patient returning for an interval visit, the physician may ask the patient specific questions about her emotional status, family or psychosocial circumstances, and her current relationships. This can be done even though her chief complaint is of a physical nature. A history of recent losses and information concerning recent or past illnesses and medication use should also be sought, as these may affect the patient's personal and family well-being.

This section discusses child physical and sexual abuse, rape, domestic violence, and grief, all of which may lead the patient to seek help under the guise of a physical problem. These conditions can also lead to a poor self-image which, in turn, frequently preprograms an individual to make poor choices in subsequent life situations. Grief stems from loss, a normal human phenomenon. However, the patient's reaction to loss may be within the limits of what is considered normal or may be exaggerated to the point where it interferes with normal functions. It may be associated with anxiety, depression, and self-destructive tendencies.

Physicians must be alert to social problems because they are extremely common. If the proper observations are made and appropriate questions are asked in a matter-of-fact, nonembarrassing, and nonjudgmental fashion, these problems can be detected in a surprisingly large number of patients. It is frequently difficult for busy physicians to counsel patients with social problems, but at least by identifying them they may be able to make referrals to appropriate individuals or agencies. Physicians should develop a referral list of agencies and individual counselors who deal with specific problems so that, when such problems are identified, the transition to such help can be made smoothly.

PHYSICAL AND SEXUAL ABUSE OF CHILDREN

Physical Abuse

The term *battered child syndrome* was introduced in 1962, and since that time public awareness of this problem has been increasing. Today, it is the major cause of death and disability among children; the incidence of reported child battering is in excess of 500,000 cases annually. It is likely that the actual rate of child abuse is even higher. If the child is returned to the home without any therapeutic intervention, at least 50%

will be battered again, and approximately 10% subsequently will be killed.

Studies have shown that less than 20% of child abuse victims are assaulted by strangers. Most attacks are by a close relative. A history of child abuse is a common finding among spouse abusers, subsequent child abusers, individuals arrested for delinquency and violent crimes, and individuals with psychosomatic problems, especially those associated with pain. Alcoholism and drug use is frequently a related condition.

All 50 states have enacted laws that require physicians to report suspected cases of child abuse or neglect. Thus, physicians should be aware of the signs and symptoms of these conditions. These signs include multiple injuries in one individual either as a present complaint or over time, cigarette burns, scaldings, fractures, tissue swelling, subdural hematomas, failure to thrive, and sexual molestation. Such phenomena are repeated within families and may occur in other children even if the child who has been a victim has been removed from the home. Although one parent may seem to be the perpetrator, the spouse is generally aware that such abuse is taking place and cannot necessarily be expected to protect the child. The local child protective services or police should be notified, even if such cases are only suspected. At high risk are children of single-parent families headed by teenaged mothers, families with a previous history of child abuse, and families in which alcohol and drug abuse occurs.

Sexual Abuse

The incidence of child sexual abuse is difficult to estimate. Some investigators claim that about 10% of the child abuse cases involve sexual abuse. Other approaches that deal with the histories of adult patients seem to imply that somewhere between one fourth and one third of women and, perhaps, one eighth of all men were sexually abused as children.

Two basic forms of sexual abuse in children are recognized. The first involves victimization by a stranger. This is usually a single act that, in most cases, is reported directly to the authorities and for which the circumstances are clearly stated by the child. The act may involve any form of sexual activity and may have been brought about by enticement, coercion, or physical force. In any case, it is the responsibility of the adult caring for the child to be supportive. The child should be interviewed carefully and allowed to tell what happened.

Active intervention consists of calling the police or protective services and evaluating the child medically, including obtaining specimens for forensic medical examination. Samples for culture for gonorrhea, chlamydia, syphilis, and HIV should be taken, and testing should be repeated at an appropriate interval. In children past menarche, pregnancy tests should be performed. Other laboratory tests should be done where appropriate. Prophylaxis for sexually transmitted diseases should be offered. Counseling with a mental health care worker should be obtained even if the child appears to be asymptomatic at the time of evaluation.

The child should be protected from recurrent acts. Plans for future medical, psychiatric, and laboratory evaluations should be made at the initial contact, and specific appointments given. In addition, the molester should be found and apprehended if possible. In many communities sexual abuse crisis-intervention centers are available and should be used as a referral source by the physician.

In every case, the child should be made to understand that the act was wrong and not the fault of the child. Statements implying that the child had something to do with causing the act or was somehow to blame are inappropriate and will frequently lead to serious problems in the development of the child's self-image. The child's long-term psychosocial adjustment may be affected.

Incest is surprisingly more common than had been previously thought. It is difficult to obtain specific data, but various studies of patients hospitalized for gynecologic or psychiatric problems tend to place the prevalence somewhere between 20% and 35% of young women. In 80% of sexual abuse cases, a parent, guardian, or male companion of the mother was involved. Incest between father (including the mother's companion) and daughter accounts for about 75% of reported cases, with mother–son, father–son, mother–daughter, and brother–sister incest or incest involving other close family members making up the remaining 25%. Incest is defined differently in each state. In some states intercourse is required, and in others it is not.

Father–daughter incest is frequently not a single occurrence. It may occur in families that appear quite normal, but frequently the family members have limited contact with the outside world. Beneath the surface, there may be chaotic family relationships. The father frequently has a passive, introspective personality and a weak sexual relationship with the mother. He may turn to a relationship with the daughter out of loneliness and dependency. The sexual activity may be quite affectionate and represent more a need for affection than intercourse. The mother is frequently aware of this situation and may actually tolerate it. Both parents thus agree consciously or subconsciously that the incestuous relationship is more acceptable than an extramarital one. The daughters frequently become little mothers around the house, fulfilling duties that the wife would ordinarily handle. In many cases, younger daughters are eventually molested as well.

Incest frequently occurs in families with other social problems, such as alcoholism, drug abuse, violence, delinquency, physical abuse, and mental illness. After reaching adolescence, the victim often feels guilty but may be afraid to withdraw from the relationship out of fear that doing so would destroy the family and the security it provides. Frequently the victim feels humiliated and develops a weak ego and self-image, making it difficult to develop appropriate relationships with members of the opposite sex and to make appropriate choices in the future. After leaving home, the victim often chooses the chaotic type of family existence he or she has known.

Among children in incestuous relationships, fewer than 10% have normal psychologic development at the time of first evaluation. Common findings are guilt, anger, behavioral problems, unexplained physical complaints, lying, stealing, failure in school, running away, sleep disturbances, and eating disturbances. Frequently, gynecologists see the individuals as either teenagers or adults, when some or all of these complaints have been more fully developed. In such women, gynecologists should seek a history of incest to fully understand the psychopathology of the patient. Questions should be specific; as an example, "Were you physically or sexually abused or raped as a child or adolescent?" An affirmative answer requires specific detailed questions about the individual involved and the circumstances of the situation. Some insight into whether any care or therapy was offered at that time may be useful. Questioning should take place in language that would be understandable by the patient and should be quite specific; for example, "What was the nature of the sexual activity? Did it include touching, genital manipulation, or intercourse?"

Frequently the individual is relieved to tell a health care professional about this experience, as it may be something that she has never discussed with anyone before. Often it helps the patient merely to know that this is a common human experience that is not limited to her alone and that she is blameless. Sharing of such experiences with a nonjudgmental individual can relieve a great deal of anxiety. Physicians must determine the current effect that these experiences have had on the individual so that they may make the appropriate referral to a counselor and treat the medically associated problems.

As adults, victims of incest frequently choose partners who have inadequate personalities and who are capable of physical and sexual violence. This may happen because they sense a familiarity in the developing relationship and gravitate to it. Another possibility is that their poor social and self-image may prevent them from achieving a more normal relationship.

RAPE AND SEXUAL ASSAULT

Sexual assault is defined as any sexual act performed by one person on another without the person's consent. Assault may occur as a result of the use or threat of force or the victim's inability to give appropriate consent. A 1987 report from the U.S. Department of Justice indicated that the annual incidence of sexual assault was 73/100,000 females, accounting for about 6% of all violent crimes. However, this figure probably reflects only a fraction of the actual incidence, since victims are often reluctant to report sexual assault because of embarrassment, fear of retribution, feelings of guilt, or simply lack of knowledge of their rights. It has been estimated that as many as 44% of all women have been victims of actual or attempted sexual assault at some time in their lives, and as many as 50% of these have been victims on more than one occasion. Males may also be the victims of sexual assault.

Society holds many misconceptions concerning the victims of sexual assault. These include the belief that women who are assaulted encourage the assault by their behavior or dress, that they did not offer sufficient resistance to the assault, and that they were promiscuous. Some believe that such victims also have an ulterior motive for pressing charges that will lead to the disgrace of the assaulter or to the victim's eventual financial gain.

Sexual assault occurs in all age, racial, and socioeconomic groups. The very young, the mentally and physically handicapped, and the very old are particularly susceptible. The act may be committed by a stranger but frequently is committed by someone who is known to the victim.

Variants of sexual assault include sexual assault in marriage, which is forced coitus or related sexual acts within a marital relationship without the consent of the partner. This often occurs in conjunction with physical abuse. An additional variant has been termed "date rape." In this situation the woman may voluntarily participate in sexual play, but coitus is performed—often forcibly—without her consent. Date rape frequently is not reported because the victim may believe that she contributed to the act by participating up to a point. However, both variants often lead to serious long-term problems with respect to the patient's self-esteem.

A third variant concerns statutes in most states that criminalize sexual intercourse with females under a specific age. This is referred to as statutory rape. The consent of the female is irrelevant in this situation because she is defined as being incapable of consenting.

When a woman is sexually assaulted she loses control over her life. Her integrity and sometimes her life are threatened, and she experiences intense anxiety and fear; as a result, after the assault a "rape trauma" syndrome often occurs. The immediate response (acute phase) may last for hours or days and is characterized by a distortion or paralysis of the individual's coping mechanism. The outward responses vary from complete loss of emotional control to an apparent well-controlled behavior pattern. The signs may include generalized pain throughout the body; eating and sleeping disturbances; physical symptoms such as vaginal discharge, itching, and rectal pain; and emotional complaints such as depression, anxiety, and mood swings. The delayed (organizational) phase is characterized by flashbacks, nightmares, phobias, and a need for the reorganization of thought processes. In addition, gynecologic and menstrual complaints may occur. This delayed phase may occur months or years after the event and may involve major life style adjustments. Counseling should be phase specific.

The physician evaluating the victim of sexual assault has several responsibilities, both medical and legal, and should be aware of the particular statutory requirements that may involve the use of kits for gathering evidence. Although specific responsibilities are determined by the needs of the patient and state law, a physician's general medical responsibilities are as follows:

- Obtain an accurate gynecologic history
- Assess and treat physical injuries
- Obtain appropriate cultures and treat any existing infections
- Provide therapy to prevent unwanted conception
- Provide or arrange for counseling
- Arrange for follow-up medical care and counseling

Legal responsibilities are as follows:

- Provide accurate recording of the events
- Document injuries
- Collect samples
- Report to the authorities as required by law

Informed consent must be obtained before the examination is begun and specimens are collected. In addition to fulfilling legal requirements, this process also helps the victim participate in regaining control over her body and her person.

With respect to the medical history involving the event, an accurate account of the event, an objective description, and documentation of what happened should be recorded. A thorough sexual and gynecologic history is important. With respect to the physical examination, the physician should collect clothing; evaluate the total body externally for evidence of cuts, bruises, and bite marks; investigate the oral cavity for secretions and injuries due to oral penetration; and examine the external and internal genitalia. Examination for areas of trauma and the presence of foreign objects should be carried out. A rectal examination should include examination for trauma.

In every situation, specimens of any cavity that may have been violated should be taken for culture for gonorrhea and chlamydia, for examination for the presence of spermatozoa (smears), and for examination for acid phosphatase or prostate-specific antigens. Pubic hair combings, fingernail scrapings, or semen may be obtained for specific DNA typing as well. Saliva may be collected from the victim to determine whether or not she is a secretor of a major blood group antigen so that this may be used in comparison with any antigen detected in materials of perpetrator origin. Hair samples of the patient to differentiate from collected hair of the perpetrator should also be obtained.

In addition to culturing specimens from the vagina and other appropriate orifices for gonorrhea and chlamydia, baseline serologic tests for syphilis should be performed. Serologic tests for HSV, hepatitis B virus, HIV, and cytomegalovirus can provide information that aids management and should be offered with proper informed consent. Vaginal smears for spermatozoa should be made. Wet mounts for *Trichomonas* and potassium hydroxide mounts for *Candida* should also be prepared.

Prophylactic antibiotics should be offered. An appropriate regimen for the prevention of gonorrhea, chlamydia, and syphilis is a single dose of ceftriaxone, 250 mg IM, plus doxycycline, 100 mg orally twice daily for 7 days. An alternative therapy would be a single dose of spectinomycin, 2 g IM, followed by doxycycline. If the patient is known to be pregnant, erythromycin may be substituted for doxycycline. The patient should be instructed to return in 3–4 weeks for repeat serologic tests, including hepatitis B and cultures. Tests for HIV serology should be repeated in 3–6 months.

The patient's menstrual history, birth control regimen, and pregnancy status should be assessed. If she is found to be at risk for pregnancy as a result of the assault, morning-after prophylaxis can be offered. The risk of pregnancy after sexual assault has been estimated to be 2–4% in victims who are not protected by some form of contraception at the time of the attack. An appropriate morning-after regimen is two combination OC tablets at the time the victim is seen and two in 12 hours. Oral contraceptives containing 50 μg of estrogen are appropriate. An alternative postcoital treatment consists of a 5-day regimen of high-dose estrogen, such as 5 mg of ethinyl estradiol per day or 20–30 mg of conjugated equine estrogen per day. A pregnancy test should be performed at the time of the return visit if conception is a possibility. If pregnancy is diagnosed, the patient should be counseled concerning all of the available options, including abortion.

All clothing, secretion samples, and smears should be labeled and turned over to the authorities, and a receipt should be obtained for the patient's chart. In order for the evidence to be used, it must be given directly to the proper authorities by the physician, along with the appropriate paperwork.

It is essential that the patient be given appropriate emotional support, and she should be invited to express her anxieties and to state her understanding of what has happened and what will happen. Misconceptions should be corrected immediately. She should be reassured about her concerns wherever possible. Other health personnel, particularly those trained to help rape trauma victims, should be consulted to facilitate counseling and follow-up. The patient should not be released from the facility until specific follow-up plans are made and explained to her. The follow-up plan should be agreed to by the patient, the physician, and the counselors who have become involved. The plan should reflect the patient's needs and may involve her desire to see her own physician for follow-up. An emergency resource should be provided in the event that acute psychologic symptoms arise before the next scheduled visit.

Because patients often do not remember what was said to them, all plans should be described in writing. The patient should be reevaluated psychologically in approximately 1–2 weeks after the initial medical evaluation. Follow-up counseling should be discussed at this visit. Future visits should be determined on the basis of the patient's individual needs. It is important at each contact to emphasize that the patient was not to blame for the attack. At each visit she should be allowed to discuss her feelings and current perceptions of her problem. Generally, the patient should be seen for medical follow-up 3–4 weeks after the first medical evaluation.

Regardless of the extent of her injuries, the victim will perceive the experience she has just suffered as life threatening. Many patients appear to be in control emotionally when first seen immediately after the sexual assault; this control simply reflects her defense mechanisms and should not be interpreted to indicate that the patient is coping with circumstances. It is best to assume that she is not, and it is important to follow the recommendations made regardless of the patient's apparent emotional state. It should be anticipated that she will demonstrate aspects of the rape trauma syndrome at some time in the future, and she should be counseled that this will probably happen. Appropriate therapy and counseling should be arranged when such behavior occurs.

DOMESTIC VIOLENCE

Domestic violence and *spouse abuse* are terms referring to violence occurring between partners in an ongoing relationship, regardless of whether they are married. The *battered woman* has been defined as any woman over the age of 16 with evidence of physical abuse on at least one occasion at the hands of her intimate male partner. The *battered wife syndrome* has been defined as a symptom complex occurring as a result of violence in which a woman has received deliberate, severe, and repeated (more than three times) physical abuse from her husband, with the minimal injury being severe bruising. Violent acts have been defined from least to most severe as verbal abuse, threat of violence, throwing an object, throwing an object at someone, pushing, slapping, kicking, hitting, beating up, threatening with a weapon, and using a weapon. Most definitions also incorporate the concept of intentionality and the repetitive nature of the assaults.

Although most definitions of violence view it as a physical abuse phenomenon, it may also include psychologic abuse; sexual assault; progressive social isolation; depriving the individual of sustenance such as food, clothing, money, transportation, and health care; and intimidation. In most situations, physical abuse, mental abuse, and other forms of intimidation are blended together as part of the syndrome.

In 1985, the Surgeon General of the United States sponsored a workshop on violence and public health in an effort to focus attention on this and similar problems in the hope of helping reduce the incidence of violence in society and providing more effective help for its victims. As a consequence, domestic violence is now considered a crime in most jurisdictions, and attention has been turned to attempting to ensure the safety of victims of domestic violence.

The actual incidence of domestic violence in the United States is not known. It has been estimated to affect about 2 million women per year, but this is probably conservative; the true incidence may be twice this number. Nearly one fourth of the women in the United States will be abused by a current or former partner sometime during their lives. In 1984, the U.S. Department of Justice, Bureau of Justice Statistics, reported that 57% of 450,000 annual cases of family violence were committed by spouses or exspouses and that the wife was the victim in 93% of the cases. In one fourth of these cases at least three similar incidents had been reported within the previous 6 months. In 1990, Federal Bureau of Investigation statistics reported similar findings. In addition, it has been estimated that between one third and one half of female homicide victims are murdered by their male partners, whereas only 12% of male homicide victims are killed by their female partners. Forty-seven percent of husbands who beat their wives do so three or more times per year. Fourteen percent of ever-married women report being raped by their current or former husband, and rape is a significant form of abuse in 54% of violent marriages.

Battered women account for 22–35% of women seeking care for any reason in emergency departments (most of whom have been seen by medical or other nontrauma services) and for 19–30% of injured women seen in emergency departments. It was noted that 14% of women seen in ambulatory care internal medicine clinics had been battered, with 28% of such women having been battered for some time. In addition, 25% of women who attempt suicide, 25% using psychiatric services, and 23% of pregnant women seeking prenatal care have been victims of domestic violence. In addition, 45–59% of mothers of abused children have been abused, and 58% of women over the age of 30 who have been raped have been abused.

In one study, 19% of battered women had received serious injuries to the head, 5% had lacerations requiring suture, and 62% had contusions and soft tissue injuries. The most common areas for injury were the head, neck, chest, abdomen, breasts, and upper extremities. The upper extremities were often fractured as the woman attempted to defend herself. In a large study reported from Denver, three fourths of the victims believed that the batterer would kill them in the relationship, and almost half felt that they might kill the batterer. Eleven percent of the victims in this study stated that they had actually tried to kill the batterer, and 87% stated that they themselves would be the one to die if someone was killed. In addition, half of the batterers and one third of the women in the series had threatened to commit suicide. Studies conclude that batterers and victims move easily between suicidal and homicidal intent. Suicide threats in a relationship on the part of the batterer or the victim may be a warning that a homicide may actually occur. This often happens when victims believe that they have no other choice in life. Counseling may help identify such choices.

The cost to society of domestic violence is difficult to establish. It includes emergency and long-term care of victims; legal expenses, including both police and court intervention; the expense of shelters and housing for abused women and their children; and the overall cost to the community for therapeutic services to the victim, the batterer, the children, and the family unit.

Physical abuse in pregnancy is quite common, with the incidence being 3–8%, depending on the population studied. In one study, 10.9% of patients stated that they had been a victim of abuse at some time in the past, and a third of these women stated that the abuse had continued into the present pregnancy.

The obstetrician–gynecologist, as the primary care provider for women, can play a vital role in detecting the woman who is a victim of abuse and offering her appropriate care. As with most psychosocial problems, the physician's ability to recognize the abused woman depends on his or her own index of suspicion. For example, one study showed that only 5% of domestic violence victims seen in emergency departments were identified by the physician on the emergency report as victims of abuse.

The profile of such women includes a history of having been beaten as a child, raised in a single-parent home, married as a teenager, and pregnant before marriage. Sixty percent of women in one study became pregnant before their current marriage. These women have frequent clinic visits and a variety of somatic complaints, including headache, insomnia, choking sensation, hyperventilation, gastrointestinal symptoms, and chest, pelvic, and back pain. There is frequently noncompliance with the advice or recommendations of the physician.

In visits to the emergency department, the patient appears shy, frightened, embarrassed, evasive, anxious, or passive, and often may cry. The batterer frequently accompanies the woman on such visits and stays close by to monitor what she says. The woman may be hesitant to give information about how she was injured, and her explanations often do not fit the injuries seen. Many have repeated visits to the emergency department, and some have been treated for drug and alcohol overdose in the past. Tranquilizers have often been prescribed.

It is appropriate for physicians to ask direct questions, such as, "Has anyone at home hit you or tried to injure you?," and, "Have you ever been physically abused either recently or in the past?" It is important for the physician to acknowledge the problem and affirm that battering is unacceptable.

Physical examination often may show evidence for previous injury, either remote or recent. It is important that the physician note these injuries and ask the patient how she got them. If the woman is wearing sunglasses, it is appropriate to ask her to remove them, as she may have an eye injury. Bruises on the breast and abdomen of a pregnant woman should certainly be discussed. Healed scarring or burns should be discussed. Obtaining informed consent and collecting and processing specimens for physical evidence of abuse (such as photos or drawings) for legal and forensic purposes should be carried out as for other types of physical or sexual assault.

In most abusive relationships, the battering acts occur in cycles consisting of three phases. The first phase, the tension-building phase, involves a gradual escalation of tension noted in discrete acts that cause family friction. These include name calling, intimidating remarks, meanness, and mild physical abuse such as pushing. The batterer expresses dissatisfaction and hostility, but this does not occur in an explosive form. The woman attempts to placate the batterer in the hopes of pleasing him or calming him down. She believes at this point that she must avoid aggravating him further. She will try not to respond to his hostile action and is often successful, at first, which only reinforces her belief that she can control him. As the tension builds she has more difficulty controlling his anger, and frequently withdraws, fearing that she will inadvertently set off his explosive behavior. Her withdrawal may be the signal for the man to become more aggressive.

The second phase occurs when anything sparks the hostile act, and the acute battering incident takes place. There is an uncontrollable discharge of tensions that have been built up through the earlier phase, and the batterer will attack the victim both verbally and physically, often leaving her injured. At this point, in self-defense, the woman may actually injure or kill the batterer. Up to two thirds of the batterers use alcohol, and the violent event may occur during a bout of heavy drinking. The victim often believes that the drinking is the cause of the beating, rather than an excuse for it. If law-enforcement officials are called, they also may conclude that this is the case.

The third phase follows, in which the batterer apologizes profusely, asks forgiveness, and may show kindness and remorse, showering the victim with gifts and promises. During this phase the victim begins to hope that the relationship can be saved and that the violence will not recur. Since many batterers seem charming and are manipulative, the victim may actually believe that the problem has passed.

With repeated cycles of violence, an increase in the first phase, a decrease in the third phase, and a tendency for the violence to become more acute and dangerous are noted. The batterer controls the victim and does not need to put much energy into obtaining forgiveness. The victim is so demoralized at this point that she finds it hard to leave the situation even though she may have the means and chances to do so.

Once it is found that a woman is living in an abusive relationship, it is important for the physician to acknowledge to the patient the seriousness of the situation. To do otherwise would give the impression that the physician approves of, or at least accepts, the violent condition. The physician should attend to specific injuries and assess the patient's emotional status from the standpoint of psychiatric conditions such as suicidal tendencies, depression, anxiety reaction, or abuse of drugs, alcohol, or other medications. The physician should estimate the woman's ability to assess her own situation and her readiness to take appropriate action. If mental illness is present, referral to an appropriate mental health worker sensitive to the issues of domestic violence should be made.

Although all states have requirements for reporting child abuse, few states have such requirements for domestic violence. However, many states have aggressive programs for intervening in domestic violence cases, and the physician should become aware of the programs in his or her state. The patient should be encouraged to leave the violent situation and live on her own, with family, or in a shelter for battered women. If she is not willing to leave the home because of economic concerns and a fear that the batterer may continue to pursue her, she should be informed of community resources that may help her. If fear of the batterer is the major reason for not leaving, her rights under the law should be reviewed, including the potential for arrest of the batterer or the issuance of restraining orders. If the victim cannot be convinced to leave the violent home, she should be given the telephone numbers of resource agencies and the police and encouraged to use them in the event of another acute outbreak of violence.

The victim should be encouraged to develop an exit plan that she and her children can practice as they would a fire drill. It should be put into effect if she senses that she or her children are in danger from her partner. The exit plan should take into consideration the following components:

- Having a change of clothes packed for herself and her children, including toilet articles, necessary medications, and an extra set of keys to the house and the car
- Placing items in a suitcase and storing it with a friend or a neighbor

- Keeping cash, checkbook, and a savings account book with the individual chosen
- Keeping identification papers such as birth certificates, social security card, voter registration card, utility bills, and a driver's license available, since children will need to be enrolled in school and financial assistance may have to be sought
- Taking something special, such as a book or a toy, for each child
- Retaining copies, if available, of financial records such as mortgage papers, rent receipts, or an auto title
- Deciding exactly where to go—a friend's or a relative's home or a shelter for battered women and children—regardless of time of day or night

If the patient is injured and is seen in an emergency facility, she should obtain a copy of her medical records, including specific injuries and medications prescribed. She is encouraged to be wary of tranquilizers, as these will not solve her problems.

Long-term aid will consist of placing the woman and her children in a violence-free setting; obtaining counseling, which will help her lessen her social isolation and rebuild her self-esteem; and obtaining mental health care, if necessary. The woman should also be encouraged to obtain legal aid and then may need help in acquiring reeducation or job skills, as well as child care. If the patient is considering returning to the violent home, the dynamics of the battering relationship should be reviewed and the available options discussed, so that all alternatives are considered before she makes the final decision.

The male batterer is often an individual who refuses to take responsibility for his behavior, blaming the victim for his violent acts. These individuals often have strong, controlling personalities and cannot tolerate autonomy in their partners. They are rigid in their expectations of marriage and sexual behavior. They consider their wives or partners as chattel, and they wish to be cared for in the most basic fashions as they were cared for by their mothers. They often make unrealistic demands and have low tolerance for stress. They may appear depressed or make suicidal gestures. Their basic behavior is aggressive and assaultive, and they often use violence to solve their problems throughout their lives. They can be charming and manipulative, especially in their relationships outside the marriage. At the same time, they frequently exhibit low self-esteem and have feelings of inadequacy and a sense of helplessness that are accentuated by the possibility of losing their wives. Batterers often exhibit contempt for women in their daily activities.

Appropriate therapy—whether individual therapy or group therapy—for the batterer focuses on finding ways to help him understand that violence is not the appropriate means of solving his problems. Later, when basic attitude changes have been achieved, family therapy may be helpful for the couple in helping them to define means of working out their problems. Often it is necessary to use the courts to get the batterer into therapeutic situations. If the male batterer has not undergone violence-elimination counseling, intervention with family counseling can be extremely dangerous, as such counseling often raises issues that both exacerbate the violence and increase the risk of serious harm to the woman and her children.

The major responsibility of a physician in managing a domestic violence situation is to recognize its existence and to help the victim obtain appropriate care and counseling to remove her from the violent situation. The physician should have available information that makes it possible for proper referrals to be made. Clinicians may contact their local Young Women's Christian Association (YWCA) chapter for information for referral for victims of domestic violence. Because many resources are publically funded, it is important to update the list of resources annually.

GRIEF AND LOSS

Grief is the universal response to loss and, as such, is a normal emotional reaction common to the human experience. It can affect women in any age group. However, as the woman ages, losses become a more common experience. These may include the loss of a spouse (as a result of death or divorce), a child, a close relative, or a friend; loss of a body part or organ; loss of a job or career; loss of the ability to perform enjoyed activities; and loss of a pet. The loss of a spouse due to either death or divorce could be equally devastating. Any of these losses may precipitate an acute grief reaction. The response is often sadness, fear, anger at having been left, despair, and multiple somatic complaints. Often an element of guilt is present.

The acute grief reaction has been described as a definite syndrome with both psychologic and somatic components. The symptomatology of normal grief is quite uniform. The individual often complains of tightness in the throat and chest, a choking sensation, and a feeling of shortness of breath; she sighs frequently. The individual often reports an empty feeling in the abdomen, muscle weakness, and a feeling of tension and mental pain. These symptoms frequently come in waves lasting for minutes to hours and are often dreaded by the sufferer. Individuals may suffer disorders of the sensorium involving a sense of unreality, a tendency to place emotional distance between themselves and other people, and a preoccupation with the imagery of the deceased if a death has occurred.

An understanding physician should ask appropriate open-ended questions and allow the patient to discuss her feelings, fears, angers, and fantasies. It can be helpful to let her know that her feelings are normal and will ease in 6–18 months. In the case of older women, the grief reaction may go on much longer, even for the rest of her life.

The patient should be encouraged not to make major decisions until the grief lessens. Grief undoubtedly affects judgment, and major life changes that she may make can have cumulative adverse effects. In severe, acute, grief reactions, mild tranquilizers may be helpful, but the physician must be certain that their use will be limited; prolonged use of tranquilizers is unnecessary and inappropriate. The grieving process ends when the individual is able to place the loss in proper overall life perspective and find new interests and activities as substitution.

Occasionally, abnormal grief responses may occur. The first of these is delay of reaction, which essentially is a postponement of grieving. This occurs often in an individual who is injured in an accident that kills the person to be grieved. The individual may be preoccupied with personal survival and recuperation and thereby may show no external evidence of grieving. Often this will surprise the physician and other care givers, or falsely reassure him or her that the individual has great strength and is handling both of her problems well. The lack of grief is noted until the individual herself is once more in good health, but sometimes the delay may be for months or years. There are many psychologic reasons why this occurs, but when grieving is finally precipitated it may appear quite pathologic and out of context of the current life situation.

A second abnormal response is the distorted reaction. In this situation the bereaved may take on the characteristics of the deceased without evidencing any sense of loss. The bereaved may even assume the symptoms of the dead person if that person had experienced a prolonged illness before death.

A third abnormal reaction may be the development of a psychosomatic condition such as ulcerative colitis, rheumatoid arthritis, or asthma. In individuals with these conditions, an exacerbation of symptoms may occur. Often the symptoms improve as the grief reaction is nearing completion.

Other types of abnormal grief reactions include pathologic alterations in relationships with friends and relatives, inappropriate hostility toward others, behavior patterns resembling psychoses, continued inability to make decisions or to take initiative, and the performance of activities that have definite destructive social or economic outcomes for the individual. Agitated depression has been called the most serious abnormal grief reaction. In this situation, the bereaved develops tensions and agitation, insomnia, feelings of worthlessness, and fantasies of a need for punishment. In such situations, suicide may be a real danger. Although this response is unusual, the physician must be alerted to it. It is most often seen when mothers lose children of any age.

Certain special situations must be recognized. The loss of a child is difficult at any time, and with the AIDS epidemic, many older mothers are facing the loss of grown children. Often they have cared for these children in the latter stages of their illness, making the situation even more serious.

The loss of an organ or body part can bring about a grief reaction with accompanying symptoms of an emotional and somatic nature. Depression is often a strong component. The loss of important structures such as limbs or eyes, or the loss of emotionally important organs such as the uterus, ovaries, or breasts may evoke an acute grief reaction. It has been shown that an individual will work through four stages of incorporation related to the acceptance of a loss of an organ. They are impact, retreat, acknowledgment, and reconstruction.

The impact stage occurs when the individual becomes aware that she has a problem with her organ (eg, uterus). If she is symptomatic this may be obvious. If she has been told that she must lose her organ because it is diseased, such as by cancer, she will need to make a mental adjustment to this fact. If she is not given an opportunity to do this, depression may occur.

The next stage of the organ loss is retreat. At this stage the patient accepts the fact that she may need to have the organ removed and begins to depersonalize it. Often she seeks second opinions to determine whether or not the operation is necessary. This is a healthy response and should be encouraged.

In the third stage, acknowledgment, the patient has accepted the need for the procedure and now discusses the meaning of the loss of the organ and the ways in which the operation will be performed. She is interested in the postoperative period, how long she will be disabled, and how she will respond postoperatively. She attempts to place the procedure and the need for the procedure within the appropriate context of her life and self-image.

In the final stage, reconstruction, she redefines her self-image without the organ. This stage requires an understanding and acceptance of the operation on the part of her spouse and significant others and by members of her circle of important individuals. The physician may need to discuss in detail with her and her spouse the reasons for the operation, its likely sequalae, and the postoperative reconstruction period, in order to help them through this stage.

Loss of a job, particularly one that the patient has experienced throughout her career, may evoke a grief reaction. Physicians should be aware of this and help the patient understand that if she is symptomatic, this loss may be the reason.

For many people the loss of a pet is a reason for bereavement. This is particularly true if the individual lives alone and the pet is the major living being in the person's life.

Grieving is a universal experience with a specific associated syndrome. A sensitive physician recognizes this when the patient has suffered a loss, and helps place her symptoms in proper perspective.

BIBLIOGRAPHY

American College of Obstetricians and Gynecologists. Sexual assault. ACOG Technical Bulletin 172. Washington, DC: ACOG, 1992

American College of Obstetricians and Gynecologists. The battered woman. ACOG Technical Bulletin 124. Washington, DC: ACOG, 1989

American Medical Association. Diagnostic and treatment guidelines on domestic violence. Chicago: AMA, 1992

Bowie SI, Silverman DC, Kalick SM, Edbril SD. Blitz rape and confidence rape: implications for clinical intervention. Am J Psychother 1990;44:180–188

Browne A, Williams KR. Gender, intimacy, and lethal violence: trends from 1976 through 1987. Gender Soc 1993;7:78–98

Cartwright PS, Moore RA. The elderly victim of rape. South Med J 1989;82:988–989

Council on Scientific Affairs, American Medical Association. Violence against women: relevance for medical practitioners. JAMA 1992;267: 3184–3189

Frazer M. Domestic violence: a medicolegal review. J Forensic Sci 1986;31:1409–1419

Gentry CE. Incestuous abuse of children: the need for an objective view. Child Welfare 1978;57:355–364

Goldberg WG, Tomlanovich MC. Domestic violence victims in the emergency department: new findings. JAMA 1984;251:3259–3264

Helton AS, McFarlane J, Anderson ET. Battered and pregnant: a prevalence study. Am J Public Health 1987;77:1337–1339

Hillard PJ. Physical abuse in pregnancy. Obstet Gynecol 1985;66:185–190

Jones JG. Sexual abuse of children: current concepts. Am J Dis Child 1982;136:142–146

Lundin T. Long term outcome of bereavement. Br J Psychiatry 1984; 145:424

Marchbanks PA, Lui KJ, Mercy JA. Risk of injury from resisting rape. Am J Epidemiol 1990;132:540–549

Renshaw DC. Treatment of sexual exploitation: rape and incest. Psychiatr Clin North Am 1989;12:257–277

Rimsza ME, Niggemann EH. Medical evaluation of sexually abused children: a review of 311 cases. Pediatrics 1982;69:8–14

Russell DE. The prevalence and incidence of forcible rape and attempted rape of females. Victimology 1982;7:81–93

U.S. Department of Health and Human Services, Public Health Services, Health Resources and Services Administration. Surgeon General's Workshop on Violence and Public Health: report. Washington DC: U.S. Government Printing Office, 1986; DHHS publication no. (HRS) D-MC 86-1

Viken RM. Family violence: aids to recognition. Postgrad Med 1982; 71:115–122

Walker LE. The battered woman syndrome. New York: Springer Publishing, 1984

Warner CG. Rape and sexual assault: management and intervention. Germantown, Maryland: Aspen Publishers, 1980:chapter 4

Ethical Issues in Obstetrics and Gynecology

Bioethics is a compilation of critical, reflective thought about the morality of what we do in medicine. The practice of obstetrics and gynecology raises ethical challenges across a wide range of issues: fetal tissue transplant, prenatal genetic manipulations, maternal–fetal conflicts, use of newly developed technologies and instruments, gender health bias, and terminal care. The ability to use critical and analytic ethics methods is essential to practitioners in a field so littered with moral quandaries. Developing such facility requires two elements. The first is the practice of a clinical method to analyze confusing cases. This establishes the domain of ethical quandaries to explore. The second is a working understanding of the basic principles and values in those domains.

ETHICAL ANALYSIS

Faced with confusing and often upsetting clinical problems, a physician may find that knowledge of principles is not in and of itself adequate to identify or deal with the underlying ethical problem. There often are multiple parties with varying points of view about basic issues surrounding a confusing patient case. Analysis in the clinical context must cut through confusing emotions and information in order to get to the ethically pertinent patient circumstance. Methods that can be used to establish a case-based philosophic analysis (casuistry) comparing similar cases with the present one (taxonomy) are of great value (see box). Disciplined use of a method that strictly adheres to delineating the "facts of the case" helps clear away the secondary issues around it. This process of identifying ethical issues and relating them to thought in literature about medical ethics helps medical caregivers make the best ethical decision possible. This reflective, researched thought about the ethics of heath care policy and individual patient care is a responsible approach to the inescapable fact that physicians and society must often make tough moral choices where no one answer is right. This type of analysis will be explored with the following sample case:

A 23-year-old, gravida 2, para 1, single woman is admitted with a bleeding placenta previa at 30 weeks of gestation. She is accompanied by her parents. There is no evidence of fetal distress or contractions. The patient's hematocrit level drops from 32% to 26% over 4 hours, with some diminution in bleeding. She refuses transfusion. She states that she and her parents are Jehovah's Witnesses. Her hematocrit level drops to 24% over the next 12 hours, with a small amount of bleeding. The medical caregivers wonder whether they can get a court order to force her to receive blood. Alternatively, should they do a cesarean delivery of a premature infant now, because delay will only further decrease the hematocrit and the patient's risk?

> **Medical Ethics Analysis**
>
> | Domains | Ethical Principles |
> |---|---|
> | I. Medical Indications: the medical facts | |
> | A. Medical conditions | |
> | B. Proposed and current interventions | |
> | 1. Outcome data | Futility |
> | a. Benefits | Beneficence |
> | b. Risks | Nonmalificence |
> | II. Patient Preferences: the patient facts | |
> | A. Patient decision making | Autonomy |
> | B. Authenticity and capacity to choose | Paternalism, competence |
> | C. Surrogate decision makers | Honesty |
> | III. Quality of Life: the patient's experience of living | Suffering |
> | A. Patient values | |
> | IV. Context | |
> | A. Family concerns | Justice |
> | B. Physician, nurse, concerns | Utility |
> | C. Legal issues | |
> | D. Financial issues | |

PRINCIPLES

There are four general domains of ethical considerations that must be addressed for every case that raises an ethical question. It is an error to assume that the "problem" is known until these four domains have been explored. Clinical ethicists and clinicians have learned from experience that the clarification of facts and the joint sharing of information often lead to conclusions quite different from the original assumptions.

Medical Indications

For this case and all of medical care, the first consideration is what the benefit of that care might be to a specific patient. From time immemorial, physicians have been urged to benefit the patient and do no harm. This is the medical equivalent of the principle of beneficence. Beneficence is the deeply ingrained principle of benefiting the patient or promoting the patient's welfare by whatever intervention offered.

The continuum between harm and benefit demands in each patient circumstance a weighing of the net benefit of an intervention against the harms. The injunction to not harm patients (nonmaleficence) is the moral principle guarding the boundary. The measure of the positive weight of the intervention is often based on its ability to meet a goal of medicine. These have been outlined by many authors and include such goals as cure of disease, promotion of health, improvement or maintenance of functional status, and relief of symptoms and pain. Hippocrates defined the goals as "to do away with the suffering of the sick, to lessen the violence of their diseases, and to refuse to treat those who are overmastered by their diseases." Clearly, the principle of benefit is a strong element of the Hippocratic tradition physicians inherit. As a corollary, physicians have no obligation to offer therapies that have no or very limited benefit and do not serve a goal of medicine.

These judgments about potential benefit also form a continuum of varying mixtures of probabilities and actual patient status. One description of "futile" therapy is therapy used to achieve a result that is possible but that reasoning or experience suggests is highly improbable and that cannot be systematically produced. Despite the uncertainty of medicine, physicians are not ethically obligated to offer such therapy. Social dialogue reflects an increasing understanding of this concern. The societal discussion of the issue of physician-assisted suicide resonates with issues of futility and criticism of medicine for the tendency to overtreat and overuse technology when those interventions are futile, and the only medical goal attainable is comfort.

In the case presented, the most direct medical benefit for mother and fetus would be achieved by transfusion and watchful waiting. This course medically has high benefit and low risks. If the physicians accept the patient's wishes, the benefit of cesarean delivery now, at a time when this mother might survive, rather than later, with increased potential for maternal death with bleeding, must be weighed against the preterm delivery of the fetus.

Autonomy

This patient refuses blood, a choice that directly affects the physicians' ability to offer the potentially most beneficial care. Autonomy describes the ethical principle of respecting the patient's right to choose his or her medical care. The question of when, if ever, it is appropriate to override patients' wishes is pertinent. The concept of a moral obligation to respect patients' wishes can be easily confused with doing anything the patient expresses as a wish. Among other obligations, caregivers must assure themselves that the patient has a capacity to make choices that goes beyond just expressing desires. The capacity to understand what is proposed, to consider the meaning of the information without coercion, and to express desires must be present.

As the medical consequences of proposed intervention or a choice for no intervention become more serious, the stringency of the obligation to assess the patients' capacity to choose becomes greater. In this case this obligation is critical, including assessing any coercion from her parents. The ability of patients to act autonomously may be seriously compromised by their disease, their treatment (especially sedating medications), and the very medical or social environments that seek to promote their welfare and respect their wishes. As an example, the depressed, confused patient who wants no treatment for a potentially curable cervical malignancy must have her uremia and depression treated before her authentic wishes can be sought and respected. Eliciting the authentic values, goals, and choices of patients is far more than doing what a patient expresses as her desire.

When a patient is *unable* to make choices about care, a surrogate decision maker must be found. In some states, statutory law describes the hierarchy of surrogate decision makers. In other cases, durable powers of attorney may direct caregivers to the appropriate person. Regardless of who the surrogate is, the obligation remains for the surrogate to reflect as accurately as possible the decisions that the patient would have made. Clinicians must assure themselves that the decisions made reflect the patient's wishes and not conflicting desires or interests of the surrogate.

Quality of Life

When asked about the consequences of receiving blood, this patient states that she will be unfaithful to God if she receives blood and that an unfaithful life is not worth living. Yet, caregivers recognize that the infant born early as a result of her choices may also bear a lifetime of sequelae that could affect both the infant's and the mother's quality of life. How each of us experiences living as meaningful frames the domains of quality of life. For both the patient and quality-of-life study contexts, the framework is the patient's—not that of the onlookers.

When practitioners begin to decide for a patient, or an infant, or for a large body of potential patients whether or not their life is or will be meaningful and satisfying, they begin to sink into moral quagmires. What ability to participate in society—mentally and physically—is a border of "quality" existence? Once onlookers try to set a standard, they impose societal and personal values and raise valid questions about discrimination from bias against such characteristics as lower intelligence, or nonmobility, or lack of monetary resources, or the presence of pain. These value judgments are highly subjective and need careful scrutiny.

Often, the border of "acceptable" quality of life is framed by the principle of nonmaleficence in an attempt to avoid the bias inherent in the subjective nature of these arguments. Continued life in a neonate who has no ability to survive infancy, to live without pain, or to participate even minimally in human existence, for example, could be argued to be of such negative nature that the principle of nonmaleficence removes the obligation to sustain life.

In this case, the patient's experience of living would be significantly diminished by the transfusion, to the point that it seems easier to her to deal with an ill—or even dead—infant than the personal consequences of transfusion.

Context

Does society have a right to intervene in this case? Elements of the social, economic, and legal context surrounding ethics cases and the issues of just care and outcomes are rarely the overriding concern in clinical ethics cases. However, this case raises the question of whether the risk of being born with the concurrent loss of a caregiver (the patient) might be of such concern to the state (which would otherwise be responsible for the infant's care) that transfusion can be forced. This has been used as an argument for treatment of pregnant Jehovah's Witness patients to ensure survival of a caregiver. The grandparents in this case are willing to be responsible for the infant, so the argument does not apply here.

The issue of the state's interest in the well-being of infants and third-trimester fetuses is an area in which law and ethics frequently overlap in obstetrics. The other contextual issue in this case would be what cost society or an individual is willing to bear for a preterm birth that potentially could be avoided. Alterations in medical reimbursement and federal law may command more ethical attention for these contextual elements in individual cases.

A broad application of the principle of justice applies to the distribution of social goods such as health care among members of the society. For example, who should be eligible for in vitro fertilization? Methods of distribution might be set by passing only a set standard of need, by lottery (fairness), by social worth (contribution to society), by queuing (get there first), by resources (having money), or by serving the greater needs of society as a whole. These are the types of choices being made as the struggle to outline a fair allocation of health care resources continues.

The ethical limitation on capitation-based allocation of resources may shift concern from overuse of technology for limited benefit of a few to underutilization of adequate technology for many. The issue of just and beneficial allocation of medical resources for all of society will remain, regardless of method of payment.

In this case, the final decision should be to respect the patient's wishes and not transfuse. A plan should be established for cesarean delivery before the blood volume diminishes to a critical level.

ETHICAL ISSUES

Obstetrics

Many of the issues in obstetrics and gynecology have raised continuous debate for centuries. New areas are also being added that were never foreseen. Consider the innovations in understanding the human genome and our increasing ability to intervene in the genetic composition of individuals.

How should *family* be defined with some of the new combinations of genetics and biology? Who is the parent when sperm were donated by one individual, the ovum was donated by another, and the pregnancy was carried out in a separate individual who may or may not raise the child? If height, color, intelligence, or sex can be chosen preconceptionally, what harm will a decreasing diversity and decreased tolerance for diversity do to society at large? Should society allow preconceptional choices or abortion for variables such as sex when no medical disease is associated? Should abortion be required for genetic defects known to be associated with an increased cost of medical care?

The debate over abortion remains a source of division of moral thought in the United States. Support for first- and early second-trimester abortion has generally fallen into ideologic groups supporting abortion as a means of alleviating burdens of mothers by protecting mental or physical health; relieving social, economic, or demographic problems; or supporting, based on the Fourteenth Amendment, rights to bodily integrity and privacy of decisions about family and parenthood.

The undue-burden language of *Roe v. Wade* was substantially altered by *Planned Parenthood v. Casey*, particularly in no longer requiring a standard of strict scrutiny for acceptance of state restrictions on abortion. These changes have raised issues of just allocation, since it will be primarily the least financially and socially endowed women who will be most affected by such restrictions.

Furthermore, individual state requirements for exposure of all patients seeking abortion to state-initiated or state-specified materials raise questions for physicians about their ability to individualize informed consent compassionately. As an example, an 18-year-old woman, pregnant and suicidal after a brutal rape, may find generic material extolling the benefits of adoption overwhelming. Intervention by state regulations in the physician–patient relationship and therapeutic alliance may have greater harm than benefit and may propel physicians to acts of conscientious objection in order to fulfill their professional obligations, despite legal retribution.

The potential use of fetal tissue obtained from elective or spontaneous abortions raises a potential for societal benefit from abortions. Fears of coercion by medical staff to obtain tissue for these uses at the time of counseling for abortion have been raised. Numerous authors stress the need for rigorous separation of the decision for abortion and for transplantation. As with many new ethical issues, the benefits and long-term outcomes of fetal tissue intervention for recipients needs to be clarified before more stringent guidelines can emerge.

An additional force in the abortion debate is the increasing access to and efficacy of therapy in the fetal stage, both before and after viability. The increasing access has led some authors to promote the idea of the fetus as a patient. Clearly, the fetus lacks an ability for decision-making and for independent survival during early gestation, so maternal decision-making regarding benefit and harm remains an essential element. The concern of coercion also exists in this setting, where parental desires for healthy offspring lend great stringency to accurate representation of the range of outcomes by medical caregivers. The changing access to the fetus challenges old definitions of fetal outcomes and raises many new frameworks in which to consider prebirth issues, regardless of the philosophical framework being used.

These changes impinge on similarly confusing cases in which maternal wishes and choices seem to be in direct opposition to the best choices for the fetus. Obstetrics and gynecology has traditionally held that the mother (as patient) has primacy in decision-making. No one else, for example, can understand the consequences of a choice on the patient's family structure, economics, or even personal health. Furthermore, the patient is the only one who can consider and choose.

Pediatrics traditionally has held a primary allegiance to the best interest of the fetus and represents the view that society must protect the best interest of children, hence its allegiance to the fetus. In fact, both viewpoints are not held in exclusion, and the anguish of having such conflicts is felt by all involved.

Even when the "facts" are clear, these choices can be confounded by issues beyond an individual case. The issue may not be what is in the best interest of this mother and this fetus but may involve the best outcome for all mothers and children. For example, the cocaine- and alcohol-abusing mother who routinely misses appointments, leaves the hospital against medical advice when in premature labor, and behaves in a fashion that puts both her and her fetus at risk is distressing to caregivers. Incarceration might control the behavior during pregnancy. But then, how likely would this and other cocaine-using mothers be to seek care? A few prenatal visits and vitamins with some connection to social help probably is a greater good than incarceration for this one patient. As with many ethical decisions, there is rarely one single right answer. A critical and reflective weighing of all outcomes and many ethical and moral considerations can help the practitioner in making the final decision.

Gynecology

For the first time in recent history, obstetricians and gynecologists have had to weigh their obligation of care and codes of professional behavior against the risk that they themselves will contract a fatal disease in the routine care of patients. The risk of contracting HIV, while statistically very small in both obstetric and gynecologic venues, illustrates a line of self-sacrifice (self-risk) to benefit patients that modern physicians have not previously had to confront. Physicians have an obligation to model behavior for the wider community that reflects the biologic reality of the disease. Such behavior should promote appropriate precautions but avoid discrimination or denial of access to care. Clearly, this is within the code of professional behavior physicians have willingly taken.

Furthermore, the positions that many health care professionals have taken over teaching their own patients and the wider society about sexual practices and contraceptive choices may have to be reexamined in light of the potential individual and social harm of the spread of the disease. The epidemic nature of the spread of HIV suggests a greater societal obligation for physicians to educate the community than is supposed in traditional medicine's focus on the single patient.

The ethical principle of honesty is raised under the larger concepts of beneficence and autonomy, but in the gynecologic sphere it has multiple areas of application of its own. Consider the use of new technology that does not clearly benefit patients economically or in outcome over traditional methods, but provides a higher compensation for the physician. Here, truth-telling to the patient in the process of informed consent should be the highest ethical principle. However, the physician's economic or research conflict-of-interest may impinge on scrupulous ethics and promote deception. Or, in another arena, a physician may deceive an insurance company in order to receive compensation for a procedure that, while medically appropriate, is not covered for a particular patient. Given the present focus on informed consent and a societal pressure for accountability, such already questionably ethical practices need to give way to physicians' social advocacy for their patients' best medical economic interests.

Gynecologic oncology continues to deal with terminal care and the issues of dignity and avoidance of futile therapies at life's end. However, the aging of the population has placed many of these same concerns and questions about reasonable allocation of medical resources and potential elder discrimination in the laps of general obstetricians and gynecologists. Discussions of choices about life support, resuscitation, and quality of life are relevant for all patients, but particularly for geriatric patients. The careful documentation of patients' values about their care at the end of life is an ethical duty of physicians that is best initiated when patients are the most able to discuss and consider what care for what outcomes are of value to them.

The passage of the Patient Self-Determination Act requires that hospitals receiving federal funds ask patients if they have advance directives, document the presence or absence of directives, and provide information regarding advance directives, if desired. These advance directives can include durable powers of attorney for health care, and directives to physicians (living wills). They can provide both clarity about whom a patient would choose as a surrogate decision maker if needed and clarity about what a patient would choose.

Terminal care, particularly around the issue of pain relief, still raises questions among caregivers about where the appropriate medical use of opioids to relieve pain crosses over to assisted suicide. The debate about assisted suicide is, in part, an expression of multiple conflicting fears of overuse of technology, lack of respect for patient wishes, and fear of financially (or otherwise) burdening the family. These concerns are pitted against intention, professional codes prohibiting killing, and concerns about coercion (financial or emotional) and benefit.

Pain relief has played a major role in the social debate, since fear of pain is the most frequently expressed reason for support of assisted suicide. Appropriate pain management in terminal care seeks to meet the goal of medicine to relieve pain and suffering by intensive palliative care. There may be a point at which the intended therapeutic effect—pain relief—is accompanied by an associated, expected side effect such as decreased respiration, which may lead to an earlier death. Both the appropriate dosage of the drug and the intent of the intervention separate this circumstance from assisted euthanasia whereby the intent of therapy is death (and the dosage increments are scaled to that outcome). This follows the rationale of the principle of double effect: the intended beneficial treatment has an undesired but recognized side effect. Inadequate pain relief due to fear of a side effect is not acceptable when the only achievable medical goal is relief of pain in a terminal patient.

The geriatric population is a good example for the final issue critical to the field of obstetrics and gynecology, that of allocation of health resources. Health care reform is focusing on cost containment through capitation. The switch from incentives to offering more care and more technology on a fee-for-service basis will lessen the conflicts that lead to deceptive reporting and the overutilization of technology at the end of life. The ethical limit of proposed new medical economics will be harmful denial of health care resources, propelled by an economic incentive to limit and deny—rather than promote—health care interventions. The physician as gatekeeper to these resources will face different conflicts of interests. The potential harms of those conflicts will need to be in the forefront of ethical reflections as a new framework of ethical challenges is faced in the future.

BIBLIOGRAPHY

American College of Obstetricians and Gynecologists. Ethical decision-making in obstetrics and gynecology. ACOG Technical Bulletin 136. Washington, DC: ACOG, 1989

American College of Obstetricians and Gynecologists. Multifetal pregnancy reduction and selective fetal termination. ACOG Committee Opinion 94. Washington, DC: ACOG, 1991

American College of Obstetricians and Gynecologists. Patient choice: maternal–fetal conflict. ACOG Committee Opinion 55. Washington DC: ACOG, 1987

Association of Professors of Gynecology and Obstetrics. Exploring issues in obstetric and gynecologic medical ethics. Washington DC: APGO, 1991

Benshoof J. Planned Parenthood v. Casey: the impact of the new undue burden standard on reproductive health care. JAMA 1993;269: 2249–2257

Brett AS, McCullough LB. When patients request specific interventions: defining the limits of the physician's obligation. N Engl J Med 1986;315:1347–1351

Byk C. The Human Genome Project and the social contract: a law policy approach. J Med Philos 1992;17:371–380

Elkins TE, Andersen HF, Barclay M, Mason T, Bowlder N, Anderson G. Court-ordered cesarean section: an analysis of ethical concerns in compelling cases. Am J Obstet Gynecol 1989;161:150–154

Gillon R. Ordinary and extraordinary means. BMJ [Clin Res] 1986; 292:259–261

Jecker NS, Schneiderman LJ. Futility and rationing. Am J Med 1992;92:189–196

Jonsen A, Siegler M, Winslade W. Clinical ethics. 3rd ed. New York: McGraw–Hill, 1992

Legal interventions during pregnancy. Court-ordered medical treatments and legal penalties for potentially harmful behavior by pregnant women. JAMA 1990;264:2663–2670

Ryan KJ. Abortion or motherhood, suicide and madness. Am J Obstet Gynecol 1991;166:1029–1036

Schneiderman LJ, Jecker NS, Jonsen AR. Medical futility: its meaning and ethical implications. Ann Intern Med 1990;112:949–954

Wertz DC, Fletcher JC. Fatal knowledge?: prenatal diagnosis and sex selection. Hastings Cent Rep 1989;19:21–27

Epidemiology and Statistical Interpretation

A basic understanding of epidemiology and biostatistics is needed to evaluate many papers in the current obstetric and gynecologic literature. Physicians should also be able to take advantage of advances in information retrieval so that they can have access to the latest scientific literature. This overview provides a brief introduction to the principles of epidemiology and biostatistics most relevant to the practicing clinician and outlines how physicians can obtain and interpret data from a broad base.

EPIDEMIOLOGY

The word *epidemiology* is derived from the Greek words *epi* (upon) and *demos* (people). Many definitions of epidemiology have been offered; one useful definition is that epidemiology is the study of the occurrence of illness. As a discipline, epidemiology is concerned with the evaluation of scientific hypotheses. The objective of any epidemiologic study should be to measure accurately the relationship between certain exposures of interest and the likelihood of developing disease. How does the science of epidemiology relate to the current obstetric and gynecologic literature? Most of the current literature consists of case reports, case series, laboratory experiments, assessments of screening and diagnostic tests, or analytic studies. An understanding of epidemiology is required to interpret only the latter two types of investigations.

Screening and Diagnostic Tests

Proper interpretation of screening and diagnostic tests requires an understanding of relevant terminology. *Sensitivity* is defined as the ability of a test to identify correctly persons who have the disease of interest. By contrast, *specificity* is defined as the ability to identify correctly persons who do not have the disease of interest (Fig. 2-1). Therefore, sensitivity and specificity deal with the extent to which persons with or without disease are correctly identified by the tests. By contrast, *predictive value* is the probability of disease, given a test result. The positive predictive value of a test deals with the likelihood that a person with a positive test is diseased; the negative predictive value deals with the likelihood that a person with a negative test is free of disease (Fig. 2-1). The predictive value of a test is influenced by the prevalence of the disease of interest in the population being tested. For example, if a disease is rare in a population, the positive predictive value of a test for the disease in that population will be low even if sensitivity and specificity are high.

Analytic Studies

The purpose of analytic epidemiologic studies is to infer or establish a causal relationship between an exposure of interest (eg, ingestion of a drug) and an outcome of interest (eg, occurrence or cure of a disease). In most epidemiologic studies, causation cannot be proven. Except in the special circumstance in which an epidemiologic study can properly be considered an experiment, causation can only be inferred. Experiments differ from nonexperimental analytic studies in that the exposure of interest can be manipulated, allowing direct estimation of the impact of the manipulation on the observed outcome.

Randomized clinical trials, in which participants are randomly assigned to exposures of interests, are the major examples of experimental epidemiologic studies in obstetric and gynecologic literature. Although randomized clinical trials usually permit stronger inference regarding causation than do nonexperimental studies, they are often difficult to conduct and are sometimes ethically unacceptable. Therefore, most of the epidemiologic studies in the literature are observational (ie, nonexperimental). In observational studies, the exposures of interest are set—one merely observes the associated outcomes.

The observational analytic epidemiologic studies in the obstetric and gynecologic literature can be classified as 1) cross-sectional, 2) case–control, or 3) cohort (follow-up) studies. The distinguishing features of these studies are generally easily recognized and often important. One useful way to appreciate the similarities and differences among the three types of studies is to consider the simple case of one exposure and

		Disease	
		Present	Absent
Test Result	Positive	a	b
	Negative	c	d

Sensitivity = a/(a + c) × 100%
Specificity = d/(b + d) × 100%
Positive Predictive Value = a/(a + b) × 100%
Negative Predictive Value = d/(c + d) × 100%

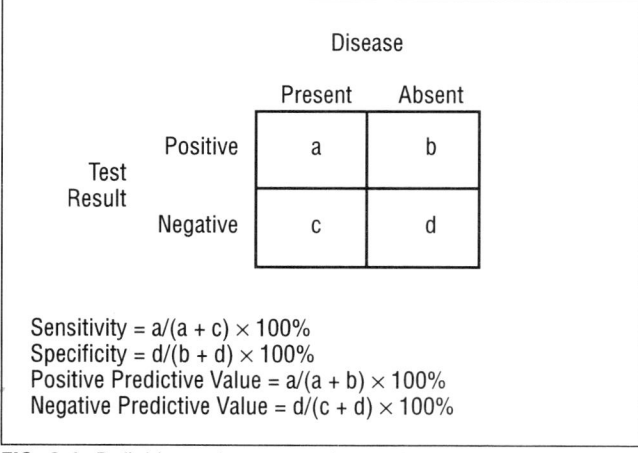

FIG. 2-1. Definitions of terms used to evaluate screening and diagnostic tests.

one outcome. The relationship between an exposure and a disease can best be determined when information is available about individuals who are exposed and not exposed and who have the disease of interest and who do not have the disease of interest. Once available, this information can be represented as a 2 × 2 table, as shown in Fig. 2-2.

The 2 × 2 table represents the final common pathway for all three types of observational analytic epidemiologic studies. The approaches to this pathway are different, however. Although a detailed description of these three types of studies is beyond the scope of this overview, some simple but important features of these studies can be discussed.

Cross-sectional studies evaluate populations of individuals, some of whom may have the disease (outcome) of interest and some of whom do not. This type of study can be thought of simplistically as taking a "snapshot" of a group of people and characterizing from the resultant view those who have and those who do not have the disease of interest at that moment and those who are and who are not exposed to the factor of interest at that moment. Individuals who have a disease at the moment the "photo" is taken are considered prevalent cases. The difference between prevalence and incidence is confusing but important. Prevalence is the proportion of individuals with disease at a specific point in time. The concept of incidence provides more information regarding the occurrence of disease. Incident cases are new cases of disease occurring over a specific period of time.

The use of incident cases, as compared with the use of prevalent cases, generally permits stronger conclusions to be made regarding the likelihood that an exposure is causally related to a disease. Thus, cross-sectional studies, which by design use prevalent cases, may not permit strong arguments for causation.

This point is best illustrated by a specific example. A cross-sectional study to evaluate the relationship between condom use and HIV transmission would evaluate a population of individuals who were and who were not diagnosed as having HIV infection at a particular point in time. Unfortunately, because this design would study only prevalent cases, the temporal association between condom use and acquisition of HIV infection could not be determined. Thus, individuals who had consistently and correctly used condoms may have done so after they became infected with HIV; and individuals who had correctly used condoms at some time in the past may have stopped using them for a brief period, become infected, and subsequently resumed their use. A cross-sectional study design does not permit assessment of the temporal relationship between condom use and HIV infection and, thus, provides little useful information regarding the etiologic relationship between condom use and HIV transmission.

Case–control and cohort studies differ from cross-sectional studies in that they can include the experience of incident cases. While case–control studies can include either prevalent or incident cases, cohort studies, by design, assess only incident cases. The major difference between case–control studies and cohort studies is that case–control studies classify study subjects on the basis of whether or not they are diseased and then determine whether or not they were previously exposed. Cohort studies, on the other hand, classify study subjects on the basis of exposure and then determine whether or not they develop disease.

The difference between case–control and cohort studies can be illustrated by using the example of condom use and HIV transmission. A case–control study would identify study subjects as having prevalent or incident cases of HIV infection and as having used or not used condoms in the recent or remote past. By contrast, a cohort study of HIV infection and condom use would identify study subjects as individuals who used or did not use condoms and would then follow these individuals over time to determine whether or not they developed HIV infection. A certain knowledge that individuals had developed HIV infection would be contingent on identifying individuals known to be seronegative for HIV at one point in time and known to have seroconverted at a subsequent time (ie, to have become seroincident cases).

As a practical matter, the distinction between case–control and cohort studies means that case–control studies are retrospective; that is, study subjects are identified as being diseased or not diseased, and then the investigator goes back in time to determine whether or not the study subject was exposed. Cohort studies, by contrast, typically involve identification of a population of individuals who are either exposed or not exposed and who are then followed prospectively to determine whether or not they develop disease. Thus, cohort studies are often called prospective studies. However, since retrospective cohort studies can also be conducted, many epidemiologists use the term *follow-up* or *longitudinal studies* when referring to those cohort studies that follow individuals over time to determine whether or not they develop disease.

Case–control studies have a number of advantages over follow-up studies. They can be completed in less time than follow-up studies. This is particularly true when the disease of interest has a long induction period. Follow-up studies would have to evaluate subjects for at least as long after exposure as the known or suspected induction period, which, for some diseases of importance to women such as cancer and cardiovascular disease, may be 10–20 years or more after exposure. Twenty-year-long studies are difficult to conduct and are generally quite expensive. Case–control studies typically are more efficient than follow-up studies, affording additional cost savings. This is particularly true when the disease being studied is uncommon.

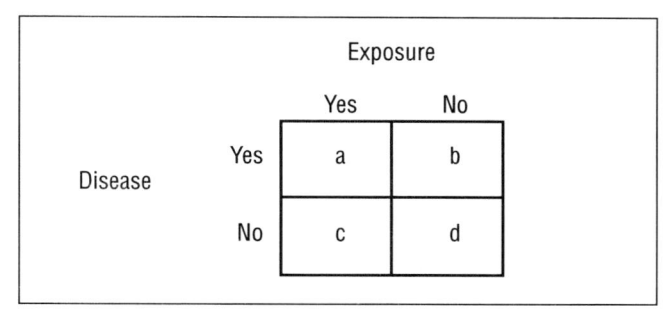

	Exposure	
	Yes	No
Disease Yes	a	b
Disease No	c	d

FIG. 2-2. Relationship between exposure and disease.

Despite these advantages, case–control studies are sometimes considered methodologically inferior to follow-up studies. This notion is debatable. From one viewpoint, a perfectly done case–control study should provide as accurate a characterization of what the investigator is trying to measure as a perfectly done follow-up study does. As a practical matter, no epidemiologic study is ever perfect. All studies have at least some methodologic limitations, and these limitations are inherently greater in case–control studies.

The limitations of case–control studies are often related to difficulties in selecting proper controls. Individuals in the control group of a case–control study should meet strict criteria including 1) being at risk of developing the disease under study; 2) being as comparable to cases as possible, except for having the disease under study; and 3) not having other conditions related to the likelihood of having the exposure of interest in the study. Despite the biases that are often inherent in the selection of study controls, a well-done case–control study may have substantially fewer methodologic limitations than a poorly done follow-up study.

Methodologic Limitations

Methodologic limitations in epidemiologic studies occur in two broad categories: precision and validity. Precision is concerned with random error or chance. More specifically, precision refers to the relative lack of random error (ie, the smallness of the variability of the estimated exposure–disease relationship). If the variability of this estimated relationship is small, then the precision is high. In general, the larger the study size, the greater the precision. Validity is concerned with systematic error or bias. When a study is invalid, it does not measure what it is supposed to measure. If a target with a bull's-eye symbolizes the occurrence being measured, then precision can be thought of simplistically as the proximity of shots to the bull's-eye (ie, how close to hitting the target the investigator comes).

Validity, by contrast, deals with whether the shots fired are directed at the right target. Biases in epidemiologic studies lead to a distortion in measurement; that is, they may lead to the wrong answer. Because of their great potential importance, biases must be identified, characterized, and, if possible, controlled. Even if biases cannot be controlled in analysis, knowledge of their magnitude and the direction in which they distort results will greatly aid in the interpretation of study findings. If biases are not so characterized, study results may be uninterpretable. There are numerous potential study biases. In broad terms, however, most biases are related to 1) how study participants are selected (ie, selection bias) 2) how study information is collected (ie, information bias, including so-called recall bias) and 3) the existence of extraneous variables.

The first two types of bias are self-explanatory, although they often are not easy to identify and control. The third type of bias requires some further explanation and deals with the concept of confounding. In simple terms, confounding can be described as the mixing of effects. Confounding results in an inaccurate measure of the effect of the study exposure, because the exposure is associated with an extraneous factor. When confounding is present, an estimate of the relationship between the exposure and the disease changes, depending on whether the suspected confounder is controlled for. To be a confounder, such an extraneous factor must be associated with both the likelihood of being exposed and the likelihood of developing disease. To obtain an accurate measure of the exposure–disease relationship, confounders must be identified and controlled for in analysis.

Both case–control and follow-up studies permit measurement of the magnitude of association between the study exposure and the disease of interest. In follow-up studies, the risk of disease, given the exposure, can be directly estimated as the relative risk (RR). In case–control studies, an approximation of this risk can be made by using the odds ratio (OR). With rare diseases, the OR is a close approximation of the RR. An RR or OR larger than 1, for example, 10, means that the risk (or odds) for exposed individuals is 10 times the risk (odds) for unexposed individuals. If the RR or OR is smaller than 1, for example, 0.1, then the risk (odds) for exposed individuals is one tenth the risk (odds) for unexposed individuals. Finally, if RR or OR is equal to 1, then the risks for exposed and unexposed individuals are the same and there is no evidence for an exposure–disease relationship.

Biostatistics

The distinction between epidemiology and biostatistics in this overview is arbitrary; these two disciplines are inextricably related. Statistical methods are required for reaching epidemiology's goal of accurate measurement.

Epidemiology is used to test hypotheses. By convention, statistical methods are used to test the null hypothesis (H_0), the hypothesis that two factors are not associated. If study findings indicate that H_0 can be rejected, then the alternative hypothesis that some association exists is accepted. It is very important to note here that "some" association means just that. It may be large or small, biologically meaningful or not. This vague area is the domain of the probability (P) value. The P value merely indicates the relative likelihood that an observation is due to chance. Typically, a P value of <0.05 is used to determine statistical significance. When H_0, the hypothesis of no association, is rejected at the P <0.05 level, it means that the observed association between two factors is unlikely due to chance. In a strict sense, a P value of >0.05 cannot be used to accept the hypothesis of no association; H_0 can only be rejected or not rejected.

Errors known as type I and type II can occur when H_0 is rejected or not rejected. A type I error occurs when H_0 is rejected incorrectly. The likelihood of a type I error is fixed when the significance level on which an observation is to be considered statistically significant or not significant is chosen. For example, if the significance level of 0.05 is chosen, then 5% of the time H_0 will be rejected when it should not be. It is useful to note here that the significance level and the P value are not the same quantities. The significance level is chosen by the investigator, ideally without looking at the data, and represents the probability of making a type I error that the investigator is willing to allow. The P value, by contrast, is a so-called posterior probability value based on one's data and represents how unlikely one's results are with respect to H_0.

A type II error occurs when H_0 is not rejected when it should have been rejected. Type II errors are quite common. To understand these errors, one needs to understand the concept of study power. In simple terms, a study's power is its ability to detect an association if it really exists. This ability is contingent on study size—the larger the study, in general, the larger the study power. A type II error occurs when a study is too small to detect an association that really exists. For example, consider the case in which maternal exposure to E truly causes birth defects in 1.0% of offspring. A study is conducted in which the rate of anomalies among 50 women with maternal exposure to E is compared with that among 50 women who are not exposed. No offspring with anomalies were reported (and with what is known, none should have been expected). The conclusion that maternal exposure to E is not associated with birth defects might be a type II error because the sample size of 50 in each group may have been too small to detect a real effect. Thus, when study findings suggest that there is no association between the factors being evaluated, it is useful to determine whether the study was large enough to have the potential to detect the association at issue.

The P value describes only the relative likelihood that chance explains study findings. Chance is only one factor to consider when determining whether an observation is likely the result of cause and effect. In the example here, the investigator does not really want to know whether maternal ingestion of E is associated with an increased risk of birth defects. The investigator wants to know whether ingestion of E causes birth defects to occur. One important means by which epidemiologists try to determine causation is to assess the strength of an observed association. This strength can be quantified by using the aforementioned OR or RR.

Calculation of an OR requires the information noted earlier in the classic 2 × 2 figure. Restated and expanded, this calculation is based on information obtained in a case–control study regarding those exposed and those not exposed to the factor of interest and those known to be diseased and not diseased. With this information the OR can be calculated, as shown in Fig. 2-3. Similarly, the RR can be calculated from follow-up studies as shown in Fig. 2-4.

Once calculated, the OR and RR provide an estimation of both the strength and direction of an association. If the OR and RR are above 1.0, then there is a positive association between the exposure and the disease, and if they are less than 1.0, then there is a negative association. The OR and RR are reported as one number and are regarded as point estimates. A confidence interval (CI) for this estimate gives an indication of the variability of the point estimate. In general, the wider the CI, the less stable the point estimate; that is, the less likely that the value of the point estimate is accurate. The 95% CI is often used. In a strict sense, if the study were to be repeated over and over again and a 95% CI was calculated each time, then 95% of these CIs would be expected to contain the true exposure–disease parameter being estimated. While this may be somewhat confusing, this interpretation of the mean-

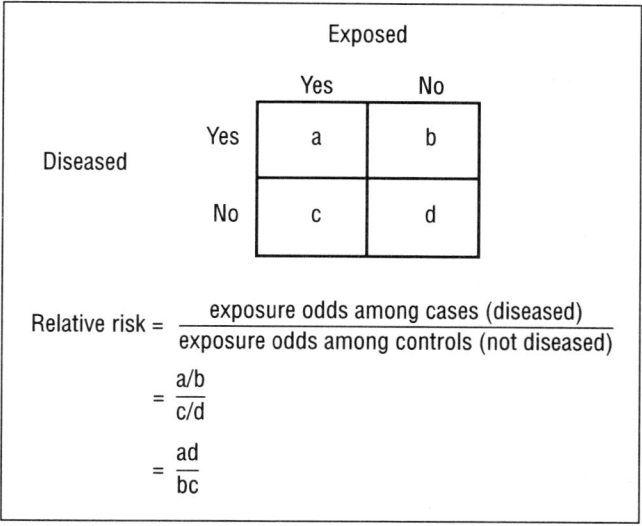

FIG. 2-3. Calculation of the odds ratio using the 2 × 2 table. a, b, c, d = the numbers of people in each of four possible combinations of exposure and disease status. (Peterson HB, Kleinbaum DG. Interpreting the literature in obstetrics and gynecology: I. Key concepts in epidemiology and biostatistics. Reprinted with permission from the American College of Obstetricians and Gynecologists [Obstetrics and Gynecology, 1991, 78, 715; correction 1992, 79, 313–314])

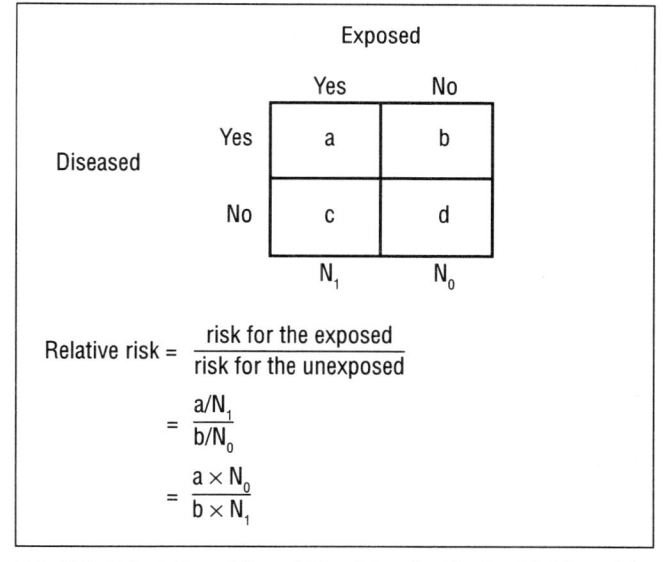

FIG. 2-4. Calculation of the relative risk using the 2 × 2 table. a, b, c, d = the numbers of people in each of four possible combinations of exposure and disease; N_1 = total number exposed; N_0 = total number unexposed. (Peterson HB, Kleinbaum DG. Interpreting the literature in obstetrics and gynecology: I. Key concepts in epidemiology and biostatistics. Reprinted with permission from the American College of Obstetricians and Gynecologists [Obstetrics and Gynecology, 1991, 78, 715])

ing of CI is correct and stands in contrast to the frequent misimpression that CI is the range of values in which the true point estimate will lie 95% of the time.

The CI for the point estimate can also be used to determine statistical significance (in a two-tailed significance test), since the confidence level used is 100 (1 − α), where α is the level set to determine statistical significance. As an example, if the 95% CI does not overlap 1.0, then one would reject the H_0 of no exposure–disease association at the 0.05 significance level ([100 (1 − α)] = 95, so α = 0.05).

Epidemiology depends on other statistical tools for its success. One such tool is mathematical modeling. The most commonly used mathematical model in the obstetric and gynecologic literature is logistic regression. Earlier in this overview, the concept of confounding was discussed. As noted, a confounder is a special type of covariate that can distort the relationship between the exposure and disease under study. To understand the true relationship between exposure and disease, confounders must be identified and controlled for in analysis. Logistic regression is a tool by which multiple confounders can be controlled simultaneously.

INTERPRETING THE LITERATURE

Each of the points discussed relates to questions the critical reader must ask. Following are a few examples:

- What is the exposure–disease relationship under study; that is, what is the hypothesis being tested? The most important question to ask initially is, "What is being measured?"
- Is the study population appropriate for testing this hypothesis?
- Is the study methodology appropriate for testing this hypothesis? What type of study was conducted, and what are its major methodologic limitations?
- What factors other than the exposure and disease under study need to be considered; for example, what study biases are likely present? Have they been adequately identified and controlled? If not, how should the interpretation of study findings be modified?
- If no association was found, was study power adequate to detect an existing important association?
- By addressing these and related questions, the reader can determine whether observed associations are likely due to 1) chance, 2) selection or information bias, 3) confounding (some epidemiologists consider confounding a bias as well), or 4) a cause-and-effect relationship.

Unfortunately, observed associations are sometimes based on studies that have such serious methodologic limitations that findings are difficult or impossible to interpret.

For clinicians, the bottom line is whether or not observed associations are important clinically. Probability values explain whether an observed association is likely due to chance, but often explain nothing about clinical relevance. Clinical utility is much more likely to be contingent on whether an observed association is causal and, if it is causal, the direction and magnitude of the observed relationship. Estimates of ORs and RRs are useful in the latter regard. Epidemiologic studies cannot, in a strict sense, prove causation. However, properly conducted and interpreted, epidemiologic studies can be used to infer causation. To determine the likelihood of causation, the critical reader must go beyond chance (P values) as an issue to consider other criteria, including the following:

- Strength of the observed association—In general, the stronger the association, the more likely it is to be real.
- Consistency of the study findings with those of other reports and all known information regarding both the exposure and outcome being investigated
- Temporality of the observed association—Does the cause precede the effect?
- Biologic plausibility of the observed association—Is there a dose–response relationship? Does the relationship make sense?

While this list of criteria to be considered is incomplete and cannot always be used to establish probable cause, these and other factors must be considered to determine whether statistically significant findings are likely to be clinically significant as well.

INFORMATION RETRIEVAL

Practicing obstetrician–gynecologists need access to current, accurate, and authoritative information to guide patient care decisions. An excellent way to gather needed information is to search an electronic database of the medical literature.

The largest and best known of these databases is MEDLINE, developed by the National Library of Medicine. MEDLINE contains more than 7 million citations to more than 3,200 biomedical journals, dating back to 1966. Hundreds of additional databases are available for searching. Reprotox, the Oxford Database of Clinical Trials, and TERIS are especially useful in obstetrics.

Physicians can perform their own MEDLINE searches or request that a professional medical librarian perform the search for them. Physicians can access MEDLINE on line via a modem or on a CD-ROM system. Access to MEDLINE is available through several commercial vendors; hospital and university librarians can provide a current listing of vendors, as well as suggestions for appropriate databases.

Members of the American College of Obstetricians and Gynecologists (ACOG) have two additional options for searching MEDLINE. They can request that the ACOG Resource Center librarians perform expert searches for them. Searches provided by the Resource Center staff include ACOG guidelines and photocopies of articles from the collection. Members can also perform their own MEDLINE searches through ACOGNET, the electronic bulletin board system provided by the College to members. One of the benefits of using ACOGNET for searching MEDLINE is that ACOGNET also contains the searchable full text of all important ACOG publications. The physician can search ACOGNET to identify and retrieve authoritative ACOG guidelines to complement MEDLINE results. ACOGNET can be accessed 24 hours per day to meet critical patient-care needs.

MEDLINE is most commonly searched to find articles on the diagnosis and management of a specific disease or use of a particular procedure. These topics can be searched by entering the official National Library of Medicine subject headings (MeSH), words in the title or abstract, or both. Results can be enhanced by checking which MeSH terms indexers used to index the retrieved citations and including some of these terms in a revised search strategy.

The National Library of Medicine has added additional MeSH terms that reflect the quality of the research described in cited articles. These terms include concepts for metaanalysis; randomized, controlled, clinical trials; and statistical bias. Use these terms in the search strategy to restrict results to quality-filtered literature. Supplement search results with records from databases that contain only controlled clinical trials and meta-analyses, such as the Oxford Database of Perinatal Trials and the Cochrane Collaboration Pregnancy and Childbirth Database.

Once the MEDLINE search is available, the next step is obtaining copies of the actual articles, as MEDLINE does not contain the complete text of the articles. ACOG members may request photocopies from the Resource Center from journals in its collection.

BIBLIOGRAPHY

Cole P. The evolving case–control study. J Chronic Dis 1979;32:15–27

Kleinbaum DG, Kupper LL, Morgenstern H. Epidemiologic research: principles and quantitative methods. Belmont, California: Lifetime Learning Publications, 1982

Kleinbaum DG, Kupper LL, Muller KE. Applied regression analysis and other multivariable methods. Boston: PWS-Kent Publishing Co, 1987

Last JM, ed. A dictionary of epidemiology. 2nd ed. New York: Oxford University Press, 1988

Peterson HB, Kleinbaum DG. Interpreting the literature in obstetrics and gynecology; I: key concepts in epidemiology and biostatistics. Obstet Gynecol 1991;78:710–717

Peterson HB, Kleinbaum DG. Interpreting the literature in obstetrics and gynecology; II: logistic regression and related issues. Obstet Gynecol 1991;78:717–720

Rothman KJ. Modern epidemiology. Boston: Little, Brown, 1986

Schlesselman JJ. Case–control studies: design, conduct, analysis. New York: Oxford University Press, 1982

Obstetrics

There has been an explosion of technology in the field of obstetrics and maternal–fetal medicine, especially in the areas of genetics and prenatal diagnosis. This technology provides valuable tools for the evaluation and monitoring of a pregnant woman and her fetus. However, it has also engendered an increase in the therapeutic limits, as well as the economic limits, for the practicing clinician. These dilemmas center on who will benefit from this technology, when it should be applied, and how often it should be used. The economics of the new technology will be of paramount importance in the future scheme of medicine, which no doubt will be centered on cost containment. It is also hoped that the information in this section of *Precis V* will provide some common-sense information in the application of the many recent advances in technology.

This section in *Precis V* is intended to provide the reader with concise and updated information in the specialty of obstetrics. It is envisioned that the information will provide a useful tool for the practicing obstetrician to maintain current knowledge in a rapidly changing field.

—*Larry C. Gilstrap III, MD*

Antepartum Care

ROUTINE CARE

The major goal of prenatal care is to ensure a healthy baby and a healthy mother. Although the pregnant woman should be aware of this goal, she should be counseled that, with current limitations in medicine and science, achievement of this goal cannot be guaranteed. Specific objectives that are an integral part of achieving this goal are as follows:

- Evaluation of the health status of both mother and fetus
- Estimation of the gestational age of the fetus
- Identification of the patient at risk for complications and minimization of that risk whenever possible
- Anticipation of problems before they occur, and prevention if possible
- Patient education and communication

In an attempt to ensure a systematic approach to prenatal care, a number of standardized prenatal forms have been developed—including that of the American College of Obstetricians and Gynecologists (ACOG)—many of which have the advantage of providing a built-in risk assessment system.

Diagnosis of Pregnancy

There is a myriad of commercial kits available for the diagnosis of pregnancy. All of the tests used in these kits depend on detection of human chorionic gonadotropin (hCG) by an antibody. The various techniques used to detect hCG include agglutination inhibition, radioimmunoassay, enzyme-linked immunosorbent assay (ELISA), and immunochromatography. Levels of hCG as low as 25 mIU/ml may be detected as early as 1 week after implantation with some tests.

There is also a wide variety of "home tests" commercially available that have relatively high positive predictive values. In addition, some of these may have high rates of false-negative results.

Initial History and Physical Examination

In addition to a general history, it is important to identify patients at significant risk of having an abnormal fetus or child. This may be accomplished by use of a prenatal questionnaire. The patient should be asked about her past medical history (eg, previous stillbirths, multiple miscarriages, congenital malformations), family history (eg, mental retardation, Down syndrome, neural tube defects [NTDs], or other genetic diseases), ethnicity (eg, Eastern European Jewish origin, Mediterranean origin, African origin), and any testing that has been accomplished (eg, Tay–Sachs disease, sickle cell disease, cystic fibrosis screening). Information about the current pregnancy should also be included (eg, medications, alcohol, tobacco, recreational or street drugs, X-rays, advanced maternal or paternal age).

The single most important part of the initial physical assessment is the pelvic examination to ascertain uterine size and gestational age and estimate the expected date of delivery. If there is a discrepancy between uterine size and the last menstrual period or if the latter is unknown, first-trimester or early second-trimester ultrasonography will help establish an expected date of delivery. Ultrasound measurement of the crown–rump length at 5–12 weeks of gestation is the most accurate technique for estimation of gestational age.

Laboratory Tests

Initial laboratory tests should include a Pap test; hemoglobin or hematocrit determination; blood group, Rh type, and antibody screen; rubella, syphilis, and hepatitis B screen; and a bacteriuria screen. Recommended intervals for routine tests and indicated tests for individual patients are summarized in Table 3-1.

Patient Education

Patients should be given information regarding the general plan of management for the pregnancy to include prenatal visits; diet, nutrition, and weight gain; signs and symptoms of potential complications; labor; plans for hospital admission; analgesic and anesthetic options; vaginal versus cesarean delivery; and exercise, travel, and work.

The initial prenatal visit is also an ideal time to discuss the frequency and types of congenital malformations occurring in the general population. Patients should be counseled against use of tobacco, alcohol, and drugs and illicit substances that might prove harmful to the fetus.

Nutrition and Weight Gain

Although there are few if any well-designed studies regarding nutrition in pregnancy, the relationship between maternal weight gain during pregnancy and newborn weight is well known. It is also generally accepted that all pregnant women should be encouraged to eat a "well-balanced" diet consisting of the dietary allowances recommended in Table 3-2. In addition to the vitamins and minerals listed, the Centers for Disease Control and Prevention (CDC) has recommended supplemental folic acid in the preconceptional and early prenatal period to prevent NTDs, although such use is controversial (see "Preconceptional Care" in the section on Office Practice).

The most recent recommendations for weight gain during pregnancy were published by the National Academy of Sciences in 1990. According to these recommendations, weight gain is based on the prepregnancy body mass index, defined as weight divided by height squared. Underweight women (body mass index < 19.8) should have a weight gain of 12.5–18 kg (28–40 lb) and overweight women (body mass index ≥ 26) should have a weight gain of 7–11.5 kg (15–25 lbs). The

Antepartum Care

TABLE 3-1. RECOMMENDED INTERVALS FOR ROUTINE AND INDICATED TESTS

Time (wk)	Assessment
Initial	Blood type
	Rh type
	Antibody screen
	Hemoglobin/hematocrit measurement
	Pap test
	Rubella antibody titer measurement
	Syphilis screen
	Gonorrhea screen
	Urine culture/screen
	Hepatitis B virus screen (HBsAg)
8–18	Ultrasonography
	Maternal serum alpha-fetoprotein
	Amniocentesis/chorionic villus sampling
	Karyotype
	Alpha-fetoprotein
24–28	Diabetes screen; glucose tolerance test (if screen abnormal)
	Repeat antibody test for unsensitized D-negative patients
	Prophylactic administration of D immune globulin
32–36	Ultrasonography
	Repeat syphilis screen
	Repeat gonorrhea screen
	Repeat hemoglobin or hematocrit measurement
Optional	Human immunodeficiency virus
	Hemoglobin electrophoresis
	Chlamydia
	Gonorrhea

Modified from American Academy of Pediatrics, American College of Obstetricians and Gynecologists. Guidelines for perinatal care. 3rd ed. Elk Grove Village, Illinois: AAP; Washington, DC: ACOG, 1992

TABLE 3-2. RECOMMENDED DAILY DIETARY ALLOWANCES FOR ADOLESCENT AND ADULT PREGNANT AND LACTATING WOMEN

Nutrient	Pregnant Women	Lactating Women
Energy (kcal)	+300	+500
Protein (g)	60	65
Fat-soluble vitamins		
Vitamin A (mg retinol equivalents)	800	1,300
Vitamin D (mg as cholecalciferol)	10	10
Vitamin E (mg α-tocopherol equivalents)	10	12
Vitamin K (mg)	65	65
Water-soluble vitamins		
Vitamin C (mg)	70	95
Thiamine (mg)	1.5	1.6
Riboflavin (mg)	1.6	1.8
Niacin (mg niacin equivalent)	17	20
Vitamin B_6	2.2	2.1
Folate (mg)	400	280
Vitamin B_{12}	2.2	2.6
Minerals		
Calcium (mg)	1,200	1,200
Phosphorus (mg)	1,200	1,200
Magnesium (mg)	300	355
Iron (mg)	30	15
Zinc (mg)	15	19
Iodine (mg)	175	200
Selenium (mg)	65	75

Adapted and reprinted with permission from Recommended Dietary Allowances: 10th Ed. Copyright 1989 by the National Academy of Sciences. Courtesy of the National Academy Press, Washington, DC

recommended weight gain for women of average weight—that is, a normal body mass index (19.8–26.0)—is 11.5–16 kg (25–35 lb).

Work During Pregnancy

A normal woman with an uncomplicated pregnancy and a normal fetus, employed where there are no greater potential hazards than those encountered in routine daily life in the community, may continue to work without interruption until the onset of labor. In addition, she may resume working several weeks after an uncomplicated delivery. Work may be limited or contraindicated during pregnancy in patients with vaginal bleeding, an incompetent cervix or uterine malformation associated with a perinatal loss, pregnancy-induced hypertension, fetal growth retardation, multiple gestations, prior history of preterm birth, or polyhydramnios. Maternal disorders that warrant special review include renal disease, diabetes mellitus with vasculopathy, heart disease with arrhythmias, pulmonary or arterial hypertension, hemoglobinopathies, a hemoglobin value below 80 g/L, seizure disorders, nerve root irritations, back problems, and uncontrolled asthma.

The Pregnancy Discrimination Act protects the right to work during pregnancy. Job discrimination on the basis of pregnancy is prohibited; the act requires that pregnancy or related disorders be considered like any other disability or medical condition. An applicant cannot be denied employment because of pregnancy. A pregnant worker cannot be excluded from any written or unwritten employment practice because of pregnancy or related medical conditions. Pregnant workers must be provided the same insurance benefits, sick leave, seniority credits, and reinstatement privileges awarded workers disabled by other causes.

The Occupational Safety and Health Act stipulates that employers maintain a safe and healthful workplace. If necessary, certain modifications may be made at the workplace that will permit pregnant patients to safely continue their employment. Some companies have adopted a "fetus protection policy" that prohibits female employees of childbearing age from holding a job that would expose them to toxic substances at levels considered to be unsafe for the fetus. Such policies have been ruled to violate the Pregnancy Discrimination Act.

Follow-up Visits

Examination at each subsequent visit should generally consist of measurement of the uterine fundus, determination of fetal heart tones, measurement of blood pressure, and determination of fetal presentation. The urine should be screened for glucose and protein at each visit. Table 3-1 lists additional laboratory tests to be done at specific times during pregnancy.

The interval for subsequent prenatal visits should be based on patient needs; in general, women with uncomplicated pregnancies should be seen every 4–5 weeks until 28 weeks of gestation, then every 2 weeks until 36 weeks, and then at least weekly until delivery. More frequent visits may be of benefit in monitoring women with diabetes, hypertension, prematurity, postterm pregnancies, or other complications.

ULTRASONOGRAPHY

Ultrasound imaging methods are based on insonation of target tissues with low-energy (<100 mW/cm^2), high-frequency (3.5–7.5 mHz) sound waves and recording of the intensity and the delay time for reflected echoes. These echo signals are converted by a digital computer to dots, the brightness of which reflects signal strength and the position of which reflects the distance of the target from the transducer. Multiple emitting crystals may be lined up and excited sequentially (linear array), a single crystal may be swept through a prescribed arc (sector array), or both may be used (curvilinear array) to produce rapidly repeating images in real time. The sector and curved linear array methods have been developed for a transvaginal probe that produces extremely high-resolution images of pelvic organs and the embryo.

There is no increased incidence of abnormalities among offspring with in utero exposure to ultrasonography, and long-term follow-up studies have also supported the safety of ultrasonography. Ultrasound techniques are within the U.S. Food and Drug Administration (FDA) guidelines of 100 mW/cm^2. Although this level for fetal safety was chosen arbitrarily, all studies to date have been conducted with equipment within this energy range and no adverse fetal effects have been shown. New Doppler methods using color-flow techniques frequently are at the upper limit of this energy range.

Technical Advances

New techniques in ultrasonography, recently introduced and commonly available, involve the increased use of Doppler methods. These include both Doppler velocimetry, particularly of the umbilical cord, and Doppler color-flow techniques. These techniques, at present, are investigational.

All transducers may be equipped with the capability of measuring Doppler shift phenomena. This is referred to as duplex Doppler, since the image and the Doppler waveform are obtained at the same time. After the area of interest is imaged, a cursor is placed on the specific point in question, usually a blood vessel, and the Doppler feature selected. At this point a plot of the pulsations through that area is recorded on the ultrasound screen. Because the same transducer is emitting as well as receiving signals, only pulses of energy are emitted. This Doppler is called pulsed-wave Doppler. Doppler velocimetry may also be performed by using a probe that transmits a continuous wave of sound. In these cases the vessel is not imaged but can be found when a recognizable, typical waveform appears on the screen. These examinations are performed with free-standing units, which are much less costly than sophisticated ultrasound units with duplex Doppler capability. They also have better resolution, with lower energy, of the sampled vessel. However, small vessels may not be found easily, since they are "visualized" by pattern recognition alone.

Velocity through vessels can be recorded by using Doppler; however, this application in obstetrics is limited by other technical considerations. Measurement of velocity is dependent on the size of the vessel involved, as well as the angle of insonance between the sampling probe and the direction of blood flow. As these angles are frequently not known and the size of the vessel is known only approximately, there are large absolute errors in calculations. Although the size of the vessel can be measured, small errors in the diameter make a large difference in the velocity calculated. To date, these technical problems have not been overcome, and therefore measures of blood flow have been with relative velocities. The most commonly used is the systole–diastole ratio, in which ratios of velocities in systole and diastole are calculated.

Color-flow Doppler may also be added to the software of existing ultrasound machines and transducers. In this case, a partial area of the field being imaged is measured for flow. The amount, velocity, and direction of flow are recorded continuously with color-graded images. Usually red indicates flow toward the transducer and blue indicates flow away from the transducer, although these designations are purely arbitrary.

Another technical advance, post-process coloring, has also become available recently. This feature substitutes a different color scheme for the more common gray scale. That is, rather than having images of black or white with shades of gray, a different base color is used. This technique occasionally may be helpful in difficult imaging situations.

Many ultrasound machines are equipped with cine-loops, which automatically store several seconds worth of images. These can then be played back after the real-time picture is frozen. This can be useful in case of a sudden fetal movement, when a good image suddenly disappears.

Development of sophisticated systems for archiving examinations, relaying images over telephone lines, and creating computer linkages have advanced quickly and will continue to modernize all forms of image management. There have also been advances in reporting software. Finally, there has been research into three-dimensional imaging, which is not commercially available.

Indications

There is considerable controversy surrounding the issue of routine ultrasound screening in pregnancy. Although this is standard practice in many countries in Western Europe, it did not receive the endorsement of the National Institutes of Health when this issue was studied in 1984 and indications were established (see box). Arguments supporting the routine use of ultrasonography include the early detection of multiple gestation, improved dating, and the detection of unsuspected fetal anomalies in low-risk patients. If performed in the first trimester, ultrasonography may be useful in finding ectopic pregnancy or missed abortion before it is apparent clinically. However, the study of the Routine Antenatal Diagnostic Imaging with Ultrasound (Radius) Study Group (involving more than 15,000 women, sponsored by the National Institute of Child Health and Human Development) reported that screening ultrasonography in low-risk pregnancies did not improve perinatal outcome. Thus, this report supports the ACOG position that ultrasonography is not necessary for every woman in early pregnancy.

Indications for Ultrasonography During Pregnancy

Estimation of gestational age for patients with uncertain clinical dates, or verification of dates for patients who are to undergo scheduled elective repeat cesarean delivery, indicated induction of labor, or other elective termination of pregnancy

Evaluation of fetal growth

Vaginal bleeding of undetermined etiology in pregnancy

Determination of fetal presentation

Suspected multiple gestation

Adjunct to amniocentesis

Significant uterine size/clinical dates discrepancy

Pelvic mass

Suspected hydatidiform mole

Adjunct to cervical cerclage placement

Suspected ectopic pregnancy

Adjunct to special procedures

Suspected fetal death

Suspected uterine abnormality

Intrauterine contraceptive device localization

Biophysical evaluation for fetal well-being

Observation of intrapartum events

Suspected polyhydramnios or oligohydramnios

Suspected abruptio placentae

Adjunct to external version from breech to vertex presentation

Estimation of fetal weight, presentation in premature rupture of membranes, premature labor

Abnormal serum alpha-fetoprotein value

Follow-up observation of identified fetal anomaly

Follow-up evaluation of placental location for identified "placenta previa"

History of previous congenital anomaly

Serial evaluation of fetal growth in multiple gestation

Evaluation of fetal condition in late registrants for prenatal care

Adapted from U.S. Department of Health and Human Services. Diagnostic ultrasound in pregnancy. Bethesda, Maryland: National Institutes of Health, 1984; National Institutes of Health publication no. 84-667

Types of Examinations

Two types of obstetric ultrasound examinations are performed. Current terminology refers to *basic* and *comprehensive* examinations, which replaces the older terminology of *level I* and *level II* examinations. A basic examination is intended to be a thorough, well-documented examination performed for any of the usual indications. A comprehensive examination may be indicated in cases where a problem is suspected. The components of a basic examination during the second and third trimesters are determination of gestational age; fetal number, viability, and lie; placental location and grade; volume of amniotic fluid; and a survey of fetal anatomy for gross malformations. Perhaps the most controversial aspect of a basic examination involves the fetal anatomic survey. Some minimal standards for anatomic survey have been proposed by ACOG and other organizations.

Brief or limited examinations are appropriate during emergencies or when ultrasonography is used as an adjunct to a procedure. In most circumstances it is recommended that the patient have a complete ultrasound examination after a limited examination unless the patient previously had one or more examinations in the second or third trimester.

Ultrasonography is also used to provide guidance during amniocentesis, chorionic villus sampling (CVS), and percutaneous umbilical cord blood sampling (PUBS). During labor and delivery it can be a useful adjunct during external cephalic version.

Basic Examinations

There has been a de facto division of examinations into early and late first trimester. In the late first trimester a large amount of anatomy may be seen in the fetus and may occasionally be difficult to interpret. For example, it is not unusual to see the physiologic herniation of bowel into the umbilical cord as late as 10 weeks of gestation. This may be mistaken for the early diagnosis of an omphalocele. On the other hand, anencephaly can certainly be excluded with a normal examination at 12 weeks, when the cranial vault is clearly seen.

First Trimester. During a basic examination in the first trimester, gestational age is estimated and the number of fetuses is recorded. This may be difficult in the very early first trimester. In the case of monochorionic twins, two sacs may not be visible until the second trimester. If the fetal pole cannot yet be distinguished, a set of twins may be missed in this circumstance. In addition, a phenomenon known as vanishing twins involves up to 15% of twin gestations. In this situation a previously healthy twin gestation results in a singleton gestation after the first trimester. Finally, small areas of bleeding or other subchorionic collections are not uncommon in the first trimester, particularly among patients who present for ultrasound examinations because of vaginal bleeding. It may be difficult to distinguish such a cystic area from a second gestational sac.

The location of the sacs is important to note in distinguishing an intrauterine gestation from an ectopic gestation. Cardiac activity should be recorded but may be difficult to see at very early gestational ages. Extremely early gestational sacs can be seen by using transvaginal ultrasound techniques.

When fetal size is measured, commonly used nomograms for crown–rump length have been extrapolated down to 5 weeks. Several authors have proposed the term *early embryonic size* to replace *crown–rump length*, and new nomograms are appearing based on transvaginal findings in very early pregnancies. In addition to the fetal pole, the sac itself may be measured and the size serially followed.

A thorough first-trimester examination should also include visualization of the maternal adnexa. At least one small ovarian cyst representing the corpus luteum is frequently seen. Any fibroids or other masses should also be noted.

Second and Third Trimesters. The basic examination in the second and third trimesters is similar to that in the first trimester, although the quality of information obtained may be quite different.

The number of fetuses should be documented, along with their cardiac motion and their lies. Multiple parameters are measured in fetuses, usually including the femur length, abdominal circumference, head circumference, and biparietal diameter. In the second trimester, combinations of these parameters may predict gestational age to as close as 10 days. More usually in the mid- to late second trimester there is up to a 2-week error in these measurements. By the end of the third trimester, the standard errors for these measurements are as high as 2½ weeks, and thus they are poor for predicting gestational age.

Fetal weight may be estimated by obtaining fetal biometry and using one of several formulas that are available to derive this calculation. Most available weight formulas have a standard deviation of approximately 10%. That is, one can expect that the fetal weight is within 10% of the estimate approximately 66% of the time.

Biometry in the third trimester is also useful for looking at patterns of fetal growth. For example, in cases of asymmetric intrauterine growth retardation (IUGR) most classically associated with uteroplacental insufficiency, the fetus will have a relatively normal head size and femur length whereas abdominal circumference will be quite a bit smaller than expected. Similarly, macrosomic babies will have large parameters throughout, but the fetal abdominal circumference will be the most affected.

Evaluation of Structures. The umbilical cord should also be examined briefly in a basic examination. The number of vessels that the cord contains can be seen after 24 weeks and frequently before this. A single umbilical artery may be associated with fetal anomalies, particularly in the genitourinary system, and may also be associated with IUGR. The placenta is easily visualized during a basic examination, and its position relative to the cervical os can be assessed in order to diagnose a placenta previa. Most of these cases do not result in a placenta previa later in gestation, however. Other patients who present with bleeding who do not have a placenta previa may well have a placental abruption. However, only 35% of patients with a significant placental abruption will have ultrasound findings that identify an area of separation or a retroplacental hematoma.

The cervix is easier to visualize early in pregnancy and becomes progressively more difficult to image as pregnancy proceeds. The advent of transvaginal ultrasonography, however, has made it easier to image the cervix at any point in pregnancy. The length, any dilatation of the endocervical canal, and the shape of the internal os may be noted. An abnormal shape includes funneling, which has been described as "beaking." Preliminary evidence suggests that beaking may be associated with cervical incompetence in the second trimester. An overall shortened or dilated cervix on ultrasonography has the same significance that it has when these findings are confirmed on a physical examination. Overall, the ultrasound-calculated length of a normal cervix is quite a bit longer than is generally determined by a vaginal examination, no doubt because of the portion of the cervix that is above the level of the vaginal fornix. The overall length obtained by transvaginal measurement is slightly longer than that obtained by transabdominal measurement, but this difference is generally only a few millimeters. Transvaginal ultrasonography of the cervix may also be useful when it is difficult to determine whether there is a placenta previa rather than a low-lying placenta.

Amniotic Fluid Volume. Amniotic fluid volume can be estimated during an ultrasound examination as normal, abnormally increased, or abnormally decreased. In an attempt to make this subjective rating more quantitative, there are two other ways of defining amniotic fluid volume. One method is to describe the largest vertical pocket of fluid free of fetal parts. A pocket greater than 8 cm defines hydramnios; if the smallest pocket is less than 2 cm, oligohydramnios is present.

A newer way to describe amniotic fluid volume is the amniotic fluid index. The amniotic fluid index is calculated by dividing the uterus into four quadrants as defined by the linea nigra and the umbilicus. In each of the four quadrants the largest vertical pocket of amniotic fluid free of umbilical cord and fetal parts is measured, and these four numbers are added together. Although the normal values vary by gestational age, 24 cm or greater is almost always abnormal and 5 cm or less is always abnormal. This method is generally reserved for the second half of the second trimester and the third trimester.

Fetal Anatomy Survey. In order for a basic examination to be complete in the second and third trimesters, a variety of fetal structures should be imaged. These structures include the head and spine, the four chambers of the heart, the stomach and kidneys, insertion of the umbilical cord into the anterior abdominal wall, and the bladder. It may be impossible to see all of this anatomy in certain situations (ie, oligohydramnios, hyperflexed position of the fetus, engagement of the head, compression of some fetal parts, and maternal obesity). If one of these structures is not clearly seen or if the image is suggestive of an abnormality, a comprehensive examination may be necessary.

Comprehensive Examinations

A comprehensive examination is generally indicated in situations in which suspicion has been raised about the pregnancy or the fetus. A common indication for a comprehensive examination is an abnormal basic examination. Patients in whom the pregnancy is at risk may be those with histories of congenital anomalies, abnormal alpha-fetoprotein test results, or previous abnormal pregnancies.

Principles behind a comprehensive examination are not very different from those behind a basic examination. Similar equipment is used, but the level of expertise of the examiner is generally higher and the center performing the examination is more specialized. General biometry is repeated, nonfetal structures such as placenta and amniotic fluid are surveyed, and the fetal anatomy is carefully reviewed. In many cases the fetal anatomy is the portion of the examination that is of concern. The anatomic survey is therefore less perfunctory and more detailed than that described for a basic examination. For example, multiple parts of the fetal intracranial anatomy would be identified in cases in which hydrocephalus is a concern. In addition, other structures in the fetus that would be expected to be affected by such a diagnosis are carefully delineated.

ANTEPARTUM TESTING

Most methods of antenatal testing have had extensive clinical trials in high-risk populations. There is a paucity of information regarding their value in low-risk populations, either as screening tools or as compared with one another. There is considerable variation in different centers regarding testing protocols, interpretation of tests, testing techniques, and testing frequency. Thus, there are no widely agreed upon standards for many of these issues.

Indications for Testing

Some common indications for testing are:

- Postterm pregnancy
- IUGR
- Hypertension
- Diabetes
- Sickle cell disease
- Premature rupture of membranes (PROM)
- Decreased fetal movement
- Maternal renal disease
- Systemic lupus erythematosus

For most fetal conditions (eg, preeclampsia, IUGR, postterm pregnancy), testing is begun when the diagnosis is established, usually in the third trimester. For long-standing fetal conditions or chronic maternal medical complications, the timing depends on the severity of the condition. Examples of indications in this category might include maternal diabetes, chronic hypertension, and D isoimmunization.

Most contraindications to testing involve fetuses in which one would not intervene based on an abnormal test result at early gestational ages, when an abnormal test result would not lead to delivery. In addition, the tests may not have the same predictive value in the late second trimester. For example, it is known that the nonstress test (NST) may not be reactive in the immature fetus. The contraction stress test (CST) may be relatively contraindicated in patients with PROM or preterm labor.

Techniques

There is considerable controversy regarding which test of antepartum fetal health is most appropriate. The NST is the easiest test to use but has a high false-positive rate. Clinical observations and laboratory studies indicate that late decelerations occur earlier than do the loss of beat-to-beat variability and accelerations from an otherwise normal heart rate tracing. Specifically, the loss of baseline variability usually occurs after fetal hypoxia has been severe enough to produce acidosis. Consequently, the CST is probably an earlier and more sensitive indicator of fetal hypoxia. In large clinical studies, however, both tests appear to be reasonably accurate predictors of fetal compromise, with low false-negative rates. False-negative rates are comparable in the NST and the CST. The biophysical profile score (BPP) is also used extensively and has advantages in certain settings. There are no contraindications to its use, and it may reveal other fetal problems not detectable through heart rate testing alone, such as multiple gestation and certain gross fetal anomalies.

Fetal Heart Rate Testing

The NST is generally accepted as the simplest screening test for fetal compromise in the antepartum period. It is best to carry out this test with the patient either in the slightly tilted, recumbent position or in the semi-Fowler position to minimize compression of the maternal vena cava by the pregnant uterus. The fetal heart rate (FHR) is recorded by using an external Doppler ultrasound device and an external tocodynamometer.

The protocol for the NST generally involves recording the FHR over 20–30 minutes, with the patient pressing a marker button when there is fetal movement. There are various criteria for the number of accelerations required during a period of time, as well as for the amplitude and duration of the accelerations. It is generally agreed that the occurrence of two accelerations of at least 10 beats per minute, lasting for 10 seconds within a 20-minute period, is a "reactive" test. Because fetuses have sleep periods of approximately 20 minutes, it is acceptable to proceed for another 20-minute observation period if movements or accelerations in the initial period are insufficient. Nonetheless, the false-positive rate for the NST is approximately 80% (ie, 80% of those fetuses that are nonreactive are, in fact, normal).

Because of the high-false positive rate for the NST, a nonreactive test is generally followed by a second test of fetal well-being rather than by delivery. There are several methods for further evaluation of a nonreactive NST. The NST may be extended; data indicate that a persistent nonreactive NST for 90 minutes or more is associated with a very high incidence of fetal compromise. Fetal stimulation by a mixed-frequency, relatively high-intensity vibroacoustic stimulator may be applied in the region of the fetal head. A fetal response to short stimulation in the form of fetal movement and heart rate acceleration suggests a noncompromised fetus. This test should be used with caution in some cases, as there is evidence that compromised, premature fetuses may not tolerate it well and may respond with profound bradycardia. An ultrasound assessment of other biophysical variables as described in the BPP may be performed. When these variables are normal, the nonreactive NST has been shown to be unrelated to an increased risk of fetal compromise. Finally, a CST may be performed.

When the NST is nonreactive but the results of the CST or BPP are normal, tests should be repeated at appropriate intervals. Most fetuses are nonreactive because of physiologic sleep or transient lack of activity, and the movements or reactivity may return before the BPP or CST is completed. No specific interval can be given for repetition of the tests; timing should be determined by the degree of concern for fetal well-being. Most clinical trials have examined weekly testing, and therefore most tests are repeated at least this often.

Biophysical Profile

The BPP combines the NST with fetal ultrasound parameters. In a 30-minute period, the fetus should exhibit movements, breathing motions, and evidence of tone as described in Table 3-3. In addition, the amniotic fluid volume is assessed and the NST results are recorded.

The total score obtained reflects the fetal status. A score of 8–10 is normal and highly correlated with normal fetal umbilical cord blood gases and a normal fetal outcome. A score of 6 is considered equivocal and generally warrants repeated testing within 24 hours or delivery if the fetus is mature. A score of 4 or less is highly predictive of fetal compromise and frequently leads to intervention. The false-positive rate (ie, a normal fetus despite an abnormal result) is much lower with this method than with other forms of heart rate testing. Large studies of the BPP as a first-line test of fetal well-being in high-risk populations have found false-negative rates (fetal death within 7 days of a normal test) similar to those with the NST or CST. There are no large-scale, randomized studies directly comparing these forms of testing.

Many centers perform a modified BPP rather than complete testing. This is accomplished in one of two ways. If the ultrasound-determined parameters (tone, breathing, amniotic fluid volume, and movements) are all normal, no NST is done and a score of 8 is assigned. Because a score of 8 is predictive of fetal well-being, an NST is not necessary to improve the score.

A different approach is to add an amniotic fluid volume determination to an NST. Most authorities agree that these are the two most significant predictors of fetal well-being. Furthermore, most would agree that in many clinical situations, such as postterm pregnancy, decreased amniotic fluid volume is an indication for delivery even if there is a reactive NST or an otherwise normal BPP.

Amniotic fluid volume is deemed adequate or inadequate in BPP scoring schemes, but the definition of *adequate* has changed. More recently, many have suggested that the amniotic fluid index should be used and that an inadequate volume of fluid as reflected by this criterion requires intervention. These individual determinations are combined to give the amniotic fluid index. For purposes of the BPP, a normal volume is greater than 5 cm. Percentiles have also been developed that would indicate that a slightly larger amount of fluid is required to define normal and that this varies by gestational age (see Table 3-4).

Contraction Stress Test

The CST attempts to mimic labor by inducing mild uterine contractions. Contractions may be spontaneous, or they may

TABLE 3-3. BIOPHYSICAL PROFILE

Biophysical Variable	Normal (Score = 2)	Abnormal (Score = 0)
Fetal breathing	At least one episode of at least 30-s duration in 30-min observation	Absent or ≤30 s of continuous breathing
Fetal body movement	Three discrete body/limb movements	Less than three body/limb movements
Fetal tone	Active extension and flexion of fetal limb or trunk	Slow extension and partial flexion of limbs; limbs in full extension or absent fetal movement
Nonstress test	Reactive	Nonreactive
Amniotic fluid volume	One vertical pocket of amniotic fluid measuring 2 cm	Less than one 2-cm pocket

TABLE 3-4. AMNIOTIC FLUID INDEX

Gestation (wk)	Fifth Percentile (mm)
36	77
37	75
38	73
39	72
40	71
41	70
42	69

Adapted from Moore TR, Cayle JE. The amniotic fluid index in normal human pregnancy. Am J Obstet Gynecol 1990;162:1168–1173

be generated either by oxytocin or by nipple stimulation. The heart rate is monitored continuously and compared with the contraction pattern. The presence of late decelerations suggests that the fetus has lost some placental reserve. However, in various studies, approximately 50% of fetuses that had abnormal responses to the CST subsequently had no demonstrable abnormality (ie, the test results were false-positive). When beat-to-beat variability is lost, the false-positive rate drops to less than 10%. The CST is frequently used if there is reason to be suspicious of other test results or if an NST is nonreactive.

Fetal Movement

It has been reported that the antepartum use of fetal movement counting (or kick counts) can decrease antepartum stillbirth rates in low-risk women. The pregnant woman records the length of time that the fetus takes to make 10 movements. She may select any period of the day to count these movements, but fetuses are generally perceived to be most active in the late evening, after the mother has had dinner. Each fetus has its own degree of activity, but most usually move 10 times in less than 40 minutes. Patients are told that if the fetus requires more than 2 hours for 10 kicks, they should contact their physicians.

Fetal Umbilical Artery Velocimetry

Recently, fetal umbilical artery velocimetry has been used to measure increased placental vascular resistance, which may potentially allow for the recognition of placental dysfunction. After 24 weeks of gestation, measurement of the relationship of peak systolic to diastolic flow velocities, with the systolic–diastolic ratio, pulsatility index, or Pourcelot index, may offer insight into fetal compromise. The absence of blood flow in diastole or reverse flow in diastole reflects extreme placental vascular resistance and is considered ominous. The value of Doppler fetal umbilical artery velocimetry is at present unclear, and this technique should be considered investigational.

FETAL THERAPY

Fetal therapy or fetal treatment is not a new concept. Corticosteroids given to the mother to hasten lung maturity and intrapartum antibiotics in intraamniotic infections are two examples of fairly routine fetal treatments.

There are also some unusual circumstances in which specific medical or invasive therapy is aimed at the fetus with a well-defined, serious condition. It is in these situations that the term *fetal therapy* is usually applied. Most such situations involve cutting-edge information, and treatment borders on experimental.

There are some principles that are important in evaluating the fetus and the proposed therapy. In general, before fetuses are considered for this sort of therapy, the fetal disease that is to be treated must be well defined. In addition, the disease or defect must have a poor prognosis if left untreated. The particular defect should be isolated rather than part of a syndrome. In general, it must be determined that interruption of the natural history of the disease or defect will improve the prognosis for the fetus. This is much less likely to be true in a fetus with multiple anomalies. Finally, treatment is offered only after the diagnosis is established. Side effects of the treatment on the mother or the fetus should be minimal and acceptable. In all cases the risks and benefits of the proposed therapy should be carefully discussed with the patient and family, as the risks may be considerable and the benefit ill defined.

Medical Therapy

There are two types of medical therapy. In the first type, medications are given to the mother solely to cross the placenta and reach the fetus. In the second type, medications are given to the mother to change her status and thus affect the fetus.

Congenital adrenal hyperplasia is a recessively inherited disorder that results in salt wasting. Glucocorticoid replacement is lifesaving, and the long-term prognosis for these children is good. Androgenic cortisol precursors build up in the fetus, and female fetuses typically present with ambiguous genitalia. Mothers of previously affected offspring may be treated with steroids in suppressive doses beginning shortly after conception, which will decrease the production of androgenic steroids in the fetus. Steroids are generally given until prenatal testing is performed. Chorionic villus sampling or amniocentesis is performed both to determine fetal sex and for DNA testing for the responsible gene. If testing shows a normal female fetus or a male fetus, the steroids can be stopped; otherwise, steroid therapy is continued through term.

In most cases of fetal tachyarrhythmia there is no underlying anatomic congenital heart disease. Children with these conditions respond well to treatment, and the long-term prognosis is good. Untreated fetuses with this condition may become hydropic, however, and the mortality under those circumstances is substantial. Digoxin is the drug of choice in children, and it may be given to the healthy mother to cross the placenta and treat the fetus. Only about one third of fetuses respond to digoxin alone, and second-line or alternative regimens such as procainamide, flecainide, and verapamil may be necessary. All of these drugs have potential side effects to both the mother and the fetus.

In neonatal alloimmune thrombocytopenia, the mother has

antibodies to fetal platelets. Unlike maternal immune thrombocytopenic purpura (ITP), these mothers themselves have normal platelet counts. These fetuses tend to have profound thrombocytopenia, which may result in spontaneous hemorrhage in utero. Various fetal therapies have been suggested, including repetitive platelet transfusions to the fetus. However, in addition to being quite invasive, circulating platelets have a short half-life in the fetus. Attempts have been made to suppress maternal antibody production by using immune globulin with or without corticosteroids, and initial results have been promising.

Invasive Fetal Therapy

Intraamniotic Injections

Attempts have been made to use the amniotic cavity as a route for treating the fetus directly. This is uncommonly used, as it has been met with limited success. Theoretically, medications that are given this way may be swallowed by the fetus and absorbed; however, this absorption is erratic compared with placental transfer after maternal administration or compared with direct intravenous fetal administration.

Intravenous Therapy

The most successful and widely used form of invasive fetal therapy is the direct transfusion of red blood cells to fetuses with red blood cell isoimmunization. A transfusion can be directed into the fetal peritoneal cavity or intravenously (IV). The latter route has been used more extensively in recent years. This is discussed in greater detail in the section on red blood cell isoimmunization.

There are other situations in which red blood cell transfusions are also given to the fetus. The most common, other than isoimmunization, is anemia, usually discovered during the workup of a fetus with nonimmune hydrops. If the fetus is found to be anemic from a reversible cause, fetal therapy may be warranted. Numerous cases of transfusion with recovery of the fetus have been reported in this situation. The most common etiologies for reversible underlying anemia are a fetal–maternal hemorrhage or parvovirus B19 infection with a resultant fetal hemolytic crisis.

Under unusual circumstances intravenous medications may be given to the fetus for treatment. Although this is technically feasible, it is warranted only in a limited number of situations. Any medication that must be administered repeatedly or continuously cannot be given in this fashion because repeatedly gaining access to the fetal circulation is far too invasive.

Stem cell transplantation has been suggested as a way of treating fetuses affected with certain genetic diseases. There have been only a limited number of successful cases of this procedure to date. Generally, stem cells are injected into the fetus in the first or early second trimester. Grafting of these cells into the fetal liver with subsequent function has been documented, although no cases of the prevention of expression of an inherited genetic disease have yet been reported.

Obstructive Uropathy

Obstructive uropathy has lent itself to early detection with ultrasonography. Posterior urethral valves or bladder outlet obstructions are the most common of these disorders, but the obstruction may be at any level of the urinary tract.

In all cases of obstructive uropathy, the rationale behind treatment is that the obstruction itself will lead to permanent renal damage in the developing fetus. Additionally, obstruction of the urinary tract will lead to oligohydramnios and pulmonary hypoplasia, which is usually the cause of death in these neonates. Thus, the rationale for invasive therapy is that it will prevent a potentially fatal sequence of events and if successful will lead to a favorable long-term prognosis. The most difficult decision in these cases is proper selection of candidates. Ideal candidates are fetuses with isolated anomalies who are found in the second or very early third trimester with progressive oligohydramnios but good remaining renal function.

Defining renal function in the fetus is a difficult task. Cystic renal parenchyma that appear abnormal on ultrasound examination, severe oligohydramnios, poor urine output, and abnormal electrolytes, osmolarity, or beta$_2$-microglobulins in a sample of aspirated fetal urine have all been suggested as prognostic indicators. However, each of these tests is difficult to interpret. Candidate selection therefore continues to be subjective and imperfect.

An obstructed urinary tract can be drained in a number of ways, depending on the level of obstruction. The most common procedure is to place a vesicoamniotic shunt to drain the fetal bladder chronically into the amniotic space. Alternatively, the shunt can be placed in a dilated renal pelvis, again to drain into the amniotic cavity. Proponents of open fetal surgery have also exteriorized the fetus and marsupialized the bladder or dilated renal pelvis to the skin, to defer definitive surgery until after delivery.

Hydrocephalus

Fetal hydrocephalus is frequently accompanied by long-term neurologic sequelae and is treated by shunting after delivery. Treatment of fetuses with in utero shunt placement has been suggested as a way to reduce brain damage by relieving pressure on the brain tissue earlier in gestation. A voluntary registry of cases of fetal surgery was created and, because of extremely poor outcome, a moratorium was placed on these procedures in 1984. These procedures had a procedure-related mortality to the fetus of approximately 10%. In addition, a large number of shunts were removed by the fetus, compared with the more commonly placed bladder shunts. The efficacy of such procedures is at best questionable.

Draining of Other Cystic Structures

A variety of other fluid collections and pathologic cystic structures in the fetus have also been drained with either serial punctures or placement of catheters. In some cases these procedures are at least partly diagnostic. For example, in the case of a large pleural effusion, an analysis of the fluid obtained by thoracentesis may differentiate a chylothorax from a pleural effusion caused by other factors. A large cyst may also impinge on adjacent structures, making them difficult to delineate ultrasonographically. For example, in the case of a large cystic mass that fills the fetal abdomen, it may be difficult to distinguish an ovarian cyst from a hugely distended bladder until the cyst is aspirated and normal adjacent structures can be seen without compression.

In addition to these diagnostic problems it may be useful to drain cystic structures for therapeutic reasons. For example, a large congenital cystic adenomatoid malformation type I in the lung may lead to nonimmune hydrops. Multiple case reports exist of serial drainage of these cysts, with resolution of hydrops, partial resolution of the size of the cyst, and the resolution of shifts of the mediastinum. Cysts in the fetal abdomen may cause soft tissue dystocia at the time of labor and delivery, and thus drainage may allow a vaginal delivery.

Open Fetal Surgery

In a small number of cases with a limited number of diagnoses, open fetal surgery has been performed to prevent lethal neonatal sequelae of a serious fetal condition. Examples of diagnoses in which open fetal surgery has been attempted include diaphragmatic hernia, congenital cystic adenomatoid malformation of the lung, sacrococcygeal teratoma, and obstructive uropathy. Each of these conditions is amenable to surgical intervention; however, without surgery these fetal conditions may have lethal consequences, usually because of pulmonary hypoplasia or nonimmune hydrops.

Open fetal surgery is complex and requires a large team experienced with a number of specialized techniques. Specialized instruments, monitoring equipment, anesthesia, and stapling devices have been developed but clearly are not routinely available. There is considerable morbidity to the mother with these procedures, and preterm labor after the surgery is an extremely frequent problem. The fetus must have enough time to recover from the insult and continue to develop normally in order for the surgery to be justified, and termination of the pregnancy within a few weeks of surgery because of progressive preterm labor is a major barrier.

In many of these cases, candidate selection is controversial. For example, neonates with sacrococcygeal teratoma do relatively well, and it is therefore not necessary in most cases to intervene during fetal life. On the other hand, in some cases nonimmune hydrops may develop, which markedly worsens the prognosis. Similarly, the prognosis for diaphragmatic hernia is the subject of considerable controversy. With developments in extracorporeal membrane oxygenation, most pediatric surgeons feel that the prognosis is much better than that quoted by obstetricians. Success rates in the clinical trials from San Francisco have been mixed, and thus this form of surgery is certainly not a panacea. Clearly, randomized trials would be helpful in sorting out many of these issues, but unfortunately these do not appear to be forthcoming.

PRENATAL DIAGNOSIS OF GENETIC DISORDERS

Two to three percent of all liveborn infants have major congenital malformations. Six to seven percent of all perinatal deaths are related to chromosomal abnormalities. Most (65–75%) congenital anomalies are described as multifactorial or of unknown etiology, and 20–25% of congenital anomalies are due to chromosomal or monogenic abnormalities.

Common indications for prenatal counseling and diagnosis are:

- Advanced maternal age
- Risk of chromosomal abnormality
- Previous child with chromosomal abnormality
- High or low maternal serum alpha-fetoprotein (MSAFP)
- Multiple spontaneous abortions
- Significant risk of single-gene defect
- Significant risk of NTD or other multifactorial disorders
- Anomalies identified on ultrasonography

Genetic Disorders

Chromosomal Abnormalities

There are a variety of chromosomal abnormalities, in both number and structure of chromosomes. Some of the most common are listed in Table 3-5.

Trisomy. The incidence of trisomy 21, as well as that of other aneuploidies such as trisomy 18, trisomy 13, and certain sex chromosomal aneuploidies, is known to increase with maternal age (Table 3-6). Trisomy 21 is the most common and clinically significant. These particular chromosomal abnormalities are frequently associated with nondisjunction during maternal meiosis I. Advanced paternal age is not a significant risk for aneuploid offspring but is a risk factor for new autosomal dominant mutations and structural chromosome rearrangements. Prenatal testing should be offered to women who will be 35 years old on the estimated date of delivery.

Antenatal chromosomal studies should be discussed with couples who have had a child with trisomy 21. Risks of up to 1% are appropriate for counseling (unless maternal age alone requires a higher risk assignment). Birth of a previous offspring with a 45,X karyotype does not increase the risk of affected siblings.

The exact recurrence risks after the birth of an infant with a de novo chromosomal abnormality other than trisomy 21 are unknown, but they may be as high as 1%. Thus, antenatal studies should also be offered to such couples. Risks in subsequent pregnancies are also uncertain after a pregnancy ending with a trisomic stillborn infant or trisomic abortus. It would be prudent, however, to assume risks of comparable magnitude and to offer antenatal studies.

Parental Translocation or Inversion. The most common parental chromosomal abnormality is a balanced translocation. Balanced translocations are of two types: Robertsonian translocations and reciprocal translocations. Robertsonian translocations are the result of centromeric fusion of two acrocentric chromosomes (chromosome 13, 14, 15, 21, or 22). A centric fusion of two acrocentric chromosomes results in a single chromosome containing the information that is ordi-

TABLE 3-5. CHROMOSOMAL ABNORMALITIES IN LIVEBORN INFANTS[*]

Type of Abnormality	Births
Numerical aberrations	
Sex chromosomes	
47,XYY	1/1,000 MB[†]
47,XXY	1/1000 MB
Other, males	1/1,350 MB
45,X	1/10,000 FB
47,XXX	1/1,000 FB
Other, females	1/2,700 FB
Autosomes	
Trisomies	
13–15 (D group)	1/20,000 LB
16–18 (E group)	1/8,000 LB
21–22 (G group)	1/800 LB
Other	1/50,000 LB
Structural aberrations	
Balanced	
Robertsonian	
t(Dq;Dq)	1/1,500 LB
t(Dq;Gq)	1/5,000 LB
Reciprocal translocations and insertional inversions	1/7,000 LB
Unbalanced	
Robertsonian	1/14,000 LB
Reciprocal translocations and insertional inversions	1/8,000 LB
Inversions	1/50,000 LB
Deletions	1/10,000 LB
Supernumeraries	1/5,000 LB
Other	1/8,000 LB
Total	1/160 LB

[*] Pooled data were tabulated by Hook EB, Hamerton JL. The frequency of chromosome abnormalities detected in consecutive newborn studies—differences between studies—results by sex and by severity of phenotypic involvement. In: Hook EB, Porter IH, eds. Population cytogenetic studies in humans. San Diego: Academic Press, 1977:63

[†] Abbreviations are as follows: LB, live births; MB, male births; FB, female births.
Gabbe SG, Niebyl JR, Simpson JL, eds. Obstetrics: normal and problem pregnancies. 2nd ed. New York: Churchill Livingstone, 1991:270

TABLE 3-6. CHROMOSOMAL ABNORMALITIES IN LIVEBORNS[*]

Maternal Age	Risk for Down Syndrome	Total Risk for Chromosomal Abnormalities[†]
20	1/1,667	1/526
21	1/1,667	1/526
22	1/1,429	1/500
23	1/1,429	1/500
24	1/1,250	1/476
25	1/1,250	1/476
26	1/1,176	1/476
27	1/1,111	1/455
28	1/1,053	1/435
29	1/1,000	1/417
30	1/952	1/385
31	1/909	1/385
32	1/769	1/322
33	1/602	1/286
34	1/485	1/238
35	1/378	1/192
36	1/289	1/156
37	1/224	1/127
38	1/173	1/102
39	1/136	1/83
40	1/106	1/66
41	1/82	1/53
42	1/63	1/42
43	1/49	1/33
44	1/38	1/26
45	1/30	1/21
46	1/23	1/16
47	1/18	1/13
48	1/14	1/10
49	1/11	1/8

[*] Because sample size for some intervals is relatively small, 95% confidence limits are sometimes relatively large. Nonetheless, these figures are suitable for genetic counseling.

[†] Karyotype 47,XXX was excluded for ages 20–32 (data not available).
Modified from Hook EB, Cross PK, Schreinemachers DM. Chromosomal abnormality rates at amniocentesis and in live-born infants. JAMA 1983; 249:2034–2038. Copyright 1983, American Medical Association; Hook EB. Rates of chromosomal abnormalities at different maternal ages. Modified with permission from the American College of Obstetricians and Gynecologists (Obstetrics and Gynecology, 1981, 58, 282–285)

narily present on two separate chromosomes; thus, the chromosome number is 45, rather than 46. The most common Robertsonian translocation is t(14q;21q). If one parent is a translocation carrier, the risk for having a child with Down syndrome is 10–15% if the translocation is maternal, and the risk is 2% or less if paternal. For other Robertsonian translocations, the risk is usually lower. For the 5% of cases of Down syndrome caused by Robertsonian translocations, about half the translocations will occur de novo (ie, neither parent carries a translocation).

Balanced reciprocal translocations involve an exchange of chromosomal material between two nonhomologous chromosomes, with no loss or gain in the total amount of DNA. Carriers of balanced reciprocal translocations can produce gametes with partial trisomies and monosomies of chromosomal material. Offspring with unbalanced karyotypes occur in approximately 11% of liveborns from all carriers of balanced reciprocal translocations.

Inversions result when two breaks occur within the same chromosome and the intervening segment is inverted prior to repair of the original breaks, with alteration of the gene sequence. In pericentric inversions, the break points occur on opposite sides of the centromere. Balanced carriers may produce unbalanced gametes. The risk for an unbalanced progeny is greater when a pericentric inversion is carried by the mother (8%) than by the father (4%).

Multiple Spontaneous Abortions. Fifty to seventy percent of early spontaneous abortions have chromosomal abnormalities. The most common single chromosomal abnormality is monosomy X, occurring in approximately 10% of cases. Autosomal trisomies, as a group, account for approximately 20–30% of cases. For habitual abortions, if the initial loss is aneuploid, subsequent losses are also likely to be aneuploid, although not necessarily for the same chromosome. A trisomy in one pregnancy may be lethal and may cause a spontaneous abortion, but subsequent pregnancies may result in a chromosomal abnormality compatible with an abnormal liveborn offspring. The birth of an aneuploid liveborn offspring apparently increases the risk in subsequent pregnancies of another aneuploid liveborn offspring. It is not clear whether aneuploidy in a spontaneous abortus increases the risk for future liveborn offspring with aneuploidy. Recurrent spontaneous abortion is an appropriate indication for prenatal diagnosis in subsequent pregnancy, and couples with recurrent abortions who have not had a phenotypically normal liveborn infant have an 8% yield of chromosome abnormalities.

Parental Aneuploidy. A parent with a numeric chromosomal abnormality is at increased risk for aneuploid offspring. Prenatal diagnosis should be offered in such cases. A woman with a karyotype of 47,XX,+21 is fertile, although few reproduce. About 30% of their conceptions would be trisomic. Men with Down syndrome are almost always sterile.

Multifactorial Abnormalities

Most single-organ-system congenital anatomic abnormalities are multifactorial, with an incidence in the general population of approximately 1:1,000. These polygenic/multifactorial traits include the following:

- Hydrocephaly (excepting some forms of aqueductal stenosis and Dandy–Walker syndrome)
- NTDs (anencephaly, spina bifida, encephalocele)
- Cleft lip, with or without cleft palate
- Cleft lip alone
- Cardiac anomalies (most types)
- Diaphragmatic hernia
- Omphalocele
- Renal agenesis (unilateral or bilateral)
- Ureteral anomalies
- Posterior urethral valves
- Hypospadias
- Müllerian fusion defects
- Limb reduction defects
- Talipes equinovarus

The recurrence risk in subsequent pregnancies in most multifactorial disorders is 1–5%, depending on the particular defect. Fetal echocardiography is recommended when a first-degree relative is affected with a congenital cardiac defect. Even though an isolated fetal anatomic defect is most likely multifactorial, it is prudent to consider cytogenetic testing because it is difficult to exclude a chromosomal cause with ultrasonography alone. Multiple fetal anomalies are frequently (5–25%) associated with an abnormal karyotype, whereas IUGR is associated with a 1–2% incidence of chromosomal abnormalities. Although early symmetric IUGR has been classically associated with an abnormal karyotype, asymmetric growth retardation may also occur. More than 90% of fetuses affected with Turner syndrome, triploidy, or trisomy 13 or 18 have ultrasonographically detected fetal anatomic malformations.

Neural tube defects are most commonly multifactorial in origin, with an overall incidence in the United States of 1–2/1,000 live births. Neural tube defects include anencephaly, encephalocele, and spina bifida. Given a proband with an NTD, the likelihood that a first-degree relative will have either anencephaly or spina bifida is 2%, although if the mother is affected the quoted risk is 5%. Maternal serum alpha-fetoprotein testing should be offered to all pregnant women between the gestational ages of 16–18 weeks.

Monogenic (Single-Gene) Disorders

Monogenic (or mendelian) disorders are responsible for phenotypic abnormalities in <1% of all liveborn infants. As of 1992, 5,710 monogenic disorders had been identified, including approximately 2,470 autosomal dominant disorders, 647 autosomal recessive disorders, and 190 X-linked disorders.

It is current practice to screen for certain disorders in selected ethnic groups, such as for sickle cell disease in the African–American population, α-thalassemia in Southeast Asians, β-thalassemia in individuals of Mediterranean extract, and Tay–Sachs and Gaucher diseases in Jewish individuals. Carrier testing and prenatal diagnosis is offered for other monogenic disorders if there is a family history of an affected relative. Common examples include cystic fibrosis, von Willebrand disease, hemophilia A and B, Duchenne/Becker muscular dystrophy, fragile X syndrome, myotonic dystrophy, adult polycystic kidney disease, 21-hydroxylase deficiency, neurofibromatosis, Huntington disease, and phenylketonuria, as well as many other metabolic disorders. In the immediate newborn period, all neonates are screened for phenylketonuria, as well as for galactosemia and congenital hypothyroidism in many states. Neonatal screening is usually limited to those inborn errors of metabolism treatable by dietary or hormonal replacement therapy. The inborn errors of metabolism, which are most commonly autosomal recessive, may be detected by either amniocentesis or CVS. An increasing number of such inborn errors of metabolism and other monogenic disorders are now amenable to diagnosis by either direct or indirect molecular techniques.

Cystic fibrosis is the most common monogenic disorder in the Caucasian population, with a carrier frequency of 1:22. General population screening is not recommended at present. The particular mutation found in approximately 75% of carriers and affected individuals is the ΔF508 mutation. More than 200 different mutations of this gene have been identified. Testing for approximately 10–12 of the more common cystic fibrosis mutations can detect about 85% of the affected alleles.

Techniques

DNA Analysis

Monogenic disorders can be diagnosed by direct molecular techniques when the gene sequence is known. Indirect techniques may be used when the exact defect is unknown or when there are multiple mutations in the gene. A tissue specimen obtained via amniocentesis, CVS, or PUBS may be evaluated in the laboratory by the following methods.

The DNA sample from the specimen is first digested by restriction endonucleases, which cleave the DNA at specific sequences. These thousands of DNA fragments of reproducible lengths are separated by agarose gel electrophoresis. These fragments are blotted to a membrane or filter and allowed to hybridize with a labeled DNA probe. The probe hybridizes with the DNA fragments containing the complementary DNA sequence and reveals a particular autoradiograph.

Polymerase chain reaction allows amplification of a defined DNA segment, even from a single cell, by 10^6–10^7 copies in about 3 hours. Thus, the polymerase chain reaction is a technique that allows minute quantities of DNA to be analyzed easily. This technique has led to the rapid characterization of disease-causing point mutations in a number of genes.

When the precise DNA sequence of a monogenic disorder is known, specific DNA probes are used to differentiate normal genes from mutant genes. Another direct technique is illustrated in the example of sickle cell anemia. In this disease, a single base in the sixth codon of the β-globin gene has undergone a change from adenine to thymine. As a result, valine rather than glutamic acid is incorporated, leading to formation of an abnormal hemoglobin. A specific restriction enzyme recognizes the normal DNA sequence at codon 6 but fails to cleave the mutant sequence. Thus, the pattern of restriction enzyme–digested DNA fragments is altered. Several conditions amenable to detection by direct DNA analysis include α- and β-thalassemia, Duchenne/Becker muscular dystrophy, hemophilia, sickle cell anemia, cystic fibrosis, and the fragile X syndrome.

If the precise DNA mutation of a particular monogenic disorder in a family is unknown, prenatal diagnosis may still be possible by taking advantage of naturally occurring differences in the DNA nucleotide sequence that exist among all individuals. This method is termed "linkage analysis" because the particular gene sequence causing the disorder is unknown, and a closely linked "marker site" is employed as the restriction endonuclease recognition site. When genomic DNA is exposed to restriction endonucleases, a characteristic cleavage pattern, which is reproducible, is obtained and is termed restriction fragment length polymorphism; this pattern is inherited in a mendelian fashion. Therefore, it is possible to obtain specimens from affected and normal family members to compare the restriction fragment length polymorphism patterns. These patterns may be compared with the DNA pattern of the proband and can thereby detect either an affected or unaffected fetus. The marker gene and the gene of interest are said to be "linked" because of their relative close proximity on a chromosome. Because of meiotic crossover, however, 100% accuracy in diagnosis is not obtainable. Restriction fragment length polymorphism analysis may not be informative in a given family.

Maternal Serum Testing

An association between Down syndrome and low MSAFP values was reported in the early 1980s. A detection rate of 45–50% of all Down syndrome fetuses could be achieved by offering prenatal diagnostic testing to all women aged 35 years and older, as well as to all women aged 34 years or younger with a "low" MSAFP value (with the risk assessment of 1:270). Once an abnormally low value is obtained, an ultrasound evaluation should be done to rule out causes of falsely low values such as a blighted ovum, fetal demise, incorrect dates, or a molar pregnancy. Most fetuses with Down syndrome may appear ultrasonographically normal.

Human chorionic gonadotropin has been reported to be significantly higher, and the unconjugated estriol levels significantly lower in pregnancies affected by Down syndrome. This has led to the use of the so-called "triple screen" or "enhanced MSAFP" composed of the MSAFP, hCG, and unconjugated estriol. Each biochemical marker is independently associated with Down syndrome, and in practice, these three markers are combined with maternal age to calculate an individual risk. Several authors have reported results that indicate that the triple screen offers improved sensitivity (60%) and fewer false-positive screens for determination of Down syndrome risk value when compared with MSAFP and maternal age. Women older than age 35 were also included in this protocol, but it is unclear at this time whether it is appropriate to downgrade an "age-related" maternal risk for Down syndrome based on the triple screen.

Low levels of all three biochemical markers may occur in pregnancies affected by trisomy 18, with a sensitivity of up to 60% for trisomy 18. The utility of the triple screen for other aneuploidies is not clear. Although the ultrasonographic stigmata of Down syndrome may be subtle, the ultrasonographic appearances of fetuses with aneuploidies such as trisomy 13 and 18 are often more obvious.

Only about 5% of NTDs occur in families with a previously affected child. Maternal serum alpha-fetoprotein screening is used to identify women with increased risk who do not have a family history. Such screening will detect approximately 80–90% of fetuses with open spina bifida or anencephaly and approximately half of fetuses affected with ventral abdominal defects. The MSAFP value is measured in nanograms and is reported as multiples of the median for the normal population. It is detectable in maternal serum at approximately 10 weeks of gestation and increases until 32 weeks of gestation, after which it plateaus. The concentration of AFP is measured in the amniotic fluid in micrograms and in the fetal blood in milligrams. The amniotic fluid and fetal blood levels increase until approximately 13 weeks of gestation and then both levels rapidly decrease in a parallel fashion through the remainder of pregnancy. Alpha-fetoprotein is a glycoprotein that is first produced in the fetal yolk sac and later in the fetal gastrointestinal tract and liver; it is the major serum protein of the embryo and early fetus. Because of the large discrepancy in AFP concentrations between fetal and maternal blood, the elevated MSAFP values have been shown to be a sensitive indicator of fetal or maternal hemorrhage.

Prior to screening, the couple should be informed of the voluntary nature, limitations, and implications of the test, as well as the need for possible further testing. Patients with an initial elevated MSAFP level can be retested at least 7 days after the initial sample was taken. Approximately 4% of the screened population have serially elevated MSAFP levels and require further evaluation.

A confirmed increase in MSAFP (ie, 2.0–2.5 multiples of the median) indicates increased risk for an NTD or other anomaly. Gestational age, maternal weight, race, and diabetes mellitus affect the interpretation of results. Elevated MSAFP levels are also associated with multifetal gestations, placental abnormalities such as chorioangiomas, fetal demise, oligohydramnios, gastroschisis, omphalocele, bladder exstrophy, sacrococcygeal teratoma, and cystic hygroma. It may also be associated with esophageal or intestinal obstruction, renal anomalies, and congenital nephrosis. After counseling, the patient should be offered a comprehensive evaluation of fetal anatomy by ultrasonography. Amniocentesis for amniotic fluid alpha-fetoprotein (AFAFP) and acetylcholinesterase measurement should also be considered.

Amniocentesis
Amniocentesis for prenatal diagnostic testing is offered between 15 and 18 weeks of gestation. Under ultrasound guidance, a 20–22-gauge spinal needle is passed into the amniotic fluid. An initial aspirate of 1–2 ml of fluid should be discarded to decrease the chance of maternal cell contamination. A total of 20–30 ml of fluid is aspirated, and the needle is removed.

Amniocentesis has greater than 99% cytogenetic diagnostic accuracy and a fetal loss rate of approximately 0.5%. The most common complications have been transient vaginal spotting or amniotic fluid leakage in approximately 1–2% of all cases. The incidence of chorioamnionitis is less than 1:1,000. Needle injuries to the fetus have been reported but are very rare. Culture failure is uncommon.

Amniocentesis with twins is possible in 95% of pregnancies. Amniotic fluid is aspirated from the first sac. Prior to removal of the needle, 2–3 ml of indigo carmine (methylene blue is not recommended) diluted 1:10 in bacteriostatic water is injected into the first sac. Amniocentesis is then performed on the second sac at a location that is selected after visualization of the separating membrane. Aspiration of clear fluid confirms that the second sac has been sampled.

Ninety percent of NTDs are associated with intracranial abnormalities or varying degrees of hydrocephaly. The value of AFAFP with an ultrasound evaluation has become increasingly controversial as ultrasound resolution has improved.

Until more data are available, analysis of AFAFP levels remains a standard method of detection of an NTD. Through AFAFP analysis, a diagnosis of an NTD is possible in all except the 5% of fetuses whose spinal defect is skin covered. The AFAFP level may be spuriously elevated if the amniotic fluid is contaminated with fetal blood. This potential error can be eliminated, however, if amniotic fluid acetylcholinesterase is assayed simultaneously. Its presence verifies that the elevated AFAFP is likely due to an NTD or other fetal defect. If fetal hemoglobin is present but acetylcholinesterase is absent, the elevated AFAFP level can be deduced to result from either the presence of fetal blood or from an anomaly other than an NTD. Failure to detect an anomaly by ultrasonography does not necessarily indicate that the elevated MSAFP was spurious. A subtle anomaly may still exist.

Chorionic Villus Sampling
Indications for CVS are essentially the same as for amniocentesis, except for analyses that require amniotic fluid rather than amniotic fluid cells. The primary advantage of CVS is that results are available much earlier in pregnancy. This allows for earlier, safer methods of pregnancy termination in cases with abnormal results and decreased parental anxiety. Earlier diagnosis may also be required for prenatal treatment (eg, prevention of female virilization in fetuses affected with 21-hydroxylase deficiency by administration of dexamethasone to the mother). Chorionic villus sampling is generally performed at 9–12 weeks of gestation. Prior to CVS, fetal viability and gestational age should be confirmed by ultrasonography.

There are three ways by which placental villi may be obtained: transcervical, transabdominal, and, less commonly, transvaginal access routes to the placenta are possible. Contraindications to transcervical CVS include active infections (eg, genital herpes, gonorrhea, chronic cervicitis, and cervical abnormalities). Later in pregnancy, when a fetal malformation or IUGR is associated with severe oligohydramnios, transabdominal CVS is an alternative method of invasive sampling.

There have been three major collaborative studies comparing CVS and amniocentesis. The National Institute of Child Health and Human Development and Canadian trials reveal similar results, with more than 99% cytogenetic analysis success and total pregnancy loss rates of 0.6–0.8% in excess of amniocentesis. A European study reported an excess loss rate in the CVS group that was different both clinically and statistically from the results of the other two large collaborative studies. This study included a large number of centers with varied levels of experience. Although the absolute pregnancy loss rates are similar for CVS and amniocentesis, patients considering CVS are counseled that there is probably a slightly higher risk of pregnancy loss from CVS than from amniocentesis, especially from the transcervical approach.

Prenatal cytogenetic diagnosis is occasionally complicated by the finding of more than one distinct cell line obtained from a single sample. When this occurs, it may be the result of fetal karyotypic mosaicism, confined placental mosaicism, or pseudomosaicism. Fetal mosaicism represents two distinct cytogenetic cell lines in the fetus. Confined placental mosaicism is defined as two cell lines that occur only in the placenta and not the fetus. Pseudomosaicism represents two or more cell lines that have arisen in cell culture but are not representative of the fetus or placenta. Most cases of true mosaicism are actually confined to the placenta. However, all mosaic findings should be analyzed by other methods of invasive prenatal diagnostic testing at a later point in pregnancy (eg, amniocentesis or PUBS). Some cytogenetic laboratories perform both direct and cultured cell karyotype analyses on villus samples. Cytotrophoblasts may be stained and analyzed directly within 24–48 hours. This method is associated with a higher incidence of apparent mosaicism; results must be considered preliminary, pending culture preparation, which can be analyzed in 7–10 days. Other centers offer only the cultured method because of the problem with mosaicism in direct preparations. Maternal cell contamination may also complicate analysis of CVS specimens.

Poor pregnancy outcome and perinatal loss have been reported in association with confined placental mosaicism. The utility and method of antepartum testing in such cases have not been established.

There have been reports of an association between CVS and limb reduction and oromandibular defects. Cavernous hemangiomas have also been reported. The risk for these anomalies is unclear. According to the World Health Organization, the global 10-year experience with CVS reveals an incidence of limb reduction defects of 6/10,000—not significantly different from that in the general population. A National Institute of Child Health and Human Development workshop on CVS and limb reduction defects concluded that the frequency of oromandibular–limb hypogenesis appeared to be more common after CVS, especially for CVS performed before 9 menstrual weeks. Women considering CVS should be informed of the present concerns about the possible association of CVS with limb and other defects.

Percutaneous Umbilical Cord Blood Sampling

Percutaneous umbilical cord blood sampling, also known as cordocentesis, in which the umbilical cord is punctured and blood is withdrawn under ultrasound guidance, was introduced in the early 1980s for the management of fetal isoimmunization. It has also been used to obtain fetal blood cells for prenatal diagnosis when a rapid diagnosis is important. The PUBS technique has also been performed when a fetal malformation or severe IUGR is detected later in pregnancy. A procedure-related pregnancy loss rate of 1% has been reported. This sample may be sent for cytogenetic analysis, metabolic and hematologic studies, acid–base analysis, viral cultures, and immunologic studies.

Fetoscopic Tissue Sampling

A condition not diagnosable by conventional modes of invasive prenatal diagnostic testing may be detected by fetal tissue sampling, either by fetoscopy with its rather high (1–3%) procedure-related pregnancy loss rate, or by ultrasound guidance. Fetal skin sampling for the diagnosis of epidermolysis bullosa and congenital ichthyosis and fetal liver biopsy to detect certain hepatic enzyme deficiencies have been described.

New Horizons

One disadvantage of amniocentesis is the need to culture cells for several days before karyotype analysis. Fluorescent in situ hybridization for the rapid detection of chromosomal aneuploidies in uncultured amniocytes has been reported. This method uses fluorescently tagged specific DNA probes to chromosomes 13, 18, 21, X, and Y. It can rapidly detect the ploidy status for these particular chromosomes. This method may not detect mosaicism and will not detect other structural chromosomal abnormalities or rare aneuploidies in other chromosomes. The method is investigational and is used only as an adjunct to the definitive cultured cytogenetic analysis. The proposed benefit of fluorescent in situ hybridization is rapid availability of preliminary results.

Experience with preimplantation diagnosis (embryo biopsy) has been reported. In a case of in vitro fertilization, a blastomere biopsy (at the eight-cell stage) was performed, with intrauterine transfer of the embryo and birth of a normal neonate. The benefits of preimplantation diagnosis are obvious.

Trisomy 21 has been diagnosed in fetal cells from maternal blood during the first trimester. Fetal cell sorting techniques may one day be developed, for example, for the diagnosis of fetal aneuploidy, by using methods such as fluorescent in situ hybridization.

TERATOGENIC AGENTS

Major congenital anomalies are observed in 2–3% of all births. Maternal exposure to drugs or environmental chemicals may be responsible for 4–6% of these anomalies, or approximately 1/400 liveborn infants.

Whether or not birth defects occur in a conceptus exposed to a potentially teratogenic agent depends in part on the genetic makeup of the conceptus and the mother. Substantial evidence suggests that the most important variable is difference in the genetically determined activity of the enzymes involved in the metabolism of drugs and chemicals. This difference is termed pharmacogenetic variation.

The stage of the organism's development is a key factor in susceptibility to a potential teratogen. Exposure to a teratogenic agent during organogenesis may result in a defect involving an organ. Conversely, exposure to such an agent during histogenesis may produce finer structural defects within the organ system. The teratogenic agent may reach the developing embryo or fetus either by direct passage through maternal tissues (eg, ionizing radiation) or by placental transfer (eg, drugs, or chemicals).

Drugs and Chemicals

Several drugs commonly used during pregnancy, such as aspirin, acetaminophen, metronidazole, caffeine, or phenothiazines, are not associated with an increased risk of congenital anomalies. However, based on anecdotal evidence, maternal hyperthermia seems to be associated with congenital anomalies when the fever persists for a protracted period of time (at least 24 hours) and is high (at least 101°F). Numerous other agents have been implicated as teratogens, including chemotherapeutic agents, which are discussed in the Oncology section.

Hormonal Agents
Androgenic hormone agents such as danazol may produce clitoral enlargement or labioscrotal fusion in the female fetus when they are given before 13 weeks of gestation. Recent studies have failed to demonstrate a significant relationship between congenital anomalies and first-trimester use of oral contraceptive agents or medroxyprogesterone acetate. In 1990, the FDA mandated a change in package labeling to reflect this.

Anticoagulants
The use of warfarin and other coumarin anticoagulants that inhibit the synthesis of vitamin K–dependent coagulation factors can produce major and minor congenital anomalies in up to 25% of fetuses exposed during the first trimester. The characteristic abnormalities include a hypoplastic nose, epiphyseal stippling, optic atrophy, microcephaly, IUGR, and other central nervous system anomalies.

Antithyroid Drugs
Medications such as propylthiouracil, methimazole, and iodide cross the placenta and may occasionally produce fetal hypothyroidism and goiter. Infants exposed to methimazole in utero may also demonstrate scalp defects, although this association is rare.

Anticonvulsants
Diphenylhydantoin may produce a syndrome characterized by abnormal facies, microcephaly, growth deficiency, mental retardation, and hypoplastic nails and distal phalanges in up to 10% of exposed offspring. As many as 30% of newborns may demonstrate some manifestations of the syndrome, however. Mild to moderate mental retardation is observed in two thirds of children who have the most severe physical stigmata. Intrauterine exposure to diphenylhydantoin is also associated with a threefold to fourfold increase in the incidence of cleft lip or cleft palate and congenital heart disease. The syndrome was recently linked to lowered maternal epoxide hydrolase activity, an enzyme involved in the metabolism of hydantoin.

In 1991 the FDA published an aggregate of data regarding carbamazepine exposure during early pregnancy and concluded that exposure to the drug during embryogenesis poses approximately a 1% risk of spina bifida to exposed fetuses. A syndrome has been proposed but has yet to be proven.

Trimethadione and paramethadione have been associated with abnormalities similar to those observed with hydantoin. The risk for defects or spontaneous abortion is 60–80% with first-trimester exposure. A syndrome including V-shaped eyebrows, low-set ears, high arched palate, and irregular dentition has been identified.

Valproic acid, when administered during the first trimester, may produce NTDs in 1–2% of exposed fetuses. A fetal valproate syndrome has also been described.

Lithium
Lithium may produce malformations in 5–10% of offspring exposed prenatally. The anomalies frequently involve the heart and great vessels, with Ebstein anomaly of the tricuspid valve being observed most frequently. Exposure late in pregnancy may produce transplacental lithium intoxication with neonatal cyanosis, hypotonia, bradycardia, goiter with hypothyroidism, diabetes insipidus, and polyhydramnios. Additionally, maternal diuresis warrants dose adjustment to avoid lithium toxicity.

Diethylstilbestrol
The synthetic estrogen diethylstilbestrol produces structural defects of the genital tract, as well as reproductive problems in prenatally exposed females. Vaginal adenosis has been detected in more than 50% of women whose mothers took this drug before the ninth week of pregnancy. A small percentage of women exposed in utero may develop clear cell adenocarcinoma of the vagina. A variety of abnormalities of the genitourinary tract have also been observed in up to 25% of males exposed in utero.

Vitamin A and Its Congeners

Isotretinoin. The vitamin A isomer isotretinoin is a potent teratogen, with serious congenital anomalies reported among approximately 35% of exposures. The specific congenital anomalies observed after oral administration of isotretinoin during early pregnancy include heart disease, thymic agenesis, microphthalmia, hydrocephalus, microtia, cleft palate, deafness and blindness, and an increased risk of spontaneous abortion.

Tretinoin. Topical tretinoin does not result in an increased risk of congenital anomalies, because skin metabolizes the drug and no detectable systemic concentrations result.

Etretinate. Etretinate is an oral agent used to treat psoriasis. Case reports link the use of this agent to birth defects similar to those observed after the use of isotretinoin during pregnancy. Unlike vitamin A and its congeners, etretinate has been detected in serum of patients at therapeutic levels for as long as 2 years after cessation of use. Infants with congenital anomalies similar to those observed with isotretinoin use have been observed when the mothers had ceased use of etretinate up to 18 months before conception.

High-Dose Vitamin A. The CDC recently evaluated the use of vitamin A during pregnancy. The recommended daily allowance of vitamin A during pregnancy is 5,000–10,000 IU. It was stated that 25,000 IU or more of this nutrient may be dangerous and that 40,000 IU or more daily during pregnancy may constitute a significant risk of congenital anomalies (eg, renal, craniofacial). This is of particular concern, because some nutritional supplements contain 50,000 IU or more in a single dose.

Occupational and Environmental Agents

A number of agents to which pregnant women may be exposed have been associated with a variety of poor reproductive outcomes, including spontaneous abortion, low birth weight, neurologic abnormalities, and congenital anomalies. These chemicals include methyl mercury, lead, polychlorinated biphenyls, polybrominated biphenyls, and organic solvents. Verified human teratogens in this class of agents include methyl mercury and organic solvents. Lead is associated with growth retardation and myelination defects but not gross congenital anomalies. Polychlorinated biphenyls and polybrominated biphenyls are associated with skin discoloration and stillbirth.

Ionizing Radiation

Embryonic or fetal radiation exposure usually results from diagnostic radiologic studies. Diagnostic radiation usually exposes the conceptus to less than 5 cGy, depending on the number of radiographs done and the maternal site examined. For example, fetal exposure from a maternal chest X-ray is 0.008 cGy. The radiation exposure associated with an upper chest or small intestinal series is approximately 0.5 cGy; that from an intravenous pyelogram is 0.4 cGy. These exposures may pose minimal increase in the risk of childhood leukemia, but the risk to the fetus is not believed to be serious until the absorbed dose is more than 10 cGy. A fertile woman who is exposed to ionizing radiation during her work should be protected by a lead apron to ensure that, should she become pregnant, her conceptus would not experience more than 0.5 cGy. Any woman who is considering pregnancy and who was exposed to irradiation on the job may wish to have her film badge evaluated more frequently to monitor radiation exposure, and she should wear a badge over the pelvic area for a more precise estimate of fetal exposure.

Therapeutic (thyrotoxic) radioisotope (^{131}I) exposure is considerably more hazardous to the fetus than diagnostic studies that use ^{125}I. The conceptus' thyroid is not susceptible to radioisotope damage prior to 9–11 weeks of gestation. Calculations of dosimetry should be made by experienced professionals, and risks may then be estimated based on isotope and biologic half-lives of the specific agents used. Generally, the use of radioisotopes should be avoided during pregnancy. The risks associated with radioisotope exposure include microcephaly, fetal growth retardation, goiter, and hypothyroidism. Postnatally, the major risk is for mental retardation and physical growth stunting.

Social and Illicit Drugs

Alcohol

Excessive maternal alcohol ingestion during pregnancy may result in a specific pattern of congenital anomalies referred to as the fetal alcohol syndrome. Major features of fetal alcohol syndrome include prenatal or postnatal growth retardation, characteristic facial anomalies (ie, short palpebral fissures, microphthalmia, indistinct/absent philtrum, thin upper lip, midfacial hypoplasia), microcephaly, joint contractures, and cardiac defects. Fetal alcohol syndrome is associated postnatally with mental retardation, hyperactivity, and developmental delays. Alcohol abuse during pregnancy is a leading cause of mental retardation. Maternal alcohol abuse is also associated with an increased risk of spontaneous abortion.

It is difficult to correlate the amount of alcohol consumed to the risk of fetal alcohol syndrome. Women who have eight or more drinks per day are at significant risk (perhaps 60% or higher) for giving birth to an infant with fetal alcohol syndrome. The American Medical Association has stated that any woman who consumes four or more alcoholic drinks per day during pregnancy is significantly endangering the health of her unborn child. One beer, one shot of liquor, one mixed drink, and one glass of wine all contain the same amount of alcohol, approximately ½ oz of absolute alcohol. Thus, all forms of alcohol are equally hazardous. Among pregnant women who consume four or more drinks per day during pregnancy, the risk for fetal alcohol syndrome may be approximately 20%, with risks increasing to about 30% with five drinks per day, and 40% with six drinks per day. The risk associated with binge drinking is unknown but likely to be substantial. No quantifiable risk has been associated with an occasional alcoholic beverage during pregnancy, but the only prudent medical advice is for pregnant women to avoid alcohol consumption completely.

Cigarette Smoking

Cigarette smoking poses a threat to reproductive function and pregnancy outcome in women. The prevalence of smoking among adults has decreased from approximately 40% in 1965 to 10–15% in 1990, with a similar decrease among women of reproductive age.

The pregnant smoker may be at increased risk for the spontaneous abortion of an otherwise normal fetus, fetal death associated with placental abruption or placenta previa, preterm delivery, and PROM. A dose–response relationship has been shown between the amount of maternal smoking and reduced birth weight. The offspring of women who smoke approximately 20 cigarettes (one pack) per day during pregnancy have birth weights that are approximately 200 g less than those of infants born to women who do not smoke. If a woman stops smoking during the last 4 months of pregnancy, the risk of delivering a baby with lowered birth weight is similar to that of a nonsmoker. The use of smokeless tobacco also increases blood levels of nicotine comparable to those associated with cigarette smoking and, based on limited data, may result in similarly decreased birth weight. The possible clinical effects of passive smoking during pregnancy have not been clearly established.

Marijuana

Marijuana, the most frequently used illicit drug, has been associated with poor perinatal outcome in some studies but not in others. It is particularly difficult to identify the effects of a single illicit drug on perinatal outcome because the life style associated with the use of any illicit drug usually includes tobacco use, alcohol consumption, and use of other psychoactive drugs.

Cocaine

Cocaine (street names "coke," "snow," "lady," and "gold dust") use is a major public health concern. Although use of cocaine in the 1970s was primarily limited to the intranasal route, a recent decrease in the street cost and availability of cocaine and an increasing prevalence of intravenous and smoked ("free-base" or "crack") routes of use have increased the prevalence of its use and the potential for medical complications. Cocaine is commonly used intranasally ("snorting"), by injection, and by smoking the free alkaloid form (crack). Crack, so named because of the cracking or popping sound that is made when the crystals are ignited in a pipe while smoking the drug, is a highly purified form of the free alkaloid. In a survey of a number of urban hospitals nationwide, positive urine toxicology for cocaine metabolites was detected among 10–48% of pregnant women. It is thought that the crack form of cocaine is more addictive than other forms. Administered systemically, cocaine blocks the presynaptic reuptake of neurotransmitters (norepinephrine and dopamine), causing these neurotransmitters to accumulate at postsynaptic receptor sites, resulting in intense vasoconstriction, acute arterial hypertension, and tachycardia.

The drug is metabolized primarily by plasma and hepatic cholinesterases to water-soluble metabolites (benzoylecgonine and ecgonine methylester). The most commonly used urine test detects benzoylecgonine at a sensitivity of 300 ng/ml. The elimination half-time of the parent drug is approximately 4–5 hours. Cocaine metabolites can be detected in urine for 24–48 hours. Pharmacokinetics of perinatal cocaine use are poorly studied, but cocaine is known to cross the placenta readily. It is thought that urine tests in neonates exposed to cocaine in utero may be positive for a similar period of time as in an adult, although benzoylecgonine has been detected in neonatal urine for up to 4 days.

Potentially lethal medical complications associated with cocaine use, directly or indirectly, seem attributable to the intense sympathomimetic effects of the drug. They include acute myocardial infarction, cardiac arrhythmias, rupture of the ascending aorta, cerebrovascular accidents, seizures, bowel ischemia, and hyperthermia.

Use or abuse of cocaine during pregnancy is a major risk factor for the mother and her unborn child. Most pregnant cocaine users are patients with unplanned pregnancies of uncertain gestational age who seek prenatal care late (if at all), have poor nutrition, and are likely to be heavy cigarette smokers. They also tend to be polydrug abusers. It seems clear that there is minimally a risk of 25% for preterm birth and 20% for small-for-gestational-age infants, but studies are confounded by these and other factors mentioned above. Studies have indicated as much as a 10-fold increase in the risk of abruption, suggesting an increase from 0.1% among all pregnancies to a 1% risk among cocaine-exposed pregnancies. Neurobehavioral abnormalities in neonates exposed to cocaine in utero have been well documented, especially the tendency for hyperirritability and a low threshold for overstimulation. A purported increased incidence of sudden infant death syndrome among cocaine-exposed infants has not been confirmed by subsequent investigations. An increased frequency of certain congenital anomalies among cocaine-exposed neonates has been reported by numerous investigators. These include congenital heart disease, intestinal atresias, cerebral infarction, brain cavitation defects, and genitourinary anomalies.

It is hypothesized that the increased risk of congenital anomalies among cocaine-exposed infants focuses upon cocaine-induced vasoconstriction that may cause infarction, severe hypoxemia, and hypoperfusion that may interrupt normal morphogenesis. A pattern of anomalies termed the "vascular disruption syndrome" has been described. The mechanism of vascular disruption is supported by animal studies that showed dose-dependent decreases in uterine blood flow and marked fetal hypoxemia, hypertension, hypoperfusion, and tachycardia in experimental animals that were administered cocaine IV.

Clinical evaluation of obstetric patients should incorporate the following protocol, which the clinician should consider for both medical and legal reasons:

1. All pregnant women should be asked about previous and current drug use at the time of the first prenatal visit.

2. The life-threatening implications of cocaine use during pregnancy for herself and for her infant should be clearly explained to the gravida admitting to cocaine use. She should be offered support services to aid in her abstinence.

3. Continued abstinence from the use of cocaine should be reinforced and encouraged. Periodic urine testing for metabolites of cocaine is one manner to discourage relapse in a pregnant woman admitting to cocaine use prior to or during pregnancy. The requirement for consent may vary from state to state.

4. Urine testing of the mother, the neonate, or both may be useful in some clinical situations, such as unexplained fetal growth retardation, unexpected prematurity, or abruption in a woman not known to have hypertensive disease, even when cocaine abuse has not been previously suspected.

Other Illicit Drugs

Maternal use of heroin, methadone, and phencyclidine may produce a neonatal withdrawal syndrome characterized by increased muscle tone, tremors, and a high-pitched cry. The teratogenicity of lysergic acid diethylamide has been suggested, but no conclusive evidence exists at present. Importantly, lysergide analogues, even those medically prescribed, may precipitate early labor.

BIBLIOGRAPHY

Routine Care

American Academy of Pediatrics, American College of Obstetricians and Gynecologists. Guidelines for perinatal care. 3rd ed. Elk Grove Village, Illinois: AAP; Washington, DC: ACOG, 1992

Institute of Medicine, Subcommittee of Nutritional Status and Weight Gain during Pregnancy. Nutrition during pregnancy. Washington, DC: National Academy Press, 1990

Ultrasonography

American College of Obstetricians and Gynecologists. Ultrasonography in pregnancy. ACOG Technical Bulletin 187. Washington, DC: ACOG, 1993

American Institute of Ultrasound in Medicine. Bioeffects and safety of diagnostic ultrasound. Rockville, Maryland: AIUM, 1993

Divon MY, ed. Abnormal fetal growth. New York: Elsevier, 1991

Ewigman BG, Crane JP, Frigoletto FD, LeFevre ML, Bain RP, McNellis D. Effect of prenatal ultrasound screening on perinatal outcome: RADIUS study group. N Engl J Med 1993;329:821–827

Lynch L, Berkowitz RL: Amniocentesis, skin biopsy, and umbilical cord blood sampling in the prenatal diagnosis of genetic diseases. In: Reece EA, Hobbins JC, Mahoney MJ, Petrie RH, eds. Medicine of the fetus and mother. Philadelphia: JB Lippincott, 1992:641–652

Moore TR, Cayle JE. The amniotic fluid index in normal human pregnancy. Am J Obstet Gynecol 1990;162:1168–1173

U.S. Department of Health and Human Services, Public Health Service, National Institutes of Health. Diagnostic ultrasound imaging in pregnancy. Washington, DC: U.S. Government Printing Office, 1984; NIH publication no. 84-667

Antepartum Testing

Druzin ML. Antepartum fetal heart rate monitoring: state of the art. Clin Perinatol 1989;16:627–642

Druzin ML, Fox A, Kogut E, Carlson C. The relationship of the nonstress test to gestational age. Am J Obstet Gynecol 1985;153:386–389

Rutherford SE, Phelan JP, Smith CV, Jacobs N. The four-quadrant assessment of amniotic fluid volume: an adjunct to antepartum fetal heart rate testing. Obstet Gynecol 1987;70:353–356

Smith CV, Phelan JP, Platt LD, Broussard P, Paul RH. Fetal acoustic stimulation testing, II: a randomized clinical comparison with the nonstress test. Am J Obstet Gynecol 1986;155:131–134

Fetal Therapy

Bussel JB, Berkowitz RL, McFarland JG, Lynch L, Chitkara V. Antenatal treatment of neonatal alloimmune thrombocytopenia. N Engl J Med 1988;319:1374–1378

Evans MI, Chrousos GP, Mann DW, Larsen JW Jr, Green I, McCluskey J, et al. Pharmacologic suppression of the fetal adrenal gland in utero: attempted prevention of abnormal external genital masculinization in suspected congenital adrenal hyperplasia. JAMA 1985;253:1015–1020

Harrison MR, Golbus MS, Filly RA, eds. The unborn patient, prenatal diagnosis and treatment. 2nd ed. Philadelphia: WB Saunders, 1991

Kleinman CS, Copel JA. Fetal cardiac arrhythmias: diagnosis and therapy. In: Creasy RK, Resnik R, eds. Maternal-fetal medicine: principles and practice. 3rd ed. Philadelphia: WB Saunders, 1994

Prenatal Diagnosis of Genetic Disorders

American College of Obstetricians and Gynecologists. Antenatal diagnosis of genetic disorders. ACOG Technical Bulletin 108. Washington, DC: ACOG, 1987

American College of Obstetricians and Gynecologists. Alpha-fetoprotein. ACOG Technical Bulletin 154. Washington, DC: ACOG, 1991

American College of Obstetricians and Gynecologists. Folic acid for prevention of recurrent neural tube defects. ACOG Committee Opinion 120. Washington, DC: ACOG, 1993

American College of Obstetricians and Gynecologists. Ultrasonography in pregnancy. ACOG Technical Bulletin 187. Washington, DC: ACOG, 1993

American College of Obstetricians and Gynecologists. Down syndrome screening. ACOG Committee Opinion 141. Washington, DC: ACOG, 1994

Cunningham FG, MacDonald PC, Gant NF, Leveno KJ, Gilstrap LC III. Genetics. In: Williams obstetrics. 19th ed. Norwalk, Connecticut: Appleton and Lange, 1993:919–938

Cunningham FG, MacDonald PC, Gant NF, Leveno KJ, Gilstrap LC III. Prenatal diagnosis and invasive techniques to monitor the fetus. In: Williams obstetrics. 19th ed. Norwalk, Connecticut: Appleton and Lange, 1993:939–957

Haddow JE, Palomaki GE, Knight GJ, Williams J, Pulkinnen A, Canick JA, et al. Prenatal screening for Down's syndrome with the use of maternal serum markers. N Engl J Med 1992;327:588–593

Handyside AH, Lesko JG, Tarin JJ, Winston RM, Hughes MR. Birth of a normal girl after in vitro fertilization and preimplantation diagnostic testing for cystic fibrosis. N Engl J Med 1992;327:905–909

Kuliev AM, Modell B, Jackson L, Simpson JL, Brambati B, Rhoads G, et al. Risk evaluation of CVS. Prenat Diagn 1993;13:197–209

Report of National Institute of Child Health and Human Development Workshop on Chorionic Villus Sampling and Limb and Other Defects, October 20, 1992. Am J Obstet Gynecol 1993;169:1–6

Simpson JL. Genetic counseling and prenatal diagnosis. In: Gabbe SG, Niebyl JR, Simpson JL, eds. Obstetrics: normal and problem pregnancies. 2nd ed. New York: Churchill Livingstone, 1991:269–298

Simpson JL, Carson SA. Preimplantation genetic diagnosis. N Engl J Med 1992;327:951–953

Simpson JL, Elias S. Prenatal diagnosis of genetic disorders. In: Creasy RK, Resnick R, eds. Maternal-fetal medicine: principles and practice. 3rd ed. Philadelphia: WB Saunders, 1994:61–88

Smidt-Jensen S, Permin M, Philip J, Lundsteen C, Zachary JM, Fowler SE, et al. Randomized comparison of amniocentesis and transabdominal and transcervical chorionic villus sampling. Lancet 1992;340:1237–1244

Ward BE, Gersen SL, Carelli MP, McGuire NM, Dackowski WR, Weinstein M, et al. Rapid prenatal diagnosis of chromosomal aneuploidies by fluorescence in situ hybridization: clinical experience with 4,500 specimens. Am J Hum Genet 1993;52:854–865

Teratogenic Agents

Buehler BA, Delimont D, van Waes M, Finell RH. Prenatal prediction of risk of the fetal hydantoin syndrome. N Engl J Med 1990;322:1567–1572

Gilstrap LC, Little BB. Drugs and pregnancy. New York: Elsevier, 1992

McDonald AD, Cherry NM, Delorme C, McDonald JC. Visual display units and pregnancy: evidence from the Montreal survey. J Occup Med 1986;8:1226–1231

McDonald AD, McDonald JC, Armstrong B, Cherry N, Nolin AD, Robert D. Work with visual display units in pregnancy. Br J Ind Med 1988;45:509–515

McDonald JC, Lavoie J, Cote R, McDonald AD. Chemical exposures at work in early pregnancy and congenital defect: a case-referent study. Br J Ind Med 1987;44:527–533

Needleman HL, Rabinowitz M, Leviton A, Linn S, Schoenbaum S. The relationship between prenatal exposure to lead and congenital anomalies. JAMA 1981;251:295–296

Rosa FW. Spina bifida in infants of women treated with carbamazepine during pregnancy. N Engl J Med 1991;324:674–677

Schardein JL. Chemically induced birth defects. 2nd ed. New York: Marcel Dekker, 1993

Schnorr TM, Grajewski BA, Hornung RW, Thun MJ, Egeland GM, Murray WE, et al. Video display terminals and the risk of spontaneous abortion. N Engl J Med 1991;324:727–733

Scialli AR. Fetal protection policies in the United States. Semin Perinatol 1993;17:50–57

Slutsker L. Risks associated with cocaine use during pregnancy. Obstet Gynecol 1992;79:778–789

Physiology of Pregancy

FETAL ACID–BASE BALANCE

The fetus forms two groups of acids—carbonic and noncarbonic—through the body's metabolic processes. Carbonic acid (H_2CO_3) is formed by the hydration of carbon dioxide (CO_2) during oxidative metabolism. Carbon dioxide rapidly diffuses across the placenta. Several noncarbonic (metabolic and fixed) acids, including lactate and hydroxybutyrate, are products of anaerobic glycolysis. These acids diffuse across the placenta much more slowly than does CO_2. Thus, metabolic acidosis takes longer to correct than does respiratory acidosis. The pH of blood or tissue is directly related to the bicarbonate buffer level and is inversely related to CO_2 levels, as is shown in the simplified equation below:

$$pH = \frac{([HCO_3] \text{ metabolic component})}{([CO_2] \text{ respiratory component})}$$

Conditions that interrupt normal blood flow to the fetus from the placenta, such as umbilical cord occlusion, may cause a rapid rise in CO_2, resulting in respiratory acidosis. Since CO_2 diffuses very quickly, respiratory acidosis is rapidly corrected once the occlusion is released. If reduced fetal perfusion persists, resulting in fetal hypoxia, the products of anaerobic metabolism, the organic acids, accumulate.

The two most important buffers in fetal blood that allow for a relatively constant pH are bicarbonate and hemoglobin. They account for approximately 70% of the total buffers in blood. Other buffers include erythrocyte bicarbonate, plasma proteins, and inorganic phosphate. The terms *base deficit* and *base excess* refer to the amount of buffer below or above normal levels.

Types of Acidemia

Fetal acidosis can be classified as respiratory, metabolic, or mixed (Table 3-7). The partial pressure of CO_2 (P_{CO_2}) is high and the base deficit is normal in respiratory acidosis. The P_{CO_2} is normal and the base deficit is increased in metabolic acidosis. In mixed acidosis, both the P_{CO_2} and the base deficit are increased. It is important to note that the maternal acid–base status may influence the acid–base status measured in fetal blood.

TABLE 3-7. CLASSIFICATION OF FETAL OR NEWBORN ACIDEMIA

Acidemia Type	P_{CO_2}	HCO_3	Base Deficit
Respiratory	High	Normal	Normal
Metabolic	Normal	Low	High
Mixed	High	Low	High

Umbilical Cord Blood Acid–Base Determinations

Umbilical cord blood acid–base analysis provides an objective method of assessing newborn conditions and is a useful adjunct to the Apgar score. It is also useful to assess retrospectively various aspects of intrapartum management. Moreover, newborn metabolic or mixed acidemia is an important component in the definition of birth asphyxia. In this context, normal umbilical cord blood gas and pH values usually eliminate the diagnosis of severe birth asphyxia, at least to a degree associated with subsequent neurologic damage.

Sample Collection

The collection of samples from the umbilical cord vessels for blood gas and pH analysis is relatively simple. Although it is not necessary to process the specimens immediately, it is of paramount importance to clamp the cord as soon after delivery as possible, as the arterial pH may change significantly by 60 seconds after birth. After clamping, blood is drawn into a 1–2-ml plastic or glass syringe that has been flushed with heparin (1,000 U/ml). Too much heparin or larger concentrations may affect the accuracy of the results.

Umbilical arterial blood best reflects the fetal condition, whereas venous blood reflects uteroplacental circulation. Moreover, it is possible to have a very low umbilical artery pH in a severely asphyxiated fetus secondary to a cord prolapse and have a relatively normal umbilical vein pH. In difficult cases such as the very premature infant, an arterial sample from the chorionic surface of the placenta (the artery crosses over the vein) will provide accurate results.

Specimens are relatively stable for 30–60 minutes at room temperature. It is important to cap the syringe immediately after obtaining the sample to avoid air contamination. The values for pH, P_{CO_2}, HCO_3, and base excess provide the most useful clinical information. The partial O_2 (P_{O_2}) value is of little, if any, clinical use.

Umbilical Cord Values

The mean "normal" values for umbilical cord pH and blood gases for term infants are summarized in Table 3-8. Umbilical artery pH and gas determinations are especially useful in the premature infant who may have low Apgar scores based solely on immaturity. The mean normal umbilical artery values for premature infants are similar to those for term infants (Table 3-9).

Although newborn acidemia has been classically defined as an umbilical artery pH of less than 7.2, it is now evident that this level is arbitrarily high. The umbilical artery level below which major neurologic morbidity occurs would appear to be closer to 7.00, and this is the cutoff currently recommended as one of the criteria necessary for defining birth asphyxia or hypoxia to a degree that might be associated with subsequent neurologic dysfunction. Interestingly, as many as two thirds of term infants with an umbilical artery pH of less than 7.00 will be admitted to the normal nursery with no apparent morbidity.

Fetal Scalp Blood Sampling

Fetal scalp blood sampling allows for determination of fetal acid–base status during labor. A specimen for acid–base determination is obtained via scalp puncture (2-ml blade); thus the cervix must be sufficiently dilated (≥ 2.5 cm). A long, heparinized, capillary tube is held with the tip just in contact with the blood as it beads from the puncture. The blood collects in the tube by capillary action. Values above 7.25 are considered normal and should be repeated as indicated by the FHR pattern and progress of labor. Values between 7.20 and 7.25 are considered to be suggestive or borderline. Results in this range must also be interpreted in light of the FHR pattern and the progress of labor and should be repeated in 15–30 minutes to detect the possibility of a downward trend in pH. A scalp blood pH of less than 7.20 is considered abnormal and is generally an indication for some type of medical or surgical intervention.

AMNIOTIC FLUID DYNAMICS

Amniotic fluid serves several functions, paramount of which is to provide a "cushion" for the fetus against trauma. Moreover, it probably plays a significant role in maintaining a stable temperature.

The production of amniotic fluid begins very early in gestation, averaging about 50 ml by the end of the first trimester and increasing to approximately 400 ml by 20 weeks of gestation. Amniotic fluid continues to increase until 36–38 weeks of gestation, when it reaches a peak volume of approximately 1,000 ml. Thereafter, it decreases and may be scant by 40 weeks and beyond. The exact mechanism for the production of amniotic fluid has not been elucidated, but it is generally accepted that in early pregnancy it is primarily produced by the amniotic membrane. During this stage of pregnancy, amniotic fluid appears to be formed as a simple ultrafiltrate of fetal plasma and has a similar osmolality. In the second half of pregnancy, the amniotic fluid osmolality decreases. Current evidence suggests that this decrease is due to the presence in

TABLE 3-9. NORMAL MEAN UMBILICAL ARTERY BLOOD pH AND BLOOD GAS VALUES IN PREMATURE INFANTS

Measurement	Ramin et al (1989) (n = 77)	Riley and Johnson (1993) (n = 1,015)
pH	7.29	7.28
P_{CO_2} (mm Hg)	49.2	50.2
HCO_3 (mEq/L)	23.0	22.4
Base excess (mmol/L)	−3.3	−2.5

TABLE 3-8. NORMAL MEAN UMBILICAL CORD BLOOD pH AND BLOOD GAS VALUES IN TERM NEWBORNS

Measurement	Yeomans et al (1985) (n = 146)	Ramin et al (1989) (n = 1,292)	Riley and Johnson (1993) (n = 3522)
Arterial			
pH	7.28	7.28	7.27
P_{CO_2} (mm Hg)	49.2	49.9	50.3
HCO_3 (mEq/L)	22.3	23.1	22.0
Base excess (mmol/L)	—	−3.6	−2.7
Venous			
pH	7.35	—	7.34
P_{CO_2} (mm Hg)	38.2	—	40.7
HCO_3 (mEq/L)	20.4	—	21.4
Base excess (mmol/L)	—	—	−2.4

amniotic fluid of fetal urine, which is more hypotonic than fetal plasma.

The fetal kidneys at term produce approximately 500–650 ml of urine per day. Another source of amniotic fluid is the fetal respiratory tract, which secretes fluid at the rate of 300–400 ml/d. Opposing this accumulation of fluid in the amniotic fluid cavity is the removal of the fluid by fetal swallowing, which may account for volumes of up to 1,500 ml/d. There may be other routes of exchange, such as the fetal skin and the chorioamniotic membrane.

An excessive amount of amniotic fluid, hydramnios, may be associated with congenital anomalies, especially those associated with gastrointestinal obstruction (ie, duodenal atresia) or those that impair fetal swallowing (ie, esophageal atresia or tumors of the neck). Other conditions that may be associated with hydramnios include diabetes, multiple gestations, fetal hydrops, and NTDs. However, progressive hydramnios may also be idiopathic, and the pregnancy may result in a normal fetus and newborn.

An abnormal reduction in the amount of amniotic fluid, oligohydramnios, may be associated with renal agenesis or obstruction to the fetal urinary tract. It may also be associated with fetal growth retardation.

IMMUNOLOGY OF PREGNANCY

The only natural grafting of tissue from one individual to another occurs during pregnancy. Understanding of the maternal–fetal parabiotic relationship has important implications in oncology, infectious diseases, and transplantation, as well as in obstetrics.

Fundamental Immunobiology

The function of the immune system is to maintain the body's integrity by repelling and destroying antigens of extrinsic origin. The body has an efficient two-part lymphatic system to deal with these invaders. For example, T cells are thymus-derived cells and are responsible for cell-mediated immunity. As such, T cells are able to mediate specific immune recognition and memory, as well as cytotoxic activity and delayed type hypersensitivity reactions. In contrast, B cells are derived from bone marrow and serve as specific antibody-producing cells. Elimination of foreign cells of any origin requires a complex interaction, primarily within the lymphatic system.

At the cellular level, T-cell or cell-mediated immunity operates through three types of T cells. These are known as helper (T4), inflammatory, and killer (T8) T cells. To become activated, the major histocompatibility complex brings the foreign antigen to the cellular surface. There, class I and II major histocompatibility complex binds with killer and helper T cells, respectively.

For example, when major histocompatibility complex brings the foreign antigen to the cellular surface, major histocompatibility complex binds in a two-step recognition process with the specific T cell to eliminate the offending antigen. In step one, the T cell binds with the outsider trapped by the macrophage. In step two, the macrophage secretes a surface-binding protein, such as B-7. B-7 then binds with a binding protein on the T cell (eg, T-28). When this recognition process is complete, the stranger cell will secrete chemicals adverse to itself, release lymphokines to promote inflammation, or assist B cells to become active, to secrete lymphokines, or to promote antibody formation. If B-7 is not found on the macrophage surface, the recognition process does not occur and the T cell will become inactive or die. This entire process serves to protect the body from self-destruction.

In contrast, humoral immunity is mediated by the sentry B cells. Here, the primary humoral antibody response to an antigen is in the immunoglobulin M (IgM) fraction, which is soon superseded by a predominantly IgG response. Antibodies produced are heterogenous proteins composed of several different classes of immunoglobulins. Four subclasses of human IgG, each with slightly different properties, can be distinguished on the basis of differences in the heavy polypeptide chain of the immunoglobin unit. Because antigens usually have multiple determinants, most humoral immune responses contain a mixture of antibodies produced from multiple clones of lymphocytes.

Cells capable of recognizing self-antigens and producing an immune response seem to be present in all normal people, but they are actively eliminated or silenced by the two-step recognition process. If the recognition process is defective, self-antigens escape to the rest of the body. The resultant self-reactive lymphocytes are responsible, in part, for autoimmune disorders (systemic lupus erythematosus, antiphospholipid antibody syndrome, autoimmune thyroid disease, myasthenia gravis, immunologic thrombocytopenic purpura) encountered in persons of reproductive age.

Maternal Immunologic Reactivity

The maternal immunologic response is altered significantly by the changing hormonal and immunologic environment of pregnancy. In fact, pregnancy is not a state of immune deficiency; rather, it is a time of sophisticated and highly specific immune regulation. During gestation, maternal T and B lymphocytes are phenotypically indistinguishable from those in the nonpregnant state. Nonetheless, for an apparently successful pregnancy, helper T cells are slightly down-regulated with respect to the fetus, while suppressor T cells remain unchanged. In contrast, B cells are very active to shield fetoplacental antigens from detection by the T-cell system. Of note, immunoglobulin levels are normal during pregnancy.

Nevertheless, it is at once apparent that the conceptus implanted into the maternal endometrium is not usually rejected like a surgically transplanted allograft. None of the many theories that have been put forward over the years adequately explains the immunologic survival of the fetoplacental unit. The most important mechanisms seem to be 1) decreased antigenicity of trophoblasts at the maternal–fetal junction, 2) separate maternal and fetal circulations and lymphatic drainage systems, 3) local decidual production of suppressive factors such as hormones and suppressor cells, and 4) perhaps, the maternal production of protective circulating blocking factors that bind and compete for receptors on trophoblasts or maternal lymphocytes.

Although survival of the fetus throughout pregnancy appears to require maternal immune tolerance, current theory suggests that the conceptus is immunogenic and evokes a response from the mother that is necessary for successful implantation and growth. However, it has recently been suggested that a defective maternal immune response and the lack of protective antibodies have been associated with recurrent spontaneous abortion. Evidence against this hypothesis are that normal pregnancies can occur in animals rendered incapable of antibody responses and in agammaglobulinemic women. Moreover, some studies have found no differences in blocking or cytotoxic antibodies in women with normal pregnancies compared with those in women who have recurrent abortions.

Fetal Immunocompetence

During the second and third weeks of gestation in the human fetus, pluripotential yolk sac cells form the precursors of all blood cell series. The thymus develops at about 6 weeks of gestation, and lymphocyte differentiation proceeds in the complete absence of foreign antigens. Small lymphocytes appear in the peripheral blood at about 7 weeks and in connective tissue around lymphocyte plexuses by 8 weeks. Primary lymph node development and lymphopoiesis do not occur until at least 12 weeks of gestation, but as early as 13 weeks of gestation, T cells that are capable of responding to mitogens and recognizing histoincompatible cells begin to appear. In the spleen, lymphocyte aggregates form at 14 weeks, and by 20 weeks of gestation the human fetus can respond to congenital infections by producing plasma cells and antibody.

Immunologic maturation in the fetus proceeds in preparation for exposure to a highly contaminated world. The transition from immunologically incompetent to immunologically competent has a profound influence on disease processes. Immunologic immaturity and susceptibility of organizing fetal tissues are factors that make first-trimester congenital rubella infection such a severe teratogenic process.

In contrast to the response in adults, the dominant humoral antibody response in the fetus is the IgM fraction. Indeed, the presence of circulating IgM of fetal origin in umbilical cord blood assists in the clinical diagnosis of such congenital infections as rubella, toxoplasmosis, syphilis, and cytomegalovirus (CMV). Since the large IgM molecule does not cross the placenta and immunoglobulins are not synthesized before antigenic stimulation, IgM is usually not detected in the fetal circulation or amniotic fluid of normal pregnancies. The smaller IgG molecule is specifically selected for placental transfer, which increases with gestational age. Fetal blood levels of IgG tend to reflect maternal levels, and specific antibody protection, in turn, depends on the mother's own total antigenic experience. To a great extent, adequate humoral immunity in the newborn period depends on the circulating antibodies that have crossed the placenta. Maternal IgG antibodies, however, in addition to their primary role of protecting the neonate from infections, can result in disease syndromes such as erythroblastosis fetalis, transient alloimmune and autoimmune neonatal thrombocytopenia, hyperthyroidism, and myasthenia gravis.

ENDOCRINOLOGY OF PREGNANCY

The hormonal changes of pregnancy and the maternal adaptations to these signals are extraordinary. These adaptations include 1) implantation and maintenance of pregnancy, 2) modification of maternal homeostasis to provide nutritional support for the developing fetus, and 3) preparation for lactation following delivery. Most of these endocrine changes during pregnancy can be directly attributed to hormonal signals emanating from the fetoplacental unit.

Implantation

Following ovulation and fertilization, the preembryo is transported from the ampullary portion of the fallopian tube to the uterine cavity, where implantation takes place 6–7 days after fertilization. Prior to implantation, the blastocyst secretes proteins and hormones that may enhance endometrial receptivity. Successful implantation requires precise synchronization between blastocyst development and endometrial maturation. At the time of implantation, the preembryo is actively secreting hCG, which can be detected in maternal serum as early as the eighth day after ovulation. The primary role of hCG is to prolong the biosynthetic activity of the corpus luteum, which allows continued progesterone production and the maintenance of the endometrium.

Between 6 and 7 weeks of gestation, corpus luteum function begins to decline. During this luteal–placental transition period, production of progesterone shifts to the developing placenta. Thus, removal of the corpus luteum before 6 weeks of gestation increases the risk of abortion. In patients with corpus luteum dysfunction or when the corpus luteum is removed surgically, exogenous progesterone supplementation treatment should be initiated and extend beyond this critical shift, until approximately 10 weeks of gestation.

Placental Compartment

The placenta has evolved into a complex structure that delivers nutrients to the fetus, produces numerous steroid and protein hormones and growth factors, removes metabolites from the fetus, and delivers them to the maternal compartment.

Progesterone

The main source of progesterone during pregnancy is the placenta. Maternal progesterone levels rise sixfold to eightfold from the luteal phase to term (Fig. 3-1). Although the placenta produces large amounts of progesterone, it has limited capacity to synthesize cholesterol de novo. It is now clear that maternal cholesterol in the form of low-density lipoprotein cholesterol is the principal source of precursor for biosynthesis of progesterone during pregnancy. The role of the large quantity of progesterone produced by the placenta includes inhibition of smooth muscle contractility, decreased prostaglandin formation leading to myometrial quiescence and prevention of uterine contractions, and inhibition of T lymphocyte cell-mediated responses involved in graft rejection.

Estrogen

During human pregnancy the rate of estrogen production and the level of estrogens in plasma increase markedly (Fig. 3-1). The corpus luteum is the principal source of estrogen during early pregnancy, but afterward nearly all of the estrogen is from the placenta, and the mechanism by which estrogen is produced is unique. The placenta is unable to convert progesterone to estrogen because of a deficiency of 17α-hydroxylase. Thus, the placenta has to rely on androgen precursors produced by the maternal and fetal adrenal glands. Almost all of the estriol is synthesized by the placenta from dehydroepiandrosterone sulfate (DHEAS) secreted by the fetal adrenal gland. The sources of estrogen biosynthesis by the maternal–fetal–placental unit are shown in Fig. 3-2. The major source

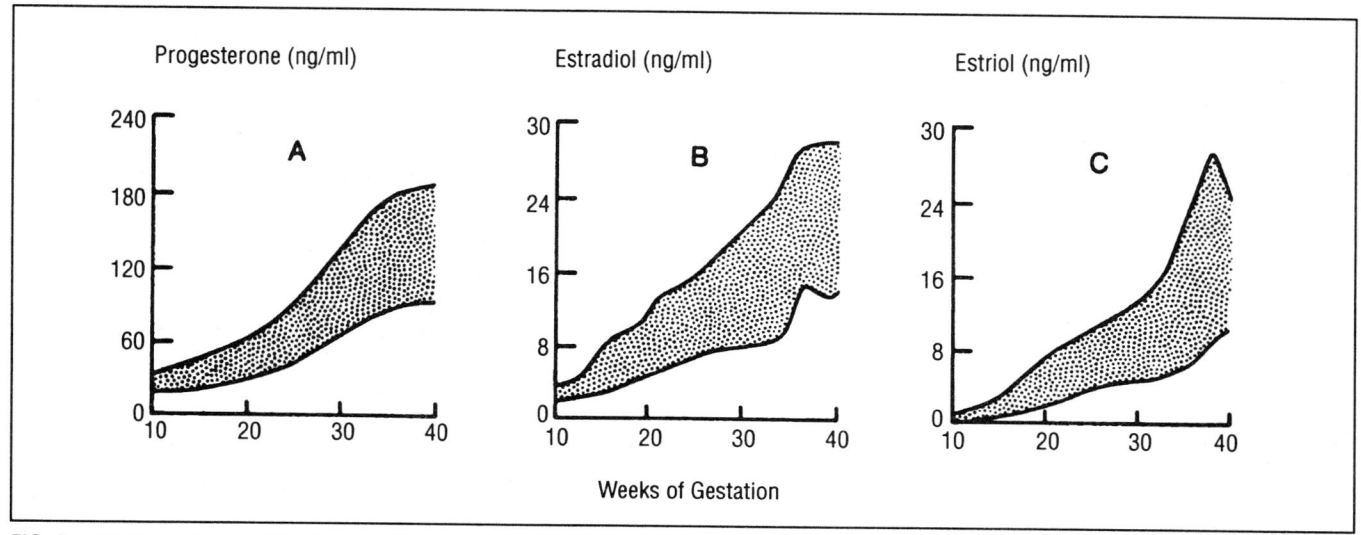

FIG. 3-1. (A) Progesterone, (B) estradiol-17β, and (C) estriol in plasma of normal pregnant women as a function of weeks of gestation (mean ± standard deviation). (Adapted from information appearing in *The New England Journal of Medicine*. Parker CR Jr, Illingsworth DR, Bissonnette J, Carr BR. Endocrine changes during pregnancy in a patient with homozygous familial hypobetalipoproteinemia. N Engl J Med 1986;314:559)

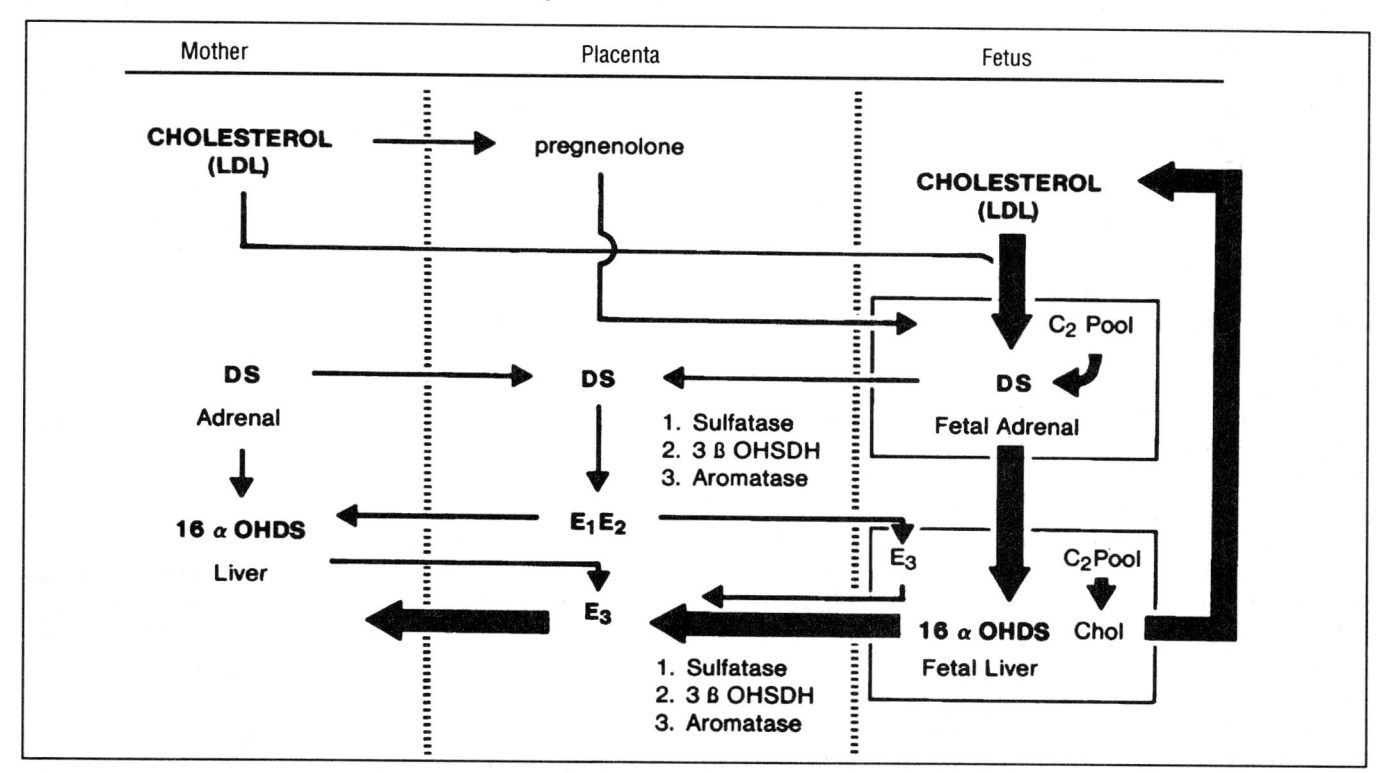

FIG. 3-2. Sources of estrogen biosynthesis in the maternal–fetal–placental unit. LDL, Low-density lipoprotein; Chol, cholesterol; C_2 pool, carbon–carbon unit; DS, dehydroepiandrosterone sulfate; E_1, estrone; E_2, estradiol-17β; E_3, estriol. (Adapted from Carr BR, Gant NF. The endocrinology of pregnancy-induced hypertension. Clin Perinatol 1983;10:737)

of fetal adrenal DHEAS is low-density lipoprotein cholesterol circulating in fetal blood. A minor source of fetal adrenal DHEAS is formed from pregnenolone secreted by the placenta. It has been reported that only 20% of fetal cholesterol is derived from the maternal compartment, and since amniotic fluid cholesterol levels are negligible, the main source of cholesterol appears to be fetal liver.

It has been proposed that the role of estrogen includes regulation of the events leading to parturition, since pregnancies are often prolonged when estrogen levels in maternal blood and urine are low, as in placental sulfatase deficiency or when associated with anencephaly. Estrogen stimulates phospholipid synthesis and turnover, increases incorporation of arachidonic acid into phospholipids, stimulates prostaglandin synthesis, and increases the number of lysosomes in uterine endometrium. Estrogens increase uterine blood flow and may also play a role in fetal organ maturation and development.

Human Chorionic Gonadotropin

Human chorionic gonadotropin is secreted by the syncytiotrophoblast of the placenta into both the fetal and maternal circulation. It is a glycoprotein with a molecular weight of about 38,000 consisting of two subunits, alpha and beta, and is similar to luteinizing hormone (LH) in structure and action. Plasma levels increase, doubling in concentration every 2–3 days until 60 and 90 days of gestation. Thereafter the concentration hCG in maternal plasma declines, plateauing at about 120 days before delivery. The most widely accepted theory of the function of hCG is support of the early corpus luteum of pregnancy to ensure continued progesterone secretion until this function is replaced by the placenta. Human chorionic gonadotropin also regulates the secretion of testosterone by the fetal testes and sexual differentiation.

Human Placental Lactogen

Human placental lactogen (hPL) is a single-chain polypeptide consisting of 191 amino acid residues with a molecular weight of about 22,000. Human placental lactogen has primarily lactogenic activity but exhibits some growth hormone–like activity and is also referred to as chorionic growth hormone or chorionic somatomammotropin. The structures of hPL, prolactin, and growth hormone are quite similar. Human placental lactogen is secreted by syncytiotrophoblasts, and levels rise with advancing gestational age, unlike hCG, and appear to plateau at term. Although the level of hPL in serum at term is the highest of all the protein hormones secreted by the placenta, the clearance rate of hPL is rapid, so it cannot be detected after the first postpartum day. Since hPL is secreted primarily into the maternal circulation, most of the proposed functions of hPL have focused on its sites of action in maternal tissues. Human placental lactogen exerts metabolic effects in pregnancy similar to those of growth hormone, by stimulation of lipolysis and increase in circulating free fatty acids, development of maternal insulin resistance, and an inhibition of gluconeogenesis, all of which favor transportation of glucose, amino acids, and fatty acids to provide nutrition to the fetus.

Fetal Compartment

The regulation of the fetal endocrine system, as is true for the placenta, is not completely independent but relies to some extent on precursor hormones secreted by the placenta or maternal tissues. As the fetus develops, its endocrine system gradually matures and becomes more independent, preparing the fetus for extrauterine existence.

Fetal Hypothalamic–Pituitary Axis

The fetal hypothalamus begins to differentiate from the forebrain during the first few weeks of fetal life, and by 12 weeks hypothalamic development is well advanced. Most of the hypothalamic-releasing hormones, including gonadotropin-releasing hormone (GnRH), thyrotropin-releasing hormone, corticotropin (ACTH)-releasing hormone, dopamine, norepinephrine, and somatostatin, have been identified as early as 6–8 weeks of fetal life (Fig. 3-3). The anterior pituitary cells that develop from the cells lining the Rathke pouch are capable of secreting growth hormone, prolactin, follicle-stimulating hormone (FSH), LH, and ACTH in vitro as early as 7 weeks of fetal life. The portal system that delivers releasing hormones to the anterior pituitary is developed by 18 weeks of gestation.

Fetal Thyroid Gland

The placenta is relatively impermeable to thyroid-stimulating hormone (TSH) and thyroid hormone, so that the fetal hypothalamic–pituitary–thyroid axis appears to develop and function independently of the mother. The levels of TSH and thyroid hormones are relatively low in fetal blood until midgestation. At 24–28 weeks of gestation, serum thyroxine (T_4) concentrations begin to rise progressively until term. At birth there is an abrupt release of TSH, T_4, and T_3, followed by a fall. The relative hyperthyroid state of the fetus is believed to facilitate thermoregulatory adjustments for extrauterine life.

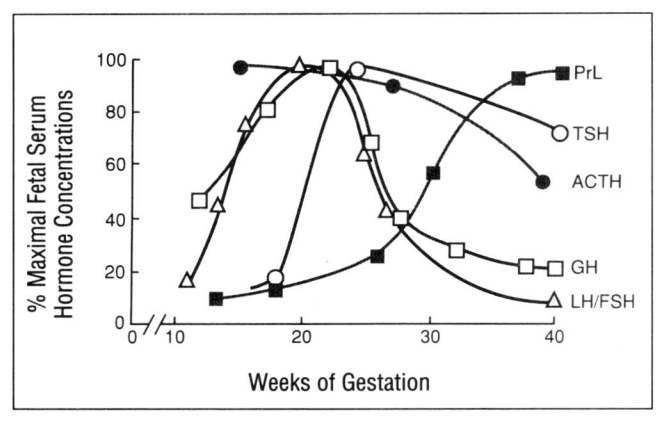

FIG. 3-3. Ontogeny of pituitary hormone levels in human fetal sera. PrL indicates prolactin; TSH, thyroid-stimulating hormone; ACTH, corticotropin; GH, growth hormone; LH/FSH, luteinizing hormone/follicle-stimulating hormone. (Parker CR Jr. The endocrinology of pregnancy. In: Carr BR, Blackwell RE, eds. Textbook of reproductive medicine. Norwalk, Connecticut: Appleton and Lange, 1993:28)

Fetal Gonads

The pattern of LH levels in fetal plasma parallels that of FSH, and the fall in gonadotropin pituitary content and plasma concentration of gonadotropins after midgestation is believed to result from the maturation of the hypothalamus (Fig. 3-3). The hypothalamus also becomes progressively more sensitive to sex steroids circulating in fetal blood, originating from the placenta. In the male, fetal testosterone secretion begins soon after differentiation of the gonad into a testis and formation of Leydig cells, which occurs at 7 weeks of life. Maximal levels of fetal testosterone are observed at about 15 weeks and decrease thereafter. The early secretion of testosterone is important in initiating sexual differentiation in the male. It is believed that the primary stimulus to the early development and growth of Leydig cells and subsequent peak of testosterone is hCG, supplemented by fetal LH. In the female, the fetal ovary is involved primarily in the formation of follicles and germ cells and less in hormone secretion.

Fetal Adrenal Gland

Of all the endocrine glands in the human fetus, the adrenal gland has aroused the greatest interest. The human fetal adrenal gland secretes large quantities of steroid hormones, up to 200 mg of steroid daily near term. This rate of steroidogenesis is five times that observed in the adrenal glands of adults at rest. The principal steroids secreted are C-19 steroids (mainly DHEAS), which serve as precursor substrate for estrogen biosynthesis by the placenta (Fig. 3-2).

The human fetal adrenal gland contains a unique fetal zone that accounts for the rapid growth of the fetal adrenal gland, and this zone regresses during the first few weeks after birth. In addition to the fetal zone, an outer layer of cells forms the neocortex or definitive zone. The fetal zone differs histologically and biochemically from the neocortex (ie, the fetal zone is deficient in 3β-hydroxysteroid dehydrogenase and secretes C-19 steroids; the neocortex secretes primary cortisol).

Studies of the fetal adrenal gland have attempted to determine what factors stimulate and regulate its growth and steroidogenesis and why the fetal zone undergoes atrophy after delivery. All investigations have shown that ACTH stimulates steroidogenesis in vitro. Furthermore, there is clinical evidence that ACTH is the major trophic hormone of the fetal adrenal gland in vivo. In anencephalic fetuses the plasma levels of ACTH are very low and the fetal zone is markedly atrophic. Maternal glucocorticosteroid therapy effectively suppresses fetal adrenal steroidogenesis by suppressing fetal ACTH secretion. Despite these observations, other ACTH-related peptides, growth factors, and other hormones have been proposed as possible trophic hormones for the fetal zone. After birth, the adrenal gland shrinks by more than 50% because of regression of fetal zone cells. This suggests that a trophic substance other than ACTH is withdrawn from the maternal or placental compartment. Following regression of the fetal zone, the neocortex zone increases to develop into the adult cortex, which secretes primarily cortisol.

Fetal Parathyroid Gland and Calcium Homeostasis

The level of calcium in the fetus is regulated by the transfer of calcium from the maternal compartment across the placenta. The maternal compartment undergoes adjustments that allow for a net transfer of sufficient calcium to the fetus to sustain fetal bone growth. Changes in the maternal compartment that permit accumulation of calcium include an increase in maternal dietary intake, increases in maternal 1,25-dihydroxyvitamin D_3 levels, and increases in parathyroid hormone levels. The levels of total calcium and phosphorus decline in maternal serum, but ionized calcium levels remain unchanged. The "placental calcium pump" allows for a positive gradient of calcium and phosphorus to the fetus. Circulating fetal calcium and phosphorus levels increase steadily throughout gestation. Fetal levels of total and ionized calcium, as well as phosphorus, exceed maternal levels at term.

The fetal parathyroid gland secretes parathyroid hormone by 10–12 weeks of gestation. Fetal plasma levels of parathyroid hormone reportedly are low but increase after delivery. The fetal thyroid gland contains calcitonin, but in contrast to unchanged maternal calcitonin, levels in the fetus are elevated. Since there is no transfer of parathyroid hormone or calcitonin across the placenta, the consequences of the observed change in these hormones on fetal calcium are consistent with an adaptation to conserve and stimulate bone growth within the fetus. After birth, serum calcium and phosphorus levels fall in the neonate. Parathyroid hormone levels begin to rise 48 hours after birth, and calcium and phosphorus levels gradually increase over the following several days, depending on dietary intake of milk.

Fetal Endocrine Pancreas

The human fetal pancreas appears during the fourth week of fetal life. The alpha cells, containing glucagon, and the delta cells, containing somatostatin, develop early, before beta-cell differentiation, although insulin can be recognized in the developing pancreas before apparent beta-cell differentiation. Total human pancreatic insulin and glucagon concentrations increase with fetal age and are higher than the concentrations of the adult human pancreas. In contrast to the pancreatic content of insulin, fetal insulin secretion is low and relatively unresponsive to acute changes in glucose in in vivo studies of umbilical cord blood at delivery and in blood samples obtained from the scalp of the fetus at term. In contrast, fetal insulin secretion in vitro is responsive to amino acids and glucagon as early as 14 weeks of gestation. In maternal diabetes mellitus, fetal islet cells undergo hypertrophy so that the rate of insulin secretion increases.

Maternal Compartment

A variety of maternal adaptations involving the endocrine system occur during pregnancy. For example, to provide effective exchange and transport of nutrients between mother and fetus, the maternal vascular system undergoes a significant increase in capacity. This is reflected by increased uterine and renal blood flow, maternal plasma and red blood cell volume, and increased cardiac output. To accommodate the increase in blood volume without a concomitant increase in blood pressure, there is a corresponding decrease in peripheral vascular resistance owing, in part, to relaxation of arteriolar smooth muscle and the development of a low-resistance uteroplacental circulation. Under the influence of estrogens, there is increased production of angiotensinogen, leading to elevations in aldosterone levels and a corresponding increase in blood volume.

Most diseases of the maternal endocrine system, if untreated, are associated with infertility and reduced conception rates. If conception occurs, the more serious the disorder, the more likely it will affect the fetus adversely, as in diabetes mellitus. Hormones or drugs used to treat the endocrine disorders may be transported across the placenta and alter the environment and development of the fetus.

Hypothalamus and Pituitary Gland

Little is known about the endocrine alterations of the maternal hypothalamus during pregnancy. Tumors or functional disorders of the hypothalamus commonly result in infertility due to amenorrhea or chronic anovulation. The anterior pituitary undergoes a twofold to threefold enlargement during pregnancy, due primarily to hyperplasia and hypertrophy of the lactotrophs thought to result from estrogen stimulation. Thus, prolactin plasma levels parallel the increase in pituitary size throughout gestation.

In contrast to lactotrophs, the number of somatotropic cells in the pituitary decreases during pregnancy. Maternal levels of growth hormone are low and do not change during pregnancy. The basal levels of gonadotropins are low, and response to an infusion of GnRH is severely blunted during pregnancy. The levels of TSH and response to thyrotropin-releasing hormone are within the normal nonpregnant adult range throughout pregnancy. Corticotropin and endorphin levels appear to increase with advancing gestations. Maternal plasma arginine vasopressin levels remain low throughout gestation and are not believed to play a role in human parturition. Maternal oxytocin levels are reported to be low and do not vary throughout pregnancy but increase during the later stages of labor.

Thyroid Gland

The thyroid gland increases slightly in size during pregnancy as a result of increased vascularity and glandular hyperplasia, but a true goiter is not present. There is a modest increase in basal metabolic rate during pregnancy secondary to fetal requirements. During pregnancy the mother is in a euthyroid state. Total T_4 and T_3 levels increase but do not result in hyperthyroidism, since there is a parallel increase in T_4-binding globulin from estrogen exposure. A similar finding is observed in women taking oral contraceptives. A reduced uptake of T_3 by renin is also observed in pregnancy and in women taking oral contraceptives. There is little if any transfer of T_4, T_3, or TSH across the placenta.

Adrenal Gland

Compared with changes in the fetal adrenal gland, the maternal adrenal gland does not change morphologically during pregnancy. During pregnancy, plasma adrenal steroid hormones increase with advancing gestation. The increase in total plasma cortisol is due principally to a concomitant increase in cortisol-binding globulin. There is a slight increase in free plasma cortisol and urinary free cortisol, but pregnant women do not exhibit any overt signs of hypercortisolism. The levels of renin and angiotensinogen rise during pregnancy, which leads to elevated angiotensin II levels and markedly elevated levels of aldosterone, as stated previously.

Endocrine Pancreas

The metabolic adaptation of pregnancy in which glucose is spared for the fetus is related to an appropriate bihormonal secretion by the maternal endocrine pancreas. In response to a glucose load there is a greater release of insulin from the beta cells and a greater suppression of glucagon release from the alpha cells, compared with the nonpregnant state. In association with the increased release of insulin, the maternal pancreas undergoes beta-cell hyperplasia and islet cell hypertrophy, accompanied by an increase in blood flow to the endocrine pancreas. During pregnancy, fasting blood glucose levels fall, but they rise more in response to a glucose load than do levels in nonpregnant women. The increased release of insulin is related to an insulin resistance due to hPL, which spares transfer of glucose to the fetus. Glucagon levels are suppressed in response to a glucose load, with the greatest suppression occurring near term.

NORMAL AND PRETERM PARTURITION

The initiation of labor in humans does not appear to be the result of increased cortisol production (as seen in the sheep model). There is also no reduction in maternal or fetal progesterone levels during spontaneous labor. It is likely, however, that prostaglandins play a critical role. It has been known for years that rupture, stripping, or infection of the fetal membranes, as well as instillation of hypertonic solutions into the amniotic fluid, results in the onset of labor. These facts and others led to the hypothesis that a fetus–amniotic fluid–fetal membrane complex is a metabolically active unit that triggers the onset of labor. Evidence in support of a causative role of prostaglandin in the labor process is provided by the fact that prostaglandins induce in vivo myometrial contractions at all stages of gestation. Despite this, direct evidence relating endogenous prostaglandins to labor is not clear. Central to this hypothesis is the understanding that at least one mechanism in the onset of parturition is the release of stored precursors of prostaglandin from the fetal membranes. The major precursor for prostaglandins is arachidonic acid, which is stored in glycerophospholipids. The fetal membranes are enriched with two major glycerophospholipids, phosphatidylinositol and phosphatidylethanolamine. As gestation advances, the progressively increasing levels of estrogen stimulate the storage, in fetal membranes, of these glycerophospholipids containing arachidonic acid in the *sn*-2 position.

The release of arachidonic acid from its storage position in fetal membrane phospholipids appears to be controlled by a series of fetal membrane lipases, including phospholipase A_2 and phospholipase C. These phospholipases are activated by a combination of the calcium ion and a new compound recently discovered in the amniotic fluid and believed to be derived from fetal urine. Once in a free state, arachidonic acid is available for conversion to prostaglandins.

Additional factors that augment and accentuate the normal process of labor include the liberation of corticosteroids by the mother or fetus, resulting in a decrease in the production of myometrial prostacyclin (a smooth muscle relaxant). Finally, active labor is characterized by a striking increase in the number of oxytocin receptors in the myometrium. Once begun, the process appears to be self-perpetuating, with an increase in the level of maternal catecholamines, resulting in the liberation of free fatty acids, which include arachidonic acid, and an increase in the level of maternal or fetal cortisol, which decreases the production of uterine smooth muscle prostacyclin. It is unlikely that oxytocin is the initiator of labor despite the facts that 1) oxytocin receptors are present in the myometrium and increase prior to labor and 2) oxytocin stimulates decidual prostaglandin E_2 and prostaglandin $F_{2\alpha}$ production. Current investigations using oxytocin antagonist to inhibit preterm labor are also inconclusive.

One possible mechanism for the preterm onset of labor can be explained by the biochemical sequence of events. Specifically, many bacteria are capable of cleaving arachidonic acid from its storage sites in fetal membrane glycerophospholipids. The liberated arachidonic acid is then available for conversion into prostaglandins, which are capable of initiating preterm labor. During the past 5 years, a growing body of evidence has accumulated suggesting a role of infection in preterm labor. Despite this, randomized, controlled investigations using antimicrobial agents have *not* shown benefit to prolonging gestation.

BIBLIOGRAPHY

Albrecht E, Pepe GJ, eds. Perinatal endocrinology. Ithaca, New York: Perinatology Press, 1985

American College of Obstetricians and Gynecologists. Utility of umbilical cord blood acid–base assessment. ACOG Committee Opinion 138. Washington, DC: ACOG, 1994

Carr BR. The maternal-fetal-placental unit. In: Becker KL, ed. Principles and practice of endocrinology and metabolism. Philadelphia: JB Lippincott, 1990:887–898

Carr BR, Simpson ER. Lipoprotein utilization and cholesterol synthesis by the human fetal adrenal gland. Endocr Rev 1981;2:306–326

Casey ML, MacDonald PC, Mitchell MD. Stimulation of prostaglandin E_2 production in amnion cells in culture by a substance(s) in human fetal and adult urine. Biochem Biophys Res Commun 1983; 11:1056–1063

Cunningham FG, MacDonald PC, Gant NF, Leveno KJ, Gilstrap LC III. Williams obstetrics. 19th ed. Norwalk, Connecticut: Appleton and Lange, 1993:184–185

Fisher DA. The unique endocrine milieu of the fetus. J Clin Invest 1986;78:603–611

Goldaber KG, Gilstrap LC 3d. Correlations between obstetric clinical events and umbilical cord blood acid-base and blood gas values. Clin Obstet Gynecol 1993;36:47–59

Goldaber KG, Gilstrap LC 3d, Leveno KJ, Dax JS, McIntire DD. Pathologic fetal acidemia. Obstet Gynecol 1991;78:1103–1107

Okazaki T, Casey ML, Okita JR, MacDonald PC, Johnston JM. Initiation of human parturition, XII: biosynthesis and metabolism of prostaglandins in human fetal membranes and uterine decidua. Am J Obstet Gynecol 1981;139:373–381

Okazaki T, Sagawa N, Bleasdale JE, Okita JR, MacDonald PC, Johnston JM. Initiation of human parturition, XIII: phospholipase C, phospholipase A_2, and diacylglycerol lipase activities in fetal membranes and decidua vera tisues from early and late gestation. Biol Reprod 1981;25:103–109

Parker CR Jr. The endocrinology of pregnancy. In: Carr BR, Blackwell RE, eds. Textbook of reproductive medicine. Norwalk, Connecticut: Appleton and Lange, 1993:17–40

Ramin SM, Gilstrap LC 3d, Leveno KJ, Burris J, Little BB. Umbilical artery acid–base status in the preterm infant. Obstet Gynecol 1989; 74:256–258

Riley RJ, Johnson JW. Collecting and analyzing cord blood gases. Clin Obstet Gynecol 1993;36:13–23

Tulchinsky D, Ryan KJ, eds. Maternal-fetal endocrinology. Philadelphia: WB Saunders, 1980

Word RA. Parturition. In: Carr BR, Blackwell RE, eds. Textbook of reproductive medicine. Norwalk, Connecticut: Appleton and Lange, 1993:41–48

Yeomans ER, Hauth JC, Gilstrap LC 3d, Strickland DM. Umbilical cord pH, PCO_2, and bicarbonate following uncomplicated term vaginal deliveries. Am J Obstet Gynecol 1985;151:798–800

Complications of Pregnancy

HYPERTENSION

There has been significant confusion over terms such as toxemia of pregnancy, pregnancy-induced hypertension (PIH), preeclampsia, and pregnancy-associated chronic hypertension. The term *toxemia* is no longer used. The following classification is currently recommended:

I. Pregnancy-induced hypertension
   A. Preeclampsia
      a. Mild
      b. Severe
   B. Eclampsia
II. Chronic hypertension preceding pregnancy (any etiology)
III. Chronic hypertension (any etiology) with superimposed PIH
   A. Superimposed preeclampsia
   B. Superimposed eclampsia

This classification has been modified from the original scheme proposed by Chesley. Pregnancy-induced hypertension is defined as a systolic blood pressure of at least 140 mm Hg or a diastolic pressure of at least 90 mm Hg on at least two occasions taken several hours apart. Preeclampsia is defined as the presence of hypertension with proteinuria or pathologic edema, or both, occurring after 20 weeks of gestation. Preeclampsia may actually occur prior to 20 weeks of gestation in patients with trophoblastic disease (ie, hydatidiform mole). Preeclampsia is defined as mild unless one or more of the signs or symptoms listed in Table 3-10 is present.

Pathophysiology

The etiology of PIH and preeclampsia is unknown. However, it is well established that the disease process occurs most often in women who are pregnant for the first time, women with multiple gestation, and women with certain vascular disorders such as those seen with insulin-dependent diabetes, lupus erythematosus, renal disease, and chronic hypertension. The major pathophysiologic derangement is vasospasm.

There are several potential maternal consequences of PIH, including cardiovascular and hematologic effects, as well as regional perfusion abnormalities. For example, cardiac output is increased 30–50% in normal pregnant women and is not decreased in pregnancies complicated by PIH. Because cardiac output is not altered significantly in patients with PIH, the control of peripheral resistance in normal and PIH-complicated pregnancies is critical to understanding blood pressure control. This is because blood pressure is the product of cardiac output times peripheral resistance, and peripheral resistance is increased in women with PIH. This likely occurs as the consequence of an increased sensitivity of the maternal vasculature to a variety of naturally occurring vasopressors, such as angiotensin II.

The increased sensitivity of the maternal vascular tree to angiotensin II precedes the development of hypertension by several weeks and results in alterations in regional perfusion and the hematologic system. The most frequently cited hematologic consequence of PIH is constriction of plasma volume, resulting in decreased perfusion of certain specific organs. Importantly, women with PIH are not hypovolemic but are, in fact, volume constricted. The vascular system is not underfilled but is constricted by virtue of the increased sensitivity of the vasculature to endogenous pressor substances. The clinical consequence is an increase in hematocrit, which worsens with increasing severity and duration of hypertension.

Thrombocytopenia is the most frequent abnormality in coagulation observed in patients with PIH. The development of disseminated intravascular coagulation, however, is rare in women with PIH, but the development of hemolytic anemia accompanied by bizarre red blood cell morphology and consumption of platelets and other coagulation factors occurs more commonly. This process is called microangiopathic hemolytic anemia and probably is the consequence of endothelial damage resulting from the arteriolar spasm that accompanies PIH.

Regional blood flows are altered by PIH in ways that are not always predictable. For example, renal and hepatic blood flows are decreased, but blood flows to the extremities and brain are unaltered by PIH.

The disease process may also be associated with adverse fetal effects. Maternal–placental perfusion is decreased in women with PIH and is believed to account for the increased perinatal morbidity and mortality that accompany pregnan-

TABLE 3-10. INDICATORS OF SEVERITY OF PREECLAMPSIA

Abnormality	Mild	Severe
Diastolic blood pressure (mm Hg)	100	≥ 110
Proteinuria	Trace to 1+	Persistent $\geq 2+$
Headache	Absent	Present
Visual disturbances	Absent	Present
Upper abdominal pain	Absent	Present
Oliguria	Absent	Present
Convulsions	Absent	Present
Serum creatinine level	Normal	Elevated
Thrombocytopenia	Absent	Present
SGOT* elevation	Minimal	Marked
Fetal growth retardation	Absent	Obvious

* SGOT is serum glutamic oxaloacetic transaminase (aspartate aminotransferase).

cies complicated by PIH. Unfortunately, diuretics and antihypertensive agents do not improve uterine blood flow in women with PIH. The failure of diuretics to increase uterine blood flow appears to be the result of the fact that these drugs further acutely decrease plasma volume and, in turn, uterine blood flow. The similar failure of antihypertensives to improve uterine blood flow and clinical outcome is the result of the fact that uterine blood flow is directly related to uterine artery blood pressure, so that uterine blood flow varies with, and in proportion to, changes in perfusion pressure.

Management

The clinical management of patients with PIH is summarized in Table 3-11. Therapy is definitive in patients with preeclampsia/eclampsia and a mature infant and in patients with preeclampsia and an immature infant and any of the signs or symptoms of severe preeclampsia, fetal growth retardation, or fetal jeopardy. Definitive therapy consists of preventing convulsions, controlling blood pressure, and instituting delivery. Prevention or treatment of convulsions is based on the parenteral use of magnesium sulfate (see box). Diuretics and hyperosmotic agents are not used.

Antihypertensive therapy is indicated for the antepartum, intrapartum, and postpartum patient with a diastolic blood pressure of 110 mm Hg or higher. In the acute therapy of intrapartum hypertension, it is *not* the goal to make the patient normotensive but rather to reduce the diastolic blood pressure to the range of 90–100 mm Hg. A too-rapid or significant drop in blood pressure may interfere with uteroplacental perfusion and result in FHR decelerations. For many years, hydralazine, given in small intravenous increments, was considered ideal for this purpose. However, the manufacturer of this antihypertensive agent has announced plans for the discontinuation of the intravenous form of the drug. Other agents such as labetalol or verapamil may prove useful, although the most efficacious dose (and the safest) for this purpose has not been established. Long-term antihypertensive medication is usually indicated for the treatment of chronic hypertension in the pregnant woman whose fetus is premature. The chronic administration of antihypertensive agents in this fashion to patients with PIH usually is not indicated.

Magnesium sulfate improves cerebral blood flow and oxygen consumption in women with PIH, while barbiturates are reported to increase cerebrovascular resistance and to decrease cerebral blood flow and oxygen consumption. Parenteral

TABLE 3-11. CLINICAL MANAGEMENT OF PATIENTS WITH PREGNANCY-INDUCED HYPERTENSION

Clinical Condition	Therapy
Mild pregnancy-induced hypertension and immature fetus	Expectant:
Compliant patient and improvement	1) Ambulatory management: a. See patient twice a week b. Fetal surveillance* c. Bed rest d. Educate about increasing severity of the disease e. Weight daily f. Home blood pressure monitoring four times a day
Noncompliant patient or lack of improvement	2) Hospitalization: a. Urine protein daily b. Fetal surveillance* c. Regular diet d. No salt restriction e. Weight daily f. Blood pressure four times a day
Severe pregnancy-induced hypertension and immature fetus in the presence of fetal growth retardation or fetal jeopardy	Definitive: 1) Prevent convulsions ($MgSO_4 \cdot 7H_2O$) 2) Control blood pressure 3) Deliver by vaginal or cesarean birth, depending on fetal and maternal conditions
Severe pregnancy-induced hypertension and mature fetus	Definitive: 1) Prevent convulsions ($MgSO_4 \cdot 7H_2O$) 2) Control blood pressure 3) Deliver by vaginal or cesarean birth, depending upon fetal and maternal conditions

* Fetal surveillance is defined as tests of fetal well-being, including but not limited to fetal movement charts, contraction stress tests, nonstress tests, and biophysical profiles. One or all of these tests may be used in a given patient.

> **Magnesium Sulfate Dosage Schedule for Severe Preeclampsia and Eclampsia**
>
> **Intravenous Regimen**
> - Give 4 g of MgSO$_4$ as 20% solution intravenously at rate not to exceed 1 g/min
> - Follow by continuous intravenous infusion of 1–3 g/h
> - Maintain plasma magnesium levels at 4–7 meq/L
>
> **Intramuscular Regimen**
> - Give 4-g intravenous loading dose as above
> - Follow promptly with 10 g of magnesium sulfate as a 50% solution, one half (5 g) injected deeply in the upper outer quadrant of both buttocks through a 7.6-cm (3-in) long 20-gauge needle (addition of 1.0 ml of 2% lidocaine minimizes discomfort).
>   If convulsions persist after 15 minutes, give up to 2 g more intravenously as a 20% solution at a rate not to exceed 1 g/min. If the woman is large, up to 4 g may be given slowly.
> - Every 4 hours thereafter, give 5 g of magnesium sulfate as a 50% solution injected deeply in the upper outer quadrant of alternate buttocks, but only after ensuring that:
>   a. The patellar reflex is present
>   b. Respirations are not depressed, and
>   c. Urine output the previous 4 hours exceeded 100 ml
> - Magnesium sulfate is discontinued 24 hours after delivery
>
> Adapted from Cunningham FG, MacDonald PC, Gant NF, Leveno KJ, Gilstrap LC III. Williams obstetrics. 19th ed. Norwalk, Connecticut: Appleton and Lange, 1993:794

magnesium sulfate therapy is believed to dilate human umbilical vessels and, possibly, increase fetoplacental blood flow. Similar therapy also has been observed to induce a transient (<15 minutes) decrease in mean arterial blood pressure and an increase in cardiac output.

Delivery is usually vaginal. The final decision as to vaginal delivery versus abdominal delivery, however, is based on obstetric indications.

In a patient with mild or early PIH with a premature fetus, therapy may be provided in either an ambulatory or a hospital setting. Ambulatory management is acceptable for women who are compliant, who can have frequent office visits, and who have access to some form of home blood pressure monitoring. For the patient who is noncompliant or who does not manifest a satisfactory response to outpatient therapy, hospitalization is indicated. The recommended regimen for the management of women, ambulatory or hospitalized, with mild PIH and an immature fetus is as follows:

- Ambulation with modified bed rest
- Regular diet
- Blood pressure measurements four times daily
- Weight and urine protein recorded two or three times weekly
- Daily urine output measurements
- Fetal surveillance
- Serial ultrasonography

Delivery is considered after 37 weeks of gestation if there is a favorable cervix, if the patient persistently has a diastolic blood pressure above 90 mm Hg, or if the patient has become normotensive but redevelops hypertension prior to delivery.

Considerable attention has been directed recently to the use of low-dose aspirin (80 mg every other day) to prevent PIH/preeclampsia. Although initial reports were encouraging, results from the recent National Institutes of Health study were somewhat disappointing in that the incidence of PIH was not decreased significantly with low-dose aspirin therapy. Moreover, the incidence of placental abruption was significantly increased. Until more information is available, it would seem prudent to restrict the use of low-dose aspirin therapy to well-designed study protocols.

BLEEDING IN THE SECOND HALF OF PREGNANCY

Third-trimester bleeding is a phrase commonly used as a "diagnosis" for bleeding occurring late in pregnancy. However, bleeding per se (in any trimester) is a sign and not a diagnosis. Moreover, significant bleeding from a variety of etiologies such as placental abruption and placenta previa may occur in the second trimester. It would be more appropriate to record the gestational age at which bleeding occurs, rather than a trimester in which it occurred.

The etiology of bleeding in many cases of bleeding in the second half of pregnancy is unknown. However, of known causes of clinically significant bleeding, placenta previa and placental abruption are the two most common etiologies.

Placenta previa occurs in approximately 0.5% of pregnancies and may be classified as follows:

- Total placenta previa—The placenta totally covers the internal cervical os.
- Partial placenta previa—The placenta partially covers the internal cervical os.
- Marginal placenta previa—The edge of the placenta extends to the margin of the internal cervical os.
- Low-lying placenta—The placenta is within reach of the examining finger introduced through the cervix.

This condition is usually associated with painless vaginal bleeding, although uterine contractions may be present. The diagnosis is best confirmed by an ultrasound scan. Factors associated with an increased risk of placenta previa include multiparity, advancing age, previous cesarean deliveries, and induced abortion. Placenta previa may be associated with placenta accreta, especially if a patient has had a previous cesarean delivery. Management depends on the amount or persistence of bleeding and the gestational age at presentation. Cesarean delivery is indicated for the patient at term, who is in labor, or whose bleeding is excessive (regardless of gestational age). Tocolytics of the beta-mimetic class are generally not recommended in women with significant bleeding, as they may be associated with tachycardia and hypotension and their efficacy is questionable. The initial episode of bleeding in patients with placenta previa is often not excessive, and it is common for patients to bleed intermittently in the third trimester. Thus, in the patient remote from term, all efforts should be directed toward conservative care with hospitalization and bed rest so that the fetus can mature. The use of conservative management, together with phospholipid analysis of the amniotic fluid to determine fetal lung maturity, has improved neonatal outcome. Because a significant number of newborns delivered after a bleeding episode caused by placenta previa have hypovolemia, anemia, or both, there is an increasing tendency to deliver them by cesarean birth once they are mature.

Premature separation of the placenta, abruptio placentae, occurs in approximately 0.5–1.5% of pregnant women. Its clinical presentation varies from minimally painful vaginal bleeding and uterine irritability to the less common severe separation with fetal demise, maternal hypotension, and disseminated intravascular coagulation.

In general, abruptio placentae must be managed with expeditious delivery and careful maternal and fetal monitoring. Following physical examination, a complete blood count and laboratory test of coagulation function, including a platelet count, fibrinogen level, and determination of partial thromboplastin time, should be performed. Urinary output should be monitored on an hourly basis, and an intravenous line large enough to allow rapid blood replacement should be placed. Invasive hemodynamic monitoring should be used as necessary.

If the fetus is alive after artificial rupture of membranes, FHR monitoring is undertaken. In the absence of a nonreassuring FHR pattern, vaginal delivery may be anticipated and is preferred. Cesarean delivery is used in the presence of an ominous FHR pattern or failure to make adequate progress in labor. Blood replacement is directed at maintaining blood pressure and urinary output, as well as keeping the hematocrit above 0.25 (25%). If a coagulopathy is present (ie, hyperfibrinogenemia), component therapy may be required in addition to blood replacement. The use of heparin to prevent intravascular coagulopathy is contraindicated in the case of abruptio placentae, as it may cause further hemorrhage.

After delivery, abnormalities of coagulation correct themselves spontaneously. These clotting factors of hepatic origin, such as fibrinogen, usually return to normal within 24–48 hours.

MULTIPLE GESTATION

Multiple gestation complicates about 1.5% of all births. Multiple pregnancy of higher order is a relatively small component of the total, but those numbers are increasing as a result of increased use of assisted reproductive technologies.

The incidence of perinatal morbidity and mortality for multiple gestation is two to five times that for singleton pregnancies; preterm births account for most of these adverse outcomes. Other complications such as fetal growth retardation, umbilical cord prolapse, and congenital malformations are also increased. The incidence of perinatal morbidity and mortality for monozygotic twins is two to three times that for dizygotic twins, with much of this being due to vascular anastomosis leading to twin–twin transfusion syndrome, abnormal amniotic fluid volumes, or altered hemodynamics leading to antenatal damage of fetal cerebral white matter. Monozygotic twins have a 1% incidence of monoamnionic sacs, which is associated with a high fetal mortality rate—up to 50% in some series—due to cord entanglement.

Causes of increased risk to the mother as a consequence of multiple pregnancy include higher incidence of PIH, anemia, abnormal placentation, hydramnios, and postpartum hemorrhage. There is also an increased risk of operative delivery with all of its associated complications.

Diagnosis of multiple gestation can be suspected based on a history of use of a fertility agent, clinical suspicions based on discrepancy between estimated gestational age and uterine size, or abnormal laboratory screening tests such as MSAFP. The most accurate method of diagnosis is ultrasound examination. All cases diagnosed should be evaluated ultrasonographically for fetal abnormalities with careful evaluation of the placenta and membranes, which will frequently determine chorionicity. Serial ultrasound evaluation to evaluate fetal growth is recommended.

Antenatal management should include attention to adequate nutrition, diminished activity, frequent prenatal visits, and ultrasound assessment of fetal growth. Other antepartum evaluations, such as genetic amniocentesis, should be performed when indicated. Elective hospitalization for prevention of preterm labor is not recommended, but prompt admission for preterm labor or other obstetric complications is generally advised. Antenatal management schemes that include frequent contacts with health care providers seem to decrease the preterm delivery rate, although the choice of an optimal management scheme remains controversial. Fetal surveillance with NST or BPP is advocated by some clinicians, but these tests are not universally performed without indication. If preterm labor occurs, the controversy continues over the safety and efficacy of the various tocolytic agents available.

Choice of route of delivery is dependent on the presentation at the time labor occurs. Most authors feel that vaginal delivery is a reasonable approach when both twins are in a vertex presentation. After delivery of twin A, and with surveillance of twin B with real-time ultrasonography or continuous monitoring, it is felt that the time interval between delivery of the twins is not important in the presence of a reassuring FHR. Management of vertex–breech or vertex–transverse presentation is more controversial. There are studies that suggest that vaginal delivery of twin B in a nonvertex presentation is a reasonable consideration for an infant with an estimated weight of more than 1,500 g. There are insufficient data to advocate a specific route of delivery when a nonvertex twin B weighs less than 1,500 g. When twin A is in a nonvertex presentation, most obstetricians would recommend cesarean delivery, since there are insufficient data to document safety of vaginal delivery.

ISOIMMUNIZATION

Despite dramatic progress in the management and prevention of hemolytic disease of the fetus and newborn caused by maternal blood group immunization, it continues to be an important cause of infant morbidity and mortality in the United States. In 1970, the incidence of hemolytic disease in newborns was approximately 45/10,000 births. In 1986, the incidence was 10.6/10,000 births, with much of this remaining incidence believed to be a gap in the appropriate use of D immune globulin when indicated during the antepartum and postpartum period. Isoimmune hemolytic disease of the fetus and newborn is caused by fetal–maternal blood group incompatibility, with maternal immunization against a fetal blood group antigen. Despite widespread use of D immune globulin, anti-D immunization remains the most common cause of erythroblastosis fetalis; however, a significant number of cases are the result of incompatibility to other blood antigens such as Kell, c, E, C, k, Fy[a], Jk[a], s, M, and many other described red blood cell antigens, both public and private. These other factors do not differ significantly from D insofar as isoimmune hemolytic disease is concerned. ABO incompatibility is a common cause of subclinical and mild hemolytic disease of the newborn, but it does not cause severe erythroblastosis or death in utero. In fact, if ABO incompatibility exists, it is known to decrease the risk to the fetus significantly.

Prenatal Screening

At the first prenatal visit, each patient's blood should be tested for ABO and Rh types and screened for antibody to these and other red blood cell antigens. Any red blood cell antibody present must be specifically identified and appropriate titers obtained to determine if there is a risk to the fetus. Antibodies of the IgM Lewis antigen type, such as anti-Le[a] and anti-Le[b], are of no clinical significance because they do not cross the placenta. When an antibody related to hemolytic disease of the fetus and newborn is identified, the patient must be considered sensitized and treated accordingly. The father's blood type and zygosity for that antigen should be determined whenever possible. If paternity is certain and the father does not have the antigen in question, no further evaluation is necessary. If this cannot be determined, it must be assumed that he is positive for the antigen in question.

Management

The antibody in the maternal circulation should be characterized and its titer determined. In general, it is believed that if the maternal titer remains less than 1:16 in an initial immunized gestation, the fetus is not in serious jeopardy. However, this value is somewhat dependent on local laboratory methods, skill of laboratory personnel, and previous experience related to titers within that institution. Once an antibody is found, titers should be obtained at regular intervals for adequate evaluation of the severity of the disease. To correct for interassay variance, serum from previous antibody titers should be preserved and used as a control with subsequent evaluations whenever possible. If the antibody titer remains less than 1:16, the fetus is at some risk but may be delivered near term if serial studies reveal no evidence of fetal compromise. Titers cannot be used as reliably during subsequent immunized pregnancies in the same woman, and individualization of the approach for management is necessary in these cases. A careful history of the outcome of previous pregnancies is important in guiding this individualized care.

In pregnancies in which the fetus is thought to be at risk by a titer of ≥1:16, or if history of a previous pregnancy suggests this, invasive testing for further fetal evaluation is indicated. Since the mid-1960s, amniocentesis with spectrophotometric examination of amniotic fluid has been the accepted method of assessing the severity of erythroblastosis in utero. This approach evaluates the difference between observed absorption in optical density at 450 nm (ΔOD_{450}) and extrapolated absorption as related to gestational age by plotting the values on a graph described by Liley. More recently, some have suggested that correlation between Liley graph values and fetal hematocrit is not as accurate prior to 26 weeks of gestation. This realization, coupled with the recently acquired ability to perform hematologic studies directly on fetal blood acquired by funipuncture, has modified evaluation and therapy of severely affected fetuses in many perinatal centers. The controversy surrounding appropriate evaluation techniques stems from the superior clinical information gained by fetal cord blood sampling by funipuncture, contrasted to the increased risk of funipuncture, which has a mortality rate estimated from 1.12% to 2.7% as a procedure-related mortality. This is compared with amniocentesis, which probably has a procedure-related mortality of less than 1/200. In addition, some authors have suggested that newer information regarding the prognostic value of amniocentesis may be important.

The above controversy notwithstanding, there are some general guidelines that may be followed. If the maternal antibody titer remains 1:8 or less, the patient may be monitored with repeated titer determinations every 2–4 weeks. These may be complemented with serial ultrasound examinations that look for evidence of hydramnios or early hydrops. If the titer is ≥1:16 but less than 1:64, the first invasive testing can probably be delayed until 25–26 weeks. If amniocentesis is chosen as a method of evaluation, the results are plotted on a Liley graph. The interval between subsequent amniocenteses depends on the ΔOD_{450}, but amniocentesis should be performed at least every 3 weeks. Obviously, if the ΔOD_{450} is very high, this may indicate fetal compromise and the need for delivery or intrauterine transfusion. If on repeated examination the ΔOD_{450} remains in Liley zone 1, either the fetus has D-negative blood or, if it is affected, the disease is mild and the fetus may be delivered close to term. In contrast, if the ΔOD_{450} is in the middle of Liley zone 2, the fetus is at moderate to severe risk and early delivery is indicated. The specific time selected for delivery depends on many factors: trend of plotted ΔOD_{450} values, the patient's previous obstetric history, evaluation of fetal well-being, assessment of fetal lung maturity, and determination of maternal cervical status. Fetuses with ΔOD_{450} in the upper portion of zone 2 require funipuncture, repeated amniocentesis, or possibly intrauterine transfusion if the ΔOD_{450} is rising rapidly. This choice will be affected by gestational age, the condition of the fetus, and the approach favored by the perinatal and neonatal team caring for the patient.

In patients with a poor obstetric history in whom the initial titer is significantly elevated, timing of the initial diagnostic procedure depends on the severity of erythroblastosis in previous pregnancies, the ultrasound findings, and the degree of titer elevation. In more severely affected patients, many experts currently recommend that funipuncture be used rather than amniocentesis in the second trimester to assess the fetus. This is particularly important if the father is heterozygotic for the offending antigen, since determination that the fetus is negative for that antigen may obviate further invasive evaluation. At the time of initial blood sampling, the fetal hematocrit, antigen status, and direct Coombs test result can be determined. If the hematocrit is less than 0.30 (30%), transfusion is indicated at that time. If the hematocrit is greater than 0.30, and the relevant antigen is found to be present in the fetal blood, the timing of future diagnostic procedures depends on the patient's history, serial ultrasound findings, and the hematocrit at the time of last sample.

Several studies have shown that ultrasonography alone is not an accurate method of diagnosing a degree of fetal anemia. Doppler waveform velocimetry of the fetus has also been disappointing in predicting the severity of fetal disease. When signs of hydrops appear on ultrasound examination, the fetus is severely compromised and usually found to have an extremely low hematocrit. While ultrasonography is, therefore, an excellent adjunctive tool to use in following the affected fetus, it cannot be relied on in lieu of invasive testing.

If a fetus is severely anemic in the second or early third trimester, transfusion in utero is necessary. These patients should be referred to individuals with significant experience, because the procedures can be technically difficult and the ongoing management requires considerable judgment. As with the techniques for fetal evaluation, the optimal technique of intrauterine transfusion has not been determined. The advent of intravascular fetal transfusion has greatly improved survival rates for severely affected fetuses, particularly those that are hydropic. Most authors feel that the intravascular transfusion approach is superior, but some suggest that a combination approach of both intraperitoneal and intravascular blood administration may be preferable. The success rates with severely affected fetuses in published series varies considerably, but with the ability to transfuse intravascularly, the successful outcome rate is approximately 90%.

Prevention

From a public health standpoint, prevention is the most important aspect of hemolytic disease. D isoimmunization is the only situation for which a preventive product is currently available. The process of prevention begins with the identification of each newly pregnant patient's major blood group and D type in early pregnancy. With respect to prophylaxis, Du positive is the equivalent of D positive except in very rare circumstances. To provide optimal prevention, the clinician should become familiar with those obstetric situations that result in sensitization and thus require prophylactic therapy:

- A D-negative woman has a slight chance of becoming sensitized in association with events that surround abortion or ectopic pregnancy. This is prevented almost completely by use of D immune globulin. A 50-mg dose is sufficient for events that occur in the first trimester.
- The risk of sensitization in association with amniocentesis is unknown. It is estimated that fetal–maternal hemorrhage occurs approximately 2.5% of the time. Prophylaxis with 300 mg of D immune globulin is recommended after amniocentesis. Prophylaxis (50 mg) is recommended after first-trimester CVS. In the presence of Rh sensitization, CVS is contraindicated.
- A D-negative woman has an approximate 1.6% chance of becoming sensitized *during* her pregnancy. This accounts for the so-called failures of postpartum prophylaxis programs. Such sensitization may be preventable with use of D immune globulin during the antepartum period, which can further reduce the incidence of D isoimmunization to 0.3%. A dose of 300 mg at approximately 28 weeks of gestation is recommended. Antibody screening should be repeated before unsensitized D-negative women receive antepartum D immune globulin at 28 weeks of gestation. It is probably not cost-effective to rescreen for irregular antibodies at that time. There is no evidence that additional prophylaxis is necessary when gestation exceeds 40 weeks, but some clinicians recommend repeating administered doses on an every-12-week basis.
- At the full-term delivery, the risk that a D-negative mother will become sensitized by her D-positive fetus is approximately 13% (16% if the fetus is ABO compatible with its mother and 1.5% if the fetus is ABO incompatible).

Postpartum administration of 300 mg of D immune globulin will almost completely prevent sensitization. This dosage will effectively treat 30 ml of fetal whole blood or 15 ml of fetal red blood cells that have entered the maternal circulation. Kleihauer–Betke or the rosette test is frequently used to determine whether fetal–maternal hemorrhage at delivery has exceeded this amount. The risk of sensitization in association with fetal–maternal hemorrhage at term is very low, perhaps on the order of 1/8,000 D-incompatible pregnancies. Therefore, the cost–benefit ratio of measuring the volume of fetal–maternal bleeding for every D-negative postpartum patient may not justify this as a routine practice; however, a quantitative Kleihauer–Betke analysis should be performed in those situations in which significant maternal bleeding may have occurred (eg, after maternal abdominal trauma, abruptio placentae, external cephalic version). If the quantitative determination is felt to be more than 30 ml, D immune globulin should be given to the mother in multiples of 300 mg for each

25 ml of estimated fetal whole blood in her circulation, unless the father of the baby is known to be D negative.

FETAL GROWTH RETARDATION

Infants born at or below the 10th percentile of mean weight for gestational age, with clinical evidence of dysfunctional or abnormal growth, are described as growth retarded. The perinatal mortality rate of these infants is 6–10 times higher than that of normal infants. Approximately one half of growth-retarded babies show wasting of soft tissue and muscle mass, especially in the cheeks, arms, buttocks, and thighs. The skin is often dry, cracked, and peeling. Intrauterine growth-retarded fetuses often aspirate meconium, are more often acidotic at birth, and are susceptible to massive pulmonary hemorrhage, convulsions, hypoglycemia, polycythemia, hypocalcemia, hypothermia, thrombocytopenia, and, if the growth retardation is severe, cerebral or renal damage.

Depending on the timing of growth retardation, as well as on its etiologic factor, infants can be either asymmetrically or symmetrically growth retarded. Asymmetric growth retardation generally occurs late in the second trimester or early in the third trimester of pregnancy. The fetal brain and heart are often spared because of nonreduced blood flow, and these fetuses usually demonstrate normal musculoskeletal growth. Asymmetric growth retardation is attributed to placental insufficiency secondary to maternal hypertensive disorders, renal disease, heavy cigarette smoking, or diabetes with vascular disease. Conversely, the symmetrically growth-retarded infant begins the process of growth retardation early, with a decrease in hyperplasia of all cells. Chromosomal abnormalities, developmental abnormalities secondary to teratogens, and intrauterine fetal infections (eg, rubella, CMV infection, hepatitis A and B, and toxoplasmosis, as well as listeriosis, syphilis, and tuberculosis) have been associated with this type of growth retardation. In addition, cyanotic heart disease, heavy cigarette smoking, and other causes of prolonged fetal hypoxia may result in a symmetrically growth-retarded infant. The fetus that is symmetrically growth retarded not only shares the growth aberration of the fetus with an asymmetric pattern but also has decreased skeletal dimensions.

The first clinical sign of fetal growth retardation may be an abnormally low increase in serial fundal height measurements. When fundal height growth is inappropriate for gestational age, an ultrasound examination should be ordered to confirm or refute the diagnosis. Most important is the evaluation of the fetal head and abdominal circumferences and their ratio, as well as femur length. Amniotic fluid volume assessment and a careful evaluation of fetal anatomy are also helpful in establishing the diagnosis. More recently, Doppler studies of umbilical arteries have shown a strong correlation between abnormal systolic–diastolic ratios and the diagnosis of fetal growth retardation. In general, however, there are no methods that allow a confident diagnosis of fetal growth retardation antenatally.

Once fetal growth retardation has been diagnosed, the fetus must be considered at risk for intrauterine hypoxia and possible death. Fetal surveillance is recommended, preferably twice a week, by use of the NST, the CST, or the BPP. Amniotic fluid volume assessment should also be performed. Although the timing of delivery is controversial, the absence of demonstrable fetal growth in association with mature fetal lungs suggests that delivery may be warranted. Furthermore, delivery may be indicated if the amniotic fluid volume is severely decreased.

PRETERM LABOR AND DELIVERY

Any birth that occurs before the 38th week of gestation is categorized as preterm. The incidence is between 8% and 10% of all births, with one third of these births indicated because of a major maternal or fetal complication and the remainder resulting from spontaneous processes, including preterm PROM and preterm labor. Preterm births account for more than 60% of nonanomalous-related neonatal mortality and morbidity. Most neonatal mortality occurs in those preterm births that occur at 20–30 weeks of gestation (or infants weighing less than 1,600 g). Survival of neonates delivered at tertiary care centers has improved yearly, particularly for those pregnancies ending at 25–32 weeks of gestation. Significant increases in survival rates occur at 25–26 weeks (20% at 24 weeks to 50% at 26 weeks). Long-term impairment has remained high for those survivors delivered at 25 weeks of gestation and earlier.

The cause of preterm labor is unknown in more than 50% of patients. Multiple factors, however, have been repeatedly reported to be associated with an increased risk of subsequent preterm labor: multiple gestation (40–50%), previous preterm labor or delivery (20–50% recurrence), diethylstilbestrol exposure, hydramnios, uterine anomalies, previous cone biopsy, previous second-trimester losses, cervical dilatation and effacement before 32 weeks of gestation, excessive preterm uterine activity, and placenta previa. In general, the lower the socioeconomic status, the higher the risk. Extremes of age (less than age 18 and greater than age 35 for first pregnancy) also present a higher risk. In addition, it is now being recognized that perhaps as many as one third of spontaneous preterm births may be complicated by intrauterine or extrauterine infections.

Subclinical chorioamnionitis has emerged as a possible significant cause of preterm birth. Many cases of preterm PROM, as well as up to one third of cases of idiopathic preterm birth, may be due to subclinical intraamnionic infection. Bacterial products such as lipopolysaccharide can be identified in the amniotic fluid without other evidence of infection. Furthermore, endogenous host products (cytokines) secreted in response to infection can also be identified in the amniotic fluid of these pregnancies. These cytokines, including interleukin-1, interleukin-6, interleukin-8, and tumor necrosis factor (cachectin), are secretory products of macrophage activation.

Numerous risk-scoring indices based on factors similar to those listed above have been proposed. In seven studies there was a positive predictive value of less than 20%. Unfortunately, only 50% of all preterm births occur in women with risk factors. There are no biochemical tests currently proven to predict preterm labor, although preliminary studies using positive cervicovaginal fetal fibronectin in preterm labor patients with intact membranes are promising. Intermittent daily monitoring of uterine activity in the outpatient setting has indicated that otherwise silent contractions of more than six per hour are associated with a positive predictive value of approximately 25–30%. The efficacy of this technology is unclear; it should be considered investigational at this time.

Although it is more desirable to prevent rather than inhibit preterm labor, methods to predict preterm labor are currently not discriminating enough to employ routine drug therapy or behavioral modifications. For selected very-high-risk patients, such as those with multiple gestations or previous recurrent preterm labor and deliveries, some physicians elect to advise bed rest or at least increased rest, cessation of coitus, or pharmacologic treatment, but the efficacy of these approaches is not proven. The use of cervical cerclage for the incompetent cervix is warranted, but it may increase the risk of subsequent preterm labor and should not be used for entities other than the incompetent cervix.

Most current preterm birth prevention programs have as an initial goal the early detection of preterm labor, so that more patients may be candidates for tocolytic therapy and the potential efficacy of tocolysis can be improved. The symptoms and signs of early preterm labor may include mild menstruallike cramps; constant low backache; uterine contractions, which are frequently painless; and a recent increase in vaginal discharge or presence of a pink-stained discharge. As these symptoms are so subtle, they may not be recognized until the labor process and cervical dilatation are in an advanced stage (>4 cm). Unfortunately, the efficacy of various preterm prevention programs is unclear.

The diagnosis of preterm labor, early in its course, is frequently difficult. If a patient is having contractions every 3–4 minutes, placebo treatment alone may be effective approximately 50% of the time, if contractions are the only criteria that are used. Thus, as with term labor, contractions plus ruptured membranes, cervical change, or a cervix effaced and dilated to at least 2 cm will improve the accuracy of diagnosis.

Initial evaluation of patients with suspected preterm labor should include determination of the presence and frequency of uterine contractions and cervical status and a reevaluation of gestational age. Before considering whether to use tocolysis, a search should be made for treatable factors of preterm labor, such as pyelonephritis, and an evaluation should be made to determine whether there are any maternal or fetal contraindications to a specific tocolytic treatment. Relative contraindications include mild hypertension, mild fetal growth retardation, and cervical dilatation greater than 4 cm. A urine culture is often useful, and cultures of the lower genital tract for group B hemolytic streptococci or *Chlamydia* species are recommended by some. Amniocentesis for fetal lung maturity and Gram stain as well as culture are frequently used, depending on the gestational age and the presenting clinical situation. Some of these relative factors may be contraindications for one drug but not for others. The risk–benefit ratio of tocolysis must be considered for each patient. Although many clinicians feel that tocolytic drugs should be used when possible, there remains considerable debate as to their efficacy and safety. Methods to arrest preterm labor include bed rest and tocolytics. The most widely used tocolytic drugs are magnesium sulfate and beta-mimetics. During the last several years an increasing interest in prostaglandin synthetase inhibitors and calcium channel blockers has emerged. The safety and efficacy of these agents are not well described.

Magnesium sulfate is frequently used as the first-line drug for tocolysis, particularly in patients with diabetes. It is initiated by a loading dose of 4–6 g IV, followed by a continuous maintenance dose of 2–4 g in an attempt to achieve serum concentrations of 6–8 mg/dl. After successful tocolysis, oral beta-adrenergic agents are usually used until near term, although a few investigators have recommended that oral magnesium be given as the gluconate or oxide, even though serum levels only reach 2–3 mg/dl. Deep-tendon reflexes should be checked routinely to ensure their presence, and fluid intake and output should be monitored as pulmonary edema can occur with this agent. Fetal serum levels equilibrate with maternal concentrations, and occasional transient depression caused by hypermagnesemia in newborns has been reported. Long-term magnesium therapy markedly increases calcium losses, which could ultimately affect bone mineralization.

Beta-adrenergic tocolysis is usually initiated by the parenteral route, either by a continuous intravenous infusion, titrating the infusion rate against contractions and side effects, or by the intermittent intramuscular or subcutaneous approach. Following cessation of uterine contractions, oral medication is often used in a dose and at a frequency that results in a mild maternal tachycardia until near term. Recent interest, based on the theory that continued exposure of the agonist results in down-regulation of the beta receptors and tachyphylaxis, has centered on intermittent administration of the agents or the use of a subcutaneous pump system to administer the drugs in bolus fashion at peak periods of uterine activity. There have been recent reports of maternal deaths secondary to use of the pump, and in one report newborn myocardial necrosis was noted.

Maternal side effects, such as hypotension, excessive tachycardia or cardiac arrhythmias, myocardial ischemia, and pulmonary edema, may be serious. Strict intake and output of fluids are necessary while on intravenous therapy and for 24 hours thereafter. Fluid restriction to less than 2,500 ml/d is recommended. Colloid osmotic pressure determinations may be useful, as pulmonary edema is rare if the colloid osmotic pressure is above 15 mm Hg. Any symptoms of significant chest pain should be evaluated by electrocardiographic studies and should lead to a search for evidence of myocardial ischemia. Hypokalemia and hyperglycemia tend to revert toward normality after 24–36 hours of treatment, but they can be a significant problem if superimposed on underlying abnormal carbohydrate metabolism.

The benefits of pregnancy prolongation with the use of betaadrenergic receptor antagonists are not clearly proven beyond the initial 24–48 hours. Data from the recent Canadian Preterm Labor Investigative Group showed that although ritodrine delayed delivery for 24 hours, its use did not improve the ultimate perinatal outcome.

Prostaglandin synthetase inhibitors have been reported to be effective tocolytic agents in isolated reports. Concern related to adverse fetal effects, however, has limited their use to very difficult patients who are early in gestation. Narrowing of the ductus arteriosus has been observed in some pregnancies during their use, and oligohydramnios may be induced after a few days. It has been suggested that the effect on the ductus is less evident prior to 32 weeks of pregnancy. Importantly, long-term use is associated with pulmonary hypertension. Thus, if these agents are used, it is recommended that they be used only at 20–32 weeks, for only 1–3 days, and that the fetus and amniotic fluid volume be evaluated daily.

Calcium channel blocking drugs are used because of their ability to cause a decrease in intracellular calcium, and hence inhibition of myometrial contractility. Only limited data are available on the calcium antagonists, although preliminary reports are encouraging. Adverse effects in experimental animal studies have necessitated caution and further careful evaluation. These adverse effects include hypercapnia, hypoxia, and acidosis.

A relatively new class of agents for inhibition of preterm labor is under investigation. Oxytocin inhibitors competitively inhibit oxytocin. Their use in humans is currently experimental, and therefore their benefit is unproven.

Maternal corticosteroid treatment with betamethasone and dexamethasone has been shown to decrease the incidence of respiratory distress syndrome in several controlled trials. Recently, the National Institute of Child Health and Human Development, together with the Office of Medical Applications of Research of the National Institutes of Health, convened a Consensus Development Conference on the effects of steroids for fetal maturation on perinatal outcomes. An independent consensus panel concluded that antenatal corticosteroid therapy decreased the risk of respiratory distress syndrome, intraventricular hemorrhage, and mortality in infants born prematurely. It recommended that antenatal therapy with corticosteroids should be considered for all fetuses at risk for preterm delivery between 24 and 34 weeks of gestational age, regardless of race, gender, or availability of surfactant therapy. It also recommended that antenatal corticosteroids should be considered in the presence of preterm PROM in pregnancies less than 30–32 weeks of gestation unless there is evidence of clinical chorioamnionitis. The incidence of intraventricular hemorrhage and neonatal mortality is high in this latter group of newborns.

There has been hesitation to use corticosteroids in some patients because of the impression that delivery will occur prior to a full course of therapy (ie, less than 24 hours). However, treatment with corticosteroids for less than 24 hours still appears to be associated with a significant reduction in neonatal mortality, respiratory distress syndrome, and intraventricular hemorrhage.

The most commonly used regimens of antenatal corticosteroids would appear to be either two doses of 12 mg of betamethasone given intramuscularly (IM) 24 hours apart or four doses of 6 mg of dexamethasone IM 12 hours apart.

Very preterm infants delivered in an intensive care setting have a greater chance for intact survival and less morbidity than those transferred for neonatal care after delivery. If it is safe and if it can be accomplished, transfer of such patients to tertiary care centers before delivery is recommended. Although controversy has existed over continuous FHR monitoring at term, most clinicians feel it is important in the preterm gestation during labor.

Retrospective studies show that the singleton breech of less than 32–34 weeks of gestation, or weighing less than 1,500 g, has less morbidity and mortality if delivered by cesarean section, particularly if the breech presents as a footling. There are no convincing data to indicate that cesarean delivery is indicated for cephalic presentations if labor is progressing in a normal fashion and if there is an absence of ominous FHR patterns. Factors associated with intraventricular hemorrhage are the prematurity of the fetus, shock, and respiratory distress syndrome but not the mode of delivery for cephalic presentations.

PREMATURE RUPTURE OF MEMBRANES

Rupture of membranes that occurs before the onset of labor is described as premature. The etiology of spontaneous PROM is not known; however, it is often suggested that uterine contractions (frequently undetected by the patient) result in cervical change and that infection of the chorioamnion leads to rupture at the site of infection. Most studies indicate the incidence of this disorder to be 7–12%.

The latent period is the interval between membrane rupture and the onset of labor. Generally, the earlier in gestational age that PROM occurs, the longer the latent period. More than 90% of patients with PROM at term begin labor within 24 hours. In preterm gestations, however, labor begins within 24 hours of rupture in only 70% of patients and within 72 hours in 90% of patients. Of patients with ruptured membranes before 34 weeks of gestation, 93% deliver in less than 1 week.

In pregnancies of less than 37 weeks of gestation, prematurity (and its sequelae) and infection are the major concerns following PROM. Because chorioamnionitis can lead to significant morbidity for both mother and fetus, once diagnosed, it must be treated aggressively with antibiotics and delivery.

Diagnosis

The diagnosis of PROM depends on history, physical examination, and laboratory information. The patient's history alone is correct for 90% of patients. Digital examination of patients who are not in labor and for whom induction is not planned should be avoided, as such examinations add no useful information and probably increase the risks for infection.

Speculum examination should be undertaken to confirm the diagnosis; evaluate the general appearance of the cervix; take appropriate samples for cultures, such as for group B streptococci, *Chlamydia* species, and *Neisseria gonorrhoeae*; and rule out prolapse of the umbilical cord.

Confirmation of the diagnosis consists of identifying a pool of fluid and testing for an alkaline pH with phenaphthazine or other appropriate indicators. A swab from the posterior fornix should be smeared on a slide, allowed to dry, and checked under a microscope for a typical "ferning" appearance, indicating amniotic fluid. In some cases the diagnosis may be difficult to confirm. A new investigative test used to identify fetal fibronectin may be useful in the diagnosis of ruptured membranes in these situations.

Ultrasound examination is often useful to support the diagnosis, but other causes of oligohydramnios could be confusing. When the diagnosis of PROM is confirmed, the gestational age must be assessed and the patient carefully evaluated for evidence of labor, chorioamnionitis, or fetal distress.

Management

Despite much controversy regarding the management of PROM, there are areas in which there is a consensus. After admission and evaluation for infection and fetal distress, management depends on gestational age. Based on these factors and individual circumstances, management in the hospital or, in compliant patients, at home with careful observation is feasible.

Term

At 36 weeks of gestation and beyond, the goal of management of PROM is delivery. Patients in active labor should be allowed to progress and be managed as any other term patient. In the absence of fetal distress or clinical infection, the patient should be observed for labor. Routine induction of labor immediately after rupture of membranes does not decrease the likelihood of such complications and may increase the cesarean delivery rate, especially if the cervix is unfavorable for induction.

Approximately 26–35 Weeks

Since the major risks to the baby following preterm PROM are related to prematurity, management is directed toward prolonging gestation when there is no labor, no infection, and no evidence of cord compression on antepartum FHR testing.

Clinical parameters, including symptoms, vital signs, uterine tenderness, and odor of the lochia, are monitored. Elevations of leukocyte count and C-reactive protein concentration may lead to an overreaction and must be interpreted and acted on only in the complete clinical context. Amniocentesis for Gram stain and culture of amniotic fluid may sometimes be helpful for identifying early or occult chorioamnionitis. An ultrasound examination should be performed to determine fetal age and lie and to detect oligohydramnios. Other recommended tests to evaluate fetal status include daily BPP. If there is absence of reactivity, fetal breathing, and fetal movement, there is a high correlation with neonatal infection.

At present, prophylactic antibiotics should not be used routinely in patients with preterm PROM. In patients with a positive cervicovaginal culture for group B streptococci or gonococci, however, it is appropriate to treat with antibiotics. Use of intrapartum ampicillin during labor in group B streptococcus-positive women with preterm PROM decreases neonatal sepsis.

In the presence of ruptured membranes, the fetus is at risk from umbilical cord compression, even in the absence of labor. Continuous FHR monitoring in the initial assessment of the patient should therefore be followed by frequent evaluation, such as daily antepartum FHR assessments.

Patients who are admitted to institutions that are not equipped to manage the expected neonatal complications of prematurity (depending on gestational age) should be transferred to a tertiary care center, if possible. The use of corticosteroids to accelerate fetal pulmonary maturity in patients with preterm PROM is controversial.

Expectant management consists of careful in-hospital observation, with delivery indicated for chorioamnionitis, fetal distress, or premature labor. Another option is to evaluate the fetus for pulmonary maturity and to expedite delivery if maturity is documented.

Less Than 25 Weeks

In patients with PROM at less than 25 weeks of gestation, there is a relatively low likelihood (approximately 40%) that a viable gestational age will be achieved or that the patient will deliver a surviving infant. Obviously this depends on the gestational age at which rupture of membranes occurs. Even in patients whose infants do survive, many of the babies suffer significant short- and long-term morbidity. Additionally, there is the problem of pulmonary hypoplasia, facial deformity, and limb contractures and deformities. If the gestational age is early enough and the patient elects to terminate her pregnancy, the option is reasonable and should be discussed. If the patient elects to continue the pregnancy, expectant management, even at home with a regimen of avoiding coitus and douching, is reasonable. Here, also, delivery is indicated for chorioamnionitis.

POSTTERM GESTATION

The average length of human pregnancy, calculated from the first day of the last menstrual period, is 280 days (ie, 40 weeks). By current definition, a postterm pregnancy is a gestation lasting 42 weeks or more (ie, 294 days from the first day of the last menstrual period), and the frequency is approximately 10%. Although the true frequency is unknown, because many cases result from the inability to time conception accurately, some pregnancies clearly proceed beyond 294 days.

The expected date of confinement is most reliably determined early in pregnancy. The date of the last menstrual period, time of quickening (first fetal movement), ability to hear the fetal heart with a stethoscope at approximately 20 weeks of gestation, and early uterine size determination are all helpful historic and physical data that help to determine the expected date of confinement. The most accurate method to determine gestational age, however, is the first-trimester measurement of the crown–rump length of the fetus. This will pinpoint true gestational age (± 4.7 days). During the second trimester, the biparietal diameter provides reasonably accurate dating (± 10 days), as does the femur length (± 6.7 days). In the third trimester, no physical findings or ultrasound measurements precisely define the estimated date of confinement (range ± 14–21 days).

Most of the complications of a postterm gestation relate to the fetus. Specifically, most studies show that at 43 weeks of gestation, the perinatal mortality rate is doubled; it is increased fourfold to sixfold by 44 weeks of gestation. Significant morbidity also results. The four problems leading to untoward outcome include oligohydramnios, which is observed in the normal course of events beyond term gestation in some pregnancies; meconium staining of the amniotic fluid, which is seen in approximately 25% of pregnancies beyond 42 weeks of gestation and which may be aspirated by the fetus in utero; macrosomia; and dysmaturity, in which the fetus undergoes a progressive diminution in subcutaneous tissue and the development of peeling, desquamating skin, and long fingernails, which occurs in approximately 20% of those pregnancies beyond 42 weeks of gestation.

If the cervix is considered ripe for induction at 41–42 weeks of gestation, it seems reasonable to do so. Considerable controversy exists as to the most judicious mode of management in the presence of an unripe cervix. At present, the use of techniques to assess fetal well-being are recommended, including the BPP, NST, and CST. There are no data from randomized trials that demonstrate the superiority of the BPP over weekly or twice-weekly FHR monitoring evaluations and estimates of amniotic fluid volume by ultrasonography. Either the NST or the CST may be used, together with studies of amniotic fluid volume. Amniotic fluid volume should be considered inadequate if vertical-diameter pockets are less than 2 cm. Currently, most investigators recommend the use of a four-quadrant amniotic fluid index, with values greater than 5 cm considered normal. Regardless of the assessment modality, delivery should be effected in the presence of an abnormal FHR tracing, oligohydramnios, or both.

During labor, umbilical cord compression may be present as a result of oligohydramnios. If macrosomia exists, careful attention should be paid to evaluating the risk of shoulder dystocia (twofold increased risk in postterm pregnancies) and its management, if it occurs. Finally, at the time of delivery, the infant's airway should be suctioned with a mechanical device after delivery of the head and before delivery of the thorax. This action, combined with immediate intubation of the infant and suction of the trachea, helps to prevent, but not eliminate, meconium aspiration. Amnioinfusion to decrease the consistency of meconium may be used. Meconium aspiration may occur even in the absence of labor.

BIBLIOGRAPHY

Hypertension

Cunningham FG, MacDonald PC, Gant NF, Leveno KJ, Gilstrap LC III. Hypertensive disorders in pregnancy. In: Williams obstetrics. 19th ed. Norwalk, Connecticut: Appleton and Lange, 1993:763–817

Gant NF, Daley GL, Chand S, Whalley PJ, MacDonald PC. A study of angiotensin II pressor response throughout primigravid pregnancy. J Clin Invest 1973;52:2682–2689

McCall ML, Sass D. The action of magnesium sulfate on cerebral circulation and metabolism in toxemia of pregnancy. Am J Obstet Gynecol 1956;71:1089–1096

Sibai BM, Caritis S, Phillips E, Klebanoff M, McNellis D, Rocco L, et al. Prevention of preeclampsia: low-dose aspirin in nulliparous women: a multicenter double-blind placebo controlled trial. Am J Obstet Gynecol 1993;168:286 (abstract 1)

Sibai BM, Caritis S, Phillips E, Klebanoff M, Witter P, Depp R, et al. Safety of low-dose aspirin in healthy nulliparous women: a double-blind placebo-controlled trial. Presented at the 40th Annual Meeting of the Society for Gynecologic Investigation; March 31–April 4, 1993; Toronto; A228

Zuspan FP, Rayburn WF. Blood pressure self-monitoring during pregnancy: practical considerations. Am J Obstet Gynecol 1991;164:2–6

Multiple Gestation

Bejar R, Vigliocco G, Gramajo H, Solana C, Benirschke K, Berry C, et al. Antenatal origin of neurologic damage in newborn infants, II: multiple gestations. Am J Obstet Gynecol 1996;162:1230–1236

Blickstein I. The twin-twin transfusion syndrome. Obstet Gynecol 1990;76:714–722

Crowther C, Chalmers I. Bed rest and hospitalization during pregnancy. In: Chalmers I, Enkin M, Keirse MJNC, eds. Effective care in pregnancy and childbirth. Oxford: Oxford University Press, 1989: 624–632

D'Alton ME, Mercer BM. Antepartum management of twin gestation: ultrasound. Clin Obstet Gynecol 1990;33:42–51

Dyson DC, Crites YM, Ray DA, Armstrong MA. Prevention of preterm birth in high-risk patients: the role of education and provider contact versus home uterine monitoring. Am J Obstet Gynecol 1991; 164:756–762

Ellings JM, Newman RB, Hulsey TC, Bivins HA Jr, Keenan A. Reduction in very low birth weight deliveries and perinatal mortality in a specialized, multidisciplinary twin clinic. Obstet Gynecol 1993;81:387–391

Evans MI, Littmann L, King M, Fletcher JC. Multiple gestation: the role of multifetal pregnancy reduction and selective termination. Clin Perinatol 1992;19:345–357

Nageotte MP. Prevention and treatment of preterm labor in twin gestation. Clin Obstet Gynecol 1990;33:61–68

Isoimmunization

Bowman JM. Maternal blood group immunization. In: Eden RD, Boehm FH, eds. Assessment and care of the fetus. Norwalk, Connecticut: Appleton and Lange, 1990

Chavez GF, Mulinare J, Edmonds LD. Epidemiology of Rh hemolytic disease of the newborn in the United States. JAMA 1991;265:3270–3274

Chitkara U, Bussel J, Alvarez M, Lynch L, Meisel RL, Berkowitz RL. High-dose intravaneous gamma globulin: does it have a role in the treatment of severe erythroblastosis fetalis? Obstet Gynecol 1990; 76:703–708

Gonsoulin WJ, Moise KJ Jr, Milam JD, Sala JD, Weber VW, Carpenter RJ Jr. Serial maternal blood donations for intrauterine transfusion. Obstet Gynecol 1990;75:158–162

Harman CR, Bowman JM, Manning FA, Menticoglou SM. Intrauterine transfusion—intraperitoneal versus intravascular approach: a case-control comparison. Am J Obstet Gynecol 1990;162:1053–1059

Ludomirsky A. Intrauterine fetal blood sampling—a multicenter registry, evaluation of 7462 procedures between 1987–1991. Am J Obstet Gynecol 1993;168(part 2):318 (abstract 69)

Spinnato JA. Hemolytic disease of the fetus: a plea for restraint. Obstet Gynecol 1992;80:873–877

Fetal Growth Retardation

Cunningham FG, MacDonald PC, Gant NF, Leveno KJ, Gilstrap LC III. Williams obstetrics. 19th ed. Norwalk, Connecticut: Appleton and Lange, 1993:853–889

Goldenberg RL, Cutter GR, Hoffman HJ, Foster JM, Nelson KG, Hauth JC. Intrauterine growth retardation: standards for diagnosis. Am J Obstet Gynecol 1989;161:271–277

Guidetti DA, Divon MY, Braverman JJ, Langer O, Merkatz IR. Sonographic estimates of fetal weight in the intrauterine growth retardation population. Am J Perinatol 1990;7:5–7

Seeds JW. Impaired fetal growth: definition and clinical diagnosis. Obstet Gynecol 1984;64:303–310

Shah DM, Brown JE, Salyer SL, Fleischer AC, Boehm FH. A modified scheme for biophysical profile scoring. Am J Obstet Gynecol 1989;160:586–591

Preterm Labor and Delivery

Boyer KM, Gadzala CA, Kelly PD, Gotoff SP. Selective intrapartum chemoprophylaxis of neonatal group B streptococcal early-onset disease, III: interruption of mother-to-infant transmission. J Infect Dis 1983;148:810–816

Creasy RK. Preterm labor and delivery. In: Creasy RK, Resnik R, eds. Maternal fetal medicine: principles and practice. 2nd ed. Philadelphia: WB Saunders, 1989:494–520

Cunningham FG, MacDonald PC, Gant NF, Leveno KJ, Gilstrap LC III. Preterm and postterm pregnancy and fetal growth retardation. In: Williams obstetrics. 19th ed. Norwalk, Connecticut: Appleton and Lange, 1993:853–859

Manning FA, Platt LD, Sipos L. Antepartum fetal evaluation: development of a fetal biophysical profile. Am J Obstet Gynecol 1980;136: 787–795

National Institutes of Health Consensus Development Conference on the Effect of Corticosteroids for Fetal Maturation on Perinatal Outcomes; February 28–March 2, 1994; Bethesda, Maryland

Rutherford SE, Smith CV, Phelan JP, Kawakami K, Ahn MO. Four-quadrant assessment of amniotic fluid volume: an adjunct to antepartum FHR testing. Obstet Gynecol 1987;70(3 part 1):353–356

Premature Rupture of Membranes

Cox SM, Williams ML, Leveno KJ. The natural history of preterm ruptured membranes: what to expect of expectant management. Obstet Gynecol 1988;71:558–562

Duff P, Huff RW, Gibbs RS. Management of premature rupture of membranes and unfavorable cervix in term pregnancy. Obstet Gynecol 1984;63:697–702

Mercer BM. Management of premature rupture of membranes before 26 weeks gestation. Obstet Gynecol Clin North Am 1992;19:33–35

Postterm Gestation

American College of Obstetricians and Gynecologists. Diagnosis and management of postterm pregnancy. ACOG Technical Bulletin 130. Washington, DC: ACOG, 1989

Cunningham FG, MacDonald PC, Gant NF, Leveno KJ, Gilstrap LC III. Williams obstetrics. 19th ed. Norwalk, Connecticut: Appleton and Lange, 1993:853–889

Hannah ME, Hannah WJ, Hellmann J, Hewson S, Miner R, Willan A. Induction of labor as compared with serial antenatal monitoring in post-term pregnancy: a randomized controlled trial. The Canadian Multicenter Post-term Pregnancy Trial Group. N Engl J Med 1992;326:1587–1592

Phelan JP, Platt LD, Yeh SY, Broussard P, Paul RH. The role of ultrasound assessment of amniotic fluid volume in the management of the postdate pregnancy. Am J Obstet Gynecol 1985;151:304–308

Medical Complications

CARDIAC DISEASE

Excluding mitral valve prolapse, which occurs in approximately 7% of the population, cardiac disease complicates approximately 1% of all pregnancies. It is a major nonobstetric cause of maternal death in the United States. With the decrease of rheumatic fever and its sequelae, congenital heart disease is now the predominant cause of most cardiac disease during pregnancy. This changing pattern has resulted from surgical advances in the treatment of congenital heart disease. Consideration of the hemodynamic effects of pregnancy becomes extremely important when planning therapy for the pregnant patient with cardiac disease.

Eisenmenger syndrome and other conditions associated with pulmonary hypertension pose a maternal risk of death as high as 50%, and death most commonly occurs in the postpartum period. Fetal growth retardation is a common finding, as well. Marfan syndrome carries a significant risk of aortic dissection during pregnancy. Patients should receive genetic counseling and be made aware of the risks of this condition. It has been suggested that a normal aortic root caliber on echocardiography is a reliable prognostic sign for such patients and that patients with a dilated aortic root (>40 mm) are at greatest risk for dissection and death.

Although most patients with mitral valve prolapse are asymptomatic, arrhythmias may be found, and bacterial endocarditis is reported to occur with increased frequency. While controversial, it has been recommended that uncomplicated patients with mitral valve prolapse be treated with prophylactic antibiotics for surgical procedures.

Prosthetic cardiac valves carry a high risk of thrombosis and subsequent embolization. Because of the significant fetal risk from warfarin anticoagulation therapy at any time during pregnancy, heparin is the anticoagulant of choice for the pregnant woman, despite the associated maternal risk. Given the teratogenic potential of warfarin and the difficulties that may arise with long-term heparin therapy, it is preferable for women of childbearing age to receive porcine valve transplants, which have a much lower propensity for thrombosis.

Pregnancy is often accompanied by physical changes that may be confused with underlying cardiac disease. The following symptoms, however, should alert the obstetrician to the presence of underlying cardiac disease: 1) any progressive limitation of physical activity due to worsening dyspnea, 2) chest pain that accompanies exercise or increased activity, and 3) syncope that is preceded by palpitations or physical exertion. Interpretation of standard techniques to investigate cardiac disease may be difficult in pregnancy. Chest films will often demonstrate cardiomegaly and venous congestion. Electrocardiographic findings in normal pregnancy may include ST–T depression and flattening of T waves. Echocardiography has therefore become the preferred technique for detection of cardiac abnormalities during pregnancy. Once a diagnosis has been established, it is clinically useful to assign a functional classification, such as the New York State Medical Association categories.

Antepartum Management

The successful management of cardiac disease during pregnancy requires close cooperation between the cardiologist and the obstetrician. Ideally, the patient's condition is evaluated by a cardiologist prior to conception so that all possible steps to ensure an adequate cardiac reserve can be taken before the physiologic changes of pregnancy have occurred. Although the type and degree of risk vary with the type of cardiac problem, certain physiologic principles are generally applicable.

Cardiac output increases 30–50% above prepregnancy values by 20–24 weeks of gestation, declining slightly during the last 10 weeks of gestation; thus, disease that tends to limit cardiac output (eg, mitral or aortic stenosis) may exert its maximal effects before the fetus is viable and may necessitate extensive limitation of physical activity to lessen demands on cardiac reserve. Conditions that tend to decrease venous return (eg, fever, hypoxia, and anemia) should be avoided. In a patient who demonstrates worsening symptoms, it is often necessary to institute changes in diet, activity, or medication. In doing so, one must carefully consider the potential for fetal effects with these therapeutic decisions. Patients with rheumatic heart disease should continue to take prescribed prophylactic antibiotics such as penicillin or erythromycin.

Intrapartum Management

Labor, delivery, and the postpartum period are critical times for patients with cardiac disease. In general, because the hemodynamic changes that occur with cesarean delivery are more rapid and dramatic than those that occur with vaginal delivery, maternal cardiac disease is not an indication for cesarean delivery. Contractions are accompanied by a significant increase in cardiac output, and the presence of pain and anxiety accentuates these changes. In addition, bearing down in the second stage of labor diminishes venous return. In cases in which tachycardia is best avoided, epidural anesthesia is recommended. Hypotension should be avoided. In patients with significant cardiac disease or high risk for failure during labor, many obstetricians use invasive central monitoring with a Swan–Ganz catheter to allow a minute-to-minute assessment of both right-sided and left-sided pressures in these patients. It is important to be alert to the possible development of arrhythmias during labor, and continuous cardiac monitoring is recommended.

Fetal Issues

There is a small increased risk of spontaneous preterm delivery in women with heart disease, particularly those with cyanotic congenital heart disease. Intrauterine growth retardation is common in these patients, as well. The incidence of congenital heart disease is about 4%; however, the disease in the offspring is not always clinically significant. High-resolution ultrasonography provides the potential for diagnosis of many fetal congenital cardiac defects and is recommended for patients who themselves have congenital cardiac disorders.

PULMONARY DISEASE

Pulmonary Embolus/Deep Vein Thrombophlebitis

Deep vein phlebitis has been estimated to occur in 0.13/1,000 antepartum women and 0.61/1,000 postpartum women. This increased incidence is believed to result both from mechanical changes in the venous system associated with pregnancy and from increases in most coagulation factors during pregnancy and the early postpartum period.

The clinical triad of *rubor, calor,* and *dolor* used to diagnose lower extremity thrombophlebitis usually does not apply during pregnancy. Most physicians, therefore, rely on such procedures as venography (with abdominal and pelvic shields), Doppler ultrasound examination, and impedance plethysmography to diagnose thrombophlebitis.

The diagnosis of pulmonary embolism is generally based on clinical suspicion and studies such as arterial blood gas determinations, electrocardiography, and chest radiography. Ventilation/perfusion lung scan and pulmonary angiography are used to make the definitive diagnosis. In skilled hands, the radiation exposure from these tests is very small and certainly well below the 0.05 Gy (5 rad) level that raises major fetal concerns. Because the mortality rate of untreated pulmonary embolism is extremely high, the benefits of these radiologic studies outweigh potential fetal risk.

The mainstay of therapy for thromboembolic disease is anticoagulation with heparin. Because of its molecular weight and negative charge, heparin does not cross the placenta. Anticoagulation should be maintained for the remainder of pregnancy and for several weeks postpartum. In the patient who has had a pulmonary embolus, the activated partial thromboplastin time should be kept at 1.5–2 times the upper limit of normal. Although warfarin anticoagulants have been used during pregnancy, their use is strongly discouraged. These agents, which are vitamin K antagonists, have been associated with fetal malformations. They have also been associated with hemorrhage in the fetus and placenta. The risk of some complications is considered to be 25% when anticoagulants are used in the first trimester, but such complications may occur at any time during pregnancy.

Asthma

Asthma occurs in 3–5% of adults. This obstructive respiratory disorder complicates 1% of pregnancies, with status asthmaticus occurring in 0.2% of all pregnancies. During pregnancy, approximately 50% of patients experience no change in the severity of their disease, 25% improve, and 25% worsen. The course of a patient's asthma in one pregnancy is not a predictor of how it will respond in other pregnancies. When asthma worsens, the physician must search for triggers such as respiratory tract infection, medications, allergens, gastrointestinal reflux, and exercise. Often, pregnant women stop taking medication when they learn they are pregnant, fearing potential fetal damage. Pregnant asthmatics must be encouraged to continue taking their medications, as most medications used by asthmatics are safe to use during pregnancy.

The degree of expiratory wheezing and the use of accessory muscles of respiration may be misleading in the pregnant woman and often do not mirror severity of disease. Although acrocyanosis is common during an asthma attack, central cyanosis warrants immediate aggressive therapy. Simple bedside or office testing of the forced vital capacity, the forced expiratory volume in 1 second, or the peak expiratory flow rate is extremely helpful to the clinician.

The goal of long-term therapy is to reduce the number and severity of attacks, and the goal of acute therapy is to alleviate hypoxia and to improve ventilation. The pharmacotherapy of asthma has greatly changed in the past few years. Whereas aminophylline and its derivatives were previously the mainstays of asthma therapy, current therapy focuses upon cytokines and other mediators of inflammation. Aerosolized beta-mimetic agents and aerosolized glucocorticoids have become the main treatments for asthma. In acute cases, subcutaneous epinephrine (0.3 ml of a diluted solution) or terbutaline (0.25 mg) can be used. Those who have previously responded well to aminophylline may be given this class of drugs. Of course, intravenous hydration is an important part of therapy. Those who do not respond rapidly should be started on intravenous glucocorticoids. If P_{CO_2} rises above 40 mm Hg or the P_{O_2} falls to less than 60 mm Hg with the oxygen saturation less than 90%, the patient may need intubation and mechanical ventilation. During pregnancy, special effort should be directed at maintaining an adequate P_{O_2}. Short courses of steroids may give the quickest relief of exacerbations with the fewest potential side effects to the fetus. Cromolyn inhibits mast cell degranulation and is most useful as single-agent treatment for young adults with exercise-induced asthma. It is not, however, useful for the acute treatment of asthma.

Adult Respiratory Distress Syndrome

The adult respiratory distress syndrome presents as acute respiratory failure caused by noncardiogenic pulmonary edema. The general pathophysiology appears to be an increased alveolar capillary permeability leading to hypoxemia secondary to decreased oxygen transport across the alveolus. In addition, there is often a significant degree of right-to-left intrapulmonary shunting. Attenuated alveolar type I cells are replaced by proliferating type II cells, and the interstitium becomes infiltrated with inflammatory cells. Pulmonary fibrosis follows rapidly, leading to obliteration of pulmonary capillaries and alveoli. During pregnancy, adult respiratory distress syndrome is seen in association with various infections, severe preeclampsia/eclampsia, disseminated intravascular coagulation, and malignancy.

Even in young, healthy women, the mortality rate from adult respiratory distress syndrome may exceed 50%. Hypoxemia is treated with O_2 in concentrations of 75–100%. If the Pa_{O_2} does not increase to above 60 mm Hg, intubation and mechanical ventilation should be used. The addition of positive end-expiratory pressure decreases both intrapulmonary shunting and capillary leak but at the expense of an increased risk of pneumothorax and a decreased cardiac output. While commonly used, high-dose corticosteroids do not appear to be of benefit in reducing the mortality rate from adult respiratory distress syndrome. In all but the mildest of cases of adult respiratory distress syndrome, the patient is best managed with invasive hemodynamic monitoring.

LIVER AND ALIMENTARY TRACT DISEASE

Cholestasis of Pregnancy

Intrahepatic cholestasis usually presents as pruritus during the third trimester of pregnancy. It begins insidiously as mild pruritus only at night and gradually increases to severe, unrelenting pruritus. It tends to recur in subsequent pregnancies. The pathophysiology remains unknown, and the histology is indistinguishable from that of other causes of cholestasis. Diagnosis is confirmed by demonstrating an increase in circulating bile acids (cholic and chenodeoxycholic acids). Generally, fasting levels three times the upper limit of normal are considered diagnostic. Additional changes include mild to moderate increases in levels of alanine aminotransferase and aspartate aminotransferase. The total bilirubin level is usually elevated but less than 86 mmol/L (5 mg/dl). Both impaired enterohepatic circulation of vitamin K and decreased production of the vitamin K-dependent clotting factors (II, VII, IX, X) may lead to prolongation of the prothrombin time in patients with severe and protracted cholestasis of pregnancy.

Intrahepatic cholestasis is associated with an increased incidence of prematurity, fetal distress, and fetal loss. The incidence of fetal compromise appears to be enough to warrant NST in the third trimester. Although deposits of bile salts have been described in the placenta, the mechanism by which they adversely affect the fetus is unknown.

Symptomatic relief may be achieved in a few patients with cornstarch baths or antihistamines such as diphenhydramine or hydroxyzine. Cholestyramine can be expected to reduce symptoms in 50% of cases, but its use is associated with mild nausea, anorexia, and bloating. Because cholestyramine may take more than 1 week to become maximally effective, therapy should be started as soon as cholestasis is diagnosed. Additionally, cholestyramine therapy interferes with the absorption of many medications and fat-soluble vitamins. Thus, the prothrombin time should be monitored periodically when this regimen is used. Also, other medications should be administered several hours after a dose of cholestyramine. Finally, high-dose S-adenosylmethionine has been reported to be very effective in reducing both symptoms and abnormal liver function tests.

Acute Fatty Liver of Pregnancy

Until recent years, acute fatty liver of pregnancy had a reported maternal mortality rate that approached 90%. Recent reports suggest, however, that with proper supportive care and early diagnosis and delivery, most patients survive. The disease presents most commonly during the third trimester in primigravidas. Initially, the patient experiences nonspecific constitutional symptoms and epigastric or abdominal pain that are followed in about a week with jaundice and neurologic symptoms. The serum amylase, creatinine, bilirubin (<171 mmol/L [<10 mg/dl]), uric acid, alanine aminotransferase, and aspartate aminotransferase levels are all elevated. The liver transaminase levels are usually in the range of 200–500 IU/L. Evidence of coagulation abnormalities, including hypofibrinogenemia, increased fibrin degradation products, thrombocytopenia, and prolongation of the prothrombin and activated partial thromboplastin times are characteristic as the disease progresses. Anemia and leukocytosis are also seen, with the anemia being caused by microangiopathic destruction of red blood cells. A liver biopsy specimen demonstrating infiltration of hepatocytes with small droplets of fat remains the definitive diagnostic study. Frozen section staining with oil red O stain gives a rapid diagnosis. Computed tomography and magnetic resonance imaging have been very helpful in establishing the diagnosis of acute fatty liver of pregnancy. The differential diagnoses include chemical hepatitis, cholangitis, hemolytic uremic syndrome, acute hepatitis, systematic lupus erythematosus, and preeclampsia/eclampsia.

Treatment of pregnant patients with acute fatty liver is immediate delivery. Multiple-system deterioration is common. Special attention should be directed to combating infection and treatment of coagulation dysfunction. Use of H_2 receptor antagonists helps reduce the incidence of gastrointestinal bleeding. While transaminase levels usually normalize promptly after delivery, other liver functions may remain abnormal for days to weeks. Patients with acute fatty liver of pregnancy often experience profound hypoglycemia, and this may be clinically helpful in making the diagnosis. There appears to be little recurrence risk for acute fatty liver.

Inflammatory Bowel Disease

Ulcerative colitis and Crohn disease are idiopathic disorders that have their peak incidence in the reproductive age group. Ulcerative colitis involves only the colon and rectum, whereas Crohn disease can be found from mouth to anus and may involve the perineum. Both disorders present with cramping pain, diarrhea, and weight loss, and in 10% of cases differentiation is impossible. Crohn disease, in contrast to ulcerative colitis, tends to run a more subacute and chronic course. Patients with colitis must be evaluated carefully for an infectious etiology before ascribing symptoms to inflammatory bowel disease. Rectal bleeding is less common in patients with Crohn disease, and the absence of rectal involvement essentially excludes ulcerative colitis. Extraintestinal manifestations of inflammatory bowel disease include arthritis of the spine, ocular inflammation, aphthous ulcers, hepatitis, and renal involvement with stones, fistula formation, and hydronephrosis.

Pregnancy has minimal, if any, increased risk to both mother and fetus. Because active disease appears to be associated with a slight increase in the spontaneous abortion rate, particularly in women with Crohn disease, these patients should delay conception until their disease is in remission. Pregnancy is associated with a 15–30% chance of exacerbation of inflammatory bowel disease. In patients with quiescent disease at conception, disease reactivation is uncommon. Treatment of inflammatory bowel disease is not altered greatly by pregnancy and includes oral sulfasalazine, oral or rectal corticosteroids, and occasionally immunosuppression and parenteral nutrition. Each of these medications can be continued during pregnancy. Surgery may be required for fistulas, bowel obstruction, hemorrhage, abscess formation, perforation, malignancy, or the failure of medical management.

Pregnancy After Gastrointestinal Bypass

After jejunoileal bypass, patients acutely lose weight and then either maintain a new lower weight or regain a small increment of the initial loss. Late complications of the procedure include diarrhea, diminished levels of folate or vitamin B_{12}, nephrolithiasis, cholelithiasis, and chronic liver dysfunction. While there are no apparent adverse effects of the surgery, evaluating glucose tolerance, liver function, and vitamin B_{12} and folate levels during early pregnancy is prudent. Water-soluble emulsions of fat-soluble vitamins should be used.

NEUROLOGIC DISEASES

Seizure Disorders

Affecting 1–2 million Americans, seizure disorders are the most common neurologic problems that coexist with pregnancy. Approximately 75% of these disorders are idiopathic in nature. In general, idiopathic seizures can be categorized into generalized tonic/clonic seizures, partial complex seizures that may or may not generalize, and absence seizures (petit mal). In general, the ability to measure and monitor drug levels has had a major impact on the effect of pregnancy on epilepsy. Some studies have shown that seizure disorders deteriorate during pregnancy. If, however, drug levels are monitored at regular intervals and the dosages adjusted accordingly, patients can achieve excellent seizure control throughout pregnancy. Drug levels will change throughout pregnancy, depending on the route of metabolism of drug taken. Hepatic microsomal enzyme levels can increase during pregnancy, making levels of medications lower and requiring that more drug be given. It is important to realize that the amount of drug given is not the important factor but rather the level of drug in the patient's blood. For example, a patient whose epilepsy is readily controlled with 300 mg of phenytoin daily when she is not pregnant may require 600 mg of phenytoin daily during gestation to keep her phenytoin levels therapeutic.

There is much debate over the effect of epilepsy on pregnancy. It appears that there may be an increase in fetal malformations in women with untreated seizure disorders. There is no doubt that some of the medications used in the treatment of epilepsy are teratogenic, but the rates of teratogenesis are controversial. Phenytoin has been associated with the fetal hydantoin syndrome. This syndrome, which was first described in 1976, consists of microcephaly, mild to moderate mental retardation, developmental delay, facial clefts, facial dysmorphisms, limb anomalies, and genital malformations. Features of this syndrome have been reported in 11% of infants; some researchers, however, feel that this is a large overestimation. The incidence of the full-blown syndrome is much lower. Phenobarbital is generally thought to be a drug that is safe to use during pregnancy. There have, however, been reports of some malformations with its use. Carbamazepine has also generally been thought to be a safe drug to use during pregnancy, although there have been reports of an increase in cranial facial defects and NTDs. Valproate has been associated with NTDs in a larger number of patients. Women taking valproate or carbamazepine should be offered assessment for NTD, including detailed ultrasonography and serum alpha-fetoprotein screening.

The risk of malformations with most of these medications, although greater than the expected rate of the general population, is still rather small. It is very important that the patient continue her medication and avoid seizures, as tonic/clonic seizures occurring during gestation can result in devastating outcomes for both mother and fetus. The role of folic acid to prevent NTDs is still somewhat controversial. Nonetheless, in patients taking anticonvulsant medications, supplemental folic acid holds no risks and may provide benefits. Fortunately, the patient with a seizure disorder most often successfully carries a pregnancy to term with no problems.

If possible, the patient should be counseled before conception. If she has not had seizures in many years, an attempt may be made to withdraw her gradually from her anticonvulsant medication. If treatment is necessary and the patient receives prepregnancy counseling, her medication may be changed to one with a smaller chance of causing a malformation. If she is taking phenytoin or valproate, it may be changed to phenobarbital, primidone, or carbamazepine. If, however, phenytoin or valproate is the only drug that controls her seizures, she should continue to take these medications.

Ultrasonography should be performed at 18–20 weeks of gestation to evaluate the fetus for possible anomalies. The patient should be monitored frequently for fetal growth; if there is evidence of poor growth, serial ultrasound examinations should be performed. Primidone, phenobarbital, and phenytoin have been shown to potentially inhibit fetal production of vitamin K. Infants exposed to these drugs in utero carry a risk of coagulopathy at birth. Some clinicians recommend giving mothers prophylactic vitamin K in the third trimester, but this is controversial. The infant should be given intramuscular vitamin K at birth. A pediatrician should be available during delivery in case an unexpected anomaly is found.

In labor, oral absorption of medication does not readily occur. If the patient appears to be having a prolonged labor, intramuscular phenobarbital or intravenous phenytoin may be used to continue anticonvulsant therapy. Anticonvulsant medication levels should be assessed often to prevent toxicity.

Myasthenia Gravis

Myasthenia gravis is an autoimmune disorder caused by antibodies directed against acetylcholine receptors on smooth muscle. Because myasthenia gravis has a predilection for women in their 20s and 30s, its occurrence in pregnant women is not rare. Pregnancy probably has no significant effect on the course of this disease, but abrupt exacerbations and remissions do occur during pregnancy. Labor and delivery, with their increased work requirements and the risks of anesthesia, are critical times for such patients.

Most myasthenic patients are treated with oral anticholinesterase drugs, which have no known adverse fetal effects. The most commonly used of these drugs is pyridostigmine. Because gastrointestinal absorption is poor during labor, it is necessary to use a parenteral preparation during labor and delivery. Anesthesia consultation is recommended. Overdosage of cholinesterase-inhibiting drugs may result in cholinergic crises. This problem may be difficult to distinguish from inadequate anticholinesterase therapy, however, because both are characterized by muscular weakness. Consequently, those caring for such patients during labor and delivery should be prepared to administer edrophonium at a test dose of 2–10 mg IV. An improvement in symptoms suggests inadequate anticholinesterase therapy, while a deterioration suggests cholinergic crisis.

Narcotic analgesics, such as meperidine, may be given, although patients may be more sensitive to their effects. The most common problems during labor, delivery, surgery, and the postoperative period are respiratory in nature and should be anticipated. Magnesium sulfate is contraindicated in patients with myasthenia gravis. Its use can lead to respiratory failure and death. Furthermore, aminoglycoside antibiotics must be used with caution in myasthenic patients. In a patient whose condition deteriorates, plasmapheresis may be used to ameliorate symptoms rapidly and effectively.

Neonatal myasthenia gravis, a transient phenomenon believed to be caused by transplacental passage of maternal antibodies against the acetylcholine receptor, occurs in approximately 10% of newborns whose mothers have myasthenia gravis. The most common symptoms are decreased neonatal tone and a poor sucking reflex.

Paraplegia–Quadriplegia

Patients with spinal cord injuries are often desirous of and able to successfully complete a pregnancy. If the patient has a cord transection above the T-6 level, she may develop a syndrome of autonomic hyperreflexia. The syndrome is characterized by headache, hypertension, reflex bradycardia, nasal congestion, and cutaneous vasodilatation and piloerection above the level of the lesion. It can be life-threatening during labor. The syndrome can be prevented by the use of lumbar epidural anesthesia, which results in effective sympathectomy. Additional complications include urinary tract infections, decubitus ulcers, anemia, and premature labor.

The uterus itself contracts normally during labor. Because patients with lesions above the T-10 level usually do not feel their uterine contractions, the cervix should be examined at each visit after week 28 of gestation. Also, the patient can be taught to palpate for uterine contractions. Most patients are not able to push effectively, and in the second stage of labor, the operator may need to use forceps or vacuum extraction.

Cerebrovascular Disease

Cerebral infarction and transient ischemic attacks are rare in young women. The most frequent site of occlusion is the middle cerebral artery. While atherosclerosis is the major cause of stroke in older patients, it is responsible for less than 25% of cases during pregnancy. Other causes such as atrial fibrillation, paradoxical embolism from deep vein thrombosis of the lower extremities, and endocarditis should be sought. Headache and seizures accompanying unilateral weakness or paralysis are often the symptoms of vasoocclusive disease. The diagnosis is made by computed tomography scanning, magnetic resonance imaging, and cerebral arteriography. Anticoagulation with heparin or antiaggregant treatment with aspirin is initiated if there is no evidence of bleeding. If the lesion is isolated and accessible, surgical removal may be considered. Vaginal delivery, unless obstetrically contraindicated, is preferable to cesarean delivery.

Subarachnoid hemorrhage is responsible for about 10% of maternal deaths. For women under age 25, arteriovenous malformations are the most common cause of hemorrhage. Berry aneurysms of the vessels of the circle of Willis are the common cause for these bleeding episodes in women over 25. The most common presenting symptom is a severe, unrelenting headache. The diagnosis of subarachnoid hemorrhage can be made by finding red blood cells in the cerebrospinal fluid upon lumbar puncture. Computed tomography scanning and cerebral arteriography are essential to clarify the diagnosis, localize the lesion, and guide therapy. Treatment consists of bed rest, analgesia, and operative correction of the lesion, if possible. Angiography is essential to determine whether any additional uncorrected lesions are present. After successful surgery, patients can undergo labor and delivery without intervention. If the lesions are uncorrected or incompletely ligated, cesarean delivery is usually recommended. If the patient is allowed to labor, elimination of the Valsalva maneuver during the second stage of labor is mandatory.

Multiple Sclerosis

Multiple sclerosis has no adverse effect on pregnancy, and pregnancy has no detrimental effect on multiple sclerosis. Subclinical disease, however, is often first discovered during pregnancy. The cause of multiple sclerosis remains unknown. Pathologically, there is focal demyelination, and clinically, there are periods of exacerbation and remission. No specific cure is available, and high-dose corticosteroids are occasionally used to treat acute exacerbations. Pregnancy appears to stabilize the disease, acute exacerbations being far less common than during a similar time period in nonpregnant women. After delivery, however, there is a twofold to threefold increase in the rate of exacerbation.

Conduction anesthesia is generally discouraged. There are no differences in the long-term disabilities of women with no, one, or two or more pregnancies.

MIGRAINE HEADACHES

Between 15% and 20% of pregnant women are affected by migraine headaches. Migraine symptoms may improve or deteriorate during pregnancy. Those patients who experience their worst headaches during the time of their menses improve the most during pregnancy. Smokers are more likely to suffer from migraine headaches during pregnancy than nonsmokers. In nonsmokers, migraines are often associated with allergies.

Supportive therapy must be used for the pregnant patient with migraines. Analgesics, including narcotic analgesics, can be used as necessary. Nonsteroidal antiinflammatory agents should be avoided in late pregnancy because of potential fetal side effects. Other serious causes of headache must be excluded, especially if the patient experiences migraines for the first time during pregnancy. Some patients benefit from beta blockers and others benefit from calcium channel blockers. Patients should look for dietary factors that trigger migraines.

DIABETES MELLITUS

Preexisting Diabetes

Preexisting diabetes mellitus complicates approximately 0.5–1.0% of pregnancies. Fetal and neonatal mortality rates have declined from approximately 65% before the discovery of insulin to 2–5% at the present time. If one excludes congenital malformations, the perinatal mortality rate for diabetic women receiving optimal care is nearly equivalent to that of the nondiabetic population. This dramatic improvement in outcome has resulted from general advances in perinatal care and primarily from a team approach stressing implementation of excellent glycemic control in pregnant diabetic women. The availability of sophisticated methods for fetal surveillance and lung maturity has also provided a rational basis for deciding the optimum timing of delivery. The general goals for management of the diabetic pregnancy include delivery, at or near term by the vaginal route if possible, of a baby who does not experience morbidity as a result of maternal diabetes mellitus.

Blood Glucose Self-Monitoring

Blood glucose self-monitoring, combined with aggressive insulin therapy, has made maintenance of maternal normoglycemia a therapeutic reality. In most institutions, patients are instructed to monitor their glucose continually by using glucose–oxidase-impregnated reagent strips and a portable reflectance meter. Glucose determinations are made in the fasting state and before meals. Postprandial and nocturnal values may be helpful, as well. Target plasma glucose values include fasting values less than 100 mg/dl, preprandial values 60–105 mg/dl, and 2-hour postprandial values less than 120 mg/dl. All patients and their families should be instructed in the use of glucagon to treat serious hypoglycemia. Patients who have achieved good glycemic control can be treated as outpatients. Early hospitalization is necessary for women whose condition is in poor control or those unfamiliar with techniques of blood glucose self-monitoring.

Insulin and Diet Therapy

Most pregnant diabetic women can be managed with an insulin regimen consisting of multiple injections of mixtures of short-acting and intermediate-acting insulin, timed to maintain the blood sugar in the normal range for pregnancy (60–120 mg/dl). The insulin pump has not been determined to be superior to the multiple-injection regimen and is generally reserved for patients whose condition is well controlled with this method prior to conception.

Diet therapy is critical to successful regulation of maternal diabetes. Most diets include 30–35 kcal/kg of ideal body weight, with a high protein intake (90–125 g) and the addition of a snack between meals. Dietary therapy must be tailored to time of day and physical activity. Flexibility is necessary to suit the patient's preferences and work schedule.

Fetal Surveillance

Early ultrasound examination to assess dating accurately is suggested for women with diabetes mellitus. A careful search for congenital malformations should be instituted when the patient is scanned between 16 and 20 weeks of gestation. Serum alpha-fetoprotein determinations should also be made at this time. There is evidence that diabetic women have lower alpha-fetoprotein values than the normal population, requiring that an adjustment be made for selection of cutoff points to screen for various defects. Repeated ultrasound examinations at monthly intervals between 28 weeks of gestation and term are useful in establishing the pattern of fetal growth and amniotic fluid volume.

Programs of fetal surveillance are initiated in the third trimester, when the risk of sudden intrauterine death appears to be greatest. The severity of the diabetes and the presence of other complicating factors (such as nephropathy, hypertension, or fetal growth disturbances) should determine the onset and frequency of fetal testing. Biophysical testing should be performed at least weekly and more often if complicating factors are present. Many centers actually prefer to perform these tests biweekly in diabetic patients. The primary benefit of normal test results is reassurance to the obstetrician and the patient, which safely allows further fetal maturation. For women with severe vascular disease, testing is often initiated at the time of potential extrauterine viability, whereas surveillance may be delayed as late as 35 weeks of gestation in patients whose diabetes is well controlled and whose pregnancy is uncomplicated. The NST, oxytocin challenge testing, nipple stimulation testing, BPP determination, and maternal assessment of fetal activity are all accepted methods of fetal evaluation.

Timing of Delivery

Prior to a decade ago, elective preterm delivery of the insulin-dependent patient to avoid sudden unexpected intrauterine fetal demise was commonplace and resulted in a high incidence of neonatal morbidity and mortality. Improved glycemic control and reliable methods of fetal surveillance now allow most diabetic women to be delivered at term. However, the rate of elective intervention at 38–39 weeks of gestation is high in insulin-dependent patients. It is critical not only to use results of fetal surveillance testing but also to recognize the clinical features of each pregnancy before making a decision to intervene. This includes evaluation of the degree of glycemic control, hypertension, nephropathy, and the patient's ophthalmologic status.

Unless excellent gestational dating has been established in a patient with good glycemic control who has reached 39 weeks of gestation, it is prudent to perform an amniocentesis prior to elective delivery to document fetal lung maturity. In patients with good glycemic control who do not have vascular disease, intervention may be delayed until the patient reaches her expected date of delivery.

The route of delivery for the diabetic patient continues to be controversial. Cesarean delivery is favored when a nonreassuring FHR pattern is present. Cesarean delivery is also reserved for cases in which the cervix cannot be ripened or excessive fetal size is suspected. Various estimated weight cutoffs ranging from 4,000 to 4,500 g have been suggested for considering a cesarean delivery, because of the increased frequency of traumatic shoulder dystocia in such cases.

Prevention of Congenital Anomalies

The incidence of congenital anomalies is increased threefold among infants of diabetic mothers, compared with the general population; congenital anomalies now account for most of the perinatal deaths in these patients. Anomalies of the cardiac, renal, vertebral, and central nervous systems arise during the first 8 weeks of gestation, a time when it is unusual for patients to seek prenatal care. Therefore, the management and counseling of women with diabetes in the reproductive age group should begin prior to conception. The high incidence of birth defects appears to be related to poor metabolic control during the periconceptional period. Poor periconceptional glycemic control may also increase the risk for spontaneous abortion. Counseling prior to conception, with improvement of glycemic status, is essential if anomalies and spontaneous abortions are to be reduced. Glycosylated hemoglobin is a commonly used marker for metabolic control over a preceding 2–3-month interval. Most authorities recommend that diabetic women be counseled to delay pregnancy until glycosylated hemoglobin is in the normal or near-normal range.

Gestational Diabetes

Gestational diabetes has been defined as a state restricted to pregnant women whose impaired glucose tolerance is discovered during pregnancy. The clinical significance of gestational diabetes continues to be challenged. This dilemma exists largely because all current studies include identified and treated women and fail to demonstrate an increase in perinatal deaths. Early studies of untreated gestational diabetes, including observations of a Pima Indian population undergoing glucose challenge testing without the assignment of any diagnosis, have demonstrated an increase in perinatal mortality rate. Morbidities such as fetal macrosomia, traumatic or operative delivery, neonatal hypoglycemia, and jaundice are all increased in such pregnancies. Recent evidence suggests that childhood and adult obesity, as well as diabetes, may be increased among offspring of gestational diabetic mothers. Survey data suggest that most clinicians in the United States consider gestational diabetes a clinical entity worth identifying and treating.

Screening

Ninety percent of cases of diabetes that complicate pregnancy are gestational diabetes. Traditionally, pregnant women with preexisting risk factors (family history of diabetes, previous macrosomic baby, poor obstetric history, history of glycosuria) were screened for gestational diabetes. It has been demonstrated that such risk factors fail to identify approximately 40–60% of women with gestational diabetes in the population. Although there is a lack of data to support the benefit of screening, many centers, but not all, have instituted universal screening of pregnant women. The most widely used screening test is the measurement of plasma glucose 1 hour after the administration of a 50-g oral glucose load. This test is generally performed at 24–28 weeks of gestation. A 3-hour 100-g oral glucose tolerance test should be performed on any patient whose screening test value exceeds 140 mg/dl.

Normal values for the glucose tolerance test differ during pregnancy from those used in the nonpregnant state. Table 3-12 lists two conversions of the O'Sullivan criteria. Any two values meeting or exceeding the threshold confirm the diagnosis of gestational diabetes.

Treatment

Women with gestational diabetes mellitus generally do not require hospitalization for dietary instruction and management. Gestational diabetic women should be counseled as to an appropriate diet, usually consisting of 2,000–2,500 kcal daily with the exclusion of simple carbohydrates. The most important intervention in gestational diabetic women is surveillance of blood glucose levels during the third trimester. Plasma glucose levels should be measured in the fasting state and postprandially at least every week. Some clinicians prefer to use daily glucose self-testing for such patients. The threshold for initiating insulin therapy in gestational diabetes is somewhat arbitrary. Many clinicians feel that if fasting plasma glucose values exceed 100 mg/dl or postprandial values exceed 120 mg/dl, the perinatal mortality rate is probably increased and that insulin therapy should be initiated to achieve euglycemia. In such cases, however, human insulin should be used. For gestational diabetic women receiving insulin, or those with hypertension or history of stillbirth, fetal evaluation should be instituted in a fashion similar to that described for women with overt diabetes. If plasma glucose levels remain in the normal range during pregnancy, perinatal mortality is probably not increased.

TABLE 3-12. DETECTION OF GESTATIONAL DIABETES

Test	Plasma Glucose Level* (mg/dl)	
50-g, 1 h, screen	130–140	
	O'Sullivan Criteria	
100-g, oral glucose tolerance test	NDDG[†] conversion	Carpenter conversion
Fasting	105	95
1 h	190	180
2 h	165	155
3 h	145	140

* Result is upper limit of normal.
[†] NDDG is the National Diabetes Data Group.
Data from Carpenter MW, Coustan DR. Criteria for screening tests for gestational diabetes. Am J Obstet Gynecol 1982;144:768–773; National Diabetes Data Group. Classification and diagnosis of diabetes mellitus and other categories of glucose intolerance. Diabetes 1979;28:1039–1057

The woman with gestational diabetes may be safely monitored until 40 weeks, as long as fasting and postprandial glucose values remain normal. As with pregestational diabetic patients, ultrasonography is used to help identify macrosomia.

THYROID DISEASE

Laboratory assessment of thyroid function is altered by the hormonal changes of pregnancy. The most significant finding is a rise in T_4-binding globulin (TBG) to levels twice normal by the end of the first trimester. Hyperestrogenic states such as pregnancy induce hepatic biosynthesis of TBG. More than 99% of thyroid hormone is bound to TBG. Measurements of total serum T_4 by radioimmunoassay include bound as well as the minute free fraction of T_4. It is this free fraction that exerts it biologic activity. Free levels of T_4 and triiodothyronine (T_3) are not significantly elevated during pregnancy. Direct measurements of free levels of T_3 and T_4 are the most accurate method for assessing thyroid function when increased TBG concentration is present. However, assays for free T_3 and T_4 are not widely available, so that an estimate of free hormone activity is generally obtained by using the resin T_3 uptake test (RT_3U).

The RT_3U serves as an indirect assay for TBG concentration. Pregnancy and other conditions in which the TBG is elevated produce more unoccupied resin-binding sites and therefore decreased resin uptake of radioiodine-labeled T_3. In pregnancy complicated by hyperthyroidism, the R_3TU is elevated. This reflects saturation of the patient's TBG with thyroid hormone, thereby allowing the resin to bind more tracer. In practice, a free T_4 index is calculated based on the R_3TU and total T_4 (free T_4 index $[FT_4I] = T_4 \times$ [patient RT_3U/normal RT_3U]). An elevated FT_4I is consistent with hyperthyroidism, just as a low value reflects hypothyroidism.

The most sensitive test for the detection of primary hypothyroidism is a measurement of serum TSH. Serum TSH concentrations remain normal during pregnancy. Elevated values in the presence of a low FT_4I reflect primary hypothy-roidism. Occasionally, elevated values are observed in the presence of a normal FT_4I. This reflects pituitary stimulation of a marginally active gland. In this case, early thyroid failure may be diagnosed and treated.

Hyperthyroidism

Thyrotoxicosis has been reported to occur in 1/500 pregnancies and may be associated with an increase in the incidence of prematurity and low birth weight. There is debate as to whether PIH is more common in hyperthyroid women. Most women with mild to moderate hyperthyroidism tolerate pregnancy well. The major threat to pregnancy is posed by thyroid storm, or uncontrolled hyperthyroidism. The diagnosis of hyperthyroidism may be difficult because symptoms may be confused with some of the normal physiologic changes of pregnancy, including tachycardia, increased cardiac output, warm skin, and heat intolerance. As noted earlier, laboratory testing during pregnancy requires calculation of FT_4I. In rare cases, FT_4I will be normal; however, free T_3 is elevated (T_3 thyrotoxicosis). Treatment during gestation involves antithyroid medication or surgery.

Radioactive ablation of the thyroid gland is contraindicated during pregnancy, as by 10 weeks of gestation the fetus may concentrate ^{131}I, resulting in hypothyroidism. Propylthiouracil is the most commonly used medication. This thioamide blocks peripheral conversion of T_4 and T_3 and inhibits thyroid hormone synthesis. The usual starting dose of 300 mg is best administered initially in divided doses every 8 hours because of its short half-life. Administration of propylthiouracil can be tapered off once improvement in symptoms such as normalization of pulse and weight gain and return to normal FT_4I occurs. These therapeutic effects do not usually occur until 2–4 weeks after the initiation of treatment. Minor side effects are frequent in patients receiving antithyroid drugs. Agranulocytosis is a serious complication, requiring leukocyte count evaluation should a patient develop fever and infection. Because propylthiouracil crosses the placenta and suppresses fetal thyroid function, maternal thyroid activity should be maintained in the upper ranges of normal, or slightly hyperthyroid, with the lowest possible dose of propylthiouracil, to avoid fetal effect (hypothyroidism). Transient mild hypothyroxinemia and elevated TSH values have been observed in the offspring of women treated with antithyroid medications. Thyroidectomy as treatment for hyperthyroidism is performed during pregnancy and should be considered for patients who do not respond to medical therapy or who exhibit excessive side effects.

Careful evaluation of the neonate for potential hyperthyroidism is also important. It is estimated that 1% of women with Graves disease will give birth to an infant with neonatal hyperthyroidism. The onset of disease may be delayed in women treated with antithyroid medication. Thyroid stimulation of the fetus probably occurs from maternal passage of thyroid-stimulating immunoglobulin. Most cases of neonatal hyperthyroidism are transient, although if progressive and unrecognized, actual nervous system damage is possible.

Hypothyroidism

Maternal hypothyroidism is rare because women with significantly reduced gland function are generally infertile. The clinical diagnosis of hypothyroidism may be extremely difficult. Nonspecific symptoms such as lethargy and weakness are often present. Weight gain and cold sensitivity may accompany physical signs, including myxedematous changes, hair loss, and cool, dry skin. The diagnosis rests on the presence of a low FT_4I and an elevated serum TSH level. Treatment consists of sufficient replacement of thyroid hormone to achieve a euthyroid state. The dosage of levothyroxine should be titrated to the serum TSH concentration. Occasionally, a pregnant patient may present taking thyroid replacement without well-documented hypothyroidism. Proper evaluation of such patients would require discontinuance of replacement for 1 month and then assaying TSH levels. Because hypothyroidism may pose a risk to mother and fetus, replacement therapy is not interrupted during pregnancy. Thyroid-stimulating hormone and FT_4I indices should be monitored to determine proper dosage to achieve a euthyroid state.

Postpartum Thyroid Disease

A form of autoimmune thyroiditis has been described, in which there is transient hyperthyroidism starting 1–3 months postpartum and progressing to hypothyroidism in one third of patients at 4–6 months postpartum, with the remainder going into remission. The temporary hyperthyroidism is thought to result from thyroiditis causing a release of stored thyroid hormone. Thioamide treatment during the hyperthyroid state is inappropriate, as it would hasten the appearance of hypothyroidism. The hypothyroidism is accompanied by the usual signs and symptoms, and it is appropriate to treat such women with adequate thyroid hormone replacement. Since few patients remain permanently hypothyroid, it is prudent to discontinue such therapy after 3 months to evaluate thyroid function. Postpartum thyroiditis may recur with subsequent pregnancies.

HEMATOLOGIC DISORDERS

Anemias

In general, anemia is defined as a hemoglobin value less than two standard deviations below the mean of a normal population. This definition for pathologic anemia does not hold true during pregnancy. With plasma volume expanding approximately 50% and red blood cell mass increasing only about 25%, many women experience a physiologic decrease in hematocrit values.

Iron deficiency anemia is the most common pathologic anemia encountered during pregnancy. An iron-replete woman has a 2-g iron store, 65% of which is found in circulating red blood cells. Ferritin, located in the liver, bone marrow, and spleen, constitutes 25% (0.5 g) of normal storage iron. If the interval between pregnancies is short, if the previous pregnancy was complicated by significant hemorrhage, or if dietary intake is poor, iron deficiency anemia readily develops.

The first pathologic change to develop is the depletion of bone marrow, liver, and spleen iron stores. The serum iron concentration falls, as does the saturation percentage of transferrin. The total iron-binding capacity, a reflection of unbound transferrin, rises and then the hematocrit falls. Because of the decrease in iron stores, hypochromic, microcytic red blood cells are released into the peripheral circulation.

In pregnancy, laboratory evaluation of iron deficiency anemia may be confusing. A peripheral smear demonstrating microcytic, hypochromic red blood cells is very suggestive of iron deficiency. Because of the normal increase of certain proteins during pregnancy, total iron-binding capacity may be elevated in 15% of pregnant women who are iron replete. In general, a serum iron concentration less than 60 mg/dl with less than 16% saturation of transferrin is diagnostic of iron deficiency anemia. Even though serum ferritin levels decrease mildly during pregnancy, a greatly depressed serum ferritin level is the best indicator of decreased iron stores. Bone marrow biopsies are rarely necessary in pregnancy to determine the adequacy of iron stores.

In pregnancy, the duodenum absorbs 1.3–2.6 mg of elemental iron daily in patients who are iron replete. Absorption increases in patients with iron deficiency. In patients who do not show signs of iron deficiency anemia, it is unclear whether iron prophylaxis increases the hematocrit at term.

Most of the common iron preparations contain 35–100 mg of elemental iron, with approximately 10% being absorbed in the duodenum. Most obstetricians prescribe one iron tablet three times daily to the patient with iron deficiency anemia, although this amount may not be necessary. Because of gastrointestinal side effects, most obstetricians have patients ingest their iron supplements with meals.

If the patient is purely iron deficient, the obstetrician should see a reticulocytosis within 2 weeks of beginning iron therapy. Iron absorption is pH dependent, so taking iron with antacids will decrease absorption.

Folic Acid Deficiency

Folic acid is a water-soluble member of the B complex group of vitamins. A woman's dietary requirement for folate is generally 0.05 mg/d, but it increases to 0.5–1.0 mg daily during normal pregnancy. Approximately 10–25% of pregnant women have low serum folate levels. Even without folic acid supplementation during pregnancy, less than 5% will develop megaloblastic anemia. Diagnostic findings include macrocytic anemia with elliptocytes, decreased white blood cell and platelet counts, low serum folate levels, and megaloblastosis on examination of the bone marrow. Hypersegmentation of polymorphonuclear leukocytes also occurs. Patients with multiple gestations, hemoglobinopathies, or those taking phenytoin are more likely to develop a folic acid deficiency. Treatment consists of the oral administration of folic acid in a dosage of 1–2 mg, up to four times daily. Folic acid supplementation has also been recommended by the CDC as a means of preventing NTDs (see "Preconceptional Care" in the section on Office Practice).

Although vitamin B_{12} deficiency is a rare cause of megaloblastic anemia in young women, it is essential to rule out vitamin B_{12} deficiency before embarking on a therapeutic course with folic acid. The inappropriate use of folic acid for the treatment of megaloblastic anemia secondary to vitamin B_{12} deficiency may result in irreversible neurologic changes.

Thalassemia

The thalassemia syndromes are characterized by defective production of hemoglobin secondary to a defect in the rate of globin synthesis. Any of the polypeptide chains can be affected. The disease may range from minimal depression of synthesis of the affected chain to its complete absence. This is an inherited condition, with the heterozygous form (thalassemia minor) being the most common. Those with β-thalassemia are usually of either Mediterranean or African ancestry, and those with α-thalassemia are usually of Oriental ancestry. The anemia of patients with thalassemia minor is mild to moderate and is of lifelong duration. Fetuses with α-thalassemia major often develop hydrops fetalis. Those who survive tend to have IUGR. β-Thalassemia major, also known as Cooley anemia, is associated with transfusion dependence, marked hepatosplenomegaly, and bone marrow changes secondary to increased hematopoiesis. These individuals usually die of cardiovascular or infectious complications before the third decade of life. However, with advances in transfusion science, many of these patients are reaching childbearing age, and successful, full-term pregnancies have been reported.

The heterozygous form of β-thalassemia can have different forms of expression. Patients with β-thalassemia minima are totally asymptomatic. Those with thalassemia intermedia exhibit splenomegaly and significant anemia and may become transfusion dependent during pregnancy. Most patients with β-thalassemia minor have the milder forms of the disease. The peripheral smear of a patient with β-thalassemia minor shows microcytic hypochromic red blood cells with increased stippling. There is also an increased number of target cells. Patients have normal or high levels of serum iron and normal total-iron binding capacities. The diagnostic test is hemoglobin electrophoresis, which shows abnormally high levels of hemoglobin A_2 or hemoglobin F, with suppressed levels of hemoglobin A_1. This is due to the fact that, although patients cannot produce adequate β chains, they can synthesize δ chains and γ chains. The peripheral smears of patients with α-thalassemia minor are similar, as are the iron studies. The hemoglobin electrophoresis, however, is normal, and the diagnosis is dependent on demonstrating the abnormal rate of α chain synthesis in comparison to that of β chains.

It is important to screen other members of the family for thalassemia once the diagnosis is made, because this is a genetic disorder. Pregnant women with thalassemia minor should see a genetic counselor, and the father of the baby should also be tested. This is important because, as previously mentioned, the homozygous form of thalassemia can result in fetal complications as well as many complications later in life.

In general, pregnancy has little effect on patients with thalassemia minor and thalassemia minima, and no treatment is indicated. These patients should not undergo iron supplementation unless serum studies show a decrease in serum iron. These patients are usually iron replete, although their hemoglobin levels are low, and may experience abnormal iron deposition in the liver and other organs if they receive much iron supplementation. Patients with thalassemia intermedia often experience symptoms similar to sickle cell anemia and should be treated like patients who have sickle cell disease.

Sickle Hemoglobinopathies

Hemoglobin S is the result of a single substitution of valine for glutamic acid in position 6 of the β chain of hemoglobin. While normal red blood cells have a half-life of 120 days, red blood cells containing predominantly hemoglobin S have a half-life of 5–10 days. These red blood cells can become sickle shaped and can sludge in small blood vessels. Sickling is usually triggered by decreased oxygen tension, acidosis, or dehydration. The sickle cell hemoglobinopathies are inherited in an autosomal codominant manner. Approximately one twelfth of African–Americans are heterozygous for hemoglobin S and thus have sickle cell trait (hemoglobin AS). These individuals are asymptomatic. The child of two individuals with sickle cell trait has a 25% risk of inheriting sickle cell anemia (hemoglobin SS). The theoretic risk of an African–American, whose parents have an unknown sickle cell status, being born with sickle cell anemia is $1/12 \times 1/12 \times 1/4 = 1/576$. In reality, the incidence among African–American pregnant women is much lower.

The diagnosis of sickle cell disease is made by hemoglobin electrophoresis, which is indicated when sickle cell screen test results are positive. Patients will show mostly hemoglobins with a little hemoglobin A_2 and hemoglobin F. Prenatal diagnosis can be performed by DNA analysis.

Painful vasoocclusive episodes secondary to sludging of red blood cells are the clinical hallmark of sickle cell anemia. These crises can affect any organ system but most commonly affect the extremities, joints, and abdomen. When they occur in the lung, they can cause pulmonary infarction. These patients are at an increased risk of pyelonephritis and lose the ability to concentrate their urine. Furthermore, they undergo infarction of the spleen and, therefore, are at an increased risk for infection with *Streptococcus pneumoniae*. They therefore should receive the vaccine against pneumococcus. Because of their constant hemolysis, patients with sickle cell disease often experience cholelithiasis with bilirubin stones.

Prepregnancy counseling is important in caring for women with sickle cell disease. Once the patient becomes pregnant, she should be screened regularly for urinary tract infections. Iron levels should be ascertained, and supplemental iron should be administered only if there is clear evidence of iron deficiency. Conversely, folic acid supplementation is essential. Blood pressures should be monitored closely because of the increased risk of preeclampsia. Sickle crises should be treated with analgesia, oxygen, and hydration. The role of prophylactic transfusion with leukocyte-poor red blood cells is controversial. Patients should, however, be transfused if the anemia becomes symptomatic or if the crises do not resolve with the previously mentioned conservative measures.

There is a high risk of poor perinatal outcome in women with sickle cell disease. There is an increased risk of spontaneous abortion, stillbirth, preterm birth, and IUGR. Because of the risk of poor perinatal outcomes, patients should be monitored with NSTs. There is a high risk of IUGR, and patients should be monitored with ultrasonography if there is any clinical evidence of fetal growth delay. Vaginal delivery is preferable in these patients; cesarean delivery should be reserved for obstetric indications.

Hemoglobin SC

Hemoglobin C is another β chain variant. Clinically significant SC disease occurs in 1 in 833 adult African–Americans in the United States. The children of these women will have either hemoglobin S or hemoglobin C, with the remaining hemoglobin chain determined by the father. The pregnancy-related morbidity rate is usually less in these patients than in those with sickle cell disease (hemoglobin SS). They do have an increased incidence of early spontaneous abortion and pregnancy-related hypertension. Whereas patients with hemoglobin SS tend to undergo splenic infarction, patients with hemoglobin SC tend to have enlarged, hyperactive spleens. They can sequester large volumes of red blood cells, causing a sudden drop in hematocrit. These patients may also be thrombocytopenic. They can readily develop urinary tract infections, which may trigger a vasoocclusive crisis. Vasoocclusive episodes are more likely to occur close to term.

Immune Thrombocytopenic Purpura

In patients with ITP, the decrease in circulating platelet count is due to peripheral destruction and sequestration of platelets, resulting from the production of antiplatelet antibodies and the clearance of these complexes by the reticuloendothelial system. Immune thrombocytopenic purpura is diagnosed by demonstrating platelet-associated antibodies in the blood, as well as increased megakaryocytes on bone marrow biopsy. It is assumed that these antiplatelet antibodies change platelet configuration, rendering them more susceptible to phagocytosis by the reticuloendothelial system.

Immune thrombocytopenic purpura has a predisposition for women, and its onset is usually before age 30. It may be the harbinger of other autoimmune diseases. Because idiosyncratic reactions to drugs also result in thrombocytopenia, a careful drug history is necessary before diagnosing ITP. Isolated thrombocytopenia can rarely be an early sign of preeclampsia, so the patient who has thrombocytopenia first diagnosed in the third trimester should be observed carefully for other signs of impending preeclampsia.

It is almost impossible to distinguish between true ITP and a declining platelet count that can occur during pregnancy and have no pathologic significance whatsoever. It is important to make the distinction, because in true ITP, there is a small but significant risk of profound neonatal thrombocytopenia. This does not appear to be the case in "gestational" thrombocytopenia. It appears that patients who have been known to have a normal platelet count before pregnancy or in a previous pregnancy who develop a platelet count of 75×10^9–150×10^9/L (75,000–150,000/mm^3) in the third trimester probably have "gestational" thrombocytopenia. It is possible that these individuals have developed ITP for the first time during pregnancy, but this is unlikely. In the patient who has had ITP antedating the pregnancy, there does appear to be a risk of neonatal thrombocytopenia. The mode of delivery in these patients remains controversial. Some feel that patients who are thought to have true ITP should undergo cordocentesis prior to delivery to make certain that the fetus has an adequate platelet count.

The goals of maternal therapy are to prevent maternal hemorrhage. Glucocorticoids are the mainstay of therapy. Patients should be started on glucocorticoids if they show any signs of hemorrhage or petechiae. The patient should be maintained on the minimal dose of glucocorticoid necessary to prevent petechiae. There is no set platelet count under which a patient should be treated.

In patients who do not respond to glucocorticoids, splenectomy should be considered and can be safely carried out in pregnancy. Splenectomy is successful in raising the platelet count in 75% of these cases. In those not responding to splenectomy, the destruction of platelets continues in the liver and bone marrow. Platelet counts can be significantly and temporarily raised using intravenous immune globulin. The usual dosage is 400 mg/kg/d for 5 days. A rise in the platelet count usually occurs by the third day. Platelet transfusions are little help in patients with ITP because the transfused platelets are almost immediately destroyed.

Platelet transfusions are reserved for cases of severe hemorrhage or intraoperative bleeding. Excessive bleeding in surgery is not generally seen unless the platelet count falls below 50×10^9/L (50,000/mm^3).

Neonatal Alloimmune Thrombocytopenia

Neonatal alloimmune thrombocytopenia is a rare disorder that is somewhat analogous to D isoimmunization. In this disorder, the mother has antibodies (usually anti-PLA 1 or BAK antibodies) that attack fetal platelets that may have these antigens. With this disorder, the mother will have a normal platelet count. These fetuses are at risk of in utero hemorrhage and usually have profoundly low platelet counts and are at high risk of hemorrhage after delivery. After birth, these infants are treated with transfusions of the mother's platelets, which are antigen negative. Present protocols to treat this disorder include intravenous immune globulins with or without dexamethasone. The results appear somewhat promising at this time. Other techniques include in utero transfusion of the mother's platelets to the fetus. The risk of recurrence with this disorder is extremely high.

RENAL DISEASE

Normal pregnancy is accompanied by anatomic changes in the urinary tract, as well as by marked alterations in renal function. Dilatation of the collecting system and ureters is present early in the second trimester and is due to a combination of both mechanical compression of the ureters by the enlarging uterus and the effect of progesterone on smooth muscle. Renal plasma flows exceeds prepregnant levels by 50–75% at the end of the first trimester, a change that is accompanied by a 30–50% rise in the glomerular filtration rate. The creatinine clearance rate, which reflects the glomerular filtration rate, usually approaches 200 ml/min. These changes produce a marked fall in blood urea nitrogen and serum creatinine.

In women with preexisting renal disease, the prognosis for a favorable pregnancy outcome is most closely related to renal function at the time of conception. When the serum creatinine level is below 1.4 mg/dl and hypertension is absent, the prognosis is excellent; a serum creatinine level above 2.0 mg/dl, a creatinine clearance less than 50 ml/min, and hypertension are associated with a much lower success rate.

Glomerulonephritis

Acute glomerulonephritis, which is usually, but not always, streptococcal in origin, is extremely rare in pregnant women. Typical findings include microscopic hematuria, red blood cell casts in the urine sediment, and low or falling serum complement levels. The usual presentation includes hypertension, edema (including periorbital), and proteinuria, making differentiation from preeclampsia difficult. Most women recover renal function postpartum, but some progress to chronic renal disease. The key to therapy is achieving normal blood pressure levels, since severe hypertension has grave implications for the fetus as well as the mother. Fluid and sodium restriction may be necessary. The presence of this condition does not dictate early delivery, since its course does not appear to be changed by pregnancy.

Chronic glomerulonephritis includes a heterogeneous group of pathophysiologic entities. While it is occasionally secondary to a known episode of acute glomerulonephritis, other causes include IgA nephropathy, membranoproliferative glomerulonephritis, focal glomerulosclerosis, and a number of other diagnoses. The natural history of this disease often results in chronic renal failure and small, scarred kidneys. Most importantly, pregnancy does not appear to affect the course of chronic glomerular disease, although urinary protein excretion may increase transiently because of the increased renal plasma flow engendered by pregnancy. It is possible that increases in proteinuria also reflect increased intraglomerular pressure, and current practice in nonpregnant individuals is to attempt to reduce such pressure with antihypertensive medications and dietary protein restriction. The course of pregnancy is most highly correlated to the degree of renal impairment and the presence of hypertension as delineated in the introduction to this section. If the patient is or becomes hypertensive or if renal function is markedly impaired, it appears that incidences of adverse outcomes such as spontaneous abortion, prematurity, IUGR, and perinatal loss are significantly higher.

Nephrotic Syndrome

Nephrotic syndrome can have a number of causes. Patients experience edema, massive proteinuria (greater than 5 g/24 h), hypoalbuminemia, and hypercholesterolemia. The most common cause in pregnant women is preeclampsia, but any type of renal disease with heavy proteinuria may eventuate in this syndrome. Lipoid nephrosis is a common cause in young women. As in chronic renal disease in general, the prognosis depends on the degree of renal dysfunction and the presence or absence of hypertension, not on the amount of proteinuria. In patients with preeclampsia, the creatinine clearance may be decreased. With other etiologies of nephrotic syndrome, the creatinine clearance may be markedly elevated.

Polycystic Disease

The adult form of polycystic kidney disease is inherited as an autosomal dominant disorder. Renal disease is typically not manifested until after childbearing but, occasionally, earlier cases are reported. The presence of renal or hepatic cysts has been used as a marker to predict this disorder in those at risk by virtue of a parent with known polycystic kidney disease. When women who were genetically at risk and who had such renal cysts were compared with those at risk but without lesions, there was no difference in rates of fertility, spontaneous abortion, or stillbirth. Hypertensive disorders of pregnancy, however, were significantly more common in those presumed to carry the dominant gene. If renal failure develops at the time of pregnancy, the prognosis is the same as for other types of chronic renal disease. Approximately 20% of these patients have intracerebral aneurysms.

Acute Renal Failure

Acute renal failure secondary to either tubular or cortical necrosis has diminished markedly as the incidence of septic abortion has declined. Pregnant women appear to be particularly susceptible, however, to renal failure secondary to necrosis. This may complicate abruptio placentae or fetal death, in which the mechanism may be disseminated intravascular coagulation or, occasionally, preeclampsia. Acute tubular necrosis is more common with preeclampsia. Renal failure may be precipitated by shock with hypoperfusion of the kidneys. In such cases, there is usually a period of oliguria or anuria, which is followed within a variable period of time by marked diuresis. Treatment is supportive, and strict attention should be given to serum electrolyte levels and restriction of fluid intake. Invasive hemodynamic monitoring is often required. Dialysis is necessary in some patients, particularly when hyperkalemia or azotemia occurs. Recovery usually occurs. In patients with cortical necrosis, however, the prognosis may not be as favorable; chronic renal insufficiency is a more likely sequela in these patients.

Lupus Nephritis

Systemic lupus erythematosus is discussed elsewhere (see "Immunologic Disorders" in this section). When lupus nephritis is present, the best predictor of the effect of pregnancy on the renal disease is the amount of activity of the disease at the time of conception. If the renal disease has been quiescent for at least 6 months, there is a decrease in the likelihood of a flare-up during pregnancy. Serial complement levels can be used to follow disease activity during pregnancy. A single level of C3, C4, or CH50 is useless, as the levels of complement, a protein, normally rise during pregnancy. Only by monitoring the trend of these levels can an obstetrician assess systemic lupus erythematosus activity during pregnancy. If levels are falling, this signals a likely increase in autoimmune activity, and treatment should be initiated or increased. Complement levels have also proven useful in differentiating lupus activity and preeclampsia. This is important because both diseases may have similar clinical manifestations, and patients with systemic lupus erythematosus are at an increased risk for developing preeclampsia.

Diabetic Nephropathy

Although clinically evident diabetic nephropathy is generally manifested as proteinuria, hypertension, declining renal function, and, ultimately, end-stage renal disease, there is an early stage of hyperfunction and hypertrophy of the glomeruli that is usually present at the time of the diagnosis of diabetes. The first clinically recognizable stage of nephropathy is that of microalbuminuria, in which urinary albumin excretion is in the range of 20–400 mg/d. This level can be detected with highly sensitive urinary dipsticks in the physician's office. Patients who have microalbuminuria or are at later stages of diabetic nephropathy almost always manifest heavier proteinuria during pregnancy. Among patients who have more than 300 mg of proteinuria per day at the beginning of pregnancy, 71% have proteinuria of more than 3 g/d by term. Approximately 50% of patients with diabetic nephropathy experience no change or an increase in serum creatinine level. The development of hypertension or the worsening of preexisting hypertension is common and generally requires hospitalization, as it represents a significant risk to the pregnancy. Perinatal survival in one study of women with diabetic nephropathy was approximately 94%, and the pregnancy appeared to have no permanent effect on renal function.

Renal Transplantation

Considerable experience has now been accumulated concerning pregnancy in renal allograft recipients, and such individuals appear to do well. Hypertensive disorders, however, occur at an increased frequency. The transplanted kidney increases its creatinine clearance in a fashion similar to that of normal kidneys. There is an increased likelihood of IUGR, presumably because of vascular compromise, and of preterm delivery. Azathioprine, cyclosporine, and prednisone, which are immunosuppressive drugs that are likely to be used in such patients, should be continued during pregnancy, since rejection of the transplanted kidney represents a life-threatening situation for both mother and fetus. Most renal allograft recipients progress normally through pregnancy and have very good maternal and perinatal outcomes.

Importantly, because the transplanted kidney is denervated, the transplant recipient can develop pyelonephritis and urosepsis with no pain. Therefore, a urine culture should be performed in these patients at least once each trimester.

HYPOADRENALISM AND PHEOCHROMOCYTOMA

The classic symptoms of hypoadrenalism include asthenia, increased pigmentation, and hypotension. Although this disease may improve spontaneously during pregnancy, adrenal crisis may occur during periods of stress, such as labor, delivery, and the postpartum period. Therefore, corticosteroids should be administered during any stress period, particularly during labor and delivery; the dosage should then be decreased gradually in the postpartum period. Because patients with Addison disease have a low tolerance for analgesics and anesthetics, the administration of these agents should be kept to a minimum.

Pheochromocytoma is a tumor of the adrenal medulla that is associated with a maternal mortality rate that approaches 50%. The diagnosis may be suspected when the patient has marked hypertension of a paroxysmal nature associated with headaches, anxiety, nausea, and vomiting. The diagnosis is confirmed by the finding of increased levels of metanephrines in the urine. This disease may sometimes be confused with preeclampsia, but it may be differentiated by the absence of both proteinuria and edema. The only treatment available is surgical extirpation of the adrenal tumor.

Adrenal insufficiency may be primary (Addison disease) or secondary to pituitary failure or adrenal suppression from chronic steroid administration. Adrenal crisis, an acute life-threatening condition, may accompany stressful conditions such as labor, the puerperium, or surgery. The clinical presentation of Addison disease during gestation is similar to that in the nonpregnant state. Fatigue, weakness, anorexia, hypotension, hypoglycemia, and increased skin pigmentation are hallmarks for this endocrinopathy. The diagnosis of adrenal insufficiency is based on laboratory findings. Plasma cortisol levels are decreased; however, because cortisol-binding globulin is increased in pregnancy, low-normal cortisol levels may reflect a state of adrenal insufficiency. Stimulation of the adrenal gland by synthetic ACTH is usually helpful in establishing a diagnosis. Failure to respond to this stimulus is characteristic of adrenal insufficiency. Pregnancy usually proceeds normally in treated patients. Maintenance replacement of adrenocortical and mineralocorticoid hormones is undertaken with careful monitoring of fluid status in those requiring mineralocorticoid therapy. Adrenal crisis is a rare, life-threatening condition that requires intensive care. Symptoms include nausea, vomiting, and profound epigastric pain accompanied by hypothermia and hypotension.

DERMATOLOGIC DISEASE

Physiologic changes in the skin during gestation may result in hyperpigmentation, hirsutism, hair loss, and several vascular abnormalities. Some of these conditions are believed to result from alterations in the hormonal milieu of pregnancy; however, for most skin changes there is little information concerning the precise etiologic factors involved.

Herpes Gestationis

Herpes gestationis is a rare pruritic bullous disease of the skin that occurs principally during pregnancy. This is no relation to herpes simplex infection. The reported incidence of herpes gestationis is 1/4,000–1/50,000 pregnancies. Herpes gestationis may recur with subsequent pregnancies and may be associated with an increased incidence of fetal growth retardation and stillbirth. The disease usually has its onset in the second trimester. Exacerbations are common during the postpartum period. The etiology of herpes gestationis is unknown, yet a genetic predisposition is suggested by the presence of certain human leukocyte antigen (HLA) haplotypes in affected persons. Clinical presentation, including past history and peripheral eosinophilia, helps secure the diagnosis. Skin biopsy with immunopathologic studies reveals complement deposition along the basement membrane between epidermis and dermis. A circulating IgG antibasement membrane antibody, along with herpes gestationis factor, has been isolated from the sera of affected patients. Treatment is aimed at controlling pruritus and reducing new vesicle formation. Corticosteroids are often required. Transient neonatal herpes gestationis has been reported; at birth, the infant may show skin lesions that are similar to those of the mother. Neonatal disease is usually mild and resolves within a short period of time.

Papular Dermatitis of Pregnancy

Papular dermatitis is characterized by a widespread pruritic papular eruption that is associated with an increased fetal mortality rate. The disease may begin at any time during gestation and may recur in subsequent pregnancies. This rare disorder may be the result of a sensitization to hCG, as increased levels have been reported in affected women. Maternal corticoid levels may be low, as well. Corticosteroid therapy controls eruptions within 24–48 hours. This condition may be a variant of prurigo gestationis.

Prurigo Gestationis

Prurigo gestationis occurs in 1/5–1/200 pregnancies. A disabling process, prurigo gestationis does not increase fetal morbidity or mortality. The etiology of this condition is unknown, and treatment is based on symptoms. It may be a variant of papular dermatitis. The lesions are small (1–2 mm), excoriated, pruritic papules that appear on the trunk and extensor surfaces of the extremities. The disease disappears after delivery.

Impetigo Herpetiformis

Impetigo herpetiformis is a rare pustular disease associated with severe constitutional symptoms and a high maternal mortality rate. The disease usually occurs in the second half of pregnancy and is marked by primary lesions consisting of painful pustules. The sites of predilection are the groin and the inner thighs, with eventual extension to the trunk and extremities. Systemic symptoms include fever, chills, arthralgias, and lymphadenopathy. Cardiac and renal failure has been reported. Corticosteroids are indicated, and early delivery or therapeutic abortion may be necessary.

Coincidental Dermatoses

Pigmented Nevi and Hyperpigmentation

The female sex hormones have a pronounced effect on melanogenesis; therefore, any existing nevi may grow and darken, and new ones may appear during pregnancy. No treatment is required. Generalized hyperpigmentation can be found in most pregnancies. Darkening of the areolae, umbilicus, vulva, and perianal skin may occur as early as the first trimester. Chloasma is a characteristic of hyperpigmentation of the face, which often prompts complaints from patients. Sunlight is thought to be necessary for its development, so that limited sun exposure and use of sunscreens are recommended for all pregnant women.

Hair Changes

Telogen effluvium, or hair loss after a shift of anagen follicles to telogens, is often seen during the postpartum period. There is generally a complete regrowth of the hair in 3–6 months. Drug therapy is seldom helpful; reassurance is the best approach. Alopecia areata may either occur or, in a preexisting case, improve during pregnancy. Intralesional corticosteroids may be helpful. Mild degrees of hirsutism are common during pregnancy. The face and extremities are primarily affected. During pregnancy, the proportion of hair in the anagen (growing) phase is increased, although elevated androgen levels from placental sources may contribute to hirsutism. Mild hirsutism rarely requires therapy. Excessive hirsutism with virilism warrants investigation for an androgen-secreting tumor.

Condylomata Acuminata

Condylomata flourish and spread in a moist medium. They often grow rapidly during pregnancy; rarely, they may attain a size that results in dystocia. As condylomata are viral in origin, they are both contagious and autoinoculable; they may be transmitted venereally. Scrupulous personal cleanliness is essential in the management of these lesions. Small lesions require no treatment and usually regress spontaneously after delivery. While podophyllum resin in a variety of forms has been the most widely used treatment for larger lesions, the systemic absorption of this agent in pregnancy may have serious teratogenic effects. During gestation, therefore, large lesions are probably best treated by surgical excision, laser therapy, or electrocauterization under general anesthesia.

Acne

The sweat and sebaceous glands are especially active during pregnancy, probably as a result of the increased progesterone secretion. Acne may become worse during pregnancy, but it usually improves. Good skin hygiene should be encouraged. Topical therapy and ultraviolet light may be used, but tetracycline should not be prescribed. Isotretinoin, an effective medication used to treat cystic acne, is a potent teratogen. Any woman contemplating pregnancy while taking this medication should be advised, and the drug should be discontinued.

Psoriasis

The effect of pregnancy on preexisting psoriasis is unpredictable. Psoriasis seldom arises de novo during gestation, and generalized lesions tend to improve. Pregnancy tends to aggravate localized lesions, however, particularly those of inverse psoriasis. Postpartum exacerbation frequently occurs and seems to be unrelated to pregnancy changes. Psoriasis has no effect on either the pregnancy or the fetus. The usual topical dermatologic treatments should be continued during gestation. Oral etretinate is a teratogen and should not be used during pregnancy.

IMMUNOLOGIC DISORDERS

Rheumatoid Arthritis

Rheumatoid arthritis is a chronic systemic disease. Although the etiology is unknown, there does appear to be a genetic predisposition. Rheumatoid arthritis affects primarily the synovial fluid–lined joints. The clinical picture is one of joint inflammation, pain, tenderness, heat, and swelling, particularly of the small and medium-sized joints (ie, the hands, wrist, knees, and feet). It is accompanied by morning stiffness and often by malaise, fatigue, and other constitutional symptoms. There are usually intermittent periods of acute exacerbations and remissions of joint inflammation; however, the disease may be of an unrelenting, progressive nature, eventually destroying the joint.

Laboratory findings in patients with rheumatoid arthritis include a normochromic, normocytic anemia, an elevated sedimentation rate, and hypergammaglobulinemia. A rheumatoid factor, an antiimmunoglobulin, is present in 75–80% of patients. Rheumatoid arthritis is diagnosed on the basis of the clinical and laboratory findings defined by the American Rheumatism Association.

Since the onset of the disease is usually toward the end of reproductive age, rheumatoid arthritis is relatively uncommon during pregnancy. However, when it is associated with pregnancy, the majority of women will experience an improvement in symptoms. In some patients the disease process may actually worsen or even appear for the first time, especially during the postpartum period.

Aspirin and nonsteroidal antiinflammatory agents are the primary therapeutic agents used for both nonpregnant and pregnant women with rheumatoid arthritis. There are no scientific data that these agents are teratogenic. However, potential adverse effects include coagulation defects and bleeding, prolongation of gestation, and premature closure of the ductus (especially if the agents are used after 34 weeks).

Corticosteroids are usually not indicated in the treatment of uncomplicated rheumatoid arthritis; however, they may provide rapid relief of pain in patients whose disease is unresponsive to other forms of therapy. This relief can usually be achieved with very low doses of corticosteroids. There is no evidence that corticosteroids are teratogenic in humans.

Several other agents have been used to treat rheumatoid arthritis in nonpregnant women, including gold salts, methotrexate, hydroxychloroquine, sulfasalazine, penicillamine, and azathioprine. There is little information regarding the use of these agents during pregnancy, and thus their safety is unknown. However, it would seem appropriate to avoid methotrexate during pregnancy, as skeletal anomalies have been reported with this agent and a related compound, aminopterin.

Systemic Lupus Erythematosus

Systemic lupus erythematosus is a chronic disease of unknown etiology. It occurs predominantly in women, with a prevalence of approximately 1/700. The disease has variable clinical and laboratory manifestations. Its clinical manifestations result from the inflammation of multiple organ systems, including the skin, joints, kidneys, nervous system, and serous membranes. The severity of the disease is variable, ranging from relatively benign skin lesions or transient polyarthritis to a fulminant, rapidly fatal condition characterized by renal failure and central nervous system, cardiac, and hematologic involvement. The diagnosis is based on the presence of any four or more of the following criteria:

- Malar rash
- Discoid rash
- Photosensitivity
- Oral ulcers
- Arthritis
- Serositis
- Renal disorder
- Neurologic disorder
- Hematologic disorder
- Immunologic disorder
- Antinuclear antibody (ANA)

Numerous antibodies have been identified in women with systemic lupus. The most common antibody identified in these patients is the ANA, which may be present in up to 95% of patients. Some other commonly found antibodies include anti-DNA, anti-Ro (SSA), anti-La (SSB), and various antiphospholipid or anticardiolipin antibodies. The presence of anti-Ro antibodies is associated with congenital heart block in the fetus and newborn. Other laboratory findings include anemia, thrombocytopenia, false-positive serologic tests for syphilis, and pneumonia.

Systemic lupus erythematosus does not appear to influence fertility; however, the incidence of spontaneous abortions, premature deliveries, and stillbirths is increased. The offspring of women with this disease have been found to have transient serologic abnormalities, skin lesions, and congenital heart block. There is some controversy concerning the incidence of exacerbated disease during pregnancy and the puerperium. In general, women in remission before conception remain in remission during pregnancy and the postpartum period.

Systemic lupus is also associated with an increased frequency of preeclampsia. Moreover, it is often impossible to distinguish severe preeclampsia/eclampsia from an exacerbation of disease in patients with lupus nephropathy. Pregnant women with either of these conditions may manifest significant hypertension, proteinuria, hemolysis, thrombocytopenia, an elevated serum creatinine level, and seizures. With the exception of corticosteroid therapy for lupus patients, the treatment is essentially the same for both conditions (ie, seizure prophylaxis, control of hypertension, and delivery).

Corticosteroid therapy is the cornerstone of treatment for patients with systemic lupus erythematosus. Generally, the lowest dosage possible should be used to control the signs and symptoms of the disease. Initial therapy in patients with active disease is generally 1–2 mg/kg. Following response, the dose should be tapered to a dosage of 10 mg/d, if possible. Other immunosuppressive agents such as azathioprine and cyclophosphamide have been used in nonpregnant women with systemic lupus. There is little information regarding their efficacy and safety during pregnancy.

Scleroderma

Also known as progressive systemic sclerosis, scleroderma is a rare connective tissue disease of unknown etiology. It is characterized by fibrosis and degenerative vascular changes in the skin, joints, esophagus, gastrointestinal tract, kidneys, and heart. Raynaud phenomenon is the most common feature of the disease and may precede other manifestations by many years. The course of the disease is extremely variable. Pulmonary hypertension and renal involvement indicate severe disease and carry a grave prognosis. There is no effective treatment of scleroderma at present. Current therapy consists of such supportive measures as the avoidance of cold, physical therapy, and patient education.

There is some debate about the effect of pregnancy on scleroderma. Some reports indicate that the condition worsens during pregnancy, but others have not demonstrated any change. When scleroderma is rapidly progressive, with hypertension and renal or cardiac involvement, pregnancy may cause a sudden deterioration in renal function that may result in death. The risk of perinatal loss appears to be increased for patients with scleroderma, especially for those with renal involvement. Esophageal dysfunction and dysphagia may worsen during pregnancy.

Antiphospholipid Antibody Syndrome

Features of the antiphospholipid antibody syndrome include recurrent fetal loss, recurrent thrombosis, thrombocytopenia, and the presence of high-titer antiphospholipid antibodies identified by either the ELISA or clotting test (ie, the lupus anticoagulant). Antiphospholipid antibodies (anticardiolipin or lupus anticoagulant) are found in up to 50% of patients with systemic lupus erythematosus but may also occur in patients without overt lupus. Various tests of clotting have been used to detect the presence of the lupus anticoagulant. Probably the most commonly used is the activated partial thromboplastin time. Approximately 70% of patients with the lupus anticoagulant will also have other antiphospholipid antibodies identified by the ELISA test.

Patients with antiphospholipid antibodies have been reported to experience other adverse pregnancy events besides recurrent fetal losses. Examples include fetal growth retardation, early-onset severe preeclampsia, and prematurity.

There is currently no unanimity of opinion regarding the most optimal therapy in women with recurrent pregnancy losses and antiphospholipid antibodies. However, there have been reports of improved pregnancy outcomes with low-dose aspirin (75–85 mg) in combination with either heparin or prednisone. It would seem reasonable to conclude that the combination of low-dose aspirin and heparin would provide the possible additional advantage of decreasing the risk of maternal thrombosis. It would also seem reasonable to use heparin in patients with a history of thrombosis and high-titer antiphospholipid antibodies or the lupus anticoagulant.

INFECTIONS

Hepatitis A

Hepatitis A is caused by an RNA virus and is responsible for approximately 30–35% of all cases of hepatitis in the United States. The virus is usually transmitted from person to person by fecal–oral contamination. Poor hygiene, poor sanitation, and intimate personal or sexual contact facilitate transmission. Epidemics frequently result from common exposure to contaminated food and water. In the United States, the incidence of acute hepatitis A in pregnancy is 1/1,000 or less.

The usual clinical manifestations of hepatitis A are malaise, fatigue, anorexia, hepatic pain and tenderness, jaundice, and clay-colored stools. The diagnosis is confirmed by identifying IgM-specific antibody in the serum.

Serious complications of hepatitis A are uncommon. A chronic carrier state does not exist, and perinatal transmission of the virus does not occur.

Hepatitis B

Hepatitis B is caused by a small DNA virus and is responsible for 40–45% of all cases of hepatitis in the United States. Acute and chronic hepatitis B occur in 1–2/1,000 and 5–15/1,000 pregnancies, respectively. Hepatitis B is transmitted by parenteral and sexual contact. Risk factors for hepatitis B are:

- History of illicit drug use
- History of sexually transmitted disease(s)
- Household contact with a hepatitis B virus carrier
- Multiple sexual partners
- Work in a health care or public safety field
- Work or residence in an institution for the developmentally disabled
- Work or residence in a detention facility
- Receipt of blood components for medical indications
- History of a tattoo
- Member of selected ethnic groups: Eskimos and Asians

Most cases of hepatitis B in the United States occur in homosexual or bisexual males, intravenous drug abusers, and heterosexual partners of infected males.

Of patients who become infected with hepatitis B, fewer than 1% develop fulminant liver failure and die. Approximately 85–90% experience complete resolution of their physical findings and develop levels of antibody that are protective against reinfection. Some (10–15%) patients fail to develop protective antibody and become chronically infected; 15–30% of these individuals subsequently develop chronic or persistent hepatitis and cirrhosis. Such complications are particularly likely to occur when superinfection with hepatitis D occurs. Patients with chronic liver disease are at increased risk of developing hepatocellular carcinoma.

In the acute stage of hepatitis B infection, the diagnosis is confirmed by identification of the surface antigen (HBsAg) and IgM antibody to the core antigen. The presence of envelope antigen (HBeAg) is indicative of an exceptionally high viral inoculum and active viral replication. Chronic hepatitis B infection is characterized by the persistence of HBsAg in the liver and serum.

The frequency of perinatal transmission of hepatitis B is dependent, in part, on the time in gestation when maternal infection occurs. When maternal infection develops in the first trimester, up to 10% of neonates will be seropositive for HBsAg if immunoprophylaxis is not administered. In women who are acutely infected in the third trimester, 80–90% of offspring will be infected in the absence of prophylaxis.

In women who are chronic carriers of hepatitis B but who are not acutely ill, the frequency of perinatal transmission is dependent on the size of the maternal viral inoculum. Approximately 10–20% of women who are seropositive only for HBsAg transmit infection to their neonates if immunoprophylaxis is not administered. In contrast, in women who are seropositive for both HBsAg and HBeAg, the frequency of vertical transmission increases to almost 90%.

Most cases of perinatal transmission occur as a consequence of intrapartum exposure of the infant to contaminated blood and genital tract secretions. The remaining cases result from hematogenous transplacental dissemination, breast-feeding, and close postnatal contact between the infant and infected parent.

The principal means of preventing hepatitis B infection in adults and neonates is immunoprophylaxis. All pregnant women should be tested for HBsAg. If they are seronegative they should be vaccinated. Two recombinant vaccines are available, and the dosage recommendations for each are listed in Table 3-13.

Individuals who have been exposed to hepatitis B before they are vaccinated should initially receive passive immunization with hepatitis B immune globulin and then undergo the vaccination series. Hepatitis B immune globulin is administered in a dosage of 0.06 ml/kg IM as soon as possible after exposure.

The CDC now recommends that all neonates be vaccinated for hepatitis B. Infants delivered to seropositive mothers also need to receive passive immunization with hepatitis B immune globulin. The recommended schedules for neonatal immunoprophylaxis are summarized in Table 3-14.

TABLE 3-13. RECOMMENDED DOSES OF HEPATITIS B VACCINE

Vaccine	Recombivax HB*	Engerix-B*
Children and adolescents 11–19 years	5 µg (0.5 ml)	20 µg (1.0 ml)
Adults ≥20 years	10 µg (1.0 ml)	20 µg (1.0 ml)
Dialysis patients and other immunocompromised persons	40 µg (1.0 ml)†	40 µg (2.0 ml)‡

* Both vaccines are routinely administered intramuscularly in a three-dose series at 0, 1, and 6 months. Engerix-B has been licensed for a four-dose series administered at 0, 1, 2, and 12 months.
† This is a special formulation.
‡ Two 1.0-ml doses are administered at one site in a four-dose schedule at 0, 1, 2, and 6 months.
Modified from Centers for Disease Control. Hepatitis B virus: a comprehensive strategy for eliminating transmission in the United States through universal childhood vaccination: recommendations of the Immunization Practices Advisory Committee. MMWR 1991;40(RR-13):7

Hepatitis D

Hepatitis D is caused by the delta agent, an RNA virus that is dependent upon coinfection with hepatitis B for replication. Hepatitis D virus has an external antigen coat of HBsAg that is encoded by the hepatitis B virus genome and an internal delta-Ag encoded by its own genome. The epidemiology of hepatitis D closely mirrors that of hepatitis B.

Acute hepatitis D may occur as a coinfection with acute hepatitis B. Coinfection is usually self-limited and rarely leads to chronic hepatitis. Hepatitis D also may develop as a superinfection in a patient who is a chronic carrier of hepatitis B. Approximately 20–25% of chronic carriers eventually become coinfected with hepatitis D. In contrast to coinfection, superinfection leads to chronic hepatitis in almost 80% of patients. Of patients with chronic infection, 70–80% ultimately develop cirrhosis and portal hypertension, and approximately 25% die of hepatic failure.

The diagnosis of hepatitis D can be confirmed by detection of D antigen in hepatic tissue or serum and identification of IgM-specific antibody. Patients with chronic hepatitis D usually have persistence of D antigenemia, and viremia and end-organ damage may continue despite the presence of antibody.

Perinatal transmission of hepatitis D infection can occur. Fortunately, however, the measures used to prevent perinatal transmission of hepatitis B are almost uniformly effective in preventing transmission of the delta agent.

Non-A, Non-B Hepatitis

Non-A, non-B hepatitis accounts for 10–20% of cases of hepatitis in the United States. The disease occurs in two distinct forms, referred to as hepatitis C and E.

Hepatitis C, or parenterally transmitted non-A, non-B hepa-

TABLE 3-14. RECOMMENDED SCHEDULES FOR IMMUNOPROPHYLAXIS OF NEONATAL HEPATITIS B INFECTION*

Infants of	Vaccine	Age
HBsAg-positive mothers	HBV 1[†]	Birth—within 12 hours
	HBIG (0.5 ml IM)	Birth—within 12 hours
	HBV 2	1 month
	HBV 3	6 months
HBsAg-unknown mothers	HBV 1[†]	Birth—within 12 hours
	HBIG (0.5 ml IM)	If mother HBsAg positive, give 0.5 ml IM as soon as possible, *not* later than 1 week after birth
	HBV 2[‡]	1–2 months
	HBV 3[‡]	6 months
HBsAg-negative mothers[§]	HBV 1[‖]	Birth—before hospital discharge
	HBV 2	1–2 months
	HBV 3	6–18 months

* HBsAg indicates hepatitis B surface antigen; HBV, hepatitis B vaccine; HBIG, hepatitis B immune globulin; IM, intramuscularly.
[†] Dose of Recombivax HB is 5 μg (0.5 ml). Dose of Engerix-B is 10 μg (0.5 ml).
[‡] If the mother is found to be HBsAg positive, use 5 μg of Recombivax HB or 10 μg of Engerix-B for second and third doses of vaccine. If mother is seronegative, use 2.5 μg of Recombivax HB. The dose of Engerix-B remains 10 μg.
[§] A second option is to administer HBV at intervals that correspond to the schedule of other childhood vaccines (ie, 1–2 months after birth, 4 months, and 6–18 months).
[‖] Dose of Recombivax HB is 2.5 μg (0.25 ml). Dose of Engerix-B is 10 μg (0.5 ml).
Modified from Centers for Disease Control. Hepatitis B virus: a comprehensive strategy for eliminating transmission in the United States through universal childhood vaccination: recommendations of the Immunization Practices Advisory Committee (ACIP). MMWR 1991;40(RR-13):12–13

titis, may result from blood transfusion, use of contaminated intravenous drug equipment, and sexual contact with an infected partner. Approximately 2.5–15% of patients who receive multiple blood transfusions subsequently develop hepatitis C. Conversely, at least 90% of cases of posttransfusion hepatitis result from hepatitis C virus infection. About 50% of patients with acute hepatitis C develop biochemical evidence of chronic liver disease. Of these individuals, up to 20% subsequently have chronic active hepatitis or cirrhosis.

The diagnosis of hepatitis C is usually made by identification of specific antibody. Antibody may not develop until 6–16 weeks after the onset of clinical illness. The present generation of serologic tests does not permit precise distinction between IgM and IgG antibody. In low-risk populations, current antibody tests may result in false-positives; thus, a positive anti-hepatitis C antibody test should be confirmed by repeat testing.

Perinatal transmission of hepatitis C has been documented. The exact frequency of transmission and the principal risk factors for perinatal infection remain to be delineated. Immunoprophylaxis for the neonate is not yet available.

Hepatitis E results from fecal–oral transmission of a viral agent. The epidemiologic features of hepatitis E are similar to those of hepatitis A. Hepatitis E is uncommon in the United States but is endemic in several developing nations, notably in Asia, Africa, the Middle East, Central America, and Mexico. It may be diagnosed by identifying viruslike particles by electron microscopy in the stool of infected patients. Recently, a serologic test for identifying antibody has been developed.

Hepatitis E is usually self-limited and does not result in a chronic carrier state. Perinatal transmission does not occur.

Rubella

Rubella is caused by an RNA virus, and only a single serotype is known. Rubella occurs primarily in young children and adolescents and is more common in the springtime. The infection is transmitted by respiratory droplets, and the incubation period is 2–3 weeks. Virus is present in the blood and nasopharyngeal secretions of the infected patient for several days before the appearance of the rash and is shed from the nasopharynx for several days after the rash is present. Immunity after natural infection is usually lifelong. Second infections have occurred after both natural infection and vaccination, but they are not associated with serious illness, viremia, or congenital infection.

Many children and adults with rubella may have minimal or no symptoms or physical findings. When present, clinical manifestations include malaise, headache, conjunctivitis, arthralgias, arthritis, postauricular adenopathy, and a diffuse, erythematous maculopapular rash.

Although rubella may be confirmed by culture of the virus from nasopharyngeal secretions, serologic tests are usually of more practical value in clinical practice. IgM-specific antibody tests typically peak at 7–10 days after the onset of the illness and persist for approximately 4 weeks. IgG antibody is usually detectable 7–14 days after the onset of symptoms and persists for life.

Rubella may severely injure the developing fetus. If a susceptible mother is infected within the first 4 weeks after conception, the risk of fetal infection is almost 50%. If infection occurs in the second 4 weeks, the risk is 25%. When maternal infection occurs in the third 4 weeks of pregnancy, the risk decreases to 10%. Beyond this point in time, the frequency of neonatal infection is less than 1%. The most frequent clinical manifestations of congenital rubella are deafness, microcephaly, mental retardation, pneumonia, congenital heart disease, ocular abnormalities, hepatosplenomegaly, hemolytic anemia, thrombocytopenia, and growth restriction.

Since the licensure of the vaccine in 1969, the incidence of rubella infection in infants, children, and adults has declined by over 95%. The present rubella vaccine, the RA 27/3 vaccine, has minimal toxicity and is highly immunogenic, resulting in seroconversion in more than 95% of recipients. New cases of rubella and congenital rubella continue to be reported, however, and appear to be due primarily to lack of vaccination in potentially susceptible individuals.

Ideally, all women of reproductive age should have a serologic test to confirm immunity to rubella before considering pregnancy. Susceptible women should be vaccinated and advised to use contraception for 3 months. There are no reports of congenital rubella as a consequence of vaccination, and the maximum theoretic risk is estimated to be 1–2%.

For the pregnant patient whose immunologic status is unknown, a rubella serologic screen should be obtained at the time of the first prenatal appointment. Susceptible patients should be counseled to avoid exposure to individuals with viral exanthems and then targeted for vaccination in the immediate postpartum period.

If a susceptible patient is exposed to rubella, she should be evaluated serially by physical examination and serologic testing to determine whether infection develops. If seroconversion occurs, she should be counseled about the risk to the fetus. When maternal infection develops within the first 12 weeks after conception, the risk of fetal infection is high enough that some women may wish to exercise their option of pregnancy termination.

For patients who elect to continue their pregnancy, ultrasound examination can identify major fetal injuries such as growth restriction, microcephaly, and cardiac malformation. It cannot, however, delineate more subtle manifestations of fetal infection such as cataracts, glaucoma, pneumonia, anemia, and thrombocytopenia.

Cytomegalovirus

Cytomegalovirus infections are caused by a double-stranded DNA herpes virus. Approximately 60–70% of adults have serologic evidence of previous CMV infection. The seroprevalence is highest in indigent patient populations. Contact with young children in the household or in day-care centers is one of the principal mechanisms of transmission of CMV infection to adults. Infection also may be transmitted by sexual contact and blood transfusion. Most CMV infections in children and adults are subclinical. Symptomatic patients typically present with a mononucleosislike illness.

Cytomegalovirus infection may be transmitted in utero to the fetus. It is the most common congenital infection in the United States, affecting approximately 1% of neonates. Congenital infection may occur with either primary or recurrent maternal infection but is much more common and serious with the former. Approximately 40% of infants delivered to mothers with primary CMV infection will become infected. On average, 10% of these neonates will have obvious clinical findings at birth, including hepatosplenomegaly, jaundice, thrombocytopenia, microcephaly, deafness, chorioretinitis, optic atrophy, cerebral calcifications, and hydrocephalus. The other infected infants will have manifestations of infection later in childhood, such as hearing impairment, learning disability, and delayed psychomotor development. Congenital infection is much less likely to occur after recurrent infection or reactivation of maternal CMV infection, and sequelae are usually limited to hearing impairment and learning disability.

The diagnosis of maternal CMV infection can be made by culturing the virus from urine or genital tract secretions. More commonly, the diagnosis is confirmed by serologic tests. The detection of IgM-specific antibody is usually indicative of acute or recent CMV infection. In addition, documentation of a positive IgG-specific antibody titer in a patient who previously was seronegative also is confirmation of infection.

There are three methodologies that are of value in diagnosing fetal CMV infection. Antibody specific for IgM may be detected by cordocentesis at approximately 21–23 weeks of gestation. The mere presence of specific antibody, however, does not necessarily correlate with severity of fetal infection. Detection of CMV in amniotic fluid and demonstration of fetal anomalies by ultrasonography actually correlate more precisely with severity of fetal infection. Characteristic findings of ultrasonography include hepatomegaly, microcephaly, periventricular calcifications, and ventriculomegaly.

At present, there is no antiviral agent that is effective in treating subclinical or mildly symptomatic CMV infection or preventing congenital infection. Ganciclovir may be of value in treating chorioretinitis caused by CMV. Such a complication is unusual in immunocompetent adults but may be evident in obstetric patients with acquired immunodeficiency syndrome (AIDS). Routine screening of asymptomatic pregnant women for CMV infection is not indicated.

Toxoplasmosis

Toxoplasmosis is caused by the protozoan parasite, *Toxoplasma gondii*. Serologic surveys have shown that up to 40–50% of adults in the United States have antibody to *T. gondii*. Seroprevalence is highest in populations of low socioeconomic status. The frequency of seroconversion during pregnancy is less than 5%, and approximately one to three infants per 1,000 show serologic evidence of congenital infection.

T. gondii has three distinct forms: trophozoite, cyst, and oocyst. The trophozoite is the invasive form of the organism. Infection of mammals occurs by ingestion of either the cyst or oocyst, which is disrupted in the host's intestine, releasing the trophozoite. Cysts are formed in the brain and muscle of mammalian hosts. Human infection occurs when meat from infected farm animals is eaten or when hands or food are contaminated by cat feces. Stray cats and domestic cats that eat raw meat are the most likely to carry the parasite. The cyst is destroyed by heat, and the practice of eating rare or raw meat in western Europe may explain the high prevalence of infection in countries such as Belgium and France.

In immunocompetent adults and children, toxoplasmosis usually causes a self-limited mononucleosislike illness. Treatment with antibiotics is usually not necessary. In immunosuppressed patients, however, toxoplasmosis can be a life-threatening disease. In these individuals, *T. gondii* has a special predilection for the central nervous system and retina and may be responsible for devastating illness.

Congenital toxoplasmosis can occur if the mother develops a primary infection during pregnancy. Approximately one third of infants born to mothers with primary infection will be affected. The frequency of fetal infection is higher when maternal infection occurs in the third trimester (60–65%) than when it occurs in the first trimester (15–20%). However, the severity of infection is greater when the mother is infected during the first trimester.

Approximately one third of infected neonates have evidence of clinical disease at birth. The characteristic triad of congenital toxoplasmosis is intracerebral calcification, chorioretinitis, and hydrocephalus. Other findings may include anemia, jaundice, splenomegaly, generalized lymphadenopathy, seizures, microcephaly, mental retardation, and hearing impairment.

The diagnosis of toxoplasmosis in adults and children may be confirmed in several ways. The organism can be detected in histologic preparations of infected tissues such as lymph nodes. The mainstay of diagnosis, however, is serologic testing. Antibodies may be detected by indirect immunofluorescence, complement fixation, and the Sabin–Feldman dye test. Patients with acute infection typically have positive assays for IgM antibody and show seroconversion in their IgG antibody test. Titers for IgM may remain positive for several months after the acute infection.

Clinicians should be aware that serologic testing for toxoplasmosis is not well standardized and that only a few reference laboratories consistently provide reliable test results. When primary toxoplasmosis during pregnancy is suspected, serum specimens should be forwarded to one of these recognized referral centers for evaluation. The state health departments and CDC can provide the names of qualified reference laboratories.

Several methodologies have been used to diagnose fetal infection. Amniotic fluid may be obtained by amniocentesis and then injected into mice or incubated in tissue culture. Fetal blood can be aspirated by cordocentesis and cultured. Fetal blood also can be assayed for total IgM concentration and IgM-specific antibody after 21–23 weeks of gestation. However, although these measures may indicate that *T. gondii* is present in the fetal and placental circulation, they do not precisely define the severity of fetal infection. Ultrasound examination is valuable in this regard. Ultrasonographic findings consistent with severe fetal infection include microcephaly, ventriculomegaly, growth restriction, visceromegaly, and hydrops.

If acute fetal infection is documented, patients may be offered pregnancy termination or antibiotic treatment. Recent investigations in France have confirmed the value of sulfadiazine, pyrimethamine, and spiramycin in treatment of fetal toxoplasmosis.

The best treatment for toxoplasmosis, of course, is prevention. Susceptible pregnant women should be advised to avoid undercooked meat. They should wash their hands after handling raw meat and thoroughly clean countertops and dishes that have come in contact with uncooked meat. If they own cats, they should be instructed to keep their cats indoors and to avoid contact with the litter box. They should not feed raw meat to their cats and should wash their hands carefully after handling the animals.

Herpes Simplex

Herpes simplex virus (HSV) is a DNA virus that has two serotypes: HSV-1 and HSV-2. The former is responsible for virtually all cases of orolabial herpes infection and for approximately 15–20% of genital infections. The principal serotype that causes genital infection is HSV-2, and it is, therefore, of greatest concern to the obstetrician–gynecologist.

Genital herpes infections may be classified into three types. Primary infection represents the patient's first exposure to the herpes virus and is characterized by constitutional symptoms and multiple painful vesicles on the vulva, vagina, and cervix. Initial, nonprimary infection is distinguished by preexisting antibody from an unrecognized earlier infection with either HSV-1 or HSV-2. Affected patients typically have minimal constitutional symptoms and fewer genital lesions than patients with primary herpes. Recurrent herpes is due to reactivation of latent viral infection and is manifested by a characteristic prodrome followed by a limited vesicular eruption.

The prevalence of herpes infection in pregnancy is ≤1%. Most affected women have recurrent rather than primary infection. Hematogenous dissemination of HSV across the placenta is extremely uncommon; however, the fetus may become infected if delivered through a colonized birth canal. The greatest risk to the fetus occurs when vaginal delivery occurs in the setting of a primary maternal infection. Approximately 40% of infants delivered vaginally under these circumstances become infected. In the absence of treatment with antiviral agents such as acyclovir, almost half of these infants die, and most of the remainder have serious neurologic morbidity. Even with treatment, the prognosis is extremely guarded.

The risk to the fetus when the mother has recurrent infection is much lower. If overt lesions are present and vaginal delivery occurs, 5% or fewer of infants become infected. If the mother has no overt lesions but is asymptomatically shedding the virus, 1% or fewer of infants are infected. The lower rates of perinatal transmission in these two situations are presumably due to the protective effects of passively acquired maternal antibody and the lower viral inoculum associated with recurrent or asymptomatic infection.

The diagnosis of primary herpes infection is made on the basis of physical examination and viral culture. Recurrent infection can usually be diagnosed simply by physical examination. Cultures are not indicated in patients with well-documented, recurrent disease. Serologic tests are rarely of value except in cases of apparent initial, nonprimary infection.

Recent investigations have demonstrated that routine surveillance cultures of obstetric patients with a history of recurrent herpes are not effective in preventing neonatal infection. They also are extremely expensive and probably lead to unnecessary cesarean deliveries. Accordingly, the following management plan is recommended for treatment of patients with herpes infections during pregnancy:

- Women who, at the time they are admitted for labor, have overt vesicular lesions from primary or recurrent infection or have a distinct prodrome, should undergo cesarean delivery regardless of time since rupture of membranes.
- Asymptomatic women who have a history of recurrent herpes should be examined carefully at the time of admission to the hospital for labor. If no prodromal symptoms or vesicular lesions are present, vaginal delivery should be anticipated. Viral cultures of the endocervix or neonate should be obtained to assist the pediatrician in planning treatment for the infant.
- Women who have genital herpetic lesions near term, but prior to labor or membrane rupture, should have viral cultures collected at 3–5-day intervals to ensure the absence of virus at the time of birth and thereby increase the likelihood of vaginal delivery.

Acyclovir should not be used routinely during pregnancy to prevent recurrent herpes infection. However, the drug should be considered in immunocompetent women who have severe symptoms due to primary infection and in immunosuppressed women who have unusual debility due to either primary or recurrent infection. To date, no teratogenic effects have been reported with acyclovir.

Urinary Tract Infections

Asymptomatic Bacteriuria and Acute Cystitis

Lower urinary tract infections in pregnancy may take two forms. Asymptomatic bacteriuria affects 4–8% of pregnant women, and all pregnant women should be screened for asymptomatic bacteriuria at the time of their first prenatal appointment. Acute cystitis occurs in 1–3% of obstetric patients. Approximately 80% of infections are caused by *Escherichia coli*; 10–15% are due to *Klebsiella pneumoniae* or *Proteus* species; 5% or less are caused by group B streptococci, enterococci, or staphylococci. Anaerobic organisms are unusual pathogens except in patients who have chronic obstructions or who undergo frequent urologic examinations or procedures.

The diagnosis of asymptomatic bacteriuria is made on the basis of a positive urine culture demonstrating ≥10^5 colonies per milliliter. This urine sample should be a midstream, clean-catch specimen, preferably after urine has incubated in the bladder for 4–6 hours. The diagnosis of acute cystitis should be suspected when patients have dysuria, frequency, and urgency. Microscopic examination of the urine typically shows white blood cells and bacteria, and the culture is subsequently positive. When urine is obtained by catheterization after a short period of incubation, a colony count ≥10^2 colonies per milliliter is considered indicative of infection.

Several oral antibiotics are effective for treatment of lower urinary tract infections: ampicillin, amoxicillin, amoxicillin–clavulanic acid, sulfisoxazole, cephalosporins, nitrofurantoin macrocrystals, trimethoprim–sulfamethoxazole, and quinolones. However, the quinolones are contraindicated in pregnancy because of their injurious effects on fetal cartilage in animals. As a general rule, trimethoprim–sulfamethoxazole and amoxicillin–clavulanic acid should be reserved for unusually refractory infections caused by resistant microorganisms. Sulfisoxazole may displace bilirubin from sites of protein binding in the neonate, but this effect is rarely a problem except in preterm infants.

Whenever possible, selection of antibiotics should be based on the result of sensitivity tests. Given equal efficacy, the agent that is least expensive and least toxic should be administered. When empirical treatment is indicated, ampicillin or amoxicillin is probably not the optimal selection because of the increasing pattern of resistance among strains of *E. coli* and *K. pneumoniae* to these two antibiotics.

The appropriate length of antibiotic treatment for uncomplicated lower urinary tract infections is controversial. In obstetric patients, single-dose therapy appears to be less effective than in nonpregnant patients. However, a 3-day course of antibiotics is usually comparable in efficacy to a 7- or 10-day course and ensures better compliance. Patients who have a poor response to this short course of therapy often have a silent upper urinary tract infection and require extended duration of treatment for 2–4 weeks.

Patients should have a repeat urine culture upon completion of treatment to be certain that the infection is eradicated. Their risk of recurrence later in pregnancy is 15–25%.

Acute Pyelonephritis

Acute pyelonephritis occurs in 1–2% of pregnant women. The single most important risk factor for pyelonephritis is previously undiagnosed or inadequately treated lower urinary tract infection. In fact, approximately 40% of women with untreated asymptomatic bacteriuria will develop pyelonephritis. Ascending infection is particularly likely in pregnancy because of the inhibitory effect of progesterone on ureteral peristalsis and the mechanical compression of the ureters by the enlarging uterus.

The principal bacteria responsible for pyelonephritis are *E. coli*, *K. pneumoniae*, and *Proteus* species. Gram-positive organisms are unlikely causes of upper urinary tract infection. The usual clinical manifestations of acute pyelonephritis are fever, chills, flank pain and tenderness, and urinary frequency and urgency. Approximately 70–75% of cases of pyelonephritis are right sided. Approximately 10–15% are left sided, and 10–15% are bilateral. Bacteremia may be present in up to 10% of infected patients, and 1–2% of patients will actually develop septic shock. A similar percentage may also manifest signs of adult respiratory distress syndrome. In patients with pyelonephritis, microscopic examination of the urine typically shows white blood cell casts and bacteria. The urine culture will be positive unless the patient has previously received antibiotic treatment.

Infected patients should be hospitalized immediately and treated with parenteral antibiotics. A first-generation cephalosporin such as cefazolin, 1–2 g every 8 hours, is an excellent empirical choice because of its uniform activity against the major uropathogens and its low expense and minimal toxicity. Patients who appear to be critically ill or who are particularly likely to have a resistant organism should be treated initially with both cefazolin and gentamicin, 1.5 mg/kg every 8 hours, or aztreonam, 2 g every 8 hours, until the sensitivity tests are completed. Parenteral antibiotics should be continued until the patient has been afebrile and asymptomatic for 24–48 hours. Once this criterion is met, the patient may be discharged from the hospital and treated with an appropriate oral antibiotic for 7–10 days. The patient subsequently needs to be assessed with periodic urine screens.

Approximately 75% of obstetric patients with pyelonephritis will become afebrile within 48 hours. Almost 95% will be afebrile within 72 hours. Patients who have a poor response to therapy are likely to have either a resistant organism or a urinary tract obstruction. If the latter condition is suspected, the patient should be evaluated with renal ultrasonography or intravenous pyelography. If obstruction is demonstrated, urologic consultation is indicated.

Group B Streptococcal Infection

The group B streptococcus, *Streptococcus agalactiae*, is an important cause of maternal and neonatal infection. Approximately 15–40% of pregnant women are colonized with this organism in either the vagina or rectum or both. The organism typically causes ascending infection following rupture of membranes.

Neonatal group B streptococcal infection may take two forms. Early-onset disease usually occurs within 7 days of delivery and has an incidence of 1–4/1,000 live births. It is characterized by overwhelming sepsis or severe pneumonia. Infection of the infant results from vertical transmission, and the overall fatality rate is approximately 10–20%. Although 60–80% of cases occur in term infants, the attack rate and subsequent morbidity and mortality rates are higher in preterm infants. Late-onset disease usually occurs after the seventh day of life and has an incidence of approximately 0.5–1.5/1,000. Late-onset disease may result from both vertical and horizontal transmission; pneumonia, bacteremia, and meningitis are the most common clinical manifestations.

The most reliable test for documenting group B streptococcal colonization is culture. Ideally, culture samples should be obtained by swab from the lower vagina and rectum and inoculated into Todd–Hewitt broth or onto selective blood agar. Failure to use selective media may substantially decrease the frequency of positive cultures.

A variety of rapid laboratory tests has been developed to identify group B streptococci. These tests include Gram stain, short incubations in starch media, latex particle agglutination, enzyme immunoassay (EIA), and DNA analysis. Of these tests the Gram stain has the least utility. The others are reasonably sensitive in identifying heavily colonized women. Only the DNA probe has acceptable sensitivity in detecting lightly colonized women.

Intrapartum chemoprophylaxis can prevent vertical transmission of infection in colonized mothers. The most extensively tested antibiotic is ampicillin; it usually is administered in a dosage of 1–2 g IV every 4–6 hours during labor. Patients who are allergic to ampicillin may be treated with erythromycin, clindamycin, or vancomycin.

The timing and selectivity of screening for group B streptococcal infection in the mother remain controversial. The American Academy of Pediatrics supports screening all pregnant women for group B streptococcal colonization as a method of preventing sequelae in their infants. ACOG does not recommend routine prenatal cultures to detect colonization because 1) colonization may be intermittent; 2) the predictive value of a single genital culture in the prenatal period is only 60–70% for a positive culture at delivery; and 3) with a low attack rate (about 1%), there is a large expense. However, administering ampicillin during labor to colonized women with high-risk factors (eg, preterm labor, preterm PROM, prolonged rupture of membranes, sibling affected by symptomatic GBS infection, or maternal fever) has been shown to decrease infection significantly in their infants.

Human Immunodeficiency Virus Infection

Human immunodeficiency virus (HIV) infection is caused by an RNA retrovirus. The principal viral strain responsible for infection in the United States is HIV type 1 (HIV-1). The virus has a unique propensity to infect CD4 lymphocytes, thus rendering the host susceptible to an extensive variety of opportunistic infections and malignancies.

Infection with HIV occurs in a continuum that begins with a transient flulike illness. Patients then enter a latent period that lasts for an average of almost 10 years. Ultimately, however, all infected individuals become overtly symptomatic and progress to the end stage of AIDS. Once a patient becomes symptomatic, average life expectancy is 5 years or less.

The prevalence of HIV infection in the general obstetric population is approximately 1/1,000. In some inner city populations, however, the prevalence is as high as 1–1.5%. Most of these women are presently in the latent phase of their illness. The two most important risk factors for HIV infection in women in the United States are intravenous drug abuse and contact with a high-risk male.

Symptomatic patients with HIV infection typically have fever, malaise, fatigue, anorexia, nausea, vomiting, diarrhea, weight loss, and generalized lymphadenopathy. Neurologic manifestations may be quite prominent and debilitating, specifically peripheral neuropathy and dementia. Opportunistic infections, of course, are the hallmark of this disease. Among the most common opportunistic infections are *Pneumocystis carinii* pneumonia, tuberculosis, toxoplasmosis, candidiasis, and CMV infection. Genital herpes; hepatitis B, C, and D; and syphilis are common concurrent sexually transmitted diseases. The two most frequent malignancies in patients with HIV infection are Kaposi sarcoma and non–Hodgkin lymphoma.

Infection with HIV may be confirmed by direct culture of virus from peripheral blood lymphocytes and by detection of viral antigen. The polymerase chain reaction test is especially valuable in amplifying low levels of viral antigen. Infected patients characteristically have a decreased number of CD4 cells and an inverted CD4:CD8 ratio.

The mainstay of diagnostic tests is identification of antibody to HIV. The initial serologic screening test is either an ELISA or an EIA. These tests are highly sensitive, easy and inexpensive to perform, and readily suited for screening large numbers of patients. Patients with a positive ELISA or EIA should have a repeat test. If the second test also is positive, a Western blot assay should be performed to identify antibody to specific viral antigens. The test is considered positive when any two of the following three antigens are detected: p 24 (viral core), gp 41 (envelope), and gp 120/160 (envelope).

As a general rule, patients in the United States should be tested only for HIV-1 infection. Testing for HIV-2 infection is indicated if the patient has had sexual or needle-sharing contact with a partner from an area of the world where HIV-2 infection is endemic (West Africa, Portugal, France).

Most cases (80–90%) of HIV infection in children result from perinatal transmission. Perinatal transmission occurs as a result of hematogenous dissemination across the placenta and as a result of intrapartum exposure to infected blood and genital tract secretions. The frequency of perinatal transmission is approximately 20–30%.

Obstetric patients with HIV infection are at increased risk for preterm delivery and delivery of a low-birth-weight infant. They also are more likely to have other problems such as inconsistent prenatal care, drug addiction, and sexually transmitted diseases, all of which increase the probability of poor perinatal outcome.

All obstetric patients should be offered voluntary screening for HIV infection. Seropositive women should be counseled about the risk of obstetric complications and perinatal transmission, and the option of pregnancy termination should be explained. Infected patients should be screened for other sexually transmitted diseases, tuberculosis, CMV infection, and toxoplasmosis. They also should be screened for cervical neoplasia and vaccinated for hepatitis B, pneumococcal infection, and influenza.

Asymptomatic seropositive patients should have CD4 counts every trimester. If the count falls below 200–500 cells per microliter or signs of overt illness develop, treatment with zidovudine (100 mg orally five times daily) is indicated. Preliminary data suggest that use of zidovudine may reduce the risk of prenatal transmission by two thirds. Patients receiving zidovudine should be monitored for marrow suppression. They also should receive double-strength trimethoprim–sulfamethoxazole, two tablets three times a week, for prophylaxis against *P. carinii* infection.

When infected women are in labor, every effort should be made to avoid instrumentation that would increase the fetus's exposure to infected blood and secretions. In the postpartum period, the mother should be advised to avoid contact between her body fluids and an open area on the skin or mucous membranes of the neonate. She should be warned that breast milk can transmit infection to her neonate and encouraged to bottle-feed. Finally, she should be urged to adopt responsible sexual practices in the future to prevent spread of infection to her partner.

Tuberculosis

Pulmonary tuberculosis is relatively rare during pregnancy but is increasing in frequency. In the United States, most cases of active tuberculosis occur during pregnancy as reactivation of old disease in immigrants from countries with endemic disease or in women with chronic diseases leading to immunosuppression, such as AIDS. At-risk populations of women should be screened with a tuberculin skin test in early pregnancy. Chest X-ray films should be obtained for tuberculin reactors with an indeterminate history of prior reactivity and for patients with a history or physical findings consistent with active disease. A definite diagnosis depends upon demonstration of *Mycobacterium tuberculosis* by culture in sputum, tissue, or other body fluids. Because culture techniques take several weeks, therapy may be started if a smear is positive for acid-fast bacilli.

While the primary goal of therapy is to eliminate the tuberculosis bacillus, it is equally important to choose agents that are not harmful to the fetus. The efficacy of short-course chemotherapy (9–12 months of isoniazid and rifampin, with ethambutol or streptomycin added for the first 1–2 months) has been well documented. Streptomycin may cause ototoxicity to both mother and fetus. Rifampin inhibits DNA-dependent RNA polymerase and readily crosses the placenta. It can, therefore, theoretically cause fetal injury. A combination of isoniazid and ethambutol is both safe and effective during pregnancy and is the therapy of choice. If a triple-drug regimen is required because of drug resistance or extrapulmonary tuberculosis, rifampin may be added after the first trimester. Rifampin can cause a reddish-orange discoloration of body fluids. When isoniazid is used during pregnancy, supplemental vitamin B_6 (pyridoxine) is recommended to prevent maternal peripheral neuropathy. Furthermore, liver transaminase levels should be assessed regularly.

Typically, patients with documented or suspected conversion of their tuberculin test are treated with isoniazid for 6 months to 1 year. However, both the CDC and the American Thoracic Society recommend that prophylactic therapy be withheld during pregnancy and then started postpartum. Any patient who has recently undergone seroconversion on the tuberculin test should be tested for HIV and should undergo isoniazid treatment if this test is positive.

Although congenital infection can occur because of either hematogenous spread or aspiration of the bacillus during the birth process, most infection comes from postpartum maternal contact. Bacillus Calmette-Guerin (BCG) vaccination of newborns of women with active tuberculosis is recommended. Theoretically, the child should be separated from the mother after vaccination until he or she develops a positive skin test. An alternative regimen is isoniazid prophylaxis; however, regularly administering this medication to a newborn is naturally associated with compliance problems.

Immunizations During Pregnancy

Four types of immunobiologic agents are currently available: toxoids, inactivated vaccines, live vaccines, and immune globulin preparations. As a general rule, only live viral or live bacterial vaccines are contraindicated during pregnancy. The most commonly used live virus vaccines in the United States are measles, mumps, and rubella. Varicella vaccine also is a live attenuated virus preparation.

Ideally, all women of childbearing age should be immune to measles, mumps, rubella, tetanus, pertussis, diphtheria, and poliomyelitis by virtue of either childhood vaccination or natural infection. Women who are susceptible to any of these infections may receive toxoids or inactivated vaccines (tetanus, pertussis, diphtheria, inactivated polio vaccine), if clinically indicated, during pregnancy. Live virus vaccinations (eg, measles, mumps, rubella, or live polio vaccine) should be deferred until after delivery.

Certain obstetric patients may merit special consideration for vaccination during pregnancy. Patients with risk factors for hepatitis B should be vaccinated with the recombinant vaccine. Patients with acute exposure to hepatitis B also should receive hepatitis B immune globulin. Patients who live in communities where hepatitis A is endemic should receive the new inactivated hepatitis A vaccine. Women who have had a splenectomy, who have sickle cell anemia, or who are immunocompromised should be vaccinated against pneumococcal infection. Pregnant women who have cardiopulmonary disease, diabetes, hemoglobinopathy, or chronic renal disease are candidates for the influenza vaccine. Susceptible women with acute exposure to varicella should receive varicella zoster immune globulin. Finally, pregnant patients who anticipate foreign travel may require special immunizations for infections such as cholera, plague, typhoid, and viral hepatitis.

BIBLIOGRAPHY

Cardiac Disease

Landon MB, Samuels P. Cardiac and pulmonary disease. In: Gabbe SG, Niebyl JR, Simpson JL, eds. Obstetrics: normal and problem pregnancies. 2nd ed. New York: Churchill Livingstone, 1991:1057–1083

Pulmonary Disease

Clark SL. Management of asthma during pregnancy. National Asthma Education Program Working Group in Asthma and Pregnancy. National Institutes of Health, National Heart, Lung and Blood Institute. Obstet Gynecol 1993;82:1036–1040

Maccato ML. Pneumonia and pulmonary tuberculosis in pregnancy. Obstet Gynecol Clin North Am 1989;16:417–430

Liver and Alimentary Tract Disease

Laifer SA, Darby MJ, Scantlebury VP, Harger JH, Caritis SN. Pregnancy and liver transplantation. Obstet Gynecol 1990;76:1083–1088

Riely CA, Latham PS, Romero R, Duffy TP. Acute fatty liver of pregnancy: a reassessment based on observation in nine patients. Ann Intern Med 1987;106:703–706

Sorokin JJ, Levine SM. Pregnancy and inflammatory bowel disease: a review of the literature. Obstet Gynecol 1983;62:247–252

Neurologic Diseases

Bag S, Behari M, Ahuja GK, Karmarkar MG. Pregnancy and epilepsy. J Neurol 1989;236:311–313

Birk K, Ford C, Smeltzer S, Ryan D, Miller R, Rudick RA. The clinical course of multiple sclerosis during pregnancy and the puerperium. Arch Neurol 1990;47:738–742

Katz VL, Peterson R, Cefalo RC. Pseudotumor cerebri and pregnancy. Am J Perinatol 1989;6:442–445

Diabetes Mellitus

Landon MB, Gabbe SG. Diabetes mellitus and pregnancy. Obstet Gynecol Clin North Am 1992;19:633–654

Metzger BE. Summary and recommendations of the Third International Workshop-Conference on Gestational Diabetes Mellitus. Diabetes 1991;40(2 suppl):197–201

Thyroid Disease

Davis LE, Lucas MJ, Hankins GDV, Roark ML, Cunningham FG. Thyrotoxicosis complicating pregnancy. Am J Obstet Gynecol 1989;160:63–70

Samuels P, Bussel JB, Braitman LE, Tomaski A, Druzin ML, Mennuti MT, et al. Estimation of the risk of thrombocytopenia in the offspring of pregnant women with presumed immune thrombocytopenia purpura. N Engl J Med 1990;323:299–235

Immunologic Disorders

Arnett FC, Edworthy SM, Bloch DA, McShane DJ, Fries JF, Cooper NS, et al. The American Rheumatism Association 1987 revised criteria for the classification of rheumatoid arthritis. Arthritis Rheum 1988;31:315–324

Branch DW, Andres R, Digre KB, Rote NS, Scott JR. The association of antiphospholipid antibodies with severe preeclampsia. Obstet Gynecol 1989;73:541–545

Cowchock FS, Reece EA, Balaban D, Branch DW, Plouffe L. Repeated fetal losses associated with antiphospholipid antibodies: a collaborative randomized trial comparing prednisone with low-dose heparin treatment. Am J Obstet Gynecol 1992;166:1318–1323

Cunningham FG, MacDonald PC, Gant NF, Leveno KJ, Gilstrap LC III. Williams obstetrics. 19th ed. Norwalk, Connecticut: Appleton and Lange, 1993:1229–1242

Hahn BH. Systemic lupus erythematosus. In: Wilson JD, Braunwald E, Isselbacher KJ, Petersdorf RG, Martin JB, Fauci AS, eds. Harrison's principles of internal medicine. 12th ed. New York: McGraw-Hill, 1991:1432–1437

Kutteh WH, Carr BR. Recurrent pregnancy loss. In: Carr BR, Blackwell RC, eds. Textbook of reproductive medicine. Norwalk, Connecticut: Appleton and Lange, 1992

Lockshin MD. Antiphospholipid antibody syndrome. JAMA 1992;268:1451–1453

Lockshin MD, Druzin ML, Goei S, Qamar T, Magid MS, Jovanovic L, et al. Antibody to cardiolipin as a predictor of fetal distress or death in pregnant patients with systemic lupus erythematosus. N Engl J Med 1985;313:152–156

Polzin WJ, Kopelman JN, Robinson RD, Read JA, Brady K. The association of antiphospholipid antibodies with pregnancies complicated by fetal growth restriction. Obstet Gynecol 1991;78:1108–1111

Silman A, Kay A, Brennan P. Timing of pregnancy in relation to the onset of rheumatoid arthritis. Arthritis Rheum 1992;35:152–155

Steen VD, Conte C, Day N, Ramsey-Goldman R, Medsger TA Jr. Pregnancy in women with systemic sclerosis. Arthritis Rheum 1989;32:151–157

Tan EM, Cohen AS, Fries JF, Masi AT, McShane DJ, Rothfield NF, et al. The 1982 revised criteria for the classification of systemic lupus erythematosus. Arthritis Rheum 1982;25:1271–1277

Triplett DA, Brandt JT, Musgrave KA, Orr CA. The relationship between lupus anticoagulants and antibodies to phospholipid. JAMA 1988;259:550–554

Varner MW. Autoimmune disorders and pregnancy. Semin Perinatol 1991;15:238–250

Infections

Adler SP. Cytomegalovirus and pregnancy. Curr Opin Obstet Gynecol 1992;4:670–675

Alford CA, Stagno S, Pass RF, Britt WJ. Congenital and perinatal cytomegalovirus infections. Rev Infect Dis 1990;12(7 Suppl):5745–5753

American Academy of Pediatrics Committee on Infectious Diseases and Committee on Fetus and Newborn. Guidelines for prevention of group B streptococcal (GBS) infection by chemoprophylaxis. Pediatrics 1992;90:775–778

Centers for Disease Control. Rubella vaccination during pregnancy—United States, 1971–1988. MMWR 1989;38:289–293

Centers for Disease Control. Rubella prevention. Recommendations of the Immunization Practices Advisory Committee (ACIP). MMWR 1990;39(RR-15):1–18

Corey L, Whitley RJ, Store EF, Mohan K. Difference between herpes simplex virus type 1 and type 2 neonatal encephalitis in neurological outcome. Lancet 1988;1:1–4

Daffos F, Forestier F, Capella-Pavlovsky M, Thulliez P, Aufrant C, et al. Prenatal management of 746 pregnancies at risk for congenital toxoplasmosis. N Engl J Med 1988;318:271–275

Dobbins JG, Stewart JA, Demmler GJ. Surveillance of congenital cytomegalovirus disease, 1990–1991. Collaborating Registry Group. MMWR CDC Surveill Summ 1992;41:35–39

Dunlow S, Duff P. Prevalence of antibiotic-resistant uropathogens in obstetric patients with acute pyelonephritis. Obstet Gynecol 1990;76:241–244

Dunn DT, Newell ML, Ades AE, Peckham CS. Risk of human immunodeficiency virus type 1 transmission through breastfeeding. Lancet 1992;340:585–588

Enders G, Nickerl-Pacher U, Miller E, Cradock-Watson JE. Outcome of confirmed periconceptional maternal rubella. Lancet 1988;1:1445–1447

European Collaborative Study: Mother-to-child transmission of HIV infection. Lancet 1988;2:1039–1043

Foulon W, Naessens A, Mahler T, de Waele M, de Catte L, de Meuter F. Prenatal diagnosis of congenital toxoplasmosis. Obstet Gynecol 1990;76:769–772

Fowler KB, Stagno S, Pass RF, Britt WJ, Boll TJ, Alford CA. The outcome of congenital cytomegalovirus infection in relation to maternal antibody status. N Engl J Med 1992;326:663–667

Gibbs RS, Mead PB. Preventing neonatal herpes—current strategies. N Engl J Med 1992;326:946–947

Gilstrap LC 3d, Cunningham FG, Whalley PJ. Acute pyelonephritis in pregnancy: an anterospective study. Obstet Gynecol 1981;57:409–413

Guinan ME, Hardy A. Epidemiology of AIDS in women in the United States, 1981 through 1986. JAMA 1987;257:2039–2042

Hohlfeld P, Vial Y, Maillard-Brignon C, Vaudaux B, Fawer CL. Cytomegalovirus fetal infection: prenatal diagnosis. Obstet Gynecol 1991;78:615–618

Italian Multicenter Study. Epidemiology, clinical features, and prognostic factors of paediatric HIV infection. Lancet 1988;2:1043–1046

Luft BJ, Remington JS. Toxoplasmic encephalitis in AIDS. Clin Infect Dis 1992;15:211–222

Lynch L, Daffos F, Emanuel D, Giovangrandi V, Meisel R, Forestier F. Prenatal diagnosis of fetal cytomegalovirus infection. Am J Obstet Gynecol 1991;165:714–718

Miles SA, Balden E, Magpantay L, Wei L, Leiblein A, Hofheinz D, et al. Rapid serologic testing with immune-complex-dissociated HIV p^{24} antigen for early detection of HIV infection in neonates. Southern California Pediatric AIDS Consortium. N Engl J Med 1993;328:297–302

Minkoff HL, DeHovitz JA. Care of women infected with the human immunodeficiency virus. JAMA 1991;266:2253–2258

Munro ND, Sheppard S, Smithells RW, Holzel H, Jones G. Temporal relations between maternal rubella and congenital defects. Lancet 1987;2:201–204

Prober CG, Hensleigh PA, Boucher FD, Yasukawa LL, Au DS, Arvin AM. Use of routine viral cultures at delivery to identify neonates exposed to herpes simplex virus. N Engl J Med 1988;318:887–891

Prober CG, Sullender WM, Yasukawa LL, Au DS, Yeager AS, Arvin AM. Low risk of herpes simplex virus infections in neonates exposed to the virus at the time of vaginal delivery to mothers with recurrent genital herpes simplex virus infections. N Engl J Med 1987;316:240–244

Roos T, Martius J, Gross U, Schrod L. Systematic serologic screening for toxoplasmosis in pregnancy. Obstet Gynecol 1993;81:243–250

Sperling RS, Stratton P. Treatment options for human immunodeficiency virus-infected pregnant women. Obstetric-Gynecologic Working Group of the AIDS Clinical Trials Group of the National Institute of Allergy and Infectious Diseases. Obstet Gynecol 1992;79:443–448

Stagno S, Pass RF, Cloud G, Britt WJ, Henderson RE, Walton PD, et al. Primary cytomegalovirus infection in pregnancy: incidence, transmission to fetus and clinical outcome. JAMA 1986;256:1904–1908

Whitley RJ, Gnann JW Jr. Acyclovir: a decade later. N Engl J Med 1992;327:782–789

Yancey MK, Armer T, Clark P, Duff P. Assessment of rapid identification tests for genital carriage of group B streptococci. Obstet Gynecol 1992;80:1038–1047

Intrapartum Management

ACTIVE MANAGEMENT OF LABOR

Cesarean deliveries in the United States have increased from 10.4% in 1975 to 23.5% in 1991. This increase is mainly due to repeat cesarean deliveries and cesarean deliveries for dystocia. Prevention of cesarean deliveries for dystocia will therefore have an impact on the two most common indications for cesarean birth. A system of labor management for nulliparous women, termed active management of labor, has been developed and practiced in Ireland. Many American obstetricians have focused on the use of "high-dose" oxytocin as the means to achieve a lower cesarean rate. High-dose oxytocin, however, is just one part of the active management of labor. Interestingly, as reported in 1993, the cesarean rate with active management of labor in Ireland has doubled, and this change has been attributed to a more widespread use of epidural analgesia.

LABOR STIMULATION

The stimulation of uterine contractions may be characterized as labor induction or labor augmentation. Induction of labor implies stimulation of uterine contractions in their previous absence, with or without ruptured fetal membranes. Labor induction may be elective or indicated. Elective induction of labor is defined as the initiation of labor solely for convenience. In general, elective induction is not recommended, and labor should be induced only when clearly indicated. Augmentation refers to stimulation of uterine contractions when spontaneous contractions have failed to result in progressive cervical dilatation or descent of the fetus.

Labor may be induced or augmented with oxytocin only after a thorough examination of both mother and fetus and indications for and methods of induction or augmentation have been documented. A physician who has privileges to perform cesarean deliveries should be readily available to respond should problems arise.

Techniques for induction of labor may be divided into surgical or medical. Surgical techniques include stripping of membranes, or amniotomy. Stripping of fetal membranes involves bluntly separating the chorioamnionic membrane from the wall of the cervix and the lower uterine segment. The efficacy of induction of labor by stripping membranes has not been established. Risks include potential infection, bleeding from previously undiagnosed placenta previa or low-lying placenta, and the accidental rupture of membranes.

Timing of amniotomy is of signal importance for maximizing the number of vaginal deliveries and for reducing the number of operative deliveries during labor induction. Induction of labor in a woman with a favorable cervix by amniotomy or a combination of amniotomy and oxytocin is widely accepted and used.

Oxytocin remains the mainstay of medical therapy for labor induction. Factors affecting the dose response to oxytocin include cervical dilatation, parity, and gestational age. Higher doses of oxytocin are generally required in a preterm nullipara with an unfavorable cervix. However, the prediction of an individual's oxytocin requirement prior to the initiation of infusion is impossible. The goal of oxytocin administration is to effect uterine activity that is sufficient to produce cervical change and fetal descent while avoiding stress to the fetus. Oxytocin is best administered in a disciplined fashion by means of an infusion pump according to established departmental protocols. Oxytocin should be diluted (10 or 20 U in 1,000 ml of balanced salt solution) and administered by personnel who have experience in its use. When oxytocin is being administered, the FHR, resting uterine tone, and frequency and duration of contractions should be monitored appropriately either by electronic fetal monitoring or palpation and auscultation every 15 minutes during the first stage of labor and every 5 minutes during the second stage of labor.

Numerous protocols, varying in the initial dose, incremental dose increases, and time intervals between dose increases have been studied and a few are listed in Table 3-15. Low-dose regimens were developed based on the knowledge that it takes oxytocin 40–60 minutes to reach a steady-state concentration in maternal serum. They are associated with a lower incidence of uterine hyperstimulation. High-dose protocols in the United States were inspired by the experience of the Irish and have been credited by their advocates with shortening time in labor and reducing cesarean deliveries for dystocia.

Recently, prostaglandin E_2 (PGE_2) gel has been approved for ripening of an unfavorable cervix in pregnant women at or near term with a medical or obstetric indication for labor induction. Prostaglandin E_2 (0.5 mg) placed intracervically

TABLE 3-15. LABOR STIMULATION WITH OXYTOCIN: EXAMPLES OF STUDIED "LOW-DOSE" AND "HIGH-DOSE" REGIMENS

Regimen and Investigator	Starting Dose (mU/min)	Incremental Increase (mU/min)	Dosage Interval (min)	Maximum Dose (mU/min)
Low-dose				
Seitchik	0.5–1	1	30–60	20
Hauth	1–2	2	15	40
High-dose				
O'Driscoll	≈ 6	≈ 6	15	≈ 36
Satin	6	6*, 3, 1	20–40	42

* Incremental increase reduced to 3 mU/min in presence of hyperstimulation; reduced to 1 mU/min with recurrent hyperstimulation.

has been shown to improve cervical favorability in women with long and closed cervixes. After gel application, the patient should remain supine for 15–30 minutes to minimize leakage of the medication from the cervical canal. Intracervical PGE_2 may induce contractions and labor and, therefore, should be administered in a monitored setting similar to that for oxytocin. It is recommended that 6–12 hours elapse before intravenous oxytocin is begun or the dose repeated. Administration of PGE_2 alone or PGE_2 followed by oxytocin does not result in a lower cesarean rate when compared to oxytocin alone.

The principles used in administering oxytocin for labor augmentation are the same as those for oxytocin labor induction. Since oxytocin for augmentation is typically prescribed in women with complete effacement and advanced cervical dilatation, it is not surprising that the maximum infusion rate required is typically lower than rates needed for induction.

INTRAPARTUM FETAL HEART RATE MONITORING

The original goal of intrapartum FHR monitoring was to detect signs of fetal compromise, hopefully in time to intervene before irreversible fetal damage occurred. However, despite the liberal use of continuous electronic fetal monitoring and operative delivery, there has been no consistent decrease in the frequency of cerebral palsy in the past two decades. Randomized, prospective trials of continuous FHR monitoring versus intermittent auscultation have shown no differences in their ability to detect fetal compromise when the following conditions are met:

- If auscultation is used as a primary surveillance technique, a 1:1 nurse-to-patient ratio is required. In certain labor and delivery circumstances, therefore, the number of nurses available may preclude monitoring FHR by auscultation.
- When intermittent auscultation is used during the active phase of the first stage of labor, the FHR should be evaluated and recorded at least every 15 minutes after a uterine contraction. If continuous electronic monitoring is used during this stage, the tracing should be evaluated at least every 15 minutes.
- When auscultation is used during the second stage of labor, the FHR should be evaluated and recorded at least every 5 minutes; when electronic monitoring is used, FHR should also be evaluated at least every 5 minutes.

Fetal heart rate should be monitored during labor by either auscultation or continuous electronic FHR monitoring (Table 3-16).

The most commonly used techniques for detection of FHR are the Doppler ultrasound transducer (external technique), and the fetal scalp electrode (internal technique). While the internal technique has been regarded as superior to the external techniques because of its ability to assess FHR variability more accurately and the fact that it is less subject to artifacts and fetal movement, the new technology of autocorrelation has resulted in significant narrowing of these differences. Uterine activity is usually measured with an externally placed tocodynamometer or an intrauterine pressure catheter. The latter is generally used when there is an abnormality of labor that requires quanti-tation of the force of contractions. Periodic auscultation of the fetal heart by either stethoscope or Doppler technique should begin immediately before a contraction and should continue for at least 30 seconds after cessation of uterine contractions.

Fetal heart rate patterns may be described in terms of baseline features and periodic changes. The normal baseline FHR is 120–160 beats per minute. A sustained FHR less than 120 beats per minute is considered bradycardia. Fetal bradycardia between 100–120 beats per minute can usually be tolerated for long periods when it is accompanied by normal FHR variability. A sustained FHR above 160 beats per minute is considered tachycardia. Fetal tachycardia usually results from chorioamnionitis but may be due to a number of fetal or maternal conditions, including maternal fever, thyrotoxicosis, medications, and fetal cardiac arrhythmias. Fetal tachycardia between 160–200 beats per minute without any other abnormalities of the FHR is usually well tolerated. The interval between successive heartbeats in the normal fetus in characterized by variability. Short-term variability is the beat-to-beat variability or the differences between adjacent beats or several beats. Beat-to-beat variability is best assessed by an internal FHR monitor. Long-term variability consists of irregular crude sine waves with a cycle of approximately three to six

TABLE 3-16. GUIDELINES FOR FETAL HEART RATE MONITORING IN LABOR

Stage	Auscultation		Continuous Electronic Monitoring	
	Low Risk	High Risk	Low Risk	High Risk
Active phase of 1st stage	FHR* evaluated and recorded every 30 minutes following a contraction	FHR evaluated and recorded every 15 minutes, preferably following a uterine contraction	Evaluate tracing at least every 30 minutes	Evaluate tracing at least every 15 minutes
2nd stage	FHR evaluated and recorded every 15 minutes	FHR evaluated and recorded at least every 5 minutes	Evaluate tracing at least every 15 minutes	Evaluate tracing at least every 5 minutes

*FHR indicates fetal heart rate.

per minute. Normal long-term FHR variability implies variability of five beats or more per minute. Decreased variability includes variability of two to six beats per minute, and less than two beats per minute (straight line) implies absence of variability. In the presence of normal FHR variability, regardless of what other FHR patterns exists, the fetus is not suffering significant cerebral tissue hypoxia.

Periodic FHR changes are changes in the FHR related to uterine contractions. Uterine contractions may cause intermittent decreases in intervillous space blood flow, may influence cerebral blood flow under certain circumstances, and, depending on the location of the umbilical cord, may cause intermittent umbilical cord occlusion. Periodic changes in FHR include early, variable, and late decelerations. Early decelerations appear mild in nature and are smooth in shape. Typically, they appear as a mirror image of the uterine contraction pattern. Early decelerations result from fetal head compression. Variable decelerations are usually abrupt in onset and cessation. The dip in the FHR differs in duration, profundity, and shape from contraction to contraction. Variable decelerations are a result of umbilical cord compression. Late decelerations are characterized by a drop in the FHR after the onset of contraction and a delay in the return of the FHR to baseline until after the contraction is completed. Late decelerations are believed to result from uteroplacental insufficiency in most cases. A combination of late decelerations and a loss of FHR variability is considered a nonreassuring FHR pattern.

The FHR pattern should be described and interpreted in terms of baseline and periodic changes. Terms such as *fetal distress* or *fetal jeopardy* should be avoided, since they are nondescriptive and difficult, if not impossible, to define. Examples of nonreassuring FHR patterns may include those with absent short-term variability, moderate or severe bradycardia, or severe repetitive variable decelerations. Absent short-term variability (beat-to-beat variability) may indicate compromise of the fetal autonomic system. Absent variability may also result from certain maternal medications. Moderate (80–100 beats per minute) or severe (<80 beats per minute for more than 3 minutes) bradycardia may indicate impending fetal loss. Variable decelerations with slow return to FHR baseline (deceleration >60 beats per minute) and severe repetitive variable decelerations (<70 beats per minute for more than 60 seconds) also represent nonreassuring FHR patterns. In the presence of nonreassuring FHR patterns, several modes of evaluation should be considered. If fetal membranes are intact, amniotomy and placement of internal electronic fetal monitors may be considered. If a nonreassuring FHR persists, initial conservative measures may include change in maternal position to the left lateral position, administration of oxygen, correction of maternal hypotension, and discontinuation of oxytocin if appropriate. Amnioinfusion, fetal scalp stimulation, or fetal scalp blood sampling for acid–base status may also be considered. If these tests remain nonreassuring, delivery should be expedited. A generalized algorithm for labor management and suggested responses to FHR patterns is depicted in Fig. 3-4. All the maneuvers described above are directed toward improving oxygen delivery to the fetus. It is important to reemphasize that the most significant prognosticator of fetal well-being is FHR variability, as FHR variability implies oxygen delivery to the fetal brain. In the presence of FHR variability, irreversible fetal hypoxia has not taken place.

OPERATIVE OBSTETRICS

Forceps Delivery

Prior to 1988, inadequate definitions were at least partially responsible for a steady decline in the use of obstetric forceps. The old definition of midforceps delivery combined relatively easy deliveries, when the head was on or very near the pelvic floor, with difficult deliveries that involved midpelvic rotation of 90 degrees or more. This situation was remedied by the adoption of the definitions put forth by ACOG in 1988 (Table 3-17). The indication, station, degree of rotation, and any difficulties encountered during the procedure should be specified in a detailed note in the patient's medical record. Station and rotation are the key elements in this classification scheme. There is preliminary evidence that the new system provides better stratification of maternal and neonatal risks associated with instrumental delivery.

A number of prerequisites should be satisfied before forceps delivery, two of which deserve special emphasis. First, accurate diagnosis of fetal position must be followed by proper application of the forceps to achieve a symmetric, bimalar, biparietal grip on the fetal head. Such an application will mini-

TABLE 3-17. CLASSIFICATION OF FORCEPS DELIVERIES ACCORDING TO STATION AND ROTATION

Type of Procedure	Classification
Outlet forceps	1) Scalp is visible at the introitus without separating labia
	2) Fetal skull has reached pelvic floor
	3) Sagittal suture is in anteroposterior diameter or right or left occiput anterior or posterior position
	4) Fetal head is at or on perineum
	5) Rotation does not exceed 45°
Low forceps	Leading point of fetal skull is at station ≥ +2 cm, and not on the pelvic floor
	a. Rotation ≤ 45° (left or right occiput anterior to occiput anterior, or left or right occiput posterior to occiput posterior)
	b. Rotation > 45°
Midforceps	Station above +2 cm but head engaged
High forceps	Not included in classification

American College of Obstetricians and Gynecologists. Operative vaginal delivery. ACOG Technical Bulletin 152. Washington, DC: ACOG, 1991

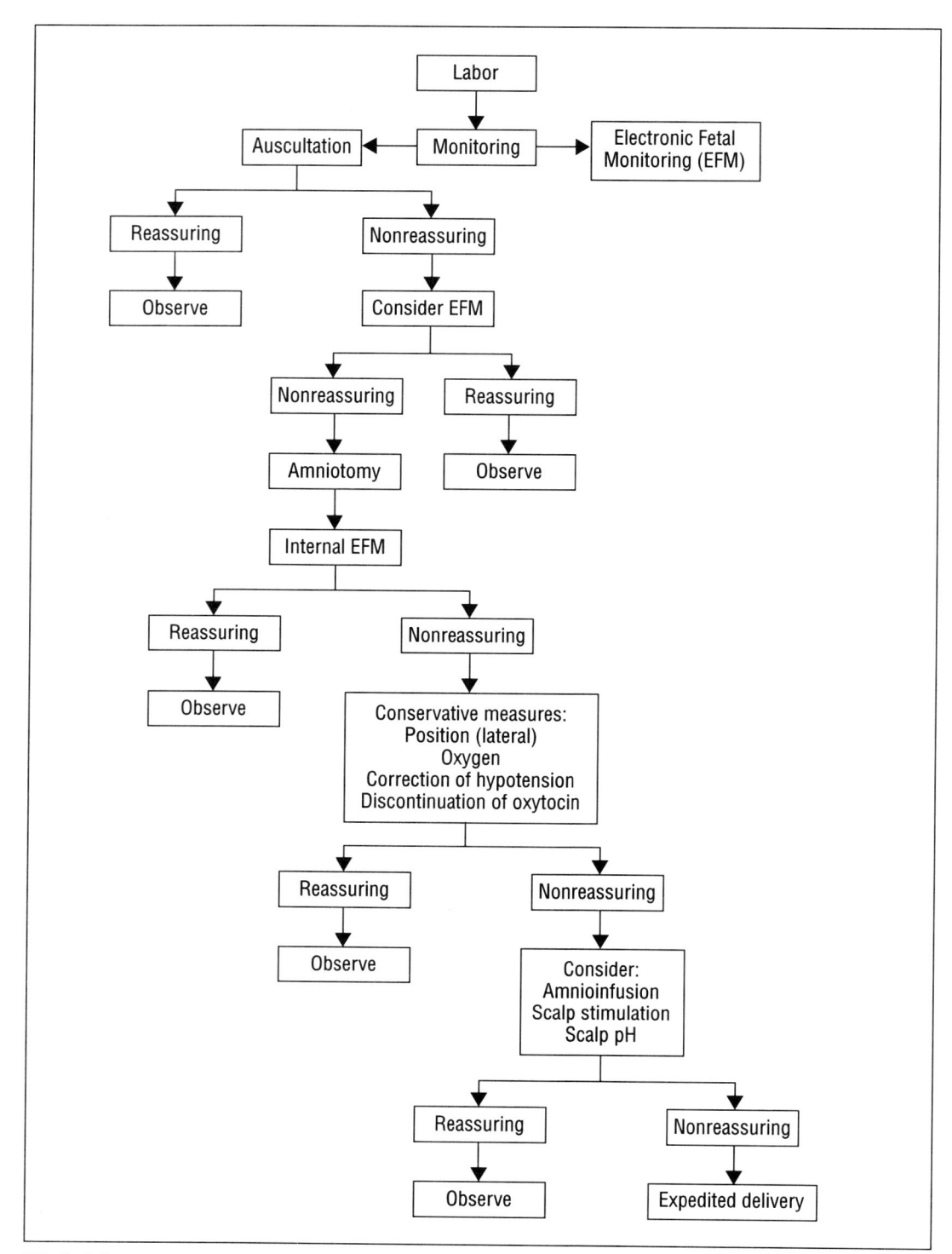

FIG. 3-4. Suggested responses to nonreassuring fetal heart rate patterns.

mize the undesirable force of compression inherent in any forceps delivery. Second, careful assessment of the fetopelvic relationship for each potential forceps delivery will enable the operator to take advantage of maximum pelvic capacity when rotating a fetal head, while simultaneously flexing the head to move the optimal diameter through the birth canal.

Safe operative vaginal delivery is preferable to cesarean delivery. Considerable training and practice during residency are required to acquire sufficient surgical judgment to be safe.

Vacuum Extraction

The definitions, indications, and prerequisites for vacuum extraction of the fetus are the same as for forceps deliveries. Application of the vacuum cup to an unengaged head or through an incompletely dilated cervix is strongly discouraged. Relative contraindications for vacuum extraction include prematurity, macrosomia, fetal coagulation defect, nonvertex presentation, and following fetal blood sampling.

A variety of devices are available for clinical use: a rigid metal cup design (Malmström), a polymeric silicone cup (Kobayashi), and several different disposable plastic cups. Proper placement of the cup over the vertex will facilitate flexion and descent when traction is applied.

Commonly cited advantages for vacuum extraction compared with forceps include decreased anesthesia requirement and reduced maternal morbidity in the form of perineal trauma (cervical and vaginal lacerations may still occur if maternal soft tissue is trapped within the cup). Disadvantages include higher failure rates and possibly increased neonatal trauma, although recent reports show little difference in injury between forceps and vacuums. The choice of instrument should be based primarily on the experience of the operator.

Cesarean Delivery

The relative safety of cesarean delivery is one of the triumphs of modern obstetrics. High forceps deliveries have long since been abandoned. Difficult midforceps deliveries no longer need be done to ensure maternal safety. Destructive operations on the fetus have been relegated to history. Placenta previa, while still a threat to maternal and fetal well-being, can be safely managed by abdominal delivery.

Beginning in 1980, however, the tripling of the cesarean delivery rate that occurred in the 1970s stimulated interest in evaluating the factors responsible for this rise. Evidence from Ireland suggested that the reduction in perinatal mortality that accompanied the increase in the cesarean delivery rate may have been coincidental. The perinatal mortality rate fell in Ireland despite a stable cesarean rate.

The four leading indications for cesarean delivery in the United States today are previous cesarean delivery, dystocia, fetal distress, and breech presentation. Interventions to lower the rate include encouraging vaginal birth after cesarean delivery, actively managing labor with proper use of oxytocin, fetal blood sampling or careful interpretation of FHR tracings, and, finally, for breech presentations, external cephalic version with selective vaginal breech delivery. Incentives to control the rate of cesarean delivery include cost-effectiveness, reduction in maternal morbidity and mortality in both the index and subsequent pregnancies, and perhaps improvement in neonatal outcome.

Low transverse uterine incisions should be almost routine. Indications for a vertical uterine incision include anterior placenta previa, back-down transverse lie, and premature breech with an undeveloped lower uterine segment. Classic cesarean deliveries are done only rarely in the 1990s. Women in labor or with ruptured membranes who require cesarean delivery should be given prophylactic antibiotics at the time of cord clamping to reduce the incidence of postoperative endometritis.

Advances in anesthetic technique, blood transfusion, and antibiotics have made the operation safe. Ten thousand cesarean deliveries without a maternal death were reported from one center. Nonetheless, when complications that led to cesarean delivery are taken into account, cesarean delivery results in a fourfold to fivefold increase in maternal mortality, compared with vaginal delivery. Therefore, each decision to perform cesarean delivery should be weighed carefully.

Cesarean and Puerperal Hysterectomy

The increase in the cesarean delivery rate over the last two decades has contributed to an increase in the incidence of placenta accreta. Therefore, the most common contemporary indication for removal of the uterus at the time of a cesarean delivery is an abnormally adherent placenta.

Other reasons to perform obstetric hysterectomy include uterine atony that does not respond to medical management, uterine rupture, and laceration of major uterine vessels that is not controlled by suture ligation. There is arguably a role for scheduled cesarean hysterectomy for women with an indication for cesarean delivery and antecedent history of dysmenorrhea, chronic pelvic pain, abnormal uterine bleeding, uterine leiomyomas, or high-grade cervical intraepithelial neoplasia. Compared with emergency peripartum hysterectomy, scheduled operations are associated with less maternal morbidity.

Notwithstanding, morbidity from the procedure is substantial and includes increased blood loss requiring transfusion, urologic injury, and pelvic cellulitis. The operation is not recommended for the sole indication of elective sterilization.

Vaginal Birth After Cesarean Delivery

In 1991, 23.5% of all live births were cesarean deliveries, of which just over one third were repeat operations. Vaginal birth after cesarean delivery is a safe approach to reducing the large number of repeat cesarean deliveries done in the United States. Throughout the 1980s vaginal births after cesarean delivery have increased in frequency from 5% to almost 20%, but there is evidence that even the 20% rate might be safely doubled.

The annual rate of vaginal births after cesarean delivery results from multiplying the percentage of women with a previous cesarean delivery who undergo a trial of labor by the success rate of such trials. The latter figure averages 70% (range 50–90%), but the former is highly variable, depending on enthusiasm for trial of vaginal delivery by the counselor, socioeconomic status of the woman, and level of service offered by the hospital.

The safety of vaginal birth after cesarean delivery should be emphasized by all counselors. Careful patient selection is essential. Vaginal delivery should not be attempted in a woman with a previous classic cesarean delivery. There are still not sufficient data to determine the safety or danger of labor for women with a previous low vertical incision. Vaginal delivery should be strongly encouraged in a woman with one previous low transverse incision and offered to women with two or more such incisions. Neither oxytocin nor epidural anesthesia should be withheld from candidates for vaginal birth after cesarean delivery. Additional data support the safety of vaginal birth for twins, breech presentation, and fetuses weighing more than 4,000 g, but the total number of patients within each category is still relatively small.

The benefits of vaginal birth after cesarean delivery include reduction of intraoperative and postoperative complications and a shorter hospital stay; the major risk is rupture of the uterus. The incidence of uterine scar interruption is not increased significantly by a trial of labor, particularly when the previous uterine incision was low transverse. Uterine scar interruption may be asymptomatic and has been found incidentally in up to 2% of patients. The incidence is similar in patients with either previous low transverse or low vertical incisions. Symptomatic uterine rupture requiring emergent intervention is infrequent (less than 1% of all attempted vaginal births after cesarean delivery), and serious maternal and fetal consequences can usually be minimized by appropriate intrapartum surveillance. The most common sign of uterine rupture is an abrupt change in FHR pattern, including bradycardia or prolonged decelerations; therefore, plans for appropriate management, rapid diagnosis, and immediate intervention should be in place prior to undertaking a trial of labor.

Vaginal Breech Delivery

Almost 90% of all fetuses with persistent breech presentations in the United States are delivered by cesarean section. Some of the remaining 10% are intentionally delivered vaginally, whereas others deliver vaginally before cesarean delivery can be performed. Selected vaginal breech delivery is therefore a seldom-used option in the 1990s. Support for this approach can still be found in contemporary literature, but there are relatively few qualified individuals to teach the procedure to residents in obstetrics. Criteria for vaginal breech delivery include fetal weight less than 4 kg and greater than 1.5 kg, frank breech presentation, adequate size pelvis, and absence of hyperextension of the fetal head. Note that nulliparity is not a contraindication. Gestational age is an important consideration. Even though conclusive evidence is lacking, most authorities recommend cesarean delivery of the preterm breech.

If fetopelvic relationships have been carefully evaluated and found to be adequate, oxytocin can be used for either induction or augmentation. Epidural anesthesia can be used but may contribute to a higher failure rate. Episiotomy prior to delivery is suggested. Manipulation of the fetus during delivery must be gentle and deliberate. The physician must avoid transverse pressure on long bones and grasping the fetus on other than bony prominences. Piper forceps are recommended for the aftercoming head.

There is substantial evidence that vaginal breech delivery of the second twin is a safe option. Whereas watchful expectancy is advocated for the singleton breech to see what the woman can accomplish on her own, total breech extraction of even a low-birth-weight second twin has been reported to be acceptable.

External Cephalic Version

Five randomized, controlled trials of external cephalic version at term have been conducted (only one in the United States) to evaluate the safety and efficacy of this intervention. All five showed a reduction in the incidence of both breech birth and of cesarean delivery for breech presentation. External cephalic version is no longer advocated prior to 37 weeks of gestation, primarily due to a high reversion rate in the preterm infant. At or beyond 37 weeks, not only is reversion uncommon but most of those fetuses destined to turn spontaneously will have already done so. External cephalic version should be performed in accordance with established guidelines:

- A reactive NST should be obtained before and after the procedure.
- Ultrasonography should be done before the procedure to confirm presentation, assess amniotic fluid volume, and exclude placenta previa.
- Ultrasonography during external cephalic version can be used to monitor both the FHR and the progress of the procedure.
- Because immediate delivery might rarely be necessary, external cephalic version should be performed in or very near the labor and delivery area.
- Most advocates of external cephalic version favor the use of tocolysis to facilitate the procedure, but this is not universal.

Recent series confirm a low incidence of perinatal morbidity associated with external cephalic version. Uncommon yet serious complications of external cephalic version include placental abruption, uterine rupture, fetomaternal hemorrhage, isoimmunization, fetal distress, and fetal death. D immune globulin should be administered to all D-negative women undergoing external cephalic version. For the fetus that reverts to breech presentation after successful external cephalic version, a second attempt may be considered.

Optimal use of external cephalic version in the management of breech presentation at term requires that the clinician accurately diagnose fetal malpresentation at 37 weeks and beyond. Ultrasound confirmation is indicated. Whether to attempt external cephalic version prior to deciding on a trial of vaginal breech delivery or to reserve it for those breech fetuses not considered suitable for vaginal delivery remains to be investigated.

Twin Gestation

When both twin A and twin B are presenting as vertex, vaginal delivery can be expected. However, there is no unanimity of opinion regarding the best route of delivery when twin A is vertex and twin B is in a nonvertex presentation (ie, breech or transverse). Many clinicians choose to perform a cesarean delivery for such a vertex, nonvertex twin presentation. Vaginal delivery is also a reasonable option if the clinician is experienced in breech extraction and internal podalic version. Although external cephalic version has been recommended for the management of the second twin after the first twin has been delivered, total breech extraction or assisted breech delivery of the second twin may be preferable for those with experience in such procedures.

When the first twin presents as nonvertex, cesarean delivery is probably the method of delivery preferred by most clinicians.

Shoulder Dystocia

True shoulder dystocia is defined as failure of the shoulders to deliver after gentle downward traction and episiotomy. Using this definition, the incidence varies from 0.15% to 0.60% of all deliveries. A number of antepartum and intrapartum risk factors for the occurrence of shoulder dystocia have been recognized. The antepartum risk factors are diabetes, postterm pregnancy, maternal obesity, and shoulder dystocia in a previous pregnancy. The intrapartum risk factors are abnormal labor, arrest or protraction disorders, midpelvic delivery, macrosomia, and oxytocin use.

However, the predictive value of these factors alone or in combination is low. Moreover, only a small percentage of cases of shoulder dystocia result in birth trauma. Intervention protocols that include induction of labor or elective cesarean delivery are likely to prevent only a few birth injuries and to increase already high cesarean delivery rates. Instead, recognition of risk factors prior to delivery should enable the clinician to anticipate the possibility of some cases of shoulder dystocia. This could lead either to early mobilization of resources or to alternative management, such as avoiding operative midpelvic delivery in a macrosomic infant of a diabetic mother.

Although the "turtle sign" (retraction of the fetal head against the vulva) has been heralded as a reliable sign of impending shoulder dystocia, maintaining the forward momentum of the fetus after either spontaneous or instrumental delivery of the head is suggested as a means of preventing such retraction.

Once shoulder dystocia is diagnosed, the following procedures are recommended:

- Obtain additional help: an anesthesiologist, a pediatrician, assistants to apply suprapubic pressure or remove the legs from the stirrups.
- Perform an adequate episiotomy if not already done.
- Flex the mother's legs against the abdomen (this requires two assistants).
- Attempt to turn the anterior shoulder to an oblique diameter by pressure on the scapula while an assistant applies suprapubic pressure.

Traction should then be directed obliquely while maintaining the head in line with the shoulders.

These simple maneuvers will resolve most cases of shoulder dystocia. Occasionally, extraordinary measures will be needed:

- Woods screw maneuver, in which the posterior shoulder is rotated anteriorly and delivered under the symphysis
- Extraction of the posterior arm across the ventral side of the fetus
- Cephalic replacement (Zavanelli maneuver) followed by cesarean delivery
- Deliberate fracture of the clavicle
- Symphysiotomy (usually reserved for medically underserved areas)

Birth Injuries and Brain Disorders

Operative deliveries, whether vaginal or abdominal, are more likely to result in birth injuries than are spontaneous deliveries. Some of these injuries are preventable with proper obstetric technique. In contrast, brain disorders in neonates and infants are only infrequently associated with intrapartum events.

The most frequently encountered birth injuries include clavicular fractures, long bone fractures, facial nerve palsy, and brachial plexus palsy. The overall incidence is approximately 7/1,000 live births.

Fractures of the clavicle may occur during delivery of a macrosomic or breech infant but also occur during spontaneous delivery of average-weight infants. Specific therapy is rarely required, and recovery is rapid and complete. The humerus and femur are the most common long bones to be fractured. Such fractures are increased with breech delivery, and cesarean delivery does not eliminate these injuries. Fracture of the humerus may also be related to shoulder dystocia, particularly during extraction of the posterior arm. To prevent fractures of long bones, pressure by the operator should always be applied parallel to long bones and never transversely.

Facial nerve palsy usually results from pressure over the stylomastoid foramen, where the nerve exits the bony skull. Forceps delivery probably increases the risk of such injury, but injury also occurs with spontaneous delivery. The outlook for complete recovery is excellent. Brachial plexus palsy occurs with shoulder dystocia and breech delivery. Injury to the upper plexus involves nerve roots C-5–C-7 and is termed Duchenne or Erb palsy. Injury to the lower plexus (Klumpke paralysis) involves roots C-8 and T-1. More than 80% of brachial plexus injuries resolve spontaneously. When shoulder dystocia is recognized, the operator should avoid excessive lateral traction. Fundal pressure is contraindicated, since it may have further impact on the anterior shoulder. During breech delivery, premature traction on the body of the infant may result in a nuchal arm, the management of which may injure the brachial plexus. The Mauriceau–Smellie–Veit maneuver involves traction on the shoulders to deliver the aftercoming head. Such traction can stretch the brachial plexus. The routine use of Piper forceps to the aftercoming head is a preferred alternative.

Cerebral palsy is a nonprogressive motor disorder that may be accompanied by epilepsy or mental retardation, or both. The incidence of 1–2/1,000 term infants has not changed in the past 20 years. There is a continuing misperception that birth asphyxia accounts for a significant portion of infants with cerebral palsy, despite a lack of supportive evidence. In a stepwise logistic regression analysis of data from the Collaborative Perinatal Project, no factor in labor or delivery was a major predictor of cerebral palsy. The leading predictors were maternal mental retardation, birth weight less than 2,000 g, fetal malformation, and breech presentation (but not breech delivery). Birth trauma, which is uncommon in modern obstetrics, apparently plays a minimal role in the development of cerebral palsy. No change in the incidence of neurologic deficit has been noted over two decades, despite a reduction in the use of forceps and an increase in the rate of cesarean delivery. For birth trauma to be implicated in the development of cerebral palsy, the trauma must cause intracranial bleeding, and the infant's course must include seizures and other signs of increased intracranial pressure. It is not known what causes most cases of cerebral palsy.

OBSTETRIC ANESTHESIA AND ANALGESIA

Relief of discomfort and pain during labor and delivery is an essential part of good obstetric care. There are several significant differences between nonobstetric or surgical and obstetric anesthesia. First and foremost, there are two patients to consider when performing anesthetic procedures in the pregnant woman. What may prove beneficial to one may actually be detrimental to the other. There are numerous physiologic changes and an increase in certain complications that occur in pregnancy that must be taken into account. For example, cardiac output, blood volume, tidal volume, minute ventilation, and creatinine clearance increase, whereas functional residual capacity and gastric emptying decrease. The most common pregnancy complications are hypertension and hemorrhage, and many have significant impact on anesthetic choice.

Systemic Agents

Although the use of regional anesthesia is increasing, obstetricians still commonly use intramuscular and intravenous injection of narcotics, barbiturates, and tranquilizers for pain relief during labor. These agents are especially useful in women who have contraindications to regional analgesia. During the past three decades, meperidine has achieved preeminence as a systemic analgesic for use during labor. It produces less nausea and vomiting than does morphine, and it appears to accumulate less readily in the fetal brain. The usual intramuscular dose is 50–100 mg, with 25 mg of promethazine every 3–4 hours. It is best to use small doses given more frequently than large doses administered less often. The intravenous route provides for more rapid onset, but in general not more than 50 mg should be given with each dose.

Butorphanol, a totally synthetic parenteral analgesic with mixed agonist–antagonist properties, appears to offer potential advantages as an analgesic for the parturient. It is 5 times as potent as morphine, 20 times as potent as pentazocine, and 40 times as potent as meperidine. The metabolites of butorphanol are inactive, and it would appear that it produces a degree of respiratory depression that is less than that caused by morphine. When given in 1–2-mg doses, butorphanol compares favorably with approximately 50 mg of meperidine. Two other narcotic analgesics that have been used for pain relief during labor are alphaprodine and nalbuphine.

The total dosage of administered narcotic and the time from administration to the time of delivery govern the transfer of the drug to the fetus. Thus, the smallest dosage possible should be administered as near to the time of delivery as practical. The number of doses should be kept to a minimum to avoid accumulation of drug and metabolites in the fetus. This is especially true for the premature infant. It should be remembered that although a drug administered to the mother may be eliminated promptly and completely from her system, levels in the newborn may be elevated for a considerable length of time.

Naloxone hydrochloride is a narcotic antagonist that is considered the drug of choice to reverse respiratory depression in the newborn associated with meperidine or other narcotics. The recommended dose for the newborn infant is 0.1 mg/kg injected into the umbilical vein.

Diazepam, a commonly used tranquilizer, is not recommended for use in laboring women, as it may cause prolonged depression, hypotonia, feeding problems, and defective temperature regulation in the newborn. Barbiturates may potentiate the sedative effects of narcotics and are used primarily in the latent phase of labor.

Regional Analgesia

Regional analgesia refers to various nerve blocks that provide pain relief without loss of consciousness. Examples include local infiltration, pudendal block, paracervical block, subarachnoid or spinal block, and lumbar epidural block. The latter two techniques are suitable for cesarean birth and are probably the two most commonly used techniques for this operation in the patient without complications.

Local, Pudendal, and Paracervical Block

A local block is infiltration of a local anesthetic, usually lidocaine, prior to performing an episiotomy or repairing genital lacerations. There are few, if any, significant complications associated with this technique.

The pudendal block is a technique of infiltration of the sacrospinous ligament near the ischial spine with a local anesthetic, usually 10 ml of 1% lidocaine. The pudendal nerve, which is blocked, provides sensory innervation to the perineum, anus, and vulva and passes close to the sacrospinal ligament. This technique usually provides adequate analgesia for spontaneous delivery, assisted breech deliveries, and outlet forceps. However, this technique may be inadequate for midpelvic delivery with forceps or vacuum. The major risk of this technique is the inadvertent intravascular injection of the local anesthetic.

Unlike the local and pudendal blocks, the paracervical block provides pain relief for uterine contractions. A local anesthetic, usually 5–10 ml of lidocaine or chloroprocaine, is infiltrated at the 3-o'clock and 9-o'clock positions next to the cervix. A major complication of this technique is fetal bradycardia, probably secondary to uterine artery vasoconstriction. Thus, this is not an ideal procedure in cases of potential fetal compromise, such as a nonreassuring FHR pattern. Moreover, inadvertent intravascular injection of the local anesthetic may result in central nervous system stimulation and convulsions.

Epidural Analgesia

Epidural analgesia can be used either to block the spinal segments that transmit pain arising from the cervix and uterus (thoracic vertebrae T-10–T-12) or to block these segments plus the segments that transmit pain arising from the lower vagina, perineum, and perianal area (sacral vertebrae S-2 and S-4). The availability of short-acting agents (eg, 2-chloroprocaine), moderately long-acting agents (eg, lidocaine), long-acting agents (eg, bupivacaine), and narcotics (eg, fentanyl and meperidine) adds to the flexibility of this method. The technique requires specialized personnel who are capable of dealing with complications, such as total spinal block and toxic reactions to local anesthetics. Because these act as depressants of the central nervous system and the cardiovascular system, their use can lead to convulsions and cardiovascular collapse. Other potential complications include inadvertent spinal blockade, hypotension, and an ineffective block.

The management of convulsions consists of controlled ventilation when needed, the administration of diazepam, and the maintenance of normal tissue perfusion. Hypotension is managed by turning the patient onto her left side and rapidly infusing 500–1,000 ml of balanced salt solution. Ephedrine may also be used as described above for spinal blocks. An epidural block should not be performed without a secure intravenous infusion and a blood pressure cuff in place.

A variety of opioids are used for injection into the epidural space. Since opioids used alone generally will not provide adequate pain relief, they are most often used in combination with a local anesthetic. However, the use of opioids allows for a much smaller dose of local anesthetic. Potential side effects or complications include pruritus, nausea and vomiting, and respiratory depression.

Contraindications to lumbar epidural analgesia are the same as those for spinal analgesia and are discussed in the following section.

Spinal Analgesia

The subarachnoid injection of local anesthetics may be used to provide analgesia for either vaginal or cesarean delivery. Low spinal block satisfactory for vaginal delivery may be obtained with a 4-mg injection of tetracaine. Lidocaine may also be used. Low spinal block is ideal for operative vaginal delivery with either forceps or vacuum extraction.

A larger dose of local anesthetic to provide a higher block is used for cesarean delivery. Either 8–10 mg of tetracaine or 50–75 mg of lidocaine may be used.

Proper monitoring of vital signs is essential lest diminished venous return (ie, sympathetic blockade combined with inferior vena cava compression) lead to diminished cardiac output, hypotension, central respiratory center ischemia, respiratory arrest, and finally cardiac arrest. Furthermore, as the systemic blood pressure drops, the gravid uterus may compress the aorta.

A secure route for the intravenous administration of fluids and medications is mandatory (16-gauge intracatheter), and measures must be taken to prevent hypotension. Such measures include the rapid administration of 500–1,000 ml of balanced salt solution immediately before and during the administration of the subarachnoid block, as well as the lifting of the gravid uterus off the inferior vena cava by placing a wedge under the patient's left buttock or placing her on her side. If, despite these measures, the systolic blood pressure drops below 100 mm Hg, 10–15 mg of ephedrine should be administered IV.

The major advantages of spinal anesthesia are that it is relatively easy to administer, the onset of action is relatively rapid, the duration of block is predictable and dependent on the specific agent, and the dose of local anesthetic is relatively small. The major complications of spinal analgesia are as follows:

- Hypotension
- Total spinal blockade
- Headache
- Convulsions
- Bladder dysfunction
- Arachnoiditis and meningitis

Treatment of hypotension consists of uterine displacement, hydration, and ephedrine. Tracheal intubation, ventilatory support, and treatment of associated hypotension are generally required when total spinal blockade occurs. The treatment of postspinal headache consists primarily of vigorous hydration. For severe headaches unresponsive to hydration, a blood patch consisting of a few milliliters of the patient's blood placed in the epidural space at the site of the lumbar puncture should be considered. Convulsions should be treated with anticonvulsants and respiratory support as necessary.

Contraindications to the administration of either spinal or lumbar epidural include:

- Hypotension
- Hypovolemia
- Infection at site where puncture is to be made
- Preexisting neurologic disease
- Patient refusal
- Absence of physician trained in regional blocks or the treatment of complications
- Unavailability of necessary drugs and equipment
- Lack of monitoring equipment
- Lack of adequate venous access
- Coagulopathy or anticoagulant therapy

Although epidural analgesia is advocated by some and apparently can be used safely in women with severe preeclampsia, spinal block is contraindicated in this scenario because of the risk of hypotension.

General Anesthesia

General anesthesia is most often used when rapid anesthesia is required, such as with an emergency cesarean delivery. Other common indications include patient desire, failed or inadequate regional blocks, need for complicated intrauterine manipulations, or conditions in which hypotension would be detrimental or life-threatening (ie, as in aortic stenosis or pulmonary hypertension).

Inhalation Agents
Inhalation analgesia consists of gas (such as nitrous oxide) and volatile anesthetic agents (such as enflurane and isoflurane). Nitrous oxide, which is the only anesthetic gas currently available, can be used for the pain of either labor or delivery.

Intravenous Agents
The most common intravenous drug used as an adjunct with inhalation agents for general anesthesia is thiopental. It is used primarily at the time of induction of anesthesia. It has a rapid onset and short duration. Ketamine is another agent that is occasionally used for the induction of general anesthesia or to produce sedation and analgesia for operative vaginal delivery. It may be the ideal agent in the woman with acute hemorrhage and significant hypotension. However, it may cause troublesome hallucinations. Moreover, it should be avoided in women with significant hypertension.

Balanced Anesthesia
The preferred method of achieving safe general anesthesia for cesarean and operative vaginal deliveries is a balanced anesthesia technique (ie, a combination of agents performing different functions). Balanced anesthesia has the advantage of preventing significant quantities of potentially dangerous drugs from reaching the fetus. At the same time, it allows a maximum flexibility of the depth of anesthesia, muscle relaxation, airway protection and management, and protection of vital functions. A commonly used protocol consists of a combination of thiopental, a muscle relaxant such as succinylcholine, nitrous oxide, and a halogenated agent such as isoflurane.

Complications
General anesthesia is still associated with a risk of maternal mortality. Fortunately, this risk would appear to be decreasing over the last one to two decades. The two major complications include failed intubation and gastric aspiration. Failed intubation would appear to be most often associated with anatomic anomalies of the neck and face, a short neck, morbid obesity, or marked tracheal edema. Thus, knowledge of and attention to these risk factors can reduce the risk of this life-threatening complication.

Aspiration pneumonitis is still a significant risk factor associated with general anesthesia and may result in maternal mortality. Steps in the prevention of this serious complication consist of fasting for 6–12 hours prior to anesthesia (often not possible with emergency procedures), use of antacids prior to anesthesia, and the use of cricoid pressure prior to intubation and extubation. An example of an effective antacid is 30 ml of sodium citrate with citric acid given 30–45 minutes before the procedure.

Treatment of aspiration consists primarily of suctioning and oxygen with ventilation when indicated. The use of either corticosteroids or antimicrobial agents is controversial, and there is no consensus as to their efficacy or safety.

BIBLIOGRAPHY

Active Management of Labor

O'Driscoll K, Meagher D. Active management of labour. 2nd ed. London: Bailliere Tindall, 1986

Centers for Disease Control and Prevention. Rates of cesarean delivery—United States, 1991. MMWR 1993;42:285–289

Labor Stimulation

Hauth JC, Hankins GD, Gilstrap LC 3d, Strickland DM, Vance P. Uterine contraction pressures with oxytocin induction/augmentation. Obstet Gynecol 1986;68:305–309

Rayburn WF. Prostaglandin E_2 gel for cervical ripening and induction of labor: a critical analysis. Am J Obstet Gynecol 1989;160:529–539

Satin AJ, Leveno KJ, Sherman ML, Brewster DS, Cunningham FG. High- versus low-dose oxytocin for labor stimulation. Obstet Gynecol 1992;80:111–116

Satin AJ, Leveno KJ, Sherman ML, McIntire DD. Factors affecting the dose response to oxytocin for labor stimulation. Am J Obstet Gynecol 1992;166:1260–1261

Intrapartum Fetal Heart Rate Monitoring

Freeman RK, Garite TJ, Nageotte MP. Fetal heart rate monitoring. 2nd ed. Baltimore: Williams and Wilkins, 1991

Operative Obstetrics

Baerthlein WC, Moodley S, Stinson SK. Comparison of maternal and neonatal morbidity in midforceps delivery and midpelvis vacuum extraction. Obstet Gynecol 1986;67:594–597

Chelmow D, Laros RK Jr. Maternal and neonatal outcomes after oxytocin augmentation in patients undergoing a trial of labor after prior cesarean delivery. Obstet Gynecol 1992;80:966–971

Chestnut DH, Eden RD, Gall SA, Parker RT. Peripartum hysterectomy: a review of cesarean and postpartum hysterectomy. Obstet Gynecol 1985;65:365–370

Christian SS, Brady K, Read JA, Kopelman JN. Vaginal breech delivery: a five-year prospective evaluation of a protocol using computed tomographic pelvimetry. Am J Obstet Gynecol 1990;163:848–855

Davison L, Easterling TR, Jackson JC, Benedetti TJ. Breech extraction of low-birth-weight second twins: can cesarean section be justified? Am J Obstet Gynecol 1992;166:497–502

Flamm BL, Fried MW, Lonky NM, Giles WS. External cephalic version after previous cesarean section. Am J Obstet Gynecol 1991;165:370–372

Flamm BL, Goings JR. Vaginal birth after cesarean section: is suspected fetal macrosomia a contraindication? Obstet Gynecol 1989;74:694–697

Flamm BL, Newman LA, Thomas SJ, Fallon D, Yoshida MM. Vaginal birth after cesarean delivery: results of a 5-year multicenter collaborative study. Obstet Gynecol 1990;76:750–754

Gonsoulin W, Kennedy RT, Guidry KH. Elective versus emergency cesarean hysterectomy cases in a residency program setting: a review of 129 cases from 1984 to 1988. Am J Obstet Gynecol 1991;165:91–94

Gross TL, Sokol RJ, Williams T, Thompson K. Shoulder dystocia: a fetal-physician risk. Am J Obstet Gynecol 1987;156:1408–1418

Hagadorn-Freathy AS, Yeomans ER, Hankins GD. Validation of the 1988 ACOG forceps classification system. Obstet Gynecol 1991;77:356–360

Jones RO, Nagashima AW, Hartnett-Goodman MM, Goodlin RC. Rupture of low transverse cesarean scars during trial of labor. Obstet Gynecol 1991;77:815–817

Mahomed K, Seeras R, Coulson R. External cephalic version at term: a randomized controlled trial using tocolysis. Br J Obstet Gynaecol 1991;98:8–13

Myers SA, Gleicher N. A successful program to lower cesarean-section rates. N Engl J Med 1988;319:1511–1516

Nelson KB, Ellenberg JH. Antecedents of cerebral palsy: multivariate analysis of risk. N Engl J Med 1986;315:81–86

Nocon JJ, McKenzie DK, Thomas LJ, Hansell RS. Shoulder dystocia: an analysis of risks and obstetric maneuvers. Am J Obstet Gynecol 1993;168:1732–1737; discussion 1737–1739

O'Driscoll K, Foley M. Correlation of decrease in perinatal mortality and increase in cesarean section rates. Obstet Gynecol 1983;61:1–5

Ophir E, Oettinger M, Yagoda A, Markovits Y, Rojansky N, Shapiro H. Breech presentation after cesarean section: always a section? Am J Obstet Gynecol 1989;161:25–28

Plauche WC. Peripartal hysterectomy. Obstet Gynecol Clin North Am 1988;15:783–795

Porreco RP. High cesarean section rate: a new perspective. Obstet Gynecol 1985;65:307–311

Pruett KM, Kirshon B, Cotton DB, Poindexter AN 3d. Is vaginal birth after two or more cesarean sections safe? Obstet Gynecol 1988;72:163–165

Robertson AW, Kopelman JN, Read JA, Duff P, Magelssen DJ, Dashow EE. External cephalic version at term: is a tocolytic necessary? Obstet Gynecol 1987;70:896–899

Rosen DJ, Illeck JS, Greenspoon JS. Repeated external cephalic version at term. Am J Obstet Gynecol 1992;167:508–509

Rosen MG. NIH Consensus development statement on cesarean childbirth: The cesarean birth task force. Obstet Gynecol 1981;57:537–545

Rosen MG, Chik L. The effect of delivery route on outcome in breech presentation. Am J Obstet Gynecol 1984;148:909–914

Rosen MG, Debanne SM, Thompson K, Dickinson JC. Abnormal labor and infant brain damage. Obstet Gynecol 1992;80:961–965

Rosen MG, Dickinson JC, Westhoff CL. Vaginal birth after cesarean: a meta-analysis of morbidity and mortality. Obstet Gynecol 1991;77:465–470

Rosen MG, Hobel CJ. Prenatal and perinatal factors associated with brain disorders. Obstet Gynecol 1986;68:416–421

Sanchez-Ramos L, Kaunitz AM, Peterson HB, Martinez-Schnell B, Thompson RJ. Reducing cesarean sections at a teaching hospital. Am J Obstet Gynecol 1990;163:1081–1087; discussion 1087–1088

Sandberg EC. The Zavanelli maneuver: a potentially revolutionary method for the resolution of shoulder dystocia. Am J Obstet Gynecol 1985;152:479–484

Scott JR. Mandatory trial of labor after cesarean delivery: an alternative viewpoint. Obstet Gynecol 1991;77:811–814

Shiono PH, McNellis D, Rhoads GG. Reasons for rising cesarean delivery rates 1978–1984. Obstet Gynecol 1987;69:696–700

Socol ML, Garcia PM, Peaceman AM, Dooley SL. Reducing cesarean births at a primarily private university hospital. Am J Obstet Gynecol 1993;168:1748–1754; discussion 1754–1758

Stanco LM, Schrimmer DB, Paul RH, Mishell DR Jr. Emergency peripartum hysterectomy and associated risk factors. Am J Obstet Gynecol 1993;168:879–883

Williams MC, Knuppel RA, O'Brien WF, Weiss A, Kanarek KS. A randomized comparison of assisted vaginal delivery by obstetric forceps and polyethylene vacuum cup. Obstet Gynecol 1991;78:789–794

Yancey MK, Harlass FE, Benson W, Brady K. The perioperative morbidity of scheduled cesarean hysterectomy. Obstet Gynecol 1993;81:206–210

Yeomans ER, Hankins GD. Operative vaginal delivery in the 1990s. Clin Obstet Gynecol 1992;35:487–493

Zelop CM, Harlow BL, Frigoletto FD Jr, Safon LE, Saltzman DH. Emergency peripartum hysterectomy. Am J Obstet Gynecol 1993;168:1443–1448

Obstetric Anesthesia and Analgesia

Abboud TK, Gangolly J, Mosaad P, Crowell D. Isoflurane in obstetrics. Anesth Analg 1989;68:388

Ackerman WE, Juneja M, Spinnato JA. Epidural opioids' ob advantages. Contemp Ob Gyn 1992;37(3):68–74

Atrash HK, Koonin LM, Lawson HE, Franks AL, Smith JC. Maternal mortality in the United States, 1979–1986. Obstet Gynecol 1990;76:1055

Cunningham FG, MacDonald PC, Gant NF, Leveno KJ, Gilstrap LC III. Analgesia and anesthesia. In: Williams obstetrics. 19th ed. Norwalk, Connecticut: Appleton and Lange, 1993:425–442

Fishburne JI Jr, Greiss FC Jr, Hopkinson R, Rhyne AL. Response of the gravid uterine vasculature to arterial levels of local anesthetic agents. Am J Obstet Gynecol 1979;133:753

Gibbs CP, Banner TC. Effectiveness of Bicitra/Pr as a preoperative antacid. Anesthesiology 1984;61:97

Gilstrap LC III, Hankins GDV. The uncomplicated patient. In: Phelan JP, Clark SL, eds. Cesarean delivery. New York: Elsevier, 1988:140

Malinow AM, Ostheimer GW. Anesthesia for the high-risk parturient. Obstet Gynecol 1987;69:951

McGrady EM. Maternal mortality. In: Ostheimer GW, ed. Manual of obstetric anesthesia. 2nd ed. New York: Churchill Livingstone, 1992:402

Rochat RW, Koonin LM, Atrash HK, Jewett JF, the Maternal Mortality Collaborative. Maternal mortality in the United States: report from the Maternal Mortality Collaborative. Obstet Gynecol 1988;72:91

The Newborn

NEONATAL RESUSCITATION

The birth of an infant is associated with a cascade of events that transform the fluid-filled lungs into an air-filled organ with establishment of functional residual volume and gas exchange. Failure of this orderly process to occur will result in cardiorespiratory failure and the necessity for resuscitation. Some of the major causes of ineffective respirations at birth are:

- Fetal hypoxemia/acidemia
- Maternal medications
- Neonatal sepsis
- Aspiration of amniotic fluid with or without meconium
- Pulmonary
  —Hypoplasia
  —Pneumothorax
- External lung compression
  —Pleural effusion
  —Congenital diaphragmatic hernia
  —Ascites
- Central nervous system
  —Central
  —Peripheral (eg, neuromuscular disease)
- Immaturity

The Apgar score was designed to be made by an independent observer at 1 minute after delivery as an indicator of immediate newborn condition, in order to guide immediate delivery room management. To this, a score at 5 minutes is added, and it is now common practice to record the score every 5 minutes while resuscitation continues. In general, an Apgar score of 7 or more indicates a newborn who requires minimal resuscitative effort other than some flow-by oxygen or warming. A score of 4–6 suggests a moderately depressed newborn who is likely to require some form of intervention (ie, bag and mask ventilation). A score of 0–3 suggests severe depression that usually requires endotracheal intubation and artificial ventilation. The application of these scores to the very preterm infant has to be interpreted with caution. Such infants frequently have lower scores, since the measures of the score (ie, reflex irritability, muscle tone, and respiratory effort) may all be less pronounced.

Proper preparation of the resuscitation area is a crucial first step for prompt, effective resuscitation of the newborn. The person responsible for resuscitation should be familiar with all equipment to be used. Most self-inflating bags provide limited pressures (40–50 mm Hg) appropriate for most infants. An anesthesia bag equipped with a manometer for measurement of inspiratory and expiratory pressures may be used to deliver higher pressures and concentrations of oxygen for infants with especially noncompliant lungs. However, the use of the anesthesia bag by an inexperienced person may be hazardous. Whenever feasible, the delivery of high-risk infants should be attended by both a physician and a nurse experienced in neonatal resuscitation, so that evaluation of the infant and, if necessary, ventilation, cardiac massage, and the administration of any drugs can be performed most effectively.

The basic principles of resuscitation in the newborn are similar to those applied to adults: 1) establish an airway; 2) provide adequate ventilation; and 3) maintain adequate circulation. It is equally important to dry the infant in order to avoid the loss of radiant heat.

MECONIUM ASPIRATION

Meconium staining of amniotic fluid complicates 10–20% of all pregnancies. Management of the infant delivered in the presence of meconium staining of amniotic fluid depends on the consistency of the meconium and the infant's arousal status. At delivery, the nostrils and oropharynx should be cleared of secretions prior to the first breath, if possible. If the meconium is thin and the infant is active and has a good heart rate, subsequent management is as for a normal delivery. If meconium is thick and the infant is depressed, intubation and suctioning are necessary before the initiation of positive-pressure ventilation. If meconium is thick and the infant is active, management is less precise; both endotracheal intubation and suctioning or observation are accepted therapeutic options.

Aspiration of meconium may be associated with pneumothorax, chemical pneumonitis, and pulmonary artery hypertension. Management strategies depend on the severity of the aspiration disease and include conventional ventilation, high-frequency ventilation, and extracorporeal membrane oxygenation.

CONGENITAL MALFORMATIONS

Recognition of congenital malformations is traumatic for physicians, nurses, and parents alike. It is important to deal with the problem immediately in a direct and supportive manner. Appropriate consultation (eg, surgical, genetic, or endocrine) should be sought as quickly as possible to deal with critical issues such as 1) the appropriate route of delivery of fetuses with certain anomalies (eg, ventral wall defects or meningomyelocele), and 2) the appropriate studies to be obtained to identify a specific syndrome or chromosomal anomaly, or to assign the sex of an infant with ambiguous genitalia. Ancillary personnel such as social workers, clinical nurse-specialists, or support groups who are experienced in dealing with such issues can be extremely helpful to families during this critical and difficult time.

COMPLICATIONS OF PRETERM BIRTH

Respiratory Distress Syndrome (Hyaline Membrane Disease)

Respiratory distress syndrome remains a common problem, occurring in approximately 10% of all premature infants, with the greatest occurrence in infants with a birth weight of less than 1,500 g. The disease is characterized by a deficiency or absence of surfactant, which is produced by type II pneumonocytes within the lung. Surfactant, a complex lipoprotein rich in phosphatidylcholine molecules, markedly lowers surface tension forces at the air–water interphase, thus reducing the pressure tending to collapse the alveolus. Absence of surfactant reduces lung compliance and increases the work of breathing.

The clinical features of respiratory distress syndrome include grunting, flaring, sternal and intercostal retractions, tachypnea, progressive hypoxia, hypercarbia, and respiratory acidosis. The chest radiograph is characterized by a ground-glass appearance with air bronchograms. The differential diagnosis of neonatal respiratory distress includes pneumonia, pulmonary hypoplasia, congenital cardiac disease, and metabolic disorders.

A major effort in treating this disease should focus on its prevention. The antenatal induction of surfactant with maternal steroids may play an important role in reducing the incidence of disease. The use of exogenous surfactant replacement therapy in preterm infants has resulted in a significant reduction in neonatal mortality (30–40%) and morbidity (reduction of pneumothorax and air leaks). Surfactants available for clinical use are of two general classes: surfactants prepared from mammalian lungs and synthetic surfactants. Two strategies for the use of surfactant have been evaluated. One strategy involves treating infants at risk for respiratory distress syndrome in the delivery room before, or concurrent with, the initiation of breathing; the second strategy involves the treatment of infants with the diagnosis of respiratory distress syndrome within 6–24 hours of birth.

Chronic Lung Disease

The problem of chronic lung disease in premature infants has increased steadily, in part because of the increased survival of low-birth-weight infants. Chronic lung disease is defined as 1) oxygen dependence with or without ventilator support beyond 28 days and the appearance of persistent infiltrates on chest radiographs, or 2) oxygen dependence beyond 36 weeks of corrected postnatal gestational age. Approximately 80% of surviving infants with a birth weight of 501–750 g, 45% of infants with a birth weight of 751–1,000 g, and 12% of infants with a birth weight of 1,001–1,500 g receive supplemental oxygen at 28 days.

The pathogenesis of chronic lung disease is unclear. Contributing factors include immaturity, oxygen toxicity, barotrauma, infections, and nutritional deficiencies. Complications of chronic lung disease include reactive airway disease, congestive heart failure, and growth failure.

Apnea of Prematurity

Apnea, defined as the complete cessation of respiration with or without bradycardia, occurs in approximately 90% of infants with a birth weight of less than 1,000 g. In most infants apnea of prematurity has resolved by 34 weeks of postconceptional age. Treatment of apnea of prematurity includes tactile stimulation, oxygen administration, medications (eg, theophylline, caffeine, doxapram), continuous positive airway pressure, or mechanical ventilation, depending on the severity of the apneic episodes.

Symptomatic Patent Ductus Arteriosus

Symptomatic patent ductus arteriosus complicates approximately 40–50% of cases of respiratory distress syndrome. Clinical manifestations include signs of congestive heart failure (tachycardia, murmur, gallop, hyperdynamic precordium, bounding pulses, cardiomegaly) and inability to wean from the ventilator. Treatment includes medical management (ie, fluid restriction, diuretics) or ductal ligation either medically (indomethacin) or surgically.

Periventricular–Intraventricular Hemorrhage

Periventricular–intraventricular hemorrhage is a significant complication of prematurity and contributes to both neonatal mortality and morbidity. The incidence ranges from 25% to 40%, with the highest occurrence in infants weighing less than 1,000 g. Hemorrhage emanates from blood vessels within the germinal matrix. Cerebral blood flow in the premature infant, particularly in the presence of hypoxia or ischemia, is pressure passive (ie, varies directly with changes in blood pressure), thereby increasing the risk for injury with systemic hypotension or hypertension. Periventricular–intraventricular hemorrhage is graded as follows: grade I, germinal matrix only; grade II, blood filling the ventricles without distention; grade III, blood filling the ventricles with distention. Intraparenchymal echodensity (the so-called grade IV) is notated separately. Fifty percent or more of neonates with grade III or grade IV periventricular–intraventricular hemorrhage will have an abnormal neurologic outcome at 2 years of age.

Periventricular Leukomalacia

Periventricular leukomalacia is a common problem of the premature infant, occurring in 5–10% of infants with a birth weight of less than 1,500 g. Periventricular leukomalacia refers to symmetric necrosis of white matter adjacent to the external angles of the lateral ventricles. The lesions are observed in border zones between the penetrating branches of the anterior, middle, and posterior cerebral arteries. The border zone regions are extremely vulnerable to decreases in cerebral blood flow. Periventricular leukomalacia occurs more frequently in twins (monozygotic), with maternal chorioamnionitis, septic shock, or drug use (eg, cocaine). Neurologic outcome is invariably poor and includes spastic diplegia, spastic quadriplegia, and cognitive deficits, depending on the extent of the injury.

Necrotizing Enterocolitis

Necrotizing enterocolitis remains the major gastrointestinal cause of morbidity and mortality, affecting approximately 10% of sick preterm infants with a birth weight of less than 1,500 g. The etiology is multifactorial, with a delicate balance between bowel perfusion, enteric organisms, and nutritional intake. The characteristic radiographic features are pneumatosis intestinalis and portal venous gas. Free peritoneal air is associated with perforation. Outcome is related to severity; approximately 25% of infants who perforate die.

Retinopathy of Prematurity

Retinopathy of prematurity is a vasoproliferative retinopathy occurring principally in approximately 20% of premature infants. Ninety percent of the cases of acute retinopathy of prematurity undergo spontaneous regression without major sequelae. Less than 10% of the involved eyes progress to significant cicatrization. The etiology of retinopathy of prematurity is unclear, but oxygen toxicity is considered to be extremely important. Management of retinopathy of prematurity includes careful monitoring of oxygen tensions.

BIBLIOGRAPHY

Fanaroff AA, Martin RJ. Neonatal-perinatal medicine. 5th ed. St Louis, Missouri: Mosby–Year Book, 1992

Hack M, Horbar JD, Malloy MH, Tyson JE, Wright E, Wright L. Very low birth weight outcomes of the National Institute of Child Health and Human Development Neonatal Network. Pediatrics 1991;87:587–597

Jobe AH. Pulmonary surfactant therapy. N Engl J Med 1993;328:861–868

Kliegman RM, Fanaroff AA. Necrotizing enterocolitis. N Engl J Med 1984;310:1093

Perlman JM. Intraventricular hemorrhage. Pediatrics 1989;84:913

The Puerperium

Classically the puerperium is that period of time from birth to the first 6 weeks postpartum. In addition to significant complications such as infection or hemorrhage, multiple anatomical and physiologic changes occur during this time.

PHYSIOLOGY

Involutional Changes

The uterus usually undergoes complete involution by 6 weeks postpartum, going from a weight of 1,000 g to one of 100 g or less. The endometrium begins to regenerate early in the postpartum period, essentially completing the regeneration by the third week. The last part of the uterus to return to normal is the placental attachment site, which may take up to 6 weeks to regenerate. The sloughed tissue becomes part of the lochia. Initially, the lochia contains blood mixed with decidua and is called the lochia rubra. By the third or fourth day, the lochia becomes pale and watery, although it is still tinged with blood; at this stage, it is termed the lochia serosa. After another 2–3 weeks, the lochia becomes yellowish white—the lochia alba. The vagina, which is dusky, engorged, spacious, and smooth after delivery, diminishes in size and regains its normal rugated, pink appearance by approximately 3 weeks postpartum.

Anatomically, the dilatation of the calyces, renal pelvis, and ureters that is characteristic of pregnancy may persist as long as 12 weeks postpartum. Functionally, the increased renal plasma flow, glomerular filtration rate, and creatinine clearance rate associated with pregnancy return to normal by 6 weeks after delivery.

The changes in the cardiovascular system that occurred during pregnancy (ie, increase in heart rate, cardiac output, and blood volume) generally return to baseline by approximately 6 weeks postpartum. Peripheral vascular resistance also returns to prepregnancy levels by this time. Most of these parameters return to normal within the first 2 weeks postpartum.

Ovulation and Menstruation

After delivery, ovulation occurs at an average of 10 weeks but may occur as early as 27 days after delivery in nonlactating women. In women who breast-feed for at least 3 months, the average time to ovulation is 17 weeks. In nonlactating women, the mean time to menstruation is 7–9 weeks after delivery, and 70% menstruate by 12 weeks after delivery. In lactating women, the return to menstruation is more gradual, so that one half to three fourths have menstruated by 36 weeks. For obvious reasons, lactation is not an ideal or necessarily effective "method" of birth control.

Lactation

Lactogenesis
One distinguishing characteristic of mammals is their capacity to nourish their young with secretions from the mammary glands. On the basis of studies in animals, lactogenesis can be arbitrarily divided into two stages. During the first stage, which

occurs during the third trimester of pregnancy, the lobular–alveolar complex is stimulated to differentiate such that there are increases in synthesis of enzymes necessary for the production of milk components. These special constituents of human milk include major proteins such as α-lactalbumin, β-lactoglobulin, and casein, as well as triglycerides and lactose. The second stage is characterized by secretion of colostrum, followed by significant milk secretion approximately 5 days after delivery.

Prolactin (PRL), in concert with cortisol, insulin, estrogen, progesterone, and placental lactogen, stimulates growth and development of the milk-secreting apparatus of the mammary gland. Prolactin, the principal hormone that stimulates lactogenesis, increases progressively throughout pregnancy from a mean level of less than 20 ng/ml in a nonpregnant woman to an average of 250–300 ng/ml during the third trimester. Prolactin exerts its principal action by binding to specific membrane receptors on mammary tissue to stimulate gene transcription of messenger RNA and subsequent synthesis of lactose, casein, milk fat, and α-lactalbumin. During pregnancy, the high estrogen levels produced by the fetal–placental unit stimulate an increase in circulating PRL; however, the high estrogen–progesterone levels also suppress the number of available PRL-binding sites in mammary tissue, such that lactogenesis is delayed until placental separation leads to a rapid decline in these steroid levels. After delivery, PRL concentrations remain elevated, and increase further during suckling. Because higher PRL levels lead to greater PRL-binding sites, PRL can induce an up-regulation of its own receptors, thereby further increasing its biologic activity.

Although both hPL and growth hormone are structurally similar to PRL and have intrinsic lactotropic properties, their role in lactogenesis in humans is unclear. During pregnancy, growth hormone is suppressed to very low levels, while placental production of hPL is parallel to the increase in placental growth during the second half of pregnancy. In animal models, hPL can mimic the biologic action of PRL by binding to the PRL receptor. Because hPL levels decline rapidly and become undetectable 24 hours after delivery, a role for hPL in the maintenance of lactation is unlikely.

In mammary tissues, cortisol induces the development of the rough endoplasmic reticulum and Golgi membranes that are necessary for increased synthesis of milk proteins. Thus, cortisol appears to be essential for PRL stimulation of casein production.

During pregnancy, estrogens promote ductal development, while progesterone stimulates lobular–alveolar maturation of the mammary gland. In addition, the high levels of estrogens present during pregnancy augment the release of PRL from the pituitary gland, while the high levels of progesterone act to suppress lactogenesis by reducing the ability of PRL to up-regulate its own receptors. Progesterone also exerts other antilactogenic effects by reducing estrogen binding to mammary tissue.

Thyroid hormones appear to play a permissive role in lactogenesis, since administration of T_4 augments mammary development and milk production. In patients with mild hypothyroidism, lactation can be maintained. Additional factors that may also influence lactogenesis but that have no clearly identifiable role include epidermal growth factor and prostaglandins.

Neuroendocrine Regulation

The production of milk is determined largely by the frequency and intensity of suckling. With suckling, a nerve reflex is initiated that causes nerve impulses to be transmitted from intercostal nerves IV–VI to the spinal cord, eventually terminating in the supraoptic and paraventricular nuclei of the hypothalamus. This stimulus induces the central release of neuronal oxytocin. In addition, there is a prompt, but not simultaneous, release of PRL from the pituitary. Once oxytocin reaches the peripheral circulation, oxytocin receptors localized on the myoepithelial cells of the breast contract, ejecting milk from the alveolus into the adjacent milk ducts. Because suckling is an intermittent stimulus, oxytocin release also exhibits an episodic pattern.

The oxytocin-mediated milk ejection reflex can also be triggered by behavioral events such as playing with the baby or hearing the baby's cry, causing a "milk letdown." This phenomenon is not associated with a concomitant PRL elevation.

The maintenance of high PRL levels during the early postpartum period appears to be directly proportional to the intensity, duration, and frequency of suckling. In the presence of high PRL levels and continued nursing, gonadotropin secretion, which is responsible for reinitiation of the menstrual cycle, remains suppressed. This period of lactational amenorrhea can be sustained for up to 4 years if suckling intensity is maintained and breast-feeding remains the sole source of nourishment for the young.

The maintenance of lactation requires the presence of PRL, cortisol, insulin, and thyroid hormone. The pivotal role of PRL in this stage of lactation is highlighted by the fact that dopamine receptor antagonists (metoclopramide and sulpiride), which increase PRL levels, can augment milk production and even induce lactation in nonpregnant women. Alternatively, the administration of the dopamine agonist bromocriptine, 2.5 mg on a twice-daily basis for 10–14 days, may prevent breast engorgement and suppress lactation. However, the FDA has recommended that no drug should be used routinely for postpartum lactation suppression.

POSTPARTUM CARE

Immediate Postpartum Period

After delivery, the placenta and membranes should be examined for completeness. The uterus should be palpated to ascertain whether the fundus is firm, with its upper margin below the umbilicus. If the uterus is not firm, it should be massaged. A dilute solution of oxytocin (20 IU in 1,000 ml of intravenous fluid) is often used to maintain a firm uterus.

The cervix and vagina should be inspected for trauma. Everything being normal, bleeding from the vagina should be slight. The episiotomy should be repaired only after all pathologic postpartum bleeding has been controlled. Even when the delivery has been uncomplicated, a trained attendant should remain with the mother for at least 1 hour after delivery.

Subsequent Postpartum Care

As a consequence of the volume of fluid infused during labor and delivery and of bladder dysfunction secondary to trauma or the effects of anesthesia, urinary retention with bladder distention is a relatively common complication of the early puerperium. Prevention of bladder overdistention requires close observation after delivery to ensure that the bladder does not overfill and that it empties adequately with each voiding.

Breast-feeding should be encouraged for several reasons. First and foremost, breast milk is the ideal source of nutrients for the neonate. Breast milk also provides some degree of immunologic protection for the neonate. Nursing is contraindicated in patients with certain viral infections such as CMV, hepatitis B, and HIV infection.

The breasts and nipples of a woman who is nursing her infant require little attention in the puerperium other than attention to cleanliness and fissures. Some parturients may request lactation suppression during the postpartum period. Lactation is suppressed in 60–70% of women who wear a tight brassiere and avoid stimulation of the nipples. Although breast engorgement may occasionally cause a temperature elevation of short duration, any rise in temperature during the puerperium might be a sign of an infection, most commonly in the genitourinary tract.

Postpartum Depression

The postpartum period may be a time of uncertainty and anxiety for new parents. Many readjustments are often necessary, and mild depression is not unusual. However, it can be a precursor of more severe depression or psychosis. Referral to a mental health professional may be required.

Postpartum blues is a transient disturbance occurring in 50–80% of puerperal women, starting within 2–3 days of delivery and remitting within a few days to 2–3 weeks. It is characterized by emotional lability, anxiety, irritability, insomnia, poor appetite, and fatigue. Postpartum depression is a major depressive disorder occurring in the first weeks to months postdelivery (occasionally starting during pregnancy) in about 10–12% of women.

Postpartum psychoses, occurring in about 1–2/1,000 births, usually start in the first 2 weeks after delivery but occasionally begin later. These are severe mental illnesses that often require hospitalization. Most (75–80%) are mood disorders, 60% of them depression. Risk factors include a history of mental illness, especially bipolar disorder, and current psychosocial stressors. Recurrence in subsequent pregnancies is about 34–38%. Treatment consists of use of antipsychotic and antidepressant medications and hospitalization (with the baby if possible). Patients at high risk should be monitored carefully in the first few weeks, with special attention to obsessive thinking about harming the baby, sleep disorders, and feelings of hopelessness and anhedonia.

Although most pregnancies end happily, occasionally the outcome is not the exciting event that a couple had anticipated. Parents who must cope with stillbirths, neonatal deaths, and infants born with congenital anomalies require sensitivity, compassion, and guidance from the medical care team.

COMPLICATIONS

The most common postpartum complications include hemorrhage, genital tract infections, urinary tract infections, and mastitis.

Hemorrhage

Obstetric hemorrhage remains one of the three leading causes of maternal mortality in the United States. The diagnosis of postpartum hemorrhage is based primarily on the estimate and judgment of the clinician. However, it generally implies bleeding to a degree associated with hemodynamic instability or that threatens to cause such. Postpartum hemorrhage is classified as either early (first 24 hours after delivery) or late (after 24 hours but before 6 weeks after delivery).

Early Hemorrhage

The etiology of early postpartum hemorrhage can be summarized as follows:

- Uterine atony
- Retained placental fragments
- Lacerations
- Uterine inversion
- Uterine rupture
- Coagulopathy

There is little question that the most common cause of postpartum hemorrhage is uterine atony, which in turn may be associated with overdistention of the uterus, protracted labor, macrosomia, high parity, chorioamnionitis, and use of uterine-relaxing agents. The most common cause of late postpartum hemorrhage is subinvolution of the placental site, infection, and retained products of conception.

Management of postpartum hemorrhage consists of ascertaining its etiology, providing volume replacement, monitoring vital signs and urine output, and treating the cause of hemorrhage by medical or surgical means or both. Appropriate laboratory tests (ie, prothrombin time, partial thromboplastin time, platelet count, and fibrinogen levels) for the diagnosis of coagulopathy should be performed.

Medical management consists primarily of drugs to treat or prevent uterine atony. Recommendations for volume replacement are summarized below:

- Large-bore intravenous line (two lines may be helpful or necessary)
- Foley catheter

- Infusion of lactated Ringer's injection or normal saline (to maintain urine output of ≥ 30 ml/h); 3 ml of crystalloid per milliliter of estimated blood loss
- Blood transfusion
- Whole blood *or* packed red blood cells
- Fresh frozen plasma, platelets, or cryoprecipitate as indicated

Surgical management is necessary for patients who fail medical management and may involve ligation of the uterine arteries, ligation of the hypogastric arteries, or hysterectomy. Uterine artery ligation is relatively simple and may convert an arterial system to a venous system with regard to bleeding. In contrast, hypogastric artery ligation is technically not easy and requires significant surgical skill. In the presence of life-threatening bleeding, hysterectomy is often the quickest and safest procedure.

Late Hemorrhage

Treatment of late postpartum hemorrhage consists of the medical modalities listed in Table 3-18 and volume replacement as previously outlined. Antibiotics should be used if infection is suspected. Curettage may lead to increased bleeding and should be used only if medical therapy fails and retained products of conception are suspected on ultrasound examination. Unless hemorrhage is profuse, angiographic embolization should also be considered prior to hypogastric artery ligation or hysterectomy.

Postpartum Infection

The most common cause of postpartum, or puerperal, fever is uterine infection. Such an infection is variably called endometritis, endomyometritis, endoparametritis, or simply metritis.

Uterine Infection

Cesarean delivery is the major predisposing clinical factor for pelvic infection. The frequency and severity of infection are greater after abdominal delivery than after vaginal delivery. The incidence of infection after vaginal delivery is only 1–3% in most studies, whereas the incidence after abdominal delivery is 5–10 times greater. The increased incidence of infection after cesarean delivery probably results from increased intrauterine manipulation, foreign-body (suture) reactions, tissue necrosis at the suture line, hematoma–seroma formation, and wound infections. Clearly, not all patients who undergo a cesarean delivery are at equal risk. Those patients who undergo elective operations (with no labor and no rupture of membranes) have lower infection rates than do those who undergo emergency or nonelective procedures (with labor, rupture of the membranes, or both).

Labor and ruptured membranes are probably the two most common risk factors associated with infection after cesarean delivery. The number of vaginal examinations, socioeconomic status, and internal fetal monitoring have also been implicated, but their independent effects are difficult to document. For example, women with internal fetal monitoring often are those with prolonged labor, frequent vaginal examinations, and ruptured membranes.

The microbiology of endometritis is polymicrobial with a mixture of aerobes and anaerobes. Commonly isolated aerobes include gram-negative bacilli (ie, *Escherichia coli*) and gram-positive cocci (ie, group B streptococcus).

Anaerobic organisms clearly have major roles in infection after cesarean delivery; they are found in 80% of properly collected and handled specimens. The most common isolate is often a species of *Bacteroides*. Anaerobic cocci are also commonly found.

Genital mycoplasmas (*Mycoplasma hominis* and *Ureaplasma urealyticum*) have been isolated in the bloodstream of women with postpartum infections, but their role is not clear. The role of *Chlamydia trachomatis* is also unclear.

The diagnosis of endometritis is based primarily on the presence of fever and the absence of other causes of fever. Uterine tenderness, especially parametrial, and purulent or foul-smelling lochia are also considered common findings. Laboratory studies, with the exception of blood cultures, are not particularly helpful. Leukocytosis is relatively common in patients with and without infection. A Gram stain of the cervical–vaginal flora may be helpful in patients suspected of having hemolytic streptococci, clostridia, or gonorrhea.

Therapy should be aimed at the wide range of aerobic and anaerobic bacteria involved in endometritis. The regimen commonly used as a standard in recent studies is clindamycin–gentamicin, a combination that is generally curative in 85–95% of patients. Treatment with a penicillin and an aminoglycoside or ampicillin alone is less effective in postcesarean endometritis. Because of the potential toxicity of clindamycin–gentamicin, as well as their combined cost, the possibility of using one of the newer penicillins or cephalosporins for single-drug therapy has attracted some interest. Good results have been reported with a number of these newer antibiotics, including cefoxitin, cefoperazone, cefotaxime, piperacillin, cefotetan, and clindamycin–aztreonam. Patients are generally treated until they have been afebrile for 24–48 hours. Further antibiotic therapy as an outpatient is generally not necessary.

TABLE 3-18. DRUGS USEFUL FOR THE TREATMENT OF POSTPARTUM HEMORRHAGE SECONDARY TO UTERINE ATONY

Drug	Protocol
Oxytocin	20 U in 1,000 ml of lactated Ringer's solution or normal saline as intravenous infusion
Methylergonovine (Methergine)	0.2 mg intramuscularly
Prostaglandin (15-methyl PGF$_{2\alpha}$ Prostin/15M)	0.25 mg as intramuscular or intramyometrial injection every 15–60 min as necessary

American College of Obstetricians and Gynecologists. Diagnosis and management of postpartum hemorrhage. ACOG Technical Bulletin 143. Washington, DC: ACOG, 1990

Causes of initial antibiotic failure include the presence of an abscess, resistant organisms, a wound infection, infection at other sites, or septic thrombophlebitis. Surgical drainage, especially for an abscess, may occasionally be necessary, although hysterectomy is rarely required. Diagnosis of a wound infection is based primarily on redness and induration of the wound, often with purulent discharge. Treatment consists of drainage and debridement. Antibiotics should be used for significant induration. A puerperal infection in the pelvis may extend along the veins, resulting in septic pelvic thrombophlebitis. Treatment is usually directed at the pelvic infection, and antibiotics are indicated for therapy. The use of anticoagulants with full heparinization is controversial but is recommended by most clinicians.

Well-designed studies have shown the efficacy of prophylactic antibiotics in patients at risk for endometritis, such as those who undergo nonelective cesarean deliveries. A short course of one to three doses of antibiotic should be used for prophylaxis. Therapy should be initiated after cord clamping. Antibiotics that are effective, safe for obstetric patients, and inexpensive are ampicillin and the older cephalosporins (eg, cephalothin and cefazolin). Although the newer, broader-spectrum antibiotics are effective for prophylaxis, there is no evidence that they are more effective than are the older, less expensive choices. Finally, the condition of patients who have received prophylactic antibiotics must be evaluated carefully if postoperative fever or other signs of infection develop.

Urinary Tract Infections
Primarily caused by coliform bacteria, urinary tract infections occur in approximately 5% of patients during the puerperium. Predisposing factors include a prolonged labor, indwelling catheters, the infusion of large amounts of intravenous fluids, and the administration of conduction anesthesia. The last two factors may result in urine retention. Upper urinary tract infections are usually characterized by chills, spiking fever, costovertebral angle tenderness, and, frequently, nausea and vomiting. Therapy for upper urinary tract infection in the puerperium should be initiated after urine and blood samples for culture have been obtained. Antibiotics of choice may be a cephalosporin, ampicillin, or gentamicin in combination with a penicillin, such as ampicillin. In many institutions, the resistance rate to ampicillin is so high as to preclude its use as an initial single agent in patients with pyelonephritis.

Mastitis
Pregnancy and lactation may be complicated by the development of mastitis. With the usual form of puerperal mastitis, there is a localized area of inflammation and tenderness and a slight elevation in temperature. Treatment includes continuation of breast-feeding or emptying the breast with a pump and the use of appropriate antibiotics. Penicillin or one of its derivatives should be administered. If the patient does not respond and if tenderness and fever persist, a breast abscess should be suspected. Because of the unique anatomy of the breast, there is far more destruction of breast tissue than a superficial physical examination would suggest. The patient is ill. The white blood cell count is elevated, and treatment requires adequate drainage under general anesthesia in an operating room setting. If possible, the incision should be circumareolar or at least follow the natural skin lines as demonstrated in the sitting position. A generous incision is made and a finger is inserted into the cavity to break up the loculations. A Penrose drain is inserted into the cavity and should remain in place for 2–3 days. Antibiotics must be continued and given in full therapeutic doses for 7–10 days after adequate drainage.

A painful infection, mastitis is most commonly caused by coagulase-positive *Staphylococcus aureus*. Other common organisms are group A or group B streptococci and *Haemophilus* species. Prevention requires meticulous breast hygiene. In the presence of mastitis, the mother may continue nursing while she receives appropriate antibiotic therapy. Drugs of choice are penicillinase-resistant penicillins (such as dicloxacillin) or a cephalosporin. If the initial cellulitis is not properly treated, an abscess may form. If so, the abscess should be incised radially in order to avoid injuring the lactiferous ducts.

Episiotomy Infection
Episiotomy infections are relatively uncommon, but when they do occur, especially if associated with a third- or fourth-degree laceration, they are often associated with significant morbidity. Diagnosis is generally based on purulent discharge in association with redness and induration. Treatment consists of opening the episiotomy and removing all sutures. The episiotomy should be irrigated with copious fluid and the wound debrided. The area should be inspected for necrotizing fasciitis. The wound should be cleaned at least twice daily, and sitz baths should be used liberally. Broad-spectrum antibiotics should also be used. A protocol for early repair of an infected episiotomy dehiscence has been described. Prior to secondary closure, the wound must be free of infection, cellulitis, and exudate.

BIBLIOGRAPHY

Physiology
Bowes WA. The puerperium. Clin Obstet Gynecol 1980;23:971

Cunningham FG, MacDonald PC, Gant NF, Leveno KJ, Gilstrap LC III. The puerperium. In: Williams obstetrics. 19th ed. Norwalk, Connecticut: Appleton and Lange, 1993:459–473

Cunningham FG, MacDonald PC, Gant NF, Leveno KJ, Gilstrap LC III. Williams obstetrics. 19th ed. Norwalk, Connecticut: Appleton and Lange, 1993:647

Liu JH, Yen SSC. Endocrinology of the postpartum state. In: Brody SA, Ueland K, eds. Endocrine disorders in pregnancy. Norwalk, Connecticut: Appleton and Lange, 1989:111–122

Tucker HA. Endocrinology of lactation. Semin Perinatol 1979;3:199–223

Postpartum Care
Lucas A, Morley R, Cole TJ, Lister G, Leeson-Payne C. Breast milk and subsequent intelligence quotient in child born preterm. Lancet 1992;329:26

Complications

American College of Obstetricians and Gynecologists. Antimicrobial therapy for obstetric patients. ACOG Technical Bulletin 117. Washington, DC: ACOG, 1988

American College of Obstetricians and Gynecologists. Diagnosis and management of postpartum hemorrhage. ACOG Technical Bulletin 143. Washington, DC: ACOG, 1990

Clark SL, Phelan JP. Surgical control of obstetric hemorrhage. Contemp Ob Gyn 1984;24(2):70–84

Clark SL, Yeh SY, Phelan JP, Bruce S, Paul RH. Emergency hysterectomy for obstetric hemorrhage. Obstet Gynecol 1984;64:376

Dinsmoor MJ, Newton ER, Gibbs RS. A randomized, double-blind placebo-controlled trial of oral antibiotic therapy following IV antibiotic therapy for postpartum endometritis. Obstet Gynecol 1991;77:60

diZerega G, Yonekura L, Roy S, Nakamura RM, Ledger WJ. A comparison of clindamycin-gentamicin and penicillin-gentamicin in the treatment of post-cesarean section endomyometritis. Am J Obstet Gynecol 1979;134:238

Duff P. Pathophysiology and management of postcesarean endomyometritis. Obstet Gynecol 1986;67:269

Gibbs RS, O'Dell TN, McGregor RR, Schwarz RH, Morton H. Puerperal endometritis: a prospective microbiologic study. Am J Obstet Gynecol 1975;121:919

Gilstrap LC III, Cunningham FG. The bacterial pathogenesis of infection following cesarean section. Obstet Gynecol 1979;53:545

Greenwood LH, Glickman MG, Schwartz PE, Morese SS, Denny DF. Obstetric and nonmalignant gynecologic bleeding: treatment with angiographic embolization. Radiology 1987;164:1557

Hankins GDV, Hauth JC, Gilstrap LC III, Hammond TL, Yeomans ER, Snyder RR. Early repair of episiotomy dehiscence. Obstet Gynecol 1990;75:48

Stiver HG, Forward KR, Livingstone RA, Fugere P, Lemay M, Verschelden G, et al. Multicenter comparison of cefoxitin versus cefozolin for prevention of infectious morbidity after nonelective cesarean section. Am J Obstet Gynecol 1983;145:158

Gynecology

The past two decades of this century will be remembered by obstetrician–gynecologists as a time of major changes. One of these changes is the ongoing nationwide downward trend in numbers of major gynecologic surgical procedures being performed. There are many explanations for this, including better diagnostic tools, greater use of medical and minor surgical alternatives that accomplish the desired results, the more effective administration of antibiotics, and the development of new therapeutic agents. Procedures such as dilation and curettage, hysteroscopy, and cone biopsy have become part of office practice.

An ever-growing array of new instruments and innovative approaches has fostered a trend toward minimally invasive surgery. Postoperative care and pain control have improved. Hospital stays are shorter. Early ambulation hastens recovery and decreases morbidity and some complications. The need for blood replacement in elective surgery is diminishing.

Reconstructive surgery of the pelvic floor has received increased recognition as an area of particular importance, especially among women with urinary or fecal incontinence. Novel concepts and principles have emerged as the result of better understanding of pelvic forces and pathophysiology. As research in this field progresses, it is anticipated that measures for preventing some pelvic floor dysfunctions will be identified.

The growing geriatric population presents a particular challenge for the gynecologic surgeon. Patients who have multiple system disorders, are taking a large array of medications, and have limited mobility are frequently encountered in practice. Some have difficulty communicating; some have impaired mentation. Even the relatively healthy elderly patient, however, is more susceptible to postoperative complications, especially cardiovascular complications, which may significantly decrease her quality of life or even be fatal. Still, advances in anesthesia permit safer interventions in older women than ever before. Gynecologists who are well informed about geriatric medical and psychosocial difficulties generally can make better choices for management of their patients' gynecologic problems.

—*Henry A. Thiede, MD*

Diagnostic and Surgical Procedures

HYSTEROSCOPY

Hysteroscopy allows direct viewing of the inside of the uterus and may be helpful in evaluating suspected uterine pathology. Its complementary procedure, hysterosalpingography, can provide information about tubal patency.

Many diagnostic studies may be performed in the office after introduction of a paracervical block. Preoperative analgesia using a prostaglandin synthetase inhibitor is used routinely. Administration of one of these drugs 30–45 minutes prior to hysteroscopy provides excellent analgesia. Operative procedures that may be completed in 15–30 minutes may also be performed under local anesthesia with the addition of a sedative such as midazolam. If possible, hysteroscopy should be performed in the early follicular phase, when the endometrium is flat. At this time tubal ostia are easy to visualize, the chance of interpreting polypoid endometrium as a true polyp is reduced, and the risk of interrupting a pregnancy is very small.

Equipment

Both rigid and flexible hysteroscopes may be used with a video camera, and the findings can be displayed on a monitor. Still or video photography can be helpful to document findings, demonstrate preoperative and postoperative differences, and explain treatment to patients. The use of video cameras permits assistants to be more helpful to the primary surgeon and facilitates teaching. If this equipment is not available, carefully drawn diagrams are an alternative.

For those who have not learned the technique in a residency program, postgraduate courses, including those with hands-on experience, are an important first step to learning. Such courses should be followed by a brief apprenticeship. Diagnostic panoramic hysteroscopy is easiest to master. Contact hysteroscopy, carbon dioxide office hysteroscopy, simple operative procedures, and finally, the use of laser or cautery should follow in that order.

Panoramic Hysteroscopy
An appropriate uterine-distending medium is necessary to permit adequate inspection of the cavity. Carbon dioxide is best suited to office procedures and requires a special insufflator. Hysteroscopy fluid (dextran 70 in dextrose) was designed specifically for this procedure and permits extensive intrauterine surgery to be performed even if the patient is bleeding. Low-viscosity fluids such as glycine, sorbitol, saline, and glucose in water may also be used, but the view becomes obscured if the patient is bleeding, because the medium and blood mix. Special pumps have been developed that instill low-viscosity fluids under controlled, high-pressure rates that vary between 60 and 120 mm Hg. Together with modifications in the sheaths of some hysteroscopes, or in other instances in combination with a special outer sheath, these pumps provide continuous irrigation of blood and cellular debris from the uterine cavity so that a clear view can be maintained even if significant bleeding occurs.

Hysteroscopes are rigid 4-mm telescopes in a diagnostic sheath that have viewing angles of between 0° and 30°; 7- and 8-mm operating sheaths are available. The 8-mm sheath has four channels for passage of the telescope, the medium, and two operating instruments. Operating instruments include scissors, grasping forceps, biopsy forceps, and a fulgurating electrode. An aspirating cannula may be used to maintain a clear field of view. After minimal cervical dilatation, the endocervical canal is inspected and the telescope is advanced up to and past the internal os. Systematic inspection of the cavity—one side wall, one ostium, the top of the fundus, the other ostium and side wall, and then both anterior and posterior walls—should be carried out before beginning any surgery.

Newly developed "flexible hysteroscopes" provide more ready access to the fallopian tubes for purposes of relieving or inducing proximal tubal obstruction. These instruments can be used with carbon dioxide as a distending medium. The images have a slight ground-glass appearance and are somewhat inferior to those provided by rigid hysteroscopes, but they are more than adequate. This type of hysteroscope is not truly flexible but has a "snout" that can be steered through a wide arc. A second site of rotation permits the operator to move the telescope throughout the cavity smoothly, increasing patient and physician comfort.

Contact Hysteroscopy
The general technique of contact hysteroscopy is similar to panoramic hysteroscopy. Because a panoramic view is not afforded, inspection of the cavity requires a meticulous approach. Gentle pressure against the mucosa permits a good view even if the patient is bleeding heavily. Contact hysteroscopes may be appropriate screening tools for office procedures due to their simplicity of equipment, setup, and procedure. They may also be used as vaginoscopes or cystoscopes.

Diagnostic Indications

Evaluation of the Endocervical Canal
Although colposcopy permits a thorough and complete assessment of neoplasia involving the ectocervix, disease that

extends into the endocervical canal often extends beyond the field of view even if an endocervical speculum is used. An extended field of view is possible, especially if a narrow-diameter panoramic hysteroscope or a small contact hysteroscope is used. The full extent of the lesion can be seen and, by using a panoramic hysteroscope, the most abnormal areas can be biopsied under direct vision. Use of the 6-mm contact hysteroscope is preferred during pregnancy because the risk of pushing a liquid or gaseous medium into the uterine cavity is obviated.

Congenital Malformations of the Uterus

Hysterosalpingography will frequently reveal a midline septal defect in women with poor reproductive histories. The depth of the defect may be difficult to ascertain if the long axis of the uterus was not maintained parallel to the film plate during the radiographic study. Hysterography affords more precise information about the size of the uterine horns than does hysteroscopy, because depth perception is absent during transcervical endoscopy. Laparoscopy is needed to distinguish the septate from the bicornuate anomaly; if the former is present, unification through hysteroscopy is possible.

Abnormal Uterine Bleeding

Polyps may be differentiated from blood clots, submucous myomas, and artifacts detected by hysterography. Simple and complex hyperplasias and endometrial cancers may be suspected by hysteroscopy, but directed biopsy is necessary before planning treatment. If hyperplasia is treated medically, follow-up hysteroscopy and biopsy can prove adequate reversal of the lesion. Adenomyosis is best detected by hysterography or contact hysteroscopy.

Patients who are at high risk for endometrial cancer are of special concern because of the unknown sequelae of disseminating malignant cells into venous and lymphatic channels and into the peritoneal cavity. The use of carbon dioxide as a uterine-distending medium for panoramic hysteroscopy or inspection with a contact hysteroscope obviates these risks and permits the diagnosis of endocervical canal involvement with greater accuracy than by fractional curettage.

Lost Intrauterine Devices

An ultrasound examination can usually detect the location of an intrauterine device (IUD) if the filaments are not visible, and removal using a blind approach is usually possible. However, verification by hysteroscopy and removal of the device or retrieval of only the filaments may be performed in the office with less endometrial trauma.

Uterine Synechiae

Even if the presence of intrauterine adhesions is suspected by history and supported by hysterosalpingography, the diagnosis of uterine synechiae may be made with certainty only by hysteroscopy. Direct inspection of the uterine cavity permits the extent of the disease to be classified, a treatment plan to be formulated, and the efficacy of different treatment regimens to be compared.

Surgical Procedures

Retrieval of Intrauterine Devices

Panoramic hysteroscopy in the office, with a mild analgesic and a paracervical block, permits location of the device, assessment of the extent of perforation, and atraumatic removal under direct vision. If the device is properly in place and the patient wishes to retain it, the filaments may be retrieved and brought back into the endocervical canal and vagina. If the device is embedded deeply, it should be removed under laparoscopic guidance to avoid intestinal or vascular injury.

Directed Biopsy and Polypectomy

One or more endometrial polyps may be missed or only partially removed by blind curettage. Panoramic hysteroscopy allows selective and complete removal. Larger polyps may be resected at their bases, which are then fulgurated to reduce the risk of recurrence. If polyps are located by hysteroscopy and then removed with polyp forceps or a curet, the hysteroscope must be reinserted before terminating the procedure, to verify that no lesions or portions thereof remain.

Resection or Excision of Submucous Myomas

Pedunculated myomas may be excised by transection of their stalks. Bleeding occurs rarely, and may be controlled by cautery or a neodymium:yttrium–aluminum–garnet (Nd:YAG) laser. If a large myoma is difficult to remove after transection of the stalk, it may be left in situ and allowed to degenerate and be passed spontaneously. If this approach is taken, the myoma must be biopsied to verify that there are no malignant changes. Myomas that have an intramural component are handled differently. A continuous-flow resectoscope with a cutting loop is used the shave off the portion of the myoma that is within the uterine cavity. The intramural component cannot be removed because the adjacent muscle would bleed profusely. Frequently, the residual intramural component is extruded into the uterine cavity and passed spontaneously 2–4 weeks after surgery. In contrast to transfundal myomectomy, cesarean delivery need not follow hysteroscopic myomectomy. Recurrence rates are low, and most recurrences occur within the first 2 years after resection.

Incision of Septa

Simultaneous laparoscopy is necessary to differentiate the bicornuate from the septate anomaly. If the latter is found, the laparoscopist must assist the hysteroscopist by guiding the depth of the uterine incision so that the risk of uterine perforation is minimized. Although a resectoscope and an Nd:YAG laser have been used to incise septa, flexible or semirigid scissors are more than adequate to achieve uterine unification. Because the septum is avascular and elastic, it retracts below the plane of the adjacent endometrium as soon as incision occurs, and therefore even the largest ones may be incised without fear of hemorrhage. Any bleeding that occurs does so because the dissection has been carried beyond the septum into normal uterine muscle. If a patient thus treated conceives, labor and vaginal delivery may be permitted. Transabdominal metroplasty for the septate uterus is now obsolete.

Intrauterine Adhesions
Following classification of the extent of disease, the hysteroscopist may decide to have an assistant perform laparoscopy and guide the adhesiolysis. However, patients with minimal or moderate disease can be treated by hysteroscopy only. Follow-up hysteroscopy or hysterography should be performed to verify that adhesions have not recurred before the patient attempts to conceive.

Endometrial Ablation
Both the Nd:YAG laser and the resectoscope have been used to destroy the endometrium in patients with excessive menstrual flow. The goal of marked hypomenorrhea or amenorrhea is achieved in three fourths of patients, and most protocols include pretreatment with a medication to induce endometrial atrophy. Appropriate candidates for this procedure include patients whose sole reason for pelvic surgery is excessive bleeding and who prefer not to have major surgery or who are at high risk for complications. Those with malignant or premalignant conditions should not undergo endometrial ablation.

Proximal Tubal Obstruction
Obstruction of the uterotubal junction is uncommon but may be secondary to inspissated mucus, adhesions, or salpingitis isthmica nodosa. After hysterosalpingography which demonstrates proximal obstruction is performed, a balloon catheter or fine wire may be placed under fluoroscopic guidance by specially trained radiologists. However, because spasm of this segment of the tube is common and true obstruction may not be present, most physicians perform laparoscopy to verify that the obstruction is real and to assess the status of the distal fallopian tubes. If they are normal and if the proximal obstruction is confirmed, a catheter may be placed in the tubal ostium under hysteroscopic guidance. These may disrupt intraluminal adhesions or dislodge mucus or cellular debris.

Complications
Complications of hysteroscopy are few. Infection is rare. Uterine perforation is an unusual complication but may be avoided by advancing the hysteroscope only when the field of view is clear and by liberally using simultaneous laparoscopy. Central uterine perforations usually require no specific treatment.

Complications related to media are more common. Carbon dioxide can be instilled only through a special insufflator. The insufflator for laparoscopy cannot be used for this purpose. Dextran 70 distending fluid may cause allergic reactions. Large volumes of dextran 70 may cause noncardiogenic pulmonary edema, pulmonary membrane damage, and prolonged clotting time. These problems occur during operative procedures when venous channels are opened and absorb dextran 70. The frequency of these problems is very low or absent if less than 500 ml is used. Dextrose (5%) in water, normal saline, glycine, and sorbitol may cause fluid overload and hyponatremia. Careful monitoring of fluid intake and output should prevent these complications.

Contraindications
Absolute contraindications to hysteroscopy include acute or subacute pelvic infection. Invasive cervical cancer should be approached with caution because of the risk of bleeding. Active uterine bleeding, endometrial cancer, pregnancy, chronic salpingitis with or without hydrosalpinges, and a recent uterine perforation are relative contraindications. The use of a medium that does not mix with blood, or a low-viscosity medium in a continuous-flow system obviates the problem of active bleeding. If carbon dioxide is used as a medium, the risk of disseminating cancer cells into lymphatic and vascular channels may be only a theoretic concern, and the ability to do selective biopsies both of the uterine cavity and above and below the internal os provides a more specific diagnosis than does fractional curettage. Contact hysteroscopy in pregnancy may be feasible but has limited use. Patients with chronic salpingitis should receive prophylactic antibiotics. Inspection of the uterine cavity with a contact hysteroscope is possible in a patient with a recent uterine perforation but panoramic hysteroscopy should be delayed until healing has occurred.

LAPAROSCOPY

Significant technical advances in the past decade have permitted an increasing number of gynecologic surgical procedures to be performed by laparoscopy. These refinements include the introduction of new laparoscope designs, improved light sources (xenon), video chip cameras, devices for rapid insufflation that permit a continuous pneumoperitoneum to be maintained, and a wider array of operative instruments. Laparoscopic suturing can be accomplished with special laparoscopic needles and needle holders. Sutures can be tied either within or outside the abdomen. Alternatively, preknotted sutures can be secured and tightened to ligate pedicles. Instruments capable of automatically stapling and dividing tissues have further facilitated dissection.

Television cameras for use in monitoring and recording the surgery have been found useful. The operating room personnel can see and participate by assisting in the surgery. Working from the screen rather than through the optics results in a normal standing posture for the surgeon, which is less strenuous for long sessions.

Attempts have been made to perform almost all gynecologic surgical procedures through the laparoscope. This has been, in part, a consumer-led phenomenon. Several advantages are perceived by the patient. They include the opportunity to have surgery performed on an outpatient basis, shorter recuperation with earlier return to work and usual activities, smaller and more cosmetically acceptable incisions, and the as yet unsupported notion that the use of more sophisticated technology confers an improved outcome. Endoscopic surgery is still undergoing considerable evolution, and most procedures can be performed endoscopically with results comparable to those achieved with laparotomy. However, current experience does not yet permit consistent identification of the endoscopic procedures that are advances from those that are technically feasible but better performed at laparotomy.

Technique

Anesthesia

Most physicians prefer general anesthesia for performing laparoscopy. Endotracheal intubation is necessary to ensure adequate ventilation in the presence of increased intraabdominal pressure (up to 20 mm Hg) and the Trendelenburg position. Full relaxation should be achieved and maintained with a succinylcholine drip to minimize "bucking" (and subsequent bowel injury) and to maximize visibility.

Local anesthesia has the advantage of greater cardiorespiratory safety. Modern analgesics such as midazolam and alfentanil allow considerable patient comfort but depress respiration and require nasal oxygen. The surgical technique must be deliberate and smooth to minimize abrupt motions that are interpreted as pain. The insufflating gas may be nitrous oxide or carbon dioxide. The use of nitrous oxide minimizes pain from peritoneal irritation by carbonic acid, which occurs with carbon dioxide. Nitrous oxide supports combustion, as does room air, but it is used safely throughout the United States for electrocoagulation. It is absorbed by the blood stream 60% as rapidly as is carbon dioxide.

Pneumoperitoneum

Blind entry into the abdomen to induce pneumoperitoneum demands strict attention to technical details. The use of a Verres needle minimizes the risk of bowel, but not large vessel, injury. The following three anatomic and surgical principles should be kept in mind simultaneously during abdominal entry:

1. Elevate the abdominal wall away from the blood vessels.
2. Aim at the uterus in the true pelvis.
3. Aim at right angles to the skin close to the umbilicus.

Correct entry can be judged by the free flow of saline or intraabdominal pressures of 5–12 mm Hg for the initial flow. The flow regulator should not allow an initial flow above 1,000 ml/min until pneumoperitoneum is established. There is general agreement that an initial volume of 2 L or an intraabdominal pressure of 15 mm Hg is a satisfactory end point prior to trocar entry. In obese patients, it is advisable to distend the abdomen maximally (to 20–25 mm Hg) just prior to trocar entry to minimize the risk of the failure of the trocar to penetrate the peritoneum. For maintenance, pressures should not exceed 20 mm Hg, since respiratory excursions may be compromised.

Trocar and Sleeve Insertion

As with Verres needle insertion, trocar and sleeve insertion requires consistent attention to surgical detail to avoid complications. Trocars should be as sharp as possible to minimize force and maximize control of entry. Disposable trocars have recently been introduced that ensure sharpness, and hence less force and greater control.

Physicians should concentrate equally on the actions of their right hand (aiming the trocar) and their left hand (elevating the abdomen). The left hand should ensure that the trocar does not push the abdominal wall down onto the vessels beneath the umbilicus. For some patients with multiple previous abdominal surgeries and in some physicians' hands, the open laparoscopy technique of Hasson minimizes the risk of large-vessel injury, although abdominal wall and bowel injuries still occur.

Uterine Manipulation

The uterus must be anteverted to ensure maximum visualization of the pelvic anatomy. When a controlling tenaculum is used, a retroverted uterus must be brought to the anteverted position before the tenaculum is held on the anterior lip. Hollow cannulas held with an intrauterine balloon or tenaculum can be used with somewhat less uterine control if tubal instillation of indigo carmine dye is planned.

Sterilization of Equipment

Although there has never been a documented case of infection transmitted from patient to patient through laparoscopic instruments, instruments should be soaked in benzalkonium chloride between cases. Some hospitals gas autoclave the laparoscopes overnight. In patients known to have acquired immunodeficiency syndrome (AIDS), hepatitis, or tuberculosis, it is prudent to gas autoclave the instruments after use as a medicolegal precaution.

Indications

Sterilization

Laparoscopic tubal ligation has been the most commonly used procedure for sterilization for more than 20 years. Sterilization performed at laparoscopy allows the opportunity to inspect and manipulate the abdominal and pelvic organs directly. There is minimal abdominal wall disruption, and it is well suited as an outpatient procedure. Postoperative scar formation and discomfort are minimal. (See "Sterilization" in this section.)

Infertility

Patients with signs and symptoms of endometriosis or tubal disease should undergo laparoscopy early in their evaluation. Patients with partial or complete tubal occlusion or evidence of loculation of dye outside of the fallopian tubes noted at hysterosalpingography benefit from laparoscopy when their diagnosis is confirmed and the extent of disease is determined. Patients completing a comprehensive infertility evaluation who still have unexplained infertility should proceed to laparoscopy. Patients with unexplained infertility have endometriosis or pelvic adhesive disease noted at laparoscopy in 30–40% of cases. If laparoscopy is indicated for infertility, the entire pelvis—including the anterior cul-de-sac and undersurfaces of both ovaries and tubes—should be thoroughly inspected. Tubal patency can be evaluated with transcervical injection of indigo carmine or methylene blue dye.

Pelvic Pain and Other Diagnostic Procedures
Laparoscopy is indicated for patients with persistent chronic pelvic pain when physical examination, radiologic studies, and other laboratory evaluations are inconclusive. An accurate diagnosis can be more consistently established with acute pelvic pain. Ectopic pregnancy, endometriosis, adnexal torsion, hemorrhagic corpus luteum, appendicitis, and chronic and acute pelvic inflammatory disease can be diagnosed. Salpingitis and ectopic pregnancy are frequently misdiagnosed when laparoscopy is delayed.

Pelvic foreign bodies, such as dislodged IUDs, can be identified and removed at laparoscopy. Laparoscopy should be used for follow-up evaluation of hysteroscopy complicated by uterine perforation. Treatment, if necessary, can frequently be performed through the laparoscope. Müllerian anomalies can be defined and their implications for fertility, menstruation, and coital function assessed with laparoscopy in conjunction with hysteroscopy and hysterosalpingography. Identification of internal genitalia may be important in the evaluation of ambiguous genitalia and permit appropriate sex assignment consistent with reproductive potential.

Endometriosis
Laparoscopy or laparotomy is the only means of definitively confirming the diagnosis of endometriosis. In addition, the extent of disease can be staged.

Laparoscopy also affords the opportunity to treat endometriosis. Individual lesions can be excised, fulgurated, or vaporized with the laser. Adhesions can be lysed or excised. Endometriomas can be resected through the laparoscope. Other ancillary procedures, including uterine suspension, presacral neurectomy, oophoropexy, and uterosacral plication, have also been performed through the laparoscope but are of less proven individual benefit.

Ectopic Pregnancy
The diagnosis of ectopic pregnancy is usually established by laparoscopy. More recently, laparoscopy has become the treatment of choice for the management of ectopic pregnancy in many locales. Patients presenting with pelvic pain, a positive pregnancy test, abnormal uterine bleeding, and ultrasound evidence of an adnexal mass or absence of an intrauterine gestation are directed to laparoscopy for diagnosis and possible treatment of ectopic pregnancy. A diagnosis can usually be established before tubal rupture, and the tube may be salvaged.

Compared with laparotomy, laparoscopic treatment of ectopic pregnancy results in shorter hospitalization, more rapid convalescence, decreased cost, and comparable fertility potential. Operating time is shorter, and a reduced need for postoperative analgesia has been reported. Patients being considered for laparoscopic treatment should be hemodynamically stable, the pelvic organs must be accessible by laparoscopy, and the affected adnexa must be fully mobile prior to initiating surgical resection. The same procedures performed at laparotomy can be undertaken through the laparoscope, including linear salpingostomy, segmental resection, and salpingectomy. Unruptured ampullary tubal pregnancies are best treated with linear salpingostomy; salpingectomy should be performed in patients with tubal rupture or other extensively damaged tubes in and those patients not desiring future fertility.

Pelvic Masses
Laparoscopy has been used for the evaluation of pelvic masses and is increasingly being used for the operative management as well. Preoperative assessment of adnexal masses is critical, and ultrasound evaluation and use of tumor markers such as CA 125 testing may be helpful in identifying malignant neoplasms preoperatively. Nevertheless, the potential for unwitting laparoscopic resection of a malignant adnexal mass exists. Those physicians skilled in operative laparoscopy have successfully approached the adnexal mass with large fenestrations, followed by examination of frozen sections of the biopsy specimen. Immediate laparotomy with appropriate staging should be performed when a malignancy is diagnosed.

Benign neoplasms such as pedunculated myomas, ovarian endometriomas, and dermoid cysts can be effectively treated through the laparoscope. Care must be undertaken in resecting the latter, since chemical peritonitis may occur in patients with incomplete resection of a dermoid cyst. Frozen-section biopsy should be performed for questionable lesions. Laparoscopic management of malignant adnexal masses is not appropriate.

Assisted Reproductive Technology
Laparoscopic aspiration of oocytes is now infrequently performed. Most centers rely on transvaginal ultrasound-directed transducers with needle guides for oocyte retrieval. However, laparoscopic oocyte aspiration can be used when the ovaries are not accessible with a transvaginal approach. Laparoscopy is used for gamete intrafallopian transfer (GIFT) and zygote intrafallopian transfer (ZIFT). Gamete intrafollicular transfer involves depositing unfertilized oocytes and sperm in the distal fallopian tube, where fertilization and subsequent embryo transfer occur. Zygote intrafallopian transfer is usually performed 1 day after oocyte retrieval, when the fertilized embryos (zygotes) are placed directly into the fallopian tube. Although the two procedures have not been compared prospectively in the same series, they appear to have comparable success rates.

Operative Laparoscopy
Laparoscopic surgery affords the surgeon the opportunity to perform tissue dissection under magnification in an environment with less potential for tissue desiccation and subsequent adhesion formation. Although de novo adhesion formation following laparoscopy is uncommon, adhesions frequently do recur after operative lysis. Instruments for grasping and dividing tissue adapted for use with the laparoscope have facilitated progress. Specially adapted lasers and electrocautery have been useful in the treatment of endometriosis and dissection of adhesions.

Photons emitted by the laser create a high-power density energy effect to incise the tissue. The power density (*PD*) produced by the laser is directly proportional to the watts (*W*) emitted by the laser and inversely proportional to the surface area (*SA*) of the laser beam squared ($PD = W \times 100/SA^2$). To minimize the zone of thermal damage with continuous waveform laser, the power density should exceed 5,000 W/cm². Lasers are usually attached to an operating laparoscope with a special channel through which the focusing lens and gas can be directed. Use of the laser creates special requirements, including the need to evacuate the laser plume rapidly from the abdomen with wall suction and to use special high-flow insufflators to maintain an adequate pneumoperitoneum.

For incising tissues, a highly focused beam with a high-power density is desirable. For tissue coagulation and hemostasis, a defocused beam with a lower-power density is preferable. Four types of lasers have been used in gynecologic endoscopy. They include the carbon dioxide, potassium–titanyl–phosphate, argon, and Nd:YAG. Each has unique properties, including differences in wavelength, beam-scattering effect, depth of penetration, and color absorption. The carbon dioxide laser has been used most extensively and is the best suited for laparoscopic use because of its wide margin of safety, lower acquisition cost, and relative ease of use. None of the lasers has been prospectively compared with conventional laparoscopic surgery, and a clear clinical advantage has not been proved. All lasers are much more expensive than conventional laparoscopic instruments.

The current generation of electrosurgical units uses low-voltage, high-frequency, and solid-state generators with insulated circuitry that are a substantial improvement over the previous "spark-gap" units. Most systems have unipolar and bipolar modes. In the unipolar system, the current passes from the generator, through the instrument, through the patient, to a ground plate, and back to the generator. Energy in the form of electrons is dissipated at the point of contact with the patient's tissues. The bipolar mode involves passage of energy from one of the blades through the patient's tissue, and the energy exits through the opposite blade, avoiding dissipation through the patient's body.

In the cutting mode, a constant, high-energy waveform is generated. In the coagulation mode there is an initial high-voltage peak that quickly dissipates. This results in desiccation of the most superficial layer of tissue, and increased tissue resistance results. Current can be blended to mix both cutting and coagulating current. Microtip cautery can be used to cut tissues in the same way as the laser, and the power density can be calculated in the same way. Laparoscopic scissors and scalpels can also be combined with unipolar electrocautery to provide simultaneous cutting and coagulation. A similar effect can be achieved as with the carbon dioxide laser, but the depth of penetration is more variable.

Absolute contraindications for operative laparoscopy include bowel obstruction, severe ileus, large undiagnosed abdominal mass, diaphragmatic or abdominal hernia, significant cardiopulmonary compromise, and uncontrolled intraabdominal bleeding with hypovolemia. Relative contraindications include severe obesity, intrauterine pregnancy, ascites, and inflammatory bowel disease.

Complications

Laparoscopy is considered to be a very safe procedure. The most common serious complications occur from placement of the insufflation needle or trocar, with major vessel injury or perforation of a viscus. Mortality rates of 2.5–8/100,000 cases have been described; mortality is associated with cardiac arrest, gas embolism, and bowel perforation. The most common complication of laparoscopy is subcutaneous emphysema from improper placement of the insufflation needle. Pelvic abscesses and wound infections can occur. Additional complications include introduction of gas into the lumen of the small or large bowel; perforation of the stomach; regurgitation of stomach contents; hemorrhage subsequent to damage of a major vessel, including the aorta, iliac arteries and veins, epigastric arteries and veins, splenic artery, and mesosalpingeal vessels; and incisional abdominal wall hematoma. Direct trauma to the liver, spleen, gallbladder, bladder, and uterus have been described. Cardiac arrest associated with arrhythmias, compression of the inferior vena cava, gas embolism, and hemorrhage have also been described. Use of instruments for electrocoagulation has been associated with electrical burns of the bowel (with necrosis, perforation, and peritonitis), skin, and abdominal wall. Similar injuries are possible with the laser.

COLPOSCOPY AND BIOPSY

Colposcopy has become the accepted method of evaluation for women with abnormalities of the lower genital tract epithelium. Originally, it was used solely for evaluation of the cervix in patients who had abnormal Pap test results. As experience has grown, it is now considered indispensable in evaluation of the entire anogenital tract.

The colposcope is an instrument that magnifies the surface epithelium under a bright light. The simplest colposcopes magnify subjects approximately 13–16 fold. A colposcope with variable magnification is preferred, as it facilitates rapid visualization of the entire anogenital tract at low-power and closer examination of the abnormal areas with higher magnification. A green filter can be interposed between the light and the viewer to give a better view of the blood vessel patterns.

Technique

The patient is placed in the normal lithotomy position, and the colposcope is brought into focus. The vulva is inspected at low power, and the speculum is inserted under direct vision. This allows the examiner to identify vulvar and vaginal abnormalities that may coexist with cervical abnormalities. The cervix is then exposed, and a cytologic smear is obtained. The cervix is first cleaned with saline and the surface examined, first at lower power and then at high power. If no ulcerations or gross lesions are seen, 4–5% acetic acid is placed, using a cotton ball or cotton-tipped applicator. The cervix should be bathed for 1–2 minutes while observing the cervix through the colposcope. The examiner should 1) identify the squamocolumnar junction, 2) examine the entire transformation zone, 3) determine whether the transformation zone is normal or abnormal, 4) perform an endocervical curettage under direct visualization, 5) perform targeted biopsies to the most abnormal areas of the transformation zone, and 6) apply Monsel solution for hemostasis.

Histopathology of the Cervix

The cervix is composed of columnar epithelium lining the endocervical canal and squamous epithelium covering the exocervix. The squamocolumnar junction is the point at which they meet and is variable, depending on age, gravidity, and hormone stimulation. The squamocolumnar junction rarely remains at the anatomic external os. In neonates, the squamocolumnar junction is located on the exocervix. During menarche, the vaginal epithelium produces glycogen, which is acted upon by lactobacilli. This reduces the vaginal pH and stimulates the subcolumnar reserve cells to undergo metaplasia. The metaplastic cells advance from the original squamocolumnar junction inward toward the external os. This establishes the transformation zone. The transformation zone extends from the original squamocolumnar junction to the active squamocolumnar junction. Once the metaplastic epithelium is matured and forms glycogen, it is called the healed transformation zone and is relatively resistant to oncogenic stimuli. Active metaplasia, with its immature cells, however, is most susceptible to oncogenic factors leading to transformation of the metaplastic cells into dysplasia.

The Bethesda System

When first introduced, cervical cytology was designed to detect cervical cancer. Soon it was realized that cytology could also detect precursor lesions of cervical cancer that, when adequately treated, would avert subsequent cancer. As a result, the objective of screening changed from finding existing cancer to preventing cancer. Gradually, the diagnostic categories for reporting cytologic abnormalities were expanded to include more lesions, many of which represented minimal changes. These expanded categories included minimal grades of cervical intraepithelial neoplasia (CIN), cytopathic effects of human papillomavirus (HPV) infection, and benign non-specific atypia secondary to inflammation. Thus, expansion of diagnostic categories actually predated the Bethesda System, which has attempted to organize the diverse cytologic changes into a coherent and logical reporting system. In the Bethesda System, potentially premalignant squamous lesions fall into three categories: atypical squamous cells of undetermined significance (ASCUS), low-grade squamous intraepithelial lesions (LSIL), and high-grade squamous intraepithelial lesions (HSIL).

Management of the Abnormal Pap Test

Atypical Squamous Cells of Undetermined Significance. Abnormal cells that do not fulfill the criteria for LSIL or HSIL are described as ASCUS. This includes many of the minor abnormalities included in the group "atypical" in the past. The ASCUS category does *not* include the condylomatous or koilocytotic atypia that was formerly included in class II of the Pap classification. Koilocytosis is now included in LSIL. The ASCUS category is restricted to those smears with abnormal cells that are truly of unknown significance. The ASCUS category was not intended to include benign, reactive, and reparative changes; these should be coded as normal in the Bethesda System.

The lack of diagnostic criteria and the fear of medicolegal action has made the ASCUS diagnosis quite common in some centers, with a range of 3–25%. It is anticipated that when standardized diagnostic criteria are used, the rate of ASCUS smears should be 3–5%.

Current management of ASCUS is controversial. Cytology is an excellent screening tool but is not an effective triage procedure since it will be negative in approximately 40% of patients who have colposcopically diagnosed squamous intraepithelial lesions. Colposcopy is a time-consuming and expensive form of triage and may result in overtreatment of patients. Nevertheless, many physicians currently manage patients with ASCUS Pap test results by colposcopically directed biopsy. Colposcopic biopsy after a single ASCUS Pap test reveals benign histology in 70% of cases, LSIL in 25%, HSIL in 5%, and cancer extremely rarely (in 0.001%). Colposcopic biopsy of persistent ASCUS lesions (using Bethesda criteria in excellent referral laboratories) reveals LSIL in 35–42% of cases, HSIL in 10–28% of cases, and invasive cancer in 0.2% of cases. The most common strategy used for ASCUS cytology is to repeat the Pap test at intervals of 3–6 months. If two consecutive test results are negative, then a return to yearly Pap tests would be indicated. If either of the tests shows a repeat ASCUS or more advanced stage, then those patients would be candidates for further testing.

Since approximately 70% of patients with ASCUS Pap tests will have a benign histologic diagnosis, simply excising the transformation zones of all of these women is not indicated. This would lead to overtreatment of most of these women, many of whom are young with active metaplasia in the transformation zone that is overcalled by cytologic examination and misinterpreted on colposcopy. If colposcopy is used as a means of evaluating the atypical Pap test, one must be cautious not to overinterpret the metaplastic areas. There is also a risk that pathologists will overinterpret the colposcopically directed biopsies and the patient will be given a diagnosis of low-grade lesion when metaplasia is the only finding.

Low-Grade Squamous Intraepithelial Lesions. The Bethesda System incorporates cellular changes associated with HPV (koilocytosis) within the category of LSIL because the natural history, distribution of various HPV types, and morphologic features of both of these lesions are the same.

Most cytologic specimens demonstrating LSIL represent processes that will spontaneously revert to normal without therapy. However, a few women in this category will have a lesion that will progress. At a minimum, patients with cytology indicating LSIL should have cervical cytologic examinations repeated at intervals of approximately 4–6 months and colposcopy performed if an abnormality persists. Because of the false-negative rate of cervical cytology, most obstetrician–gynecologists will choose to perform colposcopy after the initial LSIL test to determine whether a lesion is present. Following histologic confirmation, if the entire lesion is visualized and the limits of the transformation zone are seen, the lesion can be ablated or the patient monitored with no treatment. Management depends to a large degree on the desire and compliance of the patient. Since approximately 15% of these lesions progress to HSIL, ablation is a reasonable treatment. On the other hand, since approximately 60% of these lesions regress spontaneously, follow-up is an appropriate form of management for a compliant patient when indicated. An LSIL that is limited to the endocervical canal can be closely monitored with repeated specimens obtained with an endocervical brush and an endocervical curettage without resorting to a cone biopsy or other treatment. If follow-up and no treatment is selected and the lesion persists for a year, treatment may be indicated.

Any woman with a cytologic specimen suggesting the presence of HSIL (moderate or severe dysplasia, CIN II or CIN III, or carcinoma in situ) should undergo colposcopy and directed biopsy. Following colposcopically directed biopsy and determination of the distribution of the lesion, ablative therapy aimed at destruction or removal of the entire transformation zone should usually be performed. Outpatient management can be undertaken only if the entire lesion and limits of the transformation zone are seen and results of endocervical curettage are negative. Conization may be appropriate as outlined above.

Colposcopic Findings

The healed transformation zone will be characterized by trapped endocervical glands that form nabothian cysts. The skin may be thin and have blood vessels stretched over it. These blood vessels branch normally, and the epithelium is normal.

The columnar epithelium appears red because there is a single layer of columnar epithelium over the columnar villi that is, in turn, filled with blood from the capillaries. The metaplastic epithelium is found at the squamocolumnar junction and begins in the subcolumnar reserve cell. As the metaplastic cells replace the columnar epithelium, the central capillary of the villus regresses and the epithelium flattens out, leaving a normal maturing epithelium. Application of 4–5% acetic acid to metaplastic cells results in a thin, gray appearance. The surface is smooth, and there is no external border. Beginning colposcopists may have difficulty differentiating this metaplastic appearance from early dysplasia.

The transformation zone is called abnormal if there is 1) acetowhite epithelium, 2) punctation, 3) a mosaic pattern, 4) abnormal vasculature, or 5) leukoplakia. Acetowhite epithelium is epithelium that turns white after application of acetic acid (4–5%). Normal epithelium has mature glycogen-producing cells that are resistant to the acetic acid. Dysplastic cells, however, have no glycogen, and the acetic acid induces a white, opaque change to the epithelium. The intensity of the white depends on the thickness of the epithelium and the density of the nuclei. Lesions with higher-grade dysplasia usually have more dense nuclei and a thicker white epithelium.

Punctation refers to dilated capillaries terminating on the surface. When viewed from above, these appear as a collection of dots. When found in an area of well-demarcated acetowhite epithelium, they indicate an abnormal vascular pattern associated with cervical dysplasia. The size of the punctated vessels and their spacing on the surface epithelium are used to determine the severity of the dysplasia.

Mosaic vessels are terminal capillaries surrounding polygon-shaped blocks of acetowhite epithelium. These vessels form a basket around the blocks of abnormal epithelium and are crowded together in appearance similar to a mosaic tile. The space between mosaic vessels and the intensity of acetowhite are used to indicate the severity of dysplasia.

Atypical blood vessels can occur in three patterns: 1) hairpin or looped vessels, 2) abnormally branching vessels, or 3) abnormal network vessels. Looped vessels originate from the punctated and mosaic vessels. As the neoplastic epithelium grows, it crowds out the punctated and mosaic vessels. To maintain the blood supply, the vessels begin to tuft and then spread out along the surface of the early cancer. Their course over the surface is 2–3 mm, and they do not branch. They form a loop or a spiral and end abruptly. After application of acetic acid, they maintain their surface position and remain visible.

The abnormally branching vessels originate from the vessels of the cervical stroma. When cancer develops, the stromal vessels are pushed to the surface and the surface erodes, exposing the vessels. The cancer stimulates the growth of the vessels and causes them to branch frequently at obtuse angles, demonstrating sharp turns, dilatations, and narrowings. They bleed easily on contact and lead to postcoital bleeding.

The abnormal network vessels arise from the terminal capillaries at the junction of the epithelium with the stroma. Normal network vessels are most easily seen in postmenopausal women, whose thin epithelium allows underlying capillaries to be seen. When they become irregular in caliber, with dilatations and constrictions, or end in a "comma shape," they are considered abnormal. The abnormality may be due to cancer or simply due to erosive or atrophic cervicitis.

Leukoplakia is white epithelium that is visible on the genital tract epithelium before the application of acetic acid. It is caused by a layer of keratin on the surface of the epithelium. Since the normal genital tract is lined by glycogen cells, the production of keratin is abnormal. It is most often a marker of HPV or keratinizing dysplasia. It is rare that a keratinizing carcinoma will present in this fashion.

Selection of Treatment

Patients with abnormal transformation zones should undergo an endocervical curettage followed by a directed biopsy of the most abnormal area. Often, more than one biopsy is indicated. A cervical punch biopsy 3–5 mm in size should be used. Endocervical curettage is performed with a sharp curette designed specifically for the endocervix (see also "Hysteroscopy" in this section). The curetted epithelium collects in the mucus and coagulum at the external os. It is picked up by a forceps and placed on a paper towel or plastic film to keep it from fragmenting, then placed in formalin.

Ideally, the pathologist and colposcopist should review the cytology, colposcopic findings, cervical biopsy results, and endocervical curettage scrapings before deciding on therapy. Most patients can then be treated by outpatient modalities such as cryosurgery, laser, or electrosurgical excision. The treatment selected will depend on the equipment available to the physician, the physician's training and skills, and the desires of the patient. Cryosurgery is inexpensive, is easy to learn, and has a success rate of 90% for CIN I and CIN II lesions. Failure rates for CIN III are higher (20–30%), and other modalities should be considered. Following cryosurgery, there is a 3–4-week vaginal discharge and the scar that forms produces a small, sometimes stenotic, cervical os, making reevaluation by the colposcope very difficult. For these reasons, the carbon dioxide laser has become popular in treating CIN. It leaves a clean cervical bed that heals rapidly without significant discharge and a normal appearance that allows for future colposcopic examinations. Cure rates above 95% for all grades of CIN can be expected.

Electrosurgical excision of the transformation zone has become a standard method for treating cervical dysplasia. The equipment is cheaper than laser, the technique is easy to learn, and there is a specimen that can be sent to the pathology department. Healing is rapid, with a mild discharge, and the appearance is similar to that after laser surgery. The initial results with electrosurgical excision are comparable to those with laser vaporization. Complete removal of the transformation zone as the initial diagnostic step in colposcopy should not be practiced. It should be reserved for those patients in whom the colposcopically directed biopsy has documented a lesion that requires removal of the transformation zone.

A diagnostic conization is indicated for 1) positive endocervical curettage, 2) unsatisfactory colposcopic examination, or 3) microinvasive carcinoma on biopsy or cytologic findings. The diagnostic cone can be performed by a laser excision, electrosurgical excision, or cold knife cone. The technique selected depends on the instruments available to the physician and his or her skill.

Colposcopy of the Vagina

Colposcopy of the entire vagina with application of 4–5% acetic acid is indicated for abnormal Pap test results with normal or absent cervix, prior to cone or hysterectomy for cervical dysplasia, for all patients with vulvar intraepithelial neoplasia (VIN), and for all patients with HPV. There are generally two patterns of VIN, depending on the location of the lesion. The vaginal cuff, after hysterectomy for CIN, may have colposcopic patterns similar to those of the cervix with acetowhite epithelium, punctation, mosaic pattern, and abnormal blood vessels. The vaginal fornices after hysterectomy must be examined by pulling them into view with a vaginal hook. In the rest of the vagina, the lesions are generally multifocal, slightly raised, ovoid, and located along the ridges of the vaginal rugae. Frequently, they have surface spicules indicating HPV infection. The more advanced lesions may have a papillary surface with abnormal vessels of the loop variety. Lugol staining is necessary to more accurately and quickly identify all of the lesions. The vaginal biopsy can be done with the same instrument as is used for cervical biopsies. Treatment is determined by a review of the biopsy, cytologic, and colposcopic findings. The most common and effective treatment is laser vaporization. Excisional biopsy should be performed if carcinoma is suspected on the basis of cytologic, colposcopic, or biopsy results.

Colposcopy of the Vulva

Colposcopy of the vulva is useful in evaluating patients with VIN, invasive cancer, and HPV. The VIN lesions may be 1) white, with a thick, hyperkeratotic layer on the epithelial surface; 2) red, with the absence of a hyperkeratotic layer; or 3) pigmented, with black pigment from the basal layer carried to the surface by rapid proliferation of the cells. A single patient may exhibit one or all of these characteristics. Acetic acid (5%) should be applied to the vulva for at least 3 minutes prior to inspection with a colposcope. The thick keratin layer of the vulva is slow to react to the acetic acid effect. The mucosal surfaces of the introitus and perianal tissues will react more quickly. The mucosal surfaces may have vascular patterns of punctation, mosaic, and looped blood vessels to go along with the acetowhite epithelium, similar to the cervical lesions. Treatment depends on 1) the location of the lesions (keratinized surface versus mucosal surface), 2) the size of the lesion, 3) whether lesions are unifocal or multifocal, and 4) the age of the patient. Laser vaporization is the best treatment for mucosal lesions, since there are no hair follicles into which the VIN may extend. This allows the destruction to penetrate to the papillary dermis, where healing will be rapid (10–14 days). Large lesions on the keratinized, hair-bearing skin should be excised and closed primarily. They will heal more quickly than a laser burn that extends far enough into the dermis to destroy the hair follicles. Women over age 50 years should have the lesions excised, since up to 18% of them will have microinvasive cancer in the excised specimen. This is particularly true of unifocal lesions that have beginning ulcerations or very thick keratin layers.

ULTRASONOGRAPHY

Most use of ultrasonography in obstetrics and gynecology was in obstetrics until relatively recently, but the growing use of transvaginal scanning in the mid-1980s has permitted tremendous development of imaging in gynecology. The main advantage of transvaginal scanning is the proximity of the transducer to the organ of interest, which allows the use of higher frequency. Major improvements in resolution can be expected, since the higher the frequency, the better the resolution (but the lesser the penetration). This permits diagnosis of earlier lesions, which presumably are less advanced, with consequently better prognosis. The smaller field of view and the distance limitation are disadvantages when compared with transabdominal ultrasonography.

New technology in ultrasonography includes the use of the Doppler shift to allow quantitative flow calculation. The Doppler shift can be measured, interpreted, and processed into color images. Although this technique is considered investigational, in the future it may play a role in assessing menstrual cycles subject to hormonal manipulation and in screening for cancer of the ovary.

Diagnostic Evaluation

Accurate knowledge of pelvic anatomy is vital in performing and interpreting gynecologic ultrasonography. Bony structures, muscles (levator ani, obturator internus, iliopsoas), and blood vessels (internal iliac) are important landmarks that are helpful in localizing pelvic organs.

Transabdominal ultrasonography requires a full bladder for several reasons:

- It dislodges the uterus from behind the ultrasound-impenetrable pubic bone.
- It pushes bowel loops (and their contents) out of the field.
- It serves as a sound-enhancing window.
- It can be used as a reference in terms of tissue echogenicity.

Transvaginal ultrasonography has made the need for a full bladder obsolete because, by transducer location, transvaginal ultrasonography reduces or eliminates the problems posed by obesity or the presence of bowel.

Uterus

Uterine Anomalies. Complete absence of the uterus, as well as atresia of the cervix and vagina, is uncommon (Mayer–Rokitansky–Küster–Hauser syndrome). Other congenital anomalies of the uterus are relatively more frequent (0.1–3%). They most frequently result from defects of fusion of the paired müllerian ducts. This may take the form of complete (uterus didelphys), partial (uterus bicornis), or minimal (uterus arcuatus) failure of fusion. Lack of resorption of the septum will produce a septate uterus, often associated with recurrent pregnancy loss. Abnormal uterine shape or excessive transverse measurement should alert the examiner to the possibility of an anomaly. Two separate endometrial cavities can sometimes be identified.

Menstrual Cycle Changes. The endometrium undergoes cyclic changes during the menstrual cycle. These changes can be demonstrated by ultrasonography. No major differences have been reported in spontaneous versus induced cycles. Early in the cycle, the endometrium appears as a thin, echogenic line, 1–4-mm wide. The inner myometrium is seen as an encircling hypoechoic area, presumably due to the presence of fluid. In the proliferative phase, thickness augments to 3–10 mm, and the hypoechoic area is more pronounced. Average thickness growth of the endometrium is approximately 1 mm/d. This has been correlated to changing levels of estradiol. During the secretory phase, thickness can reach 15 mm when echogenicity is very pronounced and there is no central cavity. After menopause, the endometrium remains clearly visible and measurable for several months. It usually measures less than 5 mm in width but can be more prominent if replacement estrogens are administered.

Endometrial Hyperplasia and Carcinoma. If the central endometrial echo measures more than 10 mm or does not undergo major modifications during the menstrual cycle, hyperplasia should be suspected. Endometrial polyps and trophoblastic disease can produce similar pictures. Endometrial carcinoma or sarcoma also needs to be considered. Unfortunately, no pathognomonic findings have been described, but the addition of Doppler ultrasonography (vide infra) may heighten the sensitivity. Ovaries should also be scanned in detail for the possible presence of hormone-producing tumors. These findings, particularly in postmenopausal women, demand immediate further evaluation.

Leiomyomata. Uterine echogenicity should be homogeneous, and departure from this may suggest myomatous changes. Myomas are very common solid uterine tumors, diagnosed in 20–30% of women over age 30. Submucosal leiomyomata can distort or obliterate the uterine cavity, whereas subserous myomas may distort the outer contour and make it very irregular and bulky. A differential diagnosis to keep in mind is adenomyosis, which can also cause diffuse enlargement and irregular echoes.

Endometritis. Postpartum endometritis will often result in subinvolution. No specific ultrasonographic signs are demonstrable in postpartum or postcurettage infection, but an enlarged uterus with a dilated endometrial cavity, containing fluid or sometimes air should raise the suspicion of an infectious process. Another finding frequently described is a loss of differentiation between the endometrium and myometrium. Uterine abscesses will appear identical to those in other organs: semisolid masses with internal debris. Similar findings will be present if the infection follows other surgical intervention on the pregnant or nonpregnant uterus. Often signs of inflammation in other organs may be present (fluid in the pouch of Douglas, for instance).

Retained Products of Conception. Retained placental fragments are one of the main reasons for postpartum hemorrhage. Subinvolution needs also to be considered. Similarly, retained products of an incomplete spontaneous or therapeutic abortion can produce severe bleeding. Ultrasonography will demonstrate the presence or absence of retained tissues. Gas pockets are sometimes demonstrated. These point to the possible presence of an infection by gas-forming bacteria (*Clostridium perfringens* or *Escherichia coli*, in particular).

Postpartum and Postsurgery. The uterus returns to its prepregnancy size by approximately 6 weeks postpartum. Involution during the first 3 days is rapid, slows down for the next few days, and accelerates again during the second and third weeks postpartum. Clots are often visualized inside the uterine cavity during the first 2–3 days. This is not an abnormal finding. Normal thickness of the postpartum endometrial cavity is up to 2 cm. In assessing the uterus after surgery, one can visualize collections of blood, hematomas, and abscesses. Some authors have described the ultrasonographic assessment of a uterine scar (particularly after cesarean delivery), but this is not widely performed.

Localization of Intrauterine Devices. Ultrasonography is the first diagnostic procedure to be tried when an IUD thread cannot be visualized protruding from the cervix or cannot be retrieved with gentle probing. The presence or absence of the IUD in the uterus can be verified by ultrasonography with an accuracy of 90–100%. If the endometrial cavity and the IUD can be demonstrated separately, one can assume that the device has been displaced. Embedment within the myometrium can occur and is very difficult to diagnose by ultrasonography. When perforation occurs and the IUD becomes displaced into the peritoneal space, ultrasonography will demonstrate an empty uterus, but visualization of the IUD may be impossible. In such case, a plain anteroposterior roentgenogram of the abdomen will usually be diagnostic.

Cervix

The endocervical canal is a thin, echogenic stripe, often with a small amount of fluid, particularly in the periovulatory stage. Nabothian endocervical cysts are sometimes demonstrated, measuring 0.5–4 cm. They are of no clinical significance and should not be confused with an abnormally situated gestational sac. The cervix should be at least 3 cm long and less than 1 cm in transverse diameter. Cervical shortening and dilatation of the internal os in the nonpregnant state can occasionally be imaged by transabdominal or transvaginal ultrasonography. If this occurs when the patient is already pregnant, cerclage or serial studies may be indicated. More extreme cases will demonstrate ballooning or funneling of the sac containing amniotic fluid and occasionally umbilical cord or fetal parts into the dilated cervix, or even the vagina.

Adnexa

Fallopian tubes are not visualized on ultrasonography unless they are filled with or floating in fluid. Ultrasonography has a role in the management of ectopic pregnancy and infertility (see "Tubal and Peritoneal Factors" in this section and "Infertility" in the section on Reproductive Endocrinology and Fertility).

Cyclic Changes. Periodic changes in the ovaries are clearly demonstrable, and monitoring of follicular maturation may be the most common indication for performing gynecologic ultrasonography today. Mean daily growth is about 2–3 mm. At a mean diameter of 10 mm (on the average, on day 6), one follicle usually takes over and continues growing while the rest remain quiescent. A mature follicle measures 20–24 mm in diameter. There is a close relationship between follicular diameter and estradiol levels.

Ultrasonographic signs of imminent ovulation have been described, as well as findings after ovulation: decrease in follicular size or disappearance of the follicle with appearance of fluid in the pouch of Douglas. The corpus luteum can be demonstrated as a persistent cystic structure in the postovulatory period, especially if fertilization has occurred.

Pelvic Masses. Ultrasonography plays a major role in the evaluation of lower abdominal masses. Ultrasonography permits confirmation of the presence of an abnormal tumor and characterization of its position, size, and consistency. The main categories of pelvic masses imaged by ultrasonography are ovarian tumors (benign or malignant), tubal abnormalities (hydrosalpinx, abscess), endometriosis, ectopic pregnancy, and uterine masses.

In the ovary, the normal follicle reaches a preovulatory diameter of 20–24 mm. It then disappears or dramatically diminishes in size. Failure to rupture transforms it into a follicular cyst, which usually regresses in 6–8 weeks. This can be seen with the luteinized unruptured follicle syndrome. A corpus luteum cyst occurs when the corpus luteum fails to regress after ovulation. It may grow to 10 cm in diameter and cause symptoms. In early pregnancy, this cyst should regress by midpregnancy at the latest. Endometriosis can manifest itself as ovarian cysts. These can be completely cystic, in which case they are indistinguishable from cysts of other etiology. Mixed echoes originating in blood and clots can sometimes be demonstrated. Uniform low-level echoes can represent thickened, bloody material ("chocolate"). When more solid, this material may be difficult to differentiate from solid tumors.

One can look at ovarian masses in terms of parameters for malignancy or need for further investigation. The following criteria traditionally signify malignancy:

- Large, persistent mass (greater than 5 cm)
- Cyst with solid, irregular, internal components
- Presence of internal septations, particularly if thick (multilocular cyst)
- Fixation in the pelvis
- Large amount of intrapelvic fluid (>10–20 ml)

Some of these characteristics may be visualized with "physiologic tumors," such as a completely benign, hemorrhagic cysts, and some highly malignant lesions in their early stages may appear as "simple cysts." Paraovarian cysts arise from embryologic remnants of the Gartner ducts. They are usually single, simple, thin-walled cysts that rarely exceed 3–5 cm in diameter and do not demonstrate changes with the menstrual cycle.

Polycystic Ovaries. The classic triad associated with the polycystic ovary syndrome consists of hirsutism, oligomenorrhea, and obesity. Often, however, an ultrasound picture of polycystic ovaries will be obtained without clinical signs of the syndrome or with only partial manifestations. The ovaries are enlarged and contain multiple (usually more than 10) cysts measuring 5 mm or less in diameter. These cysts are usually peripheral but can also be scattered throughout the ovarian stroma. The typical ovarian ultrasound picture is associated with clinical syndromes in 75–95% of cases. However, the prevalence of the ultrasound findings is quite high without any biochemical or clinical signs.

Pelvic Inflammatory Disease. Ultrasound findings may sometimes be entirely normal. Fluid collections may be demonstrated in the endometrial cavity. These may be confounded with an early gestational sac or pseudogestational sac (as seen in ectopic pregnancy). Only if the fallopian tubes are distended by fluid such as blood or pus, or are "floating" in such fluid, will they be visible on ultrasonography. Percutaneous drainage under ultrasound guidance may be possible. If there is obstruction, the tubes distend and multiple loops containing clear fluid will be seen occasionally, together with a thickened wall (hydrosalpinx).

Bilateral complex adnexal masses are the most frequent finding in patients with pelvic inflammatory disease. These irregular, partly cystic, partly solid, septated, fluid-filled masses most likely represent tuboovarian abscesses. Ovaries and tubes cannot usually be separated from the mass. Ovarian torsion and neoplasm may appear somewhat similar but will rarely be bilateral. In most cases, fluid is present in the cul-de-sac. Large quantities of fluid are obviously a sign of intrapelvic pathologic lesions (infection, bleeding, tumor), but small quantities are also visible during the normal cycle, particularly during menstruation.

Kidneys, Bladder, Ureters, and Urethra

A severe degree of hydronephrosis or the presence of calcifications is relatively easy to diagnose. The normal bladder wall should be smooth and of uniform thickness. Normal ureters will not be visualized, but flow of urine can often be detected as small jets originating from one of the walls (the ureterovesical junctions, sometimes identified as a small bulge in the posterior wall). Dilated ureters are easily visualized, and Doppler sampling may help to differentiate them from blood vessels.

A quantification of residual urine is an integral part of the assessment of lower urinary tract function or of postsurgical evaluation and is a quick, easy, and accurate enough method. Intravesical neoplasms and depth of bladder wall invasion can be diagnosed by ultrasonography. Perineal ultrasongraphy can be helpful in the assessment of bladder neck position and mobility in the investigation of urinary incontinence.

Abdominal Wall

Examination of the abdominal wall may reveal pathologic lesions most often related to surgical procedures. Subfascial or subdermal fluid collection, intraperitoneal hematoma, and broad ligament hematoma are all demonstrable by ultrasonography, usually with the use of a higher-frequency transducer. In addition, bladder flap hematoma may occur after cesarean delivery. This may potentially be massive, with spread to the broad ligaments and retroperitoneum. It is practically impossible to differentiate between an organizing clot and an infectious process by ultrasonography. Fine-needle aspiration may clarify the diagnosis.

Operative Procedures

Biopsy of Pelvic Mass

Percutaneous ultrasound-guided biopsy of a pelvic mass may allow diagnosis without the need for more invasive procedures. These may include primary tumors, as well as metastases to pelvic organs or lymph nodes. Ultrasound-guided aspiration may reassure the practitioner as to the nonmalignancy of a tumor. In cases of malignant effusion (abdominal, pleural, or pericardial fluid), drainage for diagnostic or therapeutic purposes may be accomplished.

Percutaneous drainage of abnormal fluid collection may be performed transabdominally or transvaginally, according to the location. Contraindications include severe bleeding disorders (congenital or acquired), uncooperative patients, and poor visualization of the area of interest. If surgery is planned anyway, the need for ultrasound-guided biopsy is probably nonexistent. Although the risk of malignant cell seeding along the needle path is a theoretic concern, no large studies have demonstrated this to be a real issue.

Oocyte Harvesting

The transvaginal approach first described in 1985 is the preferred and most commonly used method. The choice of route depends on ovarian position:

- Choose the transabdominal route for ovaries lateral to the uterus or close to the abdominal wall. If the ovaries are adjacent to the bladder, a transabdominal–transvesical route may be selected.
- Choose the transvaginal route for low ovaries, in the pouch of Douglas.
- Choose the periurethral–transvesical route for high ovaries, lateral to the uterus and close enough to the bladder.

Postprocedural lower abdominal pain is the only common complaint. Other complications, much less commonly encountered, are infection, hematuria, puncture of vessels, and bowel injury.

Uterine Evacuation

Ultrasound visualization of the uterine cavity is extremely rewarding with new high-resolution scanners. This imaging mode can be of great help in surgical procedures in patients in whom uterine orientation is unclear, for verification of completeness of the procedure, or when a false route or perforation is suspected. This can be accomplished by following the progression of an instrument being introduced under ultrasound guidance and verifying its relation in the uterine cavity close to the posterior uterine wall or beyond it, in the abdominal cavity. Use of ultrasonography during the performance of a dilation and evacuation can actually reduce the incidence of perforation.

ANOSCOPY AND SIGMOIDOSCOPY

In 1992 in the United States, 75,000 women developed cancer of the colon and rectum, compared with 44,500 developing cancer of the uterus and 182,000 developing cancer of the breasts. Colon and rectal cancer caused the deaths of 28,200 women, compared with 46,000 deaths from breast cancer and 10,100 from uterine cancer.

Anoscopic and sigmoidoscopic procedures are performed to detect anal–rectal disease, to stage gynecologic malignancy, and to evaluate anemia. Women aged 40–49 years should have a digital rectal examination annually with fecal occult blood tests. In addition, after age 50, women should undergo flexible sigmoidoscopy every 3–5 years.

Regardless of the patient's age, these examinations should also be carried out in any patient presenting with warning signals of rectal bleeding, blood in the stool, or change in bowel habits. Increased risk of colon and rectal cancer is seen in patients with personal or family history of cancer or polyps of the colon or rectum, patients with inflammatory bowel disease, and patients with a high-fat or low-fiber diet.

Anoscopy can be performed with various types of anoscopes. Following digital examination, the lubricated anoscope with obturator in place is inserted. Removal of the obturator then allows visualization of the anus.

Flexible sigmoidoscopy, with its increased comfort over rigid proctosigmoidoscopy, can then be performed after thorough examination of the anal canal. For this, the patient should be prepared with several enemas given from 1 to 3 hours before the examination. Courses in flexible sigmoidoscopy are readily available, and the procedure is not difficult to learn, given its similarity to other endoscopic procedures.

Rectal Prolapse

Rectal prolapse is a circumferential, full-thickness intussusception of the rectum in which the intussusceptum descends through the external anal sphincter to emerge outside the anal verge. The diagnosis is frequently missed, and in many cases requires examining the patient in a squatting position. Rectal prolapse is an important cause of bleeding, mucous discharge, and fecal incontinence, and often is associated with defecation disorders. Between 90% and 98% of all patients with rectal prolapse are women, and fully one third of elderly patients with rectal prolapse are nulliparous.

When rectal prolapse occurs in younger women, there is usually an underlying predisposing cause (eg, parturition injury to pelvic floor muscles or chronic constipation and straining). Most women with prolapse are past age 50 years and generally present with fecal incontinence, lax pelvic floor, and evidence of denervation of the external anal sphincter and the puborectalis sling. Incontinence is present in up to 70% of all patients with rectal prolapse, and an even higher percentage have defecation disorders with a history of chronic straining. The anus is frequently patulous, and perineal descent is commonly seen. Many patients with this condition have proctitis, and some have solitary or multiple rectal ulcers. Therefore, proctosigmoidoscopy is indicated.

Surgical therapy of rectal prolapse usually corrects the anatomic abnormality, but many patients experience difficulty with rectal evacuation, impaired colonic transit, persistent mucous discharge, and incontinence as sequelae. The patients most likely to have these untoward and disconcerting symptoms after surgery are those with exaggerated motility, excessive perineal descent, low anal pressures, and electrophysiologic evidence of denervation. Therefore, preoperative evaluation of colonic transit, anal manometry, anal rectal sensation, electromyography, and video proctography are very helpful in predicting outcome and in modifying the type of surgical treatment.

There are many therapies for rectal prolapse. The abdominal suspension operations generally have resulted in less recurrence than the perineal and transacral procedures, although the latter are frequently preferred in debilitated, elderly patients. When combined with other pelvic floor defects such as cystocele, uterine prolapse, or enterocele, simultaneous repair of all the defects is preferable.

Fecal Incontinence

Fecal incontinence is underreported generally. In the data published, 35% of patients with bladder dysfunction have fecal incontinence, 40% being described as having major incontinence: the uncontrollable loss of formed stool. Nursing home populations have a reported fecal incontinence rate over 50%, with women more affected than men. Fecal incontinence is more prevalent in women by a ratio of 4:1. Community-dwelling women beyond age 65 have a reported incidence of 13.3/1,000, and very few of these have received advice or medical care for their disability.

Etiologies of fecal incontinence include conditions that could produce liquid stool that overwhelms normal control mechanisms. Infection, inflammatory bowel disease, rapid colon transit, or small bowel dysfunction may cause such disorders. Second, the rectal reservoir can be disturbed by inflammatory bowel disease, cancer, or pelvic masses that make the reservoir inadequate to maintain continence.

Other patients with major incontinence, however, have a significant deficit of the external anal sphincter or pelvic floor muscles, sometimes seen in addition to a weak internal sphincter. Most of these patients have denervation of the striated musculature. This denervation usually is secondary to pudendal nerve damage in the peripheral portion of the nerve, past its relatively fixed attachment at the Alcocks canal passage at the ischial spine. Such pudendal nerve denervation typically occurs with either childbirth or prolonged Valsalva attempts at defecation. Both processes lead to stretching of the distal pudendal nerve branches with subsequent demyelinization and axonal degeneration. Other causes of denervation include cauda equina disorders of peripheral neuropathies, such as diabetes mellitus, or disseminated neurologic disorders, such as multiple sclerosis. Damage to the external anal sphincter can occur with obstetric injury or with fistula or hemorrhoidal surgery.

Patients with spinal cord injury, stroke, or dementia are frequently incontinent of feces as well. With deficient cortical awareness of rectal filling, fecal impaction frequently develops, causing reflex relaxation of the internal sphincter and leakage of liquid stool.

Therapy for fecal incontinence is influenced by several factors, including the cause and severity, its impact on the patient's life, and the level of comprehension and motivation of the patient. The components of continence include 1) motor functions, with somatic innervation of the external anal sphincter and puborectalis muscle and autonomic innervation of the internal anal sphincter; 2) sensory functions, with rectal sensation (autonomic) and anal sensation (somatic); and 3) reservoir functions, consisting of autonomically regulated rectal capacity and compliance and colon motility. Clinical examination can provide a simplistic but frequently adequate appraisal of the motor, sensory, and reservoir functions of continence.

As a general rule, conservative management should be considered before surgical therapy. Treatment of fecal incontinence has one advantageous parameter that urinary incontinence does not, that is, the ability to control the consistency of the incontinence substance.

Biofeedback is available in a form for all components—motor, sensory, and reservoir function—in decreasing orders of success. The biofeedback trial is painless, inexpensive, and essentially risk free, requiring only a cooperative patient. Behavioral modification encouraging regular evacuation, sometimes to the point of using enemas to clean the left colon on a regular basis, is valuable in precluding surgery.

Surgical Therapies

Sphincter repair, unfortunately, serves only a minority of patients with fecal incontinence. Success for continence varies from 5% to 78% in published literature and is decreased in patients with evidence of extensive neuropathy. Post–anal repair had early enthusiastic reports, but prolonged follow-up studies have shown that although 60% still showed improvement, "complete continence" dropped to only 30%. Gracilis muscle transpositions have been helpful in some patients with traumatic sphincter loss, but very poor results are found in patients with neurogenic components. Electrode implantation has been used with muscle transplants as an investigational methodology that may see more use in the future.

As the population ages, the number of women affected with this terribly distressing problem is increasing. Caregivers in the past have been relatively unconcerned with fecal incontinence, and most of these patients have very little opportunity for medical intervention. Discussion with a sympathetic view can be achieved if the physician becomes comfortable with understanding the pathophysiology and methodologies of improving the patient's condition.

BIBLIOGRAPHY

Hysteroscopy

Carson SA, Hubert GD, Schriock ED, Buster JE. Hyperglycemia and hyponatremia during operative hysteroscopy with 5% dextrose in water distension. Fertil Steril 1989;51:341–343

Derman SG, Rehnstrom J, Neuwirth RS. The long-term effectiveness of hysteroscopic treatment of menorrhagia and leiomyomas. Obstet Gynecol 1991;77:591–594

Garry R, Erian J, Grochmal SA. A multi-centre collaborative study into the treatment of menorrhagia by Nd-YAG laser ablation of the endometrium. Br J Obstet Gynaecol 1991;98:357–362

Gimpelson RJ, Rappold HO. A comparative study between panoramic hysteroscopy with directed biopsies and dilatation and curettage: a review of 276 cases. Am J Obstet Gynecol 1988;158:489–492

March CM, Israel R. Hysteroscopic management of recurrent abortion caused by septate uterus. Am J Obstet Gynecol 1987;156:834–842

Seracchioli R, Possati G, Bafaro G, Cattoli M, Trevisis MR, Porcu E, et al. Hysteroscopic gamete intra-fallopian transfer: a good alternative, in selected cases, to laparoscopic intra-fallopian transfer. Hum Reprod 1991;6:1388–1390

Townsend DE, Richart RH, Paskowitz RA, Woolfork RE. "Rollerball" coagulation of the endometrium. Obstet Gynecol 1990;76:310–313

Laparoscopy

Grimes DA. Frontiers of operative laparoscopy: a review and critique of the evidence. Am J Obstet Gynecol 1992;166:1062–1071

Maiman M, Seltzer V, Boyce J. Laparoscopic excision of ovarian neoplasms subsequently found to be malignant. Obstet Gynecol 1991;77:563–565

Seltzer VL, Maiman M, Boyce J, Goldstein SR, Snyder JR, Moghissi K, et al. Laparoscopic surgery in the management of ovarian cysts. Female Patient 1992;17(6):16–23

Colposcopy and Biopsy

Benedet JL, Miller DM, Nickerson KG. Results of conservative management of cervical intraepithelial neoplasia. Obstet Gynecol 1992;79:105–110

Bigrigg MA, Codling BW, Pearson P, Read MD, Swingler GR. Colposcopic diagnosis and treatment of cervical dysplasia at a single clinic visit: experience of low-voltage diathermy loop in 1000 patients. Lancet 1990;336:229–231

Broder S. The Bethesda System for reporting cervical/vaginal cytologic diagnoses: report of the 1991 Bethesda Workshop. JAMA 1992;267:1892

Chafe W, Richards A, Morgan L, Wilkinson E. Unrecognized invasive carcinoma in vulvar intraepithelial neoplasia (VIN). Gynecol Oncol 1988;31:154–165

Jones DE, Creasman WT, Combroski RA, Lentz SS, Waeltz JL. Evaluation of the atypical Pap smear. Am J Obstet Gynecol 1987;157:544–549

Kataja V, Syrjanen K, Syrjanen S, Mantyjarvi R, Yliskoski M, Saarikoski S, et al. Prospective follow-up of genital HPV infections: survival analysis of the HPV typing data. Eur J Epidemiol 1990;6:9–14

Lorincz AT, Reid R, Jenson AB, Greenberg MD, Lancaster W, Kurman RJ. The relative prevalence of 15 major anogenital human papillomaviruses in health and disease. Human papillomavirus infection of the cervix: relative risk associations of 15 common anogenital types. Obstet Gynecol 1992;79:328–337

Luesley DM, Cullimore J, Redman CW, Lawton FG, Emens JM, Rollason TP, et al. Loop diathermy excision of the cervical transformation zone in patients with abnormal cervical smears. BMJ 1990;300:1690–1693

Nasiell K, Roger V, Nasiell M. Behavior of mild cervical dysplasia during long-term follow-up. Obstet Gynecol 1986;5:665–669

Willett GD, Kurman RJ, Reid R, Greenberg M, Jenson AB, Lorincz AT. Correlation of the histologic appearance of intraepithelial neoplasia of the cervix with human papillomavirus types: emphasis on low grade lesions including so-called flat condyloma. Int J Gynecol Pathol 1989;8:18–25

Wright TC Jr, Gagnon S, Richart RM, Ferenczy A. Treatment of cervical intraepithelial neoplasia using the loop electrosurgical excision procedure. Obstet Gynecol 1992;79:173–178

Wright VC, Davies E. Laser surgery for vulvar intraepithelial neoplasia: principles and results. Am J Obstet Gynecol 1987;156:374–378

Ultrasound

Bourne TH, Campbell S, Whitehead MI, Royston P, Steer CV, Collins WP. The detection of endometrial cancer in postmenopausal women by transvaginal ultrasonography and colour flow imaging. BMJ 1990;301:369

de Crespigny LC, Robinson HP, Davoren RA, Fortune DW. Ultrasound guided puncture for gynaecological and pelvic lesions. Aust N Z J Obstet Gynaecol 1985;25:277–229

Fleisher AC, Entman SS. Differential diagnosis of pelvic masses. In: Chervenak FA, Isaacson G, Campbell S, eds. Ultrasound in obstetrics & gynecology. Boston: Little, Brown, 1993:1643–1653

Fleischer AC, Pennell RG, McKee MS, Worrell JA, Keefe B, Herbert CM, et al. Ectopic pregnancy: features at transvaginal sonography. Radiology 1990;174:375–378

Goldstein SR. Incorporating endovaginal ultrasound into the overall gynecologic examination. Am J Obstet Gynecol 1990;162:625–632

Osmers R, Volksen M, Shauer A. Vaginosonography for early detection of endometrial carcinoma? Lancet 1990;335:1569–1571

Timor-Tritsch IE, Bar-Yam Y, Elgali S, Rottem S. The technique of transvaginal sonography with the use of a 6.5 MHz probe. Am J Obstet Gynecol 1988;158:1019–1024

Anoscopy and Sigmoidoscopy

Keighley M, Madoff RD, Watts JD, Rothenberger DA, Goldberg SM. Rectal prolapse. In: Henry MM, Swash M, eds. Coloproctology of the pelvic floor. 2nd ed. Oxford: Butterworth Heinemann, 1992:316

Leven KE, Pemberton JH. Rectal prolapse: pathogenesis and management. In: Benson JT, ed. Female pelvic floor disorders: investigation and management. New York: Norton, 1992

Preoperative Care

The purposes of the preoperative visit are 1) to obtain information that may decrease the risks of intraoperative and postoperative complications and 2) to obtain informed consent from the patient. This is a review of the components of preoperative care, including the history, physical examination, laboratory evaluation, informed consent, admission orders, and the use of prophylactic antibiotics.

HISTORY AND PHYSICAL EXAMINATION

Surgery-related morbidity and mortality are strongly correlated with preexisting medical conditions. It is essential, therefore, to review in detail the patient's complete medical history in addition to evaluating the condition for which the operation is planned. A thorough review of systems, with assessments of cardiac, pulmonary, endocrine, urologic, hepatic, reproductive, sexual, gastrointestinal, hematologic, psychiatric, social, and musculoskeletal function, often alerts the surgeon to the special needs of a patient. For example, a patient with chronic back problems may need to be positioned on the operating table while awake to avoid postoperative aggravation of this preexisting condition. The review of pulmonary function should include information on the patient's smoking status.

Included in the assessment of organ systems is a review of all medication taken by the patient within the past month. Patients must be questioned specifically about the recent use of aspirin and other nonsteroidal antiinflammatory drugs (which can acetylate platelets, leading to platelet dysfunction) and of oral contraceptives (which may increase the risk of postoperative thromboembolic disease), as many women do not know that these medications are worth mentioning. Contraceptive practices and menstrual history must be reviewed to avoid the possibility of unknowingly operating on a pregnant patient.

The physical examination should focus on the pelvic examination and the assessment of cardiovascular status (including vital signs). By performing a pelvic examination within 1 week of the proposed operation, the surgeon may finalize the surgical plan and discuss it with the patient. Routine gynecologic screening tests, such as a Pap test and mammography (when appropriate), should be brought up to date before the immediate preoperative visit. By using the information from a detailed history and physical examination, the surgeon can expect to detect approximately 90% of potential risk factors pertinent to the surgical procedure. Preoperative laboratory screening tests are used to discover the remaining 10% of these significant surgical risk factors.

LABORATORY ASSESSMENT

The general purpose of preoperative laboratory assessment is to identify and establish the extent of unsuspected and known diseases. This information will guide—and may alter—perioperative management. Unfortunately, there is currently no uniform standard for preoperative laboratory testing. However, the physician's goal should be to practice cost-effective medicine. In many instances, far too many preoperative laboratory tests are done either out of habit or because of medicolegal concerns.

A complete blood count and urinalysis are required components of the preoperative evaluation at nearly all hospitals. Anemia should be corrected, whenever possible, before an operation. In addition, asymptomatic bacteriuria, which is usually accompanied by pyuria and is common among elderly patients, should be monitored by urine culture and treated with an appropriate antibiotic to avoid bacterial dissemination after intraoperative urinary catheterization or bladder manipulation.

Levels of blood urea nitrogen or creatinine, serum glucose, and serum transaminases should be measured for women over age 40 and for those with personal or family histories of hepatic or renal disease. Assessments of renal and hepatic function are important when a patient may receive medications metabolized or excreted by these organs. Serum electrolytes should be evaluated for women taking diuretics. Finally, a sensitive test for pregnancy may be appropriate if pregnancy is suspected.

Routine chest X-rays for women under age 60 are not cost-efficient unless evidence suggesting cardiopulmonary disease is found at the physical examination. Baseline preoperative electrocardiography is a cost-efficient test for women over age 40 and for younger women with known cardiac disease. Electrocardiography may detect a recent asymptomatic myocardial infarction or potentially serious cardiac arrhythmia.

INFORMED CONSENT

Informed consent for an operation involves the education of the patient (or her family, if she is not competent to consent) about the proposed surgical procedure and the patient's granting of permission for the surgeon to perform the procedure. Informed consent is both an ethical and a legal responsibility and has more than 200 years of legal precedent. During the meeting in which informed consent is obtained, the surgeon must explain to the patient, in understandable terms, the nature and extent of the patient's disease; the nature and extent of the planned operation; the anticipated benefits and results of the surgery, including a conservative estimate of successful outcome; the risks and potential complications of the operation; and alternative methods of therapy. In addition, the surgeon should discuss with the patient what the operation will not accomplish. The possibility of discovery of unanticipated pathologic conditions during the operation should be raised before permission is obtained for the surgeon to perform a more extensive operation that may prove necessary.

ADMISSION AND PREOPERATIVE ORDERS

The surgeon's admission and preoperative orders communicate to the hospital staff the diagnosis, the planned operation, and the required preoperative preparation of the patient. In general, these orders should be subdivided into four broad categories: general measures, medications, laboratory tests, and preventive therapies. Many of these orders are self-explanatory. Patients should have nothing by mouth for 6–8 hours before the scheduled time of elective surgery to decrease the risk of vomiting and aspiration of gastric contents during the induction and reversal of anesthesia. Preventive therapies, such as the use of elastic stockings or pneumatic compression boots and the perioperative administration of heparin, may decrease the incidence of postoperative thromboembolic events in gynecologic patients. The use of enemas, with or without poorly absorbed oral antibiotics, to decrease bacterial colonization of the gastrointestinal tract may be useful when entry into the bowel is an anticipated risk or a planned part of the operation.

PROPHYLACTIC ANTIBIOTICS

The purpose of antibiotic prophylaxis is to prevent postoperative infection. Such prophylaxis should be used if risk factors for infection are documented for a given patient or if the nature of the operation itself poses a significant risk. Typically, patients who are undergoing a vaginal hysterectomy or a cesarean delivery in which labor has lasted for more than 6 hours after membrane rupture are candidates for antibiotic prophylaxis. Patients who are undergoing an abdominal hysterectomy should also receive antibiotic prophylaxis if they are obese, have a history of postoperative infection, or have cardiovascular disease, diabetes, collagen–vascular disease, or any chronic systemic disease.

Geriatric patients should receive antibiotic prophylaxis because their age places them at particularly high risk for postoperative infections. Before surgery, geriatric patients should be screened for bacteriuria; if the results are positive, treatment should be instituted. The antibiotic chosen should have a spectrum of activity that includes both gram-positive and gram-negative bacteria. Nitrofurantoin can be used empirically if the organism has been identified and if its antibiotic sensitivities are known. The antibiotic selected should be efficacious and inexpensive; its systemic and toxic effects should be minimal, so that the effect of its administration on the patient's endogenous bacterial flora will in turn be minimal. The urine should be cultured, and the bacteria found should be identified; nitrofurantoin (if selected) is not highly active against *Enterobacter* species, but it does exhibit good activity against other gram-negative facultative bacteria, as well as gram-positive cocci. Trimethoprim–sulfamethoxazole should not be used empirically for geriatric patients because of possible hematologic toxicity (eg, thrombocytopenia). A case of hepatic necrosis in an 80-year-old man has been reported.

Patients who receive prophylaxis for surgery should receive a single dose of antibiotic unless multiple doses are specifically indicated. Although data are not available on antibiotic prophylaxis for geriatric patients who are to undergo surgery, the data available from studies of patients of all ages can be extrapolated. Geriatric patients tend to have renal dysfunction (eg, decreased glomerular filtration and creatinine clearance); therefore, antibiotics that are excreted primarily by the kidneys have a longer half-life in this age group. A single dose administered when the patient is on call to the operating room or immediately preceding the operation should suffice, because the drug persists longer in the serum of geriatric patients than in that of younger patients. The antibiotic should have a spectrum of activity that includes gram-positive and gram-negative aerobes as well as anaerobes and that covers staphylococci (since geriatric patients are at risk for incision wound infection). The cephalosporins are better suited to these requirements than are the penicillins.

Combinations of antibiotics should be reserved for specific purposes, such as the prevention of endocarditis. Individuals—young and old—who have a significant murmur, a prosthesis, or a mitral valve prolapse should receive prophylaxis for endocarditis. Patients with mitral valve prolapse who are not taking specific medication and whose physical activity is not restricted should receive prophylaxis at the discretion of their cardiologist. The organisms most frequently involved in endocarditis in patients undergoing a genitourinary procedure are *Streptococcus* species, specifically *Streptococcus faecalis*. These bacteria do not respond to single-agent therapy; rather, the synergism of a penicillin (eg, ampicillin) plus an aminoglycoside is required for bactericidal activity. Patients who are allergic to ampicillin should receive vancomycin plus an aminoglycoside. If the surgical procedure is complicated or requires more than 1 hour or if there is significant blood loss (ie, 1,500 ml or more), three doses of each antibiotic should be administered every 6 hours for ampicillin and every 8 hours for aminoglycoside.

Patients who are truly allergic to penicillin and who do not require antibiotic prophylaxis for cardiac infection can be managed in either of two ways. One approach is to administer no antibiotic prophylaxis at all. If the patient subsequently develops an infection, it should be diagnosed promptly, and appropriate specimens obtained for culture (ie, samples from the suspected site, venous blood, and urine). Empirical antibiotic therapy should be administered, and the patient should be observed closely for signs of deterioration. An alternative is to administer a cephalosporin, since approximately 91–94% of patients with a history of penicillin allergy do not react to cephalosporins. The risk of cross-reactivity might be reduced by a drug such as cefoxitin, a cephamycin that is closely related in structure to the second-generation cephalosporins. A quinoline such as ciprofloxacin or ofloxacin may prove suitable for prophylaxis; although no data support the use of quinolines for this purpose, these agents have long half-lives and persist at adequate levels in serum for a prolonged period after the administration of a single dose. In addition, these antibiotics are active against gram-negative facultative anaerobes and fairly active against gram-positive aerobes.

Many studies have demonstrated the effectiveness of antibiotic prophylaxis for postoperative infections. Significant data with respect to geriatric patients are lacking, however. Single-dose antibiotic prophylaxis has been shown to be as efficacious as multiple doses, but, again, no relevant studies have been performed in the geriatric population. Despite the lack of specific data to guide antibiotic prophylaxis in geriatric patients, an antibiotic can be chosen on the basis of available data. First-generation cephalosporins have been shown to be effective against most pelvic pathogens, and their spectra of activity make them suitable prophylactic agents. Cefazolin and cephalothin are effective and inexpensive; they are active against gram-negative facultative anaerobes, some obligate anaerobes, and many gram-positive bacteria, including staphylococci. Cefazolin and cephalothin have been shown to be suitable for prophylaxis in patients undergoing gynecologic surgery. Cefazolin has a longer half-life than cephalothin and may be more suitable for this reason; that is, the longer half-life may result in higher serum concentrations for a prolonged period, which in turn may result in higher and more prolonged tissue concentrations. A 1-g dose of cefazolin, administered IV 30 minutes before the surgical procedure, should be sufficient.

Antibiotics such as moxalactam, cefoperazone, and cefotetan all have the *N*-methylthiotetrazole side chain. These antibiotics can cause hypoprothrombinemia and bleeding, as can cefamandole. This effect is thought to be due to the impairment of vitamin K synthesis. Until these antibiotics have been studied in the geriatric population, they should not be used for prophylaxis in this age group. If these agents must be used, it would be prudent to administer vitamin K concomitantly.

BIBLIOGRAPHY

Kaplan EB, Sheiner LB, Boeckmann AJ, Roizen MF, Beal SL, Cohen SN, et al. The usefulness of preoperative laboratory screening. JAMA 1985;253:3576–3581

Rucker L, Frey EB, Staten MA. Usefulness of screening chest roentgenograms in preoperative patients. JAMA 1983;250:3209–3211

Nonmalignant Disorders of the Vulva

Careful inspection of the vulva and the vagina continues to provide the best clue to the specific diagnosis of a problem involving these areas. The colposcope can be of some help in carefully examining the vulvar tissues; however, the use of a hand-held magnifying glass (magnification of two to four times) is more than adequate in most cases. Often, changes seen on the vulva are secondary to disease involving the vagina and cervix; thus, the vagina and cervix should also be examined carefully. Any discharge within the vagina should be studied for the presence of organisms that may be a cause of vaginitis resulting in secondary vulvar changes. The glabrous skin should also be examined because many dermatoses manifest themselves on the vulva (ie, psoriasis and lichen planus).

Office vulvar biopsy should be performed liberally, since adequate treatment is based on an accurate diagnosis. This simple office procedure is virtually free of complications and essentially painless when performed under local anesthesia. Small, discrete lesions are best handled by excisional biopsy. For biopsy of large or widespread skin lesions, the Keyes cutaneous punch biopsy instrument can be used. A 4-mm instrument is adequate in most instances. The area from which the biopsy specimen will be obtained is first infiltrated with lidocaine by using a small-gauge needle. The Keyes punch works like a cork borer. The sharp edges of the instrument are twisted into the anesthetized site in a circular manner. After it has cut through the epithelium and dermis, the circular portion of tissue is lifted with a small forceps and the base of the tissue is snipped off with a small scissors. The small size of the biopsy site obviates the need for sutures. Hemostasis is easily accomplished by the use of Monsel solution (ferric subsulfate) or cautery with the tip of a silver nitrate applicator.

Washing of the vulva with 4–5% acetic acid often highlights mucosal lesions such as intraepithelial neoplasia, which turn acetowhite after the application of the solution. This change is also often noted in the presence of HPV infection involving the vulvar tissues. Staining of the vulva with toluidine blue is sometimes of help in selecting a biopsy site. The vulva is covered with 1% toluidine blue. After the stain dries, the tissues are washed with 1% acetic acid, which removes the toluidine blue. Because nuclei retain toluidine blue, lesions such as invasive and intraepithelial carcinomas retain the blue color after they are washed with acetic acid.

BENIGN TUMORS

A wide spectrum of benign solid and cystic tumors involves the vulva. These tumors can easily be subclassified based on the tissue of origin, embryologic derivation, morphologic findings, or gross appearance. In most instances, if the tumor is not causing the patient discomfort and the diagnosis is quite apparent on the basis of gross inspection, it can be left alone.

Solid Tumors

The most common of the benign solid tumors affecting the vulva are the acrochordon (fibroepithelial polyp), fibroma, lipoma, neurofibroma, and solid tumors arising in the Bartholin and vestibular glands. When the diagnosis is in doubt or the tumor is causing discomfort, the tumor should be widely excised either in the office under local anesthesia or, if the lesion is of significant size, in the hospital while the patient is under general anesthesia. Wide local excision with primary closure of the defect is all that is required.

Cystic Tumors

The most common cystic tumors involving the vulva are the epidermal inclusion cyst and developmental cysts of urogenital sinus, paramesonephric duct, mesonephric duct, and ectopic mammary gland origin. As with benign solid tumors, most cystic tumors of the vulva can be left untreated if the diagnosis is apparent and they are not causing significant symptoms. If diagnosis is in doubt or the patient is uncomfortable, wide local excision is usually adequate therapy.

Hidradenoma

The hidradenoma is often a confusing tumor for clinicians as well as for pathologists. Of utmost importance is its differentiation from a primary or metastatic adenocarcinoma of the vulva—a mistake that is occasionally made. The distinction is made on the basis of the characteristic pattern of the tumor, as well as the absence of nuclear atypia and multilayering of cells. This tumor is easily removed in the office by local excision with local anesthesia.

Bartholin Duct Cyst and Abscess

Bartholin duct cysts and abscesses, seen in approximately 2% of new gynecologic patients, are probably the most significant benign cystic tumors with which clinicians deal. These cysts arise in the duct system of the Bartholin gland. Occlusion of the duct usually occurs near the opening of the main duct into the vestibule. Most cysts involve only the main duct and thus are unilocular, although occasionally one or more loculi lie deep in the main cyst. Most patients with small Bartholin duct cysts have no symptoms, although mild discomfort with sexual intercourse may be experienced. If the cyst becomes enlarged, discomfort and pressure may be experienced by the patient, as may discomfort during coitus and walking. Treatment, if necessary, is best managed by marsupialization. The line of incision for marsupialization should be made medially enough so that the new orifice is located close to the original opening of the Bartholin duct into the vestibule. The incision should be 4–6 cm in length, extending through the wall of the cyst. After evacuation of the contents of the cyst, the lining is sewn to the mucosal and skin surfaces with interrupted fine, absorbable sutures.

An acute Bartholin abscess may arise primarily or may occur in the presence of a previous Bartholin duct cyst. Most abscesses, especially if they are recurrent, develop as a consequence of a nongonococcal infection of the fluid contents of a Bartholin cyst. Cultures of Bartholin abscesses reveal a wide spectrum of organisms. The chief symptoms of a Bartholin abscess are varying degrees of pain and tenderness over the affected gland. The rapidity of development and the extent of involvement depend on the size of the infected cyst and the virulence of the infectious agent. Objective signs include unilateral swelling over the site of the affected gland, redness of the overlying skin, and frequently, edema of the labia. The abscess is a palpable and extremely tender, fluctuant mass.

An acute Bartholin abscess usually requires surgical treatment, but local application of heat in the form of hot, wet dressings or sitz baths may promote spontaneous drainage within 72 hours. Occasionally, early treatment of an obvious bartholinitis with broad-spectrum antibiotics prevents the formation of an abscess; however, this treatment could easily delay ripening of the abscess. Incision and drainage are accomplished in the physician's office. Marsupialization of the abscess by use of the Word catheter, an inflatable, bulb-tipped, closed catheter, is effective treatment. After spraying the area to be incised with ethyl chloride, the catheter is inserted into the abscess cavity after a small stab incision is made into the abscess close to the hymenal ring, and the contents of the abscess are evacuated. After insertion of the catheter, the balloon is inflated with 2 ml of saline. The small distal end of the catheter is then tucked into the vagina. It should be left in place for 4–6 weeks, after which time the balloon is deflated and the catheter is removed. The patient rarely notes the presence of the catheter and may engage in sexual activity without disturbing it.

PROLAPSE OF URETHRAL MUCOSA

Prolapse of urethral mucosa is seen in prepubertal children and postmenopausal women. It represents a sliding outward of the mucosa to the external meatus. The lesion resembles an edematous, red ring of tissue at the urinary meatus. The urethral orifice can be located in the center of the prolapsed mass of tissue. A trial of topical estrogen cream is sometimes effective in producing reduction of the prolapsed mucosa. In most instances, however, prolapse of the urethral mucosa is best treated by excision of the redundant mucosa. An incision is made around the prolapsed mucosa, and the edges of the urethral mucosa are then attached to the mucosa of the vestibule with interrupted no. 4-0 absorbable sutures. Cryocautery can be used in postmenopausal women to freeze the entire mass of prolapsed mucosa by creating an ice ball that covers the entire circumference. Refreezing is usually necessary 6–8 weeks after the initial treatment. Cryocautery can be performed on an outpatient basis without anesthesia.

VULVAR VESTIBULITIS SYNDROME

Vulvar vestibulitis syndrome is being seen and recognized with increasing frequency. The primary complaint is that of entrance dyspareunia. Patients also complain of constant vulvar burning and irritation. Examination reveals hyperemia and punctate, red areas around the openings of the paravestibular glands into the vestibule. Palpation of the vestibule with a moist, cotton-tipped applicator will elicit marked pain. Washing the vestibule with 4–5% acetic acid will often result in a diffuse acetowhite change with irregular margins. This is often seen when the vestibulitis is associated with HPV infection. There is a subset of patients with this problem related to genital HPV infection. In this group of individuals, the use of intralesional interferon is effective in relieving symptoms in approximately 50% of cases. One million units of recombinant Interferon-α diluted to 0.5 ml is injected into the vestibule just outside the hymenal ring. Usually, 1 million units is injected Monday, Wednesday, and Friday in a different site in the vestibule so that ultimately the entire vestibule has received injections in an around-the-clock fashion.

Usually, conservative measures such as warm sitz baths, topical steroids, and lubrication during coitus are of no value in relieving the symptoms of vulvar vestibulitis. Thus, if the patient is not a candidate for the use of intralesional interferon and conservative measures have not helped, consideration can be given to performing a perineoplasty. The mucosa of the vestibule is excised from the region of the opening of the Skene ducts down along the Hart line to the perineal skin midway between the vestibule and the anus. The vaginal mucosa is undermined, and the tissue is excised just inside the hymenal ring so that the entire hymenal ring is removed. The vaginal mucosa is further undermined, and the defect is then closed in two layers, using a deeper layer of interrupted no. 00 absorbable suture to take the tension off the mucosal skin closure and to help provide hemostasis. An outer layer of interrupted no. 00 absorbable suture is used to coapt the mucosal edges to the skin edges. Symptomatic relief is achieved in approximately 70–80% of properly selected individuals.

VULVAR DYSTROPHIES

At the 1987 meeting of the International Society for the Study of Vulvar Disease, a new classification of vulvar dystrophies was proposed. Unlike the previous classification, which was based purely on the histologic features of the lesions being studied, the following classification is based on a combination of gross and histopathologic changes:

- Squamous cell hyperplasia (formerly hyperplastic dystrophy)

- Lichen sclerosus et atrophicus
- Other dermatoses

Squamous cell hyperplasia includes lesions with no specific cause. In most instances, it probably represents lichen simplex chronicus. Specific lesions such as dermatoses (eg, psoriasis, lichen planus) should be diagnosed specifically. Lichen sclerosus et atrophicus with associated squamous cell hyperplasia was formerly classified as a mixed dystrophy. When these two disorders are associated, the current recommendation is to report both lichen sclerosus et atrophicus and squamous cell hyperplasia. Mixed epithelial disorders may also be associated with cellular atypia (lesions demonstrating cellular atypia are now classified under VIN). When this occurs, each diagnosis should be reported (ie, VIN types I, II, and III and lichen sclerosus et atrophicus). Since a distinction between epidermal thickening and thinning and the presence of atypia is not always possible by gross inspection alone, classification of a lesion also depends on its microscopic characteristics. Since the histologic appearance may vary in different sites on the vulva, lesions can be classified accurately only if multiple biopsy specimens are taken from several locations.

Treatment of the nonneoplastic epithelial disorders is primarily medical in nature. Squamous cell hyperplasia is best treated by the local application of corticosteroids. First, however, predisposing factors, such as vaginitis, topical irritants, and allergies, should be excluded or adequately treated. If fluorinated steroids are used as primary therapy, they should be discontinued once the pruritus is brought under control and replaced with a medication containing hydrocortisone.

Lichen sclerosus et atrophicus is most effectively treated topically with testosterone (2%) mixed in petrolatum. Initially, this medication is applied two or three times daily for at least 2–3 months or until the pruritus is relieved. Thereafter, the frequency of application is gradually reduced over 6 months to 1 year until a maintenance level of application once or twice weekly is reached. If testosterone ointment is not effective or results in disturbing side effects, progesterone (1%) in petrolatum may be effective.

Several recent studies have suggested that a new potent corticosteroid—clobetasol propionate, 0.05%—has been effective in alleviating the symptoms and occasionally resulting in regression of the skin changes in lichen sclerosus et atrophicus. The clobetasol is applied to the vulva twice daily for a period of 2 months, followed by once daily for 1–2 months and then used at a maintenance level of once or twice weekly thereafter. The use of clobetasol does not appear to result in some of the adverse changes observed after long-term use of the fluorinated corticosteroids.

Occasionally, patients complain of persistent pruritus that is unresponsive to medical management. The subcutaneous injection of alcohol may alleviate the pruritus. Once the patient stops scratching, an improvement is frequently noted in the appearance of the lesion. When the effect of the alcohol wears off, approximately 6 months later, the pruritus can be more adequately managed medically. Alcohol injection should be done with the patient in the hospital under general anesthesia. The vulva is marked in a gridlike fashion so that the lines cross at intervals of 1 cm. Absolute alcohol, 0.1–0.2 ml, is injected immediately beneath the dermis at each place where the lines cross. Following the alcohol injection, the tissues should be massaged thoroughly to obtain adequate dispersement of the alcohol. After treatment, the patient may complain of intense vulvar burning for several days, followed by a feeling of numbness of the vulvar tissues. The dramatic relief from pruritus is usually much appreciated by the patient. Some physicians continue to advocate the use of the Mehring undercutting operation to relieve persistent pruritus, but it is a somewhat radical procedure that is rarely indicated.

Erosive lichen planus is a dermatosis that not uncommonly involves the vulva and the vagina. In the past, it has been referred to as desquamative vaginitis. Patients usually complain of intense vulvar burning, dyspareunia, and a persistent vaginal discharge. Examination of the vulva will frequently reveal a hyperemic, eroded appearance to the vestibule and inner labia minora. Frequently, the vagina will be involved, demonstrating the appearance of focal areas of pronounced hyperemia usually involving the upper vagina. Biopsy usually reveals thinning or complete lack of a surface epithelium and an intense inflammatory infiltrate composed primarily of lymphocytes and plasma cells approaching the surface of the epithelium in a bandlike fashion. Approximately 60% of patients will also have or will develop similar changes in the oral cavity. In the presence of long-standing erosive lichen planus, stenosis and even obliteration of the entire vagina may occur. Management of this problem is extremely difficult. The use of 25-mg hydrocortisone suppositories inserted into the vagina will often result in relief of symptoms and regression of the physical findings. One half of a suppository is inserted twice daily for at least 2–3 months. If there is symptomatic improvement, the frequency of use of the suppositories can be gradually decreased until the patient is maintained on one-half suppository inserted into the vagina two or three times per week.

BIBLIOGRAPHY

Dalziel KL, Millard PR, Wojnarowska F. The treatment of vulval lichen sclerosus with a very potent topical steroid (clobetasol propionate 0.05%) cream. Br J Dermatol 1991;124:461–464

Kaufman RH, Friedrich EG Jr, Gardner HL, Faro S. Benign diseases of the vulva and vagina. 4th ed. St Louis: Mosby–Year Book, 1994

Liebowitch M, Neill S, Pelisse M, Moyal-Baracco M. The epithelial changes associated with squamous cell carcinoma of the vulva: a review of the clinical, histological, and viral findings of 78 women. Br J Obstet Gynaecol 1990;97:1135–1139

Mann MS, Kaufman RH. Erosive lichen planus of the vulva. Clin Obstet Gynecol 1991;34:605–613

Mann MS, Kaufman RH, Brown D, Adam E. Vulvar vestibulitis: significant variables and treatment outcome. Obstet Gynecol 1992;79:122–125

Anatomic Support Defects and Dysfunction

There are more than 6 million women over age 75 in the United States. With the expanding number of older women to whom restoration of the quality of life is increasingly important, factors related to prolapse of the pelvic organs are becoming a larger and more timely part of the total care of the patient. Practitioners may need to expand their surgical expertise to respond to the increased need for skillful surgical reconstruction.

A major cause of gynecologic complaints, particularly in older women, relates to the various types of genital prolapse. The causes of genital prolapse fall into three main groups:

1. Congenital—A careful interview often elicits a family history of a genital prolapse. This may be the consequence of a defect in the intrinsic connective tissue of the pelvis or of the innervation of pelvic musculature.
2. Acquired—Damage may arise from trauma, often obstetric; from a life style that may include a history of heavy lifting or heavy smoking or other types of chronic respiratory embarrassment; or rarely, from traumatic disruption of anatomic integrity, as from a crushing injury of the pelvis.
3. Aging—Damage to pelvic support may occur as a consequence of growing older (ie, the loss of hormone support coincident with menopause), as well as the ultimate exhaustion of the mechanism of cellular and tissue replication.

The goals of care, whether nonoperative or operative, are the same:

- Relief of symptoms
- Restoration of anatomy
- Preservation or restoration of normal function

CLASSIFICATION

Uterine Prolapse

The uterus may prolapse, but after hysterectomy the cervical stump or vagina also may prolapse. The extent of the prolapse is usually graded from 0 to 4, with 0 being normal and 4 implying complete procidentia, or prolapse through the introitus.

Cystocele

A cystocele is a type of bladder hernia that usually results from overstretching of the vagina and its supports and from damage to the deep transverse perineal musculature and the pubococcygeus portion of the levator sling, a so-called distention cystocele. Regardless of the size of the cystocele, such a hernia may or may not be associated with urinary stress incontinence. In such cases, the size of the posterior urethrovesical angle is often of importance. Herniation of the bladder posterior to the urethra results in a cystocele that is sometimes graded in severity from 1 to 3, with 3 indicating passage of the cystocele through the introitus with straining. Detachment or stretching of the vaginal sulci from their connective tissue attachment to the arcus tendineus may give rise to the lateral or paravaginal defect. Cystocele may thus result from either a midline damage to the urogenital diaphragm or a lateral damage to the paravaginal supporting tissues, or sometimes both. Cystocele may also result from displacement of the bladder coincident with prolapse of the vaginal vault, the latter bringing the bladder with it, a so-called displacement cystocele.

Enterocele

Enterocele occurs when the cul-de-sac is filled with bowel and extends between the vagina anteriorly and the rectum posteriorly through an area of weakness created by separation of the anterior musculofascial tissue in the rectovaginal septum. A sac that is empty is merely a deep cul-de-sac; when it contains bowel (usually small bowel), it is an enterocele. Simple descent of the normal cul-de-sac is not a true enterocele. There are four common causes of enterocele, each of which can be correlated with its location, which in turn correlates with the most effective treatment for each type (Table 4-1). On occasion, an enterocele may not be discovered until the posterior vaginal wall and rectum have been dissected during the course of rectocele repair.

Rectocele

Rectocele represents a rectal hernia bulging into the posterior vagina through a defect in the rectovaginal septum, usually resulting from childbirth. Rectocele represents an increase in the size of the rectal reservoir, primarily related to a deficiency in vaginal support but with secondary damage to the submucosal layer of the rectum. This defect is also graded according to its progression distally along the vaginal axis.

Perineal Defect

A perineal defect is an anatomic disturbance in the integrity and strength of the perineal body and its attachment, and is usually the consequence of obstetric damage from overstretching. It frequently, but not invariably, coexists with a rectocele.

TABLE 4-1. ENTEROCELE: DETERMINING THE RIGHT SURGICAL APPROACH

Cause	Location	Treatment
Congenital	Sac between posterior vaginal wall and anterior rectal wall	Excise the sac, with high ligation of its neck and approximation of uterosacral ligaments.
Pulsion (pushing)	Same as congenital, but with eversion of vaginal wall	Restore vault depth by shortening cardinal–uterosacral ligaments or by culdeplasty if ligaments are strong. Often, coincident hysterectomy is desirable. If ligaments are of poor quality, do sacrospinous fixation or sacrocolpopexy.
Traction (pulling)	Same as congenital, with lower eversion (cystocele and rectocele) pulling vault into eversion	Use same procedure as above, plus anterior and posterior colporrhaphy.
Iatrogenic	Anterior to vagina or (when resulting from change in vaginal axis) posterior to vagina	Excise or obliterate sac and restore normal vaginal axis if it is defective.

Nichols DH. Types of enterocele and principles underlying the choice of operation for repair. Reprinted with permission from the American College of Obstetricians and Gynecologists (Obstetrics and Gynecology, 1972, 40, 257–263)

PHYSICAL EXAMINATION

The physician should perform a careful overall assessment of the patient's general physical health, including measurement of blood pressure, weight, and height in stocking feet (noting at each annual examination any possible changes suggestive of vertebral compression); auscultation of the chest and heart; and palpation of the breast. One should note the patient's posture and the presence and width of abdominal wall striae. The latter is indicative of the patient's elastic index.

The physician should ask about the presence of backache and whether it is worse on arising and gets better during the day (suggesting an orthopedic origin) or is absent on arising, gets worse as the day goes on, and is relieved by lying down (suggesting a backache from the traction of a genital prolapse).

A large number of wide abdominal striae indicate the likelihood of a defect in the integrity of the patient's elastic tissue. The wider the striae, the lesser the elasticity of the patient's connective tissue and the greater the subsequent chances of genital prolapse.

The genitalia should be inspected, and any degree of vulvar atrophy should be noted. Any genital prolapse should be noted. Bonney described two general systems that maintain pelvic integrity—the upper suspensory system and the lower supportive system. After the prolapsed organs have been gently replaced, the patient is asked to bear down, as by the Valsalva maneuver. The site of primary damage appears first at the vulva, followed by the sites of secondary damage. When damage to the upper suspensory system is primary, the cervix or vaginal vault appears first, followed by any cystocele and rectocele. In the absence of a strong cardinal–uterosacral ligament complex, the patient with prolapse of the vaginal vault will require some form of colpopexy to suspend the vaginal vault, in addition to colporrhaphy.

With primary damage to the lower supportive system, a cystocele and rectocele appear first, followed by the cervix or vaginal vault. Such a patient as this, if a candidate for surgery, requires an extensive colporrhaphy. Culdeplasty, or shortening and fixation of the vagina to the strong uterosacral–cardinal ligament complex, will support the vault of the vagina. For those patients for whom surgery is recommended, the gynecologist should note and remember the site of primary damage, as it will aid in planning this particular patient's operation, remembering the Bonney rule: the primary site of damage should be overrepaired to lessen the chance of recurrence.

Beyond this generic classification of upper and lower factors concerned with pelvic support, seven separate anatomic systems that may be damaged either singly or in any combination can be defined. An effort should be made to determine the specific site of primary damage, as well as the nature and extent of any secondary damage. These systems are:

- The bony pelvis, to which all the soft tissues ultimately are attached
- The broad ligament, round ligament, and subperitoneal retinaculum of connective tissue
- The uterosacral and cardinal ligament complex and its attachments to the pelvic side walls and between the vaginal sulci and the arcus tendinei
- The urogenital diaphragm, including its pubourethral components
- The fascia of Denonvilliers, which is fused to the underside of the posterior vaginal wall and extends from the perineal body to the cul-de-sac of Douglas; the anterior margin of the rectovaginal space
- The pelvic diaphragm, which is made up primarily of the three parts of the levator ani and their aponeuroses and their fascial coverings
- The perineal body and the external anal sphincter

The patient is examined initially when she is in the lithotomy position, and a careful bimanual examination is performed. The general architecture of the patient's bony pelvis should be noted. The patient should be asked to voluntarily contract her pubococcygeus, thus squeezing the vagina, and the strength and symmetry of contraction should be noted. A rectal examination should be performed, noting any abnormalities, the presence of any blood on the examination finger, the strength and effectiveness of the external anal sphincter, and the presence of a rectocele or a perineal defect.

The patient should then be asked to stand, and the vaginal examination should be repeated with the patient first at rest, then while "holding," and finally, while straining, noting the presence of any vault eversion and reassessment of the posterior and anterior vaginal walls and their supports, both midline and lateral. One should observe how much the cystocele sags beneath the inferior margin of the pubis. If the patient complains of coincident urinary or rectal incontinence, this should also be evaluated carefully.

TREATMENT

Treatment may be nonsurgical or surgical; for maximal effectiveness, treatment requires precision in the diagnosis of damage, the probable etiology, and—when surgery is required—the optimal procedure with which the surgeon is comfortable. The gynecologist should have a spectrum of operations from which to choose, so that he or she may "make the operation fit the patient, not the patient fit the operation."

Although there are few things that can be done to reverse the progress of genital prolapse once it has developed, there may be steps that can be taken to slow its progress and lessen the chance of recurrence. The first of these relates to reducing pathologically increased intraabdominal pressure by adjusting the patient's weight when appropriate, and developing an alternative life style that will reduce heavy lifting. The reduction of respiratory embarrassment, such as that from smoking, asthma, and chronic bronchitis, is often effective.

Improvement in the patient's posture will be helpful, as well as learning to bend from the knees rather than from the waist. Avoidance of tight corsets and girdles will further reduce a pathologically increased intraabdominal pressure. At times estrogen replacement is recommended, and the patient may be instructed on the initiation of a long-term course of Kegel perineal resistive exercises.

Recognition and treatment of constipation is appropriate to reduce the need for frequent and excessive bearing down to achieve a bowel movement. Much of this can be relieved effectively by adding bulk to the diet, including a daily serving of some form of bran, and allowing the gastrocolic reflex to work at the same time every day. An adequate daily fluid intake is important, as an unnoticed reduction in thirst is part of the aging process.

When symptoms of pelvic fullness, pressure, and bearing down are present but are not severe enough to warrant consideration for surgery, or when for various medical or social reasons surgery is not possible, effective help can be given by these nonoperative means. Improved tissue elasticity, restoration of vaginal thickness, and improved blood supply follow long-term estrogen supplementation not only when it is given by the systemic route but also from the sustained regular use of intravaginal estrogen cream, which effectively supplies a measured dose to the target tissue. For patients with a severely atrophic birth canal, one might recommend instillation of 2 g of estrogen cream at bedtime, three times weekly for 2–4 weeks, with gradual tapering of the dosage to a maintenance level of one application at bedtime once weekly. This may lessen the speed of prolapse progression and may relieve the symptoms of urinary urgency and precipitancy in many patients.

The effective treatment of coincident medical problems improves the patient's overall and gynecologic health. The control and treatment of cardiovascular disease are helpful, and adequate attention should be given to any symptom of chronic constipation. Chronic respiratory disease, errors in carbohydrate metabolism, arthritis, and obesity are especially responsive to careful attention and follow-up.

A sustained program of voluntary exercise of the muscles of the pelvic diaphragm and pelvic sphincter system by effective isometric contractions of these pelvic muscles is helpful in strengthening tissue relationships and improving function, particularly in helping to control any urinary stress incontinence. Improvement should be seen, especially in a patient in whom, with straining, the cystocele drops to less than 4 cm beneath the lower border of the pubic symphysis, as measured when the patient strains while she is standing. An effective program of voluntary exercise of these pelvic muscles consists of 15 strong voluntary contractions in a row, each of which is of 3-second duration, six times per day (ie, on arising and at midmorning, lunchtime, midafternoon, suppertime, and bedtime). The patient should be told that these contractions can be done anywhere, even in public places, and that it makes no difference whether she is standing, sitting, or lying down. Because the muscles are deep inside the pelvic cavity, their exercise is not visible externally. For sedentary people, a general improvement in muscle tone will follow a program of brisk daily exercise, such as walking. Impact aerobics, however, should be avoided.

For those patients who require mechanical support of the prolapse, the use of a well-fitting intravaginal pessary may be helpful. Choices include a plastic ring, a plastic Gellhorn pessary, a rubber donut, or an inflatable pessary, each in an effective size. Some strength of the pelvic diaphragm, assessed at the site of the levator sling or hiatus where the levator ani crosses the sides of the vagina, is necessary for patients to be able to retain a pessary comfortably. Properly fitted, the pessary should not cause symptoms. If the patient cannot remove it nightly for cleaning, this must be done at first monthly and then quarterly by someone else, who should note and treat any effect of pessary pressure on the vagina. Since a pessary stretches the vagina in various directions and dimensions, the required size may become larger as time goes by, so that the fit must be evaluated from time to time by the examiner, and the size or style should be changed as necessary.

Operative Approach

With increased operator skill and greater safety in anesthesia during hospitalization, an operative approach to the solution of a mechanical problem is often optimal. The comfort of surgical reconstruction can be extended to increased numbers of women, with the decision based not on their age but on their general medical health and life expectancy. To be most effective, the choice of operation should be individualized to the patient. The choice may range from a perineorrhaphy to enable the patient to retain a pessary (which can be accomplished under local anesthesia if necessary), to a hysterectomy with colporrhaphy and colpopexy for patients with a prolapse who wish to retain their vaginal function. Colpocleisis or colpectomy (with hysterectomy) may be considered for patients for whom vaginal function is not a consideration.

Vaginal hysterectomy with shortening of the cardinal–uterosacral complex and with colporrhaphy is the surgical treatment that responds effectively to the goals of reconstructive surgery in most patients. When uterosacral ligaments are long and strong, the addition of a McCall or New Orleans type of culdeplasty helps to reestablish vaginal length. Careful attention must be given to the presence and correction of any enterocele, lest a posthysterectomy vaginal eversion be initiated, which would compromise a number of these patients in their postoperative years. When at the time of surgery there is insufficient cardinal–uterosacral ligament strength to which the vaginal wall can be attached with the confidence that it will remain there, the vault may be anchored to a strong nongynecologic pelvic support, such as the sacrospinous ligament or sacrum. Transvaginal sacrospinous colpopexy as part of the primary procedure in such a patient is a useful addition.

When the cervix is elongated and strong cardinal–uterosacral ligament support is evident, the Manchester operation, consisting of cervical amputation with mobilization and attachment of the cardinal ligaments anterior to the cervix, followed by appropriate colporrhaphy, supports the vagina. One must be mindful that a dropped uterus is the result and not the cause of a genital prolapse. Because uterine bleeding is sometimes subsequent to estrogen supplementation, this approach is not as popular as vaginal hysterectomy. LeFort colpocleisis is an effective, quick, and relatively simple method of vaginal obturation, but it has several notable disadvantages:

- The operation removes the coital potential, disturbing the patient's concept of her femininity.
- The operation retains the uterus, which may bleed in the future, and the diagnosis of the cause of such bleeding is difficult because of the partial vaginal obliteration.
- By fixing the base of the bladder and vesicourethral junction to the anterior rectal wall, the surgeon may create a flattening of the posterior urethrovesical angle, permitting urinary stress incontinence, which, when socially disabling, is the most difficult to treat.
- Because the LeFort operation is extraperitoneal, any enterocele remains untreated and often progresses, with relevant discomfort to both the patient and her surgeon.

For patients who have experienced previous hysterectomy, a colpectomy removes the prolapsed vagina, and although any problems with future uterine bleeding cannot occur, the other objections to colpocleisis noted above still remain. For posthysterectomy patients with vault eversion, an ideal treatment to achieve the goals of reconstructive surgery consists of effective colpopexy with appropriate colporrhaphy.

For the experienced vaginal surgeon, restorative surgery can be accomplished through a single vaginal exposure (ie, sacrospinous colpopexy with excision of any enterocele and with colporrhaphy). If the operator is more comfortable with a transabdominal method of support of the vagina or if a patient has an adnexal mass or any other indication for abdominal exploration, colporrhaphy may be followed by transabdominal sacral colpopexy. This procedure tends to restore the horizontal vaginal axis, in contrast to ventral suspension or fixation, which not only creates a permanently abnormal vaginal axis but also exposes the patient's cul-de-sac to the risk of postoperative enterocele with subsequent prolapse of the vault.

New suture materials include permanent synthetic sutures. When transabdominal sacral colpopexy is used, the distance between the vault of the vagina and the promontory of the sacrum may be bridged by permanent supportive straps of synthetic mesh, or fascia lata.

For the experienced abdominal operator, transabdominal sacrocolpopexy is indicated with appropriate transvaginal colporrhaphy. This, however, requires deeper and longer anesthesia.

Recurrent Genital Prolapse

Recurrent genital prolapse is a gynecologic tragedy, and the patient deserves special empathy and understanding. Above all, she deserves a very sophisticated reevaluation by the best and most experienced operator available, mindful that each trip to surgery tends to prejudice unfavorably the effectiveness of any subsequent operation. A special effort should be expended to identify clearly the primary weaknesses that give rise to the prolapse; reevaluation of the whole patient, including her life style and daily habits, should be accomplished. Positive ideas and findings should be noted carefully and a plan for reoperation carefully developed, making certain to allow for an appropriate time and environment for adequate postoperative convalescence. Postoperatively, adjuvant perineal resistive exercises, along with estrogen supplementation when indicated, are helpful in restoring the integrity of the pelvis.

Perineal Prolapse (Descending Perineal Syndrome)

A significant defect in the integrity or effectiveness of the pelvic diaphragm, particularly when it sags, may have a pronounced negative effect when the anus becomes the most dependent portion of the patient's intergluteal area. Although it is initially asymptomatic, progressive excessive funneling of the levator may significantly decrease the diameter of the stool and increase the difficulties of evacuation, occasionally leading to obstipation and impaction and requiring daily digital manipulation to empty the bowel. When this is left untreated, it is often associated with progressive denervation of the levator ani and external anal sphincter, first through a pudendal neuropathy and later manifested by atrophy of the neuromuscular receptors within the body of the levator ani, which may be followed by rectal incontinence.

Evacuation through a 7.6-cm hole in a board placed across a toilet seat may create effective counterpressure around the anus when this condition first becomes symptomatic, but this method is inconvenient when the patient is away from home, and laxative abuse as an alternative treatment to the point of discomfort or diarrhea may be encountered. Straining during bowel movements is to be avoided, lest it further stretch an already attenuated pelvic diaphragm and the pudendal nerves that supply it. A long-term course of isometric perineal muscle exercises is often helpful as an adjuct to treatment. A surgical treatment for this condition embraces a retrorectal levatorplasty in which an incision is made between the anus and the coccyx. The damaged levator plate is bisected, and dissection proceeds directly into the retrorectal space. The posterior surface of the rectum is attached by successive plication stitches to the periosteum of the sacrum in the hollow of the pelvis. The levator plate is reconstituted and elongated by bringing the pubococcygei together behind the rectum by a series of interrupted stitches. Any pathologic elongation of the levator ani may be shortened by appropriate Z-shaped stitches. Any coincident colporrhaphy or colpopexy as may be indicated is performed.

Lacerations of the Perineum

Lacerations of the perineum are graded 1 to 4, as follows:

1. Laceration of the hymenal ring
2. Tears extending into the perineal body but not the anal sphincter
3. Tears extending through the external sphincter but not the rectal wall
4. Tears extending through the rectal wall and exposing the mucosa

Fresh lacerations should be repaired immediately, but once infected, repair should be postponed until edema and inflammation have subsided. Each damaged layer should be recognized and repaired individually.

BIBLIOGRAPHY

Aronson MP, Lee RA, Berquist TH. Anatomy of anal sphincters and related structures in continent women: studies with magnetic resonance imaging. Obstet Gynecol 1990;76:846–851

Baden WF, Walker T. Surgical repair of vaginal defects. Philadelphia: JB Lippincott, 1992

DeLancey JO. Anatomic aspects of vaginal eversion after hysterectomy. Am J Obstet Gynecol 1992;166:1717–1724; discussion 1724–1728

Henry MM, Swash M, eds. Coloproctology of the pelvic floor. 2nd ed. Oxford: Butterworth Heinemann, 1992

Kaser O, Ikle FA, Hirsh HA, Friedman EA. Atlas of gynecological surgery. 2nd ed. New York: Thieme-Stratton, 1985

Nichols DH, ed. Gynecologic and obstetric surgery. St Louis: Mosby–Year Book, 1993

Thompson JD, Rock JA. TeLinde's operative gynecology. 7th ed. Philadelphia: JB Lippincott, 1992

Urogynecology

The field of urogynecology encompasses the evaluation and treatment of conditions that adversely affect the lower urinary tract in women and produce an array of symptoms depending on the underlying disorder. Most commonly, these urologic symptoms may be classified as due to urinary incontinence, irritative bladder complaints, urinary retention, or a combination of these problems. Over the years, there has been progressive recognition of the immense psychosocial and financial impact created by these lower urinary tract disorders on affected women and their families. Women may experience embarrassment, depression, loss of self-esteem, loss of productivity, and, at times, social isolation due to the manifestations of their disease.

URINARY INCONTINENCE

Urinary incontinence, as defined by the International Continence Society, is the "involuntary loss of urine which is objectively demonstrable and a social or hygienic problem." This definition implies that the leakage of urine must be clinically significant to the patient but not necessarily to the physician. Although studies vary, urinary incontinence has been reported to affect up to 26% of women of reproductive age and 30–42% of women in the postmenopausal years. Severe incontinence, defined as daily or weekly episodes, occurs in 4–6% of individuals.

A wide array of disorders can produce urinary incontinence, often with a myriad of overlapping and confusing symptoms. A thorough office evaluation can clarify the diagnosis in most patients and identify the remainder of women who require more sophisticated urodynamic or radiographic testing.

Diagnosis

Urinary incontinence most commonly occurs when the expulsive forces of the bladder exceed the retentive forces. Thus, active or passive increases in the expulsive forces of the bladder, decreases in the retentive forces, or anatomic conditions that bypass the normal continence mechanisms can lead to urinary leakage. The most commonly encountered disorder of expulsive forces is idiopathic detrusor instability due to uninhibited detrusor contractions, which primarily produce the symptom of urge incontinence. Underlying neurologic diseases may result in detrusor hyperreflexia. Decreased bladder wall compliance due to fibrosis from radiation or interstitial cystitis, or extrinsic pelvic disease may lead to a hypertonic bladder and urinary incontinence. Bladder atony due to neurologic disease, or bladder outlet obstruction (less common in women than men) result in urinary retention and may produce overflow urinary incontinence with elevated urinary postvoid residuals.

A decrease in retentive forces of the bladder is manifested by a decrease in urethral resistance to the flow of urine. The primary symptom associated with a decrease in retentive forces of the bladder is stress incontinence. Office and laboratory investigations are necessary to confirm the presence of stress incontinence and to establish the diagnosis of genuine stress incontinence. Genuine stress incontinence is defined by the International Continence Society as "the socially unacceptable involuntary loss of urine that occurs when intravesical pressure exceeds maximum urethral pressure in the absence of detrusor activity."

One of the most important causes of genuine stress incontinence is the anatomic relaxation of the supporting tissues of the urethra, bladder, and urethrovesical junction such that the proximal urethra is displaced outside the intraabdominal cavity. This displacement may occur due to the effects of pregnancy and delivery, or due to advancing age with its incumbent tissue changes. In this situation any increases in intraabdominal pressure with a stressful activity that normally should be transmitted equally to the urethra and bladder is transmitted appropriately only to the bladder but suboptimally to the urethra. Thus, intravesical pressure exceeds intraurethral pressure with resultant leakage of urine.

Childbirth has also been reported to produce partial denervation of the nerves supplying the urethra due to stretching of the distal portion of the pudendal nerve during the pushing stage of labor for vaginal delivery. Hypoestrogenic changes of the genitourinary system following menopause may contribute to stress incontinence by a number of mechanisms, including a decrease in the periurethral vascularity and urethral mucosal atrophy, which contributes to a loss of coaptive forces of the urethra and to relaxation of the estrogen-dependent urethral and periurethral muscular component and connective tissue.

An uncommon cause for urinary incontinence is an anatomic bypass of the normal continence mechanisms due to the presence of a urinary fistula (ureterovaginal, vesicovaginal, or urethrovaginal), an ectopic ureter, or a urinary diverticulum. Fistulae or ectopic ureters traditionally cause continuous urinary leakage or constant wetness, which is relatively easily diagnosed. Urethral diverticulum may produce postmicturition dribbling as the urine that is trapped within the diverticular sac subsequently empties on standing. A diverticulum may also be diagnosed by the discovery of a painful suburethral mass or the development of recurrent urinary tract infections from chronic infections of the diverticulum.

History

A detailed medical, gynecologic, and urologic history must be obtained in all women with lower urinary tract symptoms. A history of diabetes mellitus, thyroid disease, multiple sclerosis, cerebrovascular accidents, back pain, or back injuries suggests that the patient's symptoms may be due to an underlying neurologic abnormality. The patient's parity, mode of deliveries, and previous gynecologic procedures must be ascertained to determine their possible effects on lower urinary tract function. Commonly prescribed drugs such as alpha-methyldopa, prazosin, phenothiazines, or diazepam may precipitate stress incontinence by decreasing urethral smooth or skeletal muscle tone. Urinary retention may be a side effect of antihistamine or anticholinergic therapy. Alterations in the dosage or type of drug administered may be all that is required to alleviate the patient's symptoms.

Determination of the onset and duration of urinary symptoms is important in clarifying a patient's diagnosis. The abrupt onset of stress or urge incontinence may indicate an allergic or infectious process, whereas the gradual onset of symptoms, especially after oophorectomy or menopause, may imply estrogen deficiency.

Involuntary loss of urine prompted by coughing, laughing, sneezing, vigorous physical activity, or a change in position is consistent with the diagnosis of stress incontinence but may also be seen on occasion in patients with detrusor instability. Stress incontinence is determined to be severe historically if the patient experiences urinary leakage in the supine position, with a relatively empty bladder, or requires continuous perineal pad protection. Except in severe cases, most women with genuine stress incontinence should be able to interrupt their urinary stream voluntarily during voiding.

Associated symptoms of urgency, frequency, nocturia, or urge incontinence may be reported in women with stress incontinence, detrusor instability, or a combination of both problems. Urgency is defined as a strong desire to void accompanied by the fear of impending urinary leakage or the fear of pain. The term *urinary frequency* is used when the patient voids more than seven times in 24 hours or every 2 hours, assuming a normal fluid intake; *nocturia* is defined as being awakened from sleep by the urge to void two or more times per night. The leakage of large volumes of urine or a history of nocturnal enuresis (bed wetting) suggests the presence of an unstable bladder. Constant urinary leakage implies a functionless urethra, fistula, or ectopic ureter.

Although an accurate history is helpful in guiding the physician's diagnostic evaluation, therapeutic decisions should not be based on history alone. Lower urinary tract symptoms are notoriously nonspecific and overlapping. Patients with systemic or psychiatric disorders may present with urinary complaints without associated urologic disease. Early reports stating that a history and physical examination alone constituted a sufficient workup in the majority of patients with stress incontinence have been contradicted by numerous recent investigators who found that the diagnosis of genuine stress incontinence based on history is correct in only 50–88% of cases. Since the treatment of genuine stress incontinence may involve surgery, it is essential that each incontinent patient undergo the appropriate office evaluation to establish a correct diagnosis and to detect any alternative, nonsurgical explanations for her urinary leakage.

Urolog

A voiding diary, or urolog, is one of the most important aspects of a urogynecologic investigation. The patient is asked to record the time and volume of her spontaneous voids over a 24–72-hour time period. Additional information regarding urgency prior to voids, frequency of incontinent episodes and activity precipitating incontinence, and the type and volume of fluid intake are also recorded. From this journal vital information regarding the patient's normal voiding pattern, her functional bladder capacity, and the severity of her incontinence episodes or irritative symptoms can be obtained.

The findings from the urolog can be used to adjust fluid intake in older patients with nocturnal frequency, or to begin a timed voiding schedule in a woman with detrusor instability. Occasionally, the voiding pattern may alert the clinician to the possibility of diabetes insipidus or anxiety-related diurnal frequency in a patient who sleeps through the night without problems. Thus, a urolog is an inexpensive, noninvasive evaluation of lower urinary tract function that should be obtained early in the course of all urologic evaluations.

Physical Examination

Once a complete history is obtained and a voiding diary analyzed, clinical evaluation of the lower urinary tract should begin with a screening neurologic examination to detect sensory or motor nerve dysfunction of the bladder or urethra. The T-10–S-4 nerve roots are primarily responsible for control of micturition. Thus, an examination of the lower extremity functions dependent on these nerve roots provides indirect evidence regarding bladder function.

Motor function can be assessed by flexion and extension maneuvers against resistance at the ankle, knee, and hip. Pelvic floor muscle tone can be determined by voluntary contraction of the rectal sphincter and vaginal muscles. Normal sensation in the upper leg and perineal dermatomes confirms intact sensory innervation of the lower urinary tract. Finally, reflex contraction of the pelvic floor in response to the anal sphincter ("anal wink" reflex) and bulbocavernosus reflexes provides evidence of the integrity of the sacral reflex center. Findings suggestive of neurologic deficits should be referred for formal neurologic evaluation.

The pelvic examination should assess the patient's estrogen status and detect the presence of any concomitant pelvic relaxation. The urethra, trigone, and vagina are estrogen-dependent structures. Thus, hypoestrogenic changes of the vaginal mucosa indicate similar changes in the urethra. The resultant loss of urethral tone, which may exacerbate the symptom of stress incontinence or irritative voiding complaints in some patients, is often corrected by vaginal estrogen replacement.

Inspection of the anterior and posterior vaginal walls using a Sims retractor or the lower blade of a bivalve vaginal speculum will facilitate identification of any cystocele, rectocele, or enterocele. Although the extent of pelvic relaxation may influence the surgeon's choice of operative approach in patients with urinary leakage, a defect in the anterior vaginal wall support does not confirm the diagnosis of genuine stress incontinence. The possibility of a urethral diverticulum or urinary fistula must also be considered during the examination. Palpation of the urethra and bladder trigone may reveal tenderness consistent with acute or chronic inflammation of either structure.

A postvoid residual determination must be made to exclude the possibility of an atonic bladder and overflow incontinence. Bacteriuria must also be ruled out by obtaining a urine culture. The endotoxin produced by *Escherichia coli* may trigger abnormal detrusor activity resulting in detrusor instability, or act as an alpha-adrenergic blocker. This latter action results in loss of urethral pressure and the subsequent development of stress incontinence. In one study, four of twelve women with stress incontinence and asymptomatic bacteriuria became continent following antibiotic treatment. A urinary cytologic profile should also be obtained in older women with incontinence, to exclude the possibility of intrinsic bladder abnormalities.

Urethrovesical Junction Mobility

Since genuine stress incontinence is most often due to inadequate support of the urethrovesical junction with displacement of the proximal urethra and urethrovesical junction outside the abdominal cavity, an integral part of the workup for urinary stress incontinence is assessing the mobility of this tissue. A number of tests have been designed to ascertain the mobility of the proximal urethra and bladder base, including direct observation during pelvic examination, the cotton-tipped swab test, bead-chain cystometrography, straining cystography, and ultrasound evaluation. The cotton-tipped swab test appears to be the easiest objective method to determine this information.

The cotton-tipped swab test was initially introduced to differentiate the anatomic defects in type I and type II stress incontinence. With the patient adequately prepared and in lithotomy position, a sterile cotton-tipped swab lubricated with 2% lidocaine jelly is inserted into the urethra through the urethrovesical junction. A resting angle is determined relative to the horizontal axis, using an orthopedic goniometer. The patient is then asked to strain forcibly and to cough repetitively. A maximum straining angle of more than 30 degrees from the horizontal axis is defined as a positive test and indicates significant mobility of the urethrovesical junction but not necessarily the diagnosis of stress incontinence.

Although the cotton-tipped swab test is not a specific clinical test for predicting incompetence of the urethral sphincter or for differentiating disorders of the lower urinary tract, it does provide a simple method for demonstrating excessive mobility of the urethrovesical junction in patients with suspected stress incontinence. Since the purpose of antiincontinence procedures is to elevate the urethrovesical junction back to its normal intraabdominal position, it is essential that a defect in support of the junction be demonstrated before surgical intervention is contemplated. In patients with a negative cotton-tipped swab test result, the diagnosis of genuine stress incontinence should be seriously questioned. More sophisticated radiographic or urodynamic studies are indicated prior to undertaking surgery in this group of patients.

Stress Test

Since objective evidence of urinary leakage with stress is necessary to establish the diagnosis of genuine stress incontinence, the stress test is an integral part of the evaluation of female urinary incontinence. The patient is asked to cough repetitively with a 300-ml bladder volume or a subjectively full bladder in the supine or standing position. Simultaneous loss of urine during coughing is highly suggestive of genuine stress incontinence.

The stress test can easily be performed at the beginning of the examination if the patient is asked to arrive at the office with a full bladder. Once the test is performed, the patient is asked to void for a uroflow determination, and a postvoid residual volume is measured. Alternatively, the stress test can be done at intervals during cystometrography to determine the volume at which leakage occurs.

Several modifications of the stress test have been devised in an attempt to predict the likelihood of surgical success in patients with stress incontinence. The Bonney test simulates the results of surgical elevation of the urethrovesical junction. To perform the test, the middle and index fingers are placed 1 cm laterally on each side of the urethra, and the junction is elevated to its normal retropubic position. The Marchetti test, using Allis clamps and local anesthesia, and the Read test, using rubber-shod clamps, are performed similarly. Patients who no longer lose urine with cough during these examinations are considered to be excellent surgical candidates.

Although the reliability of these tests has been emphasized in the literature, more recent studies have questioned the validity of the Bonney test in selecting patients for surgical intervention. Using urethral pressure profilometry, investigators have demonstrated that the Bonney test restores urinary continence by external compression and occlusion of the urethra. No statistically significant difference was found in the urethral pressure recordings during the Bonney test, compared with the results obtained with deliberate urethral occlusion. Thus, although the Bonney test was originally devised to mimic preoperatively the results of surgery, most investigators have abandoned its use as a prognostic test in the evaluation of female incontinence.

Uroflowmetry

Uroflowmetry is a measurement of the urine volume voided and the time interval required for voiding. This test is used to detect preoperatively any gross voiding abnormalities that may predispose a patient to prolonged voiding after antiincontinence surgery. Obstructive voiding patterns may also be seen in women with recurrent urinary tract infections, urethral spasms, or detrusor sphincter dyssynergia, in which voiding is sporadic and the postvoid residual volume is elevated.

Although uroflowmetry may be performed by using an electronic uroflowmeter, the simplest method is to use a stopwatch and a measuring container that fits over the toilet. The patient should void at least 200 ml for the test to be accurate. The average flow rate should be at least 10 ml/s with a postvoid residual of less than 50 ml.

Cystourethroscopy

Cystourethroscopy is an endoscopic evaluation of the urethral and vesical mucosa that can be performed in the office as a screening test. The procedure may also be undertaken in the operating room to facilitate a more extensive evaluation of the bladder, including bladder biopsies or bladder hydrodistention to treat interstitial cystitis. In the incontinent woman the purpose of cystourethroscopy is to detect intrinsic bladder pathologic lesions such as fistulae or diverticula, tumors, foreign bodies, or nonfunctioning ureters. The routine use of cystourethroscopy for the evaluation of urinary incontinence has been questioned. However, this procedure should be performed in women who have failed incontinence procedures, in older incontinent women (over age 60), and in the assessment of women with irritative bladder complaints, to determine the site and possible source of inflammatory changes in the lower urinary tract. Cystourethroscopy should be avoided in women with bacteriuria.

Urethroscopy is best accomplished using a 0-degree telescope with the filling medium running to facilitate distention of the urethra. The urethrovesical junction can be visualized while the patient is asked to squeeze her vaginal muscles, bear down, and cough. This dynamic urethroscopy enables the observer to determine the integrity of the urethrovesical junction. The bladder trigone and ureteral function can be assessed with a 0-degree or—more optimally—a 30-degree endoscope. Examination of the entire bladder surface should be performed with a 30-degree or a 70-degree telescope in a systematic fashion. During cystourethroscopy, the bladder is filled with a distention medium, preferably sterile water or saline, at a rate of no more than 100 ml/min to allow sufficient time for accommodation. The volume of first sensation, fullness, and maximum bladder capacity should be recorded.

Cystometry

Cystometry is a pressure–volume relationship recorded during bladder filling. The relationship is best described in terms of compliance (C), which indicates the change in volume (V) for a given change in pressure (P): $C = V/P$. The normal bladder is compliant over a wide range of bladder volumes.

The purpose of single-channel cystometry is to detect the presence of detrusor instability, which occurs in 8–63% of incontinent women or women with a hypertonic bladder. During cystometry the first sensation, maximum bladder capacity, and the presence of uninhibited detrusor contractions should be recorded. Detrusor instability is diagnosed when a true detrusor pressure rise occurs in the presence of urgency or urinary incontinence that reproduces the patient's presenting complaint. Low-amplitude detrusor contractions of less than 15 cm H_2O may have clinical significance and have been shown to cause urinary incontinence in 10% and urgency in 85% of patients. A gradual rise in intravesical pressure of more than 15 cm H_2O at normal bladder capacity indicates a hypertonic bladder. A hypotonic bladder is diagnosed when the maximum bladder capacity exceeds approximately 800 ml H_2O.

Despite the widespread use of cystometry, the optimal technique for performing this test is unclear. Questions remain regarding positioning of the patient; antegrade versus retrograde filling of the bladder; the use of sterile water, saline, or carbon dioxide as the distention medium; the temperature of the medium; and the rate of filling. Most studies are done by using retrograde flow of water, saline, or carbon dioxide at a flow rate of 50–100 ml/min. Although carbon dioxide cystometry may be easier and cleaner, it is less physiologic than water or saline as a distention medium. Carbon dioxide may irritate the bladder mucosa and mix with urine to form carbonic acid. As a gas, carbon dioxide is compressible, which may lead to less reproducible results.

If electronic equipment is unavailable to perform a single-channel cystometrogram, a number of more simplified techniques may be substituted. A Foley catheter may be inserted into the patient's bladder and attached to a catheter-tipped syringe with the piston removed. Fluid is gradually poured into the syringe (no more than 100 ml/min) so that the fluid level is constant. A rise in the fluid level associated with urgency or leakage suggests detrusor instability. Alternatively, a spinal manometer may be used to determine intravesical pressure (Fig. 4-1). Supine single-channel cystometry will detect approximately 50–60% of patients with an unstable bladder. The accuracy of this test may be improved an additional 20–40% by performing the cystometrics 1) to maximum bladder capacity, 2) in the standing position, and 3) with the detrusor-provoking maneuvers of repetitive coughing and heel bounce.

The reliability of single-channel cystometry, compared with multichannel urodynamics, has also been debated extensively in the literature. The reported advantage of multichannel cystometry is that artifactual increases in intravesical pressure due to a rise in intraabdominal pressure (eg, Valsalva activity) can be recognized and subtracted out. This results in an accurate recording of true detrusor pressure. Thus, multichannel testing is thought to decrease the incidence of a false-positive diagnosis of detrusor instability.

Multichannel Urodynamics

Multichannel urodynamics is a group of sophisticated urologic tests using microtransducer catheters to record simultaneously urethral, vesical, and intraabdominal (through a vaginal catheter) pressures and electromyographic activity of the pelvic floor. Information can be obtained by subtracted urethrocystometry, urethral pressure profilometry, uroflowmetry, instrumented voiding studies, and electromyographic recordings of the urethral sphincter. Approximately 10% of patients with lower urinary tract dysfunction will require urodynamic testing to elucidate their diagnosis. Referral for multichannel urodynamic testing should be made for patients who have a history of:

- Incontinence and are aged 65 years or older
- Antiincontinence surgery
- Neurologic disease
- Radical pelvic surgery or radiation therapy
- Continuous urinary leakage or leakage when unaware
- Mixed stress and urge incontinence, especially with a negative simple cystometrogram
- Suspected urethral diverticulum
- Suspected urethral spasm
- Suspected intrinsic urethral dysfunction (low-pressure urethra)

Upon examination, patients with the following symptoms should also undergo multichannel urodynamic testing:

- Neurologic abnormality
- Postvoid residual greater than 100 ml
- Incontinence with negative stress test result (no demonstrable leakage), negative cotton-tipped swab test (fixed,

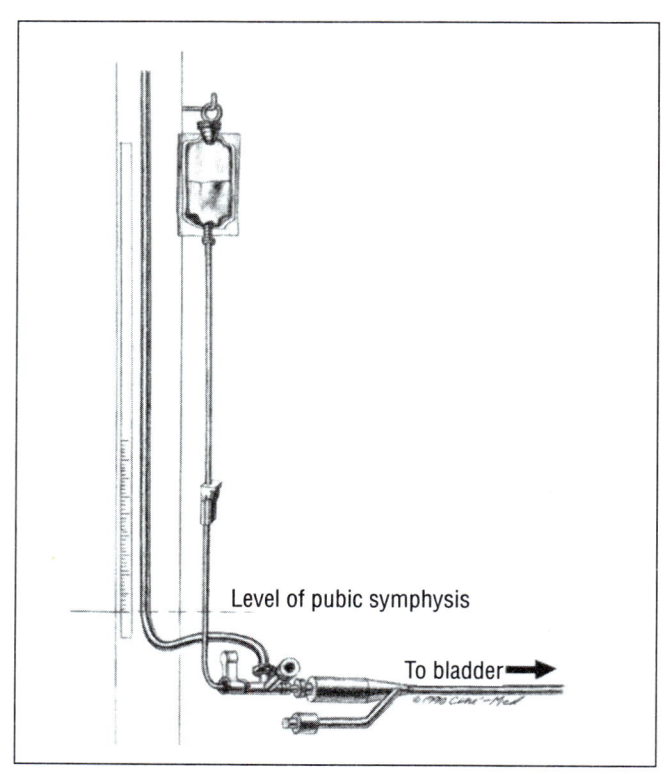

FIG. 4-1. Simple office cystometry using a Foley catheter and a meter stick with the 0 mark positioned at the upper level of the patient's pubic symphysis. Optimally the patient should be in the standing position and fluid infused at a rate of 80–100 ml/min. (American College of Obstetricians and Gynecologists. Urogynecologic evaluation, endoscopy, and urodynamic testing in the symptomatic female. ACOG Audiovisual Library. Washington, DC: ACOG, 1990)

immobile urethra), or symptoms of detrusor instability and normal simple cystometrogram
- Maximum bladder capacity less than 300 ml or greater than 800 ml on simple cystometry
- Absent sensation of filling during cystometry

Urethrocystometry. The purpose of urethrocystometry is to evaluate bladder and urethral function simultaneously during bladder filling. To improve the accuracy of the results, an intravaginal catheter is also used to record intraabdominal pressure and detect any artifactual rises in intravesical pressure that may be due to increases in intraabdominal pressure. Several pressure measurements are obtained during urethrocystometry:

- *Bladder pressure* is the pressure recorded directly from the pressure transducer within the bladder. This corresponds to the tracing generated during simple cystometry. Normal resting bladder pressure in the supine position is usually 8–12 cm H_2O and increases by 5–10 cm H_2O when standing.
- *True detrusor pressure* is the pressure generated by the detrusor muscle fibers. This pressure is determined by subtracting the recorded intraabdominal pressure from the recorded intravesical pressure. True detrusor pressure at rest is usually 0 cm of H_2O in the supine and standing positions. During bladder filling, detrusor pressure may show an increase of up to 15 cm H_2O at normal bladder capacity.
- *Intraabdominal pressure* is the pressure recorded from the intraabdominal cavity by the intravaginal or rectal catheter placed above the pelvic floor.

Urethral Pressure Profilometry. Urethral profilometry is the measure of urethral pressure obtained over the length of the urethra. This test is performed by slowly withdrawing a pressure transducer from the bladder to the external urethral meatus. A pressure curve is generated by this study (Fig. 4-2). Cough pressure profiles, which are essentially a sophisticated stress test, enable the physician to confirm the diagnosis of genuine stress incontinence and to calculate leak point pressures (the increase in intravesical pressure that overcomes urethral resistance and produces urinary leakage) and pressure transmission ratios.

Uroflowmetry and Pressure Voiding Studies. Anatomic and functional voiding abnormalities are detected by the technique of simultaneous uroflowmetry and pressure voiding studies on multichannel urodynamics. From the combined use of uroflowmetry with pressure measurements of true detrusor pressure and urethral closure pressure, both the flow rates and the mechanism of voiding can be determined. The intraabdominal lead enables one to determine whether the patient is voiding by abdominal straining. Pressure voiding studies, along with electromyography, may detect the presence of an abnormal voiding pattern called detrusor sphincter dyssynergia, in which a paradoxical increase in urethral tone is associated with a detrusor contraction during voiding.

Electromyography. Electromyography is a measure of the electrical activity of the urethral sphincter mechanism, the periurethral striated muscles, and the pelvic floor muscles. This technique is particularly important in the evaluation of the neurologically impaired patient or the woman who exhibits voiding dysfunction. A normal electromyographic pattern shows increasing activity of the pelvic floor as cystometry is performed and the patient's bladder is filled. An increase in electromyographic activity during voiding may suggest detrusor sphincter dyssynergia.

Treatment

Stress Incontinence

Genuine stress incontinence can be approached nonsurgically in some women. Candidates include women with mild symptoms, women who desire subsequent childbearing, or women who are poor surgical candidates.

Pharmacologic Agents. In postmenopausal women, topical estrogen replacement is recommended, which improves the uroepithelium, submucosal vascularity, and submucosal elastic tissues. However, these changes produce an inconsistent rise in urethral pressure, and thus it appears that the beneficial effects of estrogen are not solely dependent on augmentation of urethral pressures. The usual dosage of vaginal estrogen cream is 1–2 g three times per week for 6–12 weeks. Up to 70% of patients with mild to moderate incontinence have reported a favorable clinical response following initiation of estrogen therapy.

Alpha-adrenergic stimulation of the urethral smooth muscle with phenylpropanolamine, 75–150 mg/d, may improve the symptoms of mild to moderate stress incontinence. Many over-the-counter appetite suppressants contain phenylpropanolamine as the active ingredient, although the patient must be careful to avoid caffeine-containing medications. Some women will demonstrate better tolerance for a drug that combines 75 mg of phenylpropanolamine with 12 mg of chlorpheniramine, and is traditionally used as an antihistamine.

Imipramine hydrochloride, 50–150 mg/d, is advantageous in treating mixed stress incontinence and detrusor instability

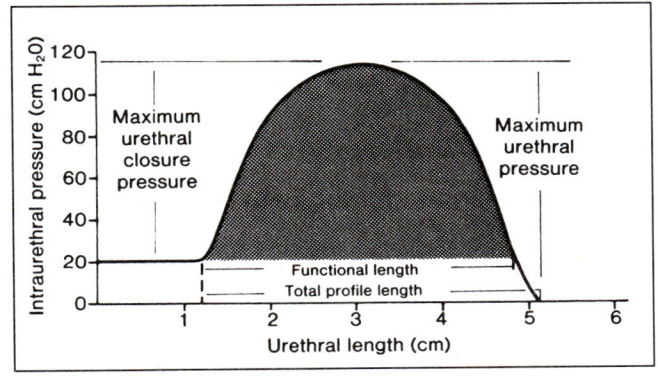

FIG. 4-2. A schematic diagram of a urethra pressure profile indicating the measurements that may be calculated from this tracing. (Ostergard DR, Bent AE. Urogynecology and urodynamics, theory and practice. Baltimore: Williams and Wilkins, 1991)

because of its combined alpha-adrenergic and anticholinergic properties. This medication must be used judiciously in the elderly, since imipramine can occasionally precipitate a dysphoric reaction at low dosages.

Pelvic Floor Rehabilitation. Kegel exercises, with or without the aid of a perineometer or vaginal weighted cones, improved urinary control in 40–75% of patients by contracting the pubococcygeus muscle and improving the tone of the voluntary external urethral musculature. The success of Kegel exercises is determined by the patient's ability to identify the correct muscle for the exercise and her commitment to perform the exercises according to the prescribed regimen.

Several approaches have been reported in the literature, including instructing the patient to execute a series of rapid pelvic floor contractions and release, followed by a contraction held for 3 seconds and released for 3 seconds for a total of 5 minutes per exercise, five or six times per day. Alternatively, patients may be requested to perform 10–20 pelvic floor contractions each for 10 seconds three times per day. Most studies indicate that a total of at least 40 pelvic floor contractions per day must be performed to see beneficial results from the exercise program. It is important to instruct the patient to perform Kegel exercises while at rest and not while voiding, to prevent the development of abnormal voiding patterns.

Several devices have been developed to assist patients in performing pelvic floor exercises. A perineometer indicates the rise in intravaginal pressure generated by the pelvic floor contraction. This device must be used carefully, since abdominal straining may also produce a rise in intravaginal pressure. Sets of weighted vaginal cones (20–100 g) are available that can be inserted into the vagina twice daily for 15 minutes. The sensation of impending slippage of the weighted cone produces a reflex contraction of the pelvic floor muscles and encourages contraction of the correct musculature. Beneficial results may be observed after 6–8 weeks of use.

Functional electrical stimulation provides stimulation of the pudendal nerve, which causes contractions of the pelvic floor and periurethral skeletal muscles. A vaginal probe that provides an electrical current to the pelvic musculature and results in a type of "electronic Kegel" exercise is inserted for 10–15 minutes twice daily. This technique has been adopted more readily in Europe than in the United States but is gaining popularity here. Improvement may be seen after 6–8 weeks of therapy. This technique also may be beneficial in women with mixed stress and urge incontinence.

Mechanical Devices. Vaginal pessaries, contraceptive diaphragms, or tampons have been used to alleviate the symptoms of pelvic relaxation with or without concomitant urinary incontinence. By compressing the urethra between the pessary ring and the pubic symphysis, urethral resistance is increased and the urethra and urethovesical junction are stabilized in an appropriate anatomic position during episodes of stress. An appropriately fitted ring or Smith–Hodge pessary may produce continence in up to 75% of women. This form of therapy is particularly well suited for older women with prolapse and incontinence who are poor surgical candidates. In addition, younger women who experience stress incontinence only during intense exercise (aerobics, tennis) may benefit from insertion of a pessary, diaphragm, or tampon temporarily just prior to exercise.

Although nonsurgical approaches to stress incontinence produce beneficial results with minimal side effects, these methods are only temporary measures to restore urinary continence. Surgical options provide a more permanent chance for cure, but they are associated with more potential complications. Thus, surgical procedures should be reserved for women who decline or fail conservative therapies and for women who have completed childbearing.

Surgical Intervention. The surgical management of genuine stress incontinence can be divided into two types of procedures: 1) procedures that restore the anatomic support of the proximal urethra and the urethrovesical junction in women with hypermobility and a normal intrinsic urethral sphincter, and 2) procedures designed to compensate for a poorly functioning intrinsic urethra. Thus, it is essential that an accurate preoperative diagnosis is established prior to surgical intervention.

The operations for hypermobility include anterior colporrhaphy, abdominal retropubic procedures, and needle urethropexies. Numerous studies have reported that the traditional anterior colporrhaphy does not provide adequate long-term support of the urethrovesical junction and has an objective cure rate of only 50–70%. The best approach for hypermobility of the urethrovescial junction appears to be the abdominal retropubic urethropexy, although some studies have found good success with the needle suspension procedures, which are particularly beneficial in the patient with significant concomitant pelvic relaxation requiring additional vaginal surgery.

Intrinsic urethral dysfunction may be treated with a suburethral sling procedure, periurethral injections to improve urethral coaptation, or an artificial urinary sphincter. All of these operations are associated with a high risk of postoperative complications, especially urinary retention. Recent studies have suggested that the cure rate of standard incontinence procedures for the treatment of intrinsic urethral dysfunction may be as high as 50–70%. Regardless of which operation is selected, adequate preoperative counseling is required for any patient prior to surgical intervention for intrinsic urethral dysfunction.

Several surgical principles should be emphasized when approaching a patient with stress incontinence with or without significant pelvic relaxation:

- All defects in pelvic support must be detected preoperatively, and the surgical procedure must be designed to correct current problems as well as to prevent iatrogenic postoperative alterations in pelvic organ support.
- Patients with severe pelvic relaxation may be continent because of the compressive effects of the proplase on the urethra. Preoperative assessment of these women should

include a stress test with the prolapse reduced, to determine whether additional support of the urethrovesical junction should be performed at the time of the prolapse surgery. Unless there is proven obstruction or kinking of the urethra caused by a severe cystocele producing urinary retention, correction of a cystocele will not improve a patient's urinary retention and elevated postvoid residual. At times, increased urethral resistance following surgery may actually worsen a patient's urinary retention.

Detrusor Instability

The treatment approaches to detrusor instability can be divided into behavioral therapy, biofeedback, medications, functional electrical stimulation, surgery, and psychologic counseling. All patients should be encouraged to void on a regular basis, avoid excess fluid intake, and restrict consumption of caffeinated beverages to one cup per day.

Behavioral therapy, referred to as bladder retraining, attempts to reestablish the cortical inhibition of reflex bladder emptying that is lost in patients with detrusor instability. Using the patient's pretreatment voiding diary as a guide, a regular voiding interval is chosen that is more often than the patient's incontinence episode frequency. The patient is instructed to void regularly during the waking hours according to the preset interval, whether or not she has the urge to void, and to ignore other desires to void even if it results in urinary leakage. She records her micturition times on a preprinted card. After 7–10 days, she should have fewer incontinent episodes, and her scheduled voiding interval can be increased by 15–30 minutes. This process is continued until the desired voiding interval of every 3–4 hours is achieved.

Success is dependent on the motivation of the patient and the physician but can approach 80%. A variation of behavioral therapy can be applied to the elderly, institutionalized patient that includes avoiding excess fluid intake, elimination of caffeine, and regular toileting or prompted voiding at 2-hour intervals.

Biofeedback facilitates the inhibition of abnormal detrusor contractions by inserting a pressure catheter into the bladder, which provides an auditory or visual stimulus when bladder pressure rises. The patient is encouraged to relax her muscles to decrease the recorded signal. Weekly sessions in a motivated patient can yield a success rate of up to 50%.

Although advocates of both bladder retraining and biofeedback report excellent success rates without side effects, the time-consuming nature of these treatments makes them unacceptable to many women. Anticholinergic and antispasmodic medications provide an excellent alternative to behavioral therapy, with a success rate of 60–80%. Preparations that have proven to be effective are shown in Table 4-2. The drug of choice is usually either oxybutynin hydrochloride, with its improved effectiveness but significant risk of side effects, or propantheline bromide, which appears to be associated with fewer adverse reactions.

Other drugs that are marketed for detrusor instability do not appear to be any more efficacious, simply more costly. These medications are associated with typical anticholinergic side effects and are contraindicated in women with narrow-angle glaucoma. In patients who experience significant untoward reactions from these drugs, the combination of low doses of more than one type of medication may produce an additive beneficial response while diminishing the reported side effects.

Surgical intervention is associated with significant morbidity and should be reserved only for severely affected individuals. These procedures may include partial denervation of the hypogastric nerve, implantation of a sacral nerve root–stimulating device, or—in extreme cases—urinary diversion.

Urethral Diverticula

The approach to patients with a urethral diverticulum varies, depending on the presenting symptoms. Some diverticula are asymptomatic and require no treatment. Acute inflammation of the diverticular sac may present as a tender suburethral swelling with purulent material being expressed from the urethral meatus upon massage of the anterior vaginal wall. Diagnosis is confirmed by urethroscopy, voiding cystourethrography, or positive pressure urethrography using a Tratner or Davis balloon catheter.

An inflamed diverticulum may be managed initially by either transvaginal aspiration of the purulent material followed by a 7–10-day course of antibiotics designed to be effective against uropathogens, or by urethral dilation with transvaginal massage to express the purulent contents of the diverticular sac. Surgical procedures to repair a diverticulum are best postponed until any acute inflammation has subsided.

TABLE 4-2. PHARMACOLOGIC MANAGEMENT OF DETRUSOR INSTABILITY

Drug	Dosage*	Comments
Propantheline bromide	15–30 mg tid–qid	Cure rates 60–80%; fewer side effects; variable gastrointestinal absorption
Oxybutynin hydrochloride	5–10 mg tid–qid	Cure rates 60–80%; side effects in up to 75% of patients
Dicyclomine hydrochloride	20 mg IM qid	Effective if used parenterally
Flavoxate hydrochloride	100–200 mg tid–qid	Limited data on efficacy; more expensive drug
Imipramine hydrochloride	25–50 mg bid–tid	Cure rates 60–74%; beneficial for childhood nocturnal enuresis or mixed stress and urge incontinence

*Abbreviations are as follows: bid, twice daily; qid, four times daily; tid, three times daily; IM, intramuscularly.

The operative approach depends on the location of the sac in relationship to the maximum urethral pressure point, which is determined by urethral pressure profilometry. Thus, preoperative urodynamics with urethral pressure profiles are essential.

A distal diverticulum may be treated with a Spence procedure, in which a marsupialization of the sac is performed by opening the sac and suturing the diverticular mucosa to the vaginal mucosa with a running locked suture. A proximal diverticulum must be isolated surgically from the surrounding tissue of the urethrovaginal septum and excised. A multilayer closure with alternating directions of the suture line is recommended to repair the defect in the urethrovaginal system.

IRRITATIVE BLADDER PROBLEMS

Although urinary incontinence primarily affects women over age 35, women of all ages may suffer from conditions that produce irritative bladder complaints. Patients typically report significant urinary urgency and frequency that may be associated with dysuria, suprapubic pressure, pain on distention of the bladder, nocturia, postvoid fullness, or dyspareunia. These symptoms may be constant, with acute exacerbations, or episodic in nature.

Many patients are treated repetitively with only temporary relief of symptoms. Alternatively, the nonspecific nature of these complaints may result in misdiagnosis when recurrent symptoms are attributed to the same condition. Thus, it is essential that the physician take a careful, detailed history and reevaluate each episode to explore the possibility of other potential causes for the patient's irritative bladder complaints. Nonurologic etiologies for these symptoms must also be considered, including vaginal infection, acute or chronic vulvitis, or atrophic vaginitis.

The conditions most commonly associated with irritative bladder symptoms are acute urinary tract infection (see "Infections" in the section on Primary and Preventive Care), acute urethritis, chronic urethritis (urethral syndrome), interstitial cystitis, or detrusor instability.

Urethral Syndrome

Urethral syndrome is an elusive chronic condition characterized by urinary urgency and frequency, and intermittent or constant dysuria, suprapubic pressure, postvoid fullness, or dyspareunia in the absence of a positive urine culture result. Symptoms appear worse during waking hours than at night and may be preceded by an actual acute urinary tract infection in some patients. Often the patient has been treated repetitively for several months with antibiotics for presumed recurrent cystitis, yielding only temporary relief of symptoms. The exact etiology of urethral syndrome remains unclear. Proposed possible causes are as follows:

- Periurethral gland inflammation due to infection or trauma
- Hypoestrogenism
- Urethral smooth or skeletal muscle spasm (functional obstruction)
- Trauma secondary to diaphragm use, tampon use, or coitus
- Allergic reactions to perfumed sanitary napkins, feminine hygiene sprays, vaginal douches, or contraceptive spermacides
- Chlamydial urethritis
- Peripheral neuropathy secondary to herpes
- Urethrohymenal fusion
- Psychogenic factors

The diagnosis of urethral syndrome is suggested in women with irritative symptoms that usually have persisted for several months and are associated with a negative urine culture. A detailed history should address the possible etiologic factors, and a thorough physical examination should exclude gynecologic sources of these symptoms. A voiding diary provides objective evidence of the severity of the patient's symptoms and often will illustrate the propensity for diurnal versus nocturnal frequency in patients with urethral syndrome.

Urethroscopy may reveal hypoestrogenic changes of the urethral mucosa or nonspecific erythema and exudate that may also be observed in asymptomatic women. Cystoscopy should be performed to exclude intrinsic bladder abnormalities, especially carcinoma in situ or bladder tumors in the older patient. Cystometry or urethral pressure profilometry may be indicated to detect the presence of low-amplitude detrusor contractions or urethral spasm, respectively.

The treatment of urethral syndrome is imprecise and frustrating, since most therapeutic options yield cure rates of only 60%, and many patients develop recurrent symptoms despite medical intervention. Treatment should begin by eliminating any potentially reversible cause of urethral syndrome, and by discontinuing the ingestion of caffeinated beverages that may aggravate the urgency symptoms. Estrogen replacement should be initiated with 1–2 g of conjugated estrogen vaginal cream two or three times per week in perimenopausal and postmenopausal women.

If urethral inflammation is suspected, urethral dilatation and massage can be performed by using a series of urethral dilators or sounds. Following antiseptic preparation of the urethral meatus and using copious amounts of 2% lidocaine jelly as a urethral lubricant and topical anesthetic, a 16-French dilator is inserted into the urethra, and gentle massage of the anterior vaginal wall over the urethral dilator is accomplished to promote drainage of infected periurethral glands. Serial dilation is continued until blanching of the external urethral meatus is observed (but only to a maximum 36 French) or the patient experiences significant discomfort. Although this procedure is generally well tolerated, some patients require a more extensive anesthetic, such as a bladder pillar block, using 10 ml of 1% lidocaine injected submucosally at the cervicovaginal junction (at the 2-o'clock and 10-o'clock positions). Urethral dilation may be repeated weekly or biweekly for two or three treatments and then episodically as necessary. Patients should be prescribed an antibiotic and phenazopyridine hydrochloride for 24 hours posttreatment to relieve discomfort and prevent the risk of iatrogenic urinary tract infection.

If urethral dilatation and massage fails, patients may be treated with periurethral steroid injections. With a urethral sound in place to guide the injection, 0.25 ml of triamcinolone acetonide (10 mg/ml) is injected submucosally along the length of the urethra at the 3-, 5-, 7-, and 9-o'clock positions, using a 30-gauge needle. Using this approach, one report found 87% of patients who were followed had relief of symptoms from 6 months to 5 years after treatment.

Pharmacologic management of urethral syndrome has been aimed at the treatment of possible chronic urethral infections with antibiotics, or relief of functional urethral spasm with muscle relaxants. Empirical treatment of chlamydia with 10–14 days of doxycycline or erythromycin is cost-effective and may be helpful. Occasionally, patients may respond to long-term therapy (3–6 months) with low-dose antibiotics designed to eradicate uropathogens. Functional urethral obstruction may be due to spasm of the urethral smooth or skeletal muscle. A skeletal muscle blocker, such as diazepam, 2 mg two to four times daily for 2–6 months, may be helpful. This drug may be used alone or in combination with a smooth muscle relaxant such as phenoxybenzamine hydrochloride, 10–40 mg/d, or prazocin, 1–2 mg two or three times daily.

Other treatment modalities that have been proven anecdotally to be effective are the Richardson urethrolysis, urethral cryotherapy, and hymenoplasty to correct urethrohymenal fusion. With any of the therapeutic approaches outlined above, one of the most essential requirements for success is a caring and supportive physician.

Interstitial Cystitis

Interstitial cystitis is a debilitating chronic inflammation of the bladder wall that is estimated to affect 1 in 350 to 1 in 415 outpatients, with a 10:1 predominance of women to men. Patients report incapacitating suprapubic pain on bladder distention that precipitates the need for frequent voids throughout the day and night. Typically, these women experience severe pain (not simply suprapubic pressure) that is usually relieved by voiding but may be exacerbated at the end of micturition in a few patients. Urge incontinence is a finding encountered in the later stages of the disease. Spontaneous remissions are uncommon, and patients may become progressively more debilitated by the frequency of voiding and the persistent pain.

Multiple theories have been proposed to explain interstitial cystitis, but no hypothesis is completely accepted at present. Infectious, allergic, autoimmune, and neurologic causes have been implicated. One theory supports the concept of a defect in the protective glycosaminoglycan layer of the bladder mucosa that allows toxins to penetrate into the submucosa and precipitate a chronic inflammatory reaction.

The diagnosis of interstitial cystitis is based on suggestive symptoms and may be further supported by cystoscopic findings. Because of the severe pain associated with bladder distention, general anesthesia may be required to ensure an adequate cystoscopic examination. A double-distention technique is used. The initial bladder distention produces the classic submucosal changes, which are then more easily visualized on the second bladder filling.

In the early stages of the disease, small, submucosal hemorrhages may be visualized without mucosal fissures, scarring, or a reduced bladder capacity. The more severe form of interstitial cystitis is characterized by submucosal petechial hemorrhages, fissures, linear scars, and the classic Hunner ulcers. Bladder capacity may be significantly reduced and gross hematuria encountered with bladder drainage.

Bladder biopsies should confirm the findings of chronic inflammation and vasodilation of the submucosa. Biopsy is also indicated to exclude other pathologic conditions, including tuberculosis, radiation cystitis, and carcinoma in situ of the bladder.

Other diagnostic tools that may be helpful are a voiding diary, which should reveal significant diurnal and nocturnal frequency with reduced functional bladder capacity, and a normal postvoid residual with negative urine culture. Urodynamic evaluation is rarely necessary except to eliminate other potential causes of the patient's symptoms, such as detrusor instability. A cystometrogram will reveal a hypertonic bladder with decreased bladder capacity.

The therapeutic approaches to interstitial cystitis can be divided into bladder instillation therapy, surgical management, or systemic agents. Bladder hydrodistention can be accomplished at the time of diagnostic cystoscopy. Distention of the bladder is believed to injure the bladder submucosal nerve plexi and destroy detrusor muscle stretch receptors, resulting in increased bladder capacity and diminished pain. To avoid the complication of bladder rupture, the bladder pressure during distention should never exceed the patient's systolic blood pressure. Other self-limited complications of hydrodistention are hematuria, backache, and urinary retention.

Dimethyl sulfoxide is the only product approved for instillation therapy in patients with interstitial cystitis. Its properties include antiinflammation, bacteriostasis, local anesthesia, cholinesterase inhibition, relaxation of skeletal and smooth muscle, and dissolution of pathologic deposits of collagen. The initial dimethyl sulfoxide treatment should be administered as 50 ml of a 25% solution through a urethral catheter after local topical urethral anesthesia has been applied. The solution is retained for 15 minutes and then released by spontaneous voiding. Subsequent instillations should be performed on a weekly or biweekly basis, using a 50% solution up to a total of four to six treatments. Cataracts are a contraindication to dimethyl sulfoxide administration.

Side effects include a garlic taste, lethargy, headache, nausea, and potentiation of the effects of ethyl alcohol. A review of several published series has found a satisfactory response rate of 53–90% over 6 months to 2 years. In patients who become refractory to dimethyl sulfoxide therapy alone, the medication may be combined with hydrocortisol to augment the antiinflammatory response. A recent retrospective report found symptomatic relief in 80% of patients treated with a combination of weekly bladder pillar block (1% lidocaine and 40 mg of triamcinolone acetonide), passive bladder distention to no more than 500 ml, and instillation of 50 ml of 50% dimethyl sulfoxide for 30 minutes.

Systemic agents with variable anecdotal effectiveness include antihistamines, azathiaprine, corticosteroids, heparin, sodium pentosan polysulfate, and tricyclic antidepressants. If these measures fail, surgical therapy to the bladder mucosa with an Nd:YAG laser has been found to be 65% effective in improving symptoms in an uncontrolled trial of 39 patients. Procedures that are reserved for the most refractory patients include selective sacral neurectomy, inferior hypogastric nerve resection, cystoplasty, cystolysis, or bladder augmentation.

Detrusor Instability

Occasionally, women with low-amplitude detrusor contractions that are insufficient to produce urge incontinence may experience significant urgency and frequency. Subthreshold detrusor contractions less than 15 cm H_2O have been shown to cause urgency in 85% of patients. However, women with detrusor instability rarely suffer from dysuria or suprapubic pain. The diagnosis is relatively easily established by a cystometrogram in which uninhibited detrusor contractions are observed that coincide with the patient's complaint of urgency. Treatment is as outlined in the previous discussion of detrusor instability.

VOIDING ABNORMALITIES

Voiding difficulties may present as urinary hesitancy, urinary retention, overflow urinary incontinence, or urgency and frequency symptoms due to the patient's inability to empty her bladder adequately with each void. Urgency and frequency symptoms not associated with an elevated postvoid residual are considered to be due to irritative bladder problems discussed in the previous section.

Normal voiding is accomplished by initial voluntary relaxation of the urethral smooth and skeletal musculature followed by the onset of a detrusor contraction of sufficient duration and amplitude to allow complete evacuation of urine. The force generated by the detrusor to expel urine may be augmented by an increase in intraabdominal pressure through voluntary straining. Thus, voiding may be facilitated in some patients by abdominal straining, which may compensate for a poorly functioning urethral sphincter or detrusor.

Urinary hesitancy, with difficulty initiating a urinary stream, may be due to inadequate urethral relaxation at the onset of voiding or due to failure of the bladder to develop a detrusor contraction in a timely fashion to initiate micturition. If these problems are overcome by the patient's consciously attempting to relax her urethral sphincter or by abdominal straining, satisfactory voiding may be accomplished with negligible postvoid residual urine volume. If, however, either process remains suboptimal, acute or chronic urinary retention may develop.

Potential causes of acute urinary retention include trauma secondary to abdominal or pelvic surgery, labor and delivery, epidural or general anesthesia, urethrocystitis, herpetic vulvitis, neurogenic disease, psychologic disorders, or urethral obstruction due to uterine myomas, ovarian masses, malignancies, an acutely retroverted uterus, or vaginal wall masses.

Chronic urinary retention may begin insidiously or as the result of an episode of acute urinary retention that leads to permanent damage to the lower urinary tract. The diagnosis of chronic retention should be reserved for patients who demonstrate elevated residual urine on at least two occasions several days apart.

Infrequent voiding in a woman with normal fluid intake may contribute to the development of chronic retention by gradual overdistention of the bladder, leading to damage or denervation of the detrusor muscle. Neurogenic factors that may be associated with progressive retention include 1) parasympathetic denervation due to radical pelvic surgery; 2) the effects of systemic diseases such as diabetes mellitus, hypothyroidism, or collagen–vascular diseases on the sensory input for bladder filling; and 3) lesions or trauma to the spinal cord. In some patients detrusor function can be lost simply as consequence of the aging process.

Anticholinergic medications may also contribute to chronic urinary retention. Retention due to chronic urethral obstruction is rare in women. It may be encountered in women with large pelvic masses or following antiincontinence surgery due to overzealous correction of the periurethral supporting tissues. The ultimate sequelae of retention are symptoms of urgency and frequency, overflow or stress incontinence, recurrent cystitis, and ureteral reflux.

Diagnosis

The hallmark of the diagnosis of urinary retention is an elevated postvoid residual usually greater than 100–200 ml. It is, however, unusual to encounter overflow incontinence unless the residual volume exceeds 300–400 ml. The subsequent evaluation of these patients should be directed at elucidating the underlying cause for the retention and correcting it. Neurologic and pelvic examination, maintenance of a voiding diary, urinalysis and urine culture, and basic uroflowmetry should be performed. Most patients, especially those with overflow incontinence, will also require referral for multichannel urodynamics testing, which should include urethrocystometry, urethral pressure profilometry (to detect urethral spasm), and electromyographic studies (to rule out detrusor sphincter dyssynergia). Intravenous pyelography and cystourethroscopy may be necessary. Finally, underlying neurologic conditions may be excluded by a computed tomographic scan or magnetic resonance imaging of the brain and spinal cord.

Treatment

Acute urinary retention should be treated by prompt urethral or suprapubic catheter drainage for 24–48 hours. Once the underlying cause of the retention has been eliminated, "tincture of time" is the most effective and well-tolerated treatment for acute urinary retention.

The use of cholinergic medications such as bethanechol chloride to improve bladder emptying has been reported to be beneficial in subjective, uncontrolled trials. However, the few blinded, well-controlled series that have been reported have found no advantage of these medications over placebo controls. If pharmacologic management is desired, alpha-adrenergic blocking agents such as phenoxybenzamine or prazocin, or skeletal muscle relaxants such as diazepam have been proven to be effective in decreasing residual urine volumes. These drugs may be used in combination as described in the previous section on the treatment of urethral spasm.

Chronic urinary retention due to poor detrusor function responds poorly to pharmacologic intervention. Some women with low urethral resistance may be taught to improve bladder emptying by a combination of Credé and Valsalva maneuvers in addition to a double-voiding technique. This approach is not recommended for patients with ureteral reflux.

A highly effective technique for the treatment of chronic retention, especially in women who have developed overflow incontinence, is clean, intermittent self-catheterization. This procedure necessitates adequate cognitive function and manual dexterity and is contraindicated in a patient with urethral strictures. Disposable, plastic catheters may be purchased inexpensively and used for 1 week before being discarded. No special antiseptic preparation is required other than regular hand-washing. Topical lubricant may be used as necessary. The patient can initially be instructed on how to insert the catheter, using a mirror to localize the urethral meatus. However, most patients are eventually able to perform the procedure without the aid of direct visualization. Once the catheterization is completed, the catheter should be washed with soap and warm water and stored in a clean plastic bag or container. Catheterization can be performed up to four to six times per day. If ureteral reflux is not a concern, asymptomatic bacteriuria does not require treatment.

BIBLIOGRAPHY

Abrams P, Blaivas JG, Stanton SL, Anderson JT. The standardisation of terminology of lower urinary tract function. The International Continence Society Committee on Standardisation of Terminology. Scand J Urol Nephrol Suppl 1988;114:5–19

Bhatia NN, Bergman A, Karram MM. Effects of estrogen on urethral function in women with urinary incontinence. Am J Obstet Gynecol 1989;160:176–181

Cardozo LD, Stanton SL. Genuine stress incontinence and detrusor instability—a review of 200 patients. Br J Obstet Gynaecol 1980; 87:184–190

Consensus conference. Urinary incontinence in adults. JAMA 1989; 261:2685–2690

Kinn AC, Lindskog M. Estrogens and phenylpropanolamine in combination for stress urinary incontinence in postmenopausal women. Urology 1988;32:273–280

Ramahi AJ, Richardson DA. A practical approach to painful bladder syndrome. J Reprod Med 1990;35:805–809

Sand PK, Brubaker LT, Novak T. Simple standing incremental cystometry as a screening method for detrusor instability. Obstet Gynecol 1991;77:453–457

Urinary Incontinence Guideline Panel. Urinary incontinence in adults: clinical practice guidelines. Rockville, Maryland: Agency for Health Care Policy and Research, Public Health Service, U.S. Department of Health and Human Services, 1992; AHCPR publication no. 92-0038

Wall LL. Diagnosis and management of urinary incontinence due to detrusor instability. Obstet Gynecol Surv 190;45(11 suppl):1S–47S

Walters MD, Diaz K. Q-tip test: a study of continent and incontinent women. Obstet Gynecol 1987;70:208–211

Wein AJ. Pharmacotherapy of the bladder and urethra. In: Stanton SL, Tanagho EA, eds. Surgery of female incontinence. 2nd ed. New York: Springer-Verlag, 1986:229–250

Disorders of the Uterus

LEIOMYOMATA UTERI

Leiomyomata uteri, also called myomata uteri, are benign neoplasms of smooth muscle cells contained within pseudocapsules of fibrous connective tissue. As the most common tumor of the uterus and female pelvis, they occur clinically in 20% of women of reproductive age and as much as 50% in autopsy series. Leiomyomata are the most common indication for pelvic surgery in women, representing the preoperative diagnosis in 30% of hysterectomies performed for nonmalignant reasons.

Etiology

Each leiomyoma is derived from a single smooth muscle cell. Each uterine myoma is monoclonal, as all cells of a particular myoma have identical electrophoretic variance of glucose-6-phosphate dehydrogenase. Two different theories exist regarding the cell of origin. One is that the cell of origin arises from persistent, small embryonic cell rests, whereas the other theory proposes that leiomyomata originate from the smooth muscle of blood vessels. The factors that induce smooth muscle cells to form leiomyomata are unknown; currently, the role of estrogens in leiomyoma growth appears central. Leiomyomata have higher levels of receptors for estradiol, progesterone, and gonadotropin-releasing hormone (GnRH) than are found in the surrounding myometrium. These tumors convert estradiol to the less potent estrone at a slower rate than a normal myometrium does, perhaps producing a local hyperestrogenic environment. Enzymes that aromatize androgens to estrogens are found in higher concentrations in leiomyomata than in a normal myometrium. Clinical evidence for the role of estrogens is found in various normal, pathologic, and therapeutic states. Leiomyomata are rare before menarche and typically diminish in size after menopause or castration. Pregnancy, oral contraceptives, and high doses of exogenous estrogens may cause leiomyoma growth. By increasing estrogen levels endogenously, ovulation induction agents such as clomiphene citrate and menotropins may be associated with myoma growth.

Another factor that may be associated with myoma growth is growth hormone, which is synergistic with estradiol in inducing uterine weight gain in rats. The growth hormone homolog human placental lactogen (hPL) may further stimulate leiomyomata.

As an antiestrogen, progesterone may inhibit the growth of leiomyomata. Relatively large doses of progestins (eg, medroxyprogesterone acetate, 20–30 mg orally) cause softening and sometimes shrinkage of leiomyomata after several weeks of therapy. In addition, both danazol and GnRH agonists can inhibit growth of leiomyomata. Preoperative use of a GnRH agonist for 3 months can produce a reduction in uterine blood flow and leiomyomata shrinkage that decreases uterine volume by as much as 51–61%.

Anatomic Classification

Ninety-five percent of leiomyomata arise in the uterine fundus; 5% originate in the cervix. The myomatous uterus may have solitary or multiple nodules ranging in size from microscopic to mammoth tumors weighing more than 45 kg (100 lb). Most tumors start intramurally and then grow toward either the serosa (subserosal leiomyomata) or the endometrium (submucosal leiomyomata). Submucosal tumors may distend, stretch, or pedunculate into the uterine cavity. Subserosal tumors may become pedunculated, with bases of various widths, and rarely, they migrate to derive their vascular support from the omentum or a viscus, the so-called parasitic leiomyoma. An intraligamentary tumor may be free of uterine vasculature, deriving its blood supply from vessels in the broad ligament.

Unusual clinical forms of leiomyomata include intravenous leiomyomatosis, which is characterized by polypoid projections of smooth muscle tumors through the veins of the parametrium and broad ligaments. This histologically benign condition has nevertheless produced death by tumor embolization and obstruction of blood flow from the right atrium. A similar histologic picture is seen with the rare disseminated intraperitoneal leiomyomatosis, which is characterized by subperitoneal implants throughout the pelvis and abdomen and is found most commonly associated with pregnancy or high-estrogen states. Usually regression is noted in both of the above conditions following cessation of estrogen stimulation.

The eventual fate of most leiomyomata is determined by their relatively poor vascularity, which is derived from one or two arteries at the base. Their arterial supply is significantly less than that of a similar-sized area of normal myometrium. Eventually, with continued growth, the leiomyoma outgrows its blood supply and degeneration occurs. As the discrepancy between the leiomyoma's growth and its blood supply worsens, so does the degree of degeneration: hyaline (mild), myxomatous, calcific, cystic, fatty, or red degeneration and necrosis (severe). The most acute form of degeneration (red or carneous) causes severe pain and localized peritoneal irritation, and occurs in 5–10% of pregnant women with leiomyomata. However, 80% of leiomyomata remain unchanged during pregnancy, and those that do enlarge are usually asymptomatic. Two thirds of all leiomyomata undergo some degeneration, with hyaline (65%), myxomatous (15%), and calcific (10%) being the most common types.

The incidence of malignant degeneration is estimated to range from 0.3% to 0.7%. However, it is unknown whether leiomyomata degenerate into sarcomas or whether sarcomas arise spontaneously in leiomyomatous uteri.

Symptoms and Signs

Leiomyomata are often asymptomatic. Symptoms and their severity depend on the number, size, and location of the tumors within the uterus. One third of women who present with leiomyomata report abnormal uterine bleeding, which is usually menorrhagia, but intermenstrual spotting can occur. The exact cause-and-effect relationship between myomas and abnormal bleeding is difficult to determine. Submucosal tumors, commonly associated with menorrhagia, have large, unprotected surface areas and fragile, thin-walled sinusoidal vessels with little or no covering endometrium. Small pressure changes within the uterine cavity, or within the vessels themselves, may induce rupture of vessel walls and promote sustained, heavy bleeding. Abnormal bleeding associated with intramural or large subserous myomata is believed to occur from impedance of venous return from the endometrium.

One third of patients with leiomyomata report pelvic pain or pressure, usually acquired dysmenorrhea or a sensation of pelvic heaviness. There is no consistent relationship between the dimensions or location of myomata with the complaints of pain or pressure. Enlarging myomata can produce pressure symptoms similar to those of an enlarging pregnant uterus (eg, increasing abdominal girth without an associated weight change). Anterior growth may create urinary frequency and urgency. Bilateral or unilateral hydroureters may occur silently from partial obstruction by large myomata. Rectal symptoms are much less common than urinary symptoms. On occasion, a submucous myoma will outgrow its blood supply, separate from the endometrium, and abort into the vagina through the endocervical canal. However, various forms of vascular compromise, either acute degeneration or pedicle torsion, usually produce severe pelvic pain. The pain associated with leiomyomata, however, is difficult to distinguish from the pain of endometriosis, pelvic infection, or sigmoid disease.

The relationship of myomata to reproductive dysfunction (eg, infertility, pregnancy loss) is poorly understood and often difficult to establish. Uterine myomata are associated with infertility in 5–10% of cases. However, when all other causes of infertility are eliminated, myomata alone are responsible for infertility in only 2–3% of cases. Several theories exist that may explain why myomata may interfere with fertility.

Submucous myomata may interfere with implantation by disrupting the overlying endometrium through vascular, endocrine, or mechanical alterations causing atrophy or ulceration. Additionally, large submucous or intramural myomata may cause tubal obstruction or distort the uterine cavity sufficiently to interfere with sperm ascension, prevent nidation, or cause spontaneous abortion. Before a myomectomy is performed for an infertile patient, a complete infertility investigation should be carried out to assess the significance of the myomata in the overall problem.

If possible, additional infertility factors should be corrected before surgery. Recurrent pregnancy loss, which is estimated to afflict 1 in 200 (0.5%) women, is caused by uterine factors (congenital anomalies, intrauterine synechiae, myomata) in approximately 15% of cases. As with infertility, other etiologies for repetitive pregnancy loss should be investigated before the myomata are blamed and removed surgically. Myomata that are in, or significantly encroach upon, the endometrial cavity may disrupt a conception.

Diagnosis

Presumptive diagnosis of myomata uteri can be made initially by abdominal or bimanual pelvic examination with the finding of an enlarged, usually irregularly shaped uterus. Errors can be made on physical examination: a retroflexed uterus may be diagnosed as a posterior uterine wall myoma projecting into the cul-de-sac; an inflammatory, neoplastic, or endometriotic mass may become adherent to the uterus and diagnosed as a myoma; and generalized uterine enlargement may be a pregnancy or adenomyosis.

Ultrasonography, magnetic resonance imaging, and hysterosalpingography have aided diagnosis, but they have limitations as well. Ultrasonography may not detect small (<1.5 cm) myomata, and an adherent solid ovarian tumor may be misdiagnosed as a myoma. Although expensive, an magnetic resonance imaging may be useful in demonstrating small myomata uteri, localizing the myomata within the uterus, and identifying whether there is impingement on the uterine cavity by the myomata. The one distinct advantage of magnetic resonance imaging over the other diagnostic modalities is its ability to differentiate adenomyosis from myomata uteri. This ability is especially helpful when myomectomy is being considered as one of the treatment options. Hysterosalpingography under fluoroscopic guidance should demonstrate intrauterine filling defects, but a myoma may be misdiagnosed as a polyp or a gestational sac.

Treatment

Just the presence of leiomyomata uteri does not require intervention. The asymptomatic patient may be managed expectantly with pelvic or ultrasound evaluation every 3–6 months to rule out rapid enlargement. After an initial follow-up visit at 3 months, if the uterine size is stable, examination every 6 months may be reasonable, unless the menstrual pattern changes or symptoms appear related to an enlarging uterine mass. If there is any question about ovarian enlargement or the uterine mass masks a good adnexal examination, pelvic ultrasonography (or, rarely, magnetic resonance imaging) should be used to identify the ovaries.

Most women will not need surgery, especially perimenopausal patients in whom diminishing levels of circulating estrogens may slow or stop the growth of myomata. If pregnancy occurs, close follow-up is recommended for the entire gestation. Early ultrasonography will indicate whether the myoma is near the implantation site.

A pregnant patient with significant leiomyomata should be informed about the potential for pain, spontaneous abortion, premature labor, placental abruption (especially with a retroplacental myoma), fetal malpresentation, uterine rupture, cesarean delivery, and postpartum hemorrhage. Occasionally during pregnancy, a myoma will undergo degeneration with localized pain, peritonitis, fever, and leukocytosis. The vast majority of these patients can be treated conservatively with analgesics, heat, and rest.

The medical modalities that can be used to treat nonpregnant women with leiomyomata who become symptomatic with enlarging tumors or excessive bleeding are danazol, progestins, or GnRH agonists. Progestins in high doses for 2–3 weeks may induce myomatous degeneration, but they are not consistent in performance and, on occasion, can lead to hemorrhage. As danazol has less estrogen suppression and more side effects, GnRH agonists are preferred. Short-term (12 weeks) GnRH agonist preoperative therapy aids surgery by producing uterine or tumor shrinkage and reducing or eliminating menstrual flow, thus allowing correction of any anemia. The mean reduction in uterine volume may be as much as 40–50%.

The profound estrogen deficiency associated with GnRH agonists that might lead to osteoporosis limits their use to 6 months. Once stopped, the leiomyomata usually return to their original size within 6 months. Therefore, at the moment, medical therapy with GnRH agonists is useful for allowing correction of anemia in the preoperative patient, reducing uterine or myoma size so that hysteroscopic myomectomy or vaginal hysterectomy may be easier to carry out, or carrying the perimenopausal patient into menopause so that surgery can be avoided.

If symptoms occur (rapid enlargement, pressure or pain, or continued or recurrent menorrhagia), operative therapy must be considered. The choice between a myomectomy and hysterectomy is usually determined by the patient's age, parity, future reproductive plans, and her own desires as to the surgical procedure.

Myomectomies may be performed endoscopically (hysteroscopy or laparoscopy) or by laparotomy. Hysteroscopic myomectomy may be considered with submucous myomas less than 3 cm. Experienced hysteroscopists may consider removing larger myomas. While laparoscopic excision of small subserous or intramural myomas may be possible, these tumors rarely cause symptoms or reproductive problems. The long-term risks and benefits of this approach are not known, and clinical trials are needed to evaluate reproductive sequelae before laparoscopic myomectomy is performed routinely in women desiring future reproduction.

Before a myomectomy is performed by laparotomy, the patient should be informed of the possible need for intraoperative blood transfusion, and a discussion concerning the option of donating autologous blood seems reasonable. There is a higher likelihood of transfusion with myomectomy (10–15%) than with hysterectomy (5–10%).

The abdominal incision may be a low vertical, Pfannenstiel, or Maylard type; a Maylard incision offers unparalleled exposure to the side walls, even in women with very large myomata. To decrease postoperative adhesion formation, single uterine incision is preferable to multiple incisions or a transcavitary approach. The optimal uterine incision for adhesion prevention and blood loss reduction is anterior and midline vertical, with the resulting closure being away from the cornu and adnexa. Posterior uterine incisions are more likely to adhere to the adnexa or bowel. All myomata should be removed. Tiny, seedling myomata of less than 1 cm may be vaporized with a laser or fulgurated by cautery. To avoid damaging the fallopian tubes, the uterine cornu must be identified and protected during surgery.

During surgery, meticulous hemostasis will help reduce blood loss. Additionally, the local injection of a solution containing 20 U of vasopressin in 40 ml of saline is usually sufficient to reduce blood loss. Other available hemostatic techniques include applying rubber-shod vascular clamps to compress the ovarian and uterine vessels and placing a catheter around the lower uterine segment to occlude the uterine vessels.

The myometrial defects should be closed carefully from the base outward to ensure that all dead space has been eliminated. The myometrium is usually approximated with two layers (sometimes one layer) of no. 2-0 absorbable, synthetic suture placed in a nonlocking, running fashion to achieve hemostasis while minimizing myometrial necrosis. Often the deeper pockets require interrupted, figure-of-eight sutures of the same material. After successful myometrial closure, a no. 4-0 synthetic absorbable suture is run in a subcuticularlike manner to approximate the serosal edges, leaving no suture material exposed in the peritoneal cavity.

Although there are no prospective, randomized studies evaluating the use of perioperative adjuvants such as broad-spectrum antibiotics and adhesion-prevention techniques, many surgeons use these modalities in an attempt to reduce postmyomectomy morbidity. At present, a small-pore-size, knitted fabric of oxidized regenerated cellulose is the resorbable barrier method of choice in hopes of reducing or preventing postmyomectomy adhesion formation. After closure of the uterine serosa, the barrier is placed over the uterine incision, moistened with saline, and left in the peritoneal cavity. It can be placed via laparoscopy or laparotomy, but, if it works, it will do so only in a completely bloodless field.

If postoperative pregnancy is desired, delaying conception depends on the number, size, and depth of the myomectomy incisions. When only the superficial myometrial layer has been entered, waiting 4–6 weeks postoperatively is reasonable. However, multiple myomectomy incisions or penetrations into, or near, the endometrial cavity necessitate a 4–6-month postoperative wait before attempting conception. Once pregnancy occurs, care can be routine unless an obstetric problem intervenes. If the myomectomy involved minimal myometrial trauma, a trial of labor should be considered. An elective cesarean delivery should be scheduled after a myomectomy in which multiple uterine incisions were made or the uterine cavity was encroached upon or entered.

The myoma recurrence rate after myomectomy is in the range of 15–20%. Following multiple myomectomy, the recurrence rate is higher than after removal of a solitary myoma. As would be expected, the likelihood of recurrence appears to increase with a lengthening follow-up period.

Hysterectomy remains the definitive treatment for leiomyomata uteri. In the United States, approximately 200,000 hysterectomies are performed each year, compared with an estimated 20,000 myomectomies. The route for hysterectomy depends on the patient's anatomy and the surgeon's experience. Vaginal hysterectomy is usually performed in women with a mobile uterus equal in size to, or smaller than, a uterus at 12 weeks of gestation, especially where there is uterine descensus. If the surgeon is experienced in techniques such as morcellation, bivalving, and coring, a larger uterus may be amendable to the vaginal approach. Additionally, presurgical therapy with GnRH agonists may produce enough uterine volume shrinkage to permit vaginal hysterectomy. If there is a reason to evaluate the adnexa, or seriously consider their removal, laparoscopically assisted vaginal hysterectomy might be considered by the endoscopically talented surgeon with smaller leiomyomatous uteri. However, the classic, definitive approach remains the abdominal hysterectomy.

ADENOMYOSIS

Adenomyosis is a benign uterine disease characterized by the presence of ectopic endometrial glands and stroma within the myometrium. It evolves spontaneously from a downward growth of the basalis layer of the endometrium; thus, the glands rarely undergo the cyclic changes seen in the more superficial layers of the endometrium, which respond to hormonal shifts. Adenomyosis is most often an incidental pathologic finding. Its frequency depends on the meticulousness of the pathologist. With multiple serial uterine wall sections, the incidence may exceed 60% in women aged 40–50 years. It is associated with leiomyomata uteri 50% of the time and with endometriosis less than 20%.

Histogenesis and Pathology

The most accepted of all the unproven theories of the origin of adenomyosis is that of basoendometrial invasion. Because adenomyosis is noted most often in parous women, one hypothesis is that chronic postpartum endometritis may create the initial break in the barrier between the endometrium and the myometrium. Initially, the stroma and then the glands begin to invade the myometrium along the path of least resistance adjacent to lymphatic and vascular channels.

Grossly, adenomyosis presents in two different ways. Most commonly, a diffuse involvement of both anterior and posterior uterine walls occurs, with greater growth seen in the posterior wall. Unlike leiomyomata uteri, the areas of adenomyomatous enlargement are not encapsulated. The second presentation occurs as focal areas known as adenomyomas. They may result in an asymmetric uterus with the involved areas surrounded by a pseudocapsule.

With diffuse enlargement, the uterus grows uniformly and can be two or three times normal size, making it difficult to distinguish grossly from leiomyomata uteri. Histologically, the ingrowing endometrial glands and stroma are usually more than one low-power field (2.5 mm) away from the basilar layer of the endometrium. Surrounding most foci of glands and stroma are localized areas of uterine smooth muscle hyperplasia. There are no progesterone receptors and few estrogen receptors in adenomyosis tissue, compared with the number of receptors found in normal endometrium. This receptor lack may help to explain the relative insensitivity of adenomyosis to hormonal suppression.

Symptoms and Signs

Eighty percent of cases occur in parous women. In one series, only 4% of women with adenomyosis had their first child after age 30. The vast majority of symptomatic cases occur in women aged 35–50 years. Adenomyosis has been reported in 5–10% of menopausal uteri and in 15% of women under age 40. There appears to be no particular racial predilection. Most women with adenomyosis are asymptomatic or have minor symptoms (eg, an increase in menstrual flow or dysmenorrhea) that they attribute to the aging process, and, therefore, they do not seek medical care.

The classic symptoms of adenomyosis are secondary dysmenorrhea (15–30%) and menorrhagia (40–50%). As the disease progresses, dysmenorrhea becomes more severe. Occasionally (7%), deep, midline dyspareunia becomes a problem. On pelvic examination, the uterus is diffusely enlarged, usually two or three times normal size. Before and during menstruation, the uterus is globular and tender. The frequency and severity of symptoms and the extent of disease appear to be positively correlated. The etiology of these symptoms is commonly ascribed to the effects of bleeding into the wall of the uterus, with the resulting edema and inflammation causing pain and abnormal uterine bleeding patterns.

Diagnosis

The presumptive diagnosis of adenomyosis is made by obtaining a typical history, along with the physical examination finding of a diffusely enlarged, soft uterus that does not contain a pregnancy. Most clinicians preoperatively diagnose adenomyosis in only 25% of the cases diagnosed postoperatively by the pathologist.

Hysterosalpingography may demonstrate intramural channels filled with dye, which suggests adenomyosis. Unfortunately, this finding may be difficult to distinguish from intravasation or intralymphatic dye. Transvaginal ultrasound examination may demonstrate irregular cystic spaces in the myometrium secondary to adenomyotic implants. Magnetic resonance imaging, although expensive, can be extremely helpful in delineating the globular enlargement due to myomata uteri. Since adenomyosis cannot be managed by conservative surgery and myomata uteri can be treated by myomectomy, preoperative differentiation by magnetic resonance imaging will prevent unnecessary, noncorrective surgery.

Treatment

There is no long-term, satisfactory medical treatment for adenomyosis. Cyclic oral contraceptives, if not contraindicated because of age or medical reasons, can be used, but success is variable and there are anecdotal reports of worsening dysmenorrhea after cessation of therapy. Prostaglandin synthetase inhibitors may relieve pain and decrease bleeding, but significant success is unlikely. While GnRH agonists may suppress adenomyosis growth, any benefit lasts only as long as the drug is continued. Recurrence of growth and symptoms occurs after drug therapy is stopped. Unlike myomata uteri, for which myomectomy can follow GnRH agonist therapy, there is no conservative surgery for adenomyosis; thus, "preoperative" treatment with GnRH agonists is nonexistent. If a patient is perimenopausal with anticipated cessation of ovarian function, medical therapy with GnRH agonists may obviate the need for hysterectomy.

If appropriate for the woman's age, parity, and future reproductive plans, hysterectomy remains the definitive treatment. Uterine size, the degree of prolapse, and the presence or absence of adnexal abnormalities will determine whether hysterectomy is performed abdominally, vaginally, or by laparoscopically assisted vaginal hysterectomy.

ENDOMETRIAL POLYPS

The second most common benign tumor of the uterus, endometrial polyps are localized overgrowths of endometrial glands and stroma that project above the endometrial surface and, on occasion, can prolapse through the endocervical canal. They are soft, pliable, single, or multiple and usually arise from the upper endometrial cavity. Their size varies from millimeters to several centimeters in diameter. They may be broad based (sessile) or attached to the endometrial wall by a pedicle (penduculated). Although the peak incidence is between 40 and 50 years of age, they occur in all age groups. The etiology of endometrial polyps is unknown, but, as they can be associated with endometrial hyperplasia, unopposed estrogen has been suggested as a possible contributing factor.

Grossly, polyps are plump and velvety and have a central vascular core. Color varies from gray-tan to red-brown. Histologically, a polyp has glands, stroma, and vessels. Like a peninsula, there is endometrium on three sides. Approximately two thirds of polyps will have immature, nonresponding endometrium that will have a cystic hyperplastic appearance no matter what the cycle phase may be. The other third will have functional endometrium that will undergo cyclic histologic change. Low-grade, low-stage, malignant transformation occurs in 0.5% of polyps, but the subsequent risk of endometrial carcinoma in women with endometrial polyps is only twofold.

Most endometrial polyps are asymptomatic. Those that are symptomatic have varied bleeding patterns. Premenstrual, postmenstrual, and intermenstrual spotting is the most common abnormality. As mentioned, occasionally a pedunculated endometrial polyp may protrude through the cervix.

Treatment of endometrial polyps can be accomplished by curettage or, preferably, by hysteroscopy. Hysteroscopy provides visual guidance to ensure that all polyps have been identified and removed. Polyps are mobile and can elude a curette, so that, without hysteroscopic help, approximately 25% of endometrial polyps may be missed.

OTHER BENIGN UTERINE DISORDERS

Adenofibromas are more common in the ovaries, but they can occur in the uterus, cervix, and fallopian tubes. Typically, the broad-based polypoid mass protrudes into the uterine cavity at the time of diagnosis. Histology demonstrates fibrous stroma and papillary structures covered by a müllerian epithelium that can be endometrial, endocervical, tubal, or mixed. The papillary cystadenofibroma is the benign counterpart to the malignant mixed müllerian tumor.

Adenomatoid tumors are small, discrete nodules that are well circumscribed, yet lack a distinct capsule. They are probably of mesothelial origin, and their histology demonstrates irregular clefts lined by mesotheliallike cells and loose stroma but no cellular anaplasia. Usually, tumors are found incidentally at surgery.

Lipomas, angiomas, lipomyomas, and neuromas may occur in the uterus. Likewise, these are typically incidental findings at surgery.

UTERINE CONSERVATION AT TIME OF ADNEXAL REMOVAL

When they are supported by exogenous hormones that mimic the endocrinology of pregnancy, women without adnexa have successfully supported implanted embryos. Therefore, in a woman faced with adnexal removal during her reproductive years, the possibility of uterine conservation should be discussed. If uterine preservation at the time of bilateral adnexectomy is elected, the patient should be made aware of the potential for future benign and malignant uterine disease; the probability that these conditions would require hysterectomy for treatment; the possibility of hysterectomy at the time of bilateral adnexectomy if the adnexa cannot be separated from the fundus secondary to severe obliterative pathologic lesions, such as an abscess or extensive endometriosis; and the distinct possibility of abnormal uterine bleeding with the use of indicated hormonal replacement therapy.

BIBLIOGRAPHY

American Fertility Society. Myomas and reproductive dysfunction: guideline for practice. Birmingham, Alabama: AFS, 1992

Coddington CC, Brzyski R, Hansen KA, Corley DR, McIntrye-Seltman K, Jones HW Jr. Short term treatment with leuprolide acetate is a successful adjunct to surgical therapy of leiomyomas of the uterus. Surg Gynecol Obstet 1992;175:57–63

Friedman AJ, Hoffman DI, Comite F, Browneller RW, Miller JD. Treatment of leiomyomata uteri with leuprolide acetate depot: a double-blind, placebo-controlled, multicenter study. The Leuprolide Study Group. Obstet Gynecol 1991;77:720–725

Herbst AL, Mishell DR Jr, Stenchever MA, Droegemueller W. Comprehensive gynecology. 2nd ed. St Louis: Mosby–Year Book, 1992

Rice JP, Kay HH, Mahony BS. The clinical significance of uterine leiomyomas in pregnancy. Am J Obstet Gynecol 1989;160:1212–1216

Smith DC, Uhlir JK. Myomectomy as a reproductive procedure. Am J Obstet Gynecol 1990;162:1476–1479; discussion 1479–1482

Verkauf BS. Myomectomy for fertility enhancement and preservation. Fertil Steril 1992;58:1–15

Tubal and Peritoneal Factors

ECTOPIC PREGNANCY

The incidence of ectopic pregnancy has increased dramatically in the United States over the past two decades. Between 1970 and 1987 the total number of ectopic pregnancies in the United States increased from 17,800 to 88,000 and the rate increased from 4.5/1,000 to 16.8/1,000 pregnancies during the same time frame. Paradoxically, the fatality rate declined 90%, from 35.5/10,000 in 1970 to 3.4/10,000 in 1987. In 1987, the mortality rate reported by the Centers for Disease Control and Prevention (CDC) was 0.034% (30 deaths in 88,000 cases). These trends have been only partially explained. The increase in sexually transmitted diseases, which began in the 1960s, has been identified as a major risk factor; the rate of increase in sexually transmitted diseases, however, does not parallel the rise in the incidence of ectopic pregnancy. Of patients with ectopic pregnancy, 50–70% have histologically normal fallopian tubes. The more prevalent application of conservative surgery, IUDs, ovulation-inducing drugs that alter estrogen and progestin levels, and previous ectopic pregnancy have all been identified as risk factors for ectopic pregnancy. The widespread application of sensitive radioimmunoassays for the serum beta subunit of human chorionic gonadotropin (β-hCG), improved resolution of ultrasonography, and the more aggressive use of laparoscopy for diagnosis and treatment have contributed to earlier and more consistent diagnosis. This, in turn, has increased the number of patients being diagnosed with ectopic pregnancy and contributed to a reduction in mortality.

Sites of Extrauterine Pregnancy

Ninety-five percent of ectopic pregnancies occur in the fallopian tube; 90% of tubal pregnancies occur within the ampullary portion of the tube; 8% occur in the isthmic segment; and the remaining 2% are interstitial, intramural, cornual, and cervical pregnancies.

Abdominal pregnancy is a rare form of ectopic pregnancy (1/15,000 deliveries), and it occurs after primary implantation in the abdomen or partial implantation of a tubal abortion. These pregnancies usually present as abdominal pain and the presence of an extrauterine mass. The diagnosis may be reliably established by ultrasound examination. Abdominal pregnancy is associated with high maternal and fetal mortality, and conservative management is not warranted. The placenta should be removed only when it is loosely attached to intraabdominal structures, the bleeding from the implantation site is minimal, and the bleeding can be easily controlled. In cases in which these criteria are not met, the umbilical cord should be trimmed and ligated and the placenta should be left in situ. The retained placenta is usually absorbed within 8–12 weeks, and prophylactic antibiotics are indicated.

Cervical pregnancy is also a rare form of ectopic pregnancy, usually associated with implantation in the lower uterine segment with prolapse into the upper portion of the cervical canal. These patients usually present with vaginal bleeding and cervical enlargement. Hysterectomy is often required for treatment. More recently, methotrexate has been successfully used in the treatment of early cervical pregnancy. The risk of massive hemorrhage exists with all conservative procedures, and they should be undertaken only under special circumstances.

Heterotopic pregnancy, combined intrauterine and ectopic pregnancy, has been reported to occur at the rate of 1/30,000 deliveries. This incidence was calculated in 1948 based on the ectopic pregnancy and dizygotic twinning rates at that time. This incidence is not reflective of current risk, since both ectopic pregnancy and dizygotic twinning (particularly in patients receiving ovulation induction therapy) have increased significantly. The current estimated incidence of heterotopic pregnancy ranges from 1/4,000 to 1/15,000, and an incidence of 1% has been described in assisted reproductive technology programs.

Subsequent Fertility

Fertility potential after treatment of ectopic pregnancy appears to have improved over the past 30 years. Approximately 30% of patients treated with salpingectomy in the 1960s had a successful intrauterine pregnancy. Fertility rates of 60–70% have been described for patients undergoing both conservative surgical procedures and salpingectomy in the past 15 years. The presence of preexisting infertility and the condition of the tubes are important determinants for future fertility. The risk of future tubal pregnancy after salpingectomy is 12–15%. The most recent studies have described a higher risk after conservative surgery. Following two ectopic pregnancies, only one third of patients achieve pregnancy without assisted reproductive technology, and the risk of ectopic pregnancy is dramatically increased.

Diagnosis

The diagnosis of ectopic pregnancy is often established in two different settings. The classic clinical presentation of pelvic pain, abnormal uterine bleeding, and a pelvic mass is commonly encountered in emergency departments and other acute care facilities. However, an increasing number of patients are diagnosed prior to clinical symptomatology by using serial serum β-hCG radioimmunoassays, ultrasonography, and laparoscopy. Patients at high risk for ectopic pregnancy, including those with a history of pelvic inflammatory disease, previous tubal surgery, and previous ectopic pregnancy can be followed prospectively from the time that pregnancy is confirmed. Although no one test will confirm the diagnosis of ectopic pregnancy with certainty, the available tests in aggregate usually permit the diagnosis to be established in a timely manner, often before laparoscopy.

The serum β-hCG radioimmunoassay remains the most valuable diagnostic test, with a sensitivity of almost 100%. Serial hCG testing will identify abnormal pregnancies, ectopic pregnancy, or those destined to abort in 85% of cases if a rate of increase less than 66% within 2 days is noted. Although recent prospective studies have failed to confirm the predictive value of serial hCG testing, most clinicians have found it useful. Serum progesterone levels are also predictive of unsuccessful pregnancy. Viable pregnancies are very rarely associated with serum progesterone levels of less than 5 ng/ml within the first 6 weeks of gestation. Most viable intrauterine pregnancies are associated with serum progesterone levels greater than 15 ng/ml, and most unsuccessful pregnancies have values less than 15 ng/ml. There is considerable overlap of ranges; 98% of patients with intrauterine pregnancies have values greater than 10 ng/ml, and 98% of patients with ectopic pregnancy not associated with ovulation induction therapy have progesterone levels less than 20 ng/ml. Although an arbitrary limit cannot be defined that will distinguish viable intrauterine pregnancies from failing pregnancies, some clinicians have used lower serum progesterone levels (5 ng/ml) as criteria for interventional therapy such as dilation and curettage.

Ultrasonography has several applications in the diagnosis of ectopic pregnancy. Once pregnancy has been confirmed, it can be used to exclude the presence of intrauterine pregnancy when the discriminatory zone is exceeded. The discriminatory zone, an hCG range above which an intrauterine pregnancy can be reliably visualized, has been reported to range from 1,200 to 1,500 IU/L, using the International Reference Preparation. Discriminatory zones will vary among institutions, depending on the particular hCG assay used, the reference standard with which it is calibrated, the available ultrasound equipment, and the skill of the ultrasonographer. If a higher discriminatory value is selected, the specificity of the test increases.

Visualization of an intrauterine pregnancy essentially rules out the presence of an ectopic pregnancy, although this clinical entity (heterotopic pregnancy) does rarely occur and should, therefore, not be neglected entirely. A normal sac should be visible at 6 weeks of gestation by transabdominal ultrasonography. Fetal cardiac activity is usually demonstrable at about the same period. These time periods are reduced by 1 week with transvaginal ultrasonography; a sac can be demonstrated in most cases of normal pregnancy at 5 weeks and fetal heart motion at about 5 weeks and 2 days. The in utero pseudogestational sac in cases of ectopic pregnancy is usually in the center of the cavity, whereas a true gestational sac is most often eccentric and usually contains an asymmetric ring produced by the early trophoblast, giving it a double sac appearance. Demonstration of fetal heart motion outside of the uterus is, naturally, the definitive ultrasound documentation of the presence of an ectopic pregnancy.

The presence of solid or cystic adnexal masses, particularly when free fluid is present in the cul-de-sac, is also highly suggestive of ectopic pregnancy. Ectopic gestational sacs can also occasionally be visualized and, with the newer 6.0–9.0-Mhz vaginal transducers, localization of ectopic gestations may be more common. Color-flow Doppler technology may also enhance diagnostic accuracy, but application of this technology is more limited because of its increased expense and more limited access. If ectopic pregnancy can be diagnosed prior to laparoscopy, there may be some advantage in considering nonoperative therapy for ectopic pregnancy. In this setting, the diagnosis may be established by direct visualization of an ectopic gestational sac with ultrasonography or if the hCG levels exceed the discriminatory zone and there is no evidence of intrauterine pregnancy. Dilation and curettage can be performed in patients with nonviable pregnancies detected by serum progesterone levels less than 5 ng/ml or with serial hCG levels failing to show an appropriate increase.

Treatment

Conservative surgery, performed at laparoscopy if possible, is the treatment of choice for ectopic pregnancy in women desiring future fertility. Patients with ruptured fallopian tubes, those who are not hemodynamically stable, and those not desirous of subsequent fertility should be treated with salpingectomy, since hemostasis can be achieved more expeditiously and future risk minimized.

If laparoscopy is required for diagnosis, treatment should be accomplished at surgery. A variety of surgical techniques can be performed through the laparoscope, including salpingectomy, partial salpingectomy, and linear salpingostomy. The last is the procedure of choice for unruptured, ampullary pregnancy. The tube is opened over the antemesenteric surface or at the point of maximum distention, using scalpel, fine cautery, or laser. The conceptus is gently expressed through the opening, and the tubal lumen is gently irrigated. Hemostasis can be achieved with point cautery or laser, injection of vasopressin, or compression of the underlying mesosalpinx. The serosal defect is usually left open to close by secondary intent (salpingostomy). Closure of the serosal defect with fine, nonreactive, interrupted sutures (salpingotomy) is more difficult to perform through the laparoscope and offers no advantage over salpingostomy. Fimbrial expression has also been used for the treatment of ampullary ectopic pregnancy and should be reserved with those pregnancies in which spontaneous tubal abortion is under way, since it otherwise unduly traumatizes the tube and is associated with higher rates of persistent and recurrent ectopic pregnancy.

Segmental resection may be performed for isthmic ectopic pregnancy, particularly when rupture has occurred. Isthmic pregnancy is more often associated with significant tubal distortion and is less amenable to linear salpingostomy. However, some early isthmic pregnancies can be treated with a simple linear incision and removal of the conceptus.

Persistent ectopic pregnancy, the continued proliferation of trophoblast after conservative surgical treatment, is a risk unique to patients undergoing conservative surgery. Approximately 5% of patients who do not have extirpative surgery have clinical evidence of a persistent ectopic pregnancy, usually presenting again with symptoms of ectopic pregnancy. Risk of persistent ectopic pregnancy may be slightly higher in patients treated at laparoscopy. Patients receiving conservative surgery should be apprised of this risk and monitored with weekly β-hCG determinations following surgery. Additional therapy, either methotrexate or additional surgery, is indicated for patients who have rising hCG levels.

Some patients with early tubal pregnancy experience spontaneous tubal abortion without clinical sequelae. Asymptomatic patients with suspected ectopic pregnancy who have declining hCG levels can be followed expectantly, provided that they remain hemodynamically stable, remain essentially pain free, and have no other findings on examination that would prompt surgical intervention.

Systemic methotrexate therapy has been documented to be effective treatment for ectopic pregnancy in several series. A variety of regimens, including 1- and 4-day courses of oral, intramuscular, or intravenous methotrexate have all proven to be effective. A simple and highly effective regimen (95% effectiveness) is a single injection of methotrexate, 50 mg/m^2, without subsequent leucovorin therapy. Patients should have a marked decline in hCG levels 7 days after therapy, or a second dose is indicated. Significant morbidity has not been described with this regimen. Preliminary results suggest that future fertility is comparable to that after surgical treatment. However, if laparoscopy is required for diagnosis, systemic methotrexate therapy offers no advantage over surgical treatment at laparoscopy.

Several compounds, including methotrexate, potassium chloride, prostaglandins, and hyperosmolar glucose, have been injected directly into the gestational sac at laparoscopy, with transvaginal ultrasound needle guidance, or by retrograde catheter placement. This technique is called salpingocentesis and appears to be somewhat less effective than systemic treatment with methotrexate.

ENDOMETRIOSIS

Endometriosis is defined as the presence of ectopic endometrial tissue, histologically confirmed by the presence of endometrial glands and stroma and often hemosiderin-laden macrophages. It is typically found on dependent surfaces in the pelvis and most often affects the posterior cul-de-sac and ovaries. Although histologically benign, it has a unique ability to invade and destroy tissues and cause severe inflammation and adhesion formation. Although the true prevalence of endometriosis is unknown, it is estimated to exist in approximately 7% of U.S. women of reproductive age. The etiologies of endometriosis include the transport theory (tubal regurgitation or lymphatic and hematogenous spread) and the coelomic metaplasia theory. Endometriosis may cause symptoms as a result of the disruption of normal tissue and the development of fibrosis and adhesions.

Diagnosis

The diagnosis of endometriosis should be suspected if a history of dysmenorrhea, dyspareunia, and premenstrual backache is noted with or without infertility. Signs include pelvic nodularity with tenderness, particularly over the uterosacral ligaments; uterine retroversion with decreased mobility; and adnexal enlargement with tenderness. Ovarian endometriomas have a characteristic appearance on ultrasonography, with irregular edges and internal echoes produced by chronic intracystic bleeding. Serum antigen CA 125 levels are helpful in detecting and monitoring more severe cases but are not specific for this condition. Computed tomography and magnetic resonance imaging have a limited role in the diagnosis of endometriosis because they usually fail to detect superficial lesions, but they may be helpful in delineating pathologic changes in more extensive cases, particularly when there is extensive fibrosis and distortion. The diagnosis can be substantiated only by laparoscopy or laparotomy. It is important to assess correctly not only the presence of but also the extent of endometriosis. Peritoneal biopsy is desirable although not necessary for the diagnosis if recognizable lesions are present. It is used for diagnostic confirmation in doubtful circumstances.

Endometriosis should be carefully documented by using the revised classification of endometriosis recommended by the American Fertility Society (Fig. 4-3). Although the current classification system does not take into account atypical presentations of the disease (ie, brown patches, petechiae, yellow-white patches, peritoneal windows, or retroperitoneal involvement), this classification does allow for a careful description of visible peritoneal disease, specific organ involvement, and adhesion formation.

Treatment

Choice of treatment of endometriosis is influenced by the patient's age, symptomatology, and goals. Although minimal and mild forms of endometriosis appear to be more prevalent in patients with infertility, a comprehensive understanding of pathogenesis is lacking. It is clear that hormonal suppression of minimal and mild disease is not effective treatment for infertility. A significant number of these patients will conceive without any therapy. Superovulation, with and without intrauterine inseminations, and assisted reproductive technology offer some promise.

Hormonal therapy is usually reserved for patients with pelvic pain due to endometriosis. Although not consistently confirmed by studies, preoperative hormonal suppression may facilitate surgical treatment for patients with extensive disease. Oral contraceptives, progestins, danazol, and GnRH agonists appear to be effective in reducing pelvic pain. Treatment may also be effective in reducing the progression of disease, but this benefit is not as well documented. Contraindications to medical therapy include hypersensitivity to any of the individual agents, undiagnosed abnormal vaginal bleeding, pregnancy, breast-feeding, and specific contraindications to oral contraceptives. Specific contraindications to danazol include impaired hepatic, renal, or cardiac function. Progestins and oral contraceptives are also contraindicated in women with a history of thromboembolic disease and in smokers over age 35. Hormonal therapy is ineffective in resolving large endometriomas and has no effect on adhesion formation. Danazol, 400–800 mg daily; GnRH agonists, including leuprolide, nafarelin, buserelin, and goserelin; or medroxyprogesterone acetate, 30 mg daily, appear to be comparably effective in relieving pain. Treatment is usually continued for 6 months. Menses usually recur within 6 weeks of stopping danazol therapy but may take 8–10 weeks to be reestablished after GnRH analogue therapy. Danazol therapy is associated with deleterious alterations in lipoprotein fractions. GnRH analogue therapy produces hypoestrogenism and modest loss of bone mineral density. This treatment should be limited to 6 months.

Surgical treatment often can be accomplished at laparoscopy. Conservative or limited surgery is appropriate for patients desiring future fertility. Conservative procedures include excision, vaporization, and coagulation of endometrial implants; excision of ovarian endometriomas; and lysis of adhesions. These techniques can be accomplished at laparoscopy with surgical excision, laser (carbon dioxide, argon, potassium–titanyl–phosphate, or Nd:YAG), and monopolar or bipolar electrocautery. Conservative surgery is most often performed through the laparoscope; with extensive disease with cul-de-sac obliteration and dense scarring of the ovaries to the pelvic sidewalls, laparotomy may be preferable. Adjunct procedures, including presacral neurectomy and uterosacral nerve ablation, have been recommended for relief of central pelvic pain. Uterosacral plication, uterine suspension, and oophoropexy have less clearly defined benefits. Patients with significant bowel involvement require resection of the affected segment and anastomosis.

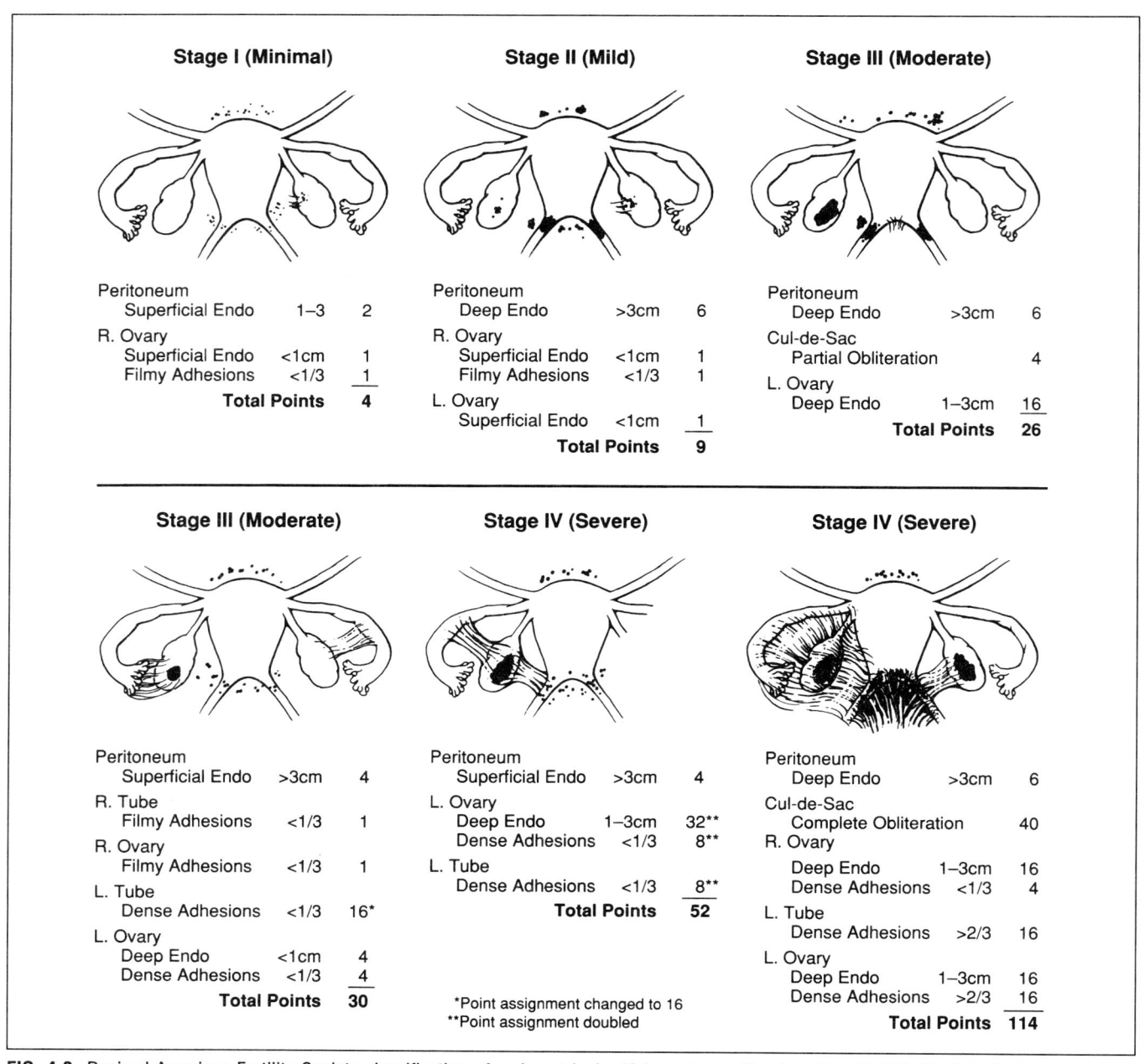

FIG. 4-3. Revised American Fertility Society classification of endometriosis. (Adapted from The American Fertility Society. Revised American Fertility Society classification of endometriosis: 1985. Fertil Steril 1985;43:351. Reproduced with permission of the publisher, The American Fertility Society.)

Definitive therapy, total abdominal hysterectomy, and bilateral salpingo-oophorectomy is indicated for patients who have completed childbearing or have significant persistent pelvic pain after conservative treatment. One or both ovaries may be spared if they are completely uninvolved and the endometriosis can be completely resected. Approximately one third of women treated conservatively will have recurrent endometriosis and require additional surgery within 5 years. After bilateral oophorectomy, estrogen replacement therapy may be initiated with little risk of reactivating residual disease. Typically, most surgeons wait 3–6 months after definitive surgery for extensive disease before initiating estrogen therapy.

BIBLIOGRAPHY

Barbieri RL. Etiology and epidemiology of endometriosis. Am J Obstet Gynecol 1990;162:565–567

Evers JL. The pregnancy rate of the no-treatment group in randomized clinical trials of endometriosis therapy. Fertil Steril 1989;52:906–907

Hull ME, Moghissi KS, Magyar DM, Hayes MF. Comparison of different treatment modalities of endometriosis in infertile women. Contrib Obstet Gynecol 1987;16:236–240

Israel R. Pelvic endometriosis. In: Mishell DR Jr, Davajan V, Lobo RA, eds. Infertility, contraception and reproductive endocrinology. 3rd ed. 1991, 723–753

Lawson HW, Atrash HK, Saftlas AF, Franks AL, Finch EL, Hughes JM. Ectopic pregnancy surveillance, United States, 1970–1987. MMWR 1988;39(SS-4):9–17

Leach RE, Ory SJ. Modern management of ectopic pregnancy. J Reprod Med 1989;34:324–333

Ory SJ. New options for diagnosis and treatment of ectopic pregnancy. JAMA 1992;267:534–537

Stovall TG, Ling FW, Buster JE. Outpatient chemotherapy of unruptured ectopic pregnancy. Fertil Steril 1989;51:435–438

Stovall TG, Ling FW, Gray LA, Carson SA, Buster JE. Methotrexate treatment of unruptured ectopic pregnancy: a report of 100 cases. Obstet Gynecol 1991;77:749–753

Vermesh M, Silva PD, Rosen GF, Stein AL, Fossum GT, Sauer MV. Management of unruptured ectopic gestation by linear salpingostomy: a prospective randomized clinical trial of laparoscopy versus laparotomy. Obstet Gynecol 1989;73:400–404

Disorders of the Ovaries

Benign ovarian processes pose one of the most common problems in gynecology. Many of these lesions occur in the reproductive years. Their proper recognition is important to allow appropriate therapy, often conservative in nature. Pain, pelvic mass, abdominal enlargement, and pressure on the rectum or bladder are common to all ovarian lesions. There are few specific symptoms that distinguish one ovarian cyst or mass from another histologic type.

NONNEOPLASTIC OVARIAN CYSTS

Follicular and Luteinized Cysts

Physiologic enlargement of the ovary may occur as a result of failure of either follicular or corpus luteum regression. These cystic changes are named according to their stage of maturation and reflect their histologic characteristics. Follicular cysts are usually thin-walled cysts with clear fluid that are 5–6 cm or less in diameter. The vast majority of these cysts regress spontaneously within 1–3 months, but they may persist and on occasion become excessively large. Occasionally, surgery is necessary because of intraperitoneal bleeding resulting from rupture of the cyst wall, persistence, symptoms, or size. At times they may be adherent to the pelvic sidewall or markedly distort the fallopian tube.

The microscopic diagnosis of the follicular cysts is usually very easy. There may be occasional difficulty with cysts of larger size, in which a single layer of cuboidal or low columnar epithelium lines the cyst wall. It is sometimes impossible to be sure whether the cyst is a follicular enlargement or a serous cyst. Demonstration of granulosa cells or theca cells permits assignment to this category. Corpus luteum cysts exhibit a convoluted lining composed of large luteinized granulosa cells and smaller luteinized theca interna cells. Involutional fibrosis of a corpus luteum or a corpus luteum cyst usually leads to formation of the corpus albicans. This entity is rarely cystic.

Multiple follicular cysts are usually secondary to elevated levels of gonadotropins and are associated with bilateral ovarian enlargement. Polycystic ovary disease is the most common cause of bilateral multiple follicular cysts, although it may also be seen in girls with juvenile hypothyroidism, 17-hydroxylase deficiency, and prematurity. Polycystic ovary disease is a spectrum of related disorders that is characterized by chronic anovulation or oligoovulation associated with increased secretion of luteinizing hormone (LH) and hyperandrogenemia or manifestations of androgen excess. It has been estimated that 3–7% of the female population may have this syndrome.

In the classic description of the syndrome, enlarged, sclerocystic ovaries with multiple follicular cysts were described. The current clinical spectrum of polycystic ovary disease does not require enlarged or polycystic ovaries for the diagnosis. In the classic form of polycystic ovary disease, the ovaries have a thickened, white cortex with numerous small follicular cysts, usually measuring 10 mm or less, and scant evidence of past ovulation (corpora lutea or albicantia). Microscopically, these cysts consist of layers of nonluteinized granulosa cells with an outer layer of theca interna cells showing varying degrees of luteinization. The deeper stroma may have an increase in volume with focal luteinization. Nests of hilar cells may be prominent.

The most common iatrogenic cause of multiple follicular cysts is ovarian hyperstimulation, which may be a consequence of ovulation induction generally with gonadotropins and rarely with clomiphene. The ovarian hyperstimulation syndrome is seen only after ovulation, most commonly 7–10 days later. Conception will worsen the syndrome because of the continued stimulation by hCG. In severe cases, the hyperstimulation syndrome may include massive ovarian enlargement, ascites, hydrothorax, and hemoconcentration. The latter may result in oliguria and a thromboembolic phenomenon that may be life threatening. Surgical intervention is very rarely necessary except in cases of torsion or rupture. Patients usually respond to conservative management with particular attention to fluid status.

Microscopically, the ovaries reveal multiple theca lutein cysts or follicular cysts with prominent luteinization of the thecal compartment. In most cases the granulosa cells are luteinized, as well. Stromal edema and stromal luteinization may be seen. Multiple theca lutein cysts may also be seen in conditions in which high levels of hCG are noted, such as hydatidiform mole, choriocarcinoma, and (rarely) multiple gestation. The frequency of this condition in gestational trophoblastic disease is approximately 10–40%, depending on whether ultrasonography is used for diagnosis. The microscopic picture is identical to that seen in the hyperstimulation syndrome and has been termed hyperreactio luteinalis.

Luteoma of Pregnancy

Although relatively rare, most patients with luteomas of pregnancy are asymptomatic and have an incidental finding at ultrasonography, cesarean delivery, or sterilization. Rarely, this ovarian enlargement may obstruct the birth canal. Approximately one fourth of these patients will experience hirsutism or virilization in the latter half of pregnancy. Maternal levels of testosterone and other androgens may be significantly elevated. Because of the rapid aromatization of androgens to estrogens by the placenta, elevated levels of androgens may be unaccompanied by maternal or fetal virilization. Rarely, mothers with signs of virilization may have female infants who show signs of virilization such as clitoromegaly and labial fusion. Regression of the ovaries begins after delivery. This is a benign, self-limited condition, and no treatment is required. The ovaries become normal within several weeks of delivery.

This nonneoplastic lesion is characterized by ovarian enlargement during pregnancy. This is generally a solid rather than cystic tumor and consists of eosinophilic, polyhedral cells that are not a part of the corpus luteum of pregnancy. These luteinized cells may grow in a diffuse, trabecular, or follicular pattern. It has been suggested that this is a profoundly exaggerated physiologic response of the ovary to the increased stimulation by hCG seen in pregnancy.

Ovarian Stromal Proliferative Disorders

Most commonly, corticostromal hyperplasia is seen in the ovaries of postmenopausal women. Although this may be an incidental finding, progressive hirsutism may be seen. Irregular bleeding may also be noted as a result of peripheral conversion of ovarian androgens to estrogens. The ovaries tend to appear somewhat enlarged but not cystic.

Stromal hyperplasia is characterized by varying degrees of nonneoplastic proliferation of stromal cells. The stromal cells in hyperplasia tend to be larger than the normal postmenopausal stromal cells. Moderate to severe stromal hyperplasia may occur in up to one third of postmenopausal women in their late sixth and seventh decades of life.

Stromal hyperplasia with focal areas of luteinized stromal cells is referred to as stromal hyperthecosis. In hyperthecosis, small clusters of polygonal cells with abundant eosinophilic or vacuolated cytoplasms are seen. These cells are commonly found in the medulla but may be seen in the cortex, as well. Although mild stromal hyperthecosis is found in one third of autopsies of women over age 50, the more severe cases are found in younger women. Stromal hyperthecosis is a disorder that clinically may be very similar to polycystic ovary disease. More severe cases may exhibit marked virilization, obesity, and insulin resistance. Some patients with hyperthecosis have the syndrome that consists of hyperandrogenism, insulin resistance, and acanthosis nigricans. Studies have noted a 50–250-fold increase in androgen secretion from the ovarian stroma of these patients when compared with normal ovarian stroma. Moreover, insulin and LH can increase the secretion of androgens into the media. It has been postulated that the primary defect is insulin resistance leading to hyperinsulinemia and that the other abnormalities are secondary. Evidence is rapidly accumulating to suggest the validity of this hypothesis.

As the name suggests, hilar or Leydig cell hyperplasia is usually found in the hilus of the ovaries and is characterized by an increase in the number of cells in a nodular or diffuse arrangement. An increase in cell size, cellular and nuclear pleiomorphism, hyperchromasia, multinucleation, and mitotic figures may be seen. Severe degrees of hyperplasia are often associated with virilization. Although most common in postmenopausal ovaries, this entity may also be seen in younger women with or without an associated pregnancy.

Germinal Epithelial Cysts

Although these lesions have no connection to the ovarian cortex, surface epithelial inclusion cysts or germinal epithelial cysts are thought to arise from invaginations of the ovarian surface epithelium. These lesions are commonly seen in postmenopausal women, although they have been demonstrated microscopically in females of all ages, including infants. Although occasionally visible to the naked eye, these lesions are usually microscopic and may be seen singly or in clusters throughout the ovarian cortex. These cysts are usually lined by a single layer of cuboidal or columnar epithelium, although other cell types such as tubal, endometrioid, or endocervical epithelium have been described. Although data are lacking, it has been proposed that these ovarian inclusion cysts give rise to most common epithelial tumors of the ovary.

BENIGN OVARIAN NEOPLASMS

Serous Cystadenomas

Serous cystadenomas are common tumors, comprising about 20% of all ovarian neoplasms. Most are found in the reproductive years, although they have been found in infancy as well. In approximately 10% of patients, the tumors are bilateral. It has been proposed that these benign lesions arise through invagination of the surface epithelium, as these tumors possess the same histologic features as epithelial inclusion cysts. These neoplasms are usually large, unilocular cysts filled with serous fluid. The cyst wall is usually smooth but may contain papillary projections that consist of a single layer of regular cuboidal epithelium, with basally arranged uniform nuclei. Mitoses are usually absent. Other epithelial cell types may be encountered. The stroma of the cyst wall consists of connective tissue with scattered blood vessels.

It is unclear whether cystadenofibromas should be included as a variant of serous cystadenomas or a separate, common, benign tumor. Cystadenofibromas make up almost half of all cystic benign serous tumors. Small papillary projections from the ovarian surface are relatively common. Although these tumors are cystic, they usually contain papillary projections and can be multiloculated. The epithelium lining the cysts is predominantly serous but may include other epithelial types such as mucinous. The stroma of the papillary projections ranges from highly cellular to hyalinized, acellular tissue. Stromal edema may be seen.

Serous adenofibromas are solid, benign tumors composed of interspersed glandular spaces of varying sizes in a dense, fibrous, connective tissue. It is thought to be a solid variant of the cystadenofibroma. The glandular spaces are lined by a variety of epithelia, with a predominance of cuboidal epithelium. Atypia and mitotic figures are not present. The cellularity of the stroma is variable, ranging from highly cellular to acellular hyalinized areas. Except for the foci of glandular tissue, these tumors are similar to ovarian fibromas. Adenofibromas are rare neoplasms. The serous proliferating tumors are usually adenofibromas in which the glandular elements show crowding.

Mucinous Cystadenomas

Mucinous cystadenomas comprise about 20% of all benign ovarian neoplasms. Although most frequent in the late reproductive years (30–50), they constitute almost 50% of benign epithelial tumors in patients less than 20 years of age. Only 5% are bilateral. Their histogenesis is controversial. Monomorphic endodermal differentiation has been suggested because of the finding of goblet cells, argentaffin cells, Paneth cells, and bile-secreting cells, which may be found in mucinous tumors. Additionally, cystic teratomas are found in 5% of mucinous neoplasms. On the other hand, the ovarian surface is known to undergo metaplasia to mucinous secreting epithelium and other epithelial types that may be seen in this tumor type.

These tumors are frequently multiloculated cysts of large size (15–30 cm on average). The cyst wall lining is usually smooth, although papillary projections can be seen. Microscopically, the lining is a single layer of tall columnar epithelium with mucin-containing cytoplasm and a basally arranged nucleus. Ultrastructurally, two cells types can be found in mucinous epithelium. One type resembles endocervix and the other gastrointestinal-type epithelium, although a mixture of both may be seen. Because of the increased frequency of the former, a metaplastic surface epithelial origin for most of these neoplasms has been favored. The stroma may vary in terms of cellularity. Pure mucinous cystadenofibromas and adenofibromas are very rare.

Pseudomyxoma peritonei is seen in 2–5% of mucinous tumors. This consists of a massive accumulation of mucinous "fluid" that accumulates in the peritoneal cavity. The gelatinous accumulation is usually loculated. The finding of mucin within the stroma of an ovarian mucinous tumor has been termed pseudomyxoma ovarii and may be associated with pseudomyxoma peritonei. The epithelial cells on the peritoneal surface appear to be mature cells with basal nuclei and cytoplasm filled with mucin. Despite their aggressive behavior, these cells rarely exhibit atypical features. It has been suggested that this peritoneal lesion may be an aggressive form of ovarian mucinous carcinoma of low malignant potential.

Endometrioid Tumors

Benign forms of endometrioid tumors include adenoma, cystadenofibroma, and adenofibroma. However, the benign and borderline forms have not been extensively described, and probably some forms of endometriosis or endometrioma qualify as such. Endometriosis and endometriomas are discussed elsewhere in this book. Adenofibroma and cystadenofibroma are similar to adenoma and cystadenoma with the exception of the prominent fibrous stroma. Their presentation and behavior are similar. Endometrioid adenofibromas comprise about 10% of all adenofibromas studied and frequently show squamous metaplasia. Proliferating endometrioid adenofibromas have histologic features similar to those of atypical endometrial hyperplasia. Besides gland crowding, there may be an increase in complexity and atypism. As their behavior is similar to that found in the uterus, they should not be classified as tumors of low malignant potential.

Clear Cell or Mesonephroid Tumors

The cell of origin for clear cell tumors has been considerably controversial. In the past these have been called mesonephroid tumors because they were thought to originate from mesonephric tissue. Primitive-appearing glomeruli can occasionally be seen. It appears that a few of these clear cell tumors were actually endodermal sinus tumors of germ cell origin. The epithelial origin of these tumors has been argued on the basis of an association of benign and malignant endometrioid and clear cell tumors, as well as the observation of clear cells arising out of endometriosis-type epithelium. Clear cells may also be noted in the endometrium. Ultrastructural studies provide additional data to support the müllerian origin of these tumors. Until recently, there were no cases of benign clear cell tumors. A few cases of clear cell cystadenofibromas have been reported that are very similar to other cystadenofibromas of other epithelial cell types.

Brenner Tumors

Numerous histogenetic theories have been postulated for Brenner tumors and include origin from granulosa cells, ovarian stroma, müllerian remnants, mesonephric elements, and teratomas. Currently, the Walthard theory is most accepted. Walthard rests are nests of epithelial cells that occur on the surface of fallopian tubes, mesosalpinx, mesovarium, and ovarian hilus. There is a striking similarity between the epithelium of the Walthard rest, Brenner tumors, and urothelium.

Continuity between the surface epithelium of the ovary and Brenner tumors has been found. It is assumed that the metaplastic process in this case forms urothelium and provides for the similarity of these seemingly unrelated elements.

Brenner tumors account for less than 2% of ovarian neoplasms and are bilateral only 5% of the time. They are more common in older women, as one third occur in postmenopausal women. These tumors appear solid and firm, with a gray-white whorled surface. Occasional cystic structures can sometimes be identified. They are composed of solid epithelial nests surrounded by tightly packed spindle-shaped stroma. The epithelial nests may also have a cystic component. Epithelial cells are squamous appearing, with oval nuclei and prominent nucleoli with longitudinal grooving, thus giving rise to the "coffee bean" appearance associated with this tumor. The association of Brenner tumors with other cystic neoplasms, especially mucinous cystadenomas and cystic teratomas, is well accepted and may be observed in the ipsilateral ovary in approximately one third of patients.

Stromal Tumors

Ovarian tumors of stromal origin are thought to include all those that contain granulosa cells, theca cells, Sertoli cells, Leydig cells, and fibroblasts of gonadal stromal origin. The components derived from the sex cords (granulosa and Sertoli) are typically arranged in epithelial configurations, whereas those derived from stroma have the appearance of cellular gonadal stroma or its specialized derivatives, the theca and Leydig cells. These tumors are generally divided into granulosa–stromal cell tumors, which are composed of cells of ovarian origin, and Sertoli–stromal cell tumors, which contain only cells of testicular types. The latter may be androgen secreting, although estrogen secretion has been reported.

Adult granulosa cell tumors account for 1–2% of all ovarian tumors and occur more often in postmenopausal women than in premenopausal women. These are the most clinically estrogenic ovarian tumors. These tumors may be associated with endometrial changes, especially cystic hyperplasia. Thecomas can be divided into typical and luteinized forms, and some are difficult to separate from fibromas. Thecomas are composed of lipid-laden stromal cells resembling theca cells with varying numbers of fibroblasts. Luteinized thecomas are predominantly fibromatous or thecomatous but also contain collections of steroid type cells. About 50% of luteinized thecomas are estrogenic. These are almost always unilateral and almost never malignant. Fibromas comprise about 4% of all ovarian tumors and are not associated with steroid hormone production. Tumors in the thecoma–fibroma group are composed of thecal cells or fibroblasts of ovarian stromal origin; therefore, fibromas are included in the granulosa–stromal cell category.

Germ Cell Tumors

Dermoids or benign cystic teratomas are among the most common ovarian tumors and make up about one quarter of benign ovarian neoplasms. They are the most common tumor found in young women and comprise 80% of tumors found before age 20. The interior is usually composed of multiloculated cysts filled with sebum, hair, bone, or teeth. Sebum can usually be identified grossly. Derivatives of any of the three germ layers (endoderm, mesoderm, and ectoderm) may be evident microscopically. The most prominent elements are stratified squamous epithelium and its appendages. Respiratory epithelium, with its associated peribronchial glands and cartilage, can be demonstrated in 50–75% of tumors. Neural elements and endodermal epithelium are recognized in many cases. Approximately 10–25% of these tumors are bilateral, so the contralateral ovary should be carefully examined but not necessarily bivalved. Malignant change in cystic teratomas is rare, and the highest incidence is in women in the fourth or fifth decade of life. The incidence of malignancy in an ovarian teratoma is 1–3%. Malignant teratomas contain immature and embryonal types of tissue, whereas benign teratomas show adult tissue.

The most generally accepted theory for the genesis of these tumors is the parthenogenic theory, which suggests an origin from the primordial germ cell. Support for the germ cell theory has come from the anatomic distribution of the tumors, which occur along the line of migration of the primoridal germ cells from the yolk sac to the primitive gonad. Pelvic pain is not uncommon, despite the fact that the ovary has no peritoneal cover. Because cystic teratomas tend to expand anteriorly and produce a large quantity of sebum, they tend to be heavy, pedunculated, and ballotable anterior to the uterus. Occasionally the cells have the capacity to produce hCG which is readily identifiable in blood or urine.

Struma ovarii is a special form of mature teratoma. It represents a teratoma in which the proliferation of the single component has overgrown other tissues. Although thyroid tissue is seen in approximately 15% of cases of mature teratoma, this does not justify the diagnosis of struma ovarii unless the thyroid tissue is dominant or there is evidence of either neoplasia or hormonal function.

DIAGNOSIS OF ADNEXAL MASSES

Diagnosis of an adnexal or ovarian mass is often made or confirmed with pelvic ultrasonography. Recently, transvaginal ultrasonography has become more popular because of the increase in sensitivity of detection as well as specificity of preoperative diagnosis. Benign follicular cysts tend to have distinct borders and no evidence of solid parts, thick septa, ascites, fixation in the pelvis, or matted bowel. Magnetic resonance imaging may provide more specific imaging, if needed. Computed tomography appears to be less useful for imaging adnexal masses and is generally avoided; however, it may provide useful information when lymph node enlargement is suspected or should be ruled out. Tumor antigens such as CA 125 can be used to aid in evaluating an adnexal mass; elevated levels can serve as a preoperative indication of possible cancer. However, many benign processes, such as endometriosis, infection, and benign ovarian cysts, may also increase CA 125 values. A negative value should not be used to delay surgical diagnosis if other clinical criteria suggest its need.

Adnexal processes that have suspicious characteristics on imaging, such as solid components, septa, or enlarged lymph nodes, should be investigated in women of any age group. Intervention should also be considered for adnexal masses in postmenopausal women and premenarcheal girls, except infants (especially premature infants). Cystic processes without the suspicious characteristics noted above can be followed conservatively for three natural or induced cycles in women of reproductive age unless signs and symptoms such as intraperitoneal bleeding suggest that conservative management should be abandoned. Very large size is a relative contraindication to conservative management, since cysts larger than 10 cm rarely regress spontaneously.

SURGICAL THERAPY

Extensive periovarian and peritubular adhesions may result from even conservative ovarian surgery and cause infertility or pelvic pain. These, among other considerations, require careful deliberation prior to operating on an adnexal mass. The following factors should be considered in deciding on observation and repeat examinations versus surgical exploration:

Observe and repeat examination in 4–6 weeks
- Reproductive age
- Mass less than 8 cm
- Simple cysts on ultrasonography
- Decreasing size
- Cystic and smooth
- Mobile
- Unilateral
- Asymptomatic
- No ascites

Surgical exploration
- Premenarcheal
- Postmenopausal
- Mass greater than 8 cm
- Complex cysts on ultrasonography
- Increase in size or persistence through two or three menstrual cycles
- Solid and irregular
- Fixed
- Bilateral
- Pain or other symptoms of acute intraabdominal process
- Ascites

In premenarcheal and postmenopausal women, simple cysts smaller than 3–5 cm may be followed closely with ultrasonography.

In ovarian reconstructive surgery, atraumatic technique cannot be overemphasized. The weight of experimental and clinical evidence suggests that ischemia, trauma, coagulation, or foreign material leads to adhesion formation. In animal models, studies suggest that external sutures are significantly more adhesiogenic than nonclosure of the ovarian cortex.

At laparotomy, an elliptical incision is made above the thin ovarian cortex in the axis of the ovary and in its most dependent area. This will facilitate reconstruction of the ovary and ensure a more "anatomic" closure. The end of the knife handle may then be inserted and a plane developed over the cyst wall. After the cyst wall has been completely separated from its adhesive attachments to the ovarian cortex, it may be shelled out without rupture. On occasion, however, because of friability of the cyst wall, rupture may occur even with the gentlest technique. It is of utmost importance prior to shelling out the cyst to surround the ovary with moist, lint-free packs so that if rupture occurs spillage will not contaminate the rest of the pelvis. After the cyst is removed, the dead space may be obliterated with internal sutures placed as pursestring, running lock, or interrupted sutures of no. 4-0 or no. 5-0 nonreactive suture material. The ovarian cortex may be approximated with subcuticular sutures of no. 5-0 or no. 6-0 nonreactive suture material. Suture of the ovarian surface should be avoided if at all possible.

Obviously, the laparoscope will be used quite often to confirm the diagnosis of ovarian or pelvic mass. However, there is currently much debate about what ovarian lesions can be approached reasonably through the laparoscope. Benign ovarian lesions can be removed through the laparoscope; however, the difficulty comes in predicting which are benign prior to pathologic examination. Ovarian cancer occurs in 1 in 95 women with an ovarian cyst between ages 20 and 35. Although recent evidence suggests that peritoneal spill does not change the prognosis of stage IA ovarian cancer, definitive data are not available. Endometriomas are almost always predictably benign, although a few cases of malignancy have been reported. Perfectly smooth cysts that are echolucent are almost always also predictably benign. However, these cysts are relatively rare as a reason for laparoscopic surgery, since they are usually functional and resolve with observation. Ovarian cysts with solid components or superficial excrescences should be approached with caution until more data are available.

Ovarian Preservation for Benign Ovarian Disease

It is imperative that surgeons consider the untoward effects that may be seen with removal of ovaries for benign processes in women of childbearing age. Oftentimes, these benign processes are bilateral (such as dermoid cysts) and recurrent (such as endometriomas, follicular cysts, and cysts with a propensity for torsion). These patients are at increased risk for surgical castration. Ovarian conservation is desirable, as pregnancy rates with assisted reproductive technologies are dependent on the number of follicles obtained. The most conservative ovarian procedure consistent with good surgical judgment should be the goal of all reproductive surgeons. Ovarian surgery, whether accomplished by laparotomy using microsurgical technique or laparoscopy, is complicated by adhesion formation in many cases. One should be as conservative as possible with functional cysts in otherwise normal ovaries, as resulting adhesion formation may compromise fertility or result in pelvic pain.

Prophylactic Oophorerectomy

The prevalence of ovarian carcinoma is 1–2%; this cancer is most common in perimenopausal and menopausal women (aged 50–60 years). Screening techniques have not proved reliable, and it is rarely diagnosed early. Bilateral oophorectomy does not eliminate the risk of ovarian cancer but substantially decreases it. Cases of mesotheliomas indistinguishable from ovarian carcinomas have been reported. Conversely, early menopause adversely affects cardiovascular and bone health, as well as symptoms such as hot flashes, vaginal dryness, urinary frequency, and mood swings. Although various hormone replacement regimens are available and offer a reasonable chance to correct the morbidity associated with the premature loss of estrogen, some women are unable to tolerate replacement therapy. Additionally, postmenopausal ovaries are not hormonally inactive in that androgens are still secreted and peripherally aromatized to estrogens.

Postmenopausal women and those over age 40 may consider it as a means of reducing their risk of ovarian carcinoma, as may younger patients with a family history of ovarian cancer. Women who are considering prophylactic oophorectomy should carefully weigh the potential benefits of reducing the cancer risk against the adverse effects of premature loss of estrogen.

BIBLIOGRAPHY

Clement PB. Nonneoplastic lesions of the ovary. In: Kurman RJ, ed. Blaustein's pathology of the female genital tract. 3rd ed. New York: Springer-Verlag, 1987:471–515

Czernobilsky B. Common epithelial tumors of the ovary. In: Kurman RJ, ed. Blaustein's pathology of the female genital tract. 3rd ed. New York: Springer-Verlag, 1987:560–606

Dembo AJ, Davy M, Stenwig AE, Berle EJ, Bush RS, Kjorstad K. Prognostic factors in patients with stage I epithelial ovarian cancer. Obstet Gynecol 1990;75:263–273

Murphy AA. Reconstructive surgery of the ovary. In: Rock JA, Murphy AA, Jones HW, eds. Female reproductive surgery. Baltimore: Williams and Wilkins, 1992:190–204

Talerman A. Germ cell tumors of the ovary. In: Kurman RJ, ed. Blaustein's pathology of the female genital tract. 3rd ed. New York: Springer-Verlag, 1987:659–721

Yen SSC. Chronic anovulation caused by peripheral endocrine disorders. In: Yen SSC, Jaffe RB, eds. Reproductive endocrinology: physiology, pathophysiology and clinical management. 3rd ed. Philadelphia: WB Saunders, 1991:576–630

Young RH, Scully RE. Sex cord-stromal, steroid cell and other ovarian tumors with endocrine, paraendocrine, and paraneoplastic manifestations. In: Kurman RJ, ed. Blaustein's pathology of the female genital tract. 3rd ed. New York: Springer-Verlag, 1987:607–658

Wound Healing: Techniques and Materials

Knowledge of the complexities of the wound healing process, as well as the basic impact of surgical manipulations on the process, enables practitioners to perform successful surgical procedures with the greatest technical ease, the lowest surgical morbidity, and the best long-term results. Today's aging population further emphasizes the need for successful long-term results, as the reconstructive procedure gynecologists perform today may need to hold for 40 years or more. Key points of wound management are as follows:

- The well-constructed wound resists infection.
- Loosely applied mass closure has the lowest complication rate in the vertical wound.
- The peritoneum is best left open.
- The best adhesion prevention is gentle tissue handling, not adhesion-prevention devices.
- The incision that heals the best is one that is least traumatically produced.
- "Approximate, don't strangulate" when tying sutures.
- Put nothing in the wound you would not put in your eye.

In the normal healing process, healthy tissue responds to injury with an inflammatory phase, a fibroblastic phase, and a remodeling phase. Cellular and biochemical messages initiate the healing response, regulate its magnitude and length, and stop the reparative process when it is complete. The pathophysiologic changes that occur during each stage of wound healing are delineated in the box.

In the inflammatory phase, from incision to day 4, blood is released in the area of injury, vessels constrict and then dilate, and leukocytes adhere to the endothelium. Red blood cells form rouleaux, fluid leaks into tissues and spaces, and the body responds with increased hemostasis. Prostaglandins E_1 and E_2, serotonins, kinins, and histamines are active. Platelets have an active and newly expanded role in wound healing. Cellular infiltrates include polymorphonuclear leukocytes,

> **Pathophysiologic Changes in the Stages of Wound Healing**
>
> **First Stage: Inflammatory Phase (Day 1 to Day 4)**
>
> *Vascular changes*
> Vasodilatation
> Slowing of blood flow
> Increased capillary permeability
>
> *Cellular events*
> Polymorphonuclear leukocytes and monocytes migrate into wound fluid
> Platelet release of chemotactic and other substances initiates and controls the early phase of healing
>
> **Second Stage: Fibroblastic Phase (Day 5 to Day 20)**
> Macrophages continue phagocytosis, control other cellular activity, and are predominant cells
> Increased numbers of fibroblasts produce ground substance and collagen
> Collagenolysis is active at wound edges
> There is new capillary formation
>
> **Third Stage: Remodeling Phase (Day 21 to 2 Years)**
> Decreased cellularity
> Decreased vascularity
> Organization and remodeling of collagen

lymphocytes, macrophages, and monocytes. The wound has practically no inherent strength without sutures during this early phase.

In the fibroblastic phase, days 5–20, fibroblasts arise locally, and capillaries containing plasminogen activators form in and around the fibroblasts. Collagen fibrils are deposited into the wound by using a fibrin scaffolding. Chemical bonds and cross-linkages occur between the fibrils of collagen, increasing its tensile strength. By day 21, the wound has regained approximately 30% of the tissue's original strength.

In the remodeling phase, the body seeks symmetry. This phase begins at day 21 and may last a year or more. The scar is essentially a reparative bridge. During this phase, the scar may resorb, constrict, and become depressed below the skin line. Most scar tissue is weaker than the normal tissue it replaces. Hence, the wider and larger the scar, the weaker the wound. The smaller the scar, the more likely the inherent original strength will be approached.

INCISIONAL AND SURGICAL INSTRUMENTS

The incision that heals the best is one that is produced least traumatically. Incisions made with a single sharp stroke of a knife produce less of a scar, heal more promptly, and are more resistant to infection than are incisions made with multiple strokes of the blade. Likewise, the effects of incisions made with the standard stainless steel scalpel are less disruptive to the wound healing process than are those made by a laser or thermal knives.

Scalpels

Knife incisions heal more promptly than scissor incisions. All incisions made with the sharper instruments heal more rapidly and with less difficulty than do those made with heated scalpels, such as the electrical cautery, the Shaw knife, or the laser. Wounds made by electrosurgery are approximately three times more susceptible to infection than are wounds made with a stainless steel scalpel. Wide zones of dissection lateral to the area of the incision likewise only increase the incidence of wound infection and do not justifiably increase exposure.

Thermal Knives

Thermal injury inflicted by thermal knives affects the overall dynamics of wound healing. Completion of epithelial migration is delayed, the average residual scar width is greater, and a lateral thermal necrotic zone is prominent. Injury patterns associated with laser incision are specific to each type of laser and vary with the energy expended into tissues. Wounds resulting from incisions made with thermal knives are weaker at 2 weeks than are those made with a scalpel.

The loop electrosurgical excision procedure recently has seen increased use in the United States. Wound healing complications after this procedure are uncommon; however, the zone of thermal injury found in electric loop specimens measuring less than 5 mm deep has been extensive. While cervical wound healing complications seem no greater than with those produced by the laser, injury to the vaginal wall, with heavy bleeding, has been noted in some studies.

METHODS OF CLOSURE

Suturing a wound gives it the support that it needs for connective tissue formation during the healing phase. Suture selection should be based on the location of the wound, the intent of the surgical procedure, healing properties of the wounded tissues, and biologic and mechanical properties of the suture material.

Because most trauma associated with suture implantation is produced by the needle, the choice of fine suture materials is wasted if a large, traumatic needle is attached. Fine-diameter intestinal needles carefully chosen to complement the suture material produce much less trauma to tissues. This becomes more important as reconstructive procedures are required by the increasing number of elderly patients.

The ultimate clinical course for the patient's wound is determined by the end of the surgical procedure. There are very few things that can done at the conclusion of the operation that will modify subsequent operative morbidity. Improperly constructed wounds with strangulating sutures, crushed tissue, or compromised blood supply will produce a higher morbidity than will properly handled wounds, regardless of postoperative care.

Selection of Suture Materials

Suture material is generally classified as absorbable and nonabsorbable or permanent. The selection of a permanent or absorbable suture depends on the length of time that the suture needs to be present to perform its selected task. Procedures such as sacrospinous fixation, suprapubic urethral suspension, and others that need to maintain the organ in apposition to a fixed area such as the sacrospinous ligament or symphysis pubis may require permanent sutures. Such sutures must continue to provide strength in the wound for many years. In contrast, suture material used to approximate episiotomy, in an area of intense blood supply and great inherent resistance to infection, should be absorbable. The absorbable chromic catgut suture loses its strength in 14–28 days, and the polyglycolic acid–type suture loses its strength in approximately 3–4 weeks and absorbs in 60–90 days.

Each surgeon should select sutures on the basis of ease of handling, absorption in tissues, lack of reactivity, radiolucency, cost, and infection potentiation. The currently available suture materials are listed in Table 4-3. Suture size as well as material appropriate to the specific gynecologic procedure must also be chosen carefully.

When suture materials are selected for closing the abdominal wall in patients who have asthma or other chronic pulmonary problems, it is probably best to choose a permanent suture such as polypropylene or polybutester. Transverse incisions need less support; therefore, delayed absorbable sutures such as polydioxanone or polyglyconate do quite well. More rapid absorption is useful in vaginal closure, and sutures of fine polyglycolic acid, polyglactin, or chromic gut are preferable for this procedure.

Placement of sutures to incorporate large "bites" of tissue, as in mass closure, produces a stronger wound. A rule of thumb is to place fascial sutures as far apart as they are from the wound edge, and in no instance should they be placed less than 1 cm from the edge. There is an area of collagenolysis that occurs up to 10 mm from the edge of incised fascia, and wounds constructed within this zone are weaker. Sutures placed in the Smead–Jones fashion are stronger than those placed with other closure techniques; therefore, a Smead–Jones suture placed 2 cm laterally produces a stronger wound and is a good choice in obese patients or in patients with chronic pulmonary disease. Giving the patient supplemental ascorbic acid inhibits the formation of collagenase, resulting in a stronger wound scar.

Use of a continuous running suture offers the advantage of speed and economy, and wound closures have superior bursting strength. A very low complication rate has been noted with the use of polyglactin, polyglyconate, and polybutester sutures. The running polyglyconate suture, size 0 or 1, and the standard or looped configuration are currently preferred for closure of the laparotomy wound. Such running closure saves 10–15 minutes of operating room time for standard laparotomy. Comparative studies of interrupted suture (polyglactin 910, size 1) and continuous suture (polyglyconate, size 0) suggest that a running polyglyconate suture is the better choice for closure of the abdominal wall fascia after midline laparotomy. The endoloop suture is useful both with the laparoscope and as a means of oophorectomy at the time of transvaginal hysterectomy, when the ovaries are not easily reached.

For closure of a uterine incision, a single-layer continuous closure with a locking stitch should be used. Comparative studies showed that this produced a stronger wound. Studies also suggest that the peritoneum is best left unsutured. To decrease the risk of adhesion formation, neither the vesicouterine nor the parietal epithelium need be closed.

The most common error made in wound construction is in tying suture materials too tightly. The loss of strength by excessively tight sutures is shown in Fig. 4-4. This is the most common error in resident surgical technique and is responsible for most dehiscences of abdominal wounds. When studied, dehiscent wounds are almost always found with the suture unbroken and the knot intact. The suture has torn through the wound because the suture was placed too near the wound edge and tied too tightly. When sutures are tied so tightly that no blood flow occurs, the tissues cannot heal effectively. One need only press one's finger on the capillary beds of the skin or the nail to recognize blanching and to understand the impact of pressure on underlying blood flow.

All sutures elicit some degree of inflammatory response regardless of the material. Just the presence of suture material potentiates the ability of the bacteria that are present in almost all wounds to cause infection. The quantity of suture material also is related directly to the magnitude of damage to host resistance. The larger the diameter of the suture and

TABLE 4-3. CURRENTLY AVAILABLE SUTURE MATERIALS

Type of Suture	In Vivo Tensile Strength (%)	
	14 Days	21 Days
Absorbable		
Synthetic		
Poliglecaprone 25	25	0
Polyglycolic acid	65	35
Polyglactin 910	65	40
Polydioxanone	86	81
Polyglyconate	74	59
Nonsynthetic		
Plain gut	0	0
Chromic gut	34	0
Nonabsorbable		
Synthetic		
Polypropylene		
Polyamide (nylon)		
Polybutester		
Polytetrafluoroethylene		
Polyester (Dacron)		
Nonsynthetic		
Silk		
Stainless Steel		

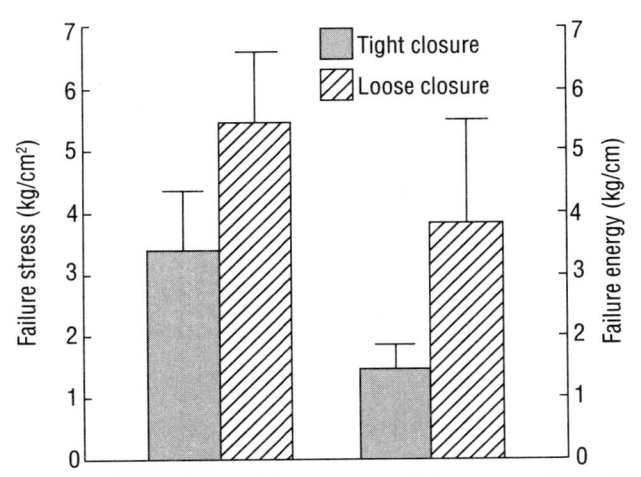

FIG. 4-4. Comparison of failure stress and failure energy for wounds closed tightly versus wounds closed loosely. (Masterson BJ. Manual of gynecologic surgery. 2nd ed. New York: Springer-Verlag, 1986:77)

the longer the suture implant, the greater the proliferation of bacteria. Multifilament sutures are infected much more easily than are monofilament sutures. The use of subcutaneous sutures to obliterate dead space has clearly been shown not only to be ineffective but also to increase the infection rate.

Although dead space is bad, suture closure of dead space is worse. Closure of dead space by sutures produces localized areas of wound ischemia and necrosis, and the presence of additional suture material adds further danger of wound complications. Suction catheters and pressure dressings provide much more efficient and less compromising methods of eliminating dead space in wounds.

Knots

The best knot is one that is stable and that uses the least amount of suture material. Sutures need to be secure and neither give nor become untied. The knot configuration needed to achieve knot stability varies with each suture material. A stable knot configuration is the number of throws required so that the suture loop breaks, but the knot does not slip and lose its strength. The surgeon must be familiar with each material and its mechanical properties to make a truly informed decision in this regard. An extra throw (1-1-1 knot) of no. 3-0 polyglycolic acid results in 85% efficiency versus 58% efficiency with a 1-1 (square) knot. A 2-1-1-1 configuration achieves knot stability for coated polyglycolic acid and coated polyglactin 910 for gauges 1-0 through 3-0. Maximal tensile strength with minimal failure by slippage in most synthetic materials requires the inclusion of a surgeon's knot and at least three square knots. Application of these broad principles depends on the technique of the surgeon.

As new synthetic textiles come into use, the surgeon must consider the specific qualities of each. The mechanical properties of elongation, friction, and tensile strength for straight and knotted sutures should be considered. Major advances continue in the manufacture of suture materials. The knot-holding properties of polyglyconate are currently superior to those of other absorbable suture. Polydioxanone has recently improved its "hand" and knot-holding properties. Polyglycolic acid is now manufactured in a tighter weave, resulting in improved strength. These tensile properties of the suture and its coatings must be clearly understood by surgeons when they choose suture material.

Staples and Absorbable Ligating Clips

Stapling devices have been available for a number of years and are most useful. An example of the low inflammatory response elicited by staples versus tape and suture is shown in Fig. 4-5. Staples are a rapid and accurate method of skin approximation. They are widely used and are most cost-effective in a high-intensity cost arena such as the operating room. Staples are also widely used in the performance of gastrointestinal surgery and are time-saving devices. Certain low anastomoses in the colon also may be performed most expediently with these devices.

Absorbable ligating clips and staples are increasingly being used in the performance of gynecologic surgery. Current absorbable clips make use of synthetic materials that have long clinical experience, such as polydioxanone, which is used for Absolok vascular ligating clips, and polyglycolic acid, which is used for Lactomer clips.

The unique properties imparted to compression of these materials produce a different impact on healing properties from those of sutures made up of the same material. Recent studies have shown that the impact of absorbable staples on tissues is also different from that of the commonly used stain-

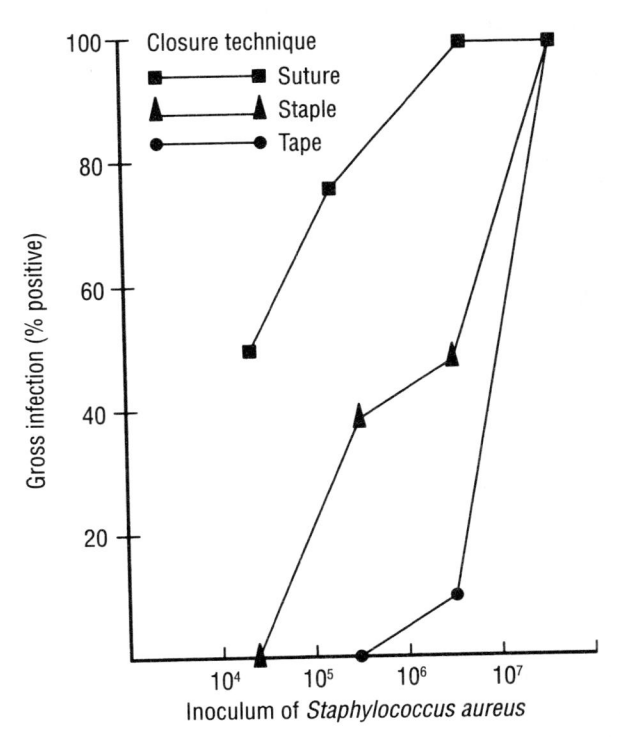

FIG. 4-5. Effect of closure technique on wound infection. (Edlich RF, Rodeheaver GT, Thacker JG. Technical factors in the prevention of wound infections. In: Howard RJ, Simmons RL, eds. Surgical infectious diseases. 2nd ed. Norwalk, Connecticut: Appleton and Lange, 1988:344)

less steel staple. The impact of infection on absorption and staple resection will require continued clinical observation and study.

Adhesion Barrier Materials

While mechanical mesh barriers have been suggested as a means of adhesion prevention, studies thus far have failed to show any independent beneficial preventive activity. Adhesion scores between ovaries treated with absorbable barrier and control ovaries were compared, and no demonstrable differences were found in postoperative adhesion formation.

PERITONEAL CONSIDERATIONS

The peritoneum heals rapidly and is generally thought to seal within 4 hours. When the peritoneum is not injured, fibrinolysis and fibrin deposition occur in balance, and there is no fibrous adhesion formation. Factors that disrupt this equilibrium elicit adhesion formation.

Surgical talc is absorbed by the peritoneal mesothelial cells within 10 minutes. Over the next 7 hours, an inflammatory reaction occurs, followed by death of the mesothelial cells over the next 10 days. The basement membrane is exposed, fibrin deposition occurs, and vascular adhesions are formed. Other items such as cornstarch powder and lint from surgical caps and gowns and laparotomy pads likewise stimulate this response, as does suture material.

Starch contamination from surgical glove powder during surgical procedures has been found to contribute to postoperative adhesion formation. The time-honored practice of washing surgical gloves is ineffective in removing starch particles. Powder-free gloves are necessary to avoid infiltration of glove powder into the wound.

The normal peritoneum has sufficient fibrinolytic activity to prevent adhesion formation. Crushing injuries from clamps, thermal injury, or sutures that produce hypoxia, however, may all induce adhesion formation. Surgeons should limit any trauma to the peritoneum, and peritoneal surfaces should be kept moist. In view of this evidence, many surgeons no longer close the peritoneum with suture material.

OTHER FACTORS AFFECTING WOUND HEALING

An appropriate clinical axiom is "put nothing in the wound you would not put in your eye." A wound is even weaker than the conjunctival sac, as it has no epithelial covering to protect itself. Careful consideration must be given to the application of topical agents and solutions that may adversely affect wound healing.

Topical Agents

In an effort to reduce infection, surgeons have historically applied topical antiseptics to wounds. Topical agents such as solutions of 1% povidine–iodine, 0.25% acetic acid, 3% hydrogen peroxide, and 0.5% sodium hypochlorite have been found to be cytotoxic when applied to human fibroblasts. Also, the mere pouring of such solutions directly into the wound has been shown not to remove bacteria but to further injure the tissues that are present. When bacteria must be removed, the wound should be irrigated under force. High-pressure irrigation with an 18-gauge needle attached to a large syringe has been found successful in cleansing wounds of small particulate matter and bacteria, thereby reducing the infection rate. However, irrigation solutions, antibiotic or saline, do not appear to be superior to primary closure in clean-contaminated (type II) or contaminated (type III) incisions.

Drainage

Surgical wound drainage is another key element that affects wound healing. The time-honored Penrose drain has now become an antique and should not be used for transfascial drainage. A Penrose drain brought through the incision quadruples the infection rate. In rare instances when use of a Penrose drain may be justified, it should always be brought out through a separate stab wound rather than the primary incision. Even then, the infection rate is likely to be higher (2.4%) than if closed-suction drainage (1.8%) is used. When drainage must be used, closed-suction drainage that comes through its own separate wound is least likely to have a negative impact on wound healing.

Catheters

The use of subcutaneous catheters continues to be investigated, and recent studies have demonstrated the value of percutaneous catheter drainage in patients with abscesses. When suction catheters have been used, they seem to reduce dead space. The addition of antibiotic solution irrigation, however, has produced conflicting data.

Antibiotics

Timing of antibiotic administration influences the success of antibiotic therapy. To be truly effective, an antibiotic needs to be in the tissue at the time of injury, because the addition of antibiotics after the wound is constructed is less useful. Antibiotics used in irrigating fluids have been shown to be less destructive to tissues than are other chemical irrigating solutions, but they are generally no more effective than systemic use. From a wound standpoint, intravenous antibiotics given immediately before the induction of anesthesia are most beneficial, and additional injections are not required, as they are much less effective when given postoperatively.

For the average gynecologic procedure, the patient need not receive an additional dose of antibiotic. Cefazolin, the standard of comparison for prophylactic antibiotics, has a half-life of 2 hours and hence covers the duration of most gynecologic procedures. In longer cases, its application can be repeated at an interval of two times the half-life, or 4 hours after the first dose was given. If the surgical procedure lasts 4 hours, one additional dose can be given and no other antibiotics are necessary. Additional coverage of 24–48 hours is not warranted, as it has no positive effect on wound infection rate. Should other antibiotics be used, their repeat dosage schedule should be at an interval of two times the half-life.

Disease Processes

Disease processes such as diabetes impair wound healing. While the infection rate for clean surgical procedures is less than 1%, the infection rate for clean surgical procedures in diabetic patients approximates 10.7%. This may be due to vascular obstruction that results in hypoxia and poor tissue nutrition. The metabolic abnormalities of diabetes also inhibit phagocytosis and the effective killing of bacteria by this process.

Vascular disease also impairs the healing process. A poor blood supply, from either partially obstructed blood vessels or compromised vessels in a reconstructive procedure or a poorly nourished flap, likewise impairs healing. Numerous clinical studies have shown the increased ease with which bacteria destroy wounds when the blood supply is compromised.

Again, the impact of the aging population on which gynecologic surgeons will be operating emphasizes the importance of an appropriate blood supply. Many elderly patients may have compromised vascular integrity because of advanced age, and the blood supply in these tissues must be carefully considered before surgery is initiated. Because of this and other factors, patients aged 65 years and older are six times more likely to develop infection in clean wounds than are patients aged 15 years or younger.

Other Factors

Many other variables have been found to adversely affect the wound infection rate, such as a prolonged length of time in the hospital prior to surgery and the duration of the operation. In general, the risk of infection doubles for every hour of the operating procedure. Preoperative shaving of patients has also been identified as a positive risk factor for wound infection and therefore should be eliminated.

As more and more patient procedures are performed in the outpatient arena, the local effects of anesthesia on wound healing must be considered. Local anesthetic uses include local infiltration, peripheral nerve blockade, and topical application. Although many studies describe no difference in wound complication rates with the use of topical agents, some suggest an increase in necrosis and infection. Caution must be used when administering epinephrine in local anesthetics, which can cause increased wound inflammation, infection rates, and uncomfortable side effects. Research to develop a nontoxic, rapidly acting topical anesthetic agent of long duration continues.

ADVANCES IN WOUND HEALING

Major advances in molecular biology are making new factors available that will modify or accelerate the wound healing process. There is now promising research in polypeptide growth factors and platelet extracts. Growth factors are active in accelerating and modulating early wound healing and scar formation and are found to promote cell division, chemotaxis, cell differentiation, and metabolic activity in target cells. Not all growth factors result in similar clinical outcomes, and early trials are currently under way. Understanding basic and applied knowledge of growth factors is essential for adapting this new technology to patient care.

A number of reconstructive pelvic procedures that use the principles described in this section are useful for the gynecologic surgeon. These procedures may be useful in both primary reparative and reoperative surgery. Full-thickness skin grafting, Z-plasty, skin flaps, and translocation island flaps are readily adaptable to gynecologic procedures.

Currently, surgeons must put their energies into those things that do not negatively affect wound healing. Surgeons must construct a wound that preserves an excellent blood supply, produce the incision with minimal injury to underlying tissues, operate expeditiously, and use the cautery and laser sparingly when performing incisions. Bleeding vessels must be isolated and tied by themselves, pedicles must be trimmed, and any trauma inflicted should be kept to a minimum.

Studies show that morbidity is not as much inherent in the gynecologic procedure as it is in the technique used by the surgeon and the length of the operation, particularly when it is more than 2 hours long. Each surgeon must therefore analyze the techniques he or she uses to construct and close wounds and then, based on an understanding of wound healing, modify those techniques to produce the minimum morbidity associated with that procedure.

BIBLIOGRAPHY

Baggish MS, Barash F, Noel Y, Brooks M. Comparison of thermal injury zones in loop electrical and laser cervical excisional conization. Am J Obstet Gynecol 1992;166:545–548

Chegini N, von Fraunhofer JA, Hay DL, Masterson BJ. Tissue reactions to absorbable ligating clips. J Reprod Med 1988;33:187–192

Cruikshank SH. Reconstructive procedures for the gynecologic surgeon. Am J Obstet Gynecol 1993;168:469–475

Durante EJ. Breaking strength of CO_2-laser and scalpel blade incisions in the dog. J S Afr Vet Assoc 1992;63:141–143

Eckersley JR, Dudley HA. Wounds and wound healing. Br Med Bull 1988;44:423–436

Ellis H. The hazards of surgical glove dusting powders. Surg Gynecol Obstet 1990;171:521–527

Hauth JC, Owen J, Davis RO. Transverse uterine incision closure: one versus two layers. Am J Obstet Gynecol 1992;167:1108–1111

Hoffman MS. Transvaginal removal of ovaries with endoloop sutures at the time of transvaginal hysterectomy. Am J Obstet Gynecol 1991;165:407–408

Howard RJ, Simmons RL. Surgical infectious diseases. 2nd ed. Norwalk, Connecticut: Appleton and Lange, 1988

Howell JM. Current and future trends in wound healing. Emerg Med Clin North Am 1992;10:655–663

Kamffer WJ, Jooste EV, Nel JT, de Wet JI. Surgical glove powder and intraperitoneal adhesion formation: an appeal for the use of powder-free surgical gloves. S Afr Med J 1992;81:158–159

Masterson BJ. Wound healing in gynecologic surgery. In: Masterson BJ, ed. Manual of gynecologic surgery. 2nd ed. New York: Springer-Verlag, 1986:71–82

Metz SA, Chegini N, Masterson BJ. In vivo tissue reactivity and degradation of suture materials: a comparison of Maxon and PDS. J Gynecol Surg 1989;5:37–46

Norris RL Jr. Local anesthetics. Emerg Med Clin North Am 1992; 10:707–718

Page CP, Bohnen JM, Fletcher JR, McManus AT, Solomkin JS, Wittman DH. Antimicrobial prophylaxis for surgical wounds: guidelines for clinical care. Arch Surg 1993;128:79–88

Sowa DE, Masterson BJ, Nealon N, von Fraunhofer JA. Effects of thermal knives on wound healing. Obstet Gynecol 1985;66:436–439

Stone IK, von Fraunhofer JA, Masterson BJ. The biomechanical effects of tight suture closure upon fascia. Surg Gynecol Obstet 1986; 163:448–452

Sutton G, Morgan S. Abdominal wound closure using a running, looped monofilament polybutester suture: comparison to Smead-Jones closure in historic controls. Obstet Gynecol 1992;80:650–654

Trimbos JB, Smit IB, Holm JP, Hermans J. A randomized clinical trial comparing two methods of fascia closure following midline laparotomy. Arch Surg 1992;127:1232–1234

von Fraunhofer JA, Storey RJ, Masterson BJ. Tensile properties of suture materials. Biomaterials 1988;9:324–327

Postoperative Care

While there have been advances in surgical technique and management, most of the principles of postoperative care have changed little since the advent of universally available intravenous fluids. In an attempt to practice more cost-effective medicine, patients are dismissed postoperatively from the hospital far sooner than in the past. Thus, the principles of postoperative care are reviewed below assuming 1) a very healthy 20–55-year-old female patient, 2) absence of intraoperative complications, 3) anticipated discharge in 24–72 hours.

BASIC CARE

All surgical procedures are body injuries. A laceration from the scalpel is no less of an injury than a laceration from a piece of glass. The difference between accidents and surgery is largely due to the controlled nature of surgery. Just as accident victims who have minor injuries recover more quickly, so also do surgical patients who have meticulous dissection and minimal muscle trauma have shorter recovery periods than those who have received less careful procedures.

When the body is recovering from any injury it is important to supply it with its basic needs: fluids, electrolytes, and calories. While it has also been assumed for centuries that injuries require "rest" to heal, scientific data to support this commonly held belief are scant. Indeed, it appears that many individuals recover faster if they are encouraged to ambulate early and return to normal daily activities as soon as possible.

Fluids and Electrolytes

In a normal woman, 50–55% of weight is composed of water. Maintenance of this fluid, with the proper amounts of electrolytes, is the primary concern in postoperative care.

For many very good reasons, patients are forced to restrict fluid intake before surgery. The typical instruction, "nothing by mouth after midnight" results in every surgical patient's being taken to the operating room in a state of relative dehydration, with an 800–1,500-ml fluid deficit, depending on the time of the patient's surgery. In order to minimize this dehydration, many operating suites now begin to infuse preoperative patients as soon as they arrive in the surgical area. This is particularly important when surgery will be delayed for many hours.

Anesthesia often is forced to make up for the patient's initial dehydration by infusing large amounts of fluids at the initiation of anesthesia. Anesthesiologists usually prefer to have patients slightly overhydrated than underhydrated, as blood pressure is easier to maintain in this condition. At the end of the procedure it is the gynecologist's responsibility to add up the amounts of fluids infused during the operation, subtract the amount of fluid denied the patient during her nothing-by-mouth period, and assess the need for additional fluids. Many surgeons use a "routine" postoperative fluid order regimen for every patient. This is inappropriate because fluids should be individualized, but in most cases a young healthy patient can manage to survive despite inappropriate fluids if they are given for a short period of time.

In general, a young woman will require 2,000–2,500 ml of water per day. This need is a result of the 800–1,200 ml of sensible water loss from breathing, skin loss, and gastrointestinal loss. Urinary losses account for another 1,200–1,500 ml/d.

Relatively few alterations in water replacement are necessary in uncomplicated patients. Febrile patients may require up to 2,000 ml of additional water per day, and patients with draining wounds or on prolonged nasogastric suction require additional fluids as well as alterations in electrolyte content.

Patients cannot be given only water postoperatively. Approximately 100–140 meq of sodium and 40–60 meq of potassium are required each day. As these electrolytes are virtually always given as a chloride salt, the body's chloride requirement is also met. The body also needs considerable amounts of magnesium and calcium, as well as minute amounts of trace minerals. However, for short recovery or short intravenous postoperative periods it is not necessary to supplement these electrolytes. Although controversial for short postoperative periods, many surgeons add vitamins C and B complex to intravenous solutions in the hope that these will aid in wound healing. There is no evidence that 1 or 2 days of intravenous administration of these vitamins is important in normal healthy women. However, patients on prolonged intravenous solutions and patients on total parenteral nutrition supplementation must receive vitamins for healing.

Two liters of dextrose (5%) in one-half normal saline will satisfy the sodium and chloride needs of a female patient for 24 hours. However, additional potassium will need to be added. Two liters of lactated Ringer's solution will provide nearly double the amount of sodium and chloride needed and can thus represent electrolyte overload. Notice also that the small amount of potassium in lactated Ringer's solution is not sufficient to cover the patient's needs; potassium supplementation of this fluid is necessary.

One measure of the effectiveness of fluid replacement is urine output. In a normal active young woman urinary output is approximately 50 ml/h, or 1,200 ml/d. Although 25–30 ml of urinary output is commonly accepted as adequate in the postoperative period, this amount is less than normal, and a 50-ml/h output is preferable. The most common cause of oliguria in a healthy postoperative patient is insufficient fluids. If urinary output is decreased, the surgeon should carefully total the amount of fluid the patient has received and subtract from this the output and the amount of dehydration from the nothing-by-mouth period preoperatively. If it is clear that the patient is lacking in fluids, the infusion rate should be increased. If the urinary output is not adequate after this increase in fluids, other sources of renal compromise (eg, acute tubular necrosis due to hypotension or hemorrhage during surgery) should be sought.

"Third spacing" refers to the loss of body water into the extracellular and extravascular spaces of the body. In gynecologic surgery this refers largely to the accumulation of fluid in the peritoneal cavity. This can occur in large amounts in patients with ovarian cancer debulking but is usually negligible in normal healthy patients who have undergone relatively little disruption of the peritoneal cavity.

Calories

The adult woman requires approximately 22 kcal/kg of body weight per day. In a 70-kg (154-lb) woman this is 1,500–1,600 kcal. A woman who is up and about and quite active will require considerably more, often 2,000–2,200 kcal/d.

It is virtually impossible to deliver basal caloric needs through simple fluid and electrolyte solutions. Most surgeons administer fluids and electrolytes in a 5% dextrose solution. Each liter of this solution provides 50 g of dextrose. If the patient received 2.5 L of this solution per day, she received 125 g of dextrose, which is approximately 500 kcal. Thus, virtually all postoperative patients are given less than their daily caloric needs, initially. Unlike fluid and electrolyte needs, which are immediate and can be life threatening if not managed correctly, the body's need for calories in the immediate postoperative period is less critical. Indeed, it has been shown that if approximately 400–500 kcal are provided to a postoperative patient per day there is very little loss of muscle mass during the first postoperative week. Although the body stores of glucose are generally small, gluconeogenesis can be accomplished from fat stores for some reasonable period of time before muscle loss occurs. Indeed, when loss of muscle mass occurs it is generally from lack of activity rather than caloric need. Patients who are bedridden for long periods of time do lose muscle mass both through inactivity and decreased caloric supplementation. Total parenteral nutrition is essential for these patients.

Based on the administration of standard fluid and electrolyte solutions containing 5% dextrose, it has been shown that the typical postoperative patient who has been maintained in fluid balance can be expected to lose approximately 300–500 g/d (assuming a short postoperative course). If fluid balance is critical or difficult to assess (eg, in a patient with a high fever) daily patient weighing can help evaluate the fluid status. The normal postoperative patient can be expected to lose ½–1 lb/d. If a postoperative patient taking nothing by mouth is gaining weight, excess fluid is being given. Daily weighing of patients is often avoided because of the "nuisance" of needing to use the same scale every day and the inconvenience to the nursing staff. However, it remains a simple and inexpensive method for assessing quickly a patient's fluid status.

In the past, patients were not fed for many days after gynecologic surgical procedures. Once bowel sounds were present, the patient was given sips of water and slowly (often over a 2–3-day period) returned to a general diet. Two things have happened that have largely changed this practice. First, studies have shown that early feeding in patients who have not undergone extensive bowel manipulation results in no problems and often hastens patient recovery. Second, early postoperative discharge is now required by virtually all insurance carriers. It is important to know, prior to discharge, whether the patient can tolerate food, and thus early feeding should be encouraged. If surgery occurs early in the morning, many surgeons will now allow patients to have a light meal the same night and have a full general diet the next morning.

BLOOD AND BLOOD PRODUCTS

Benign gynecologic surgical cases rarely require transfusion. However, all active surgeons will experience an occasional case with unexpected hemorrhage that requires transfusion. In past years, blood was replaced freely and many physicians attempted to have all patients dismissed from the hospital with their preoperative hemoglobin levels. It is now known that there are many risks associated with blood transfusion, even with today's increased surveillance. Various atypical forms of hepatitis are commonly transmitted through blood transfusions. In addition, although all blood in the United States is now screened for the human immunodeficiency virus (HIV), a negative HIV screen does not ensure that the recipient will not receive blood tainted with the virus, since the test is positive only after the donor has been infected for more than approximately 90 days. Therefore, most physicians (and certainly most patients) prefer to avoid blood transfusion whenever possible.

Normal adults tolerate acute anemia poorly. Although a patient who has a chronic slow loss of hemoglobin may feel "fine" with a hemoglobin level of approximately 80 g/L, to suddenly decrease a patient from a hemoglobin of 120 g/L to 80 g/L will result in many symptoms and overall require considerable time for compensation. The patient will feel weak and tired, will experience tachycardia with even mild exertion, and will fatigue easily. Nonetheless, it is now the practice of many surgeons not to transfuse anyone with a hemoglobin above 80 g/L (2% hematocrit). If a patient hemorrhages during surgery and is not transfused, the surgeon should explain to her that she will have symptoms of anemia for some period of time. All women with anemia should receive iron supplementation postoperatively as soon as possible. A normal adult with adequate iron stores and iron supplementation can increase her hemoglobin approximately 1 g/week. Thus, it is possible for a healthy postoperative woman to increase her hemoglobin from a level of 80 g/L to 120 g/L in approximately 1 month.

Gynecologists see many women who are relatively or absolutely anemic because of excessive menstrual blood loss. The causes of such loss are commonly leiomyomata or dysfunctional uterine bleeding from endocrine or metabolic causes. As discussed in the section on preoperative evaluation, many of these patients can be brought to nearly normal hemoglobin levels before surgery. If such action is possible it should be encouraged, as the patient's recovery from surgery will be more tolerable.

Autologous blood donation is suggested by many hospitals. Patients are requested to donate one or two units of blood prior to surgery, and this is held for them until after the procedure. While this is a reasonable plan for procedures that are likely to require blood transfusion, it is not cost-effective for most straightforward gynecologic surgical procedures, which rarely require blood transfusion. There is considerable expense involved in autologous blood collection and storage, and since transfusion is rarely required, both the blood and the expense associated with its collection are wasted. In the past it had been common practice to retransfuse patients with their donated blood at the end of a procedure even if it was not indicated because of surgical blood loss. It is now commonly recognized that this should not be standard practice. First, many patients have replaced the blood that was removed and thus transfusion really becomes "overtransfusion," with the resultant hazards of such practice. In addition, there are expenses and some risks (eg, mislabeling, contamination) associated with autologous transfusion.

PULMONARY CARE

Most surgeons have understood the need for pulmonary care for many years. Thus, it is usual to write an order such as "encourage cough and deep breathing." However, such an order may have different meanings to different hospital staff members, and it is unrealistic to expect that a nurse, in today's climate of ever-decreasing nursing staff, will be able to spend enough time with the patient to see that she performs her deep breathing, sighing, and coughing exercises several times an hour. In a normal patient the routine use of incentive spirometry devices—these "gadgets" are known by various names in various hospitals—has been shown to decrease the frequency of significant postoperative atelectasis. Fortunately, gynecologic patients with either no abdominal incision or only a lower abdominal incision are less likely to have significant splinting, and tend to be able to breathe more fully than patients with thoracotomy or upper abdominal incisions.

One of the best ways to encourage deep breathing is with early ambulation. The patient who is encouraged to walk soon after the surgical procedure is more likely to be able to breathe deeper sooner than a patient who is bedridden.

Obese patients represent a particularly difficult situation postoperatively. The weight of the fat on the chest and abdomen tends to discourage deep breathing because of the extra effort that is required. This can lead to atelectasis and eventually pneumonitis. Thus, these patients need particular attention to pulmonary care and should always have incentive spirometry devices, as well as frequent reminders from the nursing staff. Additionally, short courses of respiratory therapy may be beneficial in these patients.

The other significant pulmonary risk factor for gynecologic surgical patients is smoking. Unfortunately, nearly one third of all adult women smoke. All of these women have decreased pulmonary capacity, have increased excretions that must be eliminated, and have decreased oxygen-carrying capacity in their blood. If at all possible, these patients should be weaned from cigarette smoking for several months before any elective surgical procedure. When this is not possible, the patient will need careful and close evaluation of pulmonary status postoperatively.

BOWEL CARE

Most routine gynecologic procedures do not involve significant trauma to either the large or small bowel, and thus no preoperative bowel preparation is necessary and no postoperative bowel complications are likely to occur. However, in some cases preoperative bowel preparation is required (eg, extensive bowel adhesions). In these cases it is important to realize that such purging of the bowel results in a patient who is even more dehydrated than usual at the time of surgery, and replacement of this lost fluid should be considered.

The most common postoperative bowel problem is ileus. However, this is less likely to occur if the physician has carefully (and gently) packed the small bowel out of the way prior to the surgical procedure. In general, it is not advisable for the surgeon to "run the small bowel" at the time of surgery. An exception is a patient who has had bowel symptoms of unknown etiology and who is undergoing a gynecologic surgical procedure for some other reason.

While this is now largely a practice of the past due to recent studies and early discharge, physicians still carefully listen to the abdomen on daily rounds. In the immediate postoperative period some degree of bowel nonmotility is common due to anesthesia. The bowel appears to "wake up" less rapidly than other parts of the body. Prolonged ileus not responding to conservative measures (eg, nothing by mouth, with fluid and electrolyte administration) requires gastrointestinal drainage.

BLADDER CARE

In most gynecologic surgical procedures, bladder drainage is accomplished throughout the operative period and continues for some period of time postoperatively. In most cases of simple vaginal and abdominal hysterectomy, the catheter is removed soon after the surgical procedure. In complex urinary repair procedures, drainage is necessary for a longer period of time and may be accomplished by either urethral or suprapubic drainage. Because of short hospital stays, the patient may need to be discharged with a catheter in situ.

PAIN CONTROL

In many cases a patient's response to surgery is largely a reaction to the way she was prepared. If the patient is given to expect that she will require a prolonged hospital stay and have considerable pain, it is likely that she will. On the other hand, if a patient's discomfort postoperatively is deemphasized and she is told that early ambulation, early feeding, and early discharge are routine after her procedure, she may be expected to respond in this manner. Thus, the amount of pain a patient has postoperatively is a combination of both the extent of the injury that occurred and the patient's expectation of the pain resulting from this injury.

Patients should be prescribed adequate medications to avoid severe pain. This may be accomplished through the use of one of several commonly used injectable narcotics or through the use of ketorolac tromethamine, a nonsteroidal antiinflammatory agent known to have marked effect on postoperative pain. Regardless of the medication, a "loading dose" of either the narcotic medication or the antiprostaglandin is suggested. However, if a narcotic is used it should be administered in a dose that does not decrease respiratory effort.

For many years pain medications were given primarily by intramuscular injection. This remains the most common method of administration and largely suffices to produce satisfactory amelioration of postoperative pain. More recently, patient-controlled analgesia has become popular. These devices allow the patient to medicate herself within the limits of time intervals between injections and dosage that the device has been programmed to deliver. They have been shown to be quite safe and result in great patient satisfaction.

The downside to patient-controlled analgesia is that it is often continued longer than is necessary. Again, in keeping with the necessity to have patients up and about and ready to discharge soon after surgery, it is important that potent pain medications be held to a minimum. When patient discharge is expected within 24–48 hours it might be preferable for the patient to receive a few intramuscular injections, followed quickly by oral pain medications the morning after surgery.

It is often difficult for health care providers to know how much narcotic medication to prescribe for a patient. While there are published guidelines for amounts of these medications, patient pain tolerance varies greatly, and thus the amount of medication required after a given surgical procedure also varies greatly. In general, patients should be given the amount of analgesic necessary for them to be reasonably comfortable. Patients do not become addicted to narcotic medications when these are given short-term for pain control. Indeed, many of our commonly used narcotic medications are available over the counter in other countries without any evidence of significant abuse.

BIBLIOGRAPHY

Clarke-Pearson D, Olt G, Rodriguez G, Boente M. Preoperative and postoperative care. In: Gershenson DM, DeCherney AH, Curry SL, eds. Operative gynecology. Philadelphia: WB Saunders, 1993:29–86

Davey PG, Duncan ID, Edward D, Scott AC. Cost-benefit analysis of cephradine and mezlocillin prophylaxis for abdominal and vaginal hysterectomy. Br J Obstet Gynaecol 1988;95:1170–1177

Edwards WT. Optimizing opioid treatment of postoperative pain. J Pain Symptom Manage 1990;5(1 suppl):S24–S36

Hemsell DL. Infections after gynecologic surgery. Obstet Gynecol Clin North Am 1989;16:381–400

Lubin MF, Walker HK, Smith RB. Medical management of the surgical patient. 2nd ed. Stoneham, Massachusetts: Butterworths, 1988: 9–10

Magrina JF. Intravenous fluids and blood component therapy. Clin Obstet Gynecol 1988;31:686–689

Orr JW, Holloway RW, Orr PF. Postoperative care of the gynecologic patient. In: Copeland L, ed. Textbook of gynecology. Philadelphia: WB Saunders, 1993:670–694

Orr JW Jr, Sisson PF, Patsner B, Barrett JM, Ellington JR Jr, Jennings RH Jr, et al. Single-dose antibiotic prophylaxis for patients undergoing extended pelvic surgery for gynecologic malignancy. Am J Obstet Gynecol 1990;162:718–721

Pett SB Jr, Wernly JA. Respiratory function in surgical patients: perioperative evaluation and management. Surg Annu 1988;20:311–329

Rudolph R, Boyd CR. Massive transfusion: complications and their management. South Med J 1990;83:1065–1070

Shoemaker WC, Kram HB, Appel PL, Fleming AW. The efficacy of central venous and pulmonary artery catheters and therapy based upon them in reducing mortality and morbidity. Arch Surg 1990;125: 1332–1337; discussion 1337–1338

Smith G. Management of post-operative pain. Can J Anaesth 1989; 36:S1–S4

Summary of NIH Consensus Development Conference on perioperative red cell transfusion. Am J Hematol 1989;31:144

Warner MA, Hosking MP, Lobdell CM, Offord KP, Melton LJ 3d. Effects of referral bias on surgical outcomes: a population-based study of surgical patients 90 years of age or older. Mayo Clin Proc 1990;65:1185–1191

Wasman J, Goodnough LT. Autologous blood donation for elective surgery: effect on transfusion behavior. JAMA 1987;258:3135–3137

White PF. Patient-controlled analgesia: an update on its use in the treatment of postoperative pain. Anesthesiol Clin North Am 1989;7:63–78

Surgical Complications

Postoperative treatment of the patient should be managed as carefully as the operation itself. The major objectives are rapid healing of the wound and physiologic and psychologic restoration of the patient's health as quickly as possible. The general condition of the individual patient and the complexity of the procedure determine the type of care that is needed and the recovery course. Most patients do well following surgery, but some develop complications and must be managed accordingly. Complications of major gynecologic surgery include anesthesia-related crises, excessive bleeding, urinary and bowel injuries, infection, and thromboembolic phenomena. In elderly patients, respiratory insufficiency is the most common postoperative problem.

ANESTHESIA-RELATED PROBLEMS

Regional Anesthesia

Regional anesthesia, both spinal and more commonly epidural anesthesia, may be used for effective and safe surgical anesthesia and postoperative analgesia. The most common side effects associated with the use of regional local anesthetics are sympathetic blockade and subsequent acute hypotension. These events should be managed by immediate administration of ephedrine, 10–15 mg IV, increase in intravenous fluids, and repositioning the patient in a head-down position. Vagal overactivity is treated with atropine, 0.5–1 mg IV.

Intravenous injection of large doses of local anesthetics is manifested in the central nervous, cardiovascular, and respiratory systems. The most severe anesthetic reaction, a grand mal seizure, is often preceded by anxiousness, twitching, and mental confusion. The seizure is usually followed by depression, hypotension, vasodilatation, and inadequate perfusion as a result of the agent's toxic effects on the cardiac conduction system and myocardium. Respiratory depression occurs during and after the convulsion, and it is exacerbated by vascular collapse and depression of the central respiratory center. Once the patient has a seizure, therapy is directed toward controlling the convulsions and supporting cardiovascular and respiratory function by controlled ventilation with oxygen, as well as the intravenous administration of crystalloids and pressor drugs. If convulsions continue, it may be necessary to give succinylcholine IV to suppress muscular activity during the seizure and to permit adequate ventilation of the lungs.

Postoperative analgesia with epidural narcotics provides excellent pain control and improved respiratory capacity and function when compared with parenteral narcotics. The most serious complication of epidural analgesia is delayed respiratory depression, which may occur some 3–12 hours after the narcotic is injected. Therefore, patients should have their respiratory status evaluated frequently by the nursing staff. Respiratory support and naloxone, 0.4 mg IV, should be administered for respiratory depression. Other common side effects of epidural narcotics include pruritus and urinary retention.

Malignant Hyperthermia

Malignant hyperthermia is a life-threatening condition occurring during general anesthesia in about 1/40,000 adults. Patients appear to have a predisposed sensitivity to either the inhalation agent (particularly halothane) or the muscle relaxant succinylcholine chloride. A family history of malignant hyperthermia suggests a high-risk patient. Early diagnosis of malignant hyperthermia is essential for effective therapy. Early signs include unexplained tachycardia and an increase in core body temperature. As the syndrome progresses, acute acidosis or hyperkalemia may result in cardiac arrhythmias, which should be treated with procainamide. Treatment requires immediate discontinuation of the anesthetic agent and administration of 100% oxygen. Dantrolene sodium, 2.5 mg/kg IV, should be administered every 10 minutes, and sodium bicarbonate, 1–2 meq/kg IV, should be given to buffer the metabolic acidosis. Glucose and insulin therapy may be required for hyperkalemia.

The patient should be cooled by using cooled intravenous fluids, packing exposed surfaces in ice, and irrigating sterile cold solutions into open body cavities. Once the patient is stable, the anesthetic agent should be changed and the operation completed in an expeditious manner. Temperature, electrolytes, cardiac rhythm, and renal and hepatic function should be closely monitored in an intensive care unit. Dantrolene may be continued for 48–72 hours at a dosage of 1 mg/kg every 6 hours.

Acute Respiratory Insufficiency

Although it may have numerous causes during the immediate postoperative period, acute respiratory insufficiency is most often due to a combination of factors, such as preanesthetic medication, prolonged anesthesia, bronchial obstruction, and excessive pain medication, that lead to inadequate pulmonary ventilation. Additional attention must be paid to patients who have preexisting pulmonary disease, chronic pulmonary obstruction, or a history of long-term heavy smoking and patients who are elderly. Consultation with a specialist in pulmonary medicine, pulmonary function testing, and baseline arterial blood gas determination are important preoperative preparation for high-risk patients. Optimal preoperative preparation may include the use of chest physiotherapy, inhaled beta-adrenergic agonist, systemic steroids, antibiotics, or intravenous theophylline. Discontinuation of smoking and avoidance of environmental allergens should also be encouraged. Continued aggressive pulmonary care for these high-risk patients postoperatively is mandatory.

Cardiogenic (High-Pressure) Pulmonary Edema

Cardiogenic pulmonary edema most often results from intravascular volume overload, which most commonly results from excessive intravenous fluid replacement. Patients who have an acute myocardial infarction and those with low cardiac reserve or renal failure are at particularly high risk. Intraoperative blood loss should be measured accurately, and replace- ment of blood and fluids should be calculated to meet the patient's needs and to avoid overload. The use of a central venous pressure monitor or a Swan–Ganz catheter may aid in determining the appropriate volume of fluid replacement. Breathlessness, wheezing, and coughing with basal rales should prompt immediate chest roentgenography, electrocardiography (ECG), arterial blood gas level determinations, and initiation of therapy. The management of cardiogenic pulmonary edema includes oxygen support, aggressive diuresis, and afterload reduction to increase cardiac output. In the absence of myocardial infarction, an inotropic agent may be used. Mechanical ventilation should be instituted in the case of acute respiratory failure.

Noncardiogenic Pulmonary Edema (Adult Respiratory Distress Syndrome)

In contrast to cardiogenic pulmonary edema, in which alveolar flooding is the result of increased hydrostatic pressure of the pulmonary capillaries, adult respiratory distress syndrome (ARDS) results from increased pulmonary capillary permeability. This is due to damage to the capillary side of the alveolar–capillary membrane, thus allowing movement of fluid from the capillaries to the pulmonary interstitial space and the alveoli. Common causes of ARDS include shock, sepsis, disseminated intravascular coagulation, massive trauma, and multiple red blood cell transfusions.

Early recognition of ARDS is critical to a successful outcome. The early phase of ARDS is typified by dyspnea and tachypnea, although the partial pressure of oxygen, physical examinations, and chest X-ray are usually normal. Within 12–24 hours of onset, the patient rapidly becomes hypoxic and has a physical examination consistent with patchy consolidation, and the chest X-ray shows early infiltrates. The hypoxemia is relatively refractory to an increase in fraction of inspired oxygen. Aggressive pulmonary support and treatment of the initiating condition will commonly resolve ARDS at this phase. However, if the syndrome progresses further, acute respiratory failure will ensue. After 7 days, the syndrome becomes less reversible, as interstitial fibrosis and bacterial infection often complicate the pulmonary status. The cornerstone of treatment is to remove the source of lung injury (eg, sepsis) and provide pulmonary support. Oxygen saturation should be kept above 90%. Intubation and positive end-expiratory pressure are required for acute respiratory failure. Careful maintenance of blood volume and electrolytes is important to avoid overhydration and worsening of the edema. Swan–Ganz catheter monitoring is useful to make these determinations.

Acid Aspiration

Aspiration of gastric contents causes acute respiratory distress and is a major operative or postoperative crisis. Mortality from pulmonary aspiration is in the 20% range, and morbidity is significant, particularly when pneumonia or a lung abscess develops. Intestinal ileus, gastric dilatation, mechanical obstruction of the small bowel, and seizure disorders are common predisposing causes of pulmonary aspiration in gynecologic patients.

Appropriate anesthetic care in high-risk patients is the most important prophylactic measure. Prophylaxis should include reduction of stomach contents by having the patient ingest nothing by mouth for at least 6 hours before surgery and use of a nasogastric tube or meteclopramide. Furthermore, because the degree of injury is related to the stomach pH (a pH < 3 causes the most severe injury), the stomach contents may be neutralized by use of nonparticulate antacids (eg, sodium citrate) or an H_2 blocker. If vomiting with aspiration of solid food is recognized, the foreign material must be removed immediately to prevent asphyxiation. Smaller pieces of solid food may obstruct small bronchi and must be removed immediately by endotracheal suction or bronchoscopy to prevent absorption atelectasis. If the aspirated material is gastric fluid, chemical pneumonitis develops immediately. The acidic fluid induces bronchospasm, which is followed by atelectasis, pulmonary necrosis, and pulmonary edema.

The principles of therapy are localization of the injury, ventilation support, and intravascular fluid balance. Since the acid injury occurs within seconds to minutes after aspiration, the patient should be placed on her right side with her head down, and intratracheal suction should be started immediately. Management often requires intubation, positive end-expiratory pressure, bronchodilators, and appropriate antibiotic treatment if the patient subsequently develops a bacterial pneumonia. Fluid overload may result in worsening edema, and a pulmonary artery catheter may aid in determining appropriate fluid volume replacement. The use of steroids has not been shown to be advantageous.

Cardiac Arrest

Cardiopulmonary arrest, the unexpected cessation of effective ventilation and circulation, accounts for 10–30% of anesthesia-related fatalities. Although anesthesia-related cardiac arrest is a relatively rare occurrence, it is associated with an overall fatality rate of 50–80%. All high-risk patients, particularly those with preexisting coronary artery disease, must have a thorough medical examination and, if necessary, therapy for fluid and electrolyte imbalance, hypertension, and chronic obstructive pulmonary disease before surgery.

Anesthesia-related cardiac arrest has not been associated with any specific drug or anesthetic agent, but it does occur most often during maintenance anesthesia. The most frequent anesthetic causes of cardiac arrest are overdose, airway obstruction, deficient volume replacement, and failure to achieve effective respiration. Within minutes, upper airway obstruction, circulatory failure, and death from asphyxiation can occur. Three points must be emphasized:

1. Immediate diagnosis and institution of therapy are vital, because only 4–6 minutes of anoxia can be tolerated without cerebral damage; the time is shorter if there is preexisting hypoxia.
2. Because the arrest is cardiopulmonary, therapy must be directed toward effective oxygenation and circulatory restoration.
3. Resuscitation is a team effort and must start with basic life-support measures—airway, breathing, and circulation (ABC), in that order.

The diagnosis is clear when the patient stops breathing, has no palpable carotid or femoral pulse, and has no blood pressure. The patient quickly shows perfusion failure in skin and mucous membranes, loss of cerebral function, as demonstrated by dilated pupils (in 30–45 seconds), and loss of consciousness. Electrocardiography is valuable in the detection of arrhythmias and ventricular fibrillation; it may be misleading, however, because electrical activity can persist after cardiac arrest. Delay is catastrophic. All clinicians should have training in cardiopulmonary resuscitation (CPR).

Briefly stated, successful CPR requires a team approach to restore cardiopulmonary function promptly. The anesthesiologist immediately stops the anesthetic agent(s) and ventilates the patient with 100% oxygen. If an airway is not in place, an endotracheal tube is inserted. The anesthesiologist monitors vital signs and cardiac activity by using an ECG monitor. The surgeon gives a precordial thump and then initiates closed-chest cardiac massage. Compressions should depress the sternum 3–5 cm in the adult and should be smooth and rhythmic, with a frequency of 80–100/min, orchestrated with ventilation at a rate of one ventilation per five compressions. Optimal external cardiac massage will result in a cardiac output of 33% of normal, sufficient for adequate cerebral and coronary perfusion. Concomitant with CPR, a nurse acts as recorder while another nurse readies the necessary equipment and medication and charges the defibrillator. Specific therapy should be guided by cardiac activity as noted on the ECG monitor and judged by evidence of peripheral perfusion.

True cardiac arrest may result from 1) asystole; 2) severe bradyarrhythmias, in which the heart rate is too slow to maintain adequate cardiac output; 3) ventricular fibrillation; and 4) electromechanical dissociation, in which there is organized electrical activity without effective myocardial contraction. Asystolic cardiac arrest and bradyarrhythmias are treated pharmacologically, according to the following guidelines:

- Epinephrine (1–2 mg, 1:1,000 dilution) may be given by either intravenous or endotracheal route. Intracardiac injection in the closed-chest situation may result in pericardial tamponade, coronary artery injury, or intractable ventricular fibrillation due to intramyocardial injection and should therefore be used only if there is no other route of drug administration available. Epinephrine will increase myocardial tone, contractile force, and rate. Assuming normal acid–base status, the dose may be repeated at 5-minute intervals.

- Atropine sulfate (1 mg IV) is the drug of choice for bradyarrhythmias. Its main effects are reduction of vagal tone and reversal of the cardioinhibitory effects of acidosis. A dose may be repeated in 5 minutes, after which total vagolytic effects are encountered. Failure to restore an adequate heart rate necessitates the rapid implementation of direct ventricular pacing by either the transvenous (usually through the subclavian vein) or transthoracic approach.

Ventricular fibrillation is first treated by a precordial thump. If this maneuver is unsuccessful, direct-current asynchronous countershock with 200 J is indicated. If the initial shock fails, a second should be immediately administered at 200 J and, if necessary, a third should be given at 300 J. Delay in countershock therapy increases mortality, and countershock therapy must therefore be administered before any pause for basic life support, airway management, or medication. If the initial three shocks fail, CPR must be initiated, including pharmacologic therapy. Epinephrine should be administered (1 mg IV or endotracheally as a 1:10,000 dilution). After epinephrine, administration of defibrillation (at 360 J) should be attempted. Epinephrine must be administered every 5 minutes.

If ventricular fibrillation is resistant to electrical countershock and epinephrine, a loading dose of lidocaine (1 mg/kg) should be administered, followed by additional boluses of 0.5 mg/kg every 8–10 minutes until a total of 3 mg/kg has been given. Only bolus therapy is indicated in cardiac arrest. A single endotracheal dose (3 mg/kg) may also be effective. Bretylium should be given if lidocaine fails. Initiate treatment with 10 mg/kg by intravenous push. Additional boluses may be given every 15 minutes, up to a total of 30 mg/kg.

After successful defibrillation, the myocardium remains electrically unstable and prone to refibrillation. Therefore, all patients should be treated with full loading doses and an intravenous infusion of lidocaine. If the patient proved refractory to lidocaine during the resuscitation, an infusion of procainamide or bretylium is indicated.

In the presence of severe metabolic acidosis (pH less than 7.2) but adequate ventilation, sodium bicarbonate may be beneficial (1 meq/kg IV). In cases of refractory ventricular fibrillation, it may also be helpful to administer magnesium sulfate, 2–4 g over a period of 1 minute, particularly to patients receiving digitalis or diuretics.

After normal electrical cardiac activity is established, the adequacy of perfusion must be assessed. If perfusion is inadequate despite normal electrical activity, electromechanical dissociation exists. The prognosis for this condition is very poor. In this case, reversible causes should be sought and corrected (eg, gastrointestinal hemorrhage, ruptured aneurysm, sepsis, anaphylaxis, pulmonary embolus, cardiac tamponade). Acidemia should be corrected with sodium bicarbonate, and hyperkalemia should be corrected with calcium chloride (500 mg IV).

Guidelines for cessation of resuscitation remain controversial. The physician in charge of the patient's care, most often the surgeon, has the ultimate responsibility. The American Heart Association advocates cardiovascular unresponsiveness as a basis for termination of the resuscitative efforts.

HEMORRHAGE

Shock

During and after gynecologic surgery, blood volume deficit is usually manifested by arterial hypotension, tachycardia, weak pulse, anxiety, skin pallor, diminished urinary output, and peripheral vasoconstriction. In addition to hemorrhage, the differential diagnosis should include acute respiratory insufficiency, electrolyte imbalance, overwhelming infection, myocardial infarction, and pulmonary embolization. Appropriate studies of arterial blood gases, ECG, roentgenography of the chest, blood chemistry determinations, and blood cultures should be obtained immediately, and the patient should be prepared for blood transfusions. The degree and duration of postoperative shock determine the need for resuscitation, further central venous pressure monitoring, and Swan–Ganz catheterization.

Central Monitoring

Resuscitation of a hemorrhaging patient during or after gynecologic surgery involves stabilization of hemodynamic status and correction of the cause of blood loss. When the hemorrhage is massive, fluid, electrolyte, and hemodynamic shifts are likewise massive. Central to stabilization efforts are the replacement and maintenance of adequate intravascular volume. Coagulation factors must be assessed and replaced if they are deficient, and preparations for surgical exploration must be made if significant postoperative bleeding is suspected.

In patients with truly massive hemorrhaging or in patients who are placed at additional risk by preexisting cardiopulmonary disorders, invasive cardiovascular monitoring may be lifesaving. It allows the rational use of fluids and cardioactive medications, while it avoids their complications.

Peripheral Artery Cannulation

In patients with marked hemodynamic instability, peripheral artery cannulation allows continuous monitoring of systemic arterial pressure, as well as repeated analysis of arterial blood gases. The radial artery is usually chosen for reasons of accessibility and good collateral circulation, although the brachial and femoral arteries may be used alternatively. The complications of arterial cannulation include catheter-related septicemia (4% in one large study), local infection (up to 18%), and, rarely (0.2–0.6%), arterial embolization.

Central Venous Pressure Monitoring

The relative fluid balance of patients in shock can be assessed with a flexible catheter introduced into the great intrathoracic veins by way of the antecubital, external or internal jugular, or subclavian veins. Cannulation of the right internal jugular vein, which provides a straight course to the right atrium, has the lowest overall complication rate. While carotid artery injury is possible, the artery is usually easily palpable and less commonly injured than the subclavian artery at the time of subclavian cannulation. For long-term use, however, the subclavian approach is more comfortable for most patients.

Insertion of the catheter through the antecubital vein is associated with a higher rate of thrombophlebitis and therefore is usually only used for a duration of 48–72 hours. In all cases a chest X-ray should be obtained immediately after catheter insertion to confirm proper location and to assess for possible pneumothorax.

In patients with no cardiopulmonary disease, monitoring of central venous pressure along with monitoring of the vital signs, urine output, and other clinical signs may provide sufficient guidance for fluid resuscitation. In addition, central venous pressure monitoring may be accomplished with a simple manometer, which avoids several of the complications of a pulmonary artery (Swan–Ganz) catheter.

Swan–Ganz Catheter

The usefulness of the Swan–Ganz catheter in critically ill patients (even those without heart disease) who do not respond to therapy based on an initial noninvasive assessment has been well documented. Additional diagnostic information may be obtained concerning unsuspected cardiac dysfunction, pulmonary artery embolization, or sepsis. Patients without primary myocardial insult, but with hypotension and evidence of inadequate perfusion of vital organs (eg, oliguria, acidosis, and mental obtundation), are better managed if data are available from central monitoring. Unnecessary fluid overload can be prevented, and the risk of congestive failure and pulmonary edema can be reduced.

In patients with cardiac or pulmonary disease, cardiac output and resistance measurements allow the proper use of pressors, afterload and preload reducers, and fluids. In addition, if sepsis is part of the clinical picture, careful monitoring of pulmonary capillary wedge pressures may be necessary to prevent pulmonary edema, which is seen with even mild increases in left atrial pressures and which results from the increased permeability of the pulmonary vascular bed. This increased permeability may also be seen in patients in hypovolemic shock, again leading to pulmonary edema at relatively normal wedge pressures. Finally, invasive monitoring not only provides a direct measurement of cardiac function but also provides information within minutes of the effects of therapy.

These catheters may be placed from the antecubital fossa, although the percutaneous subclavian or internal or external jugular vein approaches are more commonly used. Complications of pulmonary artery catheters include pulmonary infarction distal to the catheter (in approximately 1–2% of cases), pulmonary artery rupture (in 0.2% of cases), balloon rupture (in 3% of cases), and sepsis (in up to 2% of cases), all of which are made more likely by prolonged placement of the catheter.

Control of Bleeding

While bleeding patients are receiving blood products, crystalloids, and colloids to attain hemodynamic and metabolic balance, the causes of bleeding must be considered. Military antishock trousers may be lifesaving for a patient who is in hemorrhagic shock before she can be fully resuscitated and the bleeding stopped. In gynecologic patients, the most common causes of postoperative life-threatening hemorrhage are retroperitoneal venous bleeding associated with radical cancer operations, retraction of ovarian or uterine vessels during hysterectomy, and bleeding from the angle of the vaginal cuff. Both immediate and delayed bleeding may be associated with cervical conization.

Whatever the cause, reoperation when the patient's condition is stable and immediate control of bleeding are essential in the treatment of blood loss shock. Under any conditions, reoperation for postoperative hemorrhage is difficult, and a highly experienced gynecologic surgeon should be present or should be standing by. Each patient is different, but experienced surgeons usually know or suspect where the bleeding originated and whether it is arterial or venous in origin. Expert administration of anesthesia, constant monitoring, and blood and fluid replacement are vital in continued emergency care.

Vaginal Bleeding

If the patient has continued vaginal bleeding following hysterectomy and is soaking several pads an hour, there is little to be gained by blind, painful, vaginal packing on a patient who is awake. After proper stabilization and preparation, she should be returned to the operating room, anesthetized, cleansed, and draped. Careful examination with anterior and posterior exposure usually reveals a vaginal angle arterial "pumper" in an unfolding convolution. A single simple suture (or mattress suture) or two below the level of the vessel usually controls the bleeding. Small, oozing vessels on the cut surface of the vaginal wall may be cauterized, but this should be done with care, to keep the point of the clamp away from the bladder or rectal wall. Compression packs in the vagina may be of value for staunching venous ooze from the vaginal wall.

Uterine or Ovarian Vessel Bleeding

Pelvic bleeding from a uterine or ovarian vessel is usually the result of a slipped ligature or retraction of an artery, particularly in large bites of tissue (eg, the uteroovarian and round ligaments sutured as a single pedicle). Compression to control bleeding, identification of the ureter, and double ligation of single bleeding vessels is the procedure of choice. When the bleeding is retroperitoneal, it is usually from the uterine artery or some of its branches; it may be difficult to identify the bleeding vessels. Hypogastric artery ligation is sometimes required, but occasionally it does not control bleeding because of the rich anastomosis of the pelvic vessels, in which case radiographically controlled arterial embolization can be used.

Retroperitoneal Venous Bleeding

Venous bleeding encountered in gynecologic patients such as that during and after radical hysterectomy and pelvic lymphadenectomy is a different and often a more difficult problem. It may appear as a boggy mass that fills the broad ligament area or as a massive hematoma that extends into the iliac fossa and that dissects to the renal area. Ultrasound studies confirm the diagnosis.

Frequently, the source of the continuous oozing is difficult to locate. Evacuating the hematoma by compression, clamping and tying off bleeding vessels, and drying the field should be performed. If the veins are in the presacral or terminal hypogastric anatomic areas, sutures tear into another vein and bleeding becomes worse. Under these circumstances, metal hemostatic clips must be used to halt the bleeding. Microfibrillar collagen, oxidized cellulose gauze, and fibrin spray may help hemostasis. Gauze packing (5 cm), carefully placed with continuous compression, is a measure of last resort; however, its use has saved many lives over the years when posterior pelvic venous bleeding was uncontrollable. When the area must be packed or drained, the exit for the pack may be through the vaginal cuff or by an extraperitoneal groin or low flank incision. Bleeding from sacral veins (such as encountered during sacral colpopexy) may be tamponaded by a sterile stainless steel thumbtack pushed into the sacrum.

INJURIES AND FISTULAS

Intestines

Small Bowel Injury and Fistulas

Injuries to the small intestine during abdominal gynecologic and obstetric surgery usually are the result of blunt or sharp dissection to release adhesions and restore normal anatomy. Adhesions are common when the patient has a history of previous surgery, acute or chronic pelvic inflammatory disease, endometriosis, malignant disease, radiation therapy, or inflammatory disease of the bowel (colitis, ileitis, appendicitis, or diverticulitis). The adhesions may be extensive or limited, fresh or old, dense or filmy. Adhesions are often found between loops of small intestines, between the small intestine and the uterine corpus and adnexal organs, between the small intestine and parietal peritoneum deep in the cul-de-sac, and especially between the small intestine and the undersurface of previous abdominal incisions.

The technique of releasing adhesions varies, depending on their character. Ordinarily, sharp scissor dissection is preferred. Dissection can be tedious and time consuming, and it should be done cautiously to avoid injury and completely to avoid leaving channels through which loops of small intestines may herniate and subsequently become obstructed. Any defects in the omentum should be closed with interrupted no. 3-0 delayed absorbable sutures. Magnification with surgical loupes can facilitate dissection and help to avoid intestinal injury when very dense adhesions are lysed.

If the serosa of the small intestine is sufficiently injured to expose the muscularis, it should be repaired promptly, since it could be more difficult to locate later. The serosa should be approximated with an appropriate number of interrupted no. 3-0 delayed absorbable sutures placed transversely to the longitudinal axis of the intestine. The sutures should approximate and not strangulate the tissue. If the defect is deeper and involves the muscularis and exposes the mucosa, interrupted no. 3-0 delayed absorbable sutures should be placed to include the serosa and muscularis of the bowel wall. Placement of the suture line transversely avoids constriction of the intestinal lumen.

If the defect exposes the lumen of the small intestine, the injured loop is mobilized and delivered through the incision, and rubber- or linen-shod clamps are placed above and below the defect to minimize leakage. Packs are placed to avoid contamination, and the area is suctioned. Assessment of the injury should include the size and location of the defect, the presence of mesenteric damage, and the health and viability of the tissues at the edge of the defect and in the adjacent field. Nonviable tags of tissue should be debrided back to healthy bleeding tissue. After debridement, if the defect is small and does not involve the entire circumference of the intestine or its mesenteric attachment, it may be closed transverse to the longitudinal axis of the intestine and interrupted no. 3-0 delayed absorbable sutures placed through all layers. This suture line is reinforced with a second layer of seromuscular-inverting interrupted no. 3-0 delayed absorbable sutures. If closure of the defect comes close to mesenteric attachments, sutures must be placed carefully in order to close the defect securely while avoiding injury to mesenteric vessels.

When the bowel wall is more extensively damaged or ischemic from an inadequate blood supply, resection of the damaged segment with end-to-end anastomosis is required. Several acceptable techniques are described in standard texts. After clamps are put into place, a small V-type incision is made in the peritoneum covering the mesentery just beneath the segment of bowel to be resected. The underlying vessels will be visible and can be exposed for ligation. Crushing clamps are placed across the intestines on each side of the defect. The clamps are placed obliquely, with the apex at the point of mesenteric attachment, to provide a larger lumen for anastomosis and to ensure a good blood supply to the intestinal wall. The defective piece is excised between these clamps. Interrupted no. 3-0 delayed absorbable or no. 3-0 silk seromuscular sutures approximate the posterior surfaces of the intestine. The crushing clamps are removed, and the ends to be approximated are freshened. The mucosal edges are approximated with a continuous or interrupted no. 3-0 delayed absorbable or silk suture with Connell sutures at the angles. A continuous mucosal suture tends to constrict the lumen more than interrupted sutures do. The anastomosis is completed by a row of interrupted no. 3-0 seromuscular delayed absorbable or silk sutures on the anterior intestinal wall. The intestinal clamps are removed, and the mesenteric defect is closed carefully to avoid injury to the mesenteric vessels.

Intravenous antibiotics and nasogastric suction should be started intraoperatively if a large defect involving the lumen has been repaired. Even without injury to the small intestine, extensive adhesiolysis may cause adynamic ileus postoperatively. This may be avoided by instituting nasogastric suction intraoperatively.

When the small intestine has been injured accidentally by a crushing clamp, the site of injury should be carefully inspected after the clamp is removed. Several interrupted no. 3-0 delayed absorbable or silk seromuscular sutures may be needed to repair the injured site. It is not necessary to excise the injured site.

A small-intestinal injury may result from laparoscopy. A segment of small intestine adherent to the undersurface of a previous incision or immobilized in some other way may be punctured when the trocar is inserted. The use of laser or electrical current through the laparoscope can injure the intestine. When injury occurs or is even suspected, laparotomy with appropriate repair is indicated to avoid fecal soilage of the peritoneal cavity, which causes peritonitis and the potential for serious illness.

If repair of injury to the small intestine does not heal primarily, a troublesome fistula may result. This is especially likely to occur if there has been a technical error in repair or anastomosis, postoperative infection or abscess formation at the repair site, or repair of intestine that was previously affected by irradiation or disease. Drainage may appear through the abdominal incision or through the incision in the vaginal vault. Sepsis may still be a problem and must be controlled by medical therapy (eg, antibiotics and hyperalimentation) or by surgical means (eg, drainage). A fistula that produces minimal drainage and that involves the lower ileum may be well tolerated. A fistula that involves the upper small bowel or that produces copious drainage may cause serious electrolyte and nutritional problems.

The care of the skin of the abdominal wall or vulva may be a major problem. Small intestinal fistulas are more likely to close spontaneously with expectant management if there is no obstruction distal to the fistula, if there is no malignancy or irradiation involved, and if there is no foreign body in the fistula tract. With appropriate management of sepsis and nutritional support, most small intestinal fistulas close spontaneously in 1–2 months. After that, if the fistula still remains open, surgery may be required to close it, to resect the intestinal segment that is involved, or to exclude the involved intestine from the remainder of the gastrointestinal tract. Sound surgical judgment is needed to pick a proper time for repair, and careful surgical technique is necessary to reconstruct the gastrointestinal tract to avoid recurrence of the fistula.

Large Bowel Injury and Fistulas
Injuries to the large intestine (usually the sigmoid colon and rectum) may occur during abdominal or vaginal gynecologic surgery or may result from obstetric delivery. Pelvic laparotomy may result in injury to the sigmoid colon or rectum in patients with extensive adhesions, endometriosis, acute or chronic pelvic inflammatory disease, benign and malignant tumors, or inflammatory bowel disease or in patients who have had previous irradiation or surgery. When extensive pelvic disease is present or an extensive pelvic dissection is anticipated, preoperative mechanical and antibiotic preparation of the bowel is advisable. Extensive disease (infection, endometriosis, or malignant disease) that obliterates the cul-de-sac may cause firm adherence of the rectum and sigmoid colon to the posterior cervix, predisposing the patient to injury of the bowel when a total abdominal hysterectomy is done. It should be possible to remove the cervix safely in almost all such cases without bowel injury. Prudent gynecologic surgeons may, on occasion, however, decide to do a subtotal rather than a total hysterectomy to avoid injury to the rectosigmoid colon, especially when the danger of removing the cervix exceeds the danger of leaving it in. Injury to the bladder and ureters may also be avoided by leaving the cervix in situ.

Injuries to the rectosigmoid colon are closed in a manner similar to the technique of closing injuries to the small intestine. If possible, the repair site should be extraperitonealized in the cul-de-sac, beneath the reflection of the cul-de-sac peritoneum and away from the vaginal vault incision. A diverting loop colostomy by use of the sigmoid or transverse colon is not often necessary but may be appropriate if the closure is not secure, the defect is large, there is fecal contamination, the bowel is unprepared, the closure cannot be extraperitonealized, or the bowel wall is unhealthy or previously irradiated.

Injury to the rectum may occur during vaginal hysterectomy, posterior colporrhaphy, posterior colpotomy, or other vaginal operations. The defect should be closed carefully with interrupted no. 3-0 delayed absorbable sutures in the rectal mucosa and should be reinforced by two additional rows of sutures. If the closure is secure and extraperitoneal, colostomy is rarely necessary, even though the bowel is unprepared.

The lower rectum and perineum may be injured by the delivery of a large infant, a difficult forceps operation, or extension of an episiotomy. It is most important that injury to the anterior rectal wall be recognized and properly repaired to avoid formation of a fistula. A continuous, no. 3-0 delayed absorbable suture should be used to approximate the rectal mucosa. This may be reinforced with several interrupted no. 3-0 delayed absorbable sutures. The repair must go beyond the superior apex of the defect in the mucosa. If the injury involves the anal sphincter, it should be approximated with several interrupted no. 2-0 delayed absorbable sutures before approximating the vaginal mucosa and perineal muscles, fascia, and skin.

Postoperatively, patients who have had colon injury repair should be placed on a limited low-residue diet with stool softeners. Enemas and rectal tubes should be withheld. Antibiotics should be continued, especially if the operative field has been contaminated with feces.

If a colon injury repaired during pelvic laparotomy does not heal primarily, the patient may exhibit peritonitis when fecal contamination of the peritoneal cavity occurs. A temporary diverting colostomy is mandatory. In several months, healing of the defect can usually be demonstrated with a barium enema and the colostomy can be closed. If the defect has not healed spontaneously, surgical repair is necessary before the colostomy is closed.

An intestinal fistula in the upper one third of the posterior vaginal wall or vaginal vault may result from abdominal or vaginal surgery and may be caused by injury to the small or large intestine. A colostomy may be required before closure is attempted, but it should not be done until one is certain as to which intestinal segment is involved. A colostomy will not help a patient whose fistula involves the small intestine.

If a colostomy is done, the fistula may be repaired at the same time after careful mechanical and antibiotic preparation of the bowel. The colon is separated from the vagina by transecting and excising the fistula tract. The orifices of the fistula are closed separately after unhealthy tissue is carefully debrided. An omental flap may be interposed between the rectosigmoid colon and vagina. The patient should be placed on a low-residue diet with stool softeners. In 2–3 months, the colostomy can be closed if a barium enema shows no defect. Very simple rectovaginal fistulas high in the vagina can sometimes be closed with a transvaginal Latzko colpocleisis without a diverting colostomy. Again, after surgery the patient should be placed on a low-residue diet with stool softeners.

When the trauma of obstetric delivery or gynecologic surgery results in a rectovaginal fistula in the lower one third of the vagina, repair must be delayed until the fistula has matured. This may take 2–3 months. A colostomy is almost never required. The repair can usually be done through a transverse incision in the perineum, dissecting between the posterior vaginal wall and the anterior rectal wall and directly through the fistula tract into the loose areolar rectovaginal space above. The vaginal orifice of the fistula is closed with interrupted no. 3-0 delayed absorbable sutures. The rectal orifice is debrided and also closed with interrupted no. 3-0 delayed absorbable sutures in the rectal mucosa. This line is reinforced with at least two more layers of sutures before the fascia and perineal skin are closed transversely. Again, the patient should be placed on a low-residue diet with stool softeners for 2–3 weeks postoperatively, and enemas should be withheld. Re-creation of the fourth-degree laceration by episioproctotomy with debridement and freshening of the edges and layered repair may be used, but this risks the integrity of the external anal sphincter if healing is delayed.

If obstetric delivery results in a complete perineal tear involving the lower posterior vaginal wall, lower anterior rectal wall, perineum, and anal sphincter, the tissues must be allowed to heal for several weeks before repair is attempted. The Noble operation is probably the best technique for surgical repair of this injury, since it does not constrict the vaginal introitus and does not leave a suture line in the anterior rectal wall approximated to the fecal stream.

Urinary Tract Injury and Fistulas

In the United States, most genitourinary fistulas are the result of pelvic surgery; the majority follow an abdominal hysterectomy performed for a benign rather than a malignant condition. Most genitourinary fistulas in the underdeveloped countries of the world are due to obstetric trauma. Some fistulas are the result of pelvic disease, irradiation therapy, or urinary tract instrumentation. Common types of genitourinary fistulas, in order of decreasing frequency, are vesicovaginal, ureterovaginal, and urethrovaginal. Patients often have multiple fistulas, some of which have very complex tracts.

The bladder and pelvic ureters are in proximity to the reproductive tract. They may be involved in primary disease of the reproductive organs and are at risk of injury with gynecologic and obstetric operations, both vaginal and abdominal. When injury to the urinary tract is recognized and repaired at the operation of injury, fistulas and other problems rarely occur. When injuries are not recognized or are improperly repaired, however, enormous disability may result.

Diagnosis

The presence of a genitourinary fistula is suggested by a watery vaginal discharge that smells like urine. Inspection of the vagina with a single-blade (ie, Sims) retractor may document urinary leakage and identify the site of the fistula. If this is not the case, it is recommended that several loosely placed cotton balls be placed sequentially throughout the length of the vagina, and at least 200 ml of dilute but intensely colored methylene blue or indigo carmine solution should be instilled into the bladder through a urethral catheter. If there is no immediate leakage of blue dye from the vagina, the patient should be allowed to ambulate for 10–15 minutes. She should then be returned to the examining table and the cotton balls should be removed from the vagina, one at a time. Blue dye on the most distal cotton ball suggests leakage from the external urethral meatus, possibly because of urinary stress incontinence or detrusor instability. Dye on the cotton balls that were in the upper vagina suggests a vesicovaginal fistula. Wet, but undyed, cotton balls in the upper vagina suggest a ureterovaginal fistula. In the latter case, if subsequent intravenous administration of indigo carmine (5 ml) results in leakage of blue dye into the vagina, the diagnosis of a ureterovaginal fistula is further substantiated.

Whenever there is leakage of dye into the vagina, it may be possible, by careful and systematic inspection of the vagina, to locate the opening of a fistula. A small malleable metal probe is helpful in exploring for fistulous openings and tracts.

An alternative method of demonstrating a vesicovaginal fistula is to place the patient in the knee–chest position, fill the vagina with water or saline, and then carefully insufflate the bladder with carbon dioxide or air through a catheter or cystoscope. Inspection of the vagina may identify a small vesicovaginal fistula as bubbles of gas escape the vaginal wall and rise through the fluid that is within the vagina.

Patients who have genitourinary fistulas should have intravenous urography and cystoscopy. The intravenous urogram is used to evaluate renal function and to detect ureteral obstruction. Cystoscopy is used to locate vesicovaginal fistulas, to determine their relationship to the ureteral orifices, and to evaluate the condition of the tissues around the fistula. Cystoscopy may also be used to determine ureteral function and to perform retrograde catheterization of the ureters.

Ureteral Injury and Fistulas

Fortunately, ureteral injury during gynecologic surgery is uncommon, occurring in approximately 0.3–0.5% of cases. It may occur with complicated and difficult operations for extensive disease, or it may occur unexpectedly in the course of simple operations for limited disease.

Understanding of the anatomy of the ureter is essential for avoiding injury. The ureter enters the pelvis by crossing over the lower common iliac artery and beneath the infundibulopelvic ligament containing the ovarian vessels. As it dips into the pelvis, it can be seen beneath the thin transparent peritoneum along the lateral pelvic sidewall. It lies between the uterosacral ligament and the hypogastric artery. It then turns anteriorly 1.5 cm lateral to the cervix and goes beneath the uterine artery. Between the uterine artery and its entrance into the bladder, the ureter goes through a tunnel in the cardinal ligament. It turns anteriorly and medially over the anterior vaginal fornix to join the bladder about 1.5 cm below the cervix. The relationship between the lower ureter and the cervix may vary on each side. A periureteral pseudosheath protects a rich anastomosis of vessels that run up and down the ureter. In mobilizing the ureter, these vessels will not be injured as long as this sheath is not damaged.

In its course through the pelvis, the ureter is susceptible to involvement, distortion, or compression by a variety of normal and pathologic conditions, including pregnancy, pelvic tumors, gynecologic malignancies, endometriosis, pelvic infection, retroperitoneal tumors, uterine procidentia, pelvic hematomas, pelvic lymphocysts, ovarian remnants, and other problems. Almost all major gynecologic operations, both abdominal and vaginal, have been implicated in ureteral injury, including total abdominal and vaginal hysterectomy, extensive hysterectomy and pelvic lymphadenectomy, suprapubic urethropexy, partial vaginectomy, anterior colporrhaphy, posterior culdeplasty, cesarean hysterectomy, and laparoscopic laser or electrocoagulation ablation of endometriosis. Subtotal abdominal hysterectomy is not often associated with ureteral injury, suggesting that removal of the cervix places the ureter at the greatest risk of injury.

Measures to prevent ureteral injury include careful preoperative evaluation and preparation of the patient, including performance of intravenous pyelography and other special imaging diagnostic studies when indicated. Occasionally, preoperative placement of ureteral catheters may be helpful.

Proper exposure is necessary in the performance of all operations. Exposure must not be limited by limited incisions. The ureter should be identified, visualized, and palpated in all gynecologic operations done abdominally; if necessary, it should be dissected, mobilized, and retracted out of harm's way.

Although the ureter can be injured at any point along its course in the pelvis, it is most vulnerable to injury in the lowest 3 cm during removal of the cervix. When total abdominal hysterectomy is done for benign disease, an intrafascial technique in which clamps are placed beneath the pubovesicocervical fascia may protect the ureter from injury. When desperate measures are needed to control intraoperative bleeding, the ureter may be accidently included in a clamp or suture. Above all, the gynecologic surgeon must be conscious of the risk of ureteral injury, especially at critical points in the pelvis: the brim, the ovarian fossa, the paracervical area, and between the vagina and bladder.

Because of the importance of detecting ureteral injuries at the time of the primary operation, gynecologic surgeons can adopt an effective and routine measure to prove ureteral integrity at the end of each operation. This may be routine visualization, palpation, and dissection of the ureter in each case. Before the incision is closed at the end of an abdominal operation, ureteral integrity can be quickly confirmed by injecting 5 ml of indigo carmine IV, placing a cystoscope in the bladder, and watching the dye spurt from each ureteral orifice. This procedure is facilitated by placing the patient in Allen universal stirrups for each laparotomy. The same procedure to prove ureteral integrity can be done easily at the end of each vaginal operation. The adoption of such a routine procedure in every operation is desirable because uncomplicated hysterectomies, and not difficult or complicated ones, are responsible for most injuries to the urinary tract.

Ureteral injuries may vary in location and type. The ureter may be kinked by a suture that was placed too close, or it may be partially or completely ligated with a suture. It may be crushed with one or more clamps. It may be cut or partially or completely resected unintentionally or, sometimes, intentionally in the course of operations for gynecologic malignancies. The ureter may undergo ischemic necrosis of the wall, usually from stripping of the blood supply for several centimeters, especially in the presence of irradiation or infection.

When the injury is minor, spontaneous healing without significant interference with kidney function may occur. More serious injuries do not disappear spontaneously and should not be expected to do so. Silent atrophy of the kidney is unusual. Superimposed infection usually produces symptoms sufficient to make ureteral ligation clinically evident. When the ureter is ligated, intraluminal pressure rises within an hour from 6–7 mm Hg to 50–75 mm Hg. Then, the pressure gradually decreases over time.

Atrophy of distal nephrons begins in the first week and extends to the cortex in the second week. Urine escapes by pyelocanalicular and pyelosinus backflow and through the venous and lymphatic systems. The afferent arterioles are constricted, and the glomerular filtration rates and total renal blood flow rates are reduced. The recovery potential following release of obstruction is dependent on many factors, including the length of time the ureter is obstructed, the completeness of obstruction, the presence or absence of infection, the degree of backflow, and the previous functional impairment of the affected and the opposite kidneys.

A ligated ureter usually does not stay ligated. An ischemic area at the point of ligation eventually ruptures, and escaped urine forms a urinoma. If a recent total hysterectomy was done, dissection of urine to the fresh incision in the vagina forms a ureterovaginal fistula. Eventually, at the site of injury, a stenosis of the ureteral lumen develops, causing dilatation of the ureter above. When the stenosis is complete, kidney function is in danger of being lost unless the obstruction is relieved.

If a suture is found around the ureter, it should be removed. A defect in the ureter usually appears. The ureter may be repaired over a double-pigtail stent, and an extraperitoneal drain can be placed to the site of repair. More extensive injuries to the lower ureter may require ureteroneocystostomy. A technique of submucosal implantation should be used. The anastomosis must be made without tension. After mobilizing the bladder away from the symphysis and the vagina, a psoas muscle hitch procedure can be used to bridge the gap to a short ureter.

Ureteroureterostomy is the procedure of choice when the ureter is injured in the upper pelvis. The anastomosis is made over a stent. A retroperitoneal suction drain is placed to the site of injury. If the ureteral injury is discovered and properly repaired at the operation of injury, percutaneous nephrostomy is not often necessary.

If the injury is not discovered at the operation of injury, the patient is likely to exhibit persistent postoperative discomfort and fever and an obstinate ileus. Eventually, transvaginal urinary incontinence may appear. Excretory urography, instillation of dye into the bladder, and cystoscopy with indigo carmine dye injection and an attempt at retrograde catheter passage are helpful in making the diagnosis of ureteral injury and in ruling out other urinary tract injuries. If the ureteral catheter can be passed, it should be left in place to encourage spontaneous healing.

When the diagnosis of ureteral injury is made in the postoperative period, the timing of repair is critical. It may be immediate or delayed, depending on the patient's condition; the extent, location, and duration of injury; the condition of periureteral tissues; and other factors. In general, it is now regarded as acceptable to attempt early repair of simple injuries in the immediate postoperative period if circumstances are ideal. Simple injuries to the lowest portion of the ureter that result from vaginal surgery may be repaired vaginally. Otherwise, if early repair is not done, percutaneous nephrostomy to preserve kidney function is the treatment of choice, with definitive repair delayed until the induration of periureteral tissues has resolved.

Very complicated ureteral injury problems may be solved by transvertebral ureteroureterostomy, autologous renal transplant, or the ingenious use of ileal segments to substitute for the damaged ureter. Intentional ureteral ligation, ureterocutaneous anastomosis, and anastomosis of the ureter to the intact functioning sigmoid colon are not usually acceptable techniques to manage ureteral injuries.

Bladder Injury and Fistulas

In developing countries throughout the world, most bladder injuries and vesicovaginal fistulas are obstetric in etiology and result from prolonged obstructed labor. In most developed countries, bladder injuries of obstetric etiology are rare; gynecologic surgery is the most important cause of bladder trauma and vesicovaginal fistula, although a rare fistula may result from other causes (such as radiation therapy for gynecologic cancer). In the United States, the most important measures for reducing the incidence of and morbidity from vesicovaginal fistulas must be directed to proper techniques of gynecologic surgery. When gynecologic surgery is performed properly, postoperative vesicovaginal fistula should be a rare occurrence.

Bladder injury occurs most commonly during total hysterectomy, both abdominal and vaginal. Prevention of bladder injury begins with thorough familiarity with the anatomy of the bladder and especially its boundaries in relation to the lower uterine isthmus, the cervix, and the upper one third of the anterior vaginal wall. The base of the bladder above the interureteric ridge rests on and is draped across the anterior lower uterine isthmus and cervix and the upper anterior vaginal wall. The bladder trigone rests on the middle third of the anterior vaginal wall and is therefore less susceptible to injury when a total hysterectomy is done. If the bladder is injured during a total hysterectomy, the injury will be above the interureteric ridge and trigone. Some injuries to the bladder base are caused by vigorous blunt dissection in the wrong plane. Injury may also result from inadequate mobilization of the bladder away from the cervix in all directions with either total abdominal or vaginal hysterectomy, so that the bladder may be accidentally caught in clamps or sutures that are placed in the cardinal ligaments or anterior vaginal cuff. Finding a proper plane for dissection may be especially difficult in patients who have had a previous low-cervical cesarean delivery.

The bladder may also be injured during operations to correct urinary stress incontinence (anterior colporrhaphy, suprapubic urethropexy, and suburethral sling operations), especially if they are repeat operations. When the bladder is mobilized away from the uterus to perform a cesarean delivery (especially an emergency or repeat cesarean delivery), abnormal adherence of the bladder and dissection in the wrong plane may result in accidental entry. Distortion of the anterior uterine isthmus by leiomyomata can cause difficulty in finding a proper plane for dissection. Dissection of the bladder from the top of the cervix after a previous subtotal hysterectomy can be especially challenging. A total of 1–3% of patients develop a vesicovaginal fistula following extensive hysterectomy as primary surgery for invasive cervical cancer. If such an operation is done after pelvic irradiation, the incidence is higher. Finally, injuries to the dome of the bladder may occur when either transverse or longitudinal incisions are made in the lower abdomen.

Practical measures to help prevent bladder injuries from gynecologic and obstetric surgery include the following:

- Empty the bladder completely before making an incision in the lower abdomen.
- Use sharp rather than blunt dissection to mobilize the bladder away from the cervix in all directions.
- Develop the pubovesicocervical fascia anterior to the cervix and place clamps beneath it.
- When difficulty is anticipated or encountered, place 5 ml of dilute indigo carmine or methylene blue in the bladder to facilitate identification of the bladder mucosa before a final entry is made.
- Place an instrument in the bladder through the urethra to identify the proper plane for dissection.
- Use an omental pedicle graft to bring new vascularity to the bladder base when hysterectomy is done after pelvic irradiation.

If an injury to the bladder is discovered at the operation of injury and properly repaired, a vesicovaginal fistula is not likely to occur. An injury to the base of the bladder (usually resulting from removal of the cervix) should be carefully assessed to determine the extent and proximity to the ureteral orifices. The first layer of closure is usually a continuous horizontal mattress suture of no. 3-0 delayed absorbable suture, which carefully approximates and inverts the bladder mucosa, making certain that the closure goes beyond the limits of the defect. The security of this first line of closure should be tested by instilling 200 ml of dilute methylene blue or sterile milk into the bladder. Any point of leakage should be closed with additional sutures. A second and possibly third layer of vertical mattress sutures approximates the bladder muscle without tension and reinforces the closure. The vesical peritoneum may be sutured to the anterior vaginal margin, thus interposing another layer between the bladder defect repair and the vaginal apex. Cystoscopy with intravenous indigo carmine dye confirms ureteral integrity.

Accidental entry into the dome of the bladder is easy to recognize and repair. A double-layered closure of continuous no. 3-0 delayed absorbable suture can be used. The site of repair should be extraperitonealized if possible.

Postoperative bladder drainage, usually with a transurethral indwelling catheter, should be maintained for 7–14 days. The length of time depends on the extent and location of the defect, the security of the closure, the condition of the tissues, and the condition of the patient.

During the course of any operation, a suspicion of weakness of the bladder wall should be confirmed by instilling 200–300 ml of sterile saline. If there is leakage of fluid or even a concern that the bladder wall is too thin at a particular point, several sutures should be placed for reinforcement.

Vesicovaginal fistulas may develop after a simple uncomplicated operation or after a difficult operation for extensive disease. The postoperative recovery is often complicated by fever, unusual discomfort, prolonged ileus, and hematuria. Transvaginal urinary incontinence usually appears sometime during the first 3 postoperative weeks. Successful treatment depends on an exact diagnosis based on speculum examination of the vagina, instillation of methylene blue in the bladder, cystoscopy, and excretory urography.

Simple vesicovaginal fistulas are those small fistulas that develop as a result of relatively minor trauma to an otherwise healthy bladder during the course of total abdominal or vaginal hysterectomy. This is by far the largest group. Although many surgeons delay repair for several months until all edema and infection have subsided, these fistulas can also be closed with a simple transvaginal Latzko partial colpocleisis as soon as the diagnosis is made. The operation should debride all indurated tissue, excise the fistula track, and mobilize the bladder base; the wound should be closed broad surface to broad surface without tension with three or four layers of interrupted no. 3-0 delayed absorbable mattress sutures. Cystoscopy should be done at the end of the repair to check ureteral integrity with intravenous indigo carmine dye. Bladder drainage should be provided for up to 10–14 days, depending on the security of the closure, the condition of the tissues, and other factors. A successful result can be expected in approximately 90% of cases. Early successful repair significantly reduces the discomfort and embarrassment experienced by the patient.

Complicated vesicovaginal fistulas are those that are large; those that have had previous unsuccessful attempts at repair; those that involve the ureter(s), vesical neck, or urethra; those that are associated with intestinal fistulas; and those that result from extensive surgery or radiation therapy for gynecologic malignancies. Such fistulas should be allowed several months to mature before repair is attempted. Some may still be closed with a transvaginal Latzko partial colpocleisis. However, a transvaginal–transvesical–transperitoneal approach may be required. Also, various techniques of autografting (eg, bulbocavernosus fat flap, gracilis muscle transplant, and omental pedicle) may be needed for neovascularization. After repair of a complicated vesicovaginal fistula, prolonged bladder drainage should be provided. When closure of a vesicovaginal fistula is considered to be technically impossible, urinary diversion above the bladder may be advisable.

Operative trauma may be responsible for other unusual fistulas, including urethrovaginal and vesicocervical fistulas. A urethrovaginal fistula may be seen after suburethral diverticulectomy or anterior colporrhaphy. A vesicocervical fistula may result from injury and necrosis of the bladder wall directly over dehiscence of a lower uterine cesarean delivery incision.

SURGICAL PELVIC INFECTIONS

Microbiology

The endogenous bacterial flora of the lower genital tract is made up of gram-positive and gram-negative aerobic, facultative, and obligate anaerobic bacteria that represent a dynamic ecosystem. Despite similarities in the kinds of microorganisms inhabiting the lower genital tract, differences exist not only among populations but also among individuals within populations. More importantly, the microbiology of the genital tract of a given individual can change over time, possibly attributable to variations within the endogenous environment (eg, metabolic byproducts, vaginal pH, hormonal status, or nutritional or other, as yet undefined, factors). Exogenous factors, for example, frequency of sexual activity, types of sexual activity, douching, and antibiotics (regardless of route of administration) can also have a significant effect on the ecosystem of the lower genital tract. An understanding of the variations that occur in the flora, as well as their interactions at the tissue and cellular levels, is essential to disease prevention.

The microflora of the healthy female genital tract is dominated by commensal bacteria, with lactobacilli being predominant. The lactobacilli were once considered to be the only organisms present on the surface of a healthy vagina. More recently, it has been shown that, while they are the predominant group of microorganisms present, they are not the sole inhabitants of the vagina. Other bacteria are often isolated at a relatively low frequency from culture material obtained from asymptomatic patients. The most common bacterial isolates are *Gardnerella vaginalis*, *Staphylococcus epidermidis*, group B streptococci (*Streptococcus agalactiae*), and *Peptostreptococcus* and *Bacteroides* species. Although most, if not all, of these organisms have the potential to cause disease, they make up the normal flora and usually live in harmony with the host.

The commensal bacteria suppress the growth of the potential pathogens. Lactobacilli, for example, maintain a healthy state by producing lactic acid and hydrogen peroxide. Lactic acid maintains the vaginal pH between 3.8 and 4.2, which favors the growth of the commensal bacteria. Hydrogen peroxide is toxic to anaerobes. If an event such as a surgical intervention occurs, the disease-causing potential of many vaginal organisms can be manifested as pelvic sepsis. It is important to recognize, however, that, because the coinhabitants of this ecosystem are constantly changing, the isolation of a particular organism from an asymptomatic patient need not cause alarm. This does not imply that organisms such as *Neisseria gonorrhoeae* or *Chlamydia trachomatis*, which are not normal flora and which cause sexually transmitted diseases, should not be treated, nor does it mean that a carrier of group B streptococci who is pregnant in preterm labor or with premature ruptured membranes should be ignored. Rather, the decision to eradicate a potential pathogen should be considered carefully, based on available scientific information and individual circumstances.

Risk Factors for Infectious Morbidity

Patients undergoing vaginal or abdominal hysterectomy or cesarean delivery following labor in the presence of ruptured membranes are at risk for postoperative infections. The factors that contribute to the potential for development of a postoperative pelvic infection can be divided into exogenous and endogenous.

Endogenous factors of importance are obesity and the presence of chronic illness (eg, diabetes, hypertension, and emphysema). Significant exogenous factors are length of hospital stay preceding surgery, preparation of the surgical site, and surgical technique. Procedures that increase the possibility of postoperative infection are inappropriate use of electrocautery, which results in tissue necrosis; excessive use of sutures, which act as foreign bodies; and the presence of large avascular pedicles, which leave necrotic tissue behind in the surgical field.

Postoperative soft tissue pelvic infections (eg, postpartum endometritis, pelvic cellulitis, and pelvic abscesses) are frequently due to mixed infections. In addition, most cases of advanced pelvic inflammatory disease are polymicrobial, reflecting the vaginal microflora. These infections involve both gram-positive and gram-negative aerobic (facultative) bacteria, as well as obligate anaerobic bacteria.

Appropriate Antibiotics

Antibiotic therapy usually commences without knowledge of the specific bacterium responsible for the infection; therefore, antimicrobial therapy must provide coverage against a wide spectrum of bacteria. Before empirical therapy is instituted, a specimen from as close to the infected site as possible should be obtained for the culture of aerobic and anaerobic bacteria. The method used depends upon the site infected (eg, an abscess or a localized collection of fluid should be aspirated). The specimen should be placed in an anaerobic transport container. An endometrial biopsy specimen obtained with a pipette and placed in an anaerobic container can serve to transport all organisms. Transporting of tissue in an anaerobic environment protects obligate anaerobes. Specimens obtained with a swab or brush require individual specific transport media.

Antibiotic treatment of postoperative infections is begun empirically. The ideal antibiotic or antibiotics will be broad in spectrum, easily administered, and relatively nontoxic. Whether one chooses a single agent or multiple agents depends on experience, the particular hospital's guidelines, and cost. There is no difference in initial effectiveness among most second- and third-generation cephalosporins (eg, cefoxitin, cefotaxime, β-lactam with lactamase inhibitors [eg, ampicillin/sulbactam], and clindamycin with an aminoglycoside). Too often antibiotics are changed too early. It is not reasonable to believe that appropriate tissue levels of any antibiotic and a response can be achieved before 48 hours. Change should not be considered until after 48–72 hours.

Failure of Antibiotic Therapy

The first step in the management of such a patient is to stop antibiotics, perform a complete physical examination, and obtain specimens 24 hours later from the infected site as well as from venous blood and urine. Blood cultures become increasingly important if the patient develops a cardiac murmur. Analysis of the available laboratory data (eg, white blood cell count, cell differential, electrolytes, and liver enzymes) can be of assistance.

The differential diagnosis should include a resistant bacterium, an abscess, septic phlebitis, and drug fever. The presence of a resistant bacterium can be determined by obtaining specimens and placing them in appropriate transport vials. The laboratory should be informed of the origin of the specimen, and the information about the specimen that is specifically desired should be requested. Once the organism has been isolated and identified, antibiotic sensitivities can be determined. This information can then be used to guide antibiotic therapy.

If the patient is suspected of having a postoperative abscess, an ultrasound examination or computed tomography scan can aid in localizing the abscess. The position of the abscess, its relationship to adjacent organs and structures, and its distance from the abdominal or vaginal walls can be determined with the aid of these imaging techniques. This information is necessary to decide whether percutaneous drainage or laparotomy should be used in the management of the abscess. The use of percutaneous drainage of an abscess avoids laparotomy and its associated morbidity. If the patient has recurring temperature elevations, tachycardia, an increasing white blood cell count, and peritonitis, however, an exploratory laparotomy should be performed. These signs, especially in the presence of an abscess, in a patient with infection are consistent with the presence of purulent material in the peritoneal cavity. Pelvic computed tomography scans are helpful in approximately half the cases of septic pelvic thrombophlebitis.

Laparoscopy

Laparoscopy in the postoperative patient with intraabdominal or pelvic infections is fraught with potential danger. A patient with an intraperitoneal infection often has inflammatory exudate disseminated throughout the cavity, resulting in the development of an adynamic ileus. Often, these adhesions are located between loops of bowel, the anterior abdominal wall, the bowel, and pelvic structures.

Insertion of the laparoscope under direct vision offers the potential for draining an abscess. Before this procedure is attempted, an ultrasound examination may be beneficial in locating the abscess and determining whether it is multiloculated or uniloculated. If the abscess is multiloculated, all cavities must be drained if resolution of the disease is to be accomplished. Abscess locations typically fall within the following categories: 1) a cul-de-sac abscess, which is a collection of pus located in the posterior cul-de-sac with borders consisting of the posterior uterine wall and bowel; 2) an abscess formed between loops of bowel; 3) a tuboovarian abscess, which is made up of purulent material contained within the walls of the ovary and fallopian tube; 4) a subhepatic abscess; and 5) a subdiaphragmatic abscess.

Surgical Drains

Drains should be used to prevent fluids from accumulating in spaces or potential spaces. The pelvis should be drained if complete hemostasis cannot be achieved or if there is free pus in the peritoneal cavity. The drain should exit through the vaginal cuff if a hysterectomy is performed. Alternately, a posterior colpotomy incision can be made. The drain, such as a mushroom or Malecot drain, should be large and should be attached to a self-contained suction device. A closed drainage system should be used to eliminate the possibility of reverse migration of fluid and bacteria.

Transabdominal drains should be used if a pelvic drain cannot exit through the vagina. In these instances, the drains should be placed in the most dependent part of the pelvis or areas requiring drainage. The drains should exit through an area distant from and not through the incision. Again, these drains should be connected to closed suction devices. The efficiency of the drain can be enhanced by keeping the connecting tube short. Double-lumen devices are more efficient than single-lumen devices. The drains should be left in place until 30 ml of fluid or less is collected over a 24-hour period. Drains also provide a means for determining blood loss and collecting specimens for the isolation and culture of bacteria. Penrose or other open drains should not be used because they provide a bidirectional flow, allowing bacteria to enter the cavity being drained.

Septic Shock (Endotoxic Shock)

Shock is marked by a disparity between circulating blood volume and vascular bed capacity. It produces hypotension and reduces tissue perfusion, leading to cellular hypoxia and, ultimately, cellular death. When it is associated with infection, it is called septic shock. By usage, this term is applied to the characteristic clinical picture of gram-negative infection and is frequently called gram-negative or endotoxic shock. Reported mortality rates range from 11% to 82%, with an average mortality rate of 40–50%. The variation may be attributed partly to differences in patients and their underlying diseases and partly to differences in the promptness of diagnosis and methods of management.

Two mechanisms have been invoked to explain the findings in endotoxic shock: 1) selective vasospasm and 2) disseminated intravascular coagulation. It has become apparent that the pathophysiology of endotoxic shock in primates can be attributed to both of these mechanisms, as well as to reduced myocardial response to sympathetic stimuli.

The gram-negative bacilli most commonly found in patients with septic shock are *Escherichia coli* and *Enterobacter, Klebsiella, Pseudomonas, Proteus,* and *Bacteroides* species. The endotoxin is liberated from the cell wall when the organisms die. This lipopolysaccharide–protein complex stimulates catecholamine production and initiates disseminated intravascular coagulation, thus leading to the shock.

Because the mortality rate in patients with septic shock is so high, prevention is particularly important. In obstetrics and gynecology, septic shock is most commonly seen in association with postabortal or postpartum endometritis, chorioamnionitis, or pyelonephritis during pregnancy.

Necrotizing Infection

Necrotizing infections are extremely serious. They usually begin as subtle infections but are associated with a high mortality rate. An error often made is a delay in diagnosis, as the condition may be of late onset. The infection often is not recognized initially and cannot be differentiated from cellulitis, induration, or abscess. This infection can be divided into necrotizing cellulitis and necrotizing fasciitis, with the difference being based upon the tissue layer that is involved. Necrotizing cellulitis involves the skin and subcutaneous tissue. Necrotizing fasciitis involves the subcutaneous tissue, fascia, and muscle. Microbiologically, the infection can be divided into those caused by clostridial and nonclostridial species, the latter of which usually involves facultative and obligate anaerobes.

The diagnosis is often difficult to establish, but aggressive evaluation is necessary. The wound may have a dark, watery, foul-smelling discharge. Frank crepitance indicates the presence of gas. Aspiration of the wound should be performed along the margin of any skin changes or directed by ultrasonography to aspirate pockets of fluid or gas.

Treatment of these infections is administration of penicillin, 20–40 million U/d. In addition, if a polymicrobial infection is suspected, clindamycin and an aminoglycoside should be added. The choice of antibiotics can be aided by Gram stain of an aspirate of the infected site. Wide surgical debridement is the hallmark of treatment. The necrotic tissue should be excised, and the margins should include healthy tissue. A good guideline is to carry out the debridement until healthy tissue bleeds. The patient should be examined for the presence of necrosis every 3 hours for the first 24 hours. If necrotic tissue is present, the patient should be taken back to surgery for more debridement. Once granulation tissue has formed, tissue grafting of defects can be considered.

DEEP VEIN THROMBOSIS AND PULMONARY EMBOLISM

Pulmonary embolism from deep vein thrombosis is the cause of 40% of the deaths in postoperative gynecologic patients, the leading nonobstetric cause of maternal mortality, and the second most common cause of death in patients who have had abortions. Overall, fatal pulmonary embolism occurs in 0.01–0.87% of patients undergoing gynecologic surgery. The incidence of venous thrombosis in patients undergoing gynecologic operations varies in the literature from 7% to 45%, with a cumulative rate of 20%, depending on the type of procedure and other associated risk factors. The clinical diagnosis is inaccurate in up to 70% of patients, with the inaccuracy equally divided between overdiagnosis and underdiagnosis. The overall incidence of postphlebitic sequelae is unknown. However, nearly two thirds of patients with proximal vessel thrombosis will have residual venous system disease with impairment of valvular function and venous return, resulting in chronic pain and lymphedema of the lower extremities.

Diagnosis

Fifty to eighty percent of pulmonary emboli occur without warning. The clinical diagnosis of deep vein thrombosis is based on nonspecific and insensitive signs and symptoms. Early detection and treatment prior to fatal embolization or the onset of complications associated with empirical therapy can be difficult. A number of diagnostic modalities, both invasive and noninvasive, currently exist for the diagnosis of deep vein thrombosis, each characterized by specific limitations. They include contrast venography, impedance plethysmography, real-time ultrasonography, fibrinogen I 125 scanning, ^{111}In-labeled platelet imaging, and magnetic resonance imaging.

Of the invasive techniques, contrast venography is the definitive reference standard for the diagnosis of deep vein thrombosis, with 95% sensitivity and specificity. However, a number of problems are associated with this technique. It is expensive and technically difficult to perform and to interpret. It is associated with a number of complications, including phlebitis, induced thrombosis, renal and systemic hypersensitivity reactions, extravasation-induced skin and tissue necrosis, and radiation exposure in pregnancy.

The minimally invasive techniques using isotope-labeled blood products have a sensitivity of greater than 90% and a specificity for acute calf vein thrombi. Disadvantages of these techniques include 1) a markedly reduced sensitivity (60–80%) in detecting proximal vein thrombi in the large vessels of the thigh and pelvis; 2) a risk of blood-borne diseases (eg, HIV and hepatitis B virus); 3) a contraindication to their use during pregnancy and lactation, since ^{125}I crosses the placenta and has been found in breast milk; 4) a duration of scanning limited by the half-life of the isotope (5–7 days for ^{125}I); and 5) accuracy to 70–80% if there are preexisting thrombi due to poor uptake of fibrinogen. A number of other radioisotopic techniques are under investigation; however, they are not in widespread use because of similar problems and lowered sensitivity or specificity when compared with the available noninvasive techniques.

Of the noninvasive diagnostic modalities, occlusive cuff impedance plethysmography has been the most thoroughly evaluated. It detects changes in blood volume, as monitored by changes in the electrical resistance of the calves, and has a sensitivity of 93% and specificity of 95% for thrombosis of the proximal veins (popliteal, femoral, or iliac veins). The major disadvantages include 1) insensitivity to calf vein thrombi; 2) detection only of thrombi producing obstruction to venous outflow, which limits the diagnosis of proximal vessel extension that is not totally occlusive in the early stages; 3) lack of differentiation between thrombotic and nonthrombotic occlusion; and 4) false-positive results obtained with unrecognized contraction of the leg muscles or any clinical condition that reduces arterial inflow to the limb (eg, congestive heart failure, compressive pelvic masses, or severe peripheral vascular disease). Accuracy can be increased if serial measurements are taken. However, a negative test result does not necessarily rule out distal disease.

Alternative noninvasive diagnostic methods include those based on ultrasonography with or without Doppler. Currently the most promising of these is the combination of real-time ultrasonography with Doppler examination, referred to as duplex B-mode imaging or duplex Doppler imaging. This technique allows simultaneous visualization of thrombi with measurement of flow velocity from changes in reflected ultrasound beam frequency (Doppler shift). Sensitivity is 100% and specificity is 78%; however, the specificity may indeed be much higher, since false-positive values may result from an incorrect reading and improper positioning of a patient with a term pregnancy. Disadvantages of this technique are similar to those associated with impedance plethysmography and include a reduced sensitivity to the presence of nonocclusive proximal thrombi and subjective interpretation requiring considerable skill and experience. Advantages over impedance plethysmography are less expense, convenience, and greater reliability in detecting proximal vein thrombosis in patients with vascular insufficiency or congestive heart failure. In addition to duplex imaging, both Doppler and real-time ultrasonography have been used as single modalities, with sensitivities and specificities greater than 90%. Additional noninvasive methods such as magnetic resonance imaging are undergoing investigation but are not currently in general use.

History

The known etiologic factors of venous thrombosis are venous stasis, vascular endothelial damage, and hypercoagulability. A number of risk factors that predispose to venous thrombosis have been identified, including age, obesity, pregnancy, immobilization, extensive varicosities, malignancy, previous thromboembolism, hypercoaguable states, estrogen therapy, myocardial infarction, congestive heart failure, and major surgery or trauma.

Of the previously mentioned etiologic factors, venous stasis is most amenable to prophylaxis and the most common inciting factor. A number of researchers have demonstrated that during an operative procedure the venous return from the lower extremities falls to half of its normal rate, due to decreased muscle and vascular tone induced by muscle relaxants and inhaled anesthetics. This results in pooling of blood in the venous sinuses. In addition to the intraoperative period, the postoperative recovery time is associated with a reduction in axial blood flow of up to 75%, which can persist for up to 14 days due to immobilization or reduced activity.

Studies using ^{125}I have demonstrated that thrombosis begins during the surgical procedure in up to 50% of patients and during the first 48 hours after surgery in 66% of those who develop postoperative deep vein thrombosis. Most commonly, venous thrombosis originates in the soleus muscle veins of the calf (up to 89%). When calf thrombosis develops, 20–25% will extend proximally into the veins of the thigh. In this group, up to 50% will experience a pulmonary embolus.

Of those who experience thromboembolic phenomena, 49% occur within 24 hours and 75% within 3 days of surgery. Rarely, late thromboembolic complications may occur after the patient has been discharged and even sometimes after negative studies performed throughout hospitalization. These data support the need for accurate diagnostic studies and therapy in the immediate postoperative period. In addition, the need for diagnosis and treatment of acute iliofemoral and iliac thrombosis is clear. Currently, however, it is believed that thrombi that are localized to the soleus veins of the calf may have little clinical significance, and some controversy exists regarding whether to initiate anticoagulant therapy or to manage with conservative observation and serial noninvasive testing.

General guidelines for assessing a patient's risk for deep vein thrombosis or pulmonary embolism prior to surgery are based on age, type and length of surgery, weight, and concurrent medical disease. Using this system, patients are assigned to low-, medium-, or high-risk categories in order to decide which prophylactic methods should be used, if any.

Patients in the low-risk group are those under the age of 40, of normal weight, and without concurrent medical disease, who are undergoing uncomplicated or minor surgery of less than 30-minute duration. These patients can be expected to have less than a 10% risk of calf thrombosis, less than a 1% risk of proximal vein deep vein thrombosis, and less than a 0.01% risk of fatal pulmonary embolism if prophylaxis is not used. Recommended prophylaxis for this group includes early ambulation and graduated compression stockings.

Patients in the medium-risk group are over 40 years of age, are moderately obese (more than 20% over ideal body weight), have minimal secondary risk factors, and are undergoing major abdominal or pelvic surgery lasting longer than 30 minutes. Without prophylaxis, this group can be expected to have a 10–40% risk of developing calf vein thrombosis, a 2–10% risk of proximal vein clot, and a 0.1–0.7% risk of fatal pulmonary embolism. Under these circumstances, prophylaxis with either systemic anticoagulants (eg, low-dose heparin, low-dose warfarin, or dextran) or intermittent pneumatic compression stockings is recommended.

The high-risk category encompasses patients over the age of 40 who are morbidly obese (more than 30% over ideal body weight), have medical disease (eg, diabetes, severe varicosities, previous venous thrombosis), and are undergoing a major operation for malignancy lasting longer than 30 minutes. This group has a 40–80% risk of calf vein thrombosis, a 10–20% risk of proximal vein thrombosis, and a 1–5% risk of fatal pulmonary embolism without prophylaxis. It is suggested that in this group multiple modalities for prophylaxis be used concurrently (for example, dextran or low-dose heparin with intermittent pneumatic compression stockings).

Treatment

Prophylactic Therapy

Early ambulation and elevation of the feet and legs while the patient is confined to bed are the most basic and easily performed prophylactic measures. A number of other modalities involving either mechanical or pharmacologic methods exist, each with its own indications, limitations, and complications.

The currently used pharmacologic agents include heparin, warfarin, and dextran. Low-dose heparin prophylaxis in selected high-risk patients has been shown to reduce the incidence of deep vein thrombosis from 35% to 45% to approximately 7%. Used properly, it does not significantly alter the clotting time or increase the amount of operative or postoperative blood loss. Some evidence suggests, however, that it may be ineffective in patients with malignant disease. It has been associated with an increase in major hemorrhagic events (from 0.8% to 1.8%), as well as a significant increase in wound hematomas (6.3%). Other complications with this type of prophylaxis include skin necrosis, thrombocytopenia, and hyperkalemia.

To reduce the associated complications, alternative regimens such as adjusted low-dose heparin therapy with or without dihydroergotamine and therapy with low-molecular-weight heparin have been investigated. Dextran 70 has also been shown to decrease the incidence of thrombosis, particularly in patients undergoing extensive surgery for pelvic malignancy, by decreasing blood viscosity and reducing platelet reactivity. The data regarding other gynecologic surgical patients are less conclusive, and the use of dextran 70 has been associated with anaphylactic reactions, heart and renal failure, and severe hemorrhage. Similarly, low-dose warfarin has been investigated for prophylactic use. However, its use is associated with significant risk of major postoperative bleeding, and it is not as easily reversible as heparin. Other drugs for experimental use only include aspirin, dihydroergotamine, and nonsteroidal antiinflammatory medications.

The most commonly used mechanical methods of prophylaxis include graduated compression stockings and intermittent pneumatic compression stockings. A number of studies have demonstrated the efficacy of graduated leg compression stockings in reducing the incidence of deep vein thrombosis by twofold to fourfold. Hence, the National Institutes of Health Consensus Development Conference on Prevention of Venous Thrombosis and Pulmonary Embolism in March 1986 concluded that in conjunction with early ambulation their use would provide sufficient prophylaxis in the low-risk surgical patient. For those patients with moderate-to-high risk of thrombosis, external pneumatic compression stockings have proven in multiple series to effectively reduce the occurrence of deep vein thrombosis and pulmonary embolism by up to 20% if used intraoperatively and for up to 5 days postoperatively or until the patient is ambulating actively. This method has many advantages over the previously mentioned pharmacologic agents, given that it is noninvasive and fairly easy to use. Problems associated with this method include occasional skin reaction, excessive sweating underneath the appliance, and difficulty in ambulation during application. For those patients who have been at bed rest or immobilized for more than 72 hours without previous prophylaxis, this device should not be used because of the possibility of disturbing an existing clot.

Deep Vein Thrombosis

The generally accepted treatment of deep vein thrombosis is full anticoagulation with intravenous heparin for a minimum of 7–10 days. This treatment should be tapered after anticoagulation has been established with an oral anticoagulant, such as coumarin. Treatment should be continued for a minimum of 6 weeks in uncomplicated deep vein thrombosis if all evidence of disease has disappeared and the inciting factor has been resolved. For patients with residual venous disease, therapy should be continued for 3–4 months; for those with pulmonary embolism, therapy for 3–6 months is recommended. This anticoagulant regimen, along with intravenous heparin, prevents further immediate thrombus formation, induces a moderate thrombolysis during the heparin phase, and allows for a prolonged natural lysis and recanalization of the major venous circulation of the legs and pelvis.

Prolonged oral administration of coumarin provides a relatively simple and inexpensive regimen to prevent relapse and to diminish postphlebitic sequelae. If further evidence of acute venous thromboembolic disease is observed, a return to intravenous heparin should be started immediately. Despite carefully controlled postoperative therapeutic anticoagulant regimens, hemorrhagic complications are a major hazard, particularly in cancer patients.

Thrombolytic Therapy

During the past decade, thrombolytic therapy has been investigated extensively in patients with clinical conditions of proximal deep vein thrombosis, pulmonary embolization, arterial thrombosis and embolism, and acute myocardial infarction. In the United States, two thrombolytic agents are available for clinical use: streptokinase and urokinase. Streptokinase and urokinase act by transforming the fibrin-bound inactive proenzyme plasminogen into the active enzyme plasmin, which has good fibrinolytic activity. Because the two drugs are therapeutically equal in effectiveness and because urokinase is several times more expensive, streptokinase is generally the thrombolytic agent of choice.

Thrombolytic therapy is effective but not without significant risk as it dissolves clots maintaining hemostasis at the operative site(s). It should be a last ditch effort in patients who are moribund and in need of relief from their antepulmonary hypertension as an alternative to surgical treatment. The safe postoperative time interval for a minor procedure is 48 hours but for a major procedure is 2 weeks.

Streptokinase is administered IV in a loading dose (to neutralize streptococcal antibodies), followed by a maintenance dose for 24–72 hours. When the thrombin time has decreased to less than twice the normal value, treatment with heparin by continuous infusion is initiated (without a loading dose) after the administration of either thrombolytic agent and is continued in the usual anticoagulant regimen. Most clinical studies have shown that thrombolytic agents, combined with heparin therapy, enhance the lysis of pulmonary thromboemboli at 24 hours, restoring pulmonary circulation and decreasing pressure on the right side of the heart. Unfortunately, combined therapy does not affect the recurrence rate of pulmonary emboli, nor does it affect the morbidity and mortality after a 2-week interval.

Present recommendations are that the use of thrombolytic agents should be limited to massive leg and pelvic deep vein thrombosis, severe pulmonary embolism with shock, and arteriovenous cannula occlusion. The intracoronary administration of thrombolytic agents in patients with severe acute myocardial infarction will be observed with interest. Their adverse effects (ie, hemorrhage in the early postoperative period and hypersensitivity reactions) exceed those of heparin alone and must be carefully weighed in the consideration of therapeutic choices.

Surgical Management

Operative procedures are not generally considered in patients with thromboembolic disease, except when heparin anticoagulant therapy fails. Venous thromboectomy is indicated only in patients with massive proximal deep vein thrombosis that is associated with severe arterial spasm and phlegmasia cerulea dolens of the leg. In these cases, the lesion must be less than 48 hours old, and despite complete excision, most thromboses recur. Interruption of the inferior vena cava is rarely performed today. Rather, percutaneous placement of a vena cava filter (eg, Greenfield) is used in patients with persistent pulmonary embolization, despite adequate heparinization; absolute contraindications to heparin; or, in rare instances, persistent showering of septic emboli after an adequate trial of antibiotic and heparin therapy. The primary indication for pulmonary embolectomy is massive embolism, documented by either lung scan or pulmonary arteriography, in patients who show persistent and refractory hypotension. An indication that seems to be increasing in frequency is chronic pulmonary embolization with development of cor pulmonale, a condition that, in the past, has shown a poor prognosis with medical therapy.

DEHISCENCE, EVISCERATION, AND INCISIONAL HERNIAS

Failure of an abdominal incision to heal may result in significant postoperative morbidity and even mortality. Early complications of abdominal wound failure include dehiscence and evisceration; late complications include incisional hernias. Disruption of abdominal incisions of some degree occurs in approximately 5% of gynecologic and obstetric laparotomies. With attention to details, these complications can be kept to a minimum, if not completely eliminated.

A variety of factors are associated with failure of wound healing. Patient factors include obesity, malnutrition, sepsis, liver disease, uremia, anemia, diabetes, corticosteroid therapy, immunodeficiency, bronchopulmonary disease, malignancy, and irradiation of the abdominal wall. Any factor that predisposes to infection in the incision (such as a prolonged surgical procedure) will also predispose to failure of wound healing. Transverse incisions (Maylard and Pfannenstiel) in the lower abdomen are thought to heal better than vertical incisions. In the postoperative period, prolonged and severe abdominal distention, vomiting, and coughing may result in wound disruption, especially if associated with other predisposing factors. However, despite the presence of factors that interfere with wound healing, primary healing will occur in most patients if the incision is properly fashioned and closed.

The strength of an incision lies mostly in the aponeurotic (fascial) coverings of the abdominal musculature. This layer requires 120 days to heal completely. In the early weeks of this healing process, wound strength depends on the strength of the fascial sutures. When suture strength is lost prematurely, before the fascia is healed securely, wound disruption is more likely to occur. Suture strength may be lost because of breakage, cutting through the tissue, knot slippage, or placement of an insufficient number of sutures.

Wound disruptions are more common when infection is present. Prophylactic perioperative antibiotics may reduce the incidence of wound infection in certain cases. More importantly, meticulous surgical technique will keep bacterial contamination of the wound at a minimum. In the presence of gross bacterial contamination, especially in obese patients with risk factors, the incision may be packed open above the fascial closure. Sutures may be placed through the skin and subcutaneous fat and tied later when the tissue appears healthy.

When superficial wound disruption occurs, usually with an infection or hematoma in the incision, careful examination should determine whether the fascial closure is intact. The wound should be irrigated and debrided of infected and devitalized tissue. This should be repeated as often as necessary until a healthy bed of granulation tissue is present. This may take several days. Systemic antibiotics may be indicated as an adjunct to surgical drainage and debridement or if systemic infection is present. The superficial disruption may then be closed with interrupted sutures, using local anesthesia. This secondary closure will reduce the time it takes for the incision to heal.

A profuse serosanguineous drainage from the incision usually during the first week after operation is an indication of impending evisceration. It may be precipitated by an episode of vomiting or coughing. The episode should be treated as an emergency, hopefully to prevent the occurrence of a complete evisceration under uncontrolled circumstances. The patient should be informed, reassured, sedated, stabilized, and transferred to the operating room with a sterile bulk dressing applied to support the incision.

Under general anesthesia, the skin sutures or staples should be removed and the fascia explored. Old suture material and infected and devitalized tissue should be removed. Number 1 polypropylene through-and-through interrupted sutures should be used to close the defect. Other interrupted sutures may also be used in the fascia and skin. The through-and-through sutures may be left in place for 14–21 days. Postoperative care should include broad-spectrum antibiotics, nasogastric suction, intravenous fluid therapy, and possibly hyperalimentation and anticoagulation. Evisceration is associated with a 15–20% mortality and a high risk of pulmonary embolization.

An incisional hernia is a late complication of incomplete or failed wound healing. Instead of complete dehiscence or evisceration of the wound, hernia formation results from incomplete dehiscence in which a defect in the fascia is present although the peritoneum, subcutaneous fat, and skin remain intact. The incidence is approximately 1% with primary incisional healing but increases greatly with infected incisions, dehiscence, and evisceration. The hernia through the fascial defect may not be apparent for several months or years later. Incisional hernias often contain incarcerated omentum and intestine. However, since the defect is usually broad or diffuse, strangulation of the contents of the hernial sac is relatively rare. Incisional hernias with small necks may be associated with intestinal obstruction.

The principles of incisional hernia repair include 1) dissection of the hernial sac from the subcutaneous fat, rectus, fascia, and peritoneal margin; 2) excision of the redundant hernial (peritoneal) sac; and 3) closure of the abdominal wound, using a layer-for-layer closure, an overlap repair of the rectus fascia, or the placement of a synthetic mesh prosthesis. The repair can be difficult, especially in obese patients. Recurrence rates of up to 40% have been reported.

BIBLIOGRAPHY

Anesthesia-Related Problems

Clarke-Pearson DL, Olt GJ, Rodriguez G, Boente M. Preoperative and postoperative care. In: Gershenson DM, DeCherney AH, Curry SL, eds. Operative gynecology. Philadelphia: WB Saunders, 1993: 29–86

Dodson ME. Post-operative pain relief. In: Nunn JF, Utting JE, Brown BR Jr, eds. General anesthesia. 5th ed. Boston: Butterworths, 1989: 1123–1140

Emergency Cardiac Care Committee and Subcommittees, American Heart Association. Guidelines for cardiopulmonary resuscitation and emergency cardiac care. I: introduction. JAMA 1992; 268: 2172–2183

Galant SP. Treatment of asthma: new and time-tested strategies. Postgrad Med 1990;87:229–236

Hotchkiss RS. Perioperative management of patients with chronic obstructive pulmonary disease. Int Anesthesiol Clin 1988;26:134–142

Mohr DN, Jett JR. Preoperative evaluation of pulmonary risk factors. J Gen Intern Med 1988;3:277–287

Hemorrhage

Harke H, Rahman S. Hemostatic disorders in massive transfusion. Bibl Haematol 1980;46:179

Stehling L. Preoperative blood ordering. Int Anesthesiol Clin 1982; 20:45

Injuries and Fistulas

Cruikshank SH. Early closure of posthysterectomy vesicovaginal fistulas. South Med J 1988;81:1525–1528

Dirksen PK, Matolo NM, Trelford JD. Complications following operation in the previously irradiated abdominopelvic cavity. Am Surg 1987;43:234–241

Elkins TE, Drescher C, Martey JO, Fort D. Vesicovaginal fistula revisited. Obstet Gynecol 1988;72:307–312

Gillenwater JY. The pathophysiology of urinary obstruction. In: Walsh PC, Gittes RF, Perlmutter AD, Stamey TA, eds. Campbell's urology. 6th ed. Philadelphia: WB Saunders, 1992:542–578

Lee RA, Symmonds RE, Williams TJ. Current status of genitourinary fistula. Obstet Gynecol 1988;72:313–319

Mann WJ, Arato M, Patsner B, Stone ML. Ureteral injuries in an obstetrics and gynecology training program: etiology and management. Obstet Gynecol 1988;72:82–85

Thompson JD, Rock JA. TeLinde's operative gynecology. 7th ed. Philadelphia: JB Lippincott, 1991

Wiskind AK, Thompson JD. Transverse transperineal repair of rectovaginal fistulas in the lower vagina. Am J Obstet Gynecol 1992; 167:694–699

Witters S, Cornelissen M, Vereecken R. Iatrogenic ureteral injury: aggressive or conservative treatment. Am J Obstet Gynecol 1986;155: 582–584

Surgical Pelvic Infections

Emmons SL, Krohn M, Jackson M, Eschenbach DA. Development of wound infections among women undergoing cesarean section. Obstet Gynecol 1988;72:559–564

Faro S. New consideration in the treatment of urinary tract infections in adults. Urology 1992;39:1–11

Faro S. Postoperative infections and thrombophlebitis. In: Nichols DH, ed. Gynecologic and obstetric surgery. St Louis: Mosby–Year Book, 1993:222–235

Faro S. Postsurgical infections: antibiotic trials. Curr Opin Obstet Gynecol 1990;2:682–689

Faro S, Phillips LE, Martens MG. Perspectives on the bacteriology of postoperative obstetric-gynecologic infections. Am J Obstet Gynecol 1988;158:694–700

Hager WD, Pascuzzi M, Vernon M. Efficacy of oral antibiotics following parenteral antibiotics for serious infections in obstetrics and gynecology. Obstet Gynecol 1989;73:326

Hemsell DL. Infections after gynecologic surgery. Obstet Gynecol Clin North Am 1989;16:381

Hemsell DL, Bowdon RE, Hemsell PG, Nobles BJ, Johnson ER, Heard MC. Single-dose cephalosporin for prevention of major pelvic infection after vaginal hysterectomy: cefazolin versus cefoxitin versus cefotaxime. Am J Obstet Gynecol 1987;156:1201–1205

Hemsell DL, Hemsell PG, Heard MC, Nobles BJ. Piperacillin and a combination of clindamycin and gentamicin for the treatment of hospital and community acquired acute pelvic infections including pelvic abscess. Surg Gynecol Obstet 1987;165:223–229

Hemsell DL, Nobles B, Heard MC. Recognition and treatment of post-hysterectomy pelvic infection. Infect Surg 1988;7:47

Loy RA, Gallup DG, Hill JA, Holzman GM, Geist D. Pelvic abscess: examination and transvaginal drainage guided by real-time ultrasonography. South Med J 1989;82:788–790

Deep Vein Thrombosis and Pulmonary Embolism

Becker DM. Venous thromboembolism: epidemiology, diagnosis, prevention. J Gen Intern Med 1986;1:402–411

Hirsh J, Hull RD, Raskob GE. Clinical features and diagnosis of venous thrombosis. J Am Coll Cardiol 1986;8(6 suppl B):114B–127B

Merli GJ. Prophylaxis for deep vein thrombosis and pulmomary embolism in the geriatric patient undergoing surgery. Clin Geriatr Med 1990;6:531–542

Mohr DN, Ryu JH, Litin SC, Rosenow ED 3d. Recent advances in the management of venous thromboembolism. Mayo Clin Proc 1988; 63:281–290

Paiement GD, Desautels C. Deep vein thrombosis: prophylaxis, diagnosis, and treatment—lessons from orthopdeic studies. Clin Cardiol 1990;13(4 suppl 6):VI19–VI22

Prevention of venous thrombosis and pulmonary embolism. NIH Consensus Development. JAMA 1986;256:744–749

Seiden AM, Pensak ML. Postoperative deep venous thrombosis and pulmonary embolism: diagnosis, management, and prevention. Am J Otol 1986;7:377–383

Thompson JD, Rock, JA. TeLinde's operative gynecology. 7th ed. Philadelphia: JB Lippincott, 1992

Dehiscence, Evisceration, and Incisional Hernias

Baggish MS, Lee WK. Abdominal wound disruption. Obstet Gynecol 1975;46:530–534

Dodson MK, Magann EF, Meeks GR. A randomized comparison of secondary closure and secondary intention in patients with superficial wound dehiscence. Obstet Gynecol 1992;80:321–324

Gallup DG, Nolan TE, Smith RP. Primary mass closure of midline incisions with a continuous polyglyconate monofilament absorbable suture. Obstet Gynecol 1990;76:872–875

Sutton G, Morgan S. Abdominal wound closure using a running, looped monofilament polybutestor suture: comparison to Smead-Jones closure in historic controls. Obstet Gynecol 1992;80:650–654

Walters MD, Dombroski RA, Davidson SA, Mandel PC, Gibbs RS. Reclosure of disrupted abdominal incisions. Obstet Gynecol 1990;76: 597–602

Sterilization

Sterilization is accepted by about 500,000 women annually in the United States. It is the most common method of maintaining family size chosen by married women over age 30. The risk of death from sterilization is less than the annual risk of death from taking oral contraceptives. Nevertheless, sterilization is the second most frequent cause of lawsuits against obstetrician–gynecologists because of operative complications and pregnancy. Attention to issues concerning documented informed consent as well as specific technical details of sterilization minimizes the legal risks.

PATIENT SELECTION AND COUNSELING

The appropriateness of the procedure depends on three judgments to be made by the surgeon. The patient should be 1) mature, 2) unpressured, and 3) informed. Women have regretted sterilization when it was performed for immature reasons or under stress (eg, during divorce or abortion). At least two states require legal compliance with federal Medicaid guidelines for all patients. These define *mature* as being over age 21, *unpressured* as having waited 30 days, and *informed* as having read the pamphlet prepared by the U.S. Department of Health and Human Services. The rest of the states have few guidelines for private patients as to age, marital status, and parity. Contraindications are few and surgically obvious: severe anesthetic risk, such as class III or class IV heart disease, or documented bowel adhesion to the abdominal wall. Obesity, diabetes, and mild heart disease may be indications that make the patient a high risk, but they are not in themselves contraindications.

It is important to ensure that the patient is aware of the nature and risks of the procedure and its alternatives. Signed documentation that the patient has seen or read these materials and has understood the contents is medicolegally prudent. The procedure should be recommended as a permanent method of contraception. The procedure may be reversible, however, if a genuine judgment error was made by the patient and her physician at the time of sterilization. This error is most commonly made by women under age 30 who seek sterilization. For this reason, a more reversible mechanical occlusive technique should be considered for women in this age group. The failure rate of sterilization should be presented as around 1%, although long-term follow-up studies of bipolar coagulation (6–10 years) suggest higher cumulative pregnancy rates. There are no consistent differences in efficacy documented among the standard techniques used today. The death rate is 2–4/100,000 procedures, a rate lower than the annual risk of death from oral contraceptives. It should be mentioned to the patient that important but uncommon complications (bowel or bladder injury and bleeding) are rare.

INVOLUNTARY STERILIZATION

Involuntary sterilization is a legal procedure in most states for patients with severe mental incompetence in whom the possibility of pregnancy, despite institutional or home care, exists. Before performing such a sterilization, the physician should be assured of the following:

- The patient is legally incompetent, as evaluated and documented by trained professionals.
- The decision makers for the patient (parents or legal guardians) have the best interest of the patient in mind.
- The technique used (medical or surgical) is the least traumatic under the particular circumstances.

Most states require a court order by a judge, which usually incorporates the considerations listed above and gives legal permission for the physician to carry out the sterilization.

TECHNIQUES

There are various means of surgical and nonsurgical techniques of sterilization. Nonsurgical methods include X-radiation of ovaries, which is noninvasive and effective but increases the risk of carcinoma. Experimental techniques are being explored in which the transuterine approach (hysteroscopic injection of occluding material) and immunologic methods (antibodies to sperm or gonadotropin) are used, but these approaches have not reached consistent levels of efficacy.

Abdominal Tubal Ligation

One of the most common forms of sterilization in the United States is the elective postpartum sterilization. This is usually accomplished with a relatively simple Pomeroy tubal ligation. The patient should make the decision during her pregnancy, well before the time of delivery. The timing for the sterilization should ensure minimal medical and anesthetic risk and ensure the survival of the infant. At the time of cesarean delivery, an Irving procedure (division and burial of the proximal stump back into the myometrium) has been associated with the lowest subsequent failure rate. Elective minilaparotomy, except postpartum, and transvaginal fimbriectomy (the Kroener procedure) are other techniques that are occasionally used in the United States.

Laparoscopic Tubal Occlusion

Single Versus Double Puncture

Very experienced physicians with an interest in laparoscopy prefer single-puncture techniques for tubal occlusion because of the relative speed and safety of abdominal entry. The view is limited, and the technique is more demanding. The double-puncture technique is preferred by most gynecologists, who do about one or two laparoscopies a week and prefer the better visibility and surgical control of the second puncture.

Unipolar

Unipolar coagulation was the originally described tubal occlusion technique and was used extensively in the 1970s. Rarely, serious and unexplained electrical burns led to general discontinuation of the teaching of this technique. It is still used safely by some experienced clinicians.

Bipolar

Bipolar coagulation is now the most common method of laparoscopic tubal occlusion. Its apparent surgical simplicity has led to underestimation of the need to pay strict attention to key technical details that the bipolar current requires:

- The design of the forceps and generator must be matched, and power cords should not be cut or taped to match existing generators. Pregnancies have been reported because of mismatching of forceps and generator.
- The end point of coagulation is a complete cessation of electron flow, as can be seen on a flow meter or heard as a decreasing pitch on an audible meter. Reliance on visual blanching of the surface of the tube can result in the preservation of a viable lumen.
- To minimize the risk of subsequent ectopic pregnancy caused by the formation of a uteroperitoneal fistula, the first 2–3 cm of isthmus next to the uterus should remain intact.
- Three contiguous areas should be coagulated by the forceps to destroy about 3–4 cm of tube lateral to this point.

Failure to destroy an adequate volume of tube may lead to spontaneous recannulation during the healing process.

Band

The Silastic band technique was widely distributed and taught by the U.S. Agency for International Development to physicians in developing countries. The technique is less destructive than bipolar coagulation but carries with it a 2% risk of transection of the tube, making coagulation equipment necessary as a backup for the management of this problem. Postoperative pain for 48 hours from gradual necrosis of the anoxic tissue in the loop is a common complaint.

Clip

The spring clip method has the advantage of having the fewest surgical complications and the most reversibility because of the minimum (0.5 cm) amount of tissue that is destroyed. Strict attention to surgical detail is required, however, to avoid misapplication and pregnancy:

- The clip should be applied within 3 cm of the uterus, onto the isthmic portion; it should not reach across the ampulla.
- To minimize the risk of tubal "roll out" from within the jaws, the tube should be up against the hinge before the jaws are closed.
- An upturning of the peritoneal fold in the hinge of the clip (Kleppinger sign) indicates that the tube is well within the upper and lower jaws during application.
- The clip should be at right angles to the isthmus of the fallopian tube and completely across it after application.
- The spring must be pressed completely forward to the point where it locks.

If the tube is not accessible, a second or third puncture is useful to grasp the tube and put it on a stretch for easier application onto the isthmus. There has been no reported medical complication from a clip that is left closed or open in the abdomen if a clip has become dislodged from the applicator and lost.

Other Techniques

The Waters cautery technique involves a 10-mm second puncture through which a loop of tube is withdrawn into a plastic sheath and is cauterized safely until division occurs. The Endotherm instrument is a slender forceps that directly heats the tube and causes occlusion through cautery. It requires 90 seconds of application and repeated adjacent applications for maximum efficacy. Other clips have been introduced: the Bleier Secuclip is no longer available and the Filshie clip has not been approved by the U.S. Food and Drug Administration (FDA).

COMPLICATIONS

Bowel Injury

Bowel injury is the most frequent major complication and occurs in about 1–2/1,000 laparoscopies. Attention to details of abdominal entry, as outlined above, should minimize these injuries. Since bowel injuries can be both traumatic (because of Verres needle or trocar insertion) and electrical, all laparoscopies have this potential complication. If a trocar injury is recognized but small (less than 2 mm) and there is no bleeding or leaking of bowel contents, it can be treated expectantly by assuming that the bowel will seal over the defect. Subsequent laparotomy would be indicated for early signs of peritonitis. If an injury is larger or is actively oozing bowel contents or blood, then laparotomy to repair the defect is indicated and should occur within 4 hours. A small bipolar burn (less than 5 mm) on the surface of the small bowel can also be treated expectantly. Patients who have had previous abdominal surgery should be specifically advised of the possible increased risk of bowel injury and the need for a possible laparotomy to correct it.

Vascular Injury

Vascular injuries are rare (approximately 1/10,000 laparoscopies) but require immediate attention. As soon as it is recognized, the patient should be transferred immediately to the operating room, after an emergency call is placed for a vascular surgeon. The best approach to management is prevention.

Cardiovascular Arrest

At laparoscopy, a combination of factors can lead to cardiac arrest. Manipulation of the uterus or cervix itself can cause a vagal reflex with hypotension, bradycardia, and hypoxia. Excessive pneumoperitoneum pressure decreases diaphragmatic excursion and ventilation and interferes with abdominal venous return. Sedation can suppress respiration, resulting in hypoxia. These factors can combine to result in cardiovascular collapse that is usually dramatic but brief. This can be successfully treated with atropine (for vagal reflex) and reversal of hypoxia by oxygen administration and intubation. Gas embolism is rare with current insufflation devices. Limitation of the rate of blind insufflation to 1,000 ml/min keeps the gas flow within the body's ability to absorb gas into the venous system at this rate.

Pregnancy

Pregnancy is a rare but consistent complication of sterilization efforts. Pregnancies at the time of sterilization can be minimized by performing the procedure within the first 2 weeks of the first day of the menstrual period. The efficacy of prophylactic curettages for all laparoscopy patients has not been sustained in the literature. In questionable cases, a pregnancy test just before surgery may be useful. Bipolar coagulation has a high risk of subsequent ectopic pregnancy: 50–75% of subsequent pregnancies are ectopic. This is thought to be due to the occurrence of uteroperitoneal fistulas that allow sperm to migrate to the released egg and fertilize it in the distal tubal stump. This risk can be minimized by allowing a 2–3-cm stump of the isthmus to remain at the uterus at the time of coagulation. The risk of subsequent pregnancies can be minimized by paying consistent attention to the details of both electrocoagulation and mechanical sterilization techniques described here.

REVERSAL

Women who had sterilization when they were younger than age 30 are most likely to request reversal by reanastomosis. This occurs in about 1% of patients, or an estimated 5,000 requests annually in the United States. The most important factor in determining the success of a subsequent reversal is the amount of tissue that remains after the initial sterilization. Isthmic–isthmic anastomoses (with less than 1 cm of tube destroyed) have the highest success rate (80–90%); ampullary–cornual anastomoses have the lowest success rate (30–50% in unselected series) and have a high risk of subsequent ectopic pregnancies. Some clinicians feel that when selecting the type of sterilization to be performed on a patient younger than age 30, the least destructive method should be recommended.

BIBLIOGRAPHY

Chi IC, Potts M, Wilkens L. Rare events associated with tubal sterilization: an international experience. Obstet Gynecol Surv 1986;41:7–19

Hulka JF, Peterson HB, Phillips JM, Surrey MW. Operative laparoscopy: American Association of Gynecologic Laparoscopists 1991 membership survey. J Reprod Med 1993;38:569–571

Makar AP, Vanderheyden JS, Schatteman EA, Albertyn GP, Verkinderen JJ, Van Marck EA. Female sterilization failure after bipolar electrocoagulation: a 6 year retrospective study. Eur J Obstet Gynecol Reprod Biol 1990;37:237–246

Peterson HB, Hulka JF, Spielman FJ, Lee S, Marchbanks PA. Local versus general anesthesia for laparoscopic sterilization: a randomized study. Obstet Gynecol 1987;70:903–908

Rulin MC, Davidson AR, Philliber SG, Graves WL, Cushman LF. Changes in menstrual symptoms among sterilized and comparison women: a prospective study. Obstet Gynecol 1989;74:149–154

Shain RN, Miller WB, Holden AE, Rosenthal M. Impact of tubal sterilization and vasectomy on female marital sexuality: results of a controlled longitudinal study. Am J Obstet Gynecol 1991;164:763–771

Wilcox LS, Martinez-Schnell B, Peterson HB, Ware JH, Hughes JM. Menstrual function after tubal sterilization. Am J Epidemiol 1992;135:1368–1381

Pregnancy Termination

Abortion should be performed only by practitioners who are qualified to identify and manage its complications. Early abortion is safely performed in an office setting, but more advanced procedures require that hospital backup facilities be immediately available. Adequate preoperative and postoperative counseling is essential. Options to pregnancy termination should be presented. Medical conditions in which termination of a desired pregnancy should be considered include cyanotic heart disease with pulmonary hypertension, severe hypertension, previous myocardial infarction or other comparable major illness, major anomalies of the fetus, and midtrimester premature rupture of membranes. In most cases of both maternal illness or fetal malformation, the woman and her partner should participate in the decision, determining how great a risk they are willing to take.

The risk of death from first-trimester abortion is less than 1/100,000 abortions. The risk of death increases with gestational age (Table 4-4). Risk of death from abortion varies by

TABLE 4-4. DEATH-TO-CASE RATE FOR LEGAL ABORTIONS BY WEEKS OF GESTATION, UNITED STATES, 1972–1980

Weeks of Gestation	No. of Deaths*	No. of Abortions	Mortality Rate[†]	Relative Risk[‡]
>8	26	5,398,877	0.5	1.0
9–10	33	3,079,493	1.1	2.2
11–12	27	1,517,986	1.8	3.7
13–15	24	555,730	4.3	9.0
16–20	59	529,698	11.1	23.1
>21	14	118,876	11.8	24.5

* Deaths from ectopic pregnancy are excluded.
[†] Deaths are per 100,000 abortions.
[‡] Relative risk is based on index rate of <8 menstrual weeks of gestation of 0.5 deaths per 100,000 abortions.
Atrash HK, MacKay T, Binkin NJ, Hogue CJR. Legal abortion mortality in the United States: 1972–1982. Am J Obstet Gynecol 1987;156:605–612

TABLE 4-5. MORBIDITY RATE AND DEATHS FOR LEGAL ABORTIONS BY TYPE OF PROCEDURE AND WEEKS OF GESTATION, UNITED STATES, 1972–1980

Type of procedure	Morbidity Rate* (No. of Deaths) at Week of Gestation						
	>8	9–10	11–12	13–15	16–20	>21	Total
Curettage[†]	0.5 (25)	1.0 (31)	1.8 (26)	0	0	0	0.8 (82)
Dilatation & evacuation	0	0	0	3.6 (14)	9.5 (12)	10.4 (2)	5.1 (28)
Instillation	0	0	0	5.0 (5)	10.9 (41)	11.7 (10)	10.1 (56)
Hysterotomy/ hysterectomy	0	48.2 (2)	33.1 (1)	62.8 (3)	80.9 (4)	115.1 (1)	44.8 (11)
Total							1.6 (177)[‡]

* Deaths are per 100,000 abortions, excluding deaths associated with ectopic pregnancy.
† First-trimester vacuum curettage plus sharp curettage was performed.
‡ Total excludes six deaths for which type of procedure was classified as "other" and three for which type of procedure was unknown.
Atrash HK, MacKay T, Binkin NJ, Hogue CJR. Legal abortion mortality in the United States: 1972–1982. Am J Obstet Gynecol 1987;156:605–612

type of procedure (Table 4-5). Dilation and evacuation (D&E) is safer than other options for the early midtrimester. Hysterotomy and hysterectomy, two procedures rarely indicated for abortion, are least safe. Risks from abortion have diminished since 1973 with improvements in technique, a shift toward earlier procedures, and the replacement of late midtrimester instillation procedures with early midtrimester D&E (Table 4-6). General anesthesia increases risk for death from vacuum curettage abortion.

MENSTRUAL EXTRACTION

Sensitive pregnancy tests allow early diagnosis of pregnancy, and many women seek abortion services within 1–2 weeks of the missed period. Abortion of these early pregnancies with a small-bore vacuum cannula is called menstrual regulation, menstrual extraction, or minisuction. The properly trained gynecologist can perform these procedures in office practice. The only instruments required are the speculum, the tenaculum, the Karman cannula, and a modified 50-ml syringe. At the end of the procedure, the tissue obtained is examined by floating it in a clear plastic dish over a light source. In this manner chorionic villi and the gestational sac are identified, ectopic pregnancy is ruled out, and incomplete abortion is detected.

FIRST-TRIMESTER VACUUM CURETTAGE

Beyond 7 menstrual weeks, larger cannulas and larger vacuum sources are required to evacuate pregnancy. This procedure, standard vacuum curettage, is the most common method of abortion in the United States. By recent convention, procedures performed prior to 13 menstrual weeks are called suction or vacuum curettage, whereas similar procedures carried out after 13 weeks as a means for midtrimester abortion are termed D&E.

Technique

Uterine size and position are noted on the pelvic examination. Ultrasonography is advised if there is a size–dates discrepancy of more than 2 weeks. If not already performed, a gonorrhea culture and chlamydia slide test are performed and the cervix and vagina are prepared with germicide. Paracervical block is established with up to 20 ml of 1% lidocaine given into the cervical stroma at the 3-, 5-, 7-, and 9-o'clock positions to form a ring of anesthetic at the junction of the cervix and lower uterine segment. The cervix is grasped with a single-toothed tenaculum placed vertically with one branch inside the canal. Optionally, the uterine depth is measured with a sound. Dilation is then carefully performed with Pratt or similar tapered dilators.

Alternatively, hygroscopic dilators can be used (synthetic versions or laminaria [*Laminaria japonicum*]) for a few hours or overnight. Hygroscopic dilators require several hours for dilation, but a fivefold reduction in cervical lacerations and a threefold reduction in uterine perforations were demonstrated when laminaria were used instead of forcible dilatation. Lami-

TABLE 4-6. RISK OF DEATH FROM ABORTION BY TYPE OF PROCEDURE, 1972–1982

Method	Risk of Death (per 100,000 procedures)	
	1972–1976	1977–1982
First-trimester vacuum curettage	1.3	0.6
Midtrimester dilation and evacuation	8.5	3.2
Saline instillation	17.8	5.1
Prostaglandin and other instillation	13.1	3.2
Hysterotomy/hysterectomy	44.7	58.5

Data from Atrash HK, MacKay T, Binkin NJ, Hogue CJR. Legal abortion mortality in the United States: 1972–1982. Am J Obstet Gynecol 1987;156:605–612

naria did not increase postabortal infection. Synthetic versions dilate faster, by either producing both dilatation and softening or primarily producing softening. In a comparative trial of a prostaglandin analogue, a synthetic hygroscopic dilator, and laminaria tents, the synthetic hygroscopic dilator was most effective for preoperative preparation of the cervix prior to first-trimester vacuum curettage. A single rod of laminaria or a synthetic hygroscopic dilator can become entrapped by a resistant cervix and fragment upon attempted removal. For first-trimester procedures, two or more laminaria or a synthetic hygroscopic dilator plus a small rod of laminaria should be used.

A vacuum cannula of diameter in millimeters one less than estimated gestational age (eg, 9-mm size for estimated 10-week gestation) is used to evacuate the cavity. After a light check with a sharp curet, the vacuum cannula is reintroduced briefly. A fresh examination of the aspirated tissue is immediately performed.

It is common for prophylactic antibiotics to be used with induced abortion. The recent literature supports this practice and confirms that morbidity is less when antibiotics are used. Tetracycline or its derivatives doxycycline and minocycline are probably the best of the current agents for this purpose because of their broad spectrum of antimicrobial effect and oral absorption.

Complications

The common postabortal triad of pain, bleeding, and low-grade fever is often managed successfully by oral antibiotics and ergot preparations, but the great majority of cases will exhibit some retained gestational tissue or clot in the uterine cavity. These symptoms are best managed by a repeat uterine evacuation, performed under local anesthesia in an ambulatory setting.

Anesthesia

Local anesthesia is preferred because general anesthesia increases the risk of perforation, visceral injury, hemorrhage, and death. There are more problems with apparent convulsions or syncope and with fever, however, when local anesthesia is used. The addition of epinephrine to the local anesthetic is now considered contraindicated. Rarely, fatal anaphylaxis has resulted from the metabisulfite preservative in epinephrine solutions.

Cervical Shock

Vasovagal syncope produced by stimulation of the cervical canal can be seen even after paracervical block. Brief tonic–clonic activity may be confused with seizure but is distinguished by the presence of a very slow pulse, the patient's rapid recovery, and the absence of any postictal state. Routine use of atropine with the paracervical anesthetic prevents cervical shock.

Perforation

The clinical syndrome produced by perforation depends on the precise anatomic location of the injury. Perforations at the junction of the cervix and lower uterine segment can lacerate the ascending branch of the uterine artery within the broad ligament, giving rise to severe pain, a broad ligament hematoma, and intraabdominal bleeding. Management requires laparotomy to ligate the severed vessels and repair the uterine injury. Hysterectomy should not be required to manage such an injury.

Low cervical perforations, on the other hand, may injure the descending branch of the uterine artery within the dense collagenous substance of the cardinal ligaments. In this case there is no intraabdominal bleeding; the bleeding is only outward, through the cervical canal, and may subside temporarily as the artery goes into spasm. Deaths have occurred as a result of bleeding several hours or even days after an unrecognized low cervical perforation. This complication has usually been managed with hysterectomy, but consideration should be given to arteriography and selective embolization of the hypogastric arteries should recurring postabortal hemorrhage suggest this diagnosis. The risk of perforation is less than 1/1,000 first-trimester abortions. It increases with gestational age and is greater for parous women than for nulliparous women. The use of laminaria reduces risk. Perforation is best managed by laparoscopy to determine the extent of the injury and complete the abortion.

Hemorrhage

Excessive bleeding may indicate uterine atony, a low-lying implantation, a pregnancy of more advanced gestational age, or perforation. Management requires a rapid reassessment of gestational age by examination of the fetal parts already extracted and gentle exploration of the uterine cavity with a curet or forceps. Intravenous oxytocin is administered, and the abortion is completed. The uterus is then massaged between two hands to ensure contraction. When these measures fail, the patient is transferred immediately to the hospital with intravenous fluids running, and blood is crossmatched. Persistent postabortal bleeding strongly suggests retained tissue or clot (hematometra) or trauma, and the patient is best managed with prompt surgical intervention: laparoscopy and repeat curettage.

Hematometra

Lower abdominal pain of increasing intensity in the half hour after an abortion suggests hematometra or the postabortal syndrome. On examination, the uterus is large, globular, and tense, and could be mistaken for a broad ligament hematoma, except that the mass is midline and arises from the cervix. The treatment is immediate reevacuation. Pretreatment with ergot, 0.1 mg IM, or the use of oxytocin reduces the incidence of this phenomenon.

Ectopic Pregnancy, Incomplete Abortion, and Failed Abortion

Early detection of ectopic pregnancy, incomplete abortion, or failed abortion is possible if the operator carefully examines the specimen immediately after the abortion. The patient may have an ectopic pregnancy if no chorionic villi are found. To detect an incomplete abortion that might result in a continued pregnancy, the actual gestational sac must be identified. Review of history, physical examination, determination of the level of β-hCG, frozen section of the aspirated tissue, and vaginal probe ultrasonography are used in an attempt to divide patients into groups at high and low risk for ectopic pregnancy. Immediate laparoscopy is performed for high-risk patients. Low-risk patients are followed closely with serial β-hCG assays until the problem is resolved.

With later gestations, all of the fetal parts must be identified to prevent incomplete abortion. It is never sufficient to send the tissue to the pathologist; a fresh examination by the surgeon is also required. Heavy bleeding or fever after abortion suggests retained tissue. If the uterus is larger than 12 weeks size, it is wise to perform preoperative ultrasonography to determine the amount of tissue remaining. When fever is present, high-dose intravenous antibiotic therapy is initiated, and curettage is performed shortly thereafter. Because of the need to cover a number of possible pathogens, combinations of two or three agents are required (eg, intravenous ampicillin, clindamycin, and gentamycin).

A small, firm uterus suggests that the uterus is empty and that curettage will not be needed. If there is a question of whether there is retained tissue, ultrasonography is useful.

SECOND-TRIMESTER ABORTION

Most abortions are performed prior to 13 menstrual weeks. Later abortions are generally performed because of fetal defects, maternal illness, or maternal age. Younger women are much more likely to need abortion after 12 weeks.

Dilation and Evacuation

Transcervical instrumental evacuation of the uterus is the method most used for midtrimester abortion prior to 21 menstrual weeks. Current techniques for D&E differ primarily in the preparatory steps that precede the evacuation. In the one-stage technique, forcible dilation is performed slowly and carefully to sufficient diameter to allow insertion of large, strong, ovum forceps for extraction. The better approach is a two-stage procedure in which multiple laminaria tents are used to achieve gradual dilatation over several hours before extraction. Overnight placement of one set of laminaria is sufficient preparation for the early midtrimester, but beyond 18–20 weeks, two sets of laminaria and 2 days of preparation are often used. Uterine evacuation is accomplished with long, heavy forceps, using the vacuum cannula to rupture the fetal membranes, drain amniotic fluid, and ensure complete evacuation. The large-bore, 16-mm vacuum system facilitates the procedure.

The procedure causes discomfort despite a paracervical block, and most patients will benefit from intravenous sedation and analgesia. Midazolam, 2 mg IV, given 1 mg at a time over 2–3 minutes, is followed with intravenous alfentanyl in 200-μg boluses at intervals of 2–4 minutes as needed. Monitoring of tissue oxygenation with a pulse oximeter is advised. If general anesthesia is elected, potent inhalation agents should be avoided or used only in low concentrations, to avoid uterine atony and increased blood loss. Combinations of oxygen, intravenous propofol, and short-acting narcotic analgesics or nitrous oxide are preferred. Standard care of the anesthetized patient must be provided, with continuous monitoring of tissue oxygenation and end-expiratory carbon dioxide and with frequent monitoring of vital signs. The patient must be closely supervised until she is fully recovered from anesthesia.

Preoperative ultrasonography is performed for all cases 14 weeks and beyond. Intraoperative real-time ultrasonography helps to locate fetal parts within the uterus. Paracervically administered vasopressin has been demonstrated to reduce bleeding significantly, but vasopressin must be used with caution. The 20-U ampule is diluted, and only 4–5 U are given. Vasopressin should not be used for women with heart disease or hypertension. Intravenous oxytocin, 40 or more units per 1,000 ml, is begun early in the procedure, just after rupture of membranes.

Coagulopathy can be seen after D&E, apparently because tissue thromboplastins have been released into maternal venous sinusoids. Use of oxytocin and intracervical vasopressin may reduce this risk. The Trendelenburg position is avoided in order to avoid negative pressure in the uterine vasculature that might increase tissue entry.

Oral tetracycline or doxycycline is begun after laminaria insertion and is continued for 2 days after uterine evacuation. An analgesic is prescribed.

After the procedure, the operator carefully examines the fetal parts to be sure that all have been evacuated. If the fetal calvaria has been retained in the uterus and gentle attempts at extraction fail, it is best to stop, administer an oxytocin infusion for 2 hours, and try again. By then, the remaining fetal parts will have been pushed down to the internal os and they can be extracted easily.

Dilation and evacuation becomes progressively more difficult as gestational age advances, and in the United States instillation techniques are more often used after 21 weeks. Dilation and evacuation can be offered in the late midtrimester, but the technique should be altered. The use of two sets of laminaria tents for a total of 36–48 hours of laminaria treatment is favored. A further modification is the Hern combination method. After multistage laminaria treatment, urea is injected into the amniotic sac. Extraction is accomplished after labor begins and after fetal maceration has occurred.

Provided that the surgeon is familiar with the procedure, fetal death in utero can be managed with D&E. Vaginal prostaglandin E_2 is highly effective for this problem, producing fetal abortion in about 10 hours, on the average, albeit with significant vomiting, diarrhea, and fever as side effects. The full dose of 20 mg should not be used beyond 28 weeks of gestation, to avoid overstimulation and uterine rupture. The suppository can be cut into quarters and administered 5 mg at a time for better control of uterine activity. Blood or amniotic fluid may impair vaginal absorption of the prostaglandin, and carboprost tromethamine, 250 μg IM at 2–3-hour intervals, may be substituted if abortion has not occurred by 24 hours or so. The same low-dose regimen can be used cautiously in patients with asthma. Coagulation studies are obtained preoperatively, as disseminated intravascular coagulopathy is a significant risk after either D&E or prostaglandin E$_2$ for fetal death.

Intrauterine Prostaglandins

Intraamniotic prostaglandin is an effective regimen, but it has disadvantages: incomplete abortion, the need for a second injection in many cases, the risk of cervical rupture in the primigravida, and the lack of a direct toxic effect on the fetus. Results with intraamniotic prostaglandin F are much improved if overnight treatment with laminaria is used prior to infusion. Mean times to abortion are reduced from 29 hours to 14 hours, and many fewer patients require a second dose. Cervical rupture is very rare. Incomplete abortion is common with prostaglandin abortion, and routine curettage is advised after all prostaglandin abortions. This can be accomplished easily under local anesthesia in a properly equipped treatment room and reduces rates of postabortal hemorrhage and infection to low levels. Failed prostaglandin abortions can be managed by D&E or by prostaglandins given IM or vaginally. There is synergism between prostaglandins and oxytocin with enhanced force of uterine contraction. To avoid uterine rupture, oxytocin should not be used until after fetal expulsion.

Prostaglandin F$_{2\alpha}$ was withdrawn by the manufacturer. An effective substitute is 2 mg of the 15-methylated analogue, carboprost tromethamine, preceded by 24 hours of treatment with multiple intracervical laminaria. In current practice, the carboprost is augmented with 64 ml of intraamniotic hypertonic saline (23.4%).

Systemic Prostaglandins

Two different prostaglandins are available for systemic administration: prostaglandin E$_2$ by vaginal suppository and carboprost tromethamine for intramuscular injection. Prostaglandin E$_2$ is given as a 20-mg vaginal suppository every 3 hours. The mean time to abortion is 13.4 hours, with 90% of patients aborting by 24 hours. When carboprost tromethamine is given as 250 µg IM every 2 hours, the mean times to abortion are 15–17 hours, with about 80% of patients aborting by 24 hours. Thirty-nine percent of patients treated with prostaglandin E$_2$ experienced vomiting, and 25% experienced diarrhea in one large trial. Eighty-three percent of patients treated with carboprost vomited, and 71% had diarrhea in the trial cited above. About one third of patients treated with prostaglandin E$_2$ will have a temperature elevation of 1° C or more. Transient fetal survival can be a problem with all prostaglandin methods. To prevent this, an ultrasound-guided fetal intracardiac injection of either potassium chloride, 3 ml of a 2-mmol solution, or 1.5 mg of digoxin may be given.

Retained placenta is common with all prostaglandin-induced abortions. If spontaneous expulsion has not occurred within 30 minutes, instrumental evacuation should be performed to prevent further blood loss. This is accomplished under low-dose intravenous sedation in a treatment room equipped with a uterine aspirator.

Urea–Prostaglandin

Hyperosmolar urea combined with low doses of prostaglandin F$_{2\alpha}$ produces abortion in a mean time of 12 hours when pretreatment laminaria tents are used. Current literature demonstrates a shorter time from instillation to abortion and fewer serious complications than with the saline method. Coagulopathy can be seen with urea–prostaglandin, but it is much less frequent than with hypertonic saline. Carboprost tromethamine, 250 µg, can be combined with the intraamniotic urea, replacing prostaglandin F$_{2\alpha}$.

High-Dose Oxytocin

Oxytocin in sufficient doses can be effective as a primary abortifacient in the midtrimester. Fifty units is given in 500 ml of 5% dextrose and normal saline over a 3-hour period. After 1 hour of rest, oxytocin infusion is repeated, adding 50 additional units to the next 500-ml infusion, and continuing with 3 hours of infusion and 1 hour of rest. This is repeated until the patient aborts or a final solution of 300 U of oxytocin in 500 ml is reached (1,667 mU/min).

Hypertonic Saline

Historically, hypertonic saline is important as the first effective labor induction method for midtrimester abortion. Hazards unique to hypertonic saline include cardiovascular collapse, pulmonary and cerebral edema, and renal failure if the solution is injected IV; all patients are at risk for serious disseminated intravascular coagulopathy. Attention to proper technique for amnioinfusion with instillation of the saline by gravity flow through connecting tubing from a single-dose bottle makes such mishaps very infrequent. The main hazards of hypertonic saline are in fact common to all of the labor induction methods: failed abortion, incomplete abortion, retained tissue, hemorrhage, infection, and embolic phenomena.

Administered by itself, hypertonic saline produces mean times from instillation to abortion of 33–35 hours. Augmentation with oxytocin reduces this to 25–26 hours and improves efficacy but at the price of increased occurrence of disseminated intravascular coagulopathy, water intoxication, and cervical or uterine rupture.

OTHER APPROACHES

Hysterotomy and Hysterectomy

Hysterotomy is essentially a cesarean delivery. There is little present indication for this procedure as the primary method for abortion, as the risk of major complications and death is greater with hysterotomy or hysterectomy for abortion than for any other technique (Tables 4-5 and 4-6). In most cases failed abortion is now managed with parenteral prostaglandins, and the only time for a hysterotomy in failed abortion is when a uterine anomaly is suspected.

The coexistence of pregnancy and a separate indication for hysterectomy, such as cervical dysplasia or enlarging myomas, have been taken as indications for gravid hysterectomy. Most patients are best served by a simpler means for pregnancy termination and a more complete evaluation of their other gynecologic problems prior to definitive therapy. In the case of myomas, the common regression in size after termination of pregnancy may obviate the need for surgery. When a physician unaccustomed to performing late abortion finds abortion indicated because of a patient's serious medical illness, the patient is better served by referral than by the addition of a major surgical procedure to her other problems.

Steroidal Abortifacients

Mifepristone (RU 486) is an analogue of norethindrone with high affinity for progesterone receptors. It acts as a false transmitter and blocks natural progesterone. It can effectively induce abortion of early gestations after a single oral dose. Effectiveness is increased to approximately 95% by the addition of a low dose of prostaglandin analogue. An alternative prostaglandin, misoprostol, given as a single oral dose of 600 mg, appears as effective and may be safer. Misoprostol is available in the United States for the treatment of peptic ulcer. Mifepristone or misoprostol could replace vacuum curettage for early pregnancy termination in the future.

Selective Reduction

In cases of multifetal pregnancies, selective reduction by means of ultrasound-guided intracardiac injection of potassium chloride (0.5–3 ml of a 2-mmol solution) has been practiced as a means of avoiding the risks of extreme prematurity for the surviving pregnancies. Coagulation surveillance is advised after second-trimester procedures. Selective reduction should not be attempted with twin–twin transfusion syndrome because of the possibility of embolic phenomena and infarction in the surviving twin.

SUBSEQUENT REPRODUCTION

Legal abortion as currently practiced in the United States has no measurable adverse effect on later reproduction. This probably reflects the safety of current abortion technology. Most abortions are performed by vacuum curettage under local anesthesia in the first trimester. The impact of midtrimester methods for later pregnancy is less well established and may vary with the method used (eg, forcible dilation of the cervix to large diameters for D&E in the late midtrimester may increase the risk of prematurity later). Laminaria tents, their synthetic alternative, or low-dose prostaglandins should be used to prepare the cervix prior to late abortion.

BIBLIOGRAPHY

Atrash HK, MacKay HT, Binkin NJ, Hogue CJ. Legal abortion mortality in the United States: 1972 to 1982. Am J Obstet Gynecol 1987:156:605–612

Darney PD, Dorward K. Cervical dilatation before first-trimester elective abortion: a controlled comparison of meteneprost, laminaria and hypan. Obstet Gynecol 1987;70:397–400

Hakim-Elahi E, Tovell HM, Burnhill MS. Complications of first-trimester abortion: a report of 170,000 cases. Obstet Gynecol 1990;76:129–135

Induced termination of pregnancy before and after Roe v. Wade. Trends in the mortality and morbidity of women. Council on Scientific Affairs, American Medical Association. JAMA 1992;268:3231–3239

Koonin LM, Smith JC, Ramick M, Lawson HW. Abortion surveillance—United States, 1989. MMWR CDC Surveill Summ 1992;41 (5):1–33

Kirz DS, Haag MK. Management of the third stage of labor in pregnancies terminated by prostaglandin E_2. Am J Obstet Gynecol 1989; 160:412–414

Levallois P, Rioux JE. Prophylactic antibiotics for suction curettage abortion: results of a clinical controlled trial. Am J Obstet Gynecol 1988;158:100–105

Osathanondh R. Conception control. In: Ryan KJ, Berkowitz R, Barbieri R, eds. Kistner's gynecology: principles and practice. 5th ed. St Louis: Mosby–Year Book, 1990:480–529

Peterson HB, Grimes DA, Cates W Jr, Rubin GL. Comparative risk of death from induced abortion at less than or equal to 12 weeks' gestation performed with local versus general anesthesia. Am J Obstet Gynecol 1981;141:763–768

Silvestre L, Dubois C, Renault M, Rezrani Y, Baulieu EE, Ulmann A. Voluntary interruption of pregnancy with mifepristone (RU 486) and a prostaglandin analogue: a large-scale French experience. N Engl J Med 1990;322:645–648

Thong KJ, Baird DT. Induction of abortion with mifepristone and misoprostol in early pregnancy. Br J Obstet Gynaecol 1992;99:1004–1007

Wapner RJ, Davis GH, Johnson A, Weinblatt VJ, Fischer RL, Jackson LG, et al. Selective reduction of multifetal pregnancies. Lancet 1990; 355:90–93

Winkler CL, Gray SE, Hauth JC, Owen J, Tucker JM. Mid second trimester labor induction: concentrated oxytocin compared with prostaglandin E_2 vaginal suppositories. Obstet Gynecol 1991;77:297–300

Oncology

Gynecologic oncology has moved in some new directions, as reflected in this section of *Precis V*. A widespread realization that the aggressiveness of our principal modalities of surgery, radiotherapy, and chemotherapy has been pushed to the limit has led to a greater emphasis on disease prevention and quality of life.

Coincident with the modified and tissue-sparing approaches to breast cancer, conservative surgical techniques have been applied to malignant neoplasms of the ovary, uterus, and vulva. This approach allows physicians to tailor surgical procedures to the disease, thus providing more information about its extent.

A cadre of drugs has been produced or is in development to ameliorate the toxicities of therapy—especially chemotherapy—including products that lessen nausea, neurotoxicity, nephrotoxicity, and bone marrow suppression. These agents will improve patients' tolerance of what is often uncomfortable therapy.

A host of tumor markers for genital tract malignancies has emerged. Some of these are now clinically useful, whereas others are still investigational. The possibilities of using these markers or similar tumor antigens as carriers of radiodiagnostic labels, or as vehicles for targeting therapy, are fields of progress that are very close to clinical application. At the same time a greater awareness of prevention has arisen, especially in conjunction with identification of high-risk groups. This type of approach has been very successful in cervical cancer and may play an important role in ovarian cancer.

Last but not least, the field of oncology, along with the entire field of medicine, has grown more aware of quality-of-life issues. The medical team must involve the patient in all decisions. For patients with incurable disease, the physician must walk the tightrope carefully between a patient's denial and a patient's complete acceptance of all the facts, answering questions truthfully but with some measure of hope. Treatment of the patient with gynecologic malignancy continues to be the greatest challenge in our specialty. At the same time, it is a rewarding endeavor, for which patients are truly grateful. I urge readers to keep this in mind as they journey through the following synopsis of a complicated area of gynecology.

Philip J. DiSaia, MD

Genetics and Gynecologic Cancer

Based on family history, cytogenetic studies, and molecular biologic analyses, there is little doubt that cancer is a disease of the genome. It has been recognized for some time that patients with hereditary diseases such as xeroderma pigmentosum, neurofibromatosis, Fanconi anemia, and Bloom syndrome exhibit an increased propensity to develop cancer. In other diseases, such as Burkitt lymphoma and chronic myelogenous leukemia, a hereditary tendency is not prominent, but consistent cytogenetic and molecular genetic alterations have been identified. Recent cytogenetic and molecular genetic studies of gynecologic malignancies provide important clues to the pathogenesis of both inherited and sporadic neoplasms of the female reproductive tract.

HEREDITARY FACTORS

It has been estimated that approximately 6% of all cancer patients have three or more relatives with cancer. Although a familial predisposition for cancers of the vulva, vagina, cervix, and fallopian tube has not been established, familial clusters of both endometrial cancer and ovarian cancer have been reported.

Endometrial Cancer

Women with endometrial cancer have a similarly affected first-degree relative in 8–13% of cases, which implies that there is a familial or genetic component. Approximately 6% of cases of endometrial adenocarcinoma are diagnosed in women grouped in the cancer family syndrome (Lynch syndrome II). This syndrome is characterized by hereditary, site-specific, nonpolyposis colon cancer in association with other multiple-site malignancies, including those of the endometrium, ovary, and breast. The trait for malignancy appears to be transmitted as an autosomal dominant one, so that the risk to first-degree relatives is 50%. In addition, individuals assigned to the cancer family syndrome demonstrate certain human leukocyte antigen gene linkage relationships. Investigations based on loss of heterozygosity indicate that tumor suppressor genes on the long arm of chromosome 17 may also play a role in the etiology of this syndrome.

Ovarian Cancer

Most cases of epithelial ovarian cancer are sporadic and exhibit no heritable or familial tendencies. However, approximately 7% of cases of ovarian cancer occur in women with a positive family history, generally defined as a proband with two or more similarly affected first-degree relatives. Within this group, three patterns of cancer occurrence have been described: site-specific ovarian cancer, familial cases of breast and ovarian cancer, and the cancer family syndrome.

CHROMOSOMAL ABNORMALITIES

Certain sex chromosome disorders are associated with an increased risk of malignancy. Turner syndrome (45,XO) is associated with an increased incidence of dysgerminoma and gonadoblastoma. Karyotype abnormalities such as 45,XO/46,XY and 46,XY streak gonads are associated with a 15–30% incidence of ovarian malignancies. The risk of neoplasia is greater in 46,XY patients with dysgenetic gonads than it is in 45,XO/46,XY mosaic patients.

Hydatidiform mole is a diagnosis associated with consistent genetic abnormalities. An incomplete hydatidiform mole, which is characterized by a haploid maternal and a diploid paternal genetic complement resulting in triploidy, is associated with negligible risks of malignant sequelae. In contradistinction, a complete hydatidiform mole, which exhibits a diploid genome of exclusive paternal origin, is associated with a 15–20% risk of malignant sequelae. Reports of molar pregnancies occurring in sisters who are monozygotic twins and of recurrent molar pregnancies in women with different partners lend credence to the suggestion that a heritable defect of the ovum may underlie the pathogenesis of complete moles.

AUTOSOMAL CHROMOSOME ALTERATIONS

Ploidy abnormalities, reflecting alterations of cellular DNA content, are found in a significant proportion of gynecologic tumors. Hereditary ovarian cancers are often hyperdiploid. Endometrial cancers are usually diploid, although pseudodiploid, triploid, and aneuploid tumors have been reported. Aneuploidy is commonly observed in cervical and ovarian carcinomas.

Cytogenetic abnormalities may occur in the absence of detectable ploidy abnormalities. The single most common abnormality reported for endometrial, ovarian, and cervical cancers involves the long arm of chromosome 1. Chromosomes 3, 5, 6, 7, 11, and 17 are also frequently abnormal. Translocations, deletions, homogeneously staining regions, and double minutes are the most frequently demonstrated alterations.

Although consistent karyotype abnormalities have been identified for hematopoietic neoplasms such as Burkitt lymphoma and chronic myelogenous leukemia, this has not been the case for most solid tumors, including those of the female reproductive tract. However, studies using molecular biologic techniques to detect the allelic loss of small amounts of genetic material have provided evidence of consistent genetic losses in both sporadic and familial ovarian cancer. The chromosomes that demonstrate frequent loss of heterozygosity include 3, 11, 17, and 18. Chromosome 17 is of particular interest because it is the location of the p53 tumor suppressor gene, the gene that encodes the epidermal growth factor receptor, and the *HER-2/neu* gene. In addition, the long arm of chromosome 17 appears to be the location of two putative tumor suppressor genes: the *BrCa1* gene and the prohibitin gene. Both genes may play a role in the initiation of familial ovarian cancer.

ABNORMALITIES OF ONCOGENE STRUCTURE AND EXPRESSION

Advances in molecular biology have provided the means with which to investigate specific genetic mutations that cannot be detected by karyotype analysis. More than 50 cancer-related genes, most of which are expressed in normal as well as neoplastic tissues, have been described. These genes play critical roles in the regulation of normal cellular growth and differentiation. To date, six cancer-related genes have been studied in detail in gynecologic neoplasms:

- The c-*myc* proto-oncogene encodes a nuclear DNA-binding protein that appears to regulate transcription. The expression of this gene increases during proliferation and returns to negligible levels when cells are quiescent.
- The c-*fms* proto-oncogene encodes the colony-stimulating factor receptor protein. Activation of this receptor signals hematopoietic precursor cells to undergo mitosis.
- The *ras* gene family includes the c-Ha-*ras*, c-Ki-*ras*, and N-*ras* genes. These genes encode signal transduction proteins that are located on the inner surface of the cell membrane.
- The *ras* p21 protein is functionally similar to the G proteins and participates in the second messenger signal transduction system.
- The *erb* B1 gene encodes the epidermal growth factor-receptor protein, which is a transmembrane protein that binds epidermal growth factor and T-cell growth factor beta and T-cell growth factor alpha, triggering a mitogenic signal that is subsequently conveyed to the nucleus.
- The *HER-2/neu* gene is structurally similar to, but distinct from, the *erb* B2 gene. The role of this gene product in normal cell growth and differentiation has not been determined.
- The p53 gene is a tumor suppressor gene. It encodes a protein that is normally present in very small amounts in the cell and functions as a negative regulator of cell growth.

In view of the roles that these genes play in the regulation of normal cell growth and differentiation, a logical corollary is that aberrant gene function may causally contribute to the neoplastic phenotype. Aberrant gene function may result from one of several alterations, including amplification, structural rearrangements, and point mutations.

Gene amplification results in an increase in the copy number of the gene and may be detected cytogenetically as double minutes or homogeneously staining regions. Amplification results in an increase in the amount of template DNA available for transcription and is frequently associated with overexpression of the gene. Gynecologic tumors as a group exhibit sporadic amplification of at least one oncogene in 10–50% of cases.

Structural rearrangements of a gene result in disruption of the normal gene product with a variety of potential consequences from loss of function or potentiation of function. Rearrangement of the *erb* B1 gene, which encodes the epidermal growth factor receptor, results in a truncated protein in which the regulatory domain is absent but some portion of the catalytic domain remains. Even in the absence of ligand binding, the mutated epidermal growth factor receptor produces a mitogenic signal.

Point mutations are single base changes that may result in significant alterations in gene product function. The clinical consequence of a point mutation is best illustrated by sickle cell disease. The mutated sickle cell protein, which results from a single base change, undergoes intracellular precipitation when subjected to low oxygen tension, with potentially devastating clinical sequelae. Similar, although less familiar, mutations are found in cancer-related genes. As an example, point mutations of codons 12, 13, and 61 of the *ras* gene family result in a protein that binds glutamyl transpeptidase in normal fashion but cannot rapidly hydrolyze it. For this reason, the mutated *ras* p21 protein remains activated for longer periods of time and therefore generates a sustained signal for cellular proliferation. Point mutations of the p53 tumor suppressor gene are among the most common genetic mutations found in human neoplasms. As a consequence of these point mutations, the p53 protein is no longer capable of functioning as an inhibitor of cellular proliferation. The normal activity of the p53 gene can also be inhibited by the human papillomavirus (HPV). In cases of cervical dysplasia and neoplasia, normal p53 protein may be inactivated by interactions with the E7 protein of HPV type 16, resulting in enhanced cellular proliferation.

Mutations of both proto-oncogenes and tumor suppressor genes have been found in gynecologic malignancies (Table 5-1). At this time, it is not clear which genetic mutations reflect important events in tumor initiation and progression versus random mutations that occur as a consequence of the inherent genomic instability associated with cancer.

POTENTIAL CLINICAL APPLICATIONS OF MOLECULAR GENETICS

Among the potential clinical applications of molecular genetics are risk assessment, the determination of prognosis, and the identification of potential therapeutic targets in women with gynecologic cancer.

Genes may exhibit restriction fragment length polymorphisms, which are hereditary differences in nucleotide struc-

TABLE 5-1. PROTO-ONCOGENE AND TUMOR SUPPRESSOR GENE ABNORMALITIES REPORTED IN GYNECOLOGIC NEOPLASMS

Site	Gene	Amplification	Structural Alterations	Overexpression	Point Mutations
Cervix	c-*myc*	Yes	Reported in only 1 study	Yes	No
	c-Ha-*ras*	No	Yes	Yes	Yes
	c-Ki-*ras*	No	No	Yes	No
	p53	No	No	Yes	Yes
Uterus	c-*myc*	Yes	No	Yes	No
	c-Ha-*ras*	No	No	Yes	No
	c-Ki-*ras*	No	No	Yes	Yes
	p53	No	No	Yes	Yes
	c-*fms*	Yes	No	Yes	No
	c-*erb* B1	Yes	Yes	Yes	No
	HER-2/neu	Yes	No	Yes	No
Ovary	c-*myc*	Yes	No	Yes	No
	c-Ha-*ras*	No	No	Yes	No
	c-Ki-*ras*	Yes	No	Yes	Yes
	p53	No	No	Yes	Yes
	c-*fms*	Yes	No	Yes	No
	c-*erb* B1	Yes	Yes	Yes	No
	HER-2/neu	Yes	No	Yes	No

ture that do not affect gene transcription or translation. Particular polymorphisms may indicate an increased risk of a specific cancer. Rare restriction fragment length polymorphisms, which appear to predict a predisposition to develop cancer of the bladder, colon, rectum, lung, breast, and skin, have been identified for select oncogenes. Conflicting results have been reported regarding the significance of rare Ha-*ras* alleles as markers of a predisposition to ovarian cancer. There are no published data regarding restriction fragment length polymorphism analysis for other malignancies of the female genital tract.

The prognostic significance of proto-oncogene and tumor suppressor genes in gynecologic malignancies has been studied to a rather limited degree. In this regard, the c-*myc* proto-oncogene in cervical cancer and the *HER-2/neu* proto-oncogene in ovarian cancer have been the most extensively studied.

Overexpression of the c-*myc* oncogene may identify a subset of patients with cervical cancer who are at increased risk for disease recurrence. In one study c-*myc* expression was measured prior to treatment in 72 stage I and stage II squamous cell carcinomas of the cervix. Elevated oncogene expression was found in 25 tumors. Of patients whose neoplasms demonstrated elevated c-*myc* expression, 49% survived without relapse for 18 months, compared with 90% for the 47 patients with normal c-*myc* expression. However, these data were not analyzed in the context of current histopathologic variables, and it is unknown whether c-*myc* is an independent prognostic variable.

Overexpression of *HER-2/neu* in epithelial ovarian cancer has been significantly, yet inconsistently, reported to be of prognostic significance. At this time, the evidence is less than convincing that *HER-2/neu* is of any prognostic significance in this disease.

Information based on the study of the molecular genetics of gynecologic neoplasms may result in new treatment strategies. Given the premise that abnormal proto-oncogene function or loss of tumor suppressor gene function may causally contribute to tumor initiation and progression, one therapeutic approach is the correction of these abnormalities.

Inhibition of abnormal proto-oncogene function can be accomplished in a variety of ways. Agents such as mithramycin, which is clinically used to treat hypercalcemia, have also been shown to inhibit selectively the expression of the c-*myc* proto-oncogene in vitro. The interferons can down-regulate the expression of *HER-2/neu* and restore sensitivity to lymphokine-activated cytolysis. Exposure of transformed cells to a monoclonal antibody specific for a proto-oncogene protein can block its function and is accompanied by loss of malignant characteristics in some cases. In addition, radioisotopes can be coupled to the monoclonal antibody in an effort to increase the specificity of treatment.

Treatment strategies to address the loss of tumor suppressor gene activity are based on the restoration of the absent function. Gene therapy, in which an abnormally functioning gene is replaced with a normal gene, has been tested in select hematopoietic malignancies and shows promise. Relatively little progress has been made toward the genetic therapy of gynecologic malignancies; however, it is anticipated that gene therapy will eventually play a role in the treatment of patients with gynecologic malignancies.

BIBLIOGRAPHY

Baker V. Oncogenes in gynecologic malignancy. Curr Opin Obstet Gynecol 1992;4:75–80

Bishop JM. Molecular themes in oncogenesis. Cell 1991;64:235–248

Druker BJ, Mamon HJ, Roberts TM. Oncogenes, growth factors, and signal transduction. N Engl J Med 1989;321:1383–1391

Stancel GM, Baker VV, Hyder SM, Kirkland JL. Oncogenes and uterine function. Oxf Rev Reprod Biol 1993;15:1–42

Cancer of the Breast

Breast cancer now represents 32% of the cancers in women and causes 18% of the deaths from cancer. The most recent figures from the National Cancer Institute reveal that after a sharp rise in the percentage of women diagnosed with breast cancer from 1980 to 1987 there has been a decline in the incidence, especially among women aged 50 years and over. The National Cancer Institute also has indicated that the lifetime risk for the development of breast cancer increased to 1/8 from 1/9 in 1992. The increase in lifetime risk reflects the increase in the life expectancy of U.S. women and the fact that breast cancer is a disease of older women. In addition, the increase in lifetime risk has resulted from the decision to include in the calculations women over age 85 years. For 1993, the American Cancer Society predicts 182,000 new cases of breast cancer and 46,000 deaths. It should be noted that lung cancer is the leading cause of death in women; however, breast cancer is still the leading cause of death among women aged 40–55 years.

EPIDEMIOLOGY

Unfortunately, the risk factors currently identified for breast cancer do not present a significant potential for control, nor are they as clear-cut as for lung and cervical cancers. Furthermore, previously identified risk factors do not hold the key to understanding the etiology of this disease. In addition, 80% of the women with breast cancer do not have any of the currently identified risk factors. Thus, from the point of view of the clinician, all women should be assumed to be at risk for breast cancer, particularly those over age 35 years. This represents approximately 56 million women in the United States. A number of other malignancies are associated with breast cancer, and multiple primary tumors involving the ovary and uterus have been reported. Patients with endometrial cancer should be carefully screened with annual mammography, and, similarly, patients with breast cancer should be carefully observed for abnormal uterine bleeding.

The biggest risk factor for breast cancer is age. Breast cancer occurs more frequently among members of upper social classes than among those in lower social classes. Whites have been more affected than African–Americans, but apparently this is true only among women over age 45. Nulliparous women are at greater risk for breast cancer. Mortality rates are higher for those who live in urban areas than for those who live in rural areas, and mortality rates are higher for those in the northeastern portions and lower for those in the southern portions of the United States. There are well-known geographic variations in breast cancer rates. Studies of migrant populations suggest that environmental rather than genetic or other factors explain the rather marked international variations. It has been suggested that dietary fat may be involved in the etiology of breast cancer; however, the most recent reports have concluded that evidence linking high dietary fat intake with an increase in breast cancer is lacking.

A number of reproductive factors have been identified with increased risk, including age at first birth. The younger a woman is at the time of her first childbirth the lower her risk of breast cancer. The reasons are unknown. A number of studies have indicated that lactation does not decrease the risk for the development of breast cancer, principally because the length of lactation has been correlated with the number of full-term pregnancies. Recent studies from South America have suggested that lactation may have an independent protective effect when other risk factors are analyzed. Early menarche and late menopause confer a greater risk. Bilateral oophorectomy before menopause reduces the risk. These data suggest that the total number of years of menstrual activity may be an etiologic factor.

Women with an affected first-degree relative have a risk of breast cancer two to three times the risk of the general population. This is particularly true with premenopausal breast cancer. Obviously, the development of breast cancer in a family group is as consistent with an environmental cause as with a genetic component. When the primary care physician discusses risks for breast cancer, it is important to place the problem in perspective. As noted previously, the lifetime risk published by the National Cancer Institute is 1/8. A more appropriate explanation is the risk by decade. For example, the risk for breast cancer for women age 30–40 years is 1/1,000; 40–50 years, 2/1,000; and 50–60 years, 3/1,000. Thus, with a threefold increase due to a first-degree relative with breast cancer, the actual risk for women age 30–40 years would be 3/1,000.

For many years, use of exogenous hormones has been linked with the later development of breast cancer, and estrogen replacement therapy has been reevaluated in this context. Some studies have suggested that long-term past use of estrogen replacement therapy is not related to the risk of breast cancer but that current use may modestly increase risk. In another study among women with a family history of breast cancer, those who had used estrogen replacement therapy had a significantly higher risk than those who had not. A meta-analysis of the literature concerning breast cancer and estrogen replacement therapy suggests that the combined results from multiple studies provide evidence that menopausal therapy consisting of 0.625 mg or less of conjugated estrogen per day does not increase breast cancer risk. Additional studies are needed to determine whether the risk of breast cancer due to estrogen replacement therapy differs in perimenopausal and postmenopausal women and whether the different estrogen preparations affect breast cancer risk.

The data supporting the use of a progesterone along with estrogen require further evaluation. Most of the studies are inconclusive, and at present, the addition of a progestational agent is not recommended as a protection against the development of breast cancer for women who have had a hysterectomy. In the past, the assumption has been that the breast responds in a manner similar to that of the endometrium, with epithelial proliferation occurring during the first part of the menstrual cycle and secretory activity following ovulation and production of the corpus luteum and progesterone. Recent data suggest that, unlike the endometrium, breast epithelial stimulation occurs following ovulation, with the production of progesterone. The thymidine labeling index is much higher during the luteal phase of the cycle. Additional studies, therefore, will be required to clarify the roles of estrogen and progesterone.

Despite a substantial overall mortality benefit associated with estrogen replacement therapy, there is still uncertainty concerning the risk–benefit ratio for hormone replacement therapy in menopausal women. The benefits and risks of estrogen replacement therapy must be discussed with the patient. Obvious benefits include reduction of the risk of osteoporosis and coronary artery disease. Before replacement therapy is instituted, some physicians obtain a mammogram to rule out an occult lesion. Mammography should be repeated on a yearly basis or as clinically indicated.

Given the uncertainty about hormone interactions and the molecular genetics of breast cancer, it seems unwise at this time to recommend that estrogen replacement therapy be routinely recommended in patients who have been treated for breast cancer. Obviously, the final decision rests with the patient and her treating physician and oncologist and is subject to medical–legal interpretation.

Soon after the approval of oral contraceptives (OCs), a number of epidemiologic studies reported on the risk of breast cancer associated with the "pill." Oral contraceptives are widely used, and any effect on the risk of breast cancer will have important public health implications. Studies suggest that overall there has been no increase in the risk of breast cancer for women who had ever used OCs; however, women who had used OCs for long periods were at higher risk of premenopausal breast cancer. This was noted among women who had used OCs before their first full-term pregnancy. It will be important to determine whether this finding in a subgroup of women using OCs is confirmed, and more importantly, whether the risk remains at advancing age.

Another study reexamined the data from the Cancer and Steroid Hormone Study to determine whether OC use had different effects on the risk of breast cancer at different ages at diagnosis. Among women age 20–34 years at diagnosis, those who had ever used OCs had a slightly increased risk of breast cancer than did women of the same ages who had never used OCs. The slightly increased risk in young women is compatible with the findings of other investigators. There appear to be no data to suggest changes in the prescribing practice for the use of OCs.

Approximately 10% of patients with breast cancer give a history of trauma to the breast. This trauma probably results in increased attention to the breast and the discovery of a tumor or other changes that initiate breast self-examination. Viruslike particles have been identified in human breast milk, but there is no evidence that viruses are involved in breast cancer risk.

A number of histologic changes have been noted in benign fibrocystic breasts, and some have been associated with the later development of breast cancer. The College of American Pathologists has published a consensus statement indicating that there is no increased risk for breast cancer in conditions such as macrocysts or microcysts, duct ectasia, fibroadenoma, mild hyperplasia, mastitis, or squamous metaplasia. There is a slight increase in risk in patients with sclerosing adenosis, biopsy-proven hyperplasia that is moderate or florid, solid or papillary, and those who had papillomas with a fibrovascular core. Finally, risk increases substantially—four- to fivefold—in women with biopsy-proven atypical hyperplasia or a ductal or lobular carcinoma in situ.

PATHOLOGY

The histologic patterns of breast cancers can be divided into two types: carcinomas of lobular epithelial origin and those of ductal epithelial origin. Carcinomas of lobular epithelial origin are generally divided on the basis of invasion, that is, lobular cancer in situ or lobular neoplasia and invasive lobular cancer. Carcinomas of ductal origin are divided into noninvasive (ie, duct cancer in situ) and invasive types.

In situ lobular carcinoma or lobular neoplasia is almost always diagnosed as an incidental finding following the biopsy of a dominant mass or an occult lesion. The most important features of this lesion when planning treatment include bilaterality, multicentricity, and the relatively low rate of development of subsequent infiltrating carcinoma. If after biopsy the margins are clear, a reasonable treatment plan includes biannual physical examination and annual mammography. The alternative is to recommend mastectomy, and because bilaterality is common, bilateral mastectomy is the treatment of choice.

In situ ductal carcinoma is an entirely different lesion and of considerably more significance. If left untreated, infiltrating carcinoma will develop in the ipsilateral breast in approximately 50% of the cases. Standard treatment has been total mastectomy with or without conventional axillary dissection. Because of the advent of conservative techniques for small, invasive cancers, there has been considerable debate about the conservative treatment for the in situ ductal carcinoma. The most recent trial has suggested that appropriate treatment consists of wide local excision or segmental mastectomy followed by radiation therapy.

STAGING

Appropriate staging includes a pretreatment chest X-ray, routine blood studies, and liver function tests. For invasive lesions, a bone scan is recommended, although the yield is low for T1 lesions. It is helpful to have the results as a baseline for later comparison during follow-up evaluations. Clinical staging by the tumor, nodes, and metastases (TNM) system is recommended (see box), although this system does not adequately segregate patients or select appropriate surgical treatment. The system was designed so that patients could be categorized, thus enabling centers to group patients similarly for intercenter comparisons. The clinical nodal status of patients often is incorrect. Patients thought to have clinically negative nodes may have histologically positive nodes, and 25% of patients who are presumed to have clinically positive nodes are found to have histologically negative nodes. In addition, it is difficult to get an accurate tumor size, from either the pathologist or the surgeon. At present, however, the TNM system is the best available and does have some value in that it requires the physician to record patient and tumor information.

TREATMENT OPTIONS

Untreated breast cancer has a surprisingly predictable 5-year survival rate. In one series, 20% of patients were still alive at 5 years and 5% survived 10 years. Thus, in discussing treatment, the surgeon must be aware of the natural history of the disease and the necessity for long-term (15–25 years) follow-up to determine the efficacy of any treatment program.

The realization that patients will not be cured even with the most extensive local treatment has resulted in a more conservative approach and the participation of the patient in the treatment planning process. Less-invasive surgical procedures, including the modified radical mastectomy and segmental resection or wide local excision combined with axillary dissection and radiotherapy, have largely replaced the classic radical mastectomy.

Alterative treatments require the expertise of not only the surgeon but also the radiation oncologist and the medical oncologist. Because of the increase in a two-stage procedure, both for diagnosis and for treatment, a number of patients are referred for a second opinion. In some states, the law mandates that the physician discuss alternative treatments with patients, and in a few states, this must be recorded in the patient's medical record. Mammography is essential even in the most obvious case. Synchronous cancer is present in 4–5% of patients, and multicentric disease may be discovered in the involved breast.

A number of factors influence the definitive surgical treatment of breast cancer. Important considerations include the size and histology of the lesion, the skill and experience of the multidisciplinary team, and the wishes of the patient. There have been a number of published reports, both from retrospective studies and from prospective randomized clinical trials, that have concluded that segmental mastectomy or wide local excision followed by axillary dissection and radiation therapy is appropriate therapy for stage I and stage II breast cancers less than 4 cm, provided the margins of the resected specimens are free of tumor. A consensus development conference on the treatment of early-stage breast cancer convened by the National Cancer Institute in 1990 concluded, "Breast conservation treatment is an appropriate method of primary therapy for the majority of women with Stage I and Stage II breast cancer and is preferable because it provides survival equivalent to total mastectomy and axillary dissection while preserving the breast."

The use of conservative surgery and radiation therapy requires consideration of four important criteria: patient selection, the surgery of the primary tumor, radiotherapy of the primary tumor, and surgery of the axilla. The principal advantage of conservative treatment is cosmetic. There are no data to indicate that the conservative approach provides improved survival when compared with the radical or modified radical mastectomy. Thus, the major criterion for patient selection is the ability to resect the primary tumor adequately without creating a cosmetic deformity. Patients who are poor candidates for breast-conserving treatment include those with widely separated primary tumors in the same breast, those whose mammograms reveal diffuse disease in many quadrants, and those with large tumors in a relatively small breast. Patients who have central lesions that involve the nipple–areolar complex can be successfully treated with the resection of the areolar with careful attention to the final cosmetic result.

Adequate surgical resection implies grossly clear margins. The surgeon must appropriately mark the specimen for orientation by the pathologist. Tissue should be removed for estrogen and progesterone receptor studies without disturbing the evaluation of the resected margins. It is generally agreed that if the microscopic margins are positive after wide local excision, further excision should be performed. This can be accomplished either at the time of the original biopsy or at the time of axillary dissection.

Radiotherapy is begun as soon as the wounds are healed. It is generally agreed that the breast should be treated with 180–200 cGy/d for a total of 4,500–5,000 cGy. Total doses in excess of 5,000 cGy result in fibrosis, retraction, and an unacceptable cosmetic result. For patients treated with wide local excision and in whom the margins of resection are close on microscopic evaluation, "boost" therapy may be recommended. If the patient requires adjuvant chemotherapy, this

DEFINITION OF TNM* STAGING SYSTEM

Stage	Definition
Primary tumor	
TX	Primary tumor cannot be assessed
T0	No evidence of primary tumor
TIS†	Carcinoma in situ: Intraductal carcinoma lobular carcinoma in situ, or Paget disease of the nipple with no tumor
T1	Tumor 2 cm or less in greatest dimension
T1a	0.5 cm or less in greatest dimension
T1b	More than 0.5 cm but not more than 1 cm in greatest dimension
T1c	More than 1 cm but not more than 2 cm in greatest dimension
T2	Tumor more than 2 cm but not more than 5 cm in greatest dimension
T3	Tumor more than 5 cm in greatest dimension
T4‡	Tumor of any size with direct extension to chest wall or skin
T4a	Extension to chest wall
T4b	Edema (including peau d'orange) or ulceration of the skin of the breast or satellite skin nodules confined to the same breast
T4c	Both (T4a and T4b)
T4d	Inflammatory carcinoma
Regional lymph nodes (N)	
NX	Regional lymph nodes cannot be assessed (eg, previously removed)
N0	No regional lymph node metastasis
N1	Metastasis to movable ipsilateral axillary lymph node(s)
N2	Metastasis to ipsilateral axillary lymph node(s) fixed to one another or to other structures
N3	Metastasis to ipsilateral internal mammary lymph node(s)
Pathologic classification (pN)	
pNX	Regional lymph nodes cannot be assessed (eg, previously removed or not removed for pathologic study)
pN0	No regional lymph node metastasis
pN1	Metastasis to movable ipsilateral axillary lymph node(s)
pN1a	Only micrometastasis (none larger than 0.2 cm)
pN1b	Metastasis to lymph node(s), any larger than 0.2 cm
pN1bi	Metastasis in 1 to 3 lymph nodes, any more than 0.2 cm and all less than 2 cm in greatest dimension

Stage	Definition
Pathologic classification (pN) (continued)	
pN1bii	Metastasis to 4 or more lymph nodes, any more than 0.2 cm and all less than 2 cm in greatest dimension
pN1biii	Extension of tumor beyond the capsule of a lymph node metastasis less than 2 cm in greatest dimension
pN1biv	Metastasis to a lymph node 2 cm or more in greatest dimension
pN2	Metastasis to ipsilateral axillary lymph nodes that are fixed to one another or to other structures
pN3	Metastasis to ipsilateral internal mammary lymph node(s)
Distant metastasis (M)	
MX	Presence of distant metastasis cannot be assessed
M0	No distant metastasis
M1	Distant metastasis (includes metastasis to ipsilateral supraclavicular lymph node[s])
Stage grouping	
Stage 0	TIS, N0, M0
Stage I	T1, N0, M0
Stage IIA	T0, N1, M0
	T1, N1,§ M0
	T2, N0, M0
Stage IIB	T2, N1, M0
	T3, N0, M0
Stage IIIA	T0, N2, M0
	T1, N2, M0
	T2, N2, M0
	T3; N1, N2; M0
Stage IIIB	T4, any N, M0
	Any T, N3, M0
Stage IV	Any T, any N, M1

* Definitions for classifying the primary tumor (T) are the same for clinical and for pathologic classification. The telescoping method of classification can be applied. If the measurement is made by physical examination, the examiner will use the major headings (T1, T2, or T3). If other measurements, such as mammographic or pathologic, are used, the telescoped subsets of T1 can be used.

† Paget disease associated with a tumor is classified according to the size of the tumor.

‡ Chest wall includes ribs, intercostal muscles, and serratus anterior muscle but not pectoral muscle.

§ The prognosis of patients with PN1a is similar to that of patients with pN0.

Modified from American Joint Committee on Cancer. Manual for staging of cancer. 4th ed. Philadelphia: JB Lippincott, 1992

treatment must be integrated with radiotherapy. There is no agreement concerning the use of chemotherapy and radiotherapy concomitantly or chemotherapy and radiotherapy in sequence. Optimal cosmesis and minimal complication risk require careful attention to the technical details of the surgery and radiotherapy. The impact of systemic therapy requires more thorough investigation.

While the conservative approach appeals to many patients, statistics clearly indicate that most patients in the United States are still treated with the modified radical mastectomy. In some cases, the conservative approach is not appropriate and some patients request removal of the breast. The modified radical mastectomy should be performed in a cosmetic manner, preferably with a transverse incision to permit later reconstruction.

There are advantages and disadvantages to the conservative and radical approaches. Obviously, the main advantage of the conservative approach is the preservation of the breast; however, the price to be paid is the extended radiation treatments and the real concern of some patients that future symptoms in the retained breast are associated with recurrent tumor. In the more radical approach, treatment is accomplished in a few days, and obviously cancer cannot recur in the breast.

Many patients elect reconstructive procedures at a later date, and some surgeons are performing reconstruction at the time of the modified radical mastectomy. The patient should see the plastic surgeon before the mastectomy. Occasionally, a support group will be available to discuss the reconstructive techniques and results. Immediate reconstruction, while appealing, has drawbacks. In some cases, following the mastectomy, it is necessary to perform a reduction mammoplasty on the opposite side. This is a lengthy procedure and more appropriately accomplished at a second operative procedure. There is also the possibility that an unexpected finding at the time of mastectomy will adversely influence the reconstruction procedure.

These options are open to question because of the recent actions of the U.S. Food and Drug Administration (FDA) regarding silicone prostheses. These are known as "preamendment devices" because they were marketed before the 1976 device law. Regulations by the FDA require manufacturers to submit data that products are safe and effective. After considerable testimony, a moratorium on the use of breast implants was announced by the FDA on January 6, 1992; on April 16, 1992, the FDA announced that breast implants filled with silicone gel would be available only through controlled clinical studies and that women who need such implants for breast reconstruction would be assured of access to these studies.

ADJUVANT TREATMENT

It must be assumed from the survival rates of even patients with the best prognosis, those with negative nodes, that some of these patients have systemic disease. There are certain major predictors of systemic recurrence, and these are the basis for recommending systemic (adjuvant) treatment. These predictors include tumor diameter and the number of involved nodes. Several less-well-defined predictors, including tumor grade, nuclear grade, DNA synthesis, and estrogen and progesterone receptors, have been described. Eventually, biochemical and immunopathologic methods may be of some value. About 16% of patients with T1,N0 disease and 26% of patients with T2,N0 disease develop recurrence in 10 years. Until recently, these patients were not treated with adjuvant therapy. This raises the question of whether perhaps it is more a matter of concern that adjuvant treatment is withheld from patients rather than that some patients are overtreated who would not have developed systemic recurrence.

A number of factors have been recognized that define high- and low-risk groups in women with node-negative breast cancer. Factors associated with low risk include ductal cancer in situ, tumor less than 1 cm, diploid tumor, low S-phase fraction, nuclear grade 1, and tumors 1–2 cm without high-risk features. Factors associated with high risk include aneuploid tumor, high S-phase fractions, high cathepsin D levels, absent estrogen receptors, and tumors greater than 3 cm in diameter. For half of the patients, the decision regarding adjuvant therapy is fairly straightforward. About 25% will have small tumors and favorable histologic types and should not be treated. Another 25% have large tumors associated with poor prognostic features and most, if not all, of these should be treated. The remaining 50%, with tumors of intermediate size, constitute the group for which it is recommended that the prognostic factors mentioned be used to help identify low- and high-risk groups so that treatment efforts can be focused on those most likely to benefit.

Several groups have developed treatment programs based on cyclic high-dose chemotherapy regimens. These programs may not require stem cell support but do use high doses of cytotoxic agents and usually require the patient to be hospitalized. The cycles are repeated as tolerated every 4–6 weeks. With short follow-up, it is clear that tumor response may be achieved, but this is of uncertain duration. High-dose chemotherapy with autologous stem cell support is effective therapy for the management of metastatic breast cancer and perhaps for patients with locally advanced disease. Because the follow-up of these programs is relatively brief, the cost and morbidity is substantial, and the long-term cost and toxicities are unknown, continuing investigation of high-dose chemotherapy and autologous stem cell support remains important.

In most treatment centers, the currently recommended adjuvant therapy consists of a standard program of either cyclophosphamide, methotrexate, and 5-fluorouracil or cyclophosphamide, doxorubicin, and 5-fluorouracil. For postmenopausal patients, tamoxifen, 10 mg twice daily, is the standard adjuvant therapy. Although postmenopausal patients may benefit from cytotoxic chemotherapy, the survival benefit is small and the cost is high. Using active life expectancy as the primary outcome reduces the benefit and adds to the cost. It has been suggested that if active life expectancy is a relevant outcome, withholding chemotherapy for patients older than age 70 is a reasonable approach.

An increasing body of evidence supports the belief that prolonged use of tamoxifen is associated with an increased incidence of endometrial hyperplasia and endometrial carcinoma. The actual risk, however, is very low, probably 0.5%. It is essential, therefore, that patients receiving tamoxifen have a complete pelvic examination on a yearly basis; some have suggested a yearly cytologic examination of endometrial aspiration.

METASTATIC DISEASE

With current treatment protocols, patients with metastatic disease are not curable. However, they may be managed with a variety of palliative therapies, and in some cases, they can be treated for many years with excellent quality of life. A local recurrence in a breast treated by wide local excision and primary radiotherapy is curable in many cases by mastectomy or even additional wide local excision and does not necessarily represent widespread metastatic disease. On the other hand, local recurrence following modified radical mastectomy is ominous and in most cases indicates systemic disease.

It is important to detect metastases as early as possible. A number of diagnostic studies are used to detect recurrent disease. Yearly liver function tests, carcinoembryonic antigen determinations, and chest X-ray are essential, although carcinoembryonic antigen levels are elevated in a number of disease states. Biopsy should be performed, if possible, to document the recurrence and hormonal receptor status. This is particularly true of lung lesions, which in fact may represent a new primary lesion. The treatment strategy depends on the extent and location of the disease, the menstrual status of the patient, and the disease-free interval.

Palliation may be achieved with hormone therapy; however, this should not be used in patients who require a rapid response, particularly those with visceral disease. Receptor status can be used to predict this response. About 60% of women with estrogen-receptive protein activity respond to hormonal manipulation, and those with progesterone receptor activity have an 80% or greater chance of hormonal response. Patients who respond to hormonal maneuvers have a subsequent median survival of more than 4 years. Tamoxifen produces a response in about one third of patients with metastatic disease and two thirds of those with estrogen receptor protein activity.

Oophorectomy may be used as an endocrine procedure for premenopausal women. The expected response is in the range of 30–40%. Patients with pathologic factors can be stabilized by appropriate orthopedic procedures, and radiotherapy can be used to prevent pathologic factors or to control pain, soft tissue disease, and brain metastasis. Occasionally, an isolated metastasis can be resected with good results.

Metastatic cancer, because of the biology of this disease, must be considered a chronic illness, and quality of life is important. Psychosocial support is required, and continuity of the health care team and a positive attitude are essential to provide the support needed for these patients.

PROGNOSIS

Prognosis is influenced by a number of factors, including histology, growth pattern, length of disease-free interval, lymphatic or blood vessel invasion, receptor status, and more recently, evaluation of flow cytometry and other prognostic indicators. Patients with negative nodes have approximately a 75% 10-year survival rate, and patients with positive nodes have a 40% absolute 10-year survival.

MEDICAL–LEGAL IMPLICATIONS

One of the most frequent causes of litigation is the failure to diagnose breast cancer. The physician must therefore document carefully the patient's chief complaint and the physical examination. This should include the chronology of the chief complaint and the use of a diagram or narrative discussion in the medical record of the patient to indicate the location and associated features of the breast lesion. If an abnormality is described as a lump or a mass or is measured or drawn, the patient by definition has a dominant three-dimensional mass, and this must be resolved by additional diagnostic studies. These include aspiration, fine-needle aspiration, or open biopsy. In some cases, resolution may include a plan of action, including reexamination after a menstrual period or at other stated intervals. The treatment plan must be carefully recorded in the patient's medical record.

It is important that the physician document the diagnosis and the disposition of the case. This may include referral, and the record should reflect to whom the patient was referred and for what purpose. If additional diagnostic studies have been ordered, including mammography, the record should indicate the result of the diagnostic study and the fact that the patient has been notified of the result. In addition, phone messages and consultation should be appropriately documented. If the patient has been admitted to the hospital for any surgical procedure, the admission history, physical examination, operative notes, and discharge summary should be reviewed carefully by the responsible physician before his or her signature is given.

BIBLIOGRAPHY

American Cancer Society. Cancer facts and figures—1994. Atlanta: ACS, 1994

Boring CC, Squires TS, Tong T. Cancer statistics, 1993. CA Cancer J Clin 1993;43:7–26

Desch CE, Hillner BE, Smith TJ, Retchin SM. Should the elderly receive chemotherapy for node-negative breast cancer? Cost-effectiveness analysis examining total and active life-expectancy outcomes. J Clin Oncol 1993;11:777–782

Kinne DW. The surgical management of primary breast cancer. CA Cancer J Clin 1991;41:71–84

Marchant DJ. Estrogen-replacement therapy after breast cancer: risks versus benefits. Cancer 1993;71(6 suppl):2169–2176

Meropol NJ, Overmoyer BA, Stadmauer EA. High-dose chemotherapy with autologous stem-cell support for breast cancer. Oncology (Huntingt) 1992;6:53–60, 63–64, 69

Miller AB, Baines CJ, To T, Wall C. Canadian National Breast Screening Study, 1: breast cancer detection and death rates among women aged 40 to 49 years. Can Med Assoc J 1992;147:1459–1476

Recht A, Come SE, Gelman RS, Goldstein M, Tishler S, Gore SM, et al. Integration of conservative surgery, radiotherapy, and chemotherapy for the treatment of early-stage node-positive breast cancer: sequencing, timing, and outcome. J Clin Oncol 1991;9:1662–1667

Winchester DP, Cox JD. Standards for breast-conservation treatment. CA Cancer J Clin 1992;42:134–162

Cancer of the Vulva

Invasive squamous cell carcinoma accounts for 90% of all invasive malignancies of the vulva, which are responsible for only 1–4% of all female cancers. Other malignant lesions of the vulva are melanoma, adenocarcinoma, and sarcoma. Over three fourths of all patients diagnosed with this disease are age 55 years or older; 30% of these cancers occur in women age 75 years or older. Approximately 500 deaths from vulvar cancer occur annually in the United States.

The cause of vulvar malignancy remains unknown. Although the association of squamous cell carcinoma of the vulva with other neoplasias of the anogenital mucosa has long suggested a common etiology, preliminary data have not been conclusive regarding the role of oncogenesis. The association of high-risk types of HPV, such as types 16, 18, 31, 33, 35, and 39, with high-grade epithelial neoplasia and invasive carcinomas of the anogenital tract has been well established. Vulvar cancer appears to have a multifactorial etiology. Human papilloma virus infection alone is probably not sufficient for malignant transformation. Primary among cofactors may be the patient's own immune competence, including conditions of local immunodeficiency, as may be represented in chronic vulvar dystrophy. While the risk of progression of vulvar dystrophy to malignancy is low, vulvar dystrophy is frequently associated with epidermoid carcinoma.

Multicentric and confluent vulvar intraepithelial neoplasia (VIN) lesions predominate among younger women, whereas the unifocal lesions, which are more likely to be associated with invasive carcinoma, are more common in older women. The lesions may appear to be white, because of thick surface keratin, or red, if hyperemia is present high within the dermal papillae. Pigmentation is common, especially with bowenoid neoplasia. Often, the appearance is of slightly raised and possibly confluent white areas resembling flat condylomata. Colposcopy with 4–5% acetic acid heightens the whitening and allows for delineation of the margins of the vulvar lesions, as well as other subclinical HPV infections over the vulva. Thickened, nodular, ulcerated areas are most suspect, as are areas of vascular prominence and atypicality. The reliability of the colposcope in ruling out the presence of invasive carcinoma on the vulva is not as great as it is in ruling out that on the vagina and cervix. A higher index of suspicion and a large number of biopsies are therefore appropriate in evaluating suggestive vulvar lesions. The potential for failure to detect early invasive carcinoma of the vulva thus limits the applicability of laser ablation for management of high-grade or extensive VIN.

CARCINOMA IN SITU

Vulvar intraepithelial neoplasia is more frequently diagnosed in younger patients. Carcinoma in situ, or VIN, has a peak onset in the fourth decade, about 10–15 years preceding the most common age for invasive epidermoid carcinoma. Vulvar intraepithelial neoplasia frequently is a multifocal disease most commonly affecting the central vulvar structures, with the posterior half of the vulva the area affected most often. The mean thickness of the epithelium for all grades of VIN is 0.52 mm. The thickness of the involved epithelium varies little, regardless of the location of the lesions. Infections caused by HPV are increasingly frequent and may be responsible for the increased frequency of diagnosis of VIN. In its most overt form, HPV causes multiple condylomata that in themselves may have a significant degree of atypia and may be associated with intraepithelial neoplasia. More subtle are the flat condylomata that may occur over the anogenital skin, producing irritative symptoms as well as atypical cytology and histology. Histologic examination of biopsies and specimens from such areas requires an experienced pathologist familiar with the subtleties of interpreting the spectra of atypia seen with intraepithelial neoplasia and HPV infection.

The histologic criteria necessary for the diagnosis of carcinoma in situ include virtual full-thickness replacement of the epithelium with atypical or immature squamous cells. Unlike the cervix, superficial layers of the vulvar epithelium are usually keratinized, thus obscuring colposcopic observation of underlying atypical patterns.

Between 20% and 40% of patients with carcinoma in situ of the vulva have previous, concurrent, or subsequent neoplasias elsewhere within the anogenital tract. Colposcopic and cytologic review of these areas is appropriate. Cases of carcinoma in situ of the vulva associated with pregnancy have been reported to regress spontaneously during the late puerperium and thus should be observed rather than treated aggressively. There have been no prospective studies to document risk and progression rates for VIN. Lesions showing characteristic Bowen cells, as well as those containing perinuclear halos suggesting HPV infection with atypia, but without full-thickness cellular atypia and abnormal mitoses, should be observed with care. They are infrequently associated with invasive carcinoma but may prove to be self-limited with spontaneous regression over a period of up to 6 months.

Because the biologic potential of VIN remains uncertain, conservative methods of therapy are appropriate. Previously, complete excision of the area at risk was recommended regardless of the size of the lesion. As it is now recognized that these lesions are only a part of the spectrum of neoplasias that occur over the entire anogenital epithelium, removal of the entire area at risk may not be feasible and would certainly be disfiguring. Rather than a routine total vulvectomy, wide excision of the intraepithelial neoplasia is more appropriate, particularly for unifocal lesions. Shallow "skinning" procedures that remove the full thickness of epithelium of the labia majora and minora and over the clitoris but leave the underlying connective tissues intact may be used for widespread multifocal involvement. Grossly, a margin of 1–1.5 cm beyond the limits of the lesion should be removed. Primary closure may be accomplished, sometimes by using rotational flaps or skin grafting.

Laser therapy for ablation of VIN is appropriate in selected cases. One of its major limitations is the loss of tissue for histologic interpretation to detect occult invasion. Laser vaporization with the carbon dioxide laser is an alternative therapy. Laser vaporization to a depth of 1.0–2.0 mm, including the zone of thermal necrosis, should be sufficient to destroy most epidermal lesions without skin appendage involvement. If the initial biopsy showed involvement of adjacent hair follicles or sebaceous glands, deeper tissue destruction is necessary to theoretically achieve greater than 90% elimination of the disease. In laser-treated patients, cosmetic results are excellent. Laser vaporization appears to be an effective and nonmutilating therapy and is preferable for young patients with VIN.

As noted previously, the colposcope is less satisfactory for detecting occult invasion on the vulva than it is for detecting that on the cervix. In addition, VIN may be present in the epithelium adjacent to the known primary lesion and may remain undetected by either gross or colposcopic visualization. Laser ablation is therefore subject to a significant failure rate because of incomplete excision, but this rate may be reduced to levels comparable to those of surgical excision if careful attention is given to adequate ablation margins and histologic study of suggestively thick lesions.

Topical chemotherapy with 5% 5-fluorouracil cream has produced a response in approximately 50% of cases in which it has been used, although recurrences have been noted. The procedure has been accompanied by significant morbidity because of local irritation and the associated ulceration and denudation. Morbidity can be reduced by weekly application over several months.

Carcinoma in situ of the vulva remains a disease whose true biologic significance, etiology, and prognosis have yet to be clarified. New questions have arisen relative to classification, virus subtyping, and diagnosis since recognition of the frequency of HPV infection. After a biopsy is performed to define precisely the histologic character of the lesion, therapy should be individualized. When feasible, the pathology of vulvar carcinoma in situ should be reviewed by a pathologist or a gynecologic oncologist familiar with the management of these lesions.

Patients of advancing age with diseases that have a raised and irregular surface pattern are more likely to have lesions with occult invasion. Treatment that uses ablative techniques cannot be recommended based on the use of preoperative representative biopsies that may miss occult invasive vulvar carcinoma.

Fewer than 10% of patients with stages I and II vulvar carcinoma have minimally invasive carcinomas diagnosed at a mean age of 60 years. Microinvasive squamous carcinoma of the vulva with 1 mm or less of stromal invasion can be treated with local resection without inguinal node dissection. Wide excision or radical wide excision of small diameter, well-differentiated lesions less than 2 cm in diameter with 1 mm or less of stromal invasion on biopsy is adequate therapy. If final pathologic review demonstrates deeper invasion, vascular involvement, or poor differentiation, selective lymph node dissection can be performed. Careful follow-up surveillance with liberal use of colposcopy and biopsies is indicated in these patients.

PAGET DISEASE

The median age of patients with Paget disease of the vulva at diagnosis is 64 years. About 10–15% of patients have an associated invasive adenocarcinoma of the vulva at the time of diagnosis. Radical surgery is the preferred treatment of patients with an associated invasive adenocarcinoma. Patients with superficial Paget disease of the vulva should be treated by local excision, using frozen sections, fluorescein, or monoclonal antibodies for margin evaluation as a guide to extent of excision. Patients can require multiple procedures for recurrent superficial Paget disease. Rarely after an initial diagnosis of superficial Paget disease of the vulva does invasive adenocarcinoma develop.

The Paget cell is of epidermal origin and represents aberrant differentiation of the epidermal multifocal stem cell. Paget cells have ultrastructural characteristics of secretory sweat gland cells and squamous cell carcinoma. Histochemical stains yield positive reactions for intracellular mucopolysaccharide in characteristic Paget cells that clearly distinguish them from cells of the even more unusual superficial amelanotic melanoma.

Paget disease of the vulva occurs most often in white, postmenopausal women. The symptoms are extreme pruritus and soreness, often of long duration. The disease appears as red or bright-pink, desquamated, eczematoid areas among which are scattered raised, white islands of hyperkeratosis. The borders appear slightly elevated and sharply demarcated. While perianal involvement is not uncommon, other areas of the anogenital tract (cervix and vagina) are involved only by continuity of the lesion rather than by multifocal primary lesions. Concomitant adenocarcinoma of the vulvar sweat glands or within the perianal glands has been noted.

The visible borders of the lesion, although seemingly sharp, are frequently misleading. Adjacent nests of Paget cells have been found deep in the epidermis or somewhat removed from these margins. Treatment encompasses wide excision of a margin of at least 2 cm in the initial definition of the lesion. These margins should be evaluated by examination of frozen sections; otherwise, the frequency of recurrence will be high. The excision should encompass more than removal of the epidermis alone; underlying fat and superficial fibromuscular tissue should also be removed because of the possibility of an underlying adenocarcinoma. Careful histologic review of the entire surgical specimen is necessary to rule out an underlying primary adenocarcinoma. When underlying adenocarcinoma is present, bilateral inguinofemoral lymphadenectomy should be considered, although the propensity for these lesions to metastasize to the nodes has not been well defined, and there are some doubts regarding the efficacy of regional lymphadenectomy in such cases. Radiotherapy and chemotherapy play no role in the primary treatment of this disease.

The corrected survival rate for all patients, including those with associated underlying adenocarcinoma, is approximately 90%, although intraepithelial recurrences have been reported following total excision in about 20% of cases. These are largely avoidable with the use of frozen-section evaluation of the margins at the time of primary treatment.

INVASIVE SQUAMOUS CELL CARCINOMA

Invasive squamous cell carcinoma of the vulva accounts for approximately 5% of all genital malignancies and 90% of vulvar malignancies. The disease occurs primarily in the sixth and seventh decades of life and is characteristically preceded by a considerable delay in diagnosis and institution of therapy on the part of both the patient and the physician, thus indicating the necessity of an early biopsy for diagnosis. The discrepancy between the extent of the lesion and its brief duration, however, can be due to rapid progression of some of the lesions that occur on the vulva and is not always simply a matter of patient denial of the existence of what appears to be a gross and obviously symptomatic lesion. There are no clear-cut precursors to carcinoma of the vulva, although women with granulomatous venereal disease and other malignancies of the lower genital tract appear to be at increased risk.

Women age 25 years or younger can have invasive squamous cell carcinoma of the vulva. An awareness of the possibility of invasive vulvar carcinoma, even in the relatively young patient, should lead to prompt and thorough histologic evaluation of any vulvar lesion. Pretreatment evaluation is particularly important when ablation of extensive lesions is planned. Although the incidence of preinvasive vulvar lesions seems to be rising in the younger population, invasive squamous cell carcinoma remains exceedingly rare. As a result, diagnostic biopsy is often delayed and ablative therapy frequently instituted without an adequate histologic diagnosis.

There is evidence that HPV types 16 and 18 are associated with the development of invasive squamous cell carcinoma of the vulva. In specimens with invasive squamous cell carcinoma, HPV type 16 or type 18, or both, can be found.

Invasive carcinoma usually presents with ulceration, friability, or induration of the surrounding tissues. While most arise in a unifocal manner, "kissing lesions" are of interest relative to the possible mechanism of contact induction of malignancy of the vulva. Most invasive carcinomas of the vulva are associated with surrounding areas of intraepithelial neoplasia and frequently are associated with vulvar dystrophy. Despite this, vulvar dystrophy is not identified as a high-risk premalignant entity, and intraepithelial neoplasia seems to have a low rate of progression into invasive carcinoma.

The most widely used system for staging invasive carcinoma of the vulva is that approved in 1988 by the International Federation of Gynecology and Obstetrics (FIGO) (see box). This is a surgical staging system. Assessment of node involvement by clinical palpation is subject to a large margin of error, with even the most experienced observers acknowledging a 25–40% error rate in such evaluation. Patients with no palpable nodes or nonsuggestive palpable nodes have as high as 25% occult metastasis. These observations do not totally undermine the validity of clinical node assessment but do emphasize the importance of avoiding overreliance on clinical assessment of the status of the inguinal nodes as an adjunct in planning appropriate therapy.

Radical surgery is the treatment of choice for this disease. Therapy should encompass adequate excision of the primary lesion, even if this includes excision of the distal urethra or necessitates colostomy for excision of the anus. Adequate control of the primary lesion is the primary objective, without which regional lymphadenectomy becomes of secondary importance.

Small lesions (less than 2 cm) with minimal stromal invasion (less than 1 mm) have prompted discussion regarding treatment by radical vulvectomy or extended local resection alone without groin dissection. Criteria have been examined by which one can define lesions that have a low incidence of positive nodes. It is reasonable to define lesions with a minimal risk of metastasis as those that extend no deeper than 1 mm below the level of the adjacent normal dermal papillae (lesion thickness no greater than 1 mm) and that are not anaplastic or associated with lymphatic permeation. These lesions should be small areas of pushing or budding rather than infiltrating or confluent patterns involving a large area of malignancy.

Current evidence indicates that one must be cautious in applying the concept of microinvasion to vulvar disease until further experience has been acquired. It does appear, however, that the pattern of lymphatic spread of primary carcinoma of the vulva is very predictable relative to its initial passage to the inguinal nodes. This has given rise to the concept of superficial inguinal lymphadenectomy as a procedure associated with decreased morbidity applicable to the man-

FIGO Staging of Vulvar Carcinoma

Stage 0
- TIS — Carcinoma in situ, intraepithelial carcinoma

Stage I
- T1 N0 M0 — Tumor confined to the vulva and/or perineum—2 cm or less in greatest dimension, no nodal metastasis

Stage II
- T2 N0 M0 — Tumor confined to the vulva and/or perineum—more than 2 cm in greatest dimension, no nodal metastasis

Stage III
- T3 N0 M0 — Tumor of any size with...
- T3 N1 M0 — (1) Adjacent spread to the lower urethra and/or the vagina, or the anus, and/or...
- T1 N1 M0 — (2) Unilateral regional lymph node metastasis
- T2 N1 M0

Stage IVA
- T1 N2 M0 — Tumor invades any of the following:
- T2 N2 M0 — Upper urethra, bladder mucosa, rectal mucosa, pelvic bone, and/or bilateral regional node metastasis
- T3 N2 M0
- T4 any N M0

Stage IVB
- Any T — Any distant metastasis including
- Any N M1 — pelvic lymph nodes

TNM Classification of Carcinoma of the Vulva (FIGO)

T	*Primary tumor*
TIS	Preinvasive carcinoma (carcinoma in situ)
T1	Tumor confined to the vulva and/or perineum—≤2 cm in greatest dimension
T2	Tumor confined to the vulva and/or perineum—>2 cm in greatest dimension
T3	Tumor of any size with adjacent spread to the urethra and/or vagina and/or to the anus
T4	Tumor of any size infiltrating the bladder mucosa and/or the rectal mucosa, including the upper part of the urethral mucosa and/or fixed to the bone
N	*Regional lymph nodes*
N0	No lymph node metastasis
N1	Unilateral regional lymph node metastasis
N2	Bilateral regional lymph node metastasis
M	*Distant metastasis*
M0	No clinical metastasis
M1	Distant metastasis (including pelvic lymph node metastasis)

Adapted from International Federation of Gynecology and Obstetrics. Annual report on the results of treatment in gynecological cancer. Int J Gynecol Obstet 1989;28:189–190

---

agement of superficially invasive carcinoma of the vulva. Patients with small lesions (less than 2 cm in diameter), limited to one side of the vulva, and not involving the clitoris, urethra, vagina, or anus, may be considered for a modified surgical procedure to include hemivulvectomy and ipsilateral inguinal lymphadenectomy. Limited and early invasive cancers of the vulva, particularly those occurring in young women, can be managed safely with a modified approach, preserving cosmetic appearance and sexual function. The intent is not to create sexual handicaps in women who can otherwise be treated safely with a less radical procedure. This type of individualized treatment is essential in all aspects of oncology but is particularly important when dealing with vulvar cancer.

The pattern of lymphatic dissemination from the primary lesion seems to be an orderly progression through the superficial inguinal nodes to the deep inguinal nodes and then through the femoral canal to the deep pelvic nodes. Theoretically, lesions involving the clitoris, urethra, vagina, and anus may have direct lymphatic communication with the pelvic lymph nodes. In practice, such direct metastasis by squamous cell carcinoma of the vulva does not occur, although with melanomas and sarcomas, patterns of lymphatic and hematogenous dissemination are less predictable. In the treatment of invasive squamous cell carcinoma, the clinical status of the inguinal nodes provides prognostic criteria regarding the risk of pelvic node metastasis, which may be improved further after removing the inguinal lymphadenectomy specimen and determining whether palpable nodes suggestive of malignancy are present. Control of regional metastases by en bloc inguinal lymphadenectomy is dependent on the number of lymph nodes positive. There is minimal risk of pelvic lymph node metastasis, particularly if the Cloquet node is uninvolved. There is significant risk of local recurrence, even with en bloc resection of the groin nodes, in patients who have a clinically suggestive or enlarged node (N2, N3).

Radical surgery, occasionally with adjunctive radiation therapy, remains the treatment of choice for this disease. With this therapy, corrected 5-year survival rates for all stages approach 90% if the nodes are negative. With positive groin nodes, approximately 40% of the patients survive for 5 years, and 15–25% survive for 5 years when the deep pelvic nodes are involved. When pelvic node metastasis is suspected or demonstrated, extraperitoneal pelvic lymphadenectomy plus radiation therapy may offer the best chance for control.

To determine whether groin irradiation is superior to and less morbid than groin dissection, the Gynecologic Oncology Group randomized patients with squamous carcinoma of the vulva and nonsuggestive inguinal nodes to receive either groin dissection or groin irradiation in conjunction with radical vulvectomy. The study was closed prematurely when interim monitoring revealed an excessive number of groin relapses on the groin irradiation regimen. Metastatic involvement of the groin nodes was projected to occur in 24% of patients. On the groin dissection regimen, patients with positive groin nodes received postoperative irradiation. There were five groin relapses among the 27 (18.5%) patients on the groin irradiation regimen and none on the groin dissection regimen. The groin dissection regimen had significantly better survival rates.

Radiation therapy with megavoltage equipment, including electron beam, has been applied as the primary treatment of extensive carcinoma of the vulva. Extended-field therapy given to the vulva and perineum, as well as the groin nodes, has resulted in control of the disease for some patients but with significant morbidity, such as a high incidence of long-term complications from fistulas, persistent vulvar ulcerations, atrophy, contractures, and pain. In cases in which surgery can be accomplished, irradiation is an unacceptable alternative. It may be considered for patients whose medical condition precludes surgery, although limited palliative surgery may be appropriate. In selected cases, radiation therapy may be given preoperatively to reduce bulky disease and define surgical margins.

Initial management with irradiation and chemotherapy offers some patients with locally advanced squamous cell cancer of the vulva an alternative to exenterative surgery and may hold curative potential for some patients with initially surgically unresectable or medically inoperable disease. External-beam radiation and synchronous radiopotentiating chemotherapy can be used to treat women with locally or regionally advanced or recurrent squamous cell cancer of the vulva. The acute toxicity is generally mild, and there are no life-threatening acute complications. The responses are usually prompt and dramatic but often not sustained. Complete clinical response is obtained in 60–80% of patients. As initial therapy, irradiation and chemotherapy may allow lesser surgery with preservation of normal anatomy in selected primary vulvar cancers in patients with vulvar cancer.

The primary morbidity of radical vulvectomy and bilateral groin dissection is lymphedema with groin wound breakdown. Few intraoperative deaths occur, but there is a postoperative mortality of up to 5%.

Acceptable survival (60% 5-year survival) for advanced or recurrent vulvar cancer can be achieved with pelvic exenteration, but the presence of metastatic disease to lymph nodes markedly decreases survival (0%). Exenteration performed for primary therapy is more successful than exenteration performed for recurrent disease.

A therapeutic alternative to exenteration for large, locally advanced vulvar carcinoma involving the rectum, anus, or vagina is the use of preoperative irradiation followed by radical surgery. Patients with stage III and stage IV vulvar carcinoma involving the rectum/anus, urethra, or vagina can be treated with 40 Gy to the vulva and 45 Gy to the inguinal and pelvic nodes, followed by a radical vulvectomy and inguinal lymphadenectomy. The overall 5-year cumulative survival rate is nearly 50%.

Carcinoma of the vulva involving perianal tissue can be resected in most cases with adequate preservation of external anal sphincter function. If the sphincter is damaged during the operation, there is a significant risk for subsequent fecal incontinence.

Exenterative procedures may be necessary for advanced vulvar lesions. Pubic bone resection can add little to surgical morbidity and gives good functional results. Pubic bone resection, in combination with radical extirpative procedures, is an option for treatment of patients with locally extensive vulvovaginal carcinomas, particularly those with previous radiation therapy.

Age alone should not be a deterrent to surgical management of gynecologic malignant disease. Morbidity or mortality cannot be predicted from age, past history, American Society of Anesthesiologists class, preoperative laboratory studies, or type of operation. With careful perioperative management and attention to the unique problems of the elderly, acceptable surgical outcomes can be achieved.

The curative potential of therapy should not be sacrificed. However, an effort must be made to determine methods that will reduce morbidity while at least retaining curative potential. Modifications that potentially may reduce the morbidity of regional nodal management include deletion of the inguinal lymphadenectomy or use of superficial inguinal lymphadenectomy in selected early lesions, the use of separate groin incisions, the selected use of unilateral inguinal lymphadenectomy, and the use of primary radiation therapy to the inguinal or pelvic nodal areas. Modifications that potentially may reduce the morbidity of the primary tumor management include wide local excision for superficial lesions, modified radical vulvectomy for regionalized lesions, the use of skin flaps in selected cases, the development of more sophisticated plastic surgical procedures for the management of posterior lesions, and the use of combined treatment modalities in the management of locally advanced disease. The outcome following triple incisions is essentially equal to that of a single incision in early-stage disease, and major morbidity is reduced.

Accounting for specimen preparation and fixation, a tumor-free surgical margin of greater than 8 mm on the vulva results in a high rate of local control, whereas a margin less than 8 mm can be associated with a 50% chance of recurrence. Depth of invasion or increasing tumor thickness is associated with local recurrence. A pushing border pattern is less likely to recur than an infiltrative growth pattern. Positive lymph–vascular space invasion is predictive of recurrence. Neither clinical tumor size nor coexisting benign vulvar pathology correlates with local recurrence.

VERRUCOUS CARCINOMA

Squamous cell carcinoma is far more common than verrucous carcinoma of the vulva. The clinical and morphologic distinctions between these neoplasms are important to understand because of their contrasting biologic behavior and treatment.

Both cancers present with symptoms of pruritus and a noticeable mass. On examination, both tumors commonly occur on the labia and are exophytic. If infection occurs in association with verrucous carcinoma, the resulting induration of the surrounding tissue, as well as reactive regional lymph node enlargement, may lead to an erroneous diagnosis of advanced squamous cell carcinoma. One third of squamous cell carcinomas are flat and ulcerated; the gross distinction from verrucous carcinoma is easy to perceive.

The microscopic analysis of squamous cell carcinomas should specify the neoplastic thickness, depth of stromal invasion, and presence or absence of lymphovascular invasion, since these parameters are important in predicting the probability of lymph node metastases in superficially invasive cancers. Verrucous carcinomas are thick neoplasms that may invade and compress the underlying stroma with "pushing" margins. It is therefore crucial to recognize the microscopic features of this well-differentiated squamous cell neoplasm in order not to mistake it for a squamous cell carcinoma, which has the capacity to metastasize to inguinal lymph nodes. Human papillomavirus has been implicated in the development of both of these tumors.

The treatment of verrucous carcinoma is wide local excision. Because recurrence may occur if the surgical resection margins are involved by the neoplasm, the pathologist must carefully evaluate these margins. Recurrence of verrucous carcinoma connotes a poor prognosis.

MELANOMA

Melanomas make up approximately 10% of all vulvar malignancies; approximately 8% of all melanomas occur on the vulva. Lesions occur most commonly after puberty, with a peak incidence after age 55. They are rare in African–American women and most frequently involve the labia minora and clitoris. The disproportionate number of melanomas that occur on the vulva, a unique skin organ, has led to emphasis on careful inspection and prophylactic excision of all darkly pigmented lesions of the vulva. Recent growth, a change in appearance, pruritus, or bleeding in a preexisting mole are all ominous clinical signs.

Considerable debate centers on the optimal treatment for vulvar melanoma, as well as those clinicopathologic factors influencing prognosis. Primary tumors can be assessed according to Chung and Breslow microstaging systems. Ten-year survival rates by Chung levels are as follows: stage I, 100%; stage II, 81%; stage III, 87%; stage IV, 11%; stage V, 33%. Tumor thickness, inguinal node metastasis, and older age at diagnosis are independent prognostic factors. Radical vulvectomy does not seem to improve survival over less radical procedures. Radical local excision for patients with malignant melanoma of the vulva is recommended. Whether patients who have more than a superficially invasive melanoma should also have inguinal lymph node dissection is controversial.

Some investigators have observed that ulceration, tumor thickness, and positive inguinal lymph nodes are the most important prognostic factors. A low-risk and a high-risk group of patients have been identified for recurrence. The low-risk patient has a nonulcerative tumor, less than 3 mm thick, without clinical evidence of inguinal lymph node metastases, and can be treated by local excision with a 2–3-cm margin. The high-risk patient has a tumor that is ulcerative or more than 3-mm thick and should also be treated by local excision without elective inguinal node dissection. If clinical suspicion of inguinal lymph node metastases exists, an inguinal node dissection is advocated for better local control of the disease.

Clear-cell hidradenocarcinoma is a malignant tumor of sweat gland origin most often found on the trunk, head, and extremities. Rarely this tumor can occur on the vulva with metastatic disease, which reflects the potentially aggressive nature of this tumor.

There is a possible origin of adenocarcinoma from mammary ectopic tissue in the vulva or from vulvar skin adnexa. The tumor can spread diffusely into the surrounding soft tissues of the vulva, as well as to the inguinal lymph nodes. Histologically, it is composed of nests, cords, and tubular formations recalling an aggressive duct carcinoma of breast. Likewise, tumor cells can exhibit positivity for common breast tumor markers, such as epithelial membrane antigen, carcinoembryonic antigen, and glandular keratins.

Bartholin gland cancer is a rare malignancy that must be considered in the differential diagnosis of a labial mass. The tentative diagnosis of adenocarcinoma of the Bartholin gland is based on the cytologic findings and location of the tumor. The nuclei are oval to oblong, and some cells have a peripherally displaced nucleus. The chromatinic material is slightly increased, and some nuclei have prominent nucleoli. The cytoplasm is basophilic and abundant. Microcalcifications and psammoma bodies are numerous. The prognosis is generally poor because of the aggressive metastatic tendencies of this cancer. The etiology of Bartholin gland cancer remains unknown, and no optimal plan of treatment has been established. Early detection followed by radical vulvectomy and bilateral inguinal–femoral node dissection may improve survival.

SARCOMA

Soft tissue sarcomas make up less than 2% of vulvar malignancies. They may occur in girls and women over a wide age range, including the pediatric population, and usually appear as a rapidly enlarging and painful mass. Most tumors on the vulva are related to the leiomyosarcoma group, although the fibrous histiocytomas, rhabdomyosarcomas, hemangiosarcomas, and the newly described epithelioid sarcomas may also occur on the vulva. The prognosis for such lesions is variable, depending on the biologic character of the individual sarcoma, but may well be related to hematogenous metastasis. Radical vulvectomy with groin dissection has yielded the lowest incidence of recurrent disease, but many patients die rapidly.

Superficial perineal leiomyosarcomas are rare and may be more aggressive than superficial leiomyosarcomas in general. The tumor is well differentiated and shows immunoreactivity for smooth muscle α-actin and α-desmin.

The natural history of vulvar leiomyosarcomas is characterized by an indolent protracted course and frequent local recurrence, followed by distant fatal metastases. Surgery, chemotherapy, and radiotherapy achieve palliation rather than cure.

The cytologic and histologic findings in extremely rare alveolar rhabdomyosarcoma of the vulva reveal round to oval nuclei, and only a few cells are multinucleated. The chromatinic material is increased in amount and finely granular. Many mitotic figures are observed. The cytoplasm is scanty in general, but some cells have abundant cytoplasm; cross-striations are not recognized. The tumor cells are positive with immunocytochemical stains for desmin, vimentin, and myoglobin.

Dermatofibrosarcoma protuberans of the vulva is an uncommon low-grade sarcoma of dermal origin. Although wide local excision is the treatment of choice, microscopic tumor projections beyond the central tumor nodule explain the tumor's propensity for local recurrence. Frozen sections of margins may be useful to ensure complete resection.

Epithelioid sarcoma typically involves the extremities of young men and may be confused histologically with various benign and malignant processes. Epithelioid sarcoma of the vulva is a soft-tissue malignancy arising from tenosynovial tissue. This can present as a painless lump of the vulva. The suggested mode of treatment can range from a wide local excision to radical vulvectomy with groin node dissection.

BASAL CELL CARCINOMA

Among the rarest of vulvar malignancies, basal cell carcinomas occur once for every 40 invasive squamous cell carcinomas. They are distinguished by cords and masses of palisading basal cells pushing into the underlying connective tissue and, like basal cell carcinomas elsewhere, do not metastasize. A history of long-standing vulvar pruritus and delay in diagnosis are common. The lesions frequently have a slightly elevated margin at their periphery. Basal cell carcinomas are most commonly found over the anterior two thirds of the labia majora and occur most frequently in white women over age 50.

The variability in clinical appearance of vulvar tumors suggests that biopsy confirmation should be obtained on all lesions for which there is the least doubt regarding the diagnosis. In addition to basal cell carcinoma, vulvar benign lesions can include epidermal inclusion cyst, lentigo, Bartholin duct obstruction, carcinoma in situ, melanocytic nevi, acrochordons, mucous cysts, hemangiomas, postinflammatory hyperpigmentation, seborrheic keratoses, varicosities, hidradenomas, verrucae, unusual neurofibromas, ectopic tissue, syringomas, and abscesses.

Basal cell carcinoma of the vulva is rare and was initially thought always to be indolent, locally invasive, and nonmetastasizing; however, there are reports of metastasis to regional lymph nodes. The metastasizing basal cell carcinoma of the vulva neoplasm manifest several features that distinguish it from most of the nonmetastasizing tumors, such as vaginal bleeding at presentation; advanced clinical stage; invasion of subcutaneous fat, urethra, and vagina; tumor thickness greater than 1 cm; and a pattern of growth like that of morphea. Vulvar basal cell carcinoma behaves much like its counterpart in sites other than the vulva, locally recurring but metastasizing only on rare occasion. Simple wide excision of the tumor is curative in most cases. More aggressive surgery may be warranted for large tumors that are locally destructive and extend into the subcutaneous fat.

BIBLIOGRAPHY

Cavanagh D, Fiorica JV, Hoffman MS, Roberts WS, Bryson SC, LaPolla JP, et al. Invasive carcinoma of the vulva: changing trends in surgical management. Am J Obstet Gynecol 1990;163:1007–1015

Heaps JM, Fu YS, Montz FJ, Hacker NF, Berek JS. Surgical-pathologic variables predictive of local recurrence in squamous cell carcinoma of the vulva. Gynecol Oncol 1990;38:309–314

Homesley HD, Bundy BN, Sedlis A, Yordan E, Berek JS, Jahshan A, et al. Assessment of current International Federation of Gynecology and Obstetrics staging of vulvar carcinoma relative to prognostic factors for survival (a Gynecologic Oncology Group study). Am J Obstet Gynecol 1991;164:997–1004

Kelley JL III, Burke TW, Tornos C, Morris M, Gershenson DM, Silva EG, et al. Minimally invasive vulvar carcinoma: an indication for conservative surgical therapy. Gynecol Oncol 1992;44:240–244

Milde-Langosch K, Becker G, Loning T. Human papillomavirus and c-myc/c-erbB2 in uterine and vulvar lesions. Virchows Arch [A] 1991; 419:479–485

Rando RF, Sedlacek TV, Hunt J, Jenson AB, Kurman RJ, Lancaster WD. Verrucous carcinoma of the vulva associated with an unusual type 6 human papillomavirus. Obstet Gynecol 1986;67(3 suppl):70S–75S

Russell AH, Mesic JB, Scudder SA, Rosenberg PJ, Smith LH, Kinney WK, et al. Synchronous radiation and cytotoxic chemotherapy for locally advanced or recurrent squamous cancer of the vulva. Gynecol Oncol 1992;47:14–20

Stehman FB, Bundy BN, Dvoretsky PM, Creasman WT. Early stage I carcinoma of the vulva treated with ipsilateral superficial inguinal lymphadenectomy and modified radical hemivulvectomy: a prospective study of the Gynecologic Oncology Group. Obstet Gynecol 1992;79:490–497

Stehman FB, Bundy BN, Thomas G, Varia M, Okagaki T, Roberts J, et al. Groin dissection versus groin radiation in carcinoma of the vulva: a Gynecologic Oncology Group study. Int J Radiat Oncol Biol Phys 1992;24:389–396

Trimble EL, Lewis JL Jr, Williams LL, Curtin JP, Chapman D, Woodruff JM, et al. Management of vulvar melanoma. Gynecol Oncol 1992;45:254–258

Cancer of the Vagina

Primary carcinoma of the vagina is a malignant lesion that arises in the vagina and does not involve the cervix or vulva. It is a rare malignancy that comprises only 1–2% of female genital tract cancers. Most primary vaginal cancers (about 80%) are squamous cell, and the mean age of patients with these lesions is between 60 and 65 years. Adenocarcinomas and other nonsquamous lesions are much rarer primary lesions; and the rare clear cell adenocarcinoma, epidemiologically related to diethylstilbestrol (DES) exposure in utero, is declining in incidence. Similarly, the incidence of squamous cell carcinomas has decreased over the past few decades, perhaps because of an increase in earlier diagnosis with cytologic screening and the more rigid criteria imposed for the diagnosis of primary vaginal malignancies.

Epidemiologically, factors noted in the past to be associated with the occurrence of preinvasive and invasive squamous cell lesions include chronic vaginal irritation, previous invasive cervical cancer, previous pelvic irradiation, long-term pessary use, long-term prolapse, excessive douching, low socioeconomic status, promiscuity, previous abnormal Pap test, hysterectomy for cervical intraepithelial neoplasia (CIN), hysterectomy for benign disease, chemotherapy, immunosuppressive treatment, and history of condyloma acuminatum. In most published series, no single predisposing factor or combination of factors could be identified. Sexually transmitted diseases, such as HPV infection, are probably not the etiologic agent for all vaginal squamous cancers.

VAGINAL INTRAEPITHELIAL NEOPLASIA

Vaginal intraepithelial neoplasia accounts for fewer than 1% of lower genital tract intraepithelial neoplasias, and generally women with vaginal intraepithelial neoplasia tend to be one to two decades younger than those with invasive squamous cell cancers. Vaginal intraepithelial neoplasia is more likely to be associated with previous irradiation, previous treatment of CIN, a history of HPV infection, and immunosuppression.

Diagnosis

Patients with vaginal intraepithelial neoplasia are usually asymptomatic, and the diagnosis is frequently made after investigation of an abnormal Pap test. The process most commonly appears in the upper one third of the vagina and frequently is multifocal. The diagnosis is usually established by colposcopically directed biopsies. During colposcopy, particular attention must be directed to pockets often present laterally in the vault after hysterectomy. Since the speculum may hide lesions, the blades should be withdrawn slowly and partially open to allow visualization of the entire length of the vaginal walls.

As in evaluating patients for CIN, application of 4–5% acetic acid will cause affected areas to appear white and well demarcated, allowing for target biopsies. The lesions may appear flat, slightly raised, or warty. Mosaic and punctation patterns may occur, but keratinization can obscure any vascular pattern. Staining of the mucosa with Lugol solution may be helpful in determining lesion location. If lesions are not readily identifiable in postmenopausal patients, a 2–4-week course of topical estrogen may help mature vaginal mucosa and allow for easier detection on reexamination.

Some patients will require local anesthesia for biopsies. A mixture of 1% lidocaine and vasopressin can be injected with a small-caliber spinal needle. Small-jawed punch biopsy forceps will obtain adequate specimens. The biopsy procedure is often facilitated by grasping adjacent to the lesion with a skin hook and pulling the tissue toward the surgeon, particularly with laterally apical vault lesions.

Treatment

Vaginal intraepithelial neoplasia is usually managed by laser vaporization or surgical excision. If the laser is used, multiple areas must be sampled by biopsy to rule out invasive carcinoma. Vaporization is carried to a depth of only 2 mm and is often facilitated by the injection of dilute vasopressin solution to the affected area. One advantage of the laser is excellent healing, without vaginal narrowing or shortening. Partial vaginectomy, particularly of the upper vagina, can be done with minimal adverse effects. Total vaginectomy for multifocal disease with split-thickness skin graft vaginoplasty is sometimes followed by scarring and stenosis. Vaginal intraepithelial neoplasia has been reported to recur in the graft, and irradiation should be considered as an alternative method, delivering 6,500–8,000 cGy by an intracavitary application.

Local application of topical 5-fluorouracil cream is efficacious in immunosuppressed patients for HPV-associated vaginal intraepithelial neoplasia and also in previously irradiated patients. To avoid severe vulvar irritation, the cream should be inserted at night with placement of a tampon and additional protection of the vulva with petrolatum jelly.

INVASIVE SQUAMOUS CELL CANCER

Primary invasive squamous carcinoma occurs in early stages I and II in only 25% of patients. In a recent collected series of 2,193 affected patients, only 10% were younger than age 40 years.

Diagnosis

Although some patients with invasive lesions are asymptomatic, and abnormal cytology leads to diagnosis, most (50–57%) present with abnormal bleeding or vaginal discharge. Less frequent presenting complaints include dysuria, urgency, constipation, and pain, all usually seen with more advanced disease. About 51% of vaginal cancers occur in the upper one third of the vagina, and about 58% occur in the posterior wall. A pelvic examination may reveal exophytic or ulcerated lesions. Most gynecologists use the FIGO clinical staging, based largely on pelvic examination (see box). Some suggest that staging pelvic examinations should be done under general anesthesia with multiple biopsies of the cervix (if present) to rule out a primary cervical lesion.

Following biopsy for histologic verification, cystoscopy and proctosigmoidoscopy are indicated in most patients because of the proximity of the vagina to adjacent organs. Chest X-ray and intravenous pyelography or computed tomography scan with contrast are standard radiographic tests, and air-contrast barium enema may be indicated for large posterior masses. Assessment of regional and distant nodes can be accomplished with a lymphangiogram or computed tomography of the pelvis and abdomen. Magnetic resonance imaging is thought to be a superior modality by some, particularly in differentiating between fibrotic tissue and tumor infiltration.

Lymphatics in the upper portion of the vagina probably drain primarily to the lymphatics of the cervix. Those in the lower portion of the vagina can follow cervical lymphatic pathways or drainage patterns of the vulva into femoral or inguinal nodes. However, the lymphatic drainage of the vagina is complex and consists of an extensive intercommunicating network.

Treatment

Radiation therapy is the preferred treatment for most vaginal carcinomas. Two groups of patients with occult or less than 1 cm stage I superficial lesions could be considered for radical surgery. Select patients with a lesion in the upper one third of the vagina and an intact cervix can be managed with a radical hysterectomy and vaginectomy, along with a bilateral pelvic node dissection. Early cancers in the lower one third of the vagina can be managed by modified radical vulvectomy, vaginectomy, and bilateral groin lymph node dissection. Patients with metastatic nodes should receive external-beam irradiation through appropriately designed ports. Patients with midvaginal cancers are probably best treated by irradiation. Women with superficial cancers who are not candidates for surgery can be treated with a combination of interstitial implants and a vaginal cylinder delivering 6,000–7,000 cGy to the vaginal mucosa, plus an additional 2,000–3,000-cGy mucosal dose to the tumor area. Use of external-beam irradiation in stage I disease is often reserved for thick, infiltrating, poorly differentiated lesions.

All other localized, advanced squamous cell vaginal cancers should be treated with individualized radiation therapy techniques. In general, 4,000 cGy to the whole pelvis, with a 5,000–6,000-cGy total parametrial dose, with midline shielding is used, along with a combination of interstitial and intracavitary insertions to deliver a total dose of 7,500–8,000 cGy to the vaginal lesion and 6,500 cGy to the parametrial and paravaginal extensions. To improve therapeutic results, a combination of irradiation and surgery has been suggested, but combined therapy may result in more complications. Exenterations are usually reserved for local, central recurrences. The use of radiation sensitizers such as hydroxyurea or 5-fluorouracil plus cisplatin has not been thoroughly evaluated in vaginal cancers but may play a future role in this disease management.

Survival for patients with stage I cancers has been reported in a range of 70–80%, whereas survival for patients with stage II is generally around 50%. About one third of stage III patients will be 5-year survivors, and survival for patients with stage IVA lesions is less than 20%. No single chemotherapeutic agent has been noted to yield significant response rates in recurrent squamous cell vaginal cancers.

DIETHYLSTILBESTROL AND ADENOCARCINOMA OF THE VAGINA

Primary adenocarcinoma of the vagina is rare, usually occurring in postmenopausal women, and it may arise from residual glands of müllerian origin. When a lesion is identified as an adenocarcinoma, a metastatic origin (from endometrium, ovary, cervix, breast, or other intraabdominal organs) must always be ruled out.

A controversial increase in the prevalence of vaginal clear cell adenocarcinoma in young women was first reported in 1971 and was possibly related to DES exposure in utero. Subsequently, a registry was established to ascertain clinical and pathologic data about patients with these unusual cancers. Millions of women were treated with DES during pregnancy, beginning in the late 1940s. Of these, 519 patients with vaginal or cervical clear cell carcinoma were registered by 1985. The risk that a DES-exposed woman will develop a clear cell lower genital tract cancer is about 0.5–2/1,000.

The registry has noted a median age of 19 for those developing clear cell carcinoma. The youngest to develop this cancer was age 7 years at the time of diagnosis. The oldest, thus far, is age 42 years. A second peak of occurrence is a concern to some. About 65% have had a documented history of DES exposure in utero. No history of exposure was noted in about

---

Modified FIGO Staging of Vaginal Carcinoma

Stage	Description
I	Carcinoma limited to vaginal mucosa (wall)
II	Submucosal infiltration into parametrium, not extending to the pelvic wall
(IIA)	Subvaginal infiltration, not to parametrium
(IIB)	Parametrial infiltration, not extending to pelvic sidewall
III	Carcinoma has extended to the pelvic wall
IV	Carcinoma has extended beyond true pelvis or involves mucosa of bladder or rectum
(IVA)	Carcinoma has spread to adjacent organs
(IVB)	Carcinoma has spread to distant organs

Modified from International Federation of Gynecology and Obstetrics. Annual report on the results of treatment in gynecological cancer. Vol 20. Stockholm: FIGO, 1988

25%. The DES-associated clear cell cancers have a predilection for the exocervix and the upper one third of the vagina, and about one third involve the cervix only.

Once an initial evaluation has been done, clear cell carcinomas are rarely detected (fewer than 10 cases) in women under surveillance. Palpation of the vagina and cervix is extremely important. Most of the lesions picked up in women under surveillance were vaginal nodules, and many clear cell cancers noted on initial examinations presented as submucosal nodules. Diethylstilbestrol-exposed adolescents who are overweight and tall may be at a relatively higher risk of developing this carcinoma.

For patients with cervical and upper vaginal cancers, a surgical approach with radical hysterectomy, upper vaginectomy, and bilateral pelvic lymphadenectomy with ovarian preservation is recommended. With small early lesions, wide local excision with or without localized interstitial irradiation has been used with preservation of reproductive potential. Since very small lesions can metastasize to regional nodes, some surgeons recommend removal of the pelvic nodes with more conservative treatments. For advanced stages, irradiation is recommended.

The 5-year survival rate for stage I clear cell cancers approaches 90%. Recommended follow-up is similar to that for patients with other cervical or vaginal cancers. However, these patients may be at risk for late recurrences 8–20 years after primary therapy. Careful attention should be given to the lungs and supraclavicular nodes, because as many as one third of recurrences will present in these areas.

BENIGN DIETHYLSTILBESTROL-RELATED ANOMALIES

Adenosis and vaginal epithelial changes are present in about 30–50% of women with intrauterine DES exposure during the first 18 weeks of gestation. Most of the abnormalities reported are associated with a large transformation zone, often extending to the vagina. The vaginal epithelial changes include cockscomb, cervical collars, hypoplastic cervices, pseudopolyps, or transverse or vertical vaginal septa. Serial examinations of DES-exposed women show that the vast majority of large transformation zones are covered with squamous metaplasia as these young women age. Furthermore, vaginal epithelial changes become less prominent and show substantial decrease with time.

The immature squamous metaplasia preceding mature squamous metaplasia in these patients often leads to erroneous colposcopic impression of neoplasia, and colposcopic evaluation of DES-exposed progeny requires special expertise. Several series have noted a very small incidence (less than 10%) of intraepithelial neoplasias in biopsy specimens, and an experienced pathologist is needed to evaluate the tissue. Aggressive treatment must be avoided. These women with large transformation zones do not appear to be at increased risk for squamous cell neoplasia. Examination with iodine staining with colposcopy and cytology should be done every 6 months. In exposed women without colposcopic changes or vaginal epithelial changes, annual examinations are sufficient. Because of the later appearance of clear cell cancers in the form of nodularity, careful palpation of the entire vagina is mandatory. The use of OCs does not place exposed patients at increased risk for developing genital tract neoplasms.

Because of vaginal epithelial changes and anatomic abnormalities of the uterus and tubes that occur in some of these exposed progeny, patients may be at risk for early pregnancy loss, ectopic pregnancy, and preterm delivery. Liberal use of ultrasonography and frequent pelvic examinations to exclude cervical incompetence should be done when these patients conceive.

Exposure to DES may place women at a small, but statistically significant, risk for developing breast cancer. The possibility of an increased risk of cancer of the uterine corpus has been raised. Exposed women should be followed for life with appropriate and cost-effective screening.

SARCOMA

The most common vaginal sarcoma occurs in children or young adolescents with a mean age of about 3. Eighty-five percent of those embryonal rhabdomyosarcomas (sarcoma botryoides) are found in children younger than age 5 years. These patients present with rapidly growing, grapelike tumors that may prolapse through the introitus. Bleeding or discharge may herald earlier lesions.

Historically, these aggressive lesions were treated with exenteration, an approach that was rarely effective, except in patients with small tumors, and an approach associated with a high complication rate. Removal of gross tumor, followed by combination chemotherapy with or without radiation therapy, has improved local control and survival and has preserved body image.

Leiomyosarcomas and mixed müllerian tumors are the most common sarcomas in adults. Most present as firm, submucosal masses. Mitotic index (more than five mitotic figures per 10 high-power fields) and nuclear atypia are associated with a malignant course. Since treatment failures initially occur in the pelvis, wide local excision with removal of closely adjacent organs is the initial treatment of choice. Local adjuvant irradiation may benefit a few patients, but the role of adjuvant chemotherapy remains to be determined.

MELANOMA

More than 100 cases of primary vaginal melanoma have been reported. Because of the rich vascular supply of the vagina, a thorough search for a primary lesion from another body organ is mandatory. Since primary melanomas of the vagina may be associated with junctional nevi or melanosis, dark lesions in the vagina should be excised prophylactically.

Local, regional control may be difficult to achieve with wide local excision alone, as adjacent organs lie in close proximity to the vaginal tube. Depending on the location, anterior or posterior exenteration might benefit a select group of patients and should be accomplished by removal of lymphatics draining the anatomic location. Irradiation may help in local control for women who are not candidates for surgery. Chemotherapy is of little value in this poor-prognosis malignancy.

BIBLIOGRAPHY

Colton T, Greenburg ER, Noller K, Resseguie L, Van Bennekom C, Heeren T, et al. Breast cancer in mothers prescribed diethylstilbestrol in pregnancy. JAMA 1993;269:2096–2100

Gallup DG, Talledo OE, Shah KJ, Hayes C. Invasive squamous cell carcinoma of the vagina: 14-year study. Obstet Gynecol 1987;69:782–785

Hoffman MS, DeCesare SL, Roberts WS, Fiorica JV, Finan MA, Cavanagh D. Upper vaginectomy for in situ and occult, superficially invasive carcinoma of the vagina. Am J Obstet Gynecol 1992;166:30–33

Holt LH, Herbst AL. DES-related female genital changes. Semin Oncol 1982;9:341–348

Kucera H, Vavra N. Radiation management of primary carcinoma of the vagina: clinical and histopathological variables associated with survival. Gynecol Oncol 1991;40:12–16

McFarlane MJ, Feinstein AR, Horwitz RI. Diethylstilbestrol and clear cell vaginal carcinoma: reappraisal of the epidemiologic evidence. Am J Med 1986;81:855–863

Perez CA, Camel HM, Galakatos AE, Grigsby PW, Kuske RR, Buchsbaum G, et al. Definitive irradiation in carcinoma of the vagina: long-term evaluation of results. Int J Radiat Oncol Biol Phys 1988;15:1283–1290

Sharp GB, Cole P. Identification of risk factors for diethylstilbestrol-associated clear cell adenocarcinoma of the vagina: similarities to endometrial cancer. Am J Epidemiol 1991;134:1316–1324

Stock RG, Mychalczak B, Armstrong JG, Curtain JP, Harrison LB. The importance of brachytherapy in the management of primary carcinoma of the vagina. Int J Radiat Oncol Biol Phys 1992;24:747–753

Sulak P, Barnhill D, Heller P, Weiser E, Hoskins W, Park R, et al. Nonsquamous cancer of the vagina. Gynecol Oncol 1988;29:309–320

Cervical Neoplasia

Invasive cervical cancer accounts for 18% of all genital cancers in women in the United States. According to American Cancer Society statistics, 13,500 new cases of invasive cervical cancer were expected to be diagnosed in the United States in 1992, and 4,400 of these women were estimated to die of their disease. From a practical point of view, this cancer appears to be nearly 100% preventable in an invasive mode when women at risk are screened with a Pap test.

A review of incidence rates for cervical cancer over the past 45 years reveals that there has been a decrease from 45/100,000 to 15/100,000 women. Along with the drop in the incidence of invasive cervical cancer, there has been a marked and exaggerated rise in the incidence of preinvasive disease.

A number of risk factors predispose women to cervical cancer. These factors include women who begin coitus early in their teenage years, have multiple sexual partners, smoke, or are infected with HPV or human immunodeficiency virus (HIV). Women without cervical neoplasia but with any one of these risk factors should be advised to have annual Pap tests. Unfortunately, women at risk typically are in lower socioeconomic groups and are less inclined to undergo recommended annual screening.

Risk of cervical cancer is increased 3.5 times among smokers, compared with nonsmokers, even when the data are adjusted for the other variables listed above. Even passive smoking increases the risk of cervical neoplasia approximately threefold if women are exposed to cigarette smoke for 3 hours daily.

SCREENING

Pap test screening of sexually active women has been based on the concept that cervical cancer is the end point of a continuum that begins with CIN grades 1, 2, and 3 and progresses to microinvasive cancer and then to invasive cancer and that both preinvasive and invasive lesions can be detected by cytologic screening.

The reliability of exfoliative cytologic analysis depends on the skill and experience of the person taking the sample, the area that is being sampled, the collection technique, and the quality control system in the laboratory. Optimally, cervical smears should be obtained from the squamocolumnar junction or the transformation zone, where the neoplastic process is known to arise. Clinical studies have shown that use of the endocervical brush increases the number of cervical smears containing endocervical cells in both premenopausal and postmenopausal women.

All women who are or who have been sexually active or who have reached age 18 should have an annual cervical Pap test and pelvic examination. After a woman has had three or more consecutive, satisfactory, normal cervical Pap tests, the cervical Pap test may be performed less frequently, for example, every 2–3 years, depending on risk factors and the discretion of the physician and the patient.

ETIOLOGY

Highly sensitive molecular techniques can detect HPV DNA in more than 90% of preinvasive and invasive cervical cancers, including both squamous carcinomas and adenocarcinomas. Human papillomavirus types 16 and 18 are found in 70% of invasive squamous cell cancers and can also be detected in many patients with low-grade squamous cell intraepithelial lesions. Because HPV can also be detected in 25–30% of women having normal cytologic test results, current forms of HPV testing lack the needed specificity to become useful screening tests for cervical neoplasia.

Human papillomavirus type 18 may be preferentially associated with adenocarcinomas or a subset of rapidly progressing cervical cancers that respond poorly to treatment. The etiology of cervical neoplasia is most likely not a single carcinogen but multiple carcinogens acting as cofactors, with HPV being just one.

DIAGNOSIS

Patients with a gross cervical lesion should undergo simple cervical biopsy of the tumor. Cold knife conization is not indicated in patients with visible or palpable lesions presumed to be cancer. Patients with an abnormal Pap test without a gross lesion need colposcopic examination. Patients with colposcopically identified abnormal epithelium should undergo biopsy and endocervical curettage. Treatment of preinvasive or invasive cervical neoplasia is based on tissue biopsy findings.

Sometimes cold knife cervical conization or loop electrosurgical excision is needed to lead to an accurate diagnosis. The following situations are the most common examples:

- Colposcopically directed biopsy that does not adequately explain abnormal cells found on a Pap test
- Atypical epithelium extending into the endocervical canal
- Abnormal cytologic findings with no visible lesion colposcopically
- Microinvasive carcinoma found on directed biopsy
- Endocervical curettings that show intraepithelial neoplasia

A second cervical Pap test within a 1–4-week interval in a patient with untreated CIN does not always identify cytologic abnormality. Cytologic tests 1–4 weeks after an abnormal test are less accurate and cannot be relied upon. For that reason, patients whose cytology predicts CIN should undergo prompt colposcopic evaluation.

Treatment of CIN with loop electrosurgical excision, carbon dioxide laser, cryosurgery, or electrocautery is safe under the following conditions: 1) invasive cancer is excluded; 2) conization is not indicated; and 3) the cytologic, colposcopic, and histologic evaluations correlate. Performed skillfully, these methods that remove or destroy an abnormal transformation zone allow success rates similar to those obtained by cold knife conization or hysterectomy.

The following guidelines must be followed before performing local destructive methods such as loop electrosurgical excision, carbon dioxide laser operation, cryosurgical procedure, or electrocautery: 1) the abnormal epithelium must be entirely visualized; 2) the endocervix must be free of any abnormal epithelium; and 3) the cytologic, colposcopic, and histologic findings must correlate. When discrepancies among cytologic, colposcopic, and histologic findings occur, further diagnostic studies such as repeat directed biopsy or conization must be performed.

Follow-up examinations after local treatment of CIN are imperative and include cervical Pap tests and, when indicated, colposcopy. Hysterectomy for the treatment of CIN is performed infrequently. In most instances there are other gynecologic indications suggesting the need for hysterectomy in patients who concomitantly have CIN.

STAGING

Clinical staging allows comparison of treatment results between treatment centers. Clinical staging for cervical cancer is based primarily on inspection and palpation of the cervix, vagina, parametrium, and pelvic sidewalls, as well as physical examination of extrapelvic areas such as the supraclavicular nodal region or the upper abdominal region. The extent of disease can be further evaluated by chest roentgenography, excretory urography, or, if appropriate, cystoscopy and flexible sigmoidoscopy.

Cystoscopy is indicated in patients with hematuria or advanced cervical cancer with involvement of the anterior vaginal wall and in those suspected to have cervical cancer extending to the bladder.

Flexible sigmoidoscopy is indicated for patients with cervical cancer that infiltrates the rectum, as determined by rectal examination, and for patients who have rectal symptoms such as bleeding, pressure, tenesmus, or excessive mucus in their stools.

Lymphangiography, computed tomography, and magnetic resonance imaging may be useful to determine the extent of disease and to assist in treatment planning but are not considered by FIGO as tools for clinical staging (see box).

TREATMENT

Gynecologic, radiation, and medical oncologists should collaborate in planning combined-modality therapy for all but the most straightforward patients with early-stage, low-volume disease. Patients with unexpected invasive cervical cancer found at total hysterectomy for benign indications can undergo postoperative irradiation or, based on more recent evidence, radical reoperation where low morbidity and excellent cure rates have been shown.

Intraoperative radiation therapy is a new treatment modality that has been used in combination with maximum surgical debulking with or without external-beam therapy in

FIGO Staging for Carcinoma of the Cervix Uteri

Stage	Description
Stage 0	Carcinoma in situ, intraepithelial carcinoma
Stage I	The carcinoma is strictly confined to the cervix (extension to the corpus should be disregarded)
Stage IA	Preclinical carcinomas of the cervix, that is, those diagnosed only by microscopy
Stage IA1	Minimal microscopically evident stromal invasion
Stage IA2	Lesions detected microscopically that can be measured. The upper limit of the measurement should not show a depth of invasion of more than 5 mm taken from the base of the epithelium, either surface or glandular, from which it originates, and a second dimension, the horizontal spread, must not exceed 7 mm. Larger lesions should be classified as stage IB
Stage IB	Lesions of greater dimensions than stage IA2, whether seen clinically or not. Preformed space involvement should not alter the staging but should be specifically recorded so as to determine whether it should affect treatment decisions in the future
Stage II	The carcinoma extends beyond the cervix but has not extended to the pelvic wall. The carcinoma involves the vagina but not as far as the lower third
Stage IIA	No obvious parametrial involvement
Stage IIB	Obvious parametrial involvement
Stage III	The carcinoma has extended to the pelvic wall. On rectal examination, there is no cancer-free space between the tumor and the pelvic wall. The tumor involves the lower third of the vagina. All cases with a hydronephrosis or nonfunctioning kidney are included unless they are known to be due to other causes.
Stage IIIA	No extension to the pelvic wall
Stage IIIB	Extension to the pelvic wall and/or hydronephrosis or nonfunctioning kidney
Stage IV	The carcinoma has extended beyond the true pelvis or has clinically involved the mucosa of the bladder or rectum. A bullous edema as such does not permit a case to be allotted to stage IV
Stage IVA	Spread of the growth to adjacent organs
Stage IVB	Spread to distant organs

Notes about the staging:
Stage IA carcinoma should include minimal microscopically evident stromal invasion as well as small cancerous tumors of measurable size. Stage IA should be divided into those lesions with minute foci of invasion visible only microscopically as stage IA1 and macroscopically measurable microcarcinomas as stage IA2, in order to gain further knowledge of the clinical behavior of these lesions. The term "IB occult" should be omitted.

The diagnosis of both stage IA1 and IA2 cases should be based on microscopic examination of removed tissue, preferably a cone, which must include the entire lesion. The lower limit of stage IA2 should be measurable macroscopically (even if dots need to be placed on the slide prior to measurement), and the upper limit of stage IA2 is given by measurement of the two largest dimensions in any given section. The depth of invasion should not be more than 5 mm taken from the base of the epithelium, either surface or glandular, from which it originates. The second dimension, the horizontal spread, must not exceed 7 mm. Vascular space involvement, either venous or lymphatic, should not alter the staging but should be specifically recorded, as it may affect treatment decisions in the future.

Lesions of greater size should be classified as stage IB.

As a rule, it is impossible to estimate clinically whether a cancer of the cervix has extended to the corpus or not. Extension to the corpus should therefore be disregarded.

A patient with a growth fixed to the pelvic wall by a short and indurated but not nodular parametrium should be allotted to stage IIB. It is impossible, at clinical examination, to decide whether a smooth and indurated parametrium is truly cancerous or only inflammatory. Therefore, the case should be placed in stage III only if the parametrium is nodular on the pelvic wall or if the growth itself extends to the pelvic wall.

The presence of hydronephrosis or nonfunctioning kidney due to stenosis of the ureter by cancer permits a case to be allotted to stage III even if, according to the other findings, the case should be allotted to stage I or stage II.

The presence of bullous edema, as such, should not permit a case to be allotted to stage IV. Ridges and furrows in the bladder wall should be interpreted as signs of submucous involvement of the bladder if they remain fixed to the growth during palpation (ie, examination from the vagina or the rectum during cystoscopy). A finding of malignant cells in cytologic washings from the urinary bladder requires further examination and a biopsy from the wall of the bladder.

International Federation of Gynecology and Obstetrics. Annual report on the results of treatment in gynecological cancer. Vol 20. Stockholm: FIGO, 1988

---

patients with periaortic or pelvic sidewall recurrences. It appears to improve long-term local control and survival. The high incidence of distant metastasis warrants the continued search for effective systemic chemotherapy.

Microinvasive Cancer

The Society of Gynecologic Oncologists has defined microinvasive carcinoma of the cervix as a lesion with an invasion depth of less than 3 mm beneath the basement membrane, with no invasion of blood or lymphatic channels, and without areas of confluence. Conservative hysterectomy is appropriate for patients who meet the definition of microinvasive cervical carcinoma.

Physicians caring for patients with carcinoma of the cervix should be aware that there is a low risk of pelvic nodal metastasis when the tumor invasion exceeds a depth of 3 mm but is less than 5 mm; therefore, pelvic lymphadenectomy should be included with hysterectomy when definitive surgical management is considered. Invasive cancer confined to the cervix that exceeds an invasion depth of 5 mm has a significant incidence of pelvic lymph node metastasis, and bilateral pelvic lymphadenectomy should also be done.

Stages IB and IIA

Early-stage invasive cancer of the cervix may be treated by either radical hysterectomy or radiation therapy. In the United States, the option between these two treatment modalities is determined individually by patients having stage IB or stage IIA disease after consultation with their physicians. Survival rates for patients with early-stage cervical cancer treated with surgery or with radiation therapy are comparable. Radiation therapy is very appropriate in the treatment of later stages of invasive cervical cancer, because increased knowledge of radiation techniques has resulted in the steady improvement of survival and control rates in patients with more advanced disease. On the other hand, improved techniques in radical surgery have established radical hysterectomy with bilateral pelvic lymphadenectomy as the preferred therapy for patients with early-stage disease.

A radical hysterectomy performed on an otherwise healthy young woman whose operative findings and postoperative course are favorable is, in terms of recovery from disease, a rewarding experience. The ovaries continue to function, and the vaginal membrane is unaltered. The patient is free of her cancer and recovers sooner and with fewer long-term side effects than if she were treated with irradiation. Likewise, the patient's history or physical status may influence the decision toward surgery. Patients with a history of ulcerative colitis, regional ileitis, or pelvic inflammatory disease, for example, may experience serious postirradiation complications.

If radical hysterectomy is determined to be the preferred treatment, the procedure must include pelvic lymphadenectomy; thorough exploration of the abdomen, including the periaortic lymph nodes; and removal of the entire uterus along with all the supporting ligaments and the upper portion of the vagina. The ovaries may be preserved if they are disease free.

Factors that adversely affect survival include the presence of metastatic nodal disease, the extent of the lesion, lymphatic or vascular space involvement, and the type of carcinoma. Small cell carcinomas are associated with the poorest outcome; adenocarcinomas frequently form bulky, barrel-shaped lesions that respond poorly to treatment; and the large cell, nonkeratinizing carcinomas are associated with the best outcome. The approximate incidence of aortic nodal metastasis based on stage is as follows: stage IB, 5%; stage IIA, 10%; stage IIB, 20%; and stages III and IV, 30%. A composite projection of reasonable expectations is shown in Table 5-2.

Positive Pelvic Nodes or Bulky Cervical Cancer

The value of postoperative pelvic irradiation in patients who have positive lymph nodes in improving survival is limited. Likewise, with very bulky, advanced cervical lesions, radiation therapy alone is of limited value. New evidence suggests that strategies combining multiagent chemotherapy and surgery in patients with high-risk, bulky cervical cancer result in improved survival rates.

Using this new approach, patients found to be at high risk of recurrence after radical hysterectomy and pelvic lymphadenectomy are likely to receive postoperative adjuvant chemotherapy designed to decrease local or distant recurrences. Likewise, in patients with local or regionally advanced cervical carcinoma, chemotherapy is being given with the aim

TABLE 5-2. PROGNOSIS FOR CERVICAL CANCER

Stage	5-Year Survival NED* (%)	Treatment	10-Year Survival NED* (%)	Treatment
0	99+	Surgery	99+	Surgery
IA (microinvasive)	98	Surgery	98	Surgery
1B	90	Surgery or irradiation	90	Surgery or irradiation
IIA	83	Irradiation	79	Irradiation
IIA	78	Surgery	75	Surgery
IIB	67	Irradiation	57	Irradiation
IIIA	45	Irradiation	40	Irradiation
IIIB	36	Irradiation	30	Irradiation
IVA	14	Irradiation	14	Irradiation

*NED indicates no evidence of disease.

of reducing the tumor bulk and allowing radical surgery in patients previously considered inoperable. Randomized, prospective trials are under way to compare neoadjuvant chemotherapy and surgery with conventional radiotherapy to determine the value of this new approach to the treatment of patients with locally advanced cervical cancer.

Persistent or Recurrent Cervical Cancer

Persistent or recurrent carcinoma of the cervix is a devastating malignant disease with a 1-year survival rate of 15% and a 5-year survival rate of less than 5%. Most recurrences can be considered to be in one of two categories: 1) those that may be treated with some hope of cure or 2) those for which only palliative treatment is available. Potentially curable lesions include isolated central pelvic recurrences, solitary lung metastasis, or perhaps lower vaginal metastases. An isolated central recurrence is the more common, potentially curable type, but few patients are candidates for curative, exenterative surgery because this type of lesion is rarely seen in the era of modern radiotherapy. Although surgical management must be tailored to suit the patient's needs and desires, in almost all cases of purely central recurrence, ultraradical surgery is necessary (ie, pelvic exenteration with removal of the bladder and rectum, in addition to the uterus, vagina, and supporting ligaments). Clinical experience has established pelvic exenteration as the best treatment for patients with advanced cancer that is not suitable for conventional treatment or that has recurred within the pelvis after irradiation.

BIBLIOGRAPHY

Bauer HM, Ting Y, Greer CE, Chambers JC, Tashiro CJ, Chimera J, et al. Genital human papillomavirus infection in female university students as determined by a PCR-based method. JAMA 1991;265: 472–477

Boring CC, Squires TS, Tong T. Cancer statistics, 1992. CA Cancer J Clin 1992;42:19–38

Changes in definitions of clinical staging for carcinoma of the cervix and ovary: International Federation of Gynecology and Obstetrics. Am J Obstet Gynecol 1987;156:263–264

Chapman JA, Mannel RS, DiSaia PJ, Walker JL, Berman ML. Surgical treatment of unexpected invasive cervical cancer found at total hysterectomy. Obstet Gynecol 1992;80:931–934

Garton GR, Gunderson LL, Webb MJ, Wilson TO, Martenson JA Jr, Cha SS, et al. Intraoperative radiation therapy in gynecologic cancer: the Mayo Clinic experience. Gynecol Oncol 1993;48:328–332

Hellberg D, Nilsson S, Haley NJ, Hoffman D, Wynder E. Smoking and cervical intraepithelial neoplasia: nicotine and cotinine in serum and cervical mucus in smokers and nonsmokers. Am J Obstet Gynecol 1988;158:910–913

Jones WB. New approaches to high-risk cervical cancer. Advanced cervical cancer. Cancer 1993;71(4 suppl):1451–1459

Lorincz AT, Temple GF, Kurman RJ, Jenson AB, Lancaster WD. Oncogenic association of specific human papillomavirus types with cervical neoplasia. J Natl Cancer Inst 1987;79:671–677

Maiman M, Fruchter RG, Serur E, Remy JC, Feuer G, Boyce J. Human immunodeficiency virus infection and cervical neoplasia. Gynecol Oncol 1990;38:377–382

Taylor PT Jr, Andersen WA, Barber SR, Covell JL, Smith EB, Underwood PB Jr. The screening Papanicolaou smear: contribution of the endocervical brush. Obstet Gynecol 1987;70:734–738

Winklesten W Jr. Smoking and cervical cancer—current status: a review. Am J Epidemiol 1990;131:945–957

Wright TC Jr, Gagnon S, Richart RM, Ferenczy A. Treatment of cervical intraepithelial neoplasia using the loop electrosurgical excisional procedure. Obstet Gynecol 1992;79:173–178

Cancer of the Uterine Corpus

Endometrial carcinoma is the most common gynecologic malignancy, accounting for approximately 7% of all cancers in women. Most of these tumors are adenocarcinomas arising from the endometrium. However, approximately 5% of corpus cancers are sarcomas, and a still smaller group are mixed tumors composed of both sarcomatous and carcinomatous elements. These are generally referred to as mixed müllerian tumors.

In the United States about 1 in every 45 women will develop endometrial cancer during her lifetime. The average age of women with endometrial cancer is 59, and the vast majority of patients are in the postmenopausal age group.

Although an increase in the incidence of endometrial carcinoma has been observed in the United States and many other countries throughout the world, in the past few years this trend has appeared to level off. This increased incidence has probably been a result of the increasing longevity of the population, increased surveillance with earlier and more accurate diagnoses, and the increased use of estrogen therapy among menopausal women in the past two decades.

In North America the incidence rates for endometrial cancer vary widely among various locations, as well as among different ethnic groups. Among white women in the San Francisco Bay area, there are approximately 40 new cases per 100,000 women, while African–American women in New Orleans have an incidence rate of only 10.5/100,000 and Native Americans in New Mexico have an incidence rate of only 3.4/100,000. White women in Iowa have an intermediate incidence rate of 21/100,000. The reason for these variations is not completely understood but probably relates in great part to the three reasons for the increased incidence rates noted above. Patients from better socioeconomic classes tend to live longer, tend to receive better medical care, and are more likely to be treated with estrogen.

The relationship between estrogens and endometrial carcinoma is now well established, and endometrial carcinoma is seen as a result of both exogenous estrogens administered as medication and endogenous estrogens produced in the ovaries or converted from adrenal androstenedione in peripheral adipose tissue.

The increased risk of endometrial carcinoma among women with estrogen-producing ovarian tumors has been observed for many years. The anovulatory patient whose endometrium is exposed to prolonged estrogen stimulation without the modifying effect of progesterone is also at an increased risk of developing endometrial cancer. Exogenous estrogen therapy given as menopausal estrogen replacement therapy or prescribed for patients with gonadal dysfunction has been shown to result in a threefold to 20-fold increase in the risk of endometrial carcinoma. This risk varies depending on the dose and duration of the hormonal therapy. It is advisable to add a progestin such as medroxyprogesterone acetate or hydroxyprogesterone caproate to the hormonal regimen of women who have a uterus and are receiving estrogen replacement therapy.

In recent years, a number of women have developed endometrial adenocarcinoma while on long-term tamoxifen therapy for breast cancer. The magnitude of this risk is low, but in one study 4 of 641 patients treated with tamoxifen for 1 year developed endometrial cancer. It is prudent to monitor closely such patients.

Several constitutional characteristics are often associated with women who are at high risk for developing endometrial carcinoma. These include obesity, nulliparity or low parity, diabetes, and hypertension. Obese women have a twofold to threefold increased risk of developing endometrial carcinoma, and it appears that this is also related to the effect of estrogens. Androstenedione produced in the adrenal glands is converted to a weak estrogen, estrone, in peripheral adipose tissue. As a result of this peripheral conversion, the endometrium of obese women is exposed to higher levels of estrogen. Although the mechanism is not well understood, the high progesterone levels that occur in women during pregnancy and the use of progestin-dominated combined OCs during the reproductive years appear to exert a protective effect on the endometrium.

DIAGNOSIS

The most common symptom associated with endometrial carcinoma is abnormal uterine bleeding. Since endometrial carcinoma occurs most frequently in postmenopausal patients, the onset of unexpected spotting or bleeding usually causes the women to seek gynecologic consultation. A careful history and physical examination may be useful in suggesting possible reasons for the bleeding. Endometrial biopsy or formal fractional dilation and curettage has been the traditional way to evaluate postmenopausal bleeding, but transvaginal ultrasonography and hysteroscopy now play important roles. If ultrasonography demonstrates a total (both front and back walls) endometrial thickness of less than 5 mm, bleeding may be ascribed to atrophy and no biopsy is needed unless bleeding persists. Most patients with endometrial adenocarcinoma will have an endometrial stripe more than 10 mm thick, and biopsy is certainly indicated in women with a thickened endometrium and those with continued bleeding. Hysteroscopy has been increasingly used in association with office endometrial biopsy or formal dilation and curettage. It may yield additional information concerning the etiology of the uterine bleeding (polyps, submucous myomas) or the extent of the endometrial cancer, but the real therapeutic value and cost-effectiveness of hysteroscopy in the evaluation of postmenopausal bleeding has still to be proven.

In perimenopausal or premenopausal patients, the risk of endometrial cancer is less, and there are many other causes for irregular bleeding. Nevertheless, the prudent clinician will use one of the simple office techniques for obtaining an endometrial tissue sample when the etiology of the bleeding is uncertain or symptoms persist.

PROGNOSTIC CHARACTERISTICS

Several clinical characteristics are important in defining the prognosis of women with endometrial adenocarcinoma. Patient age, tumor cell type, and degree of differentiation are most important. Older patients have worse survival rates. Patients with well-differentiated grade 1 adenocarcinomas have a very favorable prognosis, whereas patients with poorly differentiated grade 3 lesions have a worse prognosis. Tumors associated with squamous cell metaplasia are called adenoacanthomas. The adenocarcinoma portion of these tumors is usually well differentiated, and the prognosis for patients with these tumors is better than average. Conversely, patients with clear cell, serous papillary, and adenosquamous tumors are at high risk for early metastases and have a correspondingly poor prognosis. Measurement of progesterone receptor levels in patients with endometrial cancer may be of some prognostic value, since low levels of receptor are found in patients with a poor prognosis.

Deep myometrial invasion and extrauterine extension of carcinoma, including lymph node metastases, are also associated with a decreased survival rate. Approximately 5–10% of patients with stage I endometrial carcinoma have evidence of malignant cells in washings obtained by peritoneal lavage with normal saline. Similar to patients with gross evidence of metastatic disease, these women also have an increased risk of recurrence and a decreased 5-year survival rate.

STAGING

Many of the aforementioned prognostic characteristics require exploratory laparotomy or hysterectomy for evaluation. For this reason, in 1988 FIGO approved a new surgical/pathologic

> **FIGO Staging for Carcinoma of the Corpus Uteri**
>
> | Stage | Description |
> |---|---|
> | Stage IA G123 | Tumor limited to endometrium |
> | Stage IB G123 | Invasion to less than one-half the myometrium |
> | Stage IC G123 | Invasion to more than one-half the myometrium |
> | Stage IIA G123 | Endocervical glandular involvement only |
> | Stage IIB G123 | Cervical stromal invasion |
> | Stage IIIA G123 | Tumor invades serosa and/or adnexa, and/or positive peritoneal cytology |
> | Stage IIIB G123 | Vaginal metastases |
> | Stage IIIC G123 | Metastases to pelvic and/or paraaortic lymph nodes |
> | Stage IVA G123 | Tumor invasion of bladder and/or bowel mucosa |
> | Stage IVB | Distant metastases including intraabdominal and/or inguinal lymph nodes |
>
> **Histopathology—degree of differentiation:**
> Cases of carcinoma of the corpus should be classified (or graded) according to the degree of histologic differentiation, as follows:
>
> - G1 = 5% or less of a nonsquamous or nonmorular solid growth pattern
> - G2 = 6–50% of a nonsquamous or nonmorular solid growth pattern
> - G3 = more than 50% of a nonsquamous or nonmorular solid growth pattern
>
> **Notes on pathological grading:**
> 1) Notable nuclear atypia, inappropriate for the architectural grade, raises the grade of a grade 1 or grade 2 tumor by 1.
> 2) In serous adenocarcinomas, clear-cell adenocarcinomas, and squamous cell carcinomas, nuclear grading takes precedence.
> 3) Adenocarcinomas with squamous differentiation are graded according to the nuclear grade of the glandular component.
>
> **Rules related to staging:**
> 1) Because corpus cancer is now staged surgically, procedures previously used for determination of stages are no longer applicable, such as the findings from fractional D&C to differentiate between stage I and stage II.
> 2) It is appreciated that there may be a small number of patients with corpus cancer who will be treated primarily with radiation therapy. If that is the case, the clinical staging adopted by FIGO in 1971 would still apply, but designation of that staging system would be noted.
> 3) Ideally, width of the myometrium should be measured along with the width of tumor invasion.
>
> International Federation of Gynecology and Obstetrics. Annual report on the results of treatment in gynecological cancer. Int J Gynecol Obstet 1989;28:189–190

staging system for endometrial adenocarcinoma (see box). All patients with technically operable cancers who are medical candidates for surgery should undergo primary total abdominal hysterectomy, bilateral salpingo-oophorectomy, and appropriate staging procedures. These should include pelvic and abdominal washings for cytologic specimens on entering the abdomen, and pelvic and aortic lymph node biopsy specimens on patients with poorly differentiated or deeply invasive tumors. The indications for and extent of lymph node biopsies are currently controversial. Patients with evidence of extrauterine disease should have careful evaluation and biopsy documentation or resection of suspected metastases. Routine intravenous pyelography, barium enemas, cystoscopy, and proctosigmoidoscopy are not necessary and should be used only when the history or physical findings suggest the possible involvement of the bladder or rectum or to rule out the presence of primary conditions of the urologic or gastrointestinal tract that may complicate therapy or confuse later follow-up. Lymphangiography, computed tomography scans, and magnetic resonance imaging may be used selectively to provide important information that helps the clinician to plan treatment or evaluate prognosis.

THERAPY

The cornerstone of treatment for endometrial carcinoma is total abdominal hysterectomy and bilateral salpingo-oophorectomy. Approximately 10–12% of patients with clinical stage I endometrial carcinoma have pelvic lymph node metastasis. As many as 35% of patients with stage II disease may have involvement of the pelvic nodes. Although the incidence of aortic lymph node metastases is less well known, in as many as 8–10% of women with clinical stage I disease, tumor has already spread to the aortic nodes. One large study suggests that 60% of all patients with endometrial carcinoma who have pelvic lymph node metastasis also have involvement of the aortic nodes. The incidence of lymph node metastasis is related to tumor differentiation and depth of myometrial penetration. Pelvic and paraaortic lymph node sampling is suggested for all patients with suggestive nodes encountered at surgery and in all women with grade 3 tumors, more than superficial invasion, or evidence of cervical involvement. Preoperative ultrasonography is useful in predicting depth of myometrial invasion so that the surgeon may be prepared for appropriate staging studies.

For patients with clinical stage I disease, primary surgery with total abdominal hysterectomy and staging studies as indicated is favored by most gynecologic oncologists in the United States. Recent advances in laparoscopic techniques have prompted some gynecologists to investigate laparoscopic lymphadenectomy and laparoscopically assisted vaginal hysterectomy and bilateral salpingo-oophorectomy for the treatment of endometrial adenocarcinoma. Such an approach is still investigational.

Adjunctive irradiation with vaginal cesium, external irradiation, or both, may be added selectively, depending on the final surgical/pathologic staging. Although adjunctive irradiation in patients with stages IA and IB endometrial carcinomas appears to decrease the risk of recurrence of carcinoma in the vaginal apex, there is no conclusive evidence to suggest that overall survival is improved. Adjunctive irradiation should be used selectively, bearing in mind the potential morbidity. Patients who are unacceptable anesthetic risks or who refuse surgery may be treated for a cure with irradiation alone by both external and intracavitary techniques. The results are not as good as they are with surgery, however.

Patients with endometrial carcinoma who have gross cervical involvement have traditionally been treated with whole-pelvis external irradiation followed by total abdominal hysterectomy, bilateral salpingo-oophorectomy, and additional surgical staging done 4–6 weeks later. Treatment for clinical stage III and clinical stage IV endometrial carcinomas should be individualized, but, when possible, hysterectomy and bilateral salpingo-oophorectomy should be included. Elimination of uterine bleeding and the removal of an infected, necrotic pelvic tumor may provide a significant palliative benefit.

The treatment of patients with extrauterine disease (stage III or IV) or positive peritoneal cytologic findings (surgical stage III) is still unsatisfactory. The use of intraperitoneal radioactive colloidal chromic phosphate (^{32}P) has been suggested for those patients with positive peritoneal cytologic findings alone. This therapy consists of instilling 15 mCi of ^{32}P through an indwelling peritoneal catheter with more than 1,000 ml of normal saline to provide a uniform distribution throughout the abdominal cavity. Although satisfactory results have been reported with this technique, comparative trials are lacking, and the management of such patients remains controversial.

Both cytotoxic and hormonal chemotherapy have been effective in the treatment of patients with metastatic endometrial carcinoma. Effective cytotoxic agents include cisplatin, doxorubicin, cyclophosphamide, and 5-fluorouracil. Paclitaxel (Taxol) has recently entered trials and may be effective. When agents have been used alone or in combination, response rates of 15–35% have been reported, but complete responses are uncommon, and disease-free intervals are often short. Hormonal chemotherapy such as megestrol acetate has minimal morbidity, and response rates of 30–35% have been reported.

The results of treatment for endometrial carcinoma are shown in Table 5-3. As previously noted, results relate to both stage and grade.

ESTROGEN REPLACEMENT THERAPY AFTER ENDOMETRIAL CANCER

There are no definitive data to support specific recommendations regarding the use of estrogen in women with a history of endometrial carcinoma; however, responses from a survey of members of the Society of Gynecologic Oncologists indicate that 83% of the respondents approved the use of estrogen replacement therapy in patients with stage I, grade 1 endometrial cancer, and some would use it in higher grade lesions. The American College of Obstetricians and Gynecologists (ACOG) has concluded that in women with a history of

TABLE 5-3. TREATMENT RESULTS IN ENDOMETRIAL CARCINOMA

		5-Year Survival (%)	
Clinical Stage	% of Total	Radiation	Surgery ± Radiation
I	80	60	80–90
G1	45		88
G2	35		87
G3	20	68	
II	8	43	74
III	6	30	
IV	6	7	

endometrial carcinoma, estrogens can be used for the same indications as they are used for in any other woman, except that the selection of appropriate candidates should be based on prognostic indicators and the risk that the patient is willing to assume. Prognostic predictors (depth of invasion, degree of differentiation, and cell type) assist the physician in describing the risks of persistent tumor to the patient.

In the absence of estrogen replacement therapy:

- A well-differentiated neoplasm of the endometrioid cell type with superficial invasion would render a risk of persistent disease of approximately 5%.
- A moderately differentiated neoplasm of the endometrioid cell type with up to one-half myometrial invasion would render a 10–15% risk of persistent disease. The risk would increase to 20–30% for adenosquamous cell–type neoplasms and to approximately 50% for serous papillary tumors.
- A poorly differentiated neoplasm, regardless of cell type, with invasion of more than one half of the myometrium would render a 40–50% risk of persistent disease.

Because the metabolic changes associated with estrogen deficiency are significant, the woman should be given complete information, including counseling about alternative therapies, to enable her to make an informed decision. For some women, the sense of well-being afforded by amelioration of menopausal symptoms or the need to treat atrophic vaginitis or prevent osteoporosis and coronary artery disease may outweigh the undetermined risk of stimulating tumor growth.

ENDOMETRIAL HYPERPLASIA

Some types of endometrial hyperplasia represent a transitional or premalignant form of endometrial neoplasia. Many different classification schemes have been suggested for different degrees of hyperplasia. Current terminology favors a description of the degree of atypicality of the glandular architecture and nuclear atypia. In a series of 170 patients with all grades of endometrial hyperplasia, 29% of the patients with complex glandular patterns and cytologic atypia developed endometrial carcinoma, while only 1% of those with a simple glandular pattern and no cytologic atypia developed malignancy. When there was a complex glandular pattern without cytologic atypia the risk of cancer was low (3%), and when cytologic atypia was present but the glandular architecture was simple a relatively low risk was also observed (8%). Therefore, both cytologic atypia and complex glandular pattern are necessary to put the patient in the high-risk category of *atypical endometrial hyperplasia*. This descriptive terminology has generally replaced the older classifications of adenomatous hyperplasia and endometrial carcinoma in situ.

If endometrial hyperplasia is diagnosed, a thorough curettage and careful review of the histology are indicated to be sure the uterus has been adequately sampled and the malignant potential of the hyperplasia evaluated. Depending on other risk factors for endometrial cancer and the patient's medical condition and personal desires, endometrial hyperplasia can be managed by hysterectomy or by progestational therapy. Various hormonal regimens have been used effectively, including megestrol acetate (80–160 mg orally daily), depot medroxyprogesterone acetate (1,000 mg intramuscularly [IM] per week for 4 weeks, then 400 mg/mo), and hydroxyprogesterone caproate (500 mg orally daily for 2 weeks, then 2 g weekly). After complete discussion with the patient, if progestational therapy is selected, follow-up evaluation at 2–3 months is necessary to be sure that the hyperplasia has resolved. Long-term treatment and follow-up plans can then be developed.

SARCOMAS OF THE UTERUS

Uterine sarcomas arise from the mesenchymal tissue of the uterus and usually occur in postmenopausal women with an average age of 58. An enlarged, irregular uterus is the most common physical finding, and irregular bleeding is the most common symptom, occurring in about 85% of patients. Other, less common, complaints include abdominal pain (19%), abdominal mass (15%), weight loss (7%), and vaginal discharge (4%). It is rare to find a sarcoma that arises from within a benign leiomyoma, but it is certainly possible for these two lesions to coexist in the same uterus. Occasionally, a sarcoma may present as a pedunculated polyp prolapsing through the cervix.

Although there are multiple classifications of uterine sarcomas (see box), homologous tumors are those that arise from mesenchymal tissues that are usually found in the uterus (endometrial stroma, smooth muscle, blood vessels, fibrous tissue), whereas heterologous tumors arise from mesenchymal elements that are foreign to the uterus (bone, cartilage, striated muscle, fat). The mitotic index, or the number of mitoses per 10 high-power fields, is the chief histologic criterion of malignancy for leiomyosarcomas. Fewer than five mitoses per 10 high-power fields is usually referred to as a cellular myoma, which has little risk of metastasis or recurrence. With more than 10 mitoses per 10 high-power fields, the tumor is definitely malignant and when 5–10 mitoses per 10 high-power fields are present it is usually regarded as an intermediate or low-grade lesion.

Classification of Uterine Sarcomas

I. Pure sarcomas
  A. Pure homologous
    1. Leiomyosarcoma
    2. Stromal sarcoma
    3. Angiosarcoma
    4. Fibrosarcoma
  B. Pure heterologous
    1. Rhabdomyosarcoma
    2. Chondrosarcoma
    3. Osteogenic sarcoma
    4. Liposarcoma

II. Mixed sarcomas
  A. Mixed homologous
  B. Mixed heterologous
  C. Mixed homologous and heterologous

III. Malignant mixed müllerian tumors
  A. Malignant mixed müllerian tumor, homologous type; carcinoma plus one or more of the homologous sarcomas listed under IA above
  B. Malignant mixed müllerian tumor, heterologous type; carcinoma plus one or more of the heterologous sarcomas listed under IB; homologous sarcoma(s) may also be present

IV. Sarcoma, unclassified

V. Malignant lymphoma

Extent of disease is the most important prognostic characteristic in patients with uterine sarcoma. When sarcoma has spread beyond the uterus, only rare long-term survivors have been reported. Even when the cancer is confined to the uterus, prognosis is relatively poor, with overall 5-year survival rates of approximately 50%. There does not seem to be any prognostic difference between patients with heterologous tumors and those with homologous tumors. Metastasis to the ovaries is not uncommon, and vascular metastases to lungs and bone are also seen relatively frequently in patients with this disease.

The primary treatment for patients with uterine sarcoma is total abdominal hysterectomy and bilateral salpingo-oophorectomy. Pelvic radiation therapy may reduce the incidence of pelvic recurrence, but it has not been shown to improve overall survival. Preoperative and postoperative chemotherapy with a variety of agents has also been reported, but response rates are low, and the duration of response is short.

BIBLIOGRAPHY

American College of Obstetricians and Gynecologists. Estrogen replacement therapy and endometrial cancer. ACOG Committee Opinion 126. Washington, DC: ACOG, 1993

Abeler VM, Kjørstad KE. Endometrial adenocarcinoma in Norway. A study of a total population. Cancer 1991;67:3093–3103

Belinson JL, Lee KR, Badger GJ, Pretorius RG, Jarrell MA. Clinical stage I adenocarcinoma of the endometrium—analysis of recurrences and the potential benefit of staging lymphadenectomy. Gynecol Oncol 1992;44:17–23

Bourne TH, Campbell S, Steer CV, Royston P, Whitehead MI, Collins WP. Detection of endometrial cancer by transvaginal ultrasonography with color flow imaging and blood flow analysis: a preliminary report. Gynecol Oncol 1991;40:253–259

Chang KL, Crabtree GS, Lim-Tan SK, Kempson RL, Hendrickson MR. Primary uterine endometrial stromal neoplasms: a clinicopathologic study of 117 cases. Am J Surg Pathol 1990;14:415–438

Girardi F, Petru E, Heydarfadai M, Haas J, Winter R. Pelvic lymphadenectomy in the surgical treatment of endometrial cancer. Gynecol Oncol 1993;49:177–180

Kim YB, Niloff JM. Endometrial carcinoma: analysis of recurrence in patients treated with a strategy minimizing lymph node sampling and radiation therapy. Obstet Gynecol 1993;82:175–180

Leibsohn S, d'Ablaing G, Mishell DR Jr, Schlaerth JB. Leiomyosarcoma in a series of hysterectomies performed for presumed uterine leiomyomas. Am J Obstet Gynecol 1990;162:968–974

Sahakian V, Syrop C, Turner D. Endometrial carcinoma: transvaginal ultrasonography prediction of depth of myometrial invasion. Gynecol Oncol 1991;43:217–219

Silverberg SG, Major FG, Blessing JA, Fetter B, Askin FB, Liao SY, et al. Carcinosarcoma (malignant mixed mesodermal tumor) of the uterus. A Gynecologic Oncology Group pathologic study of 203 cases. Int J Gynecol Pathol 1990;9:1–19

Sutton GP. The significance of positive peritoneal cytology in endometrial cancer. Oncology (Huntingt) 1990;4:21–26

Cancer of the Ovary and Uterine Tube

In 1994, an estimated 74,400 new cases of gynecologic cancer will have been diagnosed and roughly 24,000 (32%) of these cancers will have originated in the ovary. Approximately 25,200 women will die of gynecologic cancer, and, of these deaths, 13,600 (54%) will be from ovarian cancer. The risk of a woman developing ovarian cancer during her lifetime is 1–2%. The incidence varies with age, being 1.4/100,000 in women less than 40 years of age and 38/100,000 in women more than 60 years of age (Fig. 5-1).

Ovarian cancer is more common in Northern European and North American countries than in Asia, developing countries, or southern continents. Although the etiology of the disease is not known, risk factors include infertility, low parity, use of talc on the perineum, high-fat diet, lactose intolerance, previous breast or colon cancer, and a family history of ovarian cancer. Smoking, alcohol use, coffee consumption, estrogen replacement therapy, and viral infections (such as mumps) have not been associated with increased risk.

Oral contraceptives appear to be protective for ovarian cancer, with an average relative risk of about 0.7 for 2 years of OC use to 0.5 relative risk for 5 years of OC use. The protective effect of OC use also appears to be long term, with some studies indicating a lifetime risk reduction.

Figure 5-2 illustrates the relationship of ovarian cancer to the other gynecologic cancers for both incidence and mortality. Table 5-4 illustrates the relative stage at diagnosis and the survival by stage for ovarian cancer in relation to the other gynecologic cancers. As can be seen, the 5-year survival for ovarian cancer by stage is not significantly different from the 5-year survival for other gynecologic cancers. However, there is a significant difference in stage at diagnosis for ovarian cancer, with about two thirds of patients having the cancer spread into the abdomen at the time of initial diagnosis. The single most important factor in the large number of deaths from ovarian cancer is the failure to diagnosis the disease at an early stage. The reasons for this relate to the growth and spread patterns of the disease. Because the ovary floats freely in the pelvic cavity, a tumor can grow for some time without producing symptoms associated with involvement of, or pressure on, other organs. At the same time, disease spread occurs not only by direct extension and through the lymphatics, but also through the exfoliation of clonagenic cells, resulting in

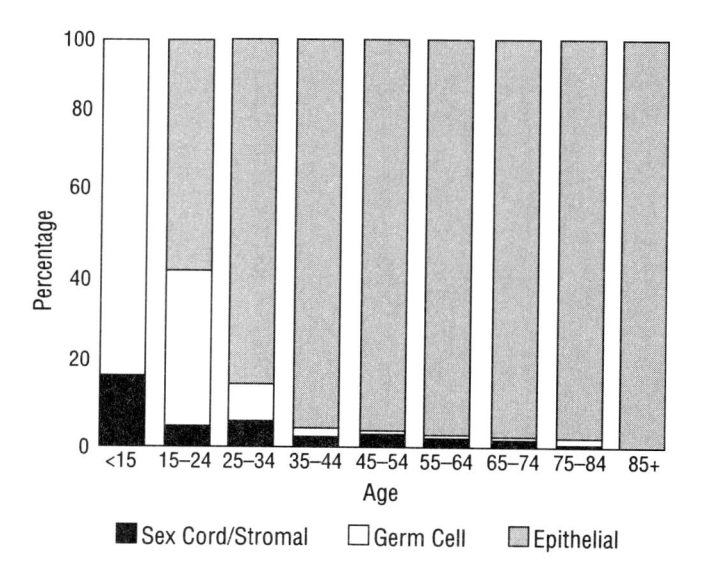

FIG. 5-1. Prevalence of different types of ovarian cancer by age.

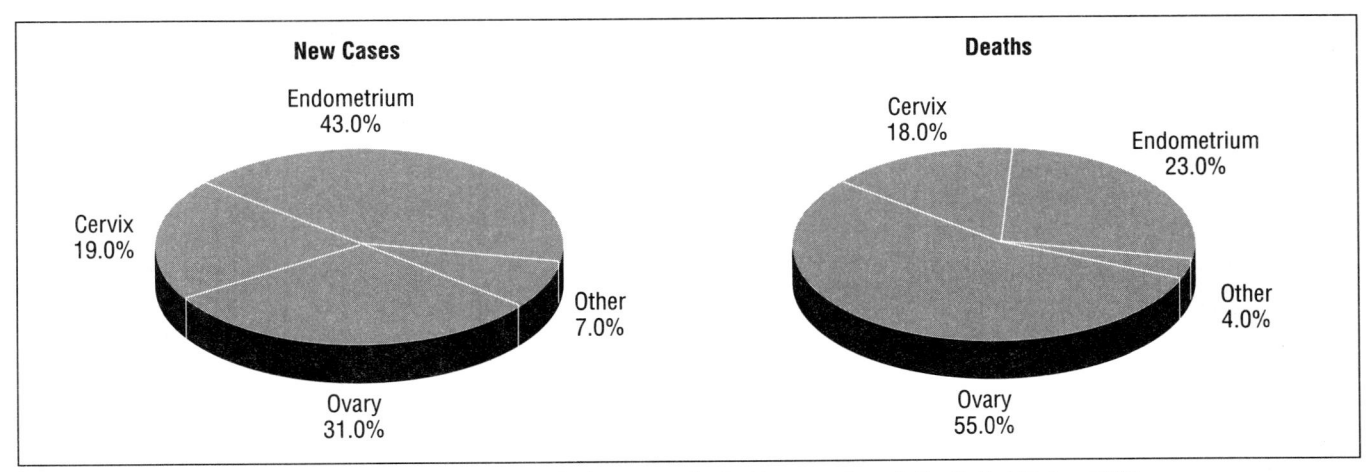

FIG. 5-2. Relationships of ovarian cancer to other gynecologic cancers for incidence and mortality, United States, 1993.

early dissemination of cancer throughout the abdominal cavity. Unlike the blood stream, which is not hospitable to tumor cells, the peritoneal cavity and the peritoneal fluid do not impede tumor growth. The symptoms of ovarian cancer, such as abdominal pain, bloating, and gastrointestinal symptoms, are usually those of advanced disease.

One of the most significant ways to improve survival for patients with ovarian cancer would be to find a way to screen patients and therefore detect the disease before its spread beyond the ovary. Methods for screening are pelvic examination, serum CA 125 levels, and pelvic or transvaginal ultrasonography. To date, there is no good evidence that routine pelvic examination has been effective in the early diagnosis of ovarian cancer. Serum CA 125 levels have also not been shown to be effective, because of the high false-negative rates. Only about 50% of patients with stage I ovarian cancer will have an abnormal serum CA 125 level. To further substantiate this point, the only study to look at CA 125 screening for ovarian cancer reported that in the six cancers of the ovary diagnosed by CA 125 screening, four of the cancers had spread beyond the ovary. On the other hand, three studies of either pelvic or transvaginal ultrasonography screened a total of 7,576 patients and diagnosed 10 cancers, all stage I. Unfortunately, this technique has a high false-positive rate, with 13–65 patients undergoing surgical exploration for each cancer detected. If some additional test could be discovered that would allow one to determine which patient with an enlarged ovary actually needs exploration, transvaginal ultrasonography might turn out to be an effective screening tool. Current research in this area centers on the use of either morphology index or color-flow Doppler as part of the ultrasound examination.

HISTOLOGY

The tumors of the ovary are usually divided by their tissue of origin: epithelial (from the coelomic epithelial cells that line the ovary), sex cord–stromal (from the mesenchymal tissue of the ovary), and germ cell (from the germinal epithelium) (see box). The most common type of malignant tumor is epithelial, accounting for approximately 85% of the ovarian cancers. Germ cell cancers account for approximately 10% of malignant tumors, and the remaining 5% are sex cord–stromal cancers.

The most common of the malignant epithelial ovarian cancers are serous (40–50%), endometrioid (15–25%), mucinous (6–16%), and clear cell (5–11%) cancers. The remainder of the cancers, such as transitional cell (Brenner), mixed epithelial, and undifferentiated carcinoma, are less frequently encountered. The epithelial tumors occur as benign tumors, tumors of low malignant potential, and frankly malignant cancer. Tumors of low malignant potential (borderline tumors) have a much better prognosis than the frankly malignant cancers but are nevertheless malignant tumors that can result in the death of the patient. Malignant tumors are further subdivided by histologic grade either into three grades based on architecture (FIGO) or into four grades based on nuclear atypia (Broders).

Of the germ cell tumors, the most common is the mature cystic teratoma, a benign tumor. The most common malignant germ cell tumor is the dysgerminoma, followed by the endodermal sinus tumor and the immature teratoma. Germ cell tumors are most commonly seen in the first two decades of life. The sex cord–stromal tumors are usually divided into

TABLE 5-4. STAGE AT DIAGNOSIS AND 5-YEAR SURVIVAL RATE OF GYNECOLOGIC CANCERS, UNITED STATES 1993

Site	Stage at Diagnosis (%)			5-Year Survival Rate (%)		
	Localized	Regional	Distant	Localized	Regional	Distant
Endometrium	74	12	10	94	71	29
Cervix	48	34	10	90	53	13
Ovary	23	26	46	89	36	17

World Health Organization Classification of Ovarian Tumors

Epithelial Tumors

Serous Tumors
Benign
    Cystadenoma and papillary cystadenoma
    Surface papilloma
    Adenofibroma and cystadenofibroma
Of borderline malignancy (carcinoma of low malignant potential)
    Cystadenoma and papillary cystadenoma
    Surface papilloma
    Adenofibroma and cystadenofibroma
Malignant
    Adenocarcinoma (papillary adenocarcinoma and papillary cystadenocarcinoma)
    Surface papillary carcinoma
    Malignant adenofibroma and cystadenofibroma

Mucinous Tumors
Benign
    Cystadenoma
    Adenofibroma and cystadenofibroma
Of borderline malignancy (carcinoma of low malignant potential)
    Cystadenoma
    Adenofibroma and cystadenofibroma
Malignant
    Adenocarcinoma and cystadenofibroma
    Malignant adenofibroma and cystadenofibroma

Endometrioid Tumors
Benign
    Adenoma and cystadenoma
    Adenofibroma and cystadenofibroma
Of borderline malignancy (carcinoma of low malignant potential)
    Adenoma and cystadenoma
    Adenofibroma and cystadenofibroma
Malignant
    Adenocarcinoma
    Adenocanthoma
    Adenosquamous carcinoma
    Malignant adenofibroma and cystadenofibroma
Epithelial–stroma and stromal
    Adenosarcoma
    Stromal sarcoma
    Mesodermal (müllerian) mixed tumors, homologous and heterologous

Clear Cell (Mesonephroid) Tumors
Benign
    Adenofibroma

Of borderline malignancy (carcinomas of low malignant potential)
Malignant
    Adenocarcinoma (carcinoma)

Transitional Cell Tumors
Benign Brenner tumor
Of borderline malignancy (proliferating)
Malignant Brenner tumor
Transitional cell carcinoma

Mixed Epithelial Tumors
Benign
Of borderline malignancy
Malignant

Undifferentiated Carcinoma

Unclassified Epithelial Tumors

Germ Cell Tumors

Dysgerminoma
    Variant: with syncytiotrophoblast cells
Yolk sac tumor (endodermal sinus tumor)
    Variants: Polyvesicular vitelline tumor
    Hepatoid
    Glandular
        Variant: "Endometrioid"
Embryonal carcinoma
Polyembryona
Choriocarcinoma
Teratomas
    Immature
    Mature
        Solid
        Cystic (dermoid cyst)
            With secondary tumor formation (specify type)
        Fetiform (homunculus)
    Monodermal and highly specialized
        Struma ovarii
            With thyroid tumor (specify type)
        Carcinoid
            Insular
            Trabecular
        Strumal carcinoid
        Mucinous carcinoid
        Neuroectodermal tumors
        Sebaceous tumors
        Others
    Mixed (specify types)
Mixed (specify types)

Sex Cord–Stromal Tumors

Granulosa–stromal cell tumors
    Granulosa cell tumor
        Juvenile
        Adult
    Tumors in the thecoma–fibroma group
        Thecoma
            Typical
            Luteinized*
        Fibroma
        Cellular fibroma
        Fibrosarcoma
        Stromal tumor with minor sex cord elements
        Sclerosing stromal tumor (Stromal luteoma)
        Unclassified (fibrothecoma)
        Others
Sertoli–stromal cell tumors; androblastomas
    Well differentiated
        Sertoli cell tumor; tabular androblastoma
        Sertoli–Leydig cell tumor (Leydig cell tumor)
    Of intermediate differentiation
        Variant
        With heterologous elements (specify types)
    Poorly differentiated (sarcomatoid)
        Variant
        With heterologous elements (specify types)
    Retiform
    Mixed
Sex cord tumor with annular tubules
Gynandroblastoma
Steroid (lipid) cell tumors
    Stromal luteoma
    Leydig cell tumor; hilus cell tumor (*Note*: A rare Leydig cell tumor is nonhilar)
    Unclassified

---

* A rare tumor has the features of luteinized thecoma and additional crystals of Reinke in the steroid cell component. This tumor has been called a stromal Leydig cell tumor.

Modified from Serov SF, Scully RE, Sobin LH. International histological classification of tumors. #9, Histological typing of ovarian tumors. Geneva: World Health Organization, 1973

the female type, characterized by the granulosa cell tumor, and the male type, characterized by the Sertoli–Leydig cell tumor. Most (over 90%) malignant stromal tumors are granulosa cell tumors. Although these tumors can occur at any age, they are more common before menopause.

STAGING AND DIAGNOSIS

The initial evaluation and therapy of ovarian cancer is surgical. The staging classification is based on surgical evaluation, and the removal of as much tumor as possible is the cornerstone of treatment. Some type of adjunctive treatment is almost always required. The proper surgical procedure and the appropriate choice of adjunctive therapy depend on the findings at initial exploration, the histologic type of the tumor, and the age and reproductive desires of the patient.

The staging classification for ovarian cancer is established by FIGO (see box). Although in advanced disease (spread throughout the abdomen) the proper staging of a patient with ovarian cancer may be obvious, the surgeon must be meticulous in the staging of early ovarian cancer.

The patterns of spread of ovarian cancer play a role in staging. The cancer can spread by direct infiltration of pelvic structures such as the pelvic peritoneum; the bladder surface; the rectal surface; or the fallopian tube, broad ligament, and uterus. Lymphatic spread occurs early in ovarian cancer, with nodal metastases in 10–12% of patients with stage I cancer and 20–25% of patients with stage II disease. In stage III and stage IV, the incidence of positive lymph nodes is 50–70%. By far the most important type of spread of ovarian cancer is the exfoliation of clonagenic cells into the peritoneal cavity. These cells are swept up the right abdominal gutter to the diaphragm and omentum by the clockwise flow of peritoneal fluid in the abdomen. The cells implant and form tumor nodules, and in turn these nodules exfoliate more cells. The normal daily activities of the patient and the normal peristalsis of the intestine result in the spread of the disease throughout the abdominal cavity. Proper staging requires a generous lower and upper midline incision and thorough exploration with multiple peritoneal and nodal biopsies.

In young patients who desire further childbearing and have epithelial, germ cell, or stromal tumors confined to one ovary, conservation of the uterus and other ovary and fallopian tube is possible, providing a full surgical staging procedure is performed. In these patients it is particularly important to perform a careful evaluation of the entire abdomen.

Unfortunately, most patients are diagnosed with ovarian cancer after the disease has spread beyond the ovary. In these patients, symptoms may be abdominal pain or a "bloated" feeling, gastrointestinal or urinary tract disturbances, or, in many cases, the onset of clinically detectable ascites. Some patients with advanced disease will have menstrual irregularity or postmenopausal bleeding, but these are not frequent symptoms. Occasionally, the patient with ovarian cancer presents with a palpable inguinal lymph node, tumor in a hernia sac, or pleural effusion. For patients with advanced disease, diagnosis is established by tissue obtained at exploratory

---

FIGO Staging for Carcinoma of the Ovary

Staging of ovarian carcinoma is based on findings at clinical examination and by surgical exploration. The histologic findings are to be considered in the staging, as are the cytologic findings as far as effusions are concerned. It is desirable that a biopsy be taken from suspicious areas outside of the pelvis.

Stage	Description
Stage I	Growth limited to the ovaries
Stage IA	Growth limited to one ovary; no ascites present containing malignant cells. No tumor on the external surface; capsule intact
Stage IB	Growth limited to both ovaries; no ascites present containing malignant cells. No tumor on the external surfaces; capsules intact
Stage IC*	Tumor classified as either stage IA or IB but with tumor on the surface of one or both ovaries; or with ruptured capsule(s); or with ascites containing malignant cells present or with positive peritoneal washings
Stage II	Growth involving one or both ovaries, with pelvic extension
Stage IIA	Extension and/or metastases to the uterus and/or tubes
Stage IIB	Extension to other pelvic tissues
Stage IIC*	Tumor either stage IIA or IIB but with tumor on the surface of one or both ovaries; or with capsule(s) ruptured; or with ascites containing malignant cells present or with positive peritoneal washings
Stage III	Tumor involving one or both ovaries with peritoneal implants outside the pelvis and/or positive retroperitoneal or inguinal nodes. Superficial liver metastasis equals stage III. Tumor is limited to the true pelvis but with histologically proven malignant extension to small bowel or omentum
Stage IIIA	Tumor grossly limited to the true pelvis with negative nodes but with histologically confirmed microscopic seeding of abdominal peritoneal surfaces
Stage IIIB	Tumor of one or both ovaries with histologically confirmed implants of abdominal peritoneal surfaces, none exceeding 2 cm in diameter; nodes are negative
Stage IIIC	Abdominal implants greater than 2 cm in diameter and/or positive retroperitoneal or inguinal nodes
Stage IV	Growth involving one or both ovaries, with distant metastases. If pleural effusion is present, there must be positive cytologic findings to allot a case to stage IV. Parenchymal liver metastasis equals stage IV.

Notes about the staging: To evaluate the impact on prognosis of the different criteria for allotting cases to stage IC or IIC, it would be of value to know whether the rupture of the capsule was spontaneous or caused by the surgeon and if the source of malignant cells detected was peritoneal washings or ascites.

International Federation of Gynecology and Obstetrics. Annual report on the results of treatment in gynecological cancer. Int J Gynecol Obstet 1989;28:189–190

laparotomy. In those rare cases in which a patient cannot undergo surgery because of medical problems, diagnosis is established by needle biopsy for either histologic or cytologic diagnosis.

Early ovarian cancer is diagnosed by the surgical evaluation of an adnexal mass. Whether to subject a patient to surgical exploration or to observe her is a difficult decision. The availability of sophisticated ultrasound evaluation of the adnexal mass has improved the ability to distinguish patients who should be explored from those that can be observed, but it has also resulted in an increasing number of occasions in which a patient is found to have an asymptomatic ovarian cyst. This is of particular concern in the postmenopausal woman. The diagnostic criteria for surgical exploration of a patient with an adnexal mass are shown in Table 5-5. As with any diagnostic or therapeutic schema, the criteria for exploration cannot be absolute. For example, a patient with known endometriosis may meet the criteria for surgical exploration when that is not the best treatment option, or a postmenopausal patient with a 4-cm simple cyst may have risk factors for surgery that make observation a more reasonable option.

The use of tumor markers to assist in the evaluation of a patient with an adnexal mass is appropriate, but one must be aware of the potential misinformation that may result from use of the test. CA 125 is the only serum marker available today with the potential accuracy to be of benefit, but even this marker is less than optimal. Approximately one half of patients with early ovarian cancer will not have an elevation of their serum CA 125 levels. Also, a variety of nonmalignant and nonovarian malignant conditions can result in an elevation of the serum CA 125 levels. Gynecologic and nongynecologic cancers that may have serum elevations of CA 125 include:

Gynecologic cancers
- Epithelial ovarian cancer
- Some germ cell tumors
- Some stromal tumors
- Fallopian tube cancer
- Endometrial cancer
- Endocervical cancer

Nongynecologic cancers
- Pancreatic cancer
- Lung cancer
- Breast cancer
- Colon cancer

A serum CA 125 elevation above 35 U may be helpful in deciding whether or not to recommend surgery in a postmenopausal patient with an ovarian mass, but a negative value is not helpful. Likewise, a serum CA 125 elevation in a woman of reproductive age with both an ovarian mass and leiomyomata or endometriosis may not be helpful.

Laparoscopic evaluation of an adnexal mass is possible. Masses too large to be removed intact through the cul-de-sac, a laparoscopy bag, or a small incision require surgical exploration. It is not appropriate to aspirate a mass or open a mass in the abdominal cavity because of the danger of seeding the abdomen with clonagenic cancer cells and because there are no data to show that the cytologic diagnosis of aspirated cyst fluid is accurate. A frozen-section diagnosis of ovarian cancer in a mass removed by laparoscopy requires surgical exploration for appropriate staging and therapy.

EPITHELIAL CANCER

Treatment

The treatment of ovarian cancer involves multimodal therapy in most cases. Although surgical therapy is the initial intervention, alone it is curative in only a small percentage of cases. In most cases, adjunctive chemotherapy or radiation therapy or both is necessary. Surgical reassessment following adjunctive therapy will be necessary in most patients who started treatment with advanced disease. In a large percentage of these patients, some type of salvage therapy will be important.

Finally, some patients apparently will be cured of their cancer while others will develop refractory disease. In the former patients, follow-up care must be provided, whereas the latter group of patients requires palliative therapy. In the following section, each of these major treatment phases is discussed. Table 5-6 outlines the current therapy and therapeutic options for epithelial ovarian cancer.

Surgical Therapy

In patients with epithelial ovarian cancer that is confined to the ovary, surgical removal of the cancer, followed by a full

TABLE 5-5. MANAGEMENT SCHEMA FOR A PATIENT WITH AN ADNEXAL MASS

Observe and Repeat Examination in 4–6 Weeks	Surgical Exploration
Reproductive age	Premenarchal*
	Postmenopausal*
Mass less than 8 cm	Mass greater than 8 cm
Simple cysts on ultrasound	Complex cysts on ultrasound
Decreasing size	Increase in size or persistence through two or three menstrual cycles
Cystic and smooth	Solid and irregular
Mobile	Fixed
Unilateral	Bilateral
Asymptomatic	Pain or other symptoms of acute intraabdominal process
No ascites	Ascites

* Simple cysts smaller than 3–5 cm may be followed closely with ultrasonography.
Modified from Young RC, Perez CA, Hoskins WJ. Cancer of the ovary. In: DeVita VT, Hellman S, Rosenberg SA, eds. Cancer: principles and practice of oncology. 4th ed. Philadelphia: JB Lippincott, 1993

TABLE 5-6. CURRENT THERAPY AND OPTIONAL THERAPY FOR EPITHELIAL OVARIAN CANCER*

Cancer	Standard Therapy	Investigational Drug Regimen
A. Early ovarian cancer		
1. Low risk (stage IA & B, grade 1[†])	TAH, BSO,[‡] full surgical staging	
2. High Risk (stage IA & B, grade 3, stage IC, IIA, B & C, no residual)	TAH, BSO,[‡] full surgical staging Adjunctive therapy with ^{32}P, single agent or combination platinum-based chemotherapy Second Look: controversial ALTERNATIVE: Whole-abdominal radiation therapy	Paclitaxel, alone or in combination
B. Advanced ovarian cancer		
1. Optimal (stage III, <1 cm residual[‡])	Maximal surgical cytoreduction Combination chemotherapy with a platinum compound and an alkylating agent Second Look: recommended ALTERNATIVE: Whole-abdominal radiation therapy for patients with no gross residual	Paclitaxel, alone or in combination
2. Suboptimal (stage III, >1 residual[§] or stage IV	Maximal surgical cytoreduction Combination chemotherapy with cisplatin and paclitaxel Second look: recommended ALTERNATIVE: None	High-dose chemotherapy
C. Recurrent and/or persistent ovarian cancer	Investigational therapy	

* TAH indicates total abdominal hysterectomy; BSO, bilateral salpingo-oophorectomy.
[†] Some investigators include grade 2 in the "low-risk" category.
[‡] Unilateral salpingo-oophorectomy permissible in patients who desire further childbearing.
[§] Stage II patients with residual disease can be either optimal or suboptimal advanced disease, depending on residual.

surgical staging procedure, may be adequate therapy. In other patients with early-stage cancer, some type of adjunctive treatment may be required. Epithelial ovarian cancer can be divided into early disease (stages I and II with no residual cancer) and advanced disease (stage II with residual cancer and stages III and IV cancer). Early ovarian cancer can be divided into low-risk and high-risk disease. For properly staged low-risk epithelial ovarian cancer, survival is approximately 95%, and no therapy has been shown to be more effective than surgical removal of the cancer. High-risk epithelial ovarian cancer requires adjuvant treatment with irradiation or chemotherapy. With adjunctive therapy, survival in this group of patients is about 75%. For patients with low-risk disease who desire further childbearing, unilateral salpingo-oophorectomy is acceptable, provided that they had a full surgical staging procedure. Most authorities would recommend removal of the retained ovary when childbearing is complete. For patients with high-risk early ovarian cancer the role of conservative surgery is more controversial, although some oncologists will preserve childbearing capability in these women despite the requirement for adjunctive chemotherapy. Patients so managed do not have the option of choosing irradiation for therapy.

Primary Reductive Surgery. Although in the late 1960s there were reports of improved survival in patients who had more extensive surgical resection followed by whole-abdomen irradiation, it was in 1975 that the exact residual diameter was first recorded and related to duration of survival in a series of patients. All of these patients had been treated postoperatively with single–alkylating agent therapy. Survival was 39 months for patients with residual diameter of 0 cm, 29 months for patients with residual diameter of 0–0.5 cm, 18 months for patients with 0.6–1.5 cm, and 11 months for patients with greater than 1.5 cm. Since then, many reports have confirmed the fact that patients whose tumors are surgically reduced to small-volume disease are more likely to have a response to chemotherapy, and the frequency of complete responses is greater. In collected literature, the overall response rate was

66.8% in patients with optimal residual disease, compared with 53.3% in patients with suboptimal residual disease. The complete response rate was 42.7% in patients with optimal residual disease, compared with 24.0% in patients with suboptimal residual disease. The larger difference in complete response rate, compared with overall response rate, is indicative of the effect of tumor-reducing surgery, because if the response rates (complete versus overall) were of the same magnitude the implication would be that those patients who can be debulked are also more likely to respond to chemotherapy. While this is probably true to some extent, it does not explain the difference in complete response rates.

There is a significant difference in the survival of patients with optimally reduced tumors, compared with patients whose tumors cannot be reduced. This difference in survival, combined with the information on response rates, seems to indicate clearly that successful initial reductive surgery is of benefit. While reductive surgery is an important factor in determining outcome, it is not the only significant factor. Also important is the age of the patient, the number of residual tumor nodules, and the grade of the tumor.

Patients with advanced ovarian cancer who begin adjunctive therapy with optimal residual disease are more likely to have a complete response and will survive longer. Performing reductive surgery is of benefit to these patients. The question of whether there is a subgroup of patients whose tumors can be reduced but who would do better even if they were not reduced has not been answered. The real answer is probably a little bit of both; the reductive surgery is important, but it is not the only factor that is important.

Although there is wide acceptance of the concept of primary reductive surgery, there have been fewer publications that address the concept of secondary reductive surgery. A review of the literature disclosed that the tumors of 32–74% of patients could be secondarily reduced to microscopic disease at second-look laparotomy and that an even greater number could be reduced to an optimal residual disease status. Improved survival rates have been demonstrated in patients whose disease was secondarily reduced to small-volume disease at second-look laparotomy.

Interval Reductive Surgery. A significant number of patients will begin initial adjunctive therapy with large-volume disease. This problem has been approached with the concept of interval disease-reducing surgery, in which patients receive a short course of chemotherapy and then undergo a second operation to surgically remove residual tumor followed by a continuation of chemotherapy. Results with this technique have been mixed, with some investigators reporting improved survival and others reporting little survival benefit. If the benefit of interval tumor reduction can be substantiated, the standard therapy of patients with suboptimal ovarian cancer may include an interval operation.

Second-Look Laparotomy. The purpose of second-look laparotomy is to identify patients who are in complete clinical remission but have minimal residual disease and would benefit from alternative therapy. Approximately 50% of patients with advanced epithelial ovarian cancer will be in complete clinical remission at the conclusion of their initial chemotherapy. At second-look laparotomy, 50% of these patients will be found to have residual disease and may benefit from additional therapy. Alternative methods of diagnosing patients with residual disease have not been successful. Diagnostic radiographs, computed tomography scan, magnetic resonance imaging, and serum markers are often not able to detect small residual disease. At present, there does not appear to be any alternative to the second-look laparotomy for the prompt diagnosis of persistent disease in the patient with a complete clinical response. The only alternative to second-look laparotomy is to monitor the patient with clinical examinations for recurrent disease. Unfortunately, the clinical diagnosis of recurrent cancer usually indicates the presence of large-volume disease.

Second-look laparotomy involves the use of a generous upper and lower midline incision and a thorough evaluation of the entire pelvic and abdominal cavity. Biopsy specimens from the pelvic sidewalls, the serosal surfaces of the rectum and bladder, and the cul-de-sac are required for adequate evaluation of the pelvis. In the upper abdomen, sites to be biopsied include both abdominal gutters, both diaphragmatic surfaces, and any residual omentum. Lymph node sampling should include the right and left paraaortic nodes and the right and left pelvic nodes. Washings for cytologic analysis should include the pelvis, both abdominal gutters, and both diaphragmatic surfaces. In addition, it is important to biopsy adhesions and any suspicious areas in the abdomen or pelvis. Most experts recommend a minimum of 25 biopsies, and often 40–50 samples are necessary.

The chance of a patient's having residual disease at second-look laparotomy is directly related to a variety of prognostic factors (stage of disease, histologic grade, and size of residual disease at initial laparotomy). Overall, 17% of patients with negative results at second-look laparotomy will develop recurrent cancer. If only patients with stage III and stage IV cancer who have grade 2 or 3 histologic features are considered, the recurrence rate approaches 50%.

Second-look laparotomy is not accepted as standard therapy by all physicians who treat ovarian cancer. Some authorities have argued that second-look laparotomy has never been proven to improve survival, while others have pointed out the lack of effective second-line therapy as a contraindication to second-look laparotomy. Although the first statement is true, in that no randomized trial has addressed the question of survival benefit in epithelial ovarian cancer, there are reports of success with salvage therapy in some series, and the major benefit appears to be in patients diagnosed as having minimal disease.

Palliative Surgery. Most patients who fail to be cured of ovarian cancer develop intestinal obstruction as the terminal event of their disease process. It appears that 50–75% of these patients can undergo some type of palliative resection of bypass surgery. Most of these patients will survive 4–6 months with the ability to take oral feedings. The mortality of such surgery is 12–30% and the rate of serious complications is 15–49%.

The patient and her family must be informed of the serious nature of the surgery and the limited success rate. However, for a great number of patients, the ability to have 4–6 months at home with the ability for a limited oral diet is sufficient reason to undertake the procedure. The recent improvements in the use of percutaneous gastrostomy are an acceptable alternative for many patients, since they can have limited oral intake supplemented by intravenous fluids administered at home.

Chemotherapy

Surgery alone is rarely curative and will by itself provide only brief palliation of advanced disease. Most patients with ovarian cancer will require adjunctive chemotherapy. Fortunately, ovarian cancer is a chemosensitive disease in most cases, with 75–80% of patients responding to chemotherapy as primary therapy. Unfortunately, many patients develop resistance to chemotherapy prior to complete eradication of the cancer. For these patients who have persistent cancer or who develop recurrent cancer, secondary, or salvage, chemotherapy is an important part of their therapy.

Primary Chemotherapy. Since the mid-1980s, the accepted standard regimen for advanced epithelial ovarian cancer has been cisplatin and cyclophosphamide, and the ideal duration of therapy is five to six courses. During the late 1980s, the first analogue of cisplatin, carboplatin, became available. Although hematologic toxicity is greater with carboplatin than with cisplatin, carboplatin produces less nausea and, because of less renal toxicity, can be given on an outpatient basis. Comparisons of cisplatin and carboplatin show similar results. Because of the ease of administration, most patients are treated with the combination of carboplatin and cyclophosphamide.

The Gynecologic Oncology Group recently reported the results of a randomized trial of a new drug, paclitaxel, in advanced epithelial ovarian cancer. In this trial, patients with suboptimal ovarian cancer (stage III disease greater than 1 cm or stage IV) received either cisplatin and cyclophosphamide or cisplatin and paclitaxel. In this trial, there was a significant improvement in complete response rate, overall response rate, and in disease-free survival for patients who received paclitaxel. Although this trial needs to be confirmed by other studies and a similar study needs to be conducted in patients with optimal disease, it appears that the standard primary chemotherapy regimen of the 1990s will be cisplatin and paclitaxel.

Salvage Chemotherapy. About 15–20% of patients with advanced epithelial ovarian cancer will be "cured" by initial surgery and primary chemotherapy, but 80–85% of patients either will have residual disease at the conclusion of initial therapy or will develop recurrent disease. For these patients, salvage therapy will be required. There are several important questions to be answered when considering the choice of salvage therapy. The two most important questions are the size and location of the persistent disease and whether the patient responds to cisplatin (or carboplatin). The definition of "platinum responder" requires that the patient had an initial response to cisplatin and did not develop regrowth of disease within 6 months.

For patients with small-volume persistent or recurrent disease that is confined to the peritoneal cavity, intraperitoneal chemotherapy may be a reasonable regimen. With large-volume disease (greater than 1 cm) or with disease located outside the peritoneal cavity, systemic chemotherapy should be chosen. Patients who are platinum responders can often be retreated with one of the platinum compounds, alone or in combination with other agents. The longer the disease-free interval from their primary chemotherapy, the better their chances of response; patients who have a disease-free interval of more than 2 years respond at a rate similar to that of newly diagnosed patients.

Patients who are platinum resistant and have not received paclitaxel should be treated with systemic paclitaxel. Paclitaxel has been shown to have a 30–35% response rate for salvage therapy and a 25–30% response rate as salvage therapy in platinum resistant patients. Other drugs that have been reported to show modest response rates are ifosfamide, hexamethylmelamine, and low-dose oral VP-16. All patients who require salvage therapy for epithelial ovarian cancer should be considered for clinical trials.

Radiation Therapy

The role of irradiation in the management of ovarian cancer remains controversial. There is little doubt that patients with early ovarian cancer and patients with microscopic residual advanced epithelial ovarian cancer can be cured with whole-abdominal radiation therapy. Although there has never been a randomized trial of modern multidrug chemotherapy and whole-abdominal radiotherapy, there are few centers using radiotherapy as primary treatment of epithelial ovarian cancer. Most specialists believe the complication rates to be higher with irradiation; however, the lack of a randomized trial does not allow that conclusion to be established.

Radiation therapy may also be used as palliative therapy for selected patients who are symptomatic from localized disease and who do not respond to conventional chemotherapy. Examples of such palliative therapy are the control of vaginal bleeding for cancer metastatic to the vagina or temporary control of persistent pelvic disease in an attempt to avoid a colostomy. Such therapy is palliative, however, since the spread pattern of the disease makes it unlikely that there are not metastases outside of the pelvis.

Follow-up Care

Patients with early ovarian cancer usually have a low recurrence rate, provided that they had full surgical staging and received appropriate therapy. Exceptions to this general statement would be patients with clear cell cancers of the ovary. Because of the low recurrence rate, follow-up recommendations are for a gynecologic examination and a serum CA 125 determination every 3 months for the first year, every 4 months for the second year, and every 6 months for the next 3 years. After 5 years, annual examinations are recommended. Annual Pap tests are recommended, but there is no proven benefit to diagnostic radiographs or computed tomography scans.

Patients with advanced ovarian cancer have a very high recurrence rate. This recurrence rate approaches 75% in patients monitored after a complete clinical response and 50% after a complete pathologic response (negative second-look laparotomy). For these patients, follow-up should be more intensive. They should have a gynecologic examination and a serum CA 125 determination every 2 months for the first 6 months and reevaluation every 3 months for the next 18 months. Follow-up at 4-month intervals is recommended for the next 3 years, after which patients should be followed at 6-month intervals. Generally, chest X-rays are indicated at 6-month intervals for the first 2 years, and then yearly until 5 years of follow-up are completed. The use of routine computed tomography scans is debatable, although many experts do recommend scans for follow-up of patients who did not have a second-look laparotomy. The optimum frequency for such scans has not been established.

The value of the serum CA 125 test in the follow-up of patients with epithelial ovarian cancer depends in large part on whether or not the patient originally had an elevated serum level (prior to therapy). The level of CA 125 does not always correlate with tumor volume, and an elevation of the CA 125 may occur after the disease has grown quite large. Nevertheless, this serum test does appear to be the best follow-up test available.

GERM CELL TUMORS

Malignant germ cell tumors of the ovary occur primarily in women in the second and third decades of life, although they will occasionally be seen in young girls and older women. Patients with one of these tumors usually present with abdominal pain, and almost 10% will present with an acute episode related to torsion, hemorrhage, or rupture of the tumor.

Germ cell tumors may have elevated serum levels of the beta subunit of human chorionic gonadotropin (β-hCG), alpha-fetoprotein, or lactic dehydrogenase. Measurement of these markers may help in the diagnosis of germ cell tumors and, when elevated, is useful in the management and follow-up of these patients. The distribution of markers is shown in Table 5-7. There is considerable variation in the production of markers, although most endodermal sinus tumors produce alpha-fetoprotein, and most choriocarcinomas and dysgerminomas produce β-hCG and lactic dehydrogenase, respectively.

With modern platinum-based multidrug chemotherapy, the prognosis for most patients with completely resected malignant germ cell tumors of the ovary is quite good. Of 85 patients given adjunctive therapy with either bleomycin, etoposide, and platinum or platinum, vinblastine, and bleomycin, 83 are progression free (98%). In comparison, patients who

TABLE 5-7. SERUM MARKERS IN MALIGNANT GERM CELL TUMORS OF THE OVARY

Malignant Germ Cell Tumor	AFP	β-hCG	LDH	CA 125
Endodermal sinus tumor	+	−	±	±
Embryonal carcinoma	+	+	±	±
Choriocarcinoma	−	+	±	±
Immature teratoma	±	−	±	±
Dysgerminoma	−	±	+	±
Mixed germ cell tumor	±[†]	±[†]	±[†]	±[†]

[†] Results depend on the type of germ cell tumors present.
* AFP indicates alpha-fetoprotein; β-hCG, beta subunit of human chorionic gonadotropin; LDH, lactic dehydrogenase.

have residual or persistent disease or who develop recurrences have a progression-free survival rate of only 59% (71/120 patients) when treated with similar regimens.

From these figures, it should be apparent that survival is enhanced by complete reduction of malignant germ cell tumors of the ovary. Every effort should be made to resect the disease completely. Despite this need for complete disease reduction, there is no need to remove reproductive organs not involved by the cancer. These tumors are virtually never bilateral. Thus, even patients with advanced disease who do not have involvement of the other ovary and the uterus should have those organs conserved. Because of the high cure rate in these patients with multidrug chemotherapy, many will retain their reproductive capability.

Patients with malignant germ cell tumors of the ovary should undergo surgical staging in a manner similar to that for patients with epithelial ovarian cancer. However, since most of these patients will require chemotherapy, reexploration for staging is not indicated unless the goal is to resect the residual cancer completely. It is best to begin chemotherapy in these patients as soon as possible, since these tumors grow and recur rapidly. The starting of chemotherapy in patients with malignant germ cell tumors is one of the few oncologic emergencies, in that every effort should be made not to delay therapy.

The potential benefit of second-look laparotomy in malignant germ cell tumors of the ovary has been debated for several years. There has been no benefit demonstrated for second-look laparotomy except in incompletely resected immature teratomas, and its routine use in other malignant germ cell tumors cannot be justified.

STROMAL TUMORS

Sex cord–stromal or sex cord–mesenchymal tumor describes a group of tumors that includes tumors of the female type (granulosa cell tumor and granulosa–theca cell tumors), tumors of the male type (Sertoli–Leydig cell tumors), and very rare tumors such as the lipid cell tumor and gynandroblastoma. Most of these rare tumors will never be seen by the practicing gynecologist, but it is important to have a basic understanding of the category of tumors and their malignant potential.

The granulosa cell tumor is the most common malignant tumor of this group of neoplasms. These tumors are seen throughout a woman's life but are more common in the first four decades. They are bilateral in about 5% of cases. All granulosa cell tumors should be considered potentially malignant, and late recurrences are common with this tumor. There are two major histologic types, the adult variety and the juvenile form. The juvenile form is much more likely to behave in a malignant fashion.

The therapy of granulosa cell tumors is surgical removal, and there is no proven benefit for adjunctive therapy. In younger patients who desire further childbearing, unilateral salpingo-oophorectomy and full surgical staging is the treatment of choice. Patients with residual or recurrent disease should receive chemotherapy. The usual choice of chemotherapy is bleomycin, etoposide, and platinum, as for germ cell tumors. There are too few reported series of granulosa cell tumors treated with chemotherapy to provide accurate figures about response rates with chemotherapy.

Young patients with granulosa cell tumors may experience precocious puberty, since these tumors may produce estrogen. In the older woman, menstrual irregularity or postmenopausal bleeding secondary to estrogen production may be the presenting symptom.

Sertoli–Leydig cell tumors occur less frequently than granulosa cell tumors and are rarely bilateral. These tumors may produce androgens and can present clinically with defeminization or masculinization. The malignant potential of these tumors is directly related to the degree of differentiation, and they are usually classified as well differentiated, moderately differentiated, and poorly differentiated. A fourth classification is Sertoli–Leydig cell tumors with heterologous elements.

The treatment of these tumors is surgical removal, and unilateral salpingo-oophorectomy is indicated for properly staged patients with tumors confined to one ovary. Little is known about the responsiveness of these tumors to modern chemotherapy, but most authors recommend bleomycin, etoposide, and platinum chemotherapy for persistent or recurrent disease.

The remainder of the various stromal tumors are very rare. In general, the therapy is total abdominal hysterectomy and bilateral salpingo-oophorectomy, with full surgical staging for patients who do not desire further childbearing. For younger patients, unilateral salpingo-oophorectomy and full surgical staging are indicated.

CANCER OF THE FALLOPIAN TUBE

The fallopian tube is the least common site of cancer in the female genital tract, accounting for fewer than 1,000 new cases each year. Histologically, these tumors resemble papillary serous carcinoma of the ovary in more than 90% of cases. The four criteria for the diagnosis of primary fallopian tube carcinoma are:

1. The main tumor is in the tube and arises from the endosalpinx.
2. The pattern histologically resembles the epithelium of the mucosa and usually shows a papillary pattern.
3. If the wall is involved, the transition between benign and malignant tubal epithelium should be demonstrable.
4. The ovaries and endometrium are either normal or contain less tumor than the tubes.

As can be seen, the major problem is to distinguish these cancers from primary ovarian cancers. The staging system used for fallopian tube cancer (see box) is modified from the current staging of ovarian cancer. This is a staging system of con-

---

Operative Staging of Fallopian Tube Carcinoma

Stage I: Growth limited to the tubes
  A. Growth limited to one tube; no ascites
  B. Growth limited to both tubes; no ascites
  C. Tumor either Stage IA or IB with malignant ascites or positive peritoneal washings

Stage II: Growth involving one or both tubes with pelvic extension
  A. Extension and/or metastases to the ovaries and/or uterus
  B. Extension to other pelvic tissues
  C. Tumor either Stage IIA or IIB with malignant ascites or positive peritoneal washings

Stage III: Tumor involving one or both tubes with peritoneal implants outside the pelvis and/or positive retroperitoneal or inguinal nodes; tumor is limited to the true pelvis but with histologically verified malignant extension to the small bowel or omentum
  A. Tumor grossly limited to the true pelvis with negative nodes but with histologically confirmed microscopic seeding of abdominal peritoneal surfaces
  B. Tumor of one or both tubes with histologically confirmed implants on abdominal peritoneal surfaces, none exceeding 2 cm in diameter; nodes negative
  C. Abdominal implants greater than 2 cm in diameter and/or positive retroperitoneal or inguinal nodes

Stage IV: Growth involving one or both tubes with distant metastases; if pleural effusion is present, positive cytologic confirmation must be made; parenchymal liver metastases equals Stage IV

Modified from Markman M, Zaino RJ, Busowski JD, Barakat RR. Carcinoma of the fallopian tube. In: Hoskins WJ, Perez CA, Young RC, eds. Principles and practice of gynecologic oncology. Philadelphia: JB Lippincott, 1992. Adapted from International Federation of Gynecology and Obstetrics. Annual report on the results of treatment in gynecological cancer. Int J Gynecol Obstet 1989;28:189–190

vention, since FIGO has not established an official staging system for fallopian tube cancer.

The pattern of spread of fallopian tube cancer is similar to that for ovarian cancer. The classic triad of colicky pain, abnormal bleeding, and leukorrhea is rarely seen in its entirety, with the most commonly seen symptom being abnormal vaginal bleeding. Pain, however, is reported frequently as an early symptom.

The therapy for fallopian tube cancer is similar to that for ovarian cancer, with the most important initial therapy being effective tumor-reducing surgery. Residual disease, as in ovarian cancer, is a good predictor of poor survival. The choice for adjuvant therapy is chemotherapy with platinum-based multidrug therapy, followed by a second-look laparotomy and second-line therapy as necessary. There are no reports of the use of paclitaxel for fallopian tube cancer, but one would surmise that this drug will have a significant role in the treatment of the disease.

BIBLIOGRAPHY

Campbell S, Bhan V, Royston P, Whitehead MI, Collins WP. Transabdominal ultrasound screening for early ovarian cancer. BMJ 1989;299:1363–1367

Colombo N, Sessa C, Landoni F, Sartori E, Pecorelli S, Mangioni C. Cisplatin, vinblastine, and bleomycin combination chemotherapy in metastatic granulosa cell tumor of the ovary. Obstet Gynecol 1986; 67:265–268

Dembo AJ, Davy M, Stenwig AE, Berle EJ, Bush RS, Kjorstad K. Prognostic factors in patients with stage I epithelial ovarian cancer. Obstet Gynecol 1990;75:263–273

DiSaia PJ, Creasman WT. Clinical gynecologic oncology. 4th ed. St Louis: Mosby–Year Book, 1993:300–466

Gershenson DM. Menstrual and reproductive function after treatment with combination chemotherapy for malignant ovarian germ cell tumors. J Clin Oncol 1988;6:270–275

Gershenson DM, Kavanagh JJ, Copeland LJ, Del Junco G, Cangir A, Saul PB, et al. Treatment of malignant nondysgerminomatous germ cell tumors of the ovary with vinblastine, bleomycin, and cisplatin. Cancer 1986;57:1731–1737

Griffiths CT. Surgery at the time of diagnosis in ovarian cancer. In: Blackledge G, Chan KK, eds. Management of ovarian cancer. London: Butterworths, 1986:60–75

Hoskins WJ, Bundy BN, Thigpen JT, Omura GA. The influence of cytoreductive surgery on recurrence-free interval and survival in small-volume stage III epithelial ovarian cancer: a Gynecologic Oncology Group study. Gynecol Oncol 1992;47:159–166

Hoskins WJ, Rubin SC, Dulaney E, Chapman D, Almadrones L, Saigo P, et al. Influence of secondary cytoreduction at the time of second-look laparotomy on the survival of patients with epithelial ovarian carcinoma. Gynecol Oncol 1989;34:365–371

Houlston RS, Collins A, Slack J, Campbell S, Collins WP, Whitehead MI, et al. Genetic epidemiology of ovarian cancer: segregation analysis. Ann Hum Genet 1991;55:291–299

Jacobs I, Bast RC Jr. The CA 125 tumor-associated antigen: a review of the literature. Hum Reprod 1989;4:1–12

Levin L, Hryniuk WM. Dose intensity analysis of chemotherapy regimens in ovarian carcinoma. J Clin Oncol 1987;5:756–767

Lynch HT, Guirgis HA, Albert S, Brennan M, Lynch J, Kraft C, et al. Familial association of carcinoma of the breast and ovary. Surg Gynecol Obstet 1974;138:717–724

Markman M, Hoskins WJ, eds. Cancer of the ovary. New York: Raven Press, 1993

McGuire WP, Rowinsky EK, Rosenshein NB, Grumbine FC, Ettinger DS, Armstrong DK, et al. Taxol: a unique antineoplastic agent with significant activity in advanced ovarian epithelial neoplasms. Ann Intern Med 1989;111:273–279

Morrow CP, Curtin JP, Townsend DE, eds. Tumors of the ovary. In: Synopsis of gynecologic oncology. 4th ed. New York: Churchill Livingstone, 1993:215–301

Neijt JP, ten Bokkel Huinink WW, ven der Burg MEL, van Oosterom AT, Willemse PH, Heintz AP, et al. Randomized trial comparing two combination chemotherapy regimens (CHAP-5 v CP) in advanced ovarian carcinoma. J Clin Oncol 1987;5:1157–1168

Ng LW, Rubin SC, Hoskins WJ, Jones WB, Hakes TB, Markman M, et al. Aggressive chemosurgical debulking in patients with advanced ovarian cancer. Gynecol Oncol 1990;38:358–363

Omura GA, Brady MF, Homesley HD, Yordan E, Major FJ, Buchsbaum HJ, et al. Long-term follow-up and prognostic factor analysis in advanced ovarian carcinoma: the Gynecologic Oncology Group experience. J Clin Oncol 1991;9:1138–1150

Omura GA, Bundy BN, Berek JS, Curry S, Delgado G, Mortel R. Randomized trial of cyclophosphamide plus cisplatin with or without doxorubicin in ovarian carcinoma: a Gynecologic Oncology Group Study. J Clin Oncol 1989;7:457–465

Ozols RF, Rubin SC, Dembo AJ, Robboy S. Epithelial ovarian cancer. In: Hoskins WJ, Perez CA, Young RC, eds. Principles and practice of gynecologic oncology. Philadelphia: JB Lippincott, 1992: 731–781

The reduction in risk of ovarian cancer associated with oral-contraceptive use. The Cancer and Steroid Hormone Study of the Centers for Disease Control and the National Institutes of Child Health and Human Development. N Engl J Med 1987;316:650–655

Reichman B, Markman M, Hakes T, Hoskins W, Rubin S, Jones W, et al. Intraperitoneal cisplatin and etoposide in the treatment of refractory/recurrent ovarian carcinoma. J Clin Oncol 1989;7:1327–1332

Rubin SC, Hoskins WJ, Saigo PE, Chapman D, Hakes TB, Markman M, et al. Prognostic factors for recurrence following negative second-look laparotomy in ovarian cancer patients treated with platinum-based chemotherapy. Gynecol Oncol 1991;42:137–141

Rubin SC, Lewis JL Jr. Second-look surgery in ovarian carcinoma. Crit Rev Oncol Hematol 1988;8:75–91

Rubin SC, Sutton GP, eds. Ovarian cancer. New York: McGraw-Hill, 1993

Scully RE. Recent progress in ovarian cancer. Hum Pathol 1970;1:73–98

Van Nagell JR Jr, DePriest PD, Puls LE, Donaldson ES, Gallion HH, Pavlik EJ, et al. Ovarian cancer screening in asymptomatic postmenopausal women by transvaginal sonography. Cancer 1991;68:458–462

Williams SD, Birch R, Einhorn LH, Irwin L, Greco FA, Loehrer PJ. Treatment of disseminated germ-cell tumors with cisplatin, bleomycin, and either vinblastine or etoposide. N Engl J Med 1987;316:1435–1440

Williams SD, Blessing JA, Hatch KD, Homesley HD. Chemotherapy of advanced dysgerminoma: trials of the Gynecologic Oncology Group. J Clin Oncol 1991;9:1950–1955

Williams SD, Blessing JA, Moore DH, Homesley HD, Adcock L. Cisplatin, vinblastine, and bleomycin in advanced and recurrent ovarian germ-cell tumors: a trial of the Gynecologic Oncology Group. Ann Intern Med 1989;111:22–27

Williams SD, Gershenson DM, Horowitz CJ, Scully RE. Ovarian germ cell and stromal tumors. In: Hoskins WJ, Perez CA, Young RC, eds. Principles and practice of gynecologic oncology. Philadelphia: JB Lippincott, 1992:715–730

Gestational Trophoblastic Disease

Gestational trophoblastic disease encompasses four clinicopathologic forms of growth disturbances of the human trophoblast: 1) hydatidiform mole, 2) invasive mole, 3) choriocarcinoma, and 4) placental site trophoblastic tumor. The term *gestational trophoblastic tumor* has been applied to the latter three conditions because the diagnosis and decision to institute treatment are often undertaken without knowledge of the precise histology. These diseases are unique because of the elaboration of the tumor marker hCG, the inherent sensitivity of trophoblastic tumors to chemotherapy, and the immunobiologic relationship between the disease and its host.

HYDATIDIFORM MOLE

Hydatidiform mole is a pregnancy that is characterized by vesicular swelling of placental villi and, usually, the absence of an intact fetus. Microscopically, there is proliferation of the trophoblast (both cytotrophoblast and syncytiotrophoblast) with varying degrees of hyperplasia and dysplasia. The chorionic villi are fluid filled and distended, and blood vessels are scanty. Two syndromes of hydatidiform mole have been described based on both cytogenetic and morphologic criteria. Complete or classic hydatidiform mole undergoes early and total hydatidiform enlargement of villi in the absence of an ascertainable fetus or embryo, and the trophoblast is consistently hyperplastic. It usually has a 46,XX karyotype derived from a paternal haploid set that totally replaces the maternal contribution and reaches the 46,XX status by its own duplication. Occasionally, a 46,XY karyotype occurs as a result of dispermic fertilization of an empty egg. Partial hydatidiform moles are characterized by slowly progressing hydatidiform change in the presence of functioning villous capillaries that affects only some of the villi. This is associated with an identifiable fetus or embryo (alive or dead), or fetal membranes or red blood cells. Trophoblastic immaturity is constant, and there is only focal hyperplasia. Partial moles have a triploid karyotype, usually 69,XXY. It may be difficult to distinguish partial moles from abortuses with hydropic degeneration. Trophoblastic sequelae (invasive mole or choriocarcinoma) follow complete hydatidiform mole in 15–20% of cases and are more commonly associated with heterozygote moles. The reported incidence of trophoblastic sequelae following partial mole varies between 4% and 11%, with metastases occurring rarely. A histopathologic diagnosis of choriocarcinoma has not been confirmed following a partial hydatidiform mole.

Incidence

The incidence of hydatidiform mole varies greatly throughout the world. In the United States and Europe the incidence is approximately 1/1,500 pregnancies. In other areas, especially the Orient, the incidence has been reported to be more than 1/100 normal pregnancies. Much of this geographic variation may in fact be due to reporting differences rather than true incidence differences. Hydatidiform moles recur in 0.5–2.6% of patients, with a subsequent greater risk of developing invasive mole or choriocarcinoma after repeated molar gestations. There is an increased risk of molar pregnancy for women more than 40 years of age and those at the younger end of the reproductive range, although there does not appear to be any significant association with gravidity.

Diagnosis

The outstanding clinical feature of hydatidiform mole is uterine bleeding, usually occurring at 6–16 weeks of gestation in over 95% of patients. About 50% of patients will have rapid uterine enlargement greater than expected for gestational dates. Preeclampsia in the first or second trimester or hyperemesis occurs in about one fourth of patients. Clinical hyperthyroidism and trophoblastic emboli with symptoms and signs of congestive heart failure and pulmonary edema occur in a small number of patients. Bilateral theca lutein cyst enlargement of the ovaries occurs in about 15% of cases. Fetal heart tones are usually absent.

Hydatidiform mole is confirmed by 1) spontaneous passage of typical molar tissue, 2) failure to visualize a fetal skeleton on X-ray after 16 weeks of gestation, 3) amniography, or 4) ultrasonography that demonstrates multiples echoes and holes within the placental mass and usually no fetus. Ultrasonography has virtually replaced all other means of preoperative diagnosis of hydatidiform mole. Human chorionic gonadotropin levels are usually, but not always, elevated above levels for normal pregnancy; therefore, a single hCG level is seldom helpful. Hydatidiform mole must be distinguished from 1) a normal intrauterine pregnancy, 2) a threatened or missed abortion, 3) an intrauterine pregnancy complicated by multiple gestation or diseases associated with an enlarged placenta and elevated hCG levels (eg, erythroblastosis fetalis and intrauterine infections), and 4) an enlarged uterus secondary to uterine leiomyomata with a small normal intrauterine pregnancy.

Treatment

When the diagnosis of hydatidiform mole is established, the molar pregnancy should be evacuated. The preoperative evaluation should consist of the history and physical examination, complete blood and platelet counts, coagulation profile, serum chemistries, thyroid panel, blood type and crossmatch, serum hCG level, urinalysis, chest X-ray, electrocardiography, and pelvic ultrasonography. The preferred method of evacuation, independent of uterine size, is suction curettage followed by gentle sharp curettage. An oxytocic agent should be infused intravenously (IV) near the end of evacuation and continued for several hours to enhance uterine contractility. Hysterectomy is an alternative to suction curettage if childbearing is complete. There is no place for hysterotomy or medical induction of labor in the management of molar evacuation, as these methods increase morbidity and the subsequent development of postmolar trophoblastic disease.

Follow-up

Follow-up of patients after evacuation of a hydatidiform mole indicates that this therapy is curative in more than 80% of patients. Incomplete involution of the uterus and vaginal bleeding may be signs of persistent trophoblastic disease, and a curettage should be performed. Clinical findings such as prompt uterine involution, ovarian cyst regression, and cessation of bleeding are all optimistic signs. Definitive follow-up, however, requires serial hCG testing using an assay of sufficient sensitivity. Quantitative serum hCG levels should be obtained every 1–2 weeks until negative for three consecutive determinations, followed by every 3 months for 6–12 months. Contraception should be maintained during this follow-up period. Oral contraceptives are acceptable, although any effective method is satisfactory.

Patients at highest risk for postmolar trophoblastic tumors are those with 1) preevacuation uterine size larger than expected for gestational duration or size greater than that at 20 weeks of gestation, 2) bilateral ovarian enlargement (theca lutein cysts) greater than 6 cm; 3) age greater than 40 years; 4) very high hCG levels; 5) medical complications of molar pregnancy such as toxemia, hyperthyroidism, and trophoblastic embolization; and 6) repeat hydatidiform mole. Prophylactic chemotherapy at the time of or immediately after molar evacuation may be considered for these high-risk patients.

Indications for treatment of postmolar trophoblastic tumor are 1) plateauing hCG levels for three consecutive weekly determinations, 2) rising hCG levels for 2 consecutive weeks, 3) high hCG levels (greater than 20,000 mIU/ml) more than 4 weeks after evacuation, 4) persistently elevated hCG levels 6 months after evacuation, 5) detection of metastases, and 6) histopathologic diagnosis of choriocarcinoma.

GESTATIONAL TROPHOBLASTIC TUMORS

Gestational trophoblastic tumors—trophoblastic diseases that can progress, invade, metastasize, and kill, if untreated—include invasive mole, choriocarcinoma, and placental site trophoblastic tumor. The overall cure rate in the treatment of gestational trophoblastic tumors now exceeds 90%. This success is the result of 1) the chemotherapy-sensitive nature of trophoblastic tumors; 2) the ability to make a diagnosis and monitor therapy effectively by using hCG as a tumor marker; 3) the referral of patients to specialized treatment centers; 4) the identification of prognostic factors, which enhances individualization of therapy; and 5) the aggressive use of combination chemotherapy, irradiation, and surgery in the care of high-risk patients.

Invasive mole, a benign tumor, arises from myometrial invasion by a hydatidiform mole, via direct extension or venous channels. It may metastasize to distant sites in about 15% of cases, most commonly to the lungs and vagina. The tumor is characterized by swollen placental villi and accompanying trophoblast with hyperplasia and usually dysplasia located in sites outside the cavity of the uterus. Invasive mole tends to undergo spontaneous regression. The overall incidence of invasive mole has been estimated to be 1/15,000 pregnancies. Approximately 10–17% of hydatidiform moles will result in invasive mole. The diagnosis is most often made clinically, based on rising or persistently elevated hCG levels after evacuation of a hydatidiform mole. Hysterectomy or biopsy of metastatic lesions in order to obtain pathologic confirmation is usually not performed because of the excellent success in treating the disease with chemotherapy.

Choriocarcinoma, a malignant disease, is characterized by abnormal trophoblastic hyperplasia and anaplasia; absence of chorionic villi; hemorrhage and necrosis; direct invasion of the myometrium; and vascular spread to the myometrium and distant sites, the most common being the lungs, brain, liver, pelvis or vagina, spleen, intestines, and kidney. Gestational choriocarcinoma may arise in association with any type of pregnancy. Approximately 2–3% of hydatidiform moles progress to choriocarcinoma, which accounts for almost 50% of cases, whereas 25% of cases follow abortion or tubal pregnancy and 25% are associated with term gestation. The incidence of choriocarcinoma is, therefore, about 1/40,000 pregnancies.

Placental site trophoblastic tumor, an extremely rare disease, arises from the placental implantation site and resembles syncytial endomyometritis. Pathologically, tumor cells infiltrate the myometrium and grow between smooth muscle cells, but, unlike syncytial endomyometritis, there is vascular invasion. Placental site trophoblastic tumor differs from choriocarcinoma primarily because of the absence of an alternating pattern of syncytiotrophoblast and cytotrophoblast, the cells being of one type called intermediate cells, and hemorrhage and necrosis are less evident. There are no placental villi. Human placental lactogen is present in the tumor cells, whereas immunoperoxidase staining for hCG is positive in only scattered cells. Serum hCG levels are relatively low compared with choriocarcinoma. Although most reports have noted a benign course for these tumors, deaths from metastatic disease have occurred. These tumors are relatively resistant to chemotherapy, and surgery has been the mainstay of treatment.

Diagnosis

Gestational trophoblastic tumor is most often diagnosed by rising or plateauing hCG levels following evacuation of a molar pregnancy. Occasionally, the diagnosis of choriocarcinoma is made based on persistent elevation of hCG levels, frequently in conjunction with the demonstration of metastases, following other pregnancy events. Pathologic diagnosis can sometimes be made by curettage, biopsy of metastatic lesions, or occasionally examination of hysterectomy specimens or placentas. Biopsy of a vaginal lesion is infrequently performed because of the massive uncontrolled bleeding that may occur.

Symptoms and Signs

The symptom most suggestive of trophoblastic tumor is continued uterine bleeding after evacuation of a hydatidiform mole or following any pregnancy event. Bleeding from uterine perforation or metastatic lesions may be expressed as abdominal pain, hemoptysis, melena, or evidence of increased intracranial pressure from intracerebral hemorrhage leading to headache, seizures, or hemiplegia. Patients may also present with pulmonary symptoms such as dyspnea, cough, and chest pain secondary to extensive lung metastases.

Signs suggestive of postmolar trophoblastic tumor are an enlarged, irregular uterus and persistent bilateral ovarian enlargement. Occasionally, a metastatic lesion is noted on examination, most commonly in the vagina. Choriocarcinoma associated with a nonmolar gestation has no characteristic physical signs but may produce findings as a result of metastatic disease.

Gestational trophoblastic tumors must be distinguished from 1) retained products of conception or endometritis as causes of postpartum uterine bleeding and subinvolution, 2) primary or metastatic tumors of other organ systems, and 3) another pregnancy occurring shortly after the first.

Classification and Staging

Once a gestational trophoblastic tumor has been diagnosed, it is necessary to determine the extent of disease. After a thorough history and physical examination, the following clinical studies should be obtained: chest X-ray with computed tomography scan of the lungs if negative, computed tomography scan of the abdomen and pelvis, computed tomography scan or magnetic resonance imaging of the brain, complete blood and platelet counts, serum chemistries (including liver and renal function studies), and a quantitative serum hCG. After these initial studies, patients are categorized based on anatomic extent of disease and likelihood of response to various chemotherapeutic protocols, and treatment is carried out accordingly.

A variety of classification and scoring systems are now used to group patients with gestational trophoblastic tumors for treatment purposes. Most major U.S. trophoblastic disease centers have used a clinical classification system, based on prognostic factors originally described by investigators at the National Cancer Institute, to determine treatment and report results (see box). An anatomic staging system conforming to those used for all other gynecologic cancers was adopted by FIGO Cancer Committee in 1982 and amended in 1992 (see box). In 1983, the World Health Organization adopted a prognostic scoring system based on a number of factors, to each of which a score is applied (Table 5-8).

Therapy

Nonmetastatic Tumors

Hysterectomy is used as primary therapy in patients with presumed nonmetastatic trophoblastic tumors who no longer wish to preserve fertility or if the diagnosis is placental site trophoblastic tumor. Adjuvant single-agent chemotherapy at

---

National Cancer Institute Prognostic Group Clinical Classification

I. Nonmetastatic Gestational Trophoblastic Tumor

II. Metastatic Gestational Trophoblastic Tumor
   A. Low-Risk
      1. hCG <100,000 IU/24-h urine or <40,000 mIU/ml serum
      2. Symptoms present for less than 4 months
      3. No brain or liver metastases
      4. No prior chemotherapy
      5. Pregnancy event is not term delivery (ie, mole, ectopic, or spontaneous abortion)
   B. High-Risk
      1. hCG > 100,000 IU/24-h urine or > 40,000 mIU/ml serum
      2. Symptoms present for more than 4 months
      3. Brain or liver metastases
      4. Prior chemotherapeutic failure
      5. Antecedent term pregnancy

FIGO Clinical Staging for Tumors

Stage I	Disease confined to uterus
Stage II	Gestational trophoblastic tumor extending outside the uterus but limited to genital structures (adnexa, vagina, broad ligament)
Stage III	Gestational trophoblastic tumor extending to lungs with or without known genital tract involvement
Stage IV	All other metastatic sites

Modified from FIGO Oncology Committee report. Int J Gynecol Obstet 1992;39:149–150

TABLE 5-8. WORLD HEALTH ORGANIZATION SCORING SYSTEM BASED ON PROGNOSTIC FACTORS

Risk Factors	Score* 0	1	2	4
Age (y)	≤39	>39		
Antecedent pregnancy	Hydatidiform mole	Abortion	Term	
Pregnancy event to treatment interval (mo)	<4	4–6	7–12	>12
hCG (IU/L)	$<10^3$	10^3–10^4	10^4–10^5	$>10^5$
ABO blood groups (female × male)		O × A A × O	B AB	
Number of metastases		1–4	4–8	>8
Site of metastases		Spleen Kidney	GI tract Liver	Brain
Largest tumor mass, including uterine (cm)		3–5	>5	
Prior chemotherapy			Single drug	Two or more drugs

* The total score for a patient is obtained by adding the individual scores for each prognostic factor. Total score: ≤4 = low-risk; 5–7 = middle-risk; ≥8 = high-risk.

the time of operation has been assumed to eradicate any occult metastases and reduce the likelihood of tumor dissemination and implantation.

Single-agent chemotherapy with methotrexate or actinomycin D is the treatment of choice for those patients wishing to preserve their fertility. Several different chemotherapy protocols have been used, all yielding excellent and fairly comparable remission rates. Methotrexate, 0.4 mg/kg IV or IM daily for 5 days per treatment course, has traditionally been the treatment of choice. Alternately, a regimen using slightly higher doses of methotrexate, 1.0–1.5 mg/kg IM every other day for four doses, with folinic acid, 0.1–0.15 mg/kg IM 24 hours after each dose of methotrexate, has been used. This protocol has the advantage of decreased toxicity, especially stomatitis, but the disadvantages of increased cost, patient inconvenience, and an increased need for a change in chemotherapy to achieve remission. These methotrexate chemotherapy courses are repeated as often as toxicity permits, usually every 12–14 days (7–9-day window). Methotrexate has also been given in single weekly doses of 30–50 mg/m² IM, for treatment of postmolar nonmetastatic disease only. Actinomycin D, 10–13 μg/kg IV daily for 5 days or as a single dose of 1.25 mg/m² IV every other week, has been used alternatively and is the appropriate therapeutic regimen for patients with hepatic or renal disease or effusions contraindicating the use of methotrexate. Chemotherapy is changed to the alternative agent if the hCG level plateaus or if toxicity precludes an adequate dose or frequency of treatment. If there is a significant elevation in hCG level or development of metastases, multiagent chemotherapy should be started. Treatment is continued until three consecutive normal hCG levels have been obtained and one or two courses have been given after the first normal hCG level.

Cure is anticipated in essentially all patients with nonmetastatic disease. Approximately 85% of patients will be cured by the initial chemotherapy regimen. Most of the remaining patients will be placed into permanent remission with additional chemotherapy. Fewer than 5% of patients will require hysterectomy for cure, resulting in preservation of reproductive function in more than 95% of patients.

Metastatic Tumors

Low-Risk Disease. Single-agent chemotherapy with 5-day dosage schedules of methotrexate or actinomycin D, as described above in the section on nonmetastatic disease, is the treatment for patients in this category. When resistance to sequential single-agent chemotherapy develops, combination chemotherapy as for high-risk disease is used. Hysterectomy may be necessary to eradicate persistent, chemotherapy-resistant disease in the uterus, or it may be performed as adjuvant treatment coincident with the institution of chemotherapy to shorten the duration of therapy.

Cure rates should approach 100% in this group of patients if treatment is administered properly. Approximately 40–50% of patients in this category will develop resistance to the first chemotherapeutic agent and require alternative treatment. It is therefore very important to carefully monitor patients undergoing treatment for evidence of drug resistance so that a change to a second agent can be made at the earliest possible time. About 10–15% of patients treated for low-risk metastatic disease with sequential single-agent chemotherapy will require combination chemotherapy with or without surgery to achieve remission.

High-Risk Disease. Patients with high-risk metastatic gestational trophoblastic tumors should be treated more aggressively with initial combination chemotherapy with or without adjuvant radiation therapy or surgery. Since the discovery of etoposide to be a very effective agent in gestational trophoblastic tumors, all currently acceptable protocols for the treatment of high-risk disease must include this drug, along with methotrexate and actinomycin D. The EMA-CO regimen uses etoposide, 100 mg/m^2 IV on days 1 and 2; high-dose methotrexate, 100 mg/m^2 IV push plus 200 mg/m^2 IV infusion over 12 hours on day 1 (with folinic acid rescue, 15 mg IM every 12 hours for four doses beginning 24 hours after starting the methotrexate); actinomycin D, 0.5 mg IV on days 1 and 2; cyclophosphamide, 600 mg/m^2 IV on day 8; and vincristine, 1.0 mg/m^2 IV on day 8. The treatment cycle is repeated every 2 weeks (ie, days 15, 16, and 22). When brain metastases are detected, the dosage of methotrexate in the EMA-CO regimen is increased to 1 g/m^2 in conjunction with folinic acid, 30 mg every 12 hours for 3 days starting 32 hours after the beginning of the infusion. This protocol has proved to be very useful and relatively nontoxic. The EMA-CO protocol or some variation of it is now the treatment of choice for high-risk patients, replacing the old triple-chemotherapy regimen of methotrexate, actinomycin D, and cyclophosphamide or chlorambucil. Cisplatin and bleomycin are other chemotherapeutic agents with proven activity in trophoblastic tumors, and combinations of these agents with etoposide have resulted in some cures in patients who have failed initial therapy. Chemotherapy is continued until three consecutive normal hCG levels are reached and two to four courses have been given after the first normal hCG level.

If central nervous system metastases are present, whole-brain irradiation (2,000–3,000 cGy) is given simultaneously with the initiation of combination chemotherapy using high-dose (1 g/m^2) infusion methotrexate with folinic acid rescue. Adjuvant surgical procedures, especially hysterectomy and thoracotomy, may be useful for the purpose of removing known foci of chemotherapy-resistant disease, controlling hemorrhage, relieving bowel or urinary obstruction, treating infection, or dealing with other life-threatening complications.

Intensive therapy with combination chemotherapy and, when indicated, adjuvant radiotherapy and surgery has resulted in cure rates of 80–90% in patients with high-risk metastatic gestational trophoblastic tumors. The factors most important in determining treatment response in these patients are 1) clinicopathologic diagnosis of choriocarcinoma, 2) metastases to sites other than the lung and vagina, 3) number of metastases, and 4) failure of previous chemotherapy. Most treatment failure can now be attributed to presence of extensive choriocarcinoma at the time of diagnosis or lack of appropriate initial treatment.

Follow-up After Successful Treatment

Trophoblastic Disease Surveillance

After chemotherapy completion, serum quantitative hCG levels should be obtained monthly for 6 months, every other month for the remainder of the first year, every 3 months during the second year, and at 6-month intervals indefinitely thereafter. Physical examinations are performed at 6–12-month intervals, and other examinations, such as chest X-rays, are performed as indicated. Contraception should be maintained during treatment and for 1 year after the completion of chemotherapy. Barrier methods and OCs are both acceptable forms of contraception; the latter have the advantage of suppressing pituitary luteinizing hormone, which may interfere with the accurate measurement of hCG levels. During a subsequent pregnancy, pelvic ultrasonography is recommended in the first trimester to confirm a normal gestation, since these patients are at increased risk for another gestational trophoblastic disease event. The products of conception or placentas from future pregnancies should be carefully examined histopathologically, and an hCG level should be obtained 6 weeks after any pregnancy event.

Reproductive Performance

The successful treatment of gestational trophoblastic tumors with chemotherapy has resulted in a large number of women whose reproductive potential has been retained despite exposure to drugs that have teratogenic potential. Many successful pregnancies have been reported in this group of patients. In general, these patients experience no increase in incidences of abortions, stillbirths, congenital anomalies, prematurity, or major obstetric complications. There has been no evidence for reactivation of disease due to a subsequent pregnancy. Patients who have had one trophoblastic disease episode are, however, at greater risk for the development of a second episode in a subsequent pregnancy, but this is unrelated to whether or not they had received chemotherapy previously. Patients are advised to delay conception for 1 year from cessation of chemotherapy. This not only allows for uninterrupted hCG follow-up to ensure cure but may permit mature ova, damaged by exposure to cytotoxic drugs, to be eliminated, thus allowing more immature oocytes to produce gametes for subsequent fertilization.

Secondary Malignancies

Because many anticancer drugs are known carcinogens, there is concern that the chemotherapy used to induce long-term remissions or cures of one cancer may induce second malignancies. Until recently, there had been no reports of increased susceptibility to the development of other malignancies after successful chemotherapy of trophoblastic tumors. This was probably due to the relatively short exposure of these patients to chemotherapeutic drugs and the infrequent use of alkylating agents. There are now a few reports of acute myelogenous leukemia developing in patients who received etoposide for treatment of gestational trophoblastic tumors.

BIBLIOGRAPHY

Berkowitz RS, Goldstein DP, eds. Clinical update on gestational trophoblastic disease. J Reprod Med 1987;32:621–684

Hammond CB, ed. Trophoblastic disease. Obstet Gynecol Clin North Am 1988;15:435–590

Hammond CB, Soper JT. Gestational trophoblastic diseases. In: Sciarra JJ, ed. Gynecology and obstetrics, vol 4. Philadelphia: JB Lippincott, 1993:1–42

Lurain JR. Chemotherapy of gestational trophoblastic disease. In: Deppe G, ed. Chemotherapy of gynecologic cancer. 2nd ed. New York: Wiley-Liss, 1990:273–301

Lurain JR, Casanova LA, Miller DS, Rademaker AW. Prognostic factors in gestational trophoblastic tumors: a proposed new scoring system based on multivariate analysis. Am J Obstet Gynecol 1991; 164:611–616

Newlands ES, Bagshawe KD, Begent RH, Rustin GJ, Holden L, et al. Results with the EMA/CO (etoposide, methotrexate, actinomycin D, cyclophosphamide, vincristine) regimen in high-risk gestational trophoblastic tumors. Br J Obstet Gynaecol 1991;98:550–557

Schink JC, Singh DK, Rademaker AW, Miller DS, Lurain JR. Etoposide, methotrexate, actinomycin D, cyclophosphamide, and vincristine for treatment of metastatic, high-risk gestational trophoblastic disease. Obstet Gynecol 1992;80:817–820

Szulman AE, Buchsbaum HJ, eds. Gestational trophoblastic disease. New York: Springer-Verlag, 1987

World Health Organization Scientific Group. Gestational Trophoblastic Disease, Technical Report Series 692. Geneva: WHO, 1983

Cancer and Pregnancy

The discovery of cancer coexisting with pregnancy creates significant uncertainty and anxiety for the physician, patient, family, and other members of the medical team. All cancer-related diagnostic or treatment decisions must consider and weigh the associated risk to both the mother and the fetus.

The obstetrician may be asked to evaluate two separate clinical situations regarding neoplasia and pregnancy. The first relates to a woman who has apparently survived her cancer and is now considering pregnancy. The second is a patient in whom a malignancy is diagnosed during pregnancy.

PREVIOUSLY TREATED CANCER

New therapies and effective support modalities have resulted in improved survival rates for many childhood and early adult malignancies. Current 5-year survival rates of 67% make childhood and adolescent cancer treatment one of the true success stories of modern cancer medicine. Consequently, the obstetrician–gynecologist must be able to render counseling and prenatal care to young women who are cancer survivors. Information should be made available so that parenthood can be planned.

Prepregnancy counseling should address the chance of recurrence, as fetal risks are potentially involved if cancer therapy is required after conception. In general, pregnancy is discouraged until the disease-free interval is at least 2 years; however, consultation with the patient's oncologist can assist in delineating an individual's risk of tumor recurrence.

Intraabdominal surgical procedures may result in adhesions that adversely affect future fertility. However, if surgical excision was the only therapy required, there should be no treatment-related risks to future pregnancies. Previous radiation therapy, chemotherapy, or combined therapy can have adverse effects on future fertility and pregnancy outcome. Ovarian irradiation results in sterilization; however, the amount of irradiation required to cause sterilization in women of reproductive age is high (≥2,000 cGy). In many cases, oophoropexy has been performed to minimize gonadal irradiation and possible later sterility. If fertility is maintained, there may be significant risk to pregnancies in women who have been treated with abdominal irradiation for certain childhood malignancies. Specifically, the risk of a pregnancy complication in women who have previously been treated with abdominal radiation for Wilms tumor is extremely high. These women have a 30% risk of an adverse pregnancy outcome with increased risks of perinatal mortality (eight times), low birth weight (four times), and abnormal pregnancy (four times). It has been suggested that pelvic irradiation damages the vascular and elastic properties of the uterus, resulting in radiation-induced intrauterine constraint and subsequent fetal malformation.

The cancer survivor previously treated with chemotherapy may also have infertility as a result of drug-related, dose-related, gonadotoxic effects (Table 5-9). Amenorrhea and anovulation may be self-limited, and patients may later conceive even after intensive therapy. The combination of chemotherapy and radiation therapy is toxic to the ovaries and has been associated with a 27-fold increase in the risk of early menopause.

Fortunately, women who remain ovulatory after cancer chemotherapy apparently do not confer a risk of congenital anomalies to their progeny. A review of pregnancy following treatment for Hodgkin disease found no increased risk of poor future pregnancy outcome with the exception of those patients who received both chemotherapy and irradiation. This finding was recently confirmed in patients previously treated for Hodgkin disease. In addition, with a mean follow-up of 11 years, there did not appear to be any adverse sequelae in offspring of these women. No increase in congenital abnormalities was reported in pregnancies following chemotherapy for trophoblastic disease. More recently, an evaluation of the potential effects of adjunctive doxorubicin given to women with breast cancer indicated no significant fetal risks in 33 subsequent pregnancies. Successful pregnancies have been reported after bone marrow transplantation.

The risk of recurrence and of accelerated tumor growth during or after pregnancy, particularly in estrogen receptor-positive tumors, is not apparently increased. There is no clini-

TABLE 5-9. DRUG-RELATED OVARIAN DYSFUNCTION

Drug	Risk of Infertility*
Bleomycin	?
Busulfan	+++
Chlorambucil	+++
Cisplatin	+
Cyclophosphamide	+++
Cytosine arabinoside	+
Doxorubicin	+
Etoposide	+
Fluorouracil	−
L-PAM	+++
M-AMSA	+
Mercaptopurine	−
Methotrexate	−
Nitrogen mustard	+++
Procarbazine	+++
Vinblastine	+
Vincristine	−

* Key: +++, definite; +, probable; −, unlikely; ?, unknown.
Modified from Orr JW Jr, Barrett JM, Holloway RW. Neoplasia in pregnancy. In: Moore TR, Reiter, RC, Rebar RW, Baker VV, eds. Gynecology and obstetrics: a longitudinal approach. New York: Churchill Livingstone, 1993

cal evidence that any of the physiologic alterations associated with pregnancy increases tumor growth dynamics. Additionally, in women with previously treated breast cancer there is no evidence that pregnancy adversely alters the future course of their malignancy, even with estrogen receptor-positive disease.

CANCER DURING PREGNANCY

Most reports suggest that cancer is coincident in approximately 1/1,000 pregnancies, although site-related risks vary dramatically. Even with these apparently small numbers, the significance of coexisting malignancy is important because it may account for as many as one third of maternal deaths.

The spectrum of common warning signs or symptoms that occur with many malignancies may be nonspecific and even overlap with symptoms of normal pregnancy. Additionally, cancer warning signs and symptoms are frequently denied or ignored. Physicians should maintain a level of clinical suspicion and institute appropriate diagnostic investigation if specific symptoms or signs persist or worsen. Failure to investigate these symptoms may result in a missed or delayed diagnosis. In fact, when evaluating specific cancer sites, the average pregnancy-associated delay in cancer diagnosis is 6–15 months longer than that of nonpregnant women.

Following diagnosis, the physician must consider both the possible direct fetal effects as well as the potential later genetic effects in making the decision to institute immediate maternal therapy. Decisions to delay therapy may adversely affect maternal and fetal prognosis in specific malignancies. Maternal concerns regarding fetal well-being must be approached cautiously. In most situations, maternal reassurance regarding the risk of fetal involvement is appropriate; however, rare fetal metastases have been reported. While it has been suggested that parental longing for a viable child should take precedence over all considerations, the potential fetal toxicity of certain cancer therapies may be significant if treatment is required during pregnancy.

Despite fears regarding the immunoregulatory effects of pregnancy, there is little evidence to suggest any adverse or accelerating effect of pregnancy on the malignant process. While some women may elect therapeutic abortion, there is little information to suggest that pregnancy interruption has a beneficial effect. Maternal–fetal management should take into consideration fetal gestational age, cancer origin, cancer extent, tumor growth potential, and proposed treatment. If pretreatment delivery is deemed necessary, short delays of therapy for specific cancers may not adversely affect maternal prognosis but may significantly improve fetal survival and decrease morbidity. Delaying delivery to 28 weeks is associated with improved fetal survival rates and lower risk of acute and long-term fetal morbidity. It is preferable to delay delivery until 32–34 weeks of gestation if possible, as fetal risks are dramatically reduced. The predelivery use of corticosteroids or the postdelivery administration of surfactant or management in a class III nursery may improve these figures.

Immunology

Women with malignancy often have evidence of depressed cellular immunity. Although conflicting data exist, pregnant women appear to have relative immunocompetence, which allows the fetal allograft to develop. An increased incidence of severe infections, depressed skin sensitivity, depressed response to mitogenic stimulation of lymphocysts, and the presence of suppressive or blocking substances may form part of a common link between cancer and pregnancy. The presence of oncofetal antigens (carcinoembryonic antigen, alpha-fetoprotein) and immunoglobulin G (which promotes nonrejection) are potentially related to the phenomenon of immune tolerance of the fetal allograft or the malignant cell.

Embryology

Even routine diagnostic studies offer potential risk to the developing fetus. The potential effects should prompt a physician to establish the presence or absence of a coexisting pregnancy in any woman of reproductive age who is suspected of having cancer or in whom cancer is diagnosed. A careful contraceptive history may suffice; however, a serum determination of hCG levels can resolve any question of a coexisting pregnancy. It is also the oncologist's or the consultant's obligation to discuss or offer contraception during treatment. In some situations, ovarian suppression may protect the ovary from the toxic effects of therapy and actually offer a benefit in regard to preserving future fertility. Although decisions regarding appropriate cancer therapy are important, once a coexistent pregnancy is recognized, it is paramount that an accurate gestational age be determined. Transabdominal or transvaginal ultrasound evaluation allows accurate pregnancy dating and may assist in excluding specific structural fetal abnormalities prior to treatment or monitoring fetal growth and development during treatment.

When comparing potential adverse effects of any diagnostic or therapeutic maneuver on pregnancy, it must be remembered that as many as 20% of all biochemically documented pregnancies result in spontaneous abortion. Analysis suggests that the predominant etiology for these losses relates to an abnormal fetal chromosome complement. Additionally, 2–3% of all live births are associated with a significant congenital abnormality.

During preimplantation, chemical or radiation insults usually result in an all-or-none phenomenon. That is, lethal insults result in pregnancy loss whereas sublethal insults have little apparent mutative effect, as the multipotentiality of embryonic cells at this gestational period allows repair of almost all sublethal cellular injury. The period during organogenesis (14–70 days) is the most potentially teratogenic period of embryonic development. Most organ systems have a specific self-limited period of teratogenic susceptibility; however, during the first 15 weeks, the central nervous system has an increased neuronal production, and migration of immature neurons to their site of cortical function occurs. While susceptibility to potential toxicity of therapy is high during this period, the central nervous system, the eyes, the genitalia, and the hematopoietic and respiratory systems remain susceptible to teratogens throughout fetal development.

Treatment

Surgery

No cancer treatment is entirely free of immediate or delayed risks; however, surgical resection of the malignant disease offers the least potential risk of direct long-term fetal sequelae. Prior to operative intervention, the cardiopulmonary physiologic changes associated with pregnancy must be considered and addressed, as fetal–placental circulation is exquisitely sensitive to hypoxemia and hypotension. Avoiding caval and aortic compression and minimizing airway closure, which occurs during tidal ventilation in 50% of pregnant women in the supine position, are imperative during preoperative, intraoperative, and postoperative care.

Lowered functional residual capacity and increased oxygen consumption renders the pregnant woman and her fetus extremely susceptible to periods of hypoxia. Careful attention prior to and during intubation of the pregnant patient is critical.

When an anesthetic is administered to a pregnant woman, the practitioner should take into account the possibility of a full stomach and risk of aspiration. The latter is thought to be responsible for approximately 25% of maternal anesthetic deaths. The administration of antacids, usually 30 ml of a nonparticulate antacid (0.3 M sodium citrate), will rapidly increase gastric pH. While this will not diminish the risk of aspiration of stomach contents, H_2 blockers decrease gastric volume and acidity production; they have little effect on those gastric contents that are already present. The potential side effects of these medications or any drugs must be considered.

The pregnancy-induced increase in blood volume may buffer clinical signs of large-volume blood loss. Alterations in mean arterial pressure may not occur until a 35% decrease in blood volume exists. In addition, catecholamine release may maintain peripheral blood pressure despite a significant decrease in uterine blood flow. Fetal monitoring should be considered an essential aspect of perioperative surgical care. Finally, any drug administered can potentially create acute or long-term fetal or infant toxicity. Consultation regarding the relative safety of all drugs administered perioperatively in the pregnant or lactating woman may be considered.

Even routine postoperative events may jeopardize the fetus. Temperature elevation (related to infection or atelectasis) requires aggressive treatment, as it has been associated with an increased risk of fetal abnormalities.

Despite concerns regarding the fetal risk of a pregnancy anesthetic, no current study of anesthetic effects has controlled for the coexisting disease process or illness that necessitated the anesthetic. Despite this shortcoming, regardless of the agent, method, or gestational age, there exists little evidence to indicate a direct fetal risk of anesthesia. One recent study reported on the risk of adverse reproductive events following anesthesia during pregnancy. In that series of 5,405 nonobstetric surgical procedures in 720,000 (0.75%) pregnant women, there was no apparent increased risk of congenital abnormalities in those women receiving anesthesia during the first trimester. Although there was an increased delivery rate of infants with low birth weight and very low birth weight and an increased rate of prematurity, neither of these events could be explained by immediate delivery in the postoperative period.

Any intraabdominal surgical procedures for the diagnosis or treatment of malignancy, particularly those requiring uterine manipulation, may theoretically increase the risk of spontaneous abortion. Surgical decisions based on clinical judgment without appropriate histologic evaluation can lead to overtreatment, with its attendant adverse maternal or fetal effects. Operations requiring adnexal removal are best performed during the second trimester, as placental progesterone production begins at 7 weeks and completely replaces the function of the corpus luteum by 12 weeks. If adnexectomy is required during the second trimester, there is little benefit to the additional use of progestogens.

On rare occasions, a previously undiagnosed intraabdominal malignant process is discovered during cesarean delivery. In that instance, appropriate surgical treatment or staging should be considered. There is no reason to abandon a properly functioning epidural anesthetic and encounter the risks of general anesthesia, as more extensive intraabdominal procedures can be completed without anesthetic induction.

Finally, surgical advisability of therapeutic abortion must be tempered by the fact that maternal morbidity and mortality from this procedure alone increase linearly with increasing gestational age.

Irradiation

There is no absolute safe amount of fetal radiation exposure. Guidelines for the probability of fetal risks do exist, and this information should be carefully discussed with the patient and her family prior to any diagnostic or therapeutic decisions.

Intensive cell proliferation, differentiation, and migration during prenatal development render the fetus susceptible to the direct effects of ionization of essential molecules and cellular components. Nuclear DNA is thought to represent the critical target for radiation damage, making the developing fetus a prime target for potential radiation injury. Obviously, the fetus is at risk when using therapeutic radiation; however, fetal risks must also be considered in those situations requiring radioisotopic diagnostic scans or radiographic studies during pretreatment evaluation.

Radiation-induced fetal injury risk can be determined by a complex formula related to gestational age, radiation dose, field size, energy source, and dose rate. The most common adverse fetal effects of radiation exposure include growth retardation, malformation, and fetal death.

Before and immediately after implantation, the developing embryo is highly susceptible to the lethal effects of irradiation. As previously noted, the multipotentiality of embryonic cells at this gestational age probably allows repair of sublethal damage, as few patients deliver a malformed infant following low-level exposure to irradiation during this time.

Radiation exposure during organogenesis may result in an infant born with congenital abnormalities of varying clinical importance. As previously noted, most organ systems become less susceptible to teratogenic effects as the pregnancy progresses. Some, such as the central nervous, hematopoietic, and respiratory systems, continue to develop and remain susceptible even to low levels of radiation therapy. Small head size and severe mental retardation have been reported at very-low-dose exposures (≤9 cGy); however, the risks are dramatically increased with intrauterine exposures of ≥10 cGy. More than 50% of those infants exposed in utero to 250 cGy at 3–10 weeks of gestation have low birth weight, microcephaly, mental retardation, retinal degeneration, cataracts, or genital or skeletal malformations. The apparent risk of these abnormalities is reduced if this level of radiation exposure occurs between 10 and 20 weeks of gestation. This amount of radiation exposure after 20 weeks results in less severe anomalies, consisting of those changes seen in postnatal life such as anemia, pigmentation changes, and erythema. The risk of severe mental retardation during the 8th to 15th postconceptional week is about 0.4%/cGy. Lesser degrees of mental deficit as related to scholastic achievement have been reported with lesser in utero radiation exposure during this sensitive time period. The overall risk of a 1-cGy exposure in utero has been calculated to be 0.003%.

The actual fetal dose, although related to gestational age, is an important factor. The lethal dose at which 50% of gestations abort (or will result in stillbirth) is 70 cGy at day 1, 150 cGy at day 18, and 300–400 cGy after the first trimester.

The potential adverse effect of 100 cGy at any gestational age is significant. Although later radiation exposure rarely results in a major congenital anomaly, the incidence of growth retardation, eye defects, and central nervous system defects is increased. In fact, fetal growth retardation may be the most sensitive indicator of intrauterine radiation exposure, and late radiation exposure results in the greatest degree of postnatal growth retardation. This problem is potentially detectable in utero with ultrasonography; therefore, any patient receiving radiation therapy during pregnancy might benefit from careful serial evaluation of the fetus and its growth. The threshold for growth retardation is less than 100 cGy; however, infants who received less than 25 cGy in utero rarely exhibit growth retardation.

Although the absolutely safe dose of radiation is unknown, it appears that exposure of less than 10 cGy may result in some subtle pathologic effects but not in gross fetal malformations or fetal growth retardation. This level is five times the current recommended dose prescribed by the National Council on Radiation Protection and Management. Doses of more than 50 cGy significantly increase the risk of central nervous system abnormality. While isolated reports of normal infants receiving in utero radiation exposure exist, therapeutic abortion should be considered and discussed if fetal radiation exposure exceeds 10 cGy.

Radioactive isotopes traverse the placenta and can cause distinct fetal complications. The most thoroughly studied of these isotopes is radioactive iodine (^{131}I). The fetal thyroid actively concentrates iodine (after the sixth gestational week), and the administration of this radioisotope can ablate the fetal thyroid and result in fetal hypothyroidism. Although successful fetal thyroid hormone replacement has been reported, all diagnostic radionuclide studies should be avoided during pregnancy. If deemed necessary, specific mechanisms to reduce fetal radiation dose include maternal hydration and bladder drainage. If possible, other diagnostic approaches (ie, ultrasonography and fine-needle aspiration) should be considered.

Women receiving therapeutic irradiation doses can expect a high rate of fetal death. In those undergoing supradiaphragmatic therapeutic radiation, appropriate shielding offers significant fetal or embryonic radiation protection from significant exposure. However, generalizations concerning radiation dose are dangerous, as uterine size may differ at different gestational ages. It is essential that the therapist and physicist attempt to calculate the actual fetal dose and communicate the possible risks to the mother. Regardless of dose level or gestational age, fetal tolerance is increased when the dose is delivered in multiple fractions.

The long-term delayed effects of fetal irradiation remain unknown. Reports indicating persistent chromosome abnormalities in children with in utero exposure at Hiroshima cause concern; however, these effects are subtle and it may be generations before they are expressed as congenital anomalies. There is little need to perform chromosomal analysis of those women with previous in utero exposure unless specific abnormalities (13q– in neuroblastoma, 11q– in Wilms tumor) are in question. The effects of intrauterine radiation exposure on future reproductive function of the fetus is also unknown. It appears that 25 cGy delivered acutely in utero will not result in fetal sterility.

During treatment, the future reproductive potential of the woman must also be considered. Although women over age 40 years may be effectively sterilized by as little as 600 cGy, women of reproductive age are not sterilized until larger doses (approaching 2,000 cGy) are delivered. Although irradiation given for pelvic tumor exceeds this dose, women treated for other tumors, such as lymphoma, may benefit from oophoropexy to minimize gonadal irradiation and the possibility of later sterility (Table 5-10).

Chemotherapy
Antineoplastic drugs are designed to destroy rapidly proliferating malignant cells. The developing fetus is a rapidly proliferating "cell line" itself, and, if exposed, becomes a potential target for the action of such drugs and their possible teratogenic effects. Although animal studies indicate a high risk of teratogenicity or mutagenicity of fetal exposure, the reported incidence of congenital abnormalities in children exposed to cytotoxic agents is small. Unfortunately, determining the exact risk of chemotherapy-related teratogenicity in humans is difficult, as most of the published literature consists of a relatively small number of individual case reports using different drugs and drug combinations, with therapy administered at different gestational ages. Pregnancy-associated physiologic alterations include alterations in oral absorption of drugs (delayed gastric emptying, altered intestinal motility), and drug binding (decreased albumin levels). Additionally, hepatic oxidation by the mixed-function oxidase system, as well as renal blood flow and glomerular filtration rate, is increased. Maternal plasma volume is increased; however, there exists little information to determine any protective or adverse effects of drug concentration (or drug gradients) related to altered vascular volume or the potential "third space" effects of amniotic fluid volume.

Chemotherapeutic drugs exert their effects through different mechanisms and at different molecular sites. Fetal consequences of cytotoxic therapy may be related to drug dosage, drug regimen, gestational age at exposure, and the possible synergism in teratogenicity when combined with irradiation. In contrast to radiation therapy, the placenta may create a biologic or pharmacologic barrier or even metabolize specific cytotoxic agents. It appears that most antineoplastic drugs possess those qualities (low molecular weight, nonionized, lipid soluble, loosely protein bound) that allow or facilitate placental passage. However, almost no information is available on actual amniotic fluid distribution.

One study reviewing 185 pregnancies of women treated prior to 1967 reported that fewer than 8% of infants exposed to chemotherapy during the first trimester had congenital malformations. Later exposure was not associated with a greater risk of congenital malformations when compared with the normal population, regardless of gestational age. Forty percent of infants exposed to cytotoxic agents were of low birth weight. Another study reached nearly the same conclusion, verifying the rarity of reported malformations in human pregnancies following in utero exposure to chemotherapy. More recently, it has been suggested that if the results of exposure to aminopterin—a known abortifacient—were excluded, the risk of malformation was about 5%, a figure not different from that for the nonexposed population. A recent review confirmed these findings, with a low risk (1.5%) of anomaly occurring if exposure occurred after the first trimester.

Antimetabolites, particularly folic acid antagonists, carry the most significant risk of producing congenital anomalies (Table 5-11). However, no drug can be considered absolutely safe. Although scattered individual case reports continue to indicate the relative fetal safety of these agents, the physician should be aware that almost any chemotherapeutic treatment regimen can be substituted with a therapeutic equivalent. If fetal status is of concern, it would appear prudent to avoid folic acid antagonists or combination therapy, particularly during the first trimester, despite recent reports of successful pregnancies.

During the administration of chemotherapy, extensive use of obstetric ultrasonography is required. In the first trimester, ultrasonography is indicated to assess fetal viability and to determine gestational age. A second-trimester detailed study should be performed to evaluate for anatomic fetal anomalies. In the second half of pregnancy, serial ultrasonography to evaluate fetal growth should be performed every 3–4 weeks.

TABLE 5-10. LIKELIHOOD OF STERILITY AND AMENORRHEA AT VARIOUS DOSES OF IRRADIATION

	Sterility		Amenorrhea	
Dose (cGy)	Age 15–40	Age >40	Age 15–40	Age >40
<60	—	—	—	—
150	—	Rare	—	Rare
250–500	60%	100%	Majority*	100%
500–800	70%	100%	Majority*	100%
>800	100%	100%	100%	100%

* Most women not sterile develop temporary amenorrhea.
Modified from Gradishar WJ, Schilsky RL. Ovarian function following radiation and chemotherapy for cancer. Semin Oncol 1989;16:425–436

TABLE 5-11. CHEMOTHERAPY DURING FIRST-TRIMESTER PREGNANCY

Drug	No. of Patients	No. of Anomalies (%)
Alkylating agents		
Busulfan	22	2 (9)
Chlorambucil	5	1 (20)
Cyclophosphamide	7	3 (43)
Mechlorethamine HCl	6	0
Triethylenemelamine	4	0
Total	44	6 (14)
Antimetabolites		
Aminopterin	52	10 (19)
Methotrexate	3	3 (100)
Mercaptopurine	20	0
Cytarabine	1	1 (100)
Fluorouracil	1	1 (100)
Total	77	15 (19)
Antibiotics		
Daunorubicin	1	0
Alkaloids		
Vinblastine	14	1 (7)
Others		
Procarbazine	1	1 (100)
Amsacrine	1	1 (100)
Cisplatin	1	0
All chemotherapy	139	24 (17)
Combination	30	7 (23)

Modified from Doll DC, Ringenberg QS, Yarbro JW. Management of cancer during pregnancy. Arch Intern Med 1988;148:2058–2064. Copyright 1988, American Medical Association

Early in the third trimester, weekly fetal biophysical profile testing to assess fetal status should be considered.

Regardless of the presence or absence of congenital abnormality at birth, infants exposed in utero to chemotherapy should be screened for possible drug-specific deleterious effects such as low birth weight, marrow suppression, and cardiac or pulmonary toxicity. Since fetal hepatic and renal metabolic pathways may be immature at birth, acute drug toxicity may be highest if recent treatment occurred in close proximity to delivery. Breast-feeding by mothers receiving cytotoxic agents (particularly those with oral cytotoxic activity) should be discouraged, as these drugs are probably excreted in breast milk, placing the infant at potential risk of neutropenia or other toxicity.

Intensive cytotoxic treatment of young women—whether or not they are pregnant—may place them at risk of the later development of another malignancy; however, this risk may relate to the initial tumor type or therapy. To date, there exist few reports of apparent transplacental carcinogenesis; however, continued close observation is necessary to delineate possible late effects such as those reported with in utero DES exposure.

Timing of delivery for the pregnant patient receiving intensive antineoplastic chemotherapy is important. If possible, delivery at the time of maternal leukocyte or platelet nadir should be avoided to minimize the maternal and fetal risks associated with delivery. The neonate should be evaluated for thrombocytopenia or neutropenia. Care to monitor mother and newborn is also important. Specific cytotoxic drugs may be excreted in breast milk and potentially may be absorbed.

Fetal–Placental Metastasis

Although extremely rare, placental metastases have been described in more than 50 women, with melanoma being the most common metastasizing tumor. Fewer than 25% of infants with placental metastatic melanoma succumb to disease. Only 50% of placental metastases are visible. Careful visual and microscopic evaluation of the placenta from any patient recently treated or undergoing treatment for malignancy during pregnancy is advised. The microscopic finding of intervillous space involvement portends a poor maternal prognosis and should prompt fetal evaluation for metastatic disease.

To date, fewer than 25 cases of fetal metastases have been reported, most being melanoma or choriocarcinoma. The rarity of this situation suggests the possibility of a protective placental barrier or function. Features that are associated with an unfavorable fetal or infant prognosis with metastatic melanoma include maternal age less than 30 years, primiparity, leg primary site, maternal disease onset less than 3 years prior to pregnancy, node metastatic status prior to pregnancy, M4 metastatic status in the third trimester, and male gender.

Reproductive Tract Cancer

Cervical Cancer

Premalignant or malignant cervical changes represent the most common reproductive-tract cancer associated with pregnancy. While reported incidence rates vary in relation to population base and referral bias, it appears that invasive cervical cancer may be present in 1/2,000 pregnancies. As many as 7% of patients with cervical cancer are pregnant or immediately postpartum at the time of diagnosis. Carcinoma in situ coexists in approximately 1/770 pregnancies. As many as 2% of women have abnormal cytology of some degree, even in a private-practice population.

Cervical abnormalities are usually diagnosed during pregnancy by routine screening cytology. An endocervical brush can be safely used and may increase the yield of abnormalities, compared with use of cotton-tipped swabs. Atypical glandular cells require specific evaluation, as adenocarcinoma may be particularly difficult to diagnose during pregnancy. Persistent symptoms such as vaginal bleeding (which occurs in as many as 87% of women with invasive disease) should prompt revisualization and reevaluation of the cervix. Unfortunately, these symptoms tend to be dismissed as pregnancy-related bleeding, and this delay in diagnosis may be longer than 4 months. Regardless of cytologic findings, a visually abnormal cervix should prompt further investigation, including colposcopy and biopsy.

All pregnant women with squamous cell intraepithelial lesions should undergo colposcopy. Most practicing physicians will diagnose invasive coexisting cervical cancer only once or twice during their careers, so they must be prepared to recognize the associated epithelial and vascular changes. Colposcopic visualization of the squamocolumnar junction is generally easier during pregnancy because of cervical hypertrophy and dilatation. However, the hyperemic, redundant vagina occasionally obscures adequate visualization. Vaginal retraction using a vaginal retractor, tongue blades, or a condom over the speculum may improve visualization. Although cervical biopsy is associated with bleeding, a histologic diagnosis is usually necessary unless colposcopic expertise is available. One study indicated that 2 of 969 pregnant patients with CIN I to CIN II cytology will have invasive disease. If the presence of invasive disease is excluded, the need for further diagnostic or therapeutic intervention is delayed until after delivery, because there is little risk of progression of premalignant lesions during pregnancy.

There is little indication for antepartum therapy of the squamous cell intraepithelial lesion of the cervix, although cryotherapy (for benign lesions) has been performed during pregnancy with little apparent adverse effect on delivery or prematurity. Therapeutic cervical conization is not advised during pregnancy; however, diagnostic conization may be necessary to exclude invasive cancer. This procedure significantly increases maternal and fetal complications. At least 1 in 10 women experiences significant bleeding after conization, and this risk apparently increases with gestational age. Cervical stenosis or intrapartum lacerations occur in 3–8% of pregnant women after conization. The fetal risk of abortion or premature delivery is quoted as 3–8% but approaches 50% after first-trimester conization. Although term infants are delivered in 80% of pregnancies after conization and fetal salvage approaches 90%, the physician should be hesitant to perform conization unless an invasive lesion is indicated by cytologic or colposcopic evaluation and immediate therapeutic action is anticipated. Additionally, the risk of residual premalignant or malignant cervical disease may be increased after the narrow, shallow cone performed during pregnancy.

Noninvasive lesions can be followed with a repeat colposcopic evaluation during the third trimester, although one recent report questions the need for this repeat procedure once invasion has been excluded. Although reports of malignant progression of dysplasia during pregnancy are uncommon, this noninvasive reevaluation adds little fetal or maternal risk. All patients with abnormal cytology should be reevaluated and treated (if deemed clinically necessary) during the postpartum period. Cesarean hysterectomy as treatment of cervical dysplasia is not advised, as this procedure is associated with increased blood loss, risk of ovarian removal, and urinary tract injury. Additionally, removing the cervix through an abdominal approach, particularly with cervical dilatation, may compromise surgical margins.

If the diagnosis of an invasive lesion is established, treatment-related options revolve around gestational age, disease extent, and maternal desires. While progression can occur, therapeutic delays of up to 17 weeks are not associated with an adverse maternal prognosis in low-volume, early-stage disease. One study recently reported the significant adverse fetal effects of early delivery and recommended the consideration of relatively long delays to avoid fetal problems, including intraventricular hemorrhage associated with prematurity.

If the decision to delay therapy is reached after careful physician–patient discussion and documentation, the method of delivery should be chosen primarily by obstetric indications. Despite theoretic considerations, stage-controlled studies indicate no adverse maternal effect of a vaginal delivery. It would be preferable to avoid cervical dilation in the presence of a large cervical tumor because of a significant risk of bleeding and potential difficulty with cervical dilatation. However, careful postpartum evaluation is necessary, as recurrent cervical cancer has been reported in an episiotomy scar.

With the decision to institute treatment, consideration of surgical versus radiation therapy is related to the disease extent and actually differs little from consideration for the non-pregnant woman. There have been reports suggesting a pregnancy-associated altered tissue tolerance during irradiation, with intestinal and urinary injuries more likely. This fact should not bias the selection of treatment regimen, but it serves to alert the physician and staff to possible problems. There appears to be little benefit of a pretreatment induced abortion prior to radiation therapy. Spontaneous abortion usually occurs between the third and sixth weeks of treatment. More than 70% occur prior to the delivery of 4,000 cGy.

While concerns exist regarding the effect of delayed diagnosis or postpartum therapy on survival, clinical stage appears to be the most important prognostic variable. Extensive reviews suggest that 5-year survival in patients with stage I or stage II disease is not different as related to the trimester of the treatment. One recent report suggested an increased risk of lymph vascular space involvement and macrometastasis in patients treated during the postpartum interval. However, patients diagnosed during the postpartum interval apparently have more advanced disease than those diagnosed during pregnancy.

While serum tumor markers may aid in the evaluation and follow-up for squamous cancers, their use in pregnant women remains to be defined. It has been suggested that 0.9% of pregnant women with normal Pap test results have an elevated serum squamous cell antigen level.

Ovarian and Tubal Malignancy

Adnexal masses are frequently encountered during pregnancy. Although ovarian cancer occurs in only 1/18,000–1/25,000 pregnancies, the risk of ovarian malignancy in a gravid patient with an adnexal mass ranges from 2.2% to 8%. The most common coexisting adnexal abnormality includes benign cystic teratomas (45%), mucinous cystadenomas (40%), and serous cystadenomas. Dysgerminomas represent the most common ovarian cancer coexisting with pregnancy, representing nearly 35% of ovarian malignancies. Tubal cancers are extremely rare, with fewer than five reported cases to date.

Prior to prenatal ultrasound evaluation, most ovarian masses remained unrecognized until cesarean delivery or a postpartum evaluation. The early use of prenatal vaginal or abdominal ultrasonography for gestational dating causes many asymptomatic adnexal masses to be recognized early in pregnancy. Current protocol requires exploration and histologic evaluation of any mass (particularly with a complex ultrasound evaluation) greater than 5 cm if it persists into the second trimester.

The diagnostic role of tumor markers can be complicated. Alpha-fetoprotein levels may be elevated in those pregnancies with neural tube defects, twin gestations, or other fetal or placental conditions. However, elevated maternal levels have been described with hepatic metastases. CA 125 levels increase during the first trimester (mean, 71.7 U/ml) but normalize during the second trimester (<35 U/ml). Serum levels following second-trimester abortion (mean, 447 U/ml) and term delivery (mean, 204 U/ml) hamper the usefulness of CA 125 during pregnancy. Careful preoperative explanation and documentation of all options of the surgical algorithm as it relates to maternal or fetal well-being is necessary.

Whether an adnexal mass is discovered unexpectedly (at cesarean delivery) or during a planned pregnancy-related laparotomy, several questions should be addressed before the procedure is completed. A rapid histologic diagnosis is imperative prior to "radical" extirpative surgery, as several benign entities may clinically resemble a malignancy. If a malignant diagnosis is confirmed, the decisions concerning what constitutes an optimal procedure may be difficult. Not infrequently, the primary operative procedure is undertaken without prior knowledge of adnexal pathologic lesions. Conservative surgery should be considered for apparent stage I ovarian malignancy or tumors of borderline malignant potential when preservation of fertility is of prime concern. At a minimum, peritoneal cytologic tests and careful visual examination and palpation of the mesenteric surfaces, colic gutters, subdiaphragmatic spaces, omentum, and retroperitoneal areas should be performed and recorded. If any doubt exists intraoperatively, a lesser procedure should be performed, with the realization that a second, more definitive procedure may be necessary.

The use of adjunctive chemotherapy for women with ovarian cancer is based entirely on surgical and histologic findings. In specific situations, particularly with a coexisting ovarian germ cell malignancy, there may be a role for conservative surgical therapy and chemotherapy to allow later delivery of a viable infant. Surgeons should remember that women of childbearing age are at greater risk for harboring either low-malignant-potential ovarian tumors, which can often be treated conservatively with an excellent prognosis, or germ cell tumors, which can also be conservatively managed with surgery and adjuvant chemotherapy.

While the overall long-term prognosis of women with ovarian cancer remains poor, there is little evidence to suggest an adverse effect of a coexisting or subsequent pregnancy.

Vulvar or Vaginal Malignancy

Fewer than 50 documented cases of vulvar or vaginal malignancy coexisting with pregnancy have been reported. With the exception of DES-associated vaginal adenocarcinomas, neither of these two malignancies would be expected with pregnancy, as they usually occur during or after the sixth decade of life.

The diagnosis of an early vaginal cancer during pregnancy would be fortuitous, as pregnancy-associated vaginal changes frequently render visualization and bimanual examination difficult. When screening cervical cytology suggests an invasive lesion and colposcopy fails to delineate a cervical lesion, the vagina should be thoroughly evaluated prior to considering conization.

Treatment of a cancer in the upper one third of the vagina parallels that of cancer of the cervix, with essentially the same indications for surgery or radiation therapy. Fetal implications are not different. Local vaginal irradiation has been used in very specific situations in which dosimetry allows a low fetal exposure; however, its routine use during pregnancy is not advocated. Although clinical experience is limited, pregnancy has no apparent adverse effect on the clinical course or prognosis of vaginal carcinoma (squamous or adenocarcinoma).

Invasive vulvar lesions during pregnancy are rare and may be associated with condylomata. While condylomata may not require treatment, careful vulvar inspection during the initial prenatal or subsequent pelvic examinations should allow the astute physician to establish the diagnosis of coexisting intraepithelial or invasive disease. If a vulvar lesion is encountered during pregnancy, a histologic diagnosis is necessary prior to ablative surgery. Colposcopic evaluation allows directed biopsy; however, the presence of hyperkeratosis and a heavy, white, vulvar epithelium may require an excisional biopsy to preclude the diagnosis of invasive vulvar disease. Delaying treatment of VIN into the postpartum period should be considered.

The surgical approach to treatment of vulvar carcinoma in the pregnant woman parallels that of the nongravid patient, and there is little justification for a therapeutic abortion to improve disease prognosis. Early lesions do not require a classic radical vulvectomy, as the surgical procedure can be modified according to lesion size and depth of invasion. If indicated, unilateral operations or wide radical resection with or without inguinal node dissection are more cosmetic and do not compromise cure. Inguinal node dissections may be necessary in patients with deeply invasive tumors and can be completed through separate incisions with less apparent morbidity. There appears to be little benefit of pelvic node dissection. In the presence of involved inguinal nodes, the delivery of pelvic irradiation is associated with equal survival rates and less morbidity than pelvic node dissection. As with cervical cancer, fetal considerations should dictate the timing of pelvic radiation in node-positive patients.

Uterine Carcinoma

Fewer than 5% of patients with endometrial adenocarcinoma are younger than age 40 years. Pregnancy and uterine cancer are rarely associated (10 reported cases), and this low risk may be explained by age, the increased rate of infertility of patients with uterine cancer (related to anovulation), the antimitotic inhibitory effects on the endometrium of high pregnancy-related progesterone levels, and an altered internal uterine environment (inhibiting implantation) associated with premalignant endometrium.

The diagnosis of endometrial cancer in most (60%) pregnant women has been established after curettage for presumed spontaneous abortion, although two cases of coexisting uterine cancer and a viable infant have been reported. There has been no reported case of uterine cancer in an asymptomatic pregnant woman. However, with the evolving sophistication of routine prenatal ultrasonography, this diagnosis may be established in the future.

Surgical staging of endometrial cancer allows the best use of histologic findings to determine the role of adjunctive radiotherapy or chemotherapy.

Breast Cancer

Breast cancer may occur in 1/3,000 pregnancies. The average age of pregnant women with breast cancer is 34, and this malignancy has been diagnosed in a 16 year old. As many as 3.8% of women diagnosed with breast cancer are pregnant or lactating. This problem may become more common as women intentionally delay their childbearing.

During prenatal evaluation, a careful breast examination is imperative. Tense, nodular breast hypertrophy and other physiologic changes secondary to the hormonal stimulation necessary for lactation frequently render breast examination difficult and probably contribute to the delay in cancer diagnosis during pregnancy. Pregnancy-associated increase in breast water density creates a loss of the contrasting fatty tissue necessary for mammographic evaluation, resulting in a less-definitive study and a 50% false-negative rate. With appropriate precautions, mammography is safe. In 368 mammographic exams performed during pregnancy, there was no associated fetal abnormality. Therefore, biopsy of palpable abnormalities is essential regardless of mammographic findings. Fine-needle aspiration carries a 66% diagnostic rate, and a negative aspirate does not preclude the need for biopsy. Biopsy of either benign or malignant lesions during pregnancy is not associated with a significant risk of milk fistula, fetal, or maternal problems. In fact, the risk of pregnancy loss is 1/86–1/135. Epidemiologic studies suggest that diagnostic delays of 6 months or less are associated with an adverse effect on survival. Physicians need not ignore a palpable nodule to allow postpartum evaluation. The practice of observing a breast lump during pregnancy is risky.

When controlled for stage and patient age, pregnancy does not worsen the prognosis for breast cancer. However, pregnancy-associated breast cancers are less likely to be estrogen-receptor positive (30%) and are more likely to be node-positive, particularly if diagnosis is delayed.

Once the diagnosis, histology, and lesion size of breast cancer are established, the approach to treatment is not different from that in nonpregnant women. Pretreatment diagnostic evaluation may differ. Evaluation for distal metastatic sites normally includes brain, bone, and liver studies. In the absence of physical or historic evidence of distal disease, the liver can usually be adequately evaluated with determination of serum liver enzymes and ultrasonography. If indicated, the fetal radiation exposure from a bone scan can be decreased by one third (76 mrem) with adequate maternal hydration and a Foley catheter to decrease bladder accumulation. However, the incidence of truly positive bone scans in stage I (3%) or stage II (7%) is relatively small.

Appropriate fetal precautions are required for primary or adjunctive irradiation that can be completed prior to delivery. If used, the mother should be warned that the irradiated breast likely will not lactate. Decisions concerning the necessity of adjunctive chemotherapy for treatment of systemic disease require appropriate consultation regarding possible fetal effects. There is a paucity of information regarding the concurrent use of the antiestrogen tamoxifen. However, the use of other hormonal agents is contraindicated during pregnancy.

There is no apparent negative survival effect of a concurrent or subsequent pregnancy. However, some have suggested waiting 5 years in the presence of involved nodes and 3 years if nodes are negative because of concerns about the stimulation risks of elevated estrogen levels associated with pregnancy.

Non–Reproductive Tract Cancer

Melanoma

Melanoma represents approximately 1% of all cancer diagnosed in the United States, and because most affected women are ages 30–60 years, the incidence of coexisting melanoma in pregnancy is significant. It is estimated that the average individual has 15 nevi, all capable of developing into melanoma. Malignant melanoma is quite uncommon prior to puberty. Unfortunately, it appears that the frequency of this malignancy is doubling every decade.

Following surgical excision and histopathologic evaluation, a careful examination and routine diagnostic studies, including hematologic profile, urinalysis, and serum liver function, are important. Specific scans of the liver, bone, and brain should be performed only if there are signs or symptoms suggesting metastatic disease in one of these organ sites. Because of the predilection for intestinal metastasis, stool should be tested for the presence of blood. Prominent sites of metastatic involvement in melanoma, in decreasing order, are lungs, liver, adrenal glands, brain, kidneys, bone, intestines, pancreas, spleen, stomach, and urinary bladder.

Histologic microstaging of melanoma to evaluate the depth of invasion is important for clinical management. Tumor thicknesses as described in anatomical levels are currently in use.

If the histologic microstaging indicates a thin melanoma (less than 0.076 mm), there is an extremely low (less than 5%)

risk of developing regional or distant metastatic disease, and therefore wide resection alone is indicated. Patients with intermediate-thickness melanoma (0.76–3.99 mm) have a 50–60% risk of micrometastasis in the regional nodes but less than a 20% risk of distant disease. Treatment by wide local resection and regional lymphadenectomy is beneficial, because resection of all disease remains the best chance for cure. Patients with thick melanomas (greater than 4 mm) are not likely to benefit from lymphadenectomy, as they have a greater than 80% chance of harboring distant metastatic disease, although it may be undetectable at initial clinical presentation.

Regardless of tumor depth of invasion, surgical margins of 1–2 cm seem adequate. Classic radical vulvectomy is rarely indicated for vulvar melanoma. Other prognostic factors, including ulceration and growth pattern, must be considered. While current information suggests that the previously noted adverse effect of ulceration and tumor type (nodular, superficial spreading) is not as important after controlling for tumor thickness, bodily location of the melanoma may be of prognostic importance. Patients with melanomas of the extremities have an improved survival, compared with patients with head and neck disease. Patients with truncal melanomas have the worst prognosis. The presence of nodal metastasis is associated with a worsening prognosis in direct proportion to the number of nodes involved. All of these facts suggest that early recognition of melanoma remains absolutely critical and that changes in skin nevi during pregnancy should not be casually dismissed as "related to estrogen levels."

Patients with distant metastasis may benefit from systemic chemotherapy, particularly if the disease is in skin, soft tissue, and lymph nodes, where response rates approach 50%. Unfortunately, response rates where liver and bone metastases are present are less than 10%. Immunotherapy or isolated limb perfusion chemotherapy remains investigational.

The possible hormonal effect on melanoma creates a concern that pregnancy may exert an adverse effect on melanoma. Theoretic concerns are based on the pigmentation changes that occur in existing nevi at puberty, the hyperpigmentation associated with pregnancy, the pregnancy-associated increase in melanin-stimulating hormone, the detection of estrogen receptors in 46% of melanomas, and reports of melanoma regression following hormonal manipulation. While individual reports might suggest an adverse effect of pregnancy on melanoma, most reports do not confirm this notion. The current consensus is that abortion should not be considered therapeutic and that when controlled for stage, site, and age, the 3- and 5-year survival rates are not affected by pregnancy termination.

Consequently, treatment of melanoma during pregnancy should be similar to that for the nonpregnant woman, proceeding immediately with appropriate surgical staging and diagnostic evaluation.

Hematologic Cancer

Non-Hodgkin lymphoma or Hodgkin disease coexists with pregnancy in 1/1,000–1/6,000 deliveries, making this disease the fourth most common cancer diagnosed during pregnancy. Most women (80%) with lymphoma are asymptomatic and present with lymphadenopathy. Symptoms of night sweats, pruritus, or weight loss are associated with a poor prognosis.

Hodgkin disease usually occurs in younger women (average age 32), is more likely to be localized, and is more likely to be cured than non-Hodgkin lymphoma (average age 42). Clinical staging for lymphoma necessitates the systematic evaluation of history, laboratory findings, bone marrow, and radiographic imaging. Clinical staging and treatment should be individualized. Pathologic staging for Hodgkin disease may involve laparotomy and splenectomy; however, this is not usually necessary for non-Hodgkin lymphoma, as disseminated disease can usually be documented without surgery. Aggressive therapy with nodal irradiation and multiple-agent therapy results in a 70% cure rate for patients with Hodgkin disease and a 50% cure rate for patients with non-Hodgkin lymphoma. Therapeutic irradiation usually involves a supradiaphragmatic field with fetal radiation related to dose, energy, and gestational age.

Current recommendations suggest the possible benefit of therapeutic abortion (to allow complete staging) in those patients with a first-trimester pregnancy and Hodgkin disease. However, others have limited the role of therapeutic abortion to those women requiring infradiaphragmatic irradiation, or those with systemic symptoms or visceral disease that are best treated with multiagent systemic chemotherapy.

Observation alone results in less than 10% 5-year survival. Delayed treatment in most situations is unacceptable. However, in patients with apparently localized upper abdominal disease and a gestation of less than 20 weeks, therapy delays should be considered. For women with late gestations and infradiaphragmatic or advanced disease, combination chemotherapy is probably preferred and should be instituted as soon as possible.

Indolent forms of non-Hodgkin lymphoma constitute a minority of disease coexisting with pregnancy. While therapy delay or local treatment may suffice in this subgroup, those with unfavorable histology (Burkitt disease, lymphoblastic lymphoma) require aggressive therapy and consideration of abortion if fetal risks warrant. The institution of lesser therapies, including single-drug vinblastine, seems unjustified.

There is no apparent increased risk of spontaneous abortion; however, non-Hodgkin lymphoma may adversely affect pregnancy outcome. Burkitt lymphoma may represent the one situation that is potentially adversely affected by pregnancy, as this disease is rapidly fatal. Short delays in those women with good prognostic factors may be appropriate. However, if lymphoma is diagnosed early in pregnancy, patients should be treated with multiple-agent chemotherapy. If therapeutic irradiation is considered, the fetal consequences must be recognized and outlined. It has been suggested that subsequent pregnancy be considered only after 2 years of remission, as the long-term prognosis of early recurrence is poor in non-Hodgkin lymphoma.

Acute leukemia represents 90% of leukemias coexisting with pregnancy, and most cases (78%) are diagnosed after the first trimester. With the institution of aggressive therapy, complete remission rates approach 75%, and 40% of these are durable. There exists no evidence that pregnancy adversely affects the incidence, natural history, or prognosis of acute leukemia; however, there have been spontaneous remissions after pregnancy termination.

Pregnant patients with chronic leukemia have a median survival time of 38 months, which is not different from that for nonpregnant women. Although aggressive combination chemotherapy forms the cornerstone of acceptable medical therapy for leukemia patients, the periodic episodes of myelosuppression increase the risk of placental injury, sepsis, spontaneous abortion, and premature delivery.

Chronic myelogenous leukemia occurs as frequently as chronic lymphocytic leukemia. It is not uncommon for these patients to have serious clinical infections or a bleeding diathesis at the time of diagnosis. Pregnancy itself does not alter the incidence, natural history, or prognosis, with obtainable cure rates of greater than 70% in acute myelogenous lymphocytic leukemia.

Urinary Tract Malignancies
Carcinoma of the upper or lower urinary tract is rarely diagnosed during pregnancy. To date, fewer than 50 cases of renal cell carcinoma and fewer than 10 cases of coexisting bladder carcinoma have been documented. Only two pregnant women with urethral carcinoma have been reported. Just as in the nongravid state, the most common symptom of urinary tract cancer is hematuria. While the risk of having a coexisting malignancy is low, persistent hematuria during pregnancy should prompt additional investigation, which might include intravenous pyelography or cystoscopy. The potential adverse fetal effects of these radiologic studies must be considered, and the number of X-ray exposures should be limited. At least one report indicates the presence of a renal cell carcinoma diagnosed at 29 weeks of gestation in a gravida with severe hypertensive disease that did not respond to delivery of the fetus.

It is thought that therapy in pregnant women with a renal malignancy should be instituted shortly after diagnosis, avoiding long delays in treatment. Survival rates with the treatment of localized disease exceed 50%. The treatment of upper urinary tract malignancies remains surgical; however, adjunctive irradiation either preoperatively or postoperatively may be needed pending tumor size and vascularity.

Bladder cancer, if superficial and well differentiated, can be treated with local fulguration. More deeply invasive tumors or recurrent tumors may require partial or total cystectomy, often preceded by external radiotherapy. These findings suggest that treatment of the pregnant woman with bladder carcinoma must be individualized based on estimated fetal risks and extent of disease. There is no known adverse effect of pregnancy on transitional cell carcinoma of the bladder.

Urethral carcinoma may be treated by excision, brachytherapy, teletherapy, or some combination of these treatments. While the choice of treatment depends on the size and location of the cancer, implanted radium seeds have been used during pregnancy in at least two reported cases, with no observable harm to the fetus.

The relatively low number of reported genitourinary tract malignancies and pregnancy preclude any well-founded statement regarding prognosis. It is thought that renal cell carcinomas have an overall 5-year survival rate of 45%. Women with bladder cancers that exhibit no invasion, invasion of the submucosa, or superficial muscles have a 54% 3-year survival, while those with deep invasion have a 3-year survival of 42%. Bone metastases are the most common type of distal spread; liver, lung, or kidney metastases are rare.

Gastrointestinal Malignancies
Gastrointestinal malignancies are rare in women of reproductive age, with only 5–8% of all patients with colorectal carcinoma being under age 40. The incidence of coexisting colorectal carcinoma in pregnancy is estimated to be 0.002–0.02%. Fewer than 200 cases of rectal cancer associated with pregnancy have been reported. Only three cases of pregnancy and carcinoma of the stomach have been reported in the English literature. In fact, cancer of the stomach is rarely diagnosed in U.S. women under age 35. Obviously, this risk is increased in Asian populations, related to environment, with 44 cases of stomach cancer in pregnant women having been reported from Japan alone.

Hepatocellular carcinoma is predominantly a malignancy of males; most female cases are in the postmenopausal age group. While an increased incidence of liver tumors has been associated with the use of OCs, there has been no increased incidence of coexisting malignant hepatic cancers.

Only five pregnant women have been reported to have coexisting carcinoma of the pancreas, and only a single case of extrahepatic biliary tract carcinoma has been reported.

An overall delay in diagnosis of colorectal carcinoma is common, since symptoms may be overshadowed by those typical of pregnancy. Persistent or significant rectal bleeding, abdominal pain, markedly altered bowel habits, weight loss, nausea, and vomiting in late pregnancy should alert the obstetrician to the possibility of lower gastrointestinal malignancy. Sigmoidoscopy, proctoscopy, or colonoscopy can be performed but must be undertaken with caution since the enlarged uterus may exert extrinsic pressure on the colon. The routine use of a barium enema during pregnancy is of little benefit because of its poor sensitivity and fetal radiation exposure.

Surgery for colon and rectal carcinoma entails anterior resection with reanastomosis or abdominoperineal resection, depending on the position of the malignant lesion. In early pregnancy the gestation itself may be ignored in favor of surgically treating the malignancy. In some instances the uterus may be retracted out of the pelvis, allowing the operation to proceed and the pregnancy to continue. Tumors located deep in the pelvis may obstruct labor and therefore may have bearing on decisions regarding delivery. Short therapeutic delays may allow delivery of a viable infant by cesarean delivery with concomitant resection of the bowel tumor. In the second trimester, uterine evacuation may be required to facilitate or allow bowel resection. It would appear that there is no evidence of adverse hormonal effect during pregnancy either to increase or to decrease the rate of growth of colorectal or colonic tumors. As in other types of malignancy, delay in diagnosis and treatment is probably a more important factor affecting survival than the effects of the hormonal milieu of pregnancy.

Protracted symptoms referable to the upper intestinal tract are common during pregnancy, making the diagnosis of an upper intestinal tumor extremely difficult. If necessary, radiologic evaluation or gastroduodenoscopy should be considered for those patients with severe protracted symptomatology. Curative resection of stomach cancer is possible in less than 50% of patients, with the remainder of patients invariably succumbing to malignancy. Because of the poor prognosis and importance of surgical resection, treatment should not be delayed.

One third of hepatic tumors are discovered accidentally by the patient or by the physician on routine examination. Another one third are discovered intraoperatively at the time of surgery for some other indication, and one third present as acute life-threatening intraabdominal hemorrhage from liver rupture. Review of 54 patients with subcapsular hemorrhage with or without liver rupture during pregnancy indicated a maternal mortality of 70% and a fetal mortality of 77%. If a liver mass is discovered during pregnancy, diagnostic procedures such as ultrasonography, computed tomography scanning, and perhaps arteriography should be considered.

Hepatocellular tumors should be resected, if possible, during pregnancy. There is no known adverse effect of pregnancy, and there is no increased vascularity of the liver. High levels of sex steroids during pregnancy theoretically may predispose the tumor to rupture. Therapeutic abortion may be indicated if pregnancy occurs in a patient with a hepatoma that is either unresectable or only partially resectable.

Miscellaneous Tumors

Malignancies of the central nervous system and spinal cord rarely complicate pregnancy; however, they carry a 60% mortality rate when present. The usual symptoms of headache and visual disturbance are common, with seizures being relatively rare. Diagnosis of central nervous system malignancy is best established by computerized tomography or magnetic resonance imaging. Infratentorial tumors are associated with a particularly poor prognosis. Therapeutic abortion may be considered for women with poor-prognosis tumors discovered in the first trimester, because of the likelihood that neither mother nor fetus will survive. All patients should receive steroids, osmotic agents, and timely surgical decompression in the presence of central nervous system symptoms.

Fewer than 10 cases of soft tissue sarcoma and fewer than six patients with malignant bone sarcomas have been reported. There appears to be no adverse effect of pregnancy, and all considerations regarding maternal and fetal prognosis related to disease should be undertaken prior to treatment. Obstetrician–gynecologists frequently have good opportunity to detect thyroid nodules. Although 2,000–3,000 cases of thyroid cancer are found yearly, fewer than half of these are diagnosed in women of childbearing age. Patients who have a history of thyroid irradiation for benign conditions (use of radioactive iodine for diagnosis) appear to be at decreased risk of thyroid cancer. If thyroid nodules are found on routine examination, a radioactive scan must be used to determine the nature of the enlargement. Surgery remains the primary treatment for thyroid carcinoma, with irradiation reserved for unresectable primary tumors or metastatic lesions. Abortion has not been found to have an ameliorating effect on this malignancy.

Although scans are important diagnostic tools, the use of radioactive iodine in diagnostic scans for pregnant women carries a considerable risk of fetal injury and is contraindicated during pregnancy.

BIBLIOGRAPHY

Aisner J, Wiernik PH, Pearl P. Pregnancy outcome in patients treated for Hodgkin's disease. J Clin Oncol 1993;11:507–512

Anderson JF, Kent S, Machin GA. Maternal malignant melanoma with placental metastasis: a case report with literature review. Pediatr Pathol 1989;9:35–42

Antunez de Mayolo J, Ahn YS, Temple JD, Harrington WJ. Spontaneous remission of acute leukemia after the termination of pregnancy. Cancer 1989;63:1621–1623

Baltzer J, Regenbrecht ME, Kopcke W, Zander J. Carcinoma of the cervix and pregnancy. Int J Gynaecol Obstet 1990;31:317–323

Ben-Baruch G, Menczer J, Goshen R, Kaufman B, Gorodetzky R. Cisplatin excretion in human milk. J Natl Cancer Inst 1992; 84:451–452

Caligiuri MA, Mayer RJ. Pregnancy and leukemia. Semin Oncol 1989; 16:388–396

Christman JE, Teng NNH, Lebovic GS, Sikic BI. Delivery of a normal infant following cisplatin, vinblastine, and bleomycin (PVB) chemotherapy for malignant teratoma of the ovary during pregnancy. Gynecol Oncol 1990;37:292–295

Dildy GA III, Moise Jr KJ, Carpenter Jr RJ, Kilma T. Maternal malignancy metastatic to the products of conception: a review. Obstet Gynecol Surv 1989;44:535–540

Doll DC, Ringenberg QS, Yarbro JW. Antineoplastic agents and pregnancy. Semin Oncol 1989;16:337–346

Giuntoli R, Yeh IT, Bhuett N, Chu W, Van Leewen K, Van der Lans P. Conservative management of cervical intraepithelial neoplasia during pregnancy. Gynecol Oncol 1991;42:68–73

Gonsoulin W, Mason B, Carpenter RJ Jr. Colon cancer in pregnancy with elevated maternal serum alpha-fetoprotein level at presentation. Am J Obstet Gynecol 1990;163:1172–1173

Gordon AN, Jensen R, Jones HW III . Squamous carcinoma of the cervix complicating pregnancy: recurrence in episiotomy after vaginal delivery. Obstet Gynecol 1989;73:850–852

Greer BE, Easterling TR, McLennan DA, Benedetti TJ, Cain JM, Figge DC, et al. Fetal and maternal considerations in the management of stage I-B cervical cancer during pregnancy. Gynecol Oncol 1989;34: 61–65

Hannigan EV. Cervical cancer in pregnancy. Clin Obstet Gynecol 1990;33:837–845

Holloway RW, To A, Moradi M, Boots L, Watson N, Shingleton HM. Monitoring the course of cervical carcinoma with the squamous cell carcinoma serum radioimmunoassay. Obstet Gynecol 1989;74:944–949

Kobayashi F, Sagawa N, Nakamura K, Nonugaki M, Ban C. Mechanism and clinical significance of elevated CA 125 levels in the sera of pregnant women. Am J Obstet Gynecol 1989;160:563–566

Malfetano JH, Goldkrand JW. Cis–platinum combination chemotherapy during pregnancy for advanced epithelial ovarian carcinoma. Obstet Gynecol 1990;75:545–547

Mazze RI, Kallen B. Reproductive outcome after anesthesia and operation during pregnancy: a registry study of 5405 cases. Am J Obstet Gynecol 1989;161:1178–1185

Orr Jr JW, Shingleton HM. Cancer in pregnancy. Curr Probl Cancer 1993;8:1–50

Parente JT, Amsel M, Lerner R, Chinea F. Breast cancer associated with pregnancy. Obstet Gynecol 1988;71:861–864

Patsner B. Management of low-grade cervical dysplasia during pregnancy. South Med J 1990;83:1405–1406, 1412

Patsner B, Baker DA, Orr Jr JW. Human papillomavirus genital tract infections during pregnancy. Clin Obstet Gynecol 1990;33:258–267

Schwartz P. Cancer in pregnancy. In: Gusberg SB, Shingleton HM, Deppe G, eds. Female genital cancer. New York: Churchill Livingstone, 1988:725–754

van der Vange N, van Dongen JA. Breast cancer and pregnancy. Eur J Surg Oncol 1991;17:1–8

VanVoorhis B, Cruikshank DP. Colon carcinoma complicating pregnancy: a report of two cases. J Reprod Med 1989;34:923–927

Ward FT, Weiss RB. Lymphoma and pregnancy. Semin Oncol 1989; 16:397–409

Wong DJ, Strassner HT. Melanoma in pregnancy. Clin Obstet Gynecol 1990;33:782–791

Quality of Life Considerations

Quality of life is a judgment that compares one status against another, for example, the patient's condition versus what it could be, what it was, or what the patient would like it to be. Quality of life is also multidimensional, embracing physical well-being, psychologic well-being, social well-being, spiritual well-being, and financial well-being.

Addressed here are three issues that warrant a physician's attention regarding quality of life in the management of the cancer patient: 1) the grieving process, 2) cancer pain control, and 3) the use of patient-controlled directives.

THE GRIEVING PROCESS

The problem of the management of the dying cancer patient is one that concerns all physicians. In medical school, students' first confrontation with death is in the anatomy laboratory, where they are quickly desensitized to the cadaver, thus objectifying death. As clinical training proceeds, the patient becomes a collection of symptoms representing a pathologic state. Medical students are confronted with more information than can possibly be assimilated and are socialized to simulate more knowledge and greater mastery of the situation than actually possible at this stage. This encourages a kind of counterphobic bravado when dealing with situations in which physicians are faced with a patient's death. Physicians must remember that help does not necessarily mean cure.

Preparation for caring for dying patients is learned from the dying themselves—but only if they are viewed with respect and never merely with pity and if allowed to teach such care. Being with the dying can be a humbling and yet an ennobling experience. Whatever else it is, it is an intensely human event.

Death and dying are often avoided, not simply because they do not fit into the world of death-denying, pleasure-seeking attitudes, but also because of a lack of experience or learning about interaction with the dying. A lack of normative expectations for a situation leaves one with no understanding of how to behave. This leads to a tendency to withdraw from or avoid the dying.

Avoidance of the dying is demonstrated by the aversion of hospital personnel to discussing death when that topic is raised by the dying patient. Several strategies have been identified as ones that are used by staff members in responding to a patient's desire to discuss death: 1) reassurance ("You're doing so well."), 2) denial ("Oh, you'll live to be a hundred."), 3) changing the subject ("Let's talk about something more cheerful."), 4) fatalism ("Well, we all have to die sometime."), and 5) discussion ("What happened to make you feel that way?"). Few choose to discuss death with the patient. The typical response tends to be evasion.

It is often not death that the cancer patient fears, but dying. The struggle to gain control over an uncertain future takes many forms. The literature uses the words *bereavement, grief,* and *mourning* interchangeably to explain this phenomenon. Definitions of these terms help to place them in a useful perspective.

Bereavement comes from a root word meaning shorn off or torn up—as if something has been suddenly yanked away. The word thus conveys a sense of being deprived, of having something stripped away against one's will, of being robbed. Bereavement signifies a force that comes from outside as a violent, destructive action taken. Bereavement can be defined as the event of loss. A form of bereavement might be when a patient is given the diagnosis of cancer.

Grief is a person's emotional response to the event of a loss. Like bereavement, grief has usually been thought of in negative terms: heartbreak, anguish, distress, suffering—a burdensome emotional state. Yet grief can be considered as the total emotional response to loss. Among the range of emotions that might be present are not only sorrow and sadness, but also anger, disgust, and self-pity. Limiting the definition of grief reduces the chance of accepting all of the emotions that may be present.

Mourning is the process of incorporating the experience of loss into daily life. This process deals with the question: How does one carry on? Mourning is also the outward acknowledgment of loss.

In discussing the trinity of bereavement, grief, and mourning as it relates to the cancer patient, it is impossible to account for the entire range of possible idiosyncratic manifestations of a patient. Cancer alters an individual's self-concept. The illusion of immortality is forever lost. The patient is made aware of how little control she has and of the fact that unless she assumes some responsibility for her choices and for how she lives today, she may never again be given the opportunity to do so. Tomorrow may bring sudden death, loss of function, or changes in dependency on social systems, such as the family and health care system. She undergoes a change, and change always means loss. This is the bereavement experience.

The diagnosis of cancer is heard by many patients as a death sentence, which produces a kind of "ego chill." Initial grief reactions include shock, disbelief, dismay, self-pity, bitterness, anger, fear, anxiety, and depression. These are usually followed by some form of acceptance or resolution to do whatever is deemed necessary to fight for life. Mourning follows, hopefully as a basis for a healing process.

Elisabeth Kubler-Ross, in her pioneering work on death and dying, concluded that when one is aware that death is imminent, one experiences a relatively predictable pattern of responses of denial, anger, bargaining, depression, and acceptance. Although Kubler-Ross's work has been at once cherished, challenged, added to, and disregarded as rationally ordered scientific data demanded by the nature of the medical model, it can serve as a basis for understanding and enhancing further self-study and observation.

Denial, the defense mechanism by which a person unconsciously fails to perceive reality accurately, acts as a buffer after unexpected, shocking news. It has both positive and negative aspects. It is a destructive mechanism to the extent that failure to recognize the full implications of a diagnosis of cancer or the actual diagnosis leads to failure to seek consultation and obtain effective or palliative therapy. Denial is positive in that it allows the reality to be integrated without too much disturbance to the individual's psychic equilibrium. Denial, in addition, may lead to a fight to survive that facilitates longevity. It may help to create the balance so poignantly expressed in the statement, "We cannot look at the sun all the time; we cannot face death all the time."

This does not mean that a patient in the denial stage will not in time be willing or even happy and relieved to sit and talk with someone about her impending death. Human beings have a magnificent filtering system built into their perceptual senses. When discussing any delicate subject, this system sifts out any data the mind is not ready to know. No matter how loud, how clear, or how often the speaker communicates an unwanted fact, the mind resists acceptance until it is ready.

However, such a dialogue will and must take place at the convenience of the patient—not the convenience of the listener. This exchange must also be terminated when the patient can no longer tolerate it, and she must be allowed to resume her previous denial.

Depending very much on how a patient is told of her cancer diagnosis, how much time she has to gradually acknowledge that the inevitable is happening, and how she has been prepared throughout her life to cope with stressful situations, she will gradually drop her denial and use less radical defense mechanisms.

Kubler-Ross's second stage is anger. When denial can no longer be maintained, it is replaced by feelings of rage, envy, and resentment. The question becomes, "Why me?" This stage can be very difficult to cope with from the point of view of family and staff because the anger is displaced in various directions and projected onto the environment almost at random. In short, no one and no thing is beyond reproach in the mind of the patient. Wherever the patient looks she will find grievances. Her lashing out begins a cycle of avoidance and returned anger on the part of the family and caregivers, which only increases the patient's discomfort and anger, and so the cycle goes.

The challenge here is for the caregivers and loved ones to place themselves in the patient's position. Might we not all be angry if all of our life's dreams and activities were prematurely interrupted?

The greatest regrets are for what might have been. Cancer confronts the patient with her own mortality and with the need for taking responsibility for how she lives her own life. This may be the first time that she reevaluates with whom she chooses to live, what she will tolerate in a relationship, and how she spends her time and money.

Bargaining, the third stage, occurs as the patient seeks to delay the terrible fate that awaits. If she has been unable to face the sad facts in the first period and has been angry at people and God in the second phase, maybe she can succeed in entering into some sort of agreement that may postpone her worst fears. An example is that of a child who does not accept the parents' "no" to a request to spend the night at a friend's house. The child becomes angry, pouts, and withdraws. Eventually, the child will reconsider this approach and volunteer to complete chores or any parent-pleasing behavior in return for a "yes" answer to a request.

The cancer patient might use the same maneuvers. She knows from past experience that there is a slim chance that she might be rewarded for good behavior and be granted a wish. Her wish is almost always for an extension of life—followed, perhaps, by the wish for a few days without pain, or a self-imposed deadline (to live long enough to see her child graduate or marry)—and it usually includes an implicit promise that she will not ask for more if this one reprieve is granted.

The fourth stage, depression, comes when the patient can no longer deny her illness, when she is forced to undergo more surgery or hospitalization, when she begins to have more symptoms or becomes weaker and thinner. Her numbness, stoicism, anger, and rage will be replaced with a sense of a great loss. Kubler-Ross maintains that there are two kinds of depression. Reactive depression is the response to the loss of physical well-being, autonomy, finances, a job, etc. Preparatory depression is the emotional response to the impending loss of one's life.

Finally, Kubler-Ross identifies acceptance as the final stage. It seems to be "the point toward the end of the long dark hours when the new reality registers as clearly in her inner images as in her outer adjustment." Kubler-Ross describes the patient as contemplating "[her] coming end with a certain degree of quiet expectation." This stage may be somewhat neutral in emotion, and the patient's interest in the rest of the world may seem diminished.

Difficulties in dealing with the dying patient tend to spring from personal fears and anxieties. We can work to balance our fears with openness, our anxieties with trust. As valuable as our physical help and education can be, it is the emotional interchange that we have with the dying patient and her family that is, in the long run, the most effective care. Through our capacity and willingness to comfort, reassure, and hearten, we reaffirm to our patients and ourselves that we are also members of the human race and no less mortal than those we treat. The patient is oddly comforted by the finiteness that we have in common with them.

CANCER PAIN CONTROL

Pain is a common and overwhelming symptom of cancer that greatly affects the quality of life of both the patient and her family. It is one of the most feared consequences of cancer.

Cancer pain can be managed effectively for most patients. Integration of pain assessment and treatment into overall cancer care depends on understanding the goals of pain therapy, knowing the most effective use of all available drugs and modalities, and eliminating the barriers to effective management.

Patients with cancer have two types of pain: acute and chronic. Acute pain is characterized by a well-defined temporal pattern of onset. It is generally associated with the autonomic nervous system. These signs serve as objective evidence to the physician, substantiating the patient's report of pain. Chronic pain is pain that persists longer than 6 months, in which adaptation of the autonomic nervous system occurs. Patients with chronic pain lack the objective signs common to acute pain. Chronic pain leads to marked changes in personality, life style, and functional attitudes. Such pain requires an approach that includes both treatment of the cause of pain and treatment of its psychologic and social consequences.

Because pain is a subjective experience, evaluation of it is difficult. The patient and the physician are best served if the physician believes the patient's report.

Nonnarcotic, narcotic, and adjuvant analgesic drugs are the mainstays of therapy for patients with cancer pain. Effective use of these drugs requires an understanding of their clinicopharmacologic characteristics. Although opiates are often the keystone of cancer pain management, noninvasive measures can enhance pain relief and improve sleep, mood, and mobility. These measures include relaxation, guided imagery, cognitive intervention, music, massage, and heat.

Novel routes and methods of administration have been established and warrant further study beyond the constraints of this material. They include oral, intranasal, transdermal, sublingual, continuous infusion by intravenous or subcutaneous routes, epidural and intrathecal, and patient-controlled analgesia pumps.

It is estimated that 80% of patients do not receive adequate pain relief. The barrier that most undermines pain relief is the erroneous belief that long-term use or high doses of opiates inevitably lead to substance abuse and addiction. This belief leads professionals to underprescribe and underuse opiates for pain relief, causes patients and families to limit or underuse medications that have been prescribed, and influences legislative and regulatory initiatives that purport to control illegal substance use, yet severely limit the legitimate medical use of opiates.

Inherent in legislative initiatives is the government's requirement that physicians complete lengthy and fee-imposing forms each year that certify them to prescribe narcotic analgesics. This is a discouraging deterrent to adequate patient management. In California, only 5% of surgeons are certified to prescribe opiate analgesia, presumably because of these complexities. Physicians have a moral responsibility to treat all aspects of a disease, including controlling pain, either by conforming to the current legislation or by involving themselves in change that would simplify the certification process.

Studies of the patterns of chronic narcotic drug use in patients with cancer have demonstrated that tolerance and physical dependence occur, but that the psychologic dependence (addiction) is rare (less than 0.1%). Pain relief is possible when available knowledge and technologies are applied.

Ethical principles of autonomy, beneficence, nonmaleficence, and justice provide a framework within which to examine clinical issues in pain management practice:

- *Autonomy* is based on respect for the individual and suggests that patients must be informed of all treatments and associated outcomes. Conflict-of-interest issues arise when physicians and hospitals own infusion treatment or equipment companies. Decisions must not be based on revenue.
- *Beneficence* asserts that health care providers have a responsibility to benefit the patient. Common threats to beneficence to the patient in pain include undermedication, health care providers' misconception of the nature of cancer pain, and failure of the medical profession to provide adequate pain education in schools of medicine.
- *Nonmaleficence* states that physicians should avoid causing harm and should strive to protect the patient from harm. Research has documented that pain treatments may decrease pain intensity while decreasing other aspects of quality of life.
- The principle of *justice* contends that scarce resources should be distributed fairly and that individuals should have equal access to care. Access to pain treatment is a serious concern

for the future, and a system whereby only the wealthy can afford comfort must be avoided.

The most important reassurance a physician can give a patient is that she will not be abandoned in her suffering and that both patient and physician will work together to find out what will best alleviate her pain. This kind of statement and its follow-through relieves anxiety, calms fears, and may have a placebo effect of its own.

PATIENT-CONTROLLED DIRECTIVES

People have become increasingly concerned that the dying process is oftentimes needlessly protracted by medical technology. This attention comes on the heels of a dramatic shift in the places where people die. Sixty years ago, most deaths occurred at home. Now most deaths occur in hospitals or long-term care facilities.

In a public opinion poll, 68% of the respondents believed that "people dying of an incurable painful disease should be allowed to end their lives before the disease runs its course." However, the development of sophisticated life-support technologies now enable medicine to intervene and delay death for most patients. These developments have brought many ethical issues to the forefront of the practice of medicine.

Biomedical ethics, the concept of a person as an autonomous agent, places an obligation on physicians to respect the values of patients and not let their own values influence decision-making about life-sustaining treatment. Life-sustaining treatment is any medical treatment that serves to prolong life without reversing the underlying medical condition. Life-sustaining treatment may include, but is not limited to, mechanical ventilation, renal dialysis, chemotherapy, antibiotics, and artificial nutrition and hydration.

The conflict between autonomy and medical judgment is extremely complex and strongly warrants intense study by every physician. The dilemma of patient values versus physician values becomes most troublesome when a patient refuses treatment needed to sustain life and a physician believes that the patient should be treated. The patriarchal notion of "what the doctor thinks is best" is now challenged by the consumer-minded patient and family, as well as by the private and federally funded insurance providers.

Some quality of care guidelines for moral and ethical dilemmas are documents that are referred to as advance directives. They deal with such issues as "do not resuscitate" orders, durable power of attorney for health care, and the Patient Self-Determination Act.

An order not to resuscitate means specifically that in the event of a cardiopulmonary arrest there should be no blow to the chest, artificial ventilation, electric shock, or cardiac drugs administered to the patient. A writing of a "do not resuscitate" order should initiate a rethinking of all the goals of therapy and a discussion of these goals with the patient or her family, or both. Consideration should also be given to other therapeutic modalities (concurrent care concerns) that stop short of resuscitative orders but that offer some type of relief or comfort and assure the patient that she will not be abandoned. Concurrent care concerns include intubation, dialysis, blood product support, antibiotics, pressor drugs, vital sign frequency, adjustment of sedatives and analgesics, discharge or hospice planning, spiritual needs, nutrition, and hydration.

The durable power of attorney for health care is a legal document that allows the signer to appoint an agent to make health care decisions if the signer is unable to do so. It also allows the patient to explore and express specific preferences regarding medical treatment that she may wish the agent to choose. Uses and specifics of this durable power of attorney vary nationwide and must be studied by physicians in each state.

The Patient Self-Determination Act of 1990 was passed by Congress as part of the Omnibus Budget Reconciliation Act, and it became effective on December 1, 1991. The Patient Self-Determination Act applies to all hospitals, home health agencies, skilled nursing facilities, hospices, and health maintenance organizations that are federally funded. The Patient Self-Determination Act requires that providers do several things: 1) give adult patients written information about their rights under state law to make medical decisions, including the right to create advance directives; 2) have written institutional policies and procedures about advance directives and about patients' rights to consent to or refuse treatment and inform patients about these policies; 3) document in the medical record whether a patient has executed an advance directive; and 4) provide education about advance directives for staff and the community.

Providers must comply with state law regarding advance directives in order to receive care. The Patient Self-Determination Act requires that this information be given upon admission as an inpatient. The patient brochure can be given to a family member or a surrogate decision maker if it looks as if the patient will not quickly be capable of making his or her own decisions, or it can be given to the patient as soon as the patient has been stabilized enough to receive information.

The specifics of the Patient Self-Determination Act vary from state to state and from facility to facility. Every physician needs to educate himself or herself accordingly.

Physicians will continue to face the formidable ethical frontier. They have an obligation to relieve pain and suffering and to promote the dignity and autonomy of dying patients under their care. Support, comfort, respect for autonomy, good communication, and adequate pain control may dramatically alter the patient's quality of life.

Physicians should strive to develop their own philosophies and beliefs about death and dying, and about choosing the time of death. Such views are unique to each person, may not be held consistently by the same person from time to time, are highly complex, and may coexist with contradictory beliefs within the same individual.

BIBLIOGRAPHY

DeSpelder LA, Strickland AL. The last dance: encountering death and dying. Palo Alto, California: Mayfield Publishing, 1983

Foley KM. The treatment of cancer pain. N Engl J Med 1985;313: 84–95

Kavanaugh RE. Facing death. Los Angeles: Nash, 1972

Kubler-Ross E. On death and dying. New York: Macmillan, 1969

Porter J, Jick H. Addiction rare in patients treated with narcotics. N Engl J Med 1980;302:123

Saunders C. The moment of truth. In: Perason L, ed. Death and dying: current issues in the treatment of the dying person. Cleveland: Press of Case Western Reserve University, 1969

Sheehy G. Pathfinders. New York: Bantam Books, 1981

Slaby AE, Glicksman AS. Adapting to life and threatening illness. New York: Praeger Publishers, 1985

Spross JA. Pain management: issues in the hospital setting. In: American Cancer Society. Pain management issues in research and practice. New York: ACS, 1992

Sulmasy DP, Geller G, Faden R, Levine DM. The quality of mercy: caring for patients with "do not resuscitate" orders. JAMA 1992; 267:682–686

Whedon M, Ferrell BR. Professional and ethical considerations in the use of high-tech pain management. Oncol Nurs Forum 1991; 18:1135–1143

Reproductive Endocrinology and Fertility

Since the publication of *Precis IV*, the pace of progress in reproductive endocrinology and infertility has accelerated. In fact, few areas in obstetrics and gynecology have witnessed such rapid advances. Developments in reproductive biology, neuroendocrinology, and molecular biology have provided new insight into the regulation of hypothalamic–pituitary–ovarian function and better understanding of many reproductive disorders. New research into the role of growth factors in ovarian function and ovulatory disorders has identified promising therapeutic avenues.

Assisted reproductive technology has become routine and has continued its own explosive progress. Preservation of embryos and oocytes by freezing, implantation of embryos in recipients with no ovarian function, microinjection of sperm into the oocyte, assisted hatching, and preimplantation biopsy for diagnosing genetic disorders are but a few of such advances that have profoundly affected clinical practice.

Clinical studies of new drugs have also had an impact on the management of patients in reproductive medicine. Expanded clinical applications of gonadotropin-releasing hormone analogues have revolutionized the treatment of a larger number of endocrine and gynecologic conditions. Beneficial effects of hormone replacement therapy have been found to include protection against cardiovascular disease, a major cause of mortality in elderly women.

Infertility surgery has become more refined and is performed principally by laparoscopy and pelviscopy. The introduction of new and sophisticated instrumentation, laser technology, and refined optics has enabled us to perform complicated procedures via hysteroscopy or laparoscopy.

The content of *Precis V* has been updated to reflect these and many other innovations and discoveries in this field. Once again the reader is reminded that this text is not intended to represent a comprehensive review of reproductive endocrinology and infertility or to replace standard textbooks. Rather, it is meant to provide a concise description of new and relevant information that exerts an impact on clinical practice. When necessary, basic sciences are discussed merely as a prelude to clinical recognition and appropriate management of various disorders. Throughout the text, generally accepted concepts and therapeutic modalities are recommended. Advocacy of extreme views and untried or experimental management regimens is avoided.

Kamran S. Moghissi, MD

Receptor Physiology

All hormonal signals known to date require that the hormone be recognized by a specific cellular receptor. That recognition results in profound changes in cellular function that lead to the end hormonal effect. Although hormones enter the bloodstream and are circulated throughout the body, only those cells possessing hormone-specific receptors are capable of responding to the hormone. Receptors are generally found in large excess on hormonally responsive cells, only a small fraction of which (1–3%) need to be occupied to produce a maximal hormonal response. This excess of receptors allows the cell to be exquisitely sensitive to the low concentrations (typically 10^{-11}–10^{-9} mol/L) at which most hormones are found in the bloodstream. Furthermore, the cell can "adjust" its sensitivity to the hormone in question by altering the number of receptors available, a process known as up-regulation or down-regulation.

Receptors for protein hormones are located on the cell surface, where they form an integral part of the cell wall structure. In contrast, receptors for steroid hormones are located intracellularly.

CELL SURFACE RECEPTORS

The essence of a hormone's action is its effect on the cellular machinery of the target cell. All cell surface receptors for which the mechanism of action is known exert their effects via the activation of various enzymes, resulting in an enhanced (or diminished) ability to catalyze various molecular transformations. The binding of the hormone to the specific receptor is only the first step in a cascade of reactions and conformational changes that use one or more intermediary molecules (so-called second messengers) to relay the information to the intracellular machinery.

MECHANISM OF PROTEIN HORMONE ACTION

Receptors for the glycoprotein hormones thyroid-stimulating hormone (TSH), follicle-stimulating hormone (FSH), luteinizing hormone (LH), and human chorionic gonadotropin (hCG) (LH and hCG use a common receptor) have been isolated and sequenced, and their primary structures have been determined. These receptors belong to a large superfamily of hormone receptors characterized by hydrophilic sequences on each end flanking seven hydrophobic regions, presumed to be membrane-spanning areas. The N-terminus is located extracellularly and comprises the hormone-binding site. The C-terminus is located intracellularly and is probably involved in relaying the hormonal signal to the second messenger.

Common to all receptors in the superfamily containing seven transmembrane domains is the use of a specialized membrane-associated guanine nucleotide–binding protein (G protein). The G protein has three subunits, alpha, beta, and gamma. In the inactive state, guanosine diphosphate (GDP) is bound to the alpha subunit. The binding of hormone to receptor promotes dissociation of GDP from the alpha subunit and its replacement by guanosine triphosphate (GTP). When GTP is bound to the alpha subunit, the alpha subunit–GTP complex can associate with the catalytic subunit of the enzyme adenylate cyclase to activate it. The activated catalytic subunit then converts Mg^{++}–ATP to cyclic adenosine monophosphate (cyclic AMP). Activated alpha subunit contains guanosine triphosphatase activity, which hydrolyzes GTP to GDP and terminates the adenylate cyclase activation. In addition to the stimulatory alpha subunit, there exists an inhibitory alpha subunit, the activation of which inhibits adenylate cyclase activity. There are many hormones that activate the inhibitory alpha subunit. Therefore, the net adenylate cyclase activity depends on the relative input from both inhibitory and stimulatory G proteins.

Cyclic AMP performs its role in the cell by binding to a cyclic AMP-dependent protein kinase (protein kinase A). This holoenzyme is composed of a regulatory subunit dimer and two catalytic subunits. Each of the regulatory subunits binds four molecules of cyclic AMP, which when bound causes dissociation of the two catalytic subunits from the regulatory subunits and the expression of protein kinase activity. Protein kinase A catalyzes the transfer of a phosphate from ATP to the hydroxyl groups of serine and threonine residues of cellular proteins. This phosphorylation results in altered enzymatic activity. The specific responses of various cell types to an increase in cyclic AMP and protein kinase A activation is determined by the cellular phenotype and, therefore, by the enzymes and substrates available for regulation.

Another recently appreciated action of cyclic AMP is the transcriptional regulation of specific genes within the cell nucleus. A cyclic AMP response element–binding protein has been identified as the mediator of cyclic AMP action on gene regulation. Cyclic AMP activates cyclic AMP response element–binding protein via protein kinase A–mediated phosphorylation of specific serine residues. As a dimer, cyclic AMP response element–binding protein binds to a specific DNA sequence located on cyclic AMP-regulated genes called the cyclic AMP response element and regulates transcription of those genes.

The hormones TSH, FSH, LH, hCG, and corticotropin (ACTH) are examples of cyclic AMP-mediated activity. However, not all protein hormone–G protein interactions use cyclic AMP as the second messenger. Examples of second messengers produced by G protein activation with other ligands include diacylglycerol, inositol triphosphate, and intracellular Ca^{++}.

Yet other protein hormones use systems independent of G proteins. An example is the family of receptors with tyrosine kinase activity. Binding of ligand to these receptors results in G protein–independent phosphorylation of tyrosine residues of various cellular signaling proteins.

INTERCELLULAR RECEPTORS

Receptors for a number of regulatory molecules such as steroid hormones, thyroid hormone, vitamin D, and retinoic acid are localized within the target cells, primarily within the nucleus. In general, these are hormones that exert long-term effects on the cells, such as growth and differentiation. The hormone–receptor complex acts by altering the rate of transcription of specific genes. Thus, these receptors properly belong to the class of molecules known as transcription factors.

MECHANISM OF STEROID HORMONE ACTION

Steroids travel in the circulation largely bound to several classes of serum proteins, predominantly sex hormone–binding protein and, to a lesser extent, albumin. Unbound steroids are freely transported into cells by simple diffusion but are sequestered only in those cells that express specific intracellular receptors. Recent studies have shown conclusively that, with the possible exception of the glucocorticoids, both free and occupied receptors are localized to the nucleus.

The ligand-binding domain of the steroid hormone receptor is located at the C-terminus. The DNA-binding region is located within the central portion of the molecule and contains two repeated sequences rich in cysteine, lysine, and arginine residues. Each of these units is folded such that a Zn^{++} ion is held within a fingerlike projection protruding from the main portion of the molecule. These "zinc fingers" can insert into a half-turn of DNA and are a common finding in a variety of transcription factors. The transcriptionally active forms of these molecules are dimers produced between leucine-rich regions ("leucine zippers") resulting from steroid–receptor interaction. The conformational changes that result produce an active transcription factor.

The dimerized steroid hormone–receptor complex binds to its specific *cis*-acting element (the nucleotide base sequence of the target regulatory gene), also known as the steroid response element to regulate gene transcription. Different hormones may share common response elements; thus, the response elicited is determined by what receptors are presently expressed within the cell.

BIBLIOGRAPHY

Evans RM. The steroid and thyroid hormone receptor superfamily. Science 1988;240:889–895

Forman BM, Samuels HH. Interactions among a subfamily of nuclear hormone receptors: the regulatory zipper model. Mol Endocrinol 1990;4:1293–1301

Merz WE. Properties of glycoprotein hormone receptors and postreceptor mechanisms. Exp Clin Endocrinol 1992;100:4–8

Montminy MR, Gonzalez GA, Yamamoto KK. Characteristics of the cAMP response unit. Recent Prog Horm Res 1990;46:219–229; discussion 29–30

O'Malley BW, Tsai M-J. Molecular pathways of steroid receptor action. Biol Reprod 1992;46:163–167

Segaloff DL, Sprengel R, Nikolics K, Ascoli M. Structure of the lutropin/choriogonadotropin receptor. Recent Prog Horm Res 1990; 46:261–301; discussion 301–303

Simpson ER, Mendelson CR. The molecular basis of hormone action. In: Carr BR, Blackwell RE, eds. Textbook of reproductive medicine. Norwalk, Connecticut: Appleton and Lange, 1993:121–139

Neuroendocrinology

Normal reproductive development and function require the complex interaction of higher brain centers, the hypothalamus, pituitary gland, gonads, and target organs. Within this framework it has become clear that the hypothalamus serves as the central conduit that sends appropriate signals to control the secretion of the peptide hormones of the anterior pituitary gland, including the three essential for coordinated reproductive function: LH, FSH, and prolactin. In turn, the neurons within the hypothalamus receive signals from the periphery and higher brain centers. These signals between neurons take the form of chemicals and form the basis for the concept of neurosecretion.

NEUROSECRETION

The distinctions among neurotransmitters, neurohormones, paracrine mediators, and hormones circulating in the peripheral circulation have blurred. Neurotransmitters differ from other chemical messengers only in that they are released from neurons and act over relatively short distances. Classically, neurotransmitters had been thought to be released only at synapses between neurons. Thus, released from one neuron, transmitters classically act on adjacent neurons. However, in the brain it now seems that some cells release their transmitters into the cerebrospinal fluid to act on large numbers of other neurons in a paracrine fashion. Other neurons release their chemical messengers into the blood stream to act as neurohormones. Although these neurohormones function identically to hormones secreted by glandular endocrine organs, they are subject to more complex regulation. Several molecules function in different ways. Epinephrine, for example, serves as both a neurotransmitter and a neurohormone. Vasopressin acts as a neurotransmitter, a neurohormone, and a paracrine agent.

To be considered a neurotransmitter or a neurohormone, the specific molecule must be synthesized by the neurons in which it is found. Each transmitter or hormone has its own unique distribution, presumably reflecting its function, among cells within the nervous system. Many cells contain more than one chemical messenger; these different molecules are often stored in the same storage granules, indicating simultaneous release.

Neurotransmitters and neurohormones initiate their effects by binding to protein receptors in the cell membrane of target cells. Presumably the conformation of the receptor is altered by binding, leading to changes in the conformation and function of neighboring proteins. In some cases receptor occupancy causes opening or closing of specific ion channels, while in others the effect of the intercellular chemical messenger is to mobilize intracellular "second messengers" (such as cyclic AMP).

Neurohormones synthesized within the hypothalamus at the base of the brain adjacent to the third ventricle are released in response to received neurotransmitter signals. The various neurohormones, each of which is produced within specific hypothalamic nuclei, reach the pituitary gland by way of the infundibular or pituitary stalk, which contains defined neural tracts and a rich capillary plexus known as the portal system.

HYPOTHALAMIC SECRETION OF GONADOTROPIN-RELEASING HORMONE

Within the median eminence of the hypothalamus is a cluster of neurons called the arcuate nucleus. Gonadotropin-releasing hormone (GnRH), a 10–amino acid peptide that stimulates the anterior pituitary gland to release LH and FSH, is synthesized in these neurons. Like most brain peptides, GnRH is synthesized as part of a much larger precursor peptide 92 amino acids in length. This precursor is enzymatically cleaved to yield the smaller, more biologically active decapeptide. Upon its release into the circulation, the degradation of GnRH is quite rapid, with a half-life of 2–4 minutes. The physiologic importance of these GnRH-containing neurons is obvious from observations that specific anatomic lesions within the arcuate nucleus result in hypogonadotropic hypogonadism because of absent or deficient gonadotropin secretion. Of particular interest is experimental evidence that the GnRH-containing neurons originate outside the central nervous system within the otic bulb and migrate to their site in the hypothalamus very early in fetal development. The ontogeny of these cells explains the association of anosmia, sexual infantilism, and hypogonadotropic hypogonadism observed clinically in Kallmann syndrome (also known as isolated gonadotropin deficiency).

Classic neurotransmitters, including norepinephrine, dopamine, and serotonin, as well as more recently defined transmitters, including endogenous opiates and prostaglandins, appear to influence secretion of GnRH from the hypothalamus (Fig. 6-1). Norepinephrine appears to stimulate GnRH release, whereas dopamine and serotonin probably exert inhibitory effects. The endogenous opioids also inhibit gonadotropin secretion by suppressing the hypothalamic secretion of GnRH. In addition, both estrogens and androgens bind to neurons within the hypothalamus and the anterior pituitary, and progestins bind to cells within the hypothalamus, apparently to modulate GnRH release. The GnRH secreted in the arcuate nucleus is transported in high concentrations to the anterior pituitary via the pituitary portal vascular system. Because of the rapidity with which GnRH is degraded, as well as its dilution within the circulation, peripheral levels of GnRH are extremely low and do not reflect hypothalamic–pituitary interaction accurately. Very high levels of GnRH may be present in the portal circulation when peripheral levels are undetectable.

Gonadotropin-releasing hormone binds to specific receptors located on the cell membranes of pituitary gonadotropes. When these receptors are activated by GnRH, there is a rapid influx of calcium into the cell through calcium channels, resulting in a rapid release of LH and FSH.

Since the gonadotropins are secreted in a pulsatile manner, GnRH also must be secreted in discrete pulses. Based on the observation that the pulses of gonadotropin coincide with the coordinated depolarization of many arcuate neurons, it appears that the pulse generator for the regulation of the reproductive system resides within the arcuate nucleus. In the human, the average frequency of GnRH released, based on measurements of LH secretion, varies from 60 minutes in the follicular phase to 4 hours during the midluteal phase of the menstrual cycle. Presumably, it is the nearby neuronal systems that modify the pulsatile release of GnRH.

With constant exposure to high doses of GnRH, LH and FSH levels first increase and then begin to decrease progressively over time. This biphasic response ultimately results in hypogonadotropic hypogonadism, with markedly reduced LH and FSH secretion, resultant decreased gonadal steroid secretion, and effective "medical castration."

Two separate mechanisms are believed to play roles in this biphasic gonadotropin response: desensitization and down-regulation. Desensitization refers to the uncoupling of the activated GnRH–receptor binding complex from intracellular events normally set in motion after receptor binding. Down-regulation refers to a decrease in the number of unoccupied GnRH receptors. Following GnRH binding, internalization of GnRH-receptor complexes leads to a decrease in the number of receptors. Continuous exposure to high doses of GnRH does not allow adequate replenishment of unoccupied receptors on the cell surface. Thus, continuous exposure

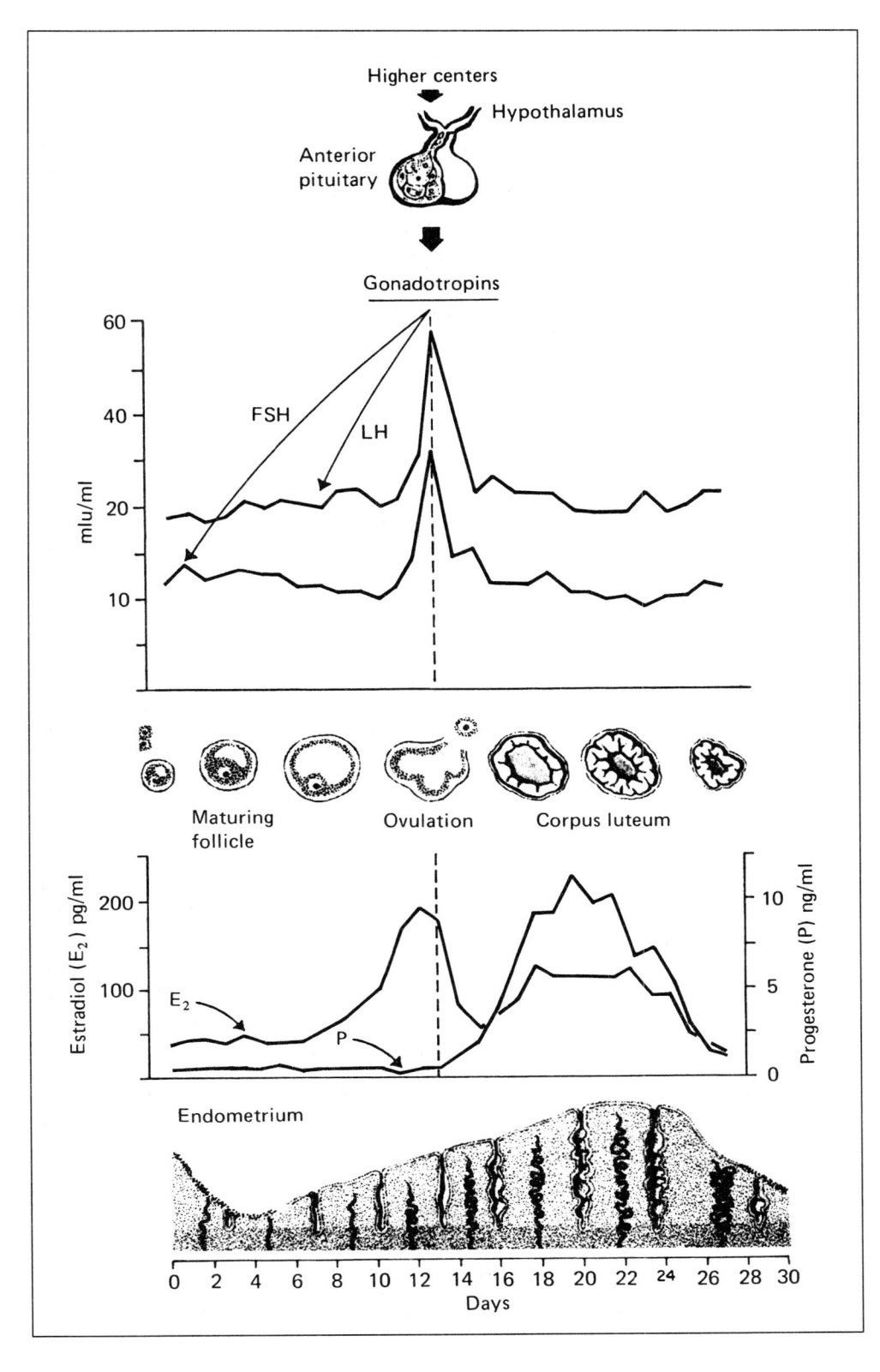

FIG. 6-1. Diagrammatic representation of events of pituitary, ovarian, and menstrual cycles. Note that the plasma estradiol level peaks about day 12, plasma follicle-stimulating hormone (FSH) and luteinizing hormone (LH) levels peak about day 13, and ovulation occurs about day 14. (Couchman GM, Hammond CB. Physiology of reproduction. In: Scott JR, DiSaia PJ, Hammond CB, Spellacy WN, eds. Danforth's obstetrics and gynecology. 7th ed. Philadelphia: JB Lippincott, 1994:30)

to GnRH will lead to a dose-dependent reduction in the number of unoccupied GnRH receptors by 1) increased receptor occupancy (accounting for perhaps two thirds of the reduction in GnRH receptors) and 2) receptor loss. Despite the high percentage of occupied receptors, pituitary gonadotropin content decreases, suggesting that the occupied GnRH receptors are functionally uncoupled from the intracellular mechanisms for normal hormone synthesis and release. Although desensitization is not understood, it is presumed that conformational changes in the gonadotrope surface membrane occur. Down-regulation and desensitization may represent the mechanisms by which pituitary gonadotropes protect themselves from excessive stimulation.

Down-regulation and desensitization also occur with administration of long-acting synthetic GnRH agonists. Thus, any disorder in women dependent on ovarian steroid secretion can be treated effectively with GnRH agonists, including uterine leiomyomata, endometriosis, dysmenorrhea, hirsutism, premenstrual syndrome, anovulatory bleeding, and precocious puberty. Gonadotropin-releasing hormone analogues are approved for only a few of their possible uses. Because the profound hypoestrogenism associated with treatment with these analogues results in accelerated bone loss, these drugs currently are approved for use for only 6 continuous months in any given individual. Studies are under way to determine whether the addition of various agents, such as progestins alone or with estrogen or bisphosphonates, termed "add back" therapy, may prevent or reduce this bone loss.

Long-acting agonists initially stimulate gonadotropin secretion for perhaps 1–2 weeks before down-regulation leads to very low levels of LH and FSH. Because of the early stimulatory effects of GnRH agonists, efforts to develop effective antagonists of GnRH that will cause only inhibition are continuing. Development of antagonists has been hampered by accompanying histamine release.

Pulsatile GnRH, administered at 5-μg doses every 60–120 minutes, can be used to induce ovulation in women with an intact pituitary gland. Human chorionic gonadotropin can be administered at a dose of 1,500 IU intramuscularly (IM) every 3–4 days to support the corpus luteum after ovulation. Alternatively, the GnRH can be continued. Hyperstimulation is very uncommon with GnRH. As might be expected, it is highly effective in women with hypothalamic amenorrhea in which pulsatile secretion of GnRH is diminished. Even in such amenorrheic women, however, pregnancy rates have been no greater than those achieved with menotropin therapy.

POSTERIOR PITUITARY HORMONES

Antidiuretic hormone (ADH, vasopressin) and oxytocin are released from the posterior pituitary gland, or neurohypophysis. These peptide hormones, each containing nine amino acids, are actually synthesized within separate cells in both the supraoptic and paraventricular nuclei of the hypothalamus. Each is synthesized as part of a larger precursor peptide and remains bound to a portion of the precursor, termed neurophysin, with which it is transported down axons from cell bodies within the hypothalamus to nerve terminals within the posterior pituitary. Both ADH and oxytocin are secreted in response to neural impulses, rapidly dissociate from their neurophysins, and are rapidly removed from the circulation with half-lives of about 10 minutes. No functions for the neurophysins have been established.

Antidiuretic hormone is secreted to promote water conservation by the kidney. At high concentrations it also causes vasoconstriction. Vasopressin release is stimulated by an increase in blood osmolality, sensed by osmoreceptors in the hypothalamus, or volume depletion, sensed by baroreceptors in the left atrium, pulmonary veins, carotid sinus, and aortic arch. Release of ADH is also stimulated by a number of other factors, including pain, fear, stress, exercise, hypoglycemia, cholinergic agonists, beta-adrenergic agonists, angiotensin, and prostaglandins. Alcohol, alpha-adrenergic agonists, and glucocorticoids inhibit ADH secretion. Antidiuretic hormone plays an important role in the regulation of ACTH secretion.

Diabetes insipidus results from deficient ADH synthesis and secretion (termed central diabetes mellitus) or from inability of the kidney to respond normally to ADH (termed nephrogenic diabetes insipidus). Hypophysectomy usually does not result in permanent diabetes insipidus, even though it commonly occurs immediately after surgery, because many ADH-containing neurons terminate not in the posterior pituitary, but in the median eminence of the hypothalamus and continue to function.

Oxytocin secretion occurs in response to suckling (the milk letdown reflex) and cervical or vaginal stimulation (the Ferguson reflex). Oxytocin receptors are found in the myoepithelial cells of the breast, which surround the alveoli of the mammary gland, and in the smooth muscle cells of the uterus. In response to oxytocin released with suckling, the myoepithelial cells contract and milk is expelled from the large alveoli to large sinuses for ejection. Oxytocin also stimulates contraction of uterine smooth muscle cells, and uterine sensitivity to oxytocin increases throughout pregnancy, but circulating concentrations do not increase sharply even during labor. Thus, any role for oxytocin in the initiation of parturition is uncertain even if exogenous oxytocin is useful to augment or initiate uterine contractions in pregnant women. Because of the structural similarity of oxytocin and ADH, oxytocin has intrinsic vasopressinlike activity. Water intoxication can occur if fluid intake is not restricted and monitored during oxytocin augmentation or induction of labor. No known disorder has been documented in the absence of oxytocin.

ANTERIOR PITUITARY HORMONES

In contrast to the posterior pituitary, there are no direct neuronal connections between the hypothalamus and the anterior pituitary gland, or adenohypophysis. Specific neurohormones that stimulate release or inhibition of the anterior pituitary hormones are secreted into and reach the anterior pituitary through the hypothalamic–pituitary portal capillary plexus. In response to these neurohormones, the cells of the anterior lobe of the pituitary, which comprises 80% of the pituitary by weight and is derived from an outpouching of oral ectoderm, synthesize and secrete several peptide hormones required for normal growth and development, as well as stimulation of several target organs (Table 6-1).

The pituitary glycoprotein hormones—LH, FSH, and TSH —and the placental hormone hCG are each composed of a common alpha and a unique beta subunit. As noted, the synthesis and secretion of LH and FSH is stimulated by the secretion of a common hypothalamic neurohormone, GnRH.

TABLE 6-1. ANTERIOR PITUITARY HORMONES AND THEIR ASSOCIATED HYPOTHALAMIC NEUROHORMONES

Anterior Pituitary Hormone	Neurohormone	Effect on Pituitary Hormone Secretion
Luteinizing hormone	Gonadotropin-releasing hormone Dopamine	Stimulates* Inhibits
Follicle-stimulating hormone	Gonadotropin-releasing hormone Dopamine	Stimulates* Inhibits
Thyroid-stimulating hormone	Thyrotropin-releasing hormone Dopamine Somatostatin	Stimulates Inhibits Inhibits
Prolactin	Dopamine Thyrotropin-releasing hormone Gonadotropin-releasing hormone (?)†	Inhibits Stimulates Stimulates* (?)†
Corticotropin	Corticotropin-releasing hormone Vasopressin	Stimulates Stimulates
Growth hormone	Growth hormone-releasing hormone Somatostatin	Stimulates Inhibits

* The effect is obtained under physiologic conditions and when the hypothalamic neurohormone is administered exogenously in intermittent pulses.
† The question mark refers to suspected or questionable action.

Ovarian inhibin may be important in the differential suppression of FSH. The synthesis and secretion of TSH is controlled by the hypothalamic hormone, thyrotropin-releasing hormone (TRH), and by circulating thyroid hormone from the pituitary. Thyroid-stimulating hormone is involved primarily in regulating the function of the thyroid gland. In primary hypothyroidism, increased TRH stimulation results in increased TSH secretion. Because TRH also stimulates secretion of prolactin, hyperprolactinemia and galactorrhea may be present in individuals with this disorder.

Prolactin is the only anterior pituitary hormone primarily under the control of a hypothalamic inhibitory transmitter, dopamine. Circumstantial data suggest the possibility of another hypothalamic stimulating hormone in addition to TRH. In the nonpregnant woman, lactotropes producing prolactin generally comprise about 30% of the cells of the anterior pituitary. The anterior pituitary doubles in size during pregnancy, largely because of hypertrophy and hyperplasia of the lactotropes. In humans, the major function of prolactin is the regulation of milk production in the puerperium. Prolactin is also released in response to stress, food, sleep, and sexual activity, but its specific functions are unknown. Prolactin is the most frequent hormone produced in excess by pituitary tumors, with most affected women presenting with amenorrhea and galactorrhea. In general, these prolactinomas can be treated effectively by dopamine agonists, but details of therapy are beyond the scope of this discussion.

Corticotropin, a single-chain polypeptide of 39 amino acids formerly known as adrenocorticotropin hormone, is secreted primarily in response to hypothalamic ACTH-releasing hormone and stimulates cortisol secretion by the adrenal cortex. The ACTH-releasing hormone–ACTH–cortisol axis is a primary component of the response to stress. Corticotropin release is also modulated by vasopressin through separate pathways.

In the absence of ACTH, the adrenal cortex atrophies and secretion of cortisol almost stops. Resulting symptoms include weakness, hypoglycemia, weight loss, and diminished axillary and pubic hair. Corticotropin deficiency is exceedingly rare but occurs most commonly in women with pituitary necrosis (Sheehan syndrome). It may also occur as a result of a variety of tumors involving the anterior pituitary or following sudden withdrawal of exogenous corticosteroids after more than 4 weeks of continuous use. Cushing disease occurs as a result of excess cortisol secretion in response to a pituitary adenoma. Prominent clinical features include a rounded "moon" face with plethora, truncal obesity with prominent supraclavicular and dorsal fat pads ("buffalo hump"), muscle wasting and weakness, purple striae on the abdomen, easy bruisability, hypertension, glucose intolerance, oligomenorrhea or amenorrhea, hirsutism, osteoporosis, and psychiatric disturbances.

Corticotropin is one of several distinct peptide hormones derived from a large common precursor, proopiomelanocortin. Proopiomelanocortin is synthesized in both the anterior and intermediate lobes of the pituitary, the hypothalamus, the placenta, the adrenal medulla, and other areas of the brain. The active hormones formed from proopiomelanocortin differ in each site where it is synthesized, depending on variations in enzymatic processing. In the anterior, pituitary ACTH is the principal product, whereas in the arcuate nucleus of the hypothalamus endorphin is produced in the greatest quantity. Proopiomelanocortin is the source of endorphins (α, β, and γ), β-lipotropin, α- and β-melanocyte–stimulating hormone, enkephalins, and dynorphins. In the intermediate lobe of the pituitary, ACTH is cleaved to form ACTH-like intermediate lobe (corresponding to ACTH 18–39) and α-melanocyte–stimulating hormone (corresponding to ACTH 1–13). In addition, the formation of proopiomelanocortin within the intermediate lobe appears to be regulated primarily by dopamine and serotonin, whereas ACTH-releasing hormone is the important regulatory agent in the anterior lobe. Proopiomelanocortin and melanocyte-stimulating hormone can cause hyperpigmentation of the skin and are only of significance in disorders such as Addison and Nelson disease associated with markedly increased secretion of ACTH-releasing hormone and ACTH.

Growth hormone (GH) is a single-chain polypeptide that is structurally similar to the placental hormone human chorionic somatomammotropin (also known as human placental lactogen) and somewhat less similar to prolactin. Growth hormone-releasing hormone is the major hypothalamic hormone stimulating GH secretion, and somatostatin is the major neurohormone inhibiting GH secretion. Growth hormone stimulates somatic growth and is also important in several metabolic processes. Growth is mediated in large measure by insulinlike growth factor I ([IGF-I] also known as somatomedin C), whose synthesis is controlled by GH. The liver is the major source of IGF-I. The metabolic effects of GH are complex and biphasic. Acutely, GH has insulinlike effects, increasing glucose uptake in muscle and fat, stimulating amino acid uptake and protein synthesis in muscle and liver, and inhibiting lipolysis in adipose tissue. The longer, more profound antiinsulin type of effects of GH begin several hours later. Glucose uptake and use are then inhibited, causing plasma glucose levels to rise, and lipolysis increases, causing plasma free fatty acids to rise. Growth hormone secretion increases during fasting and is important in adaptations to lack of food and starvation. Along with cortisol, epinephrine, and glucagon, GH maintains blood glucose levels for use by the brain and mobilizes fat as an alternative metabolic fuel source.

STEROID HORMONE FEEDBACK

Gonadal steroids can exert both negative and positive feedback effects on gonadotropin secretion. The feedback effects are both time and dose dependent. Estradiol is the most potent steroid inhibitor of gonadotropin secretion. Bilateral oophorectomy results in rapid increases in both LH and FSH, and infusion of 17β-estradiol into hypoestrogenic women leads to rapid decreases in circulating levels of both LH and FSH. Elevated levels of gonadotropins in castrated women cannot be suppressed to the levels observed in normal premenopausal women by gonadal steroids alone, suggesting that peptide factors from the gonads, such as inhibin, are also important in feedback regulation of gonadotropin secretion. Although relatively low concentrations of estradiol inhibit secretion of gonadotropins, estradiol simultaneously stimulates both synthesis and storage of the gonadotropins in the gonadotropes.

In order for women to ovulate, estradiol also must elicit an appropriate positive feedback effect on gonadotropin secretion. Positive feedback requires an estrogenic stimulus of increasing levels and duration. The high concentrations of estradiol secreted just before ovulation stimulate synthesis and storage of gonadotropins but also augment the effect of GnRH in eliciting release of LH and FSH. Thus, in the normal menstrual cycle, the positive feedback action of high levels of estradiol in eliciting the midcycle LH surge is preceded by a period of time when lower estradiol levels are present with their negative feedback effects. Progesterone levels also begin to increase before ovulation and appear to play a role in eliciting the midcycle LH surge as well.

It is not clear whether pulsatile secretion of GnRH is increased at midcycle. Experimental studies have proven that the midcycle LH surge can occur without any increase in GnRH secretion. The surge might occur because of a rapid increase in the number of GnRH receptors on the gonadotropes and the release of LH from cells in which synthesis and storage have resulted in accumulation of large quantities of LH and FSH that are available for secretion.

The ovary may be considered as the *zeitgeber,* or clock, for the timing of ovulation, with the hypothalamic pulse generator stimulating pulsatile release of LH and FSH. The follicular complex and the corpus luteum develop in response to gonadotropin stimulation. It appears that, for appropriate regulation of reproductive function in women, there must be 1) appropriate negative and positive feedback actions of gonadal steroids, 2) differential feedback effects on the release of LH and FSH, and 3) local intraovarian controls on follicular growth and maturation that are distinguishable from but interrelated to the effects of gonadotropins on the ovaries.

PUBERTY: MATURATION OF THE HYPOTHALAMIC–PITUITARY AXIS

The fetal hypothalamus begins to synthesize GnRH as early as 10 weeks of gestation, with gonadotropin secretion increasing soon thereafter. Levels of both LH and FSH increase steadily until about 20–24 weeks of fetal life. Beginning at midgestation there is increasing sensitivity to the negative feedback inhibition of placental steroids, with a gradual decline in gonadotropin secretion. After another transient increase in circulating FSH and LH levels in both boys and girls at birth, presumably due to the loss of feedback inhibition of placental steroids at delivery, these hormones fall to low levels within a few months and remain low during the prepubertal years. Serum FSH concentrations are typically somewhat higher than LH levels in children. The hypothalamic–pituitary unit appears to be exquisitely sensitive to extremely low levels of gonadal steroids, and negative feedback influences predominate. That the prepubertal gonad does suppress gonadotropin secretion is documented by the observation that gonadotropin levels increase after gonadectomy in children.

Puberty may be defined as the period in life beginning with the earliest physical signs of sexual maturation and concluding with the attainment of physical, mental, and emotional maturity. The changes occurring at puberty result directly or indirectly from maturation of the hypothalamic–pituitary unit, gonadotropin stimulation of the gonads, and the secretion of sex steroids. Hormonally, puberty is characterized by the resetting of the negative gonadal steroid feedback loop, the establishment of new circadian and ultradian (frequent) gonadotropin rhythms, and the acquisition in the female of a positive estrogen feedback loop controlling the monthly rhythm as an interdependent expression of the interaction between gonadotropins and ovarian steroids.

Early in puberty there is increased sensitivity of LH to GnRH. Sleep-associated secretion of both LH and FSH occurs in both sexes and is associated with increased gonadal sex steroid secretion. In boys, the nighttime increases in LH are accompanied by nocturnal increases in testosterone. In girls, the nighttime increases in LH are followed by increased secretion of estradiol the following morning. The delay observed in girls most likely reflects the additional time and metabolic steps necessary to synthesize estradiol by aromatization from androgens.

The net result is that basal levels of both FSH and LH increase through puberty, with the patterns differing in boys and girls and with LH levels eventually becoming greater than FSH levels. Although it seems likely that there is a pulsatile pattern to the secretion of the very small quantities of gonadotropin released in childhood, the pulsatile secretion of gonadotropins is more easily documented as puberty progresses and basal levels increase.

The mechanisms responsible for the numerous hormonal changes occurring during puberty are poorly understood, but the central nervous system must be involved in the initiation of puberty. In women there is evidence that hypothalamic–pituitary gonadotropin maturation occurs in two stages at puberty. First, sensitivity to the negative or inhibitory feedback effects of the low quantities of circulating estrogen present in girls decreases. Second, there is maturation of the positive stimulatory feedback response to estrogen, which is responsible for the midcycle ovulatory LH surge.

It is currently believed that the central nervous system exercises the only major restraint to the onset of puberty. The neuroendocrine control of puberty appears to be mediated by the hypothalamic GnRH-secreting neurons of the arcuate nucleus, which function as the pulse generator. At puberty there appears to be reactivation (or disinhibition) of the suppressed GnRH pulse generator characteristic of childhood, leading to an increased amplitude and frequency of GnRH pulsatile discharges, to increased stimulation of the pituitary gonadotropes, and to gonadal maturation.

Supporting evidence for the primacy of the pulse generator and of GnRH secretion in pubertal maturation may be found in two very different experiments of nature. Even in the absence of functional gonads, as occurs in Turner syndrome (45,X gonadal dysgenesis), an increase in gonadotropin secretion and changes in sensitivity to exogenous GnRH and gonadal steroids can be documented at the expected age of puberty. Children with hypothalamic hamartomas, which have been shown to secrete GnRH, presumably in a pulsatile fashion, undergo precocious pubertal development.

BIBLIOGRAPHY

Brownstein MJ. Neurotransmission and endocrinology. In: Becker KL, ed. Principles and practice of endocrinology and metabolism. Philadelphia: JB Lippincott, 1990:52–56

Casper RF. Disorders of the hypothalamic pulse generator: insufficient or inappropriate gonadotropin-releasing hormone release. Clin Obstet Gynecol 1990;33:611–621

Friedman AJ. The biochemistry, physiology, and pharmacology of gonadotropin releasing hormone (GnRH) and GnRH analogs. In: Barbieri RL, Friedman AJ, eds. Gonadotropin releasing hormone analogs: applications in gynecology. New York: Elsevier Science Publishing Inc, 1991:1–15

Grumbach MM, Kaplan SL. The neuroendocrinology of human puberty: an ontogenetic perspective. In: Grumbach MM, Sizonenko PC, Aubert ML, eds. Control of the onset of puberty. Baltimore: Williams and Wilkins, 1990:1–62

Knobil E. The neuroendocrine control of the menstrual cycle. Recent Prog Horm Res 1980;36:53–88

LaBarbera AR, Rebar RW. Reproductive peptide hormones: generation, degradation, reception, and action. Clin Obstet Gynecol 1990; 33:576–590

Miller DS, Reid RR, Cetel NS, Rebar RW, Yen SSC. Pulsatile administration of low-dose gonadotropin-releasing hormone: ovulation and pregnancy in women with hypothalamic amenorrhea. JAMA 1983;250:2937–2941

Pohl CR, Knobil E. The role of the central nervous system in the control of ovarian function in higher primates. Annu Rev Physiol 1982;44:583–593

Robertson GL. Physiology of vasopressin, oxytocin, and thirst. In: Becker KL, ed. Principles and practice of endocrinology and metabolism. Philadelphia: JB Lippincott, 1990:222–230

Veldhuis JD. The hypothalamic pulse generator: the reproductive core. Clin Obstet Gynecol 1990;33:538–550

Yen SSC. The hypothalamic control of pituitary hormone secretion. In: Yen SSC, Jaffe RB, eds. Reproductive endocrinology—physiology, pathophysiology and clinical management. 3rd ed. Philadelphia: WB Saunders, 1991:65–104

The Menstrual Cycle

Events in the normal menstrual cycle are the result of highly coordinated interactions among the hypothalamus, the pituitary, the ovaries, and the endometrium. A thorough understanding of the mechanisms regulating the cycle is essential for the accurate diagnosis of common menstrual irregularities, as well as for planning rational management of disordered ovulatory function in women of reproductive age.

Most cycles fall between 25 and 30 days in length, the model 28-day cycle being the exception rather than the rule. Greatest variability is found in the years following menarche and those ushering in menopause. Cycle length is most consistent between the ages of 20 and 30 years. The postovulatory or luteal phase of the ovarian cycle is remarkably constant in duration and lasts approximately 14 days; the follicular or preovulatory phase is more variable. Luteal phase duration is between 10 and 16 days in 95% of cycles, whereas the follicular phase falls in this same interval in only 80% of cycles overall.

It is the orderly sequence of hormonal events leading to approximately monthly ovulation that is responsible for the normally consistent and predictable nature of the menstrual cycle. During each cycle, a single ovarian follicle emerges as dominant over all others in its cohort and subsequently directs the sequence and timing of events leading to its ovulation. Thereafter, the corpus luteum, which is itself derived from the same selected follicle, governs events in the latter half of the cycle designed to mature and prepare the endometrium for implantation of a fertilized ovum.

The weight of available evidence, most of it derived from studies in nonprimate species, indicates that estrogen produced by the ovary, or more specifically by the selected follicle, is the essential hormonal signal on which most events in the normal menstrual cycle in some way depend. However, more recent studies in nonhuman primates and women, many using new and very powerful molecular techniques, strongly suggest that autocrine and paracrine actions of various locally produced intraovarian peptide hormones and growth factors play a major role. Indeed, the normal menstrual cycle may ultimately depend as much on local regulatory mechanisms as on the feedback actions of ovarian steroid hormones, if not more. Knowledge of the mechanisms involved in the production of ovarian steroid and peptide hormones and the development of their source, the ovarian follicle, is therefore key to understanding the menstrual cycle.

THE PRIMORDIAL FOLLICLE

Primordial germ cells arise in the yolk sac in the region of the fetal hindgut, migrate into the genital ridge, and there undergo successive mitotic divisions to give rise to oogonia that continue to proliferate and ultimately number 6–7 million by 20 weeks of gestation. Between the 8th and 13th weeks of fetal life, some of the oogonia leave the mitotic cycle and enter the first meiotic division. This change marks their conversion to primary oocytes, which become surrounded by a single layer of flattened pregranulosa cells to form primordial follicles. The primary oocyte reaches the first meiotic prophase, where it remains suspended until the time of ovulation. The exact mechanism responsible for oocyte meiotic arrest remains uncertain, but it appears to involve local paracrine control, probably mediated by a granulosa cell–derived meiosis inhibitor.

Those oocytes that fail to enter meiosis and become incorporated into primordial follicles are destined to degenerate. As a result, only approximately 2 million persist at birth. Evidence from studies in nonhuman primates suggests that gonadotropins influence even this earliest stage of follicular development; experimental hypophysectomy of the fetal monkey results in waves of atresia that dramatically reduce the number of primordial follicles present at term.

THE PREANTRAL FOLLICLE

All preovulatory follicles ultimately derive from the large pool of inactive primordial follicles. Follicular growth is a continuous process; it occurs throughout life, without interruption, until the pool of available follicles is exhausted. It occurs, to a limited extent, in prepubertal girls, persists during pregnancy, and continues inexorably to the point of complete follicular depletion that marks menopause. The rate at which inactive follicles begin to grow is governed, in some way, by the number of follicles remaining. This phenomenon has important clinical implications. It explains the smaller size of follicular cohorts observed with advancing age. It explains why women having only a single ovary do not experience premature menopause. It should also remind us that any remnant of normal ovary that can be preserved during adnexal surgery may serve the patient well for quite some time.

The precise stimulus for the initiation of follicular growth remains unclear. Observations in patients with "resistant ovary" syndrome suggest that even the earliest stages of further development may require gonadotropin support; the ovaries of such patients are small and contain many primordial follicles but virtually no follicles in more advanced stages of maturation. The mechanisms that determine which specific follicles will participate in each wave of follicular growth are even more obscure; why some are recruited while the rest of the pool remains dormant, awaiting an invitation to join a later cohort, is a mystery. Since the entire follicular pool is theoretically exposed to the same cyclic fluctuations in gonadotropin secretion, the mechanisms responsible for initiating or suppressing the growth of any one individual or group of follicles seem likely to include some form of intraovarian signaling, probably involving one or more of the many putative intraovarian regulators recently described. These include a variety of growth factors and cytokines. The potential importance of such local control mechanisms is suggested by the relatively advanced stages of gonadotropin-independent follicular growth that accompany isosexual precocious pubertal development in the McCune–Albright syndrome.

Whatever the mechanisms responsible, once stimulated, the follicle enters a preantral growth phase. The oocyte enlarges and becomes surrounded by a layer of glycoprotein, called the zona pellucida, secreted by its investment of granulosa cells. Cytoplasmic processes of the granulosa cells extend through the zona to maintain close contact with the oocyte and provide a channel for direct transfer of information and nutrients to the oocyte. Cellular differentiation begins; the granulosa undergoes a multilayer proliferation, and a thecal layer organizes from the surrounding ovarian stroma. Combined, these processes cause a progressive increase in the diameter of the follicle. With development of the theca, the follicle also acquires a blood supply; arterioles penetrate the theca and terminate in a network of capillaries adjacent to the basement membrane lying just beneath the granulosa layer. At this point, the development of LH receptors in the theca and FSH receptors in the granulosa secures the formation of a functional follicular unit responsive to gonadotropin stimulation.

Even at this early stage of development, the enzymes necessary for steroid hormone production are in place; the preantral follicle can effectively synthesize all three classes of sex steroids (androgens, progestogens, and estrogens). The most important of these steroids, estrogens, are produced through the action of an enzyme complex known as aromatase, which converts androgens to estrogens. This conversion, called aromatization, is induced by FSH, which first binds to specific, membrane-bound protein receptors on the surface of granulosa cells. The amount of estrogen produced is determined to a large extent by the number of FSH receptors in the follicle. Importantly, in addition to aromatase activity, FSH stimulates synthesis of its own cell surface receptor. This action is enhanced by estrogens (an autocrine function within the follicle) generated through FSH-induced aromatization and further modulated by growth factors.

At least in nonprimate species, FSH and estrogen also combine to stimulate mitosis and thereby promote granulosa cell proliferation. Whether the same or another mechanism operates to stimulate granulosa proliferation in primates is not entirely clear. Early follicular growth thus becomes somewhat self-sustaining, as long as adequate FSH is available. Follicle-stimulating hormone stimulates aromatization, which results in the production of estrogen. Estrogen then teams with FSH to increase both the number of FSH receptors per cell and the total number of granulosa cells. These mechanisms combine to expand gradually the follicle's capacity to produce estrogen which, in turn, supports and promotes continued follicular growth.

Androgens play a complex role in early follicular development. Androgens serve as the substrate for aromatization and estrogen production in the granulosa. They may also exert a direct paracrine effect and stimulate aromatase activity. However, at high concentrations or in the absence of adequate FSH, androgens may also be converted to other, more potent, 5α-reduced androgens such as androstanedione and dihydrotestosterone. In this form, androgens cannot be converted to estrogen and, in fact, inhibit aromatase activity and other FSH- and estrogen-mediated processes. Whether androgens produced in the follicle are converted to estrogen or to more potent androgens depends on the hormonal environment surrounding the young follicle. Its ultimate fate hangs in a rather delicate balance. At low concentrations, androgens are readily converted to estrogen, but at higher levels, the still-limited capacity for aromatization may be overwhelmed. If so, the follicle becomes profoundly androgenic and, consequently, atretic because continued growth and maturation depend on its ability to maintain an estrogenic nature.

Clearly, the androgen-rich environment of the polycystic ovary is not conducive to either aromatization or granulosa proliferation. In fact, high local androgen concentrations may be responsible for the aborted follicular development characteristically seen in these patients. Because FSH receptor development and estrogen production are limited under these conditions, rather than developing normally, follicles in the polycystic ovary may be prone to atresia; thus they contribute to further enlargement of the stromal compartment, driven, in turn, to produce still more androgen by often elevated LH concentrations.

THE ANTRAL FOLLICLE

Under the continuing influence of estrogen and FSH, there is an increase in the production of follicular fluid that accumulates in the intercellular spaces of the granulosa, eventually coalescing to form a cavity as the follicle makes its gradual transition to the antral stage. This phase of development clearly requires gonadotropins, but relatively low circulating levels appear sufficient to support follicular growth to diameters of approximately 2 mm; small antral follicles can be identified in the ovaries of prepubertal females, in the ovaries of women with other hypogonadotropic conditions such as anorexia nervosa and Kallmann syndrome (hypogonadotropic hypogonadism and anosmia), and in the ovaries of women using oral contraceptives. With formation of the antrum, the follicular fluid provides a means whereby the oocyte and surrounding granulosa cells can be nurtured in a hormonal environment unique to each follicle.

Follicular fluid contains protein-bound and free sex steroids, plasma-derived and locally derived proteins, and electrolytes, all in amounts that vary with the age, size, and relative health of the follicle. Plasma proteins, gonadotropins, and prolactin reach the antrum by diffusion from the vasculature spaces surrounding the follicle; the origin of steroid hormones found in antral fluid is less clear. Undoubtedly, some are produced locally and diffuse or are secreted into the antrum. Antral fluid steroid hormone concentrations are often vastly higher than those in plasma and, to some extent, reflect the functional capacity of the surrounding granulosa and thecal cells.

As the antral follicle develops, the synthesis of steroid hormones becomes functionally compartmentalized within the follicle. Granulosa cells are the principal source of estrogen. Because thecal cells have no FSH receptors, steroid biosynthesis in this compartment is shunted toward the production of androgens. However, both cell layers are equally important, and their functions are complementary. Androgens produced in the theca serve as substrate for estrogen production in the granulosa. This cooperative effort toward steroid hormone production has come to be known as the "two-cell, two-gonadotropin concept" of ovarian follicular steroidogenesis. Luteinizing hormone stimulates thecal cells to produce androgens that diffuse to the granulosa, where they are converted to estrogens through FSH-induced aromatization.

The functional significance of the two-cell, two-gonadotropin system is illustrated by the response of gonadotropin-deficient women to treatment with pure FSH; follicles develop, but estradiol production is severely limited. Whereas only FSH may be required for folliculogenesis, without LH to stimulate synthesis of substrate androgens in the theca, granulosa cells cannot generate estrogen levels much beyond those seen in the early follicular phase. This remarkably efficient local interaction between the granulosa and thecal compartments of the follicle is not fully operational until the later stages of antral development. Granulosa cells from smaller antral follicles still exhibit the tendency to convert androgens to their more potent, inhibitory 5α-reduced forms. In contrast, granulosa cells from larger, more mature, antral follicles readily and preferentially metabolize androgens to estrogen.

Early on, the balance between these two alternative routes of metabolism determines whether the follicle can generate the local estrogenic environment essential for continued growth. Later, the rapid, progressive accumulation of FSH receptors in the granulosa and continued FSH stimulation drive aromatase activity to ever-increasing levels of efficiency. Ultimately, the follicle's expanding capacity for estrogen production generates rising plasma estrogen concentrations; levels increase gradually at first, then exponentially, and finally exceed the threshold required to trigger the midcycle LH surge. Thus, the follicle remains dependent on a supportive gonadotropin environment throughout its development, but given that support, it may ultimately grow and develop sufficient steroidogenic capacity to allow it to dictate the pattern of gonadotropin secretion itself.

Development through the early antral stages may require only tonic levels of gonadotropin support, but the final stages of follicular development are clearly heavily dependent on gonadotropins. In all probability, each new cohort of follicles is effectively recruited during intervals when FSH is elevated and LH levels are relatively low, conditions that arise during the late luteal phase of each cycle. This last, exponential, growth phase takes place during the follicular phase of the ovulatory cycle; mean follicular diameter increases from about 5 mm at recruitment to approximately 20 mm just prior to ovulation. These final stages of growth require that high local estrogen concentrations be maintained, conditions that support continued granulosa proliferation and high levels of aromatase activity. Antral follicles that have high estrogen concentrations and low androgen–estrogen ratios in their follicular fluid will likely contain a healthy oocyte; oocytes that give rise to successful pregnancies after in vitro fertilization (IVF) most often come from follicular fluid aspirates having these characteristics.

Privileged by its greater sensitivity to declining levels of FSH and thus its unique ability to maintain the high local estrogen concentrations required for continued growth, the dominant follicle enjoys conditions that are optimal for the final stages of development. In such large antral follicles, FSH induces the appearance of specific LH receptors on granulosa cells. This action, like the FSH-induced synthesis of its own receptor, is further enhanced by estrogen. Thus, the dominant follicle's own accelerating estrogen production, which later acts centrally to stimulate the LH surge, first acts locally to promote induction of the receptor population required to mediate luteinization and the ovulatory response.

SELECTION OF THE DOMINANT FOLLICLE

If a group of follicles participates in each new cycle, how is it that, with rare exceptions, only a single follicle is selected, emerges as dominant, and goes on to ovulate? What mechanisms underlie the selection process, and when does it occur? In contrast to the normal cycle in which only one follicle typically reaches maturity, multiple follicular development is almost universal, and multiple gestations are common in cycles induced with exogenous gonadotropins. Obviously, such treatment often effectively overrides the mechanisms that normally conspire to yield only a single preovulatory follicle. This suggests that modulation of gonadotropin secretion is somehow involved in selection of the dominant follicle.

The interactions of estrogen and FSH, so crucial to promote and support gradual maturation of the antral follicle, also play a role in determining which follicle will finally ovulate. Whereas estrogen exerts a positive influence on FSH actions within the maturing follicle, its classic negative feedback relationship with FSH at the hypothalamic–pituitary level may also be the key to a natural selection process that ends in survival of the fittest follicle. As circulating estrogen levels rise, reflecting increasing estrogen production in the maturing antral follicles, they inhibit FSH release centrally. Accordingly, peripheral FSH concentrations decline and the gonadotropin support required for continued follicular growth is gradually withdrawn. The FSH-dependent aromatase activity and estrogen synthesis slow to a halt, thereby interrupting the many estrogen-dependent processes in all but the selected follicle. The inevitable consequence is a loss of developmental momentum and irreversible atretic change.

The gradual fall in FSH levels corresponds with the rise in circulating estradiol concentrations during the midfollicular phase. The principal source of this rising tide of estrogen is the dominant follicle, already selected and expressing its dominance by days 5–7 of the cycle. Although it is not yet clearly the largest follicle in the cohort, the functional dominance of the selected follicle can be clearly recognized even at this early point in time; estrogen concentrations in the venous blood draining the ovary containing the selected follicle are higher than those on the contralateral side. Rising levels of estrogen produced by the dominant follicle inhibit pituitary FSH secretion, which, in turn, interrupts the growth of less-developed follicles.

Under experimental conditions, exogenous estrogen treatment causes a fall in circulating FSH levels and invariably disrupts folliculogenesis. Clinically, attempts to improve cervical mucus and postcoital test results through empirical, late follicular phase exogenous estrogen administration, a common clinical practice, may have unintended consequences; if indicated, the lowest effective dose for the shortest possible interval seems prudent. Once selected, the dominant follicle is the only member of the cohort in that cycle that can ovulate. If the dominant follicle is removed or destroyed, no other follicle in the cohort can take its place to allow timely ovulation; instead, the process of selection begins anew.

Whereas the negative feedback relationship between estrogen and FSH may serve to effectively withdraw gonadotropin support for continued growth of other, less well-developed follicles in the cohort, evidence suggests that survival of even the dominant follicle depends on FSH, right up to ovulation. If so, the dominant follicle must somehow retain a unique responsiveness to FSH and complete development while plasma FSH concentrations are declining.

How can the selected follicle escape the consequences of falling FSH levels brought about by its own ever-increasing estrogen production? Two different, but complementary, mechanisms are involved. First, the dominant follicle has a larger mass of granulosa cells and therefore a greater number of FSH receptors. This gives it the advantage of a greater sensitivity to FSH actions and allows it to maintain its developmental momentum while, at the same time, gonadotropin support is withdrawn from less mature follicles. Second, because of the local actions of potent growth factors that stimulate angiogenesis, development of the thecal vasculature is also more advanced in the dominant follicle. Increased vascularity offers the added advantage of preferential delivery of both gonadotropins and low-density lipoprotein (LDL), a source of steroidogenic substrate.

In this view of the selection process, smaller members of the follicular cohort fall victim to a deteriorating endocrine environment orchestrated by the dominant follicle and in which it alone can survive; less mature follicles starve for lack of support and their growth is arrested. In addition to the negative feedback actions of estrogen, timely and effective withdrawal of gonadotropin support almost certainly requires the actions of inhibin and follistatin, two of a growing family of ovarian peptide hormones. Both are produced by granulosa cells in response to FSH, and like estrogen, inhibin and follistatin exert negative feedback effects on pituitary FSH secretion. Inhibin blocks both synthesis and secretion of FSH, inhibits up-regulation of pituitary GnRH receptors by GnRH, and at high concentrations, can even promote intracellular degradation of gonadotropins. These effects are at least additive to, if not synergistic with, those of estrogen; taken together, they likely serve to seal the fate of smaller, unselected follicles. Plasma inhibin concentrations rise slowly in parallel with estradiol during the follicular phase to reach a peak at midcycle that coincides with the LH surge. Large follicles make more inhibin than small follicles, probably because of their greater mass of granulosa cells. In IVF cycles, peak serum concentrations correlate with the number of mature follicles that arise during controlled ovarian hyperstimulation.

Whereas the gradual withdrawal of gonadotropin support caused by the feedback inhibition of estrogen, inhibin, and, to a lesser extent, follistatin is an important part of the selection process, this mechanism alone cannot explain how the follicle destined to ovulate is initially selected. After all, the dominant follicle cannot produce sufficient estrogen and inhibin to influence gonadotropin secretion until after it is already selected. The earliest elements of the selection process, indeed many aspects of normal follicular growth and development, appear to involve a complex system of intraovarian signals.

INTRAOVARIAN SIGNALING SYSTEMS

A number of putative intraovarian regulators have now been described, and the vital roles they play are just beginning to be appreciated. In addition to its negative feedback effects on pituitary FSH secretion, inhibin has important actions within the ovary, where it regulates androgen production in the theca by enhancing the actions of LH and other growth factors. Inhibin consists of two distinct peptides (designated as alpha and beta subunits) linked by disulfide bonds. Two forms exist, inhibin A and inhibin B; each contains the same alpha subunit and one of two distinct but related beta subunits (β_A, β_B). These same two subunits, when combined (β_A-β_A, β_A-β_B, β_B-β_B), form other peptides known as activins (activin A, activin AB, and activin B, respectively) having actions that oppose those of inhibin. In the follicle, activin increases FSH binding by regulating receptor concentrations. It enhances FSH-stimulated estrogen and inhibin secretion but interferes with inhibin's ability to potentiate LH-stimulated thecal androgen production. Activin also suppresses granulosa cell progesterone synthesis, an action that may prevent premature luteinization. Follistatin is yet another of the peptides in this family; it too modulates FSH actions in the ovary, by binding and thus inhibiting the actions of activin.

There is now considerable evidence that events within the ovary are also regulated by various growth factors. These ubiquitous polypeptide molecules operate through local autocrine and paracrine mechanisms to modulate cell proliferation and functions. There are many different growth factors; among the more important are the insulinlike growth factors (IGFs), IGF-I and IGF-II, also known as somatomedins. Their physiologic effects are mediated by specific transmembrane receptors; in the ovary, those for IGF-I can be found on both granulosa and theca cells, whereas IGF-II receptors are plentiful in luteinized granulosa cells and in the corpus luteum.

As their name implies, these peptides are structurally similar to insulin. In fact, insulin cross-reacts with the IGF-I receptor; conversely, IGF-I binds the insulin receptor, albeit with limited affinity.

By themselves, IGF-I and IGF-II have only modest effects, but in synergy with gonadotropins, their effects are quite dramatic. Insulinlike growth factor I teams with FSH to stimulate granulosa proliferation, aromatase activity, LH receptor synthesis, and inhibin secretion; because IGF-I is produced in the theca, these effects appear to be paracrine in nature. In contrast, autocrine mechanisms operate in the theca, where IGF-I combines with LH to stimulate androgen production. Another family of peptides known as IGF-binding proteins regulates the tissue effects of these growth factors by binding them and preventing their access to membrane surface receptors. The main binding protein in serum is IGF-binding protein 3; its synthesis in the liver is primarily dependent on GH, and circulating levels reflect the total IGF concentration (IGF-I plus IGF-II). These binding proteins are also synthesized in the ovary, where they inhibit IGF actions. Their synthesis, in turn, is inhibited by FSH and both IGF-I and IGF-II, actions that maximize growth factor availability. Evidence suggests that IGF-binding proteins 1 and 3 play an important role in growing follicles, whereas IGF-binding proteins 2, 4, and 5 are expressed primarily in atretic and regressing follicles.

Other growth factors and peptides may also be important intraovarian regulators. Epidermal growth factor is a potent granulosa cell mitogen. Transforming growth factors a and b (derived from the same gene family as activin and inhibin), fibroblast growth factor, and platelet-derived growth factor are others that exhibit regulatory actions in vitro. Cytokines such as interleukin-1, derived from resident ovarian macrophages, may also be operating. Evidence suggests that there is an intraovarian renin–angiotensin system that may be involved in angiogenesis. Another peptide, endothelin-1, has been implicated as the putative luteinization inhibitor. Whether GnRH-like peptides and oxytocin, also found in preovulatory follicles, have any specific functions is unknown.

Current speculation favors the notion that intraovarian signals provided by growth factors and other peptides play a crucial role in normal follicular growth and development in primates. Acting locally via autocrine and paracrine mechanisms, they exert subtle but distinct influences on many ovarian cell functions by amplifying or otherwise modulating the effects of gonadotropins and steroid hormones. The precise role that each may have is not yet certain, but it is likely that these locally produced peptides serve to fine-tune and coordinate events among the various ovarian cellular compartments. Deficiencies, excesses, or otherwise abnormal patterns of production may ultimately explain some of the more enigmatic reproductive disorders.

FEEDBACK MECHANISMS

The mechanisms involved in the control of follicular development involve complex hormonal interactions within the ovary, but the feedback relationships between ovarian steroids and gonadotropins are what allow events in the ovary to be coordinated with higher centers in the hypothalamus and pituitary. By way of its own estrogen and inhibin production, the dominant follicle effectively assumes control of its own destiny. By altering gonadotropin secretion through feedback mechanisms, it can optimize its own environment to the detriment of other follicles.

A key feature of the selection process is the negative feedback of estrogen on pituitary FSH release. At all levels, FSH secretion is exquisitely sensitive to estrogen inhibition. In contrast, the effect of estrogen on LH release varies with concentration and duration of exposure. For the most part, estrogen has the same negative feedback effect on LH as it does on FSH. However, at very high levels, estrogen also exerts a positive feedback effect on LH release. In fact, estrogen positive feedback is the mechanism responsible for the preovulatory LH surge. In women, the required threshold concentration of estrogen is approximately 200 pg/ml; estradiol levels must exceed this threshold for 50 hours or more to trigger the LH surge. If estradiol levels fail to reach threshold concentrations or cannot be sustained for the requisite time, the LH surge, and therefore ovulation, will not occur.

THE PREOVULATORY FOLLICLE

As the follicle enters the final stages of maturation, its granulosa cells enlarge and acquire lipid inclusions. The thecal layer develops vacuoles and becomes richly vascular. The oocyte within resumes meiosis and approaches completion of its reduction division.

Now clearly singular and dominant, the preovulatory follicle produces ever-increasing amounts of estrogen. Levels rise rapidly, surging to a peak approximately 24–36 hours prior to ovulation. At full maturity, estrogen production in the dominant follicle becomes sufficient to reach and exceed the required threshold concentration and stimulate the LH surge. Recall that mature antral follicles acquire LH receptors in response to the combined effects of estrogen and FSH. As the principal source of this rising tide of estrogen and the only follicle capable of responding to declining FSH levels, the dominant (now preovulatory) follicle is also the only one able to respond appropriately to the LH surge.

In follicles that have been deprived of adequate FSH and estrogen, the LH surge induces atresia, not ovulation. This phenomenon is another that has important clinical implications. Neither a natural nor an exogenous surrogate LH surge will induce ovulation unless the follicle has achieved sufficient size and maturity to respond; it will, instead, disrupt preovulatory development and drive the follicle into atresia. Consequently, in cycles induced with clomiphene or exogenous gonadotropins, hCG should be withheld until ultrasonography demonstrates that there is a follicle capable of responding. The LH surge induces ovulation and, in all but the selected preovulatory follicle, a wave of atresia that seals the fate of less mature follicles.

Acting through its receptor, LH promotes luteinization and

the appearance of progesterone receptors in granulosa cells. There is an increase in the activity of enzymes that convert cholesterol to pregnenolone, the immediate steroidogenic precursor of progesterone. Circulating progesterone levels first increase on the day of the LH peak, 12–24 hours prior to ovulation. This modest increase in periovulatory progesterone concentrations has immense physiologic importance. Acting in an autocrine fashion in the luteinized granulosa, progesterone directly inhibits cell mitosis; this probably explains why granulosa proliferation slows as cells gain LH receptors.

Progesterone also synergizes with estrogen to initiate the LH surge. In the presence of otherwise subthreshold concentrations of estrogen, progesterone treatment can stimulate an LH surge; above the estradiol threshold, progesterone advances surge onset, LH levels reach greater amplitude, and the surge is shorter in duration. Moreover, evidence suggests that without the preovulatory rise in progesterone, the midcycle FSH peak, which normally accompanies the LH surge, may not occur. However, if levels rise prematurely or reach too high a concentration, progesterone can block the LH surge. Taken together, these observations suggest that by sending the appropriate sequence of feedback signals, the preovulatory follicle communicates its full maturity to higher centers and coordinates its final development with a timely ovulatory stimulus.

OVULATION

It seems clear that the preovulatory follicle, through its steroid hormone production, can initiate and control the dimensions of its own ovulatory stimulus. The sequence of events that follows is not fully defined but appears to be initiated by the massive release of LH triggered by sustained threshold levels of estradiol (Fig. 6-1).

Considerable variation in the timing of ovulation exists from cycle to cycle, even in the same patient. Ovulation occurs approximately 12–24 hours after the LH peak and 24–48 hours after peak estradiol levels are attained. The most reliable indicator of impending ovulation appears to be onset of the LH surge, occurring some 28–32 hours before actual follicle rupture. In addition to inducing luteinization in granulosa cells, the LH surge stimulates the resumption of meiosis in the oocyte and promotes other local events essential to follicle rupture.

Within the follicle, LH actions are mediated by a second messenger, cyclic AMP, which appears to act not directly, but to overcome the local inhibition of both meiosis and luteinization. Oocyte maturation inhibitor and luteinization inhibitor are two of the putative, locally produced, regulatory peptides alluded to earlier. Their existence has been inferred from observations that oocytes resume meiosis and granulosa cells luteinize spontaneously, once they are removed from the follicle. A specific meiosis inhibitor has so far eluded investigators, but a growing body of evidence suggests that interleukin-1, a polypeptide cytokine produced and secreted by resident ovarian macrophages, may be the long-sought putative suppressor of premature follicular luteinization. Research continues, and a better understanding of the actions and mechanisms involved is likely soon to be forthcoming.

With the LH surge, progesterone levels in the preovulatory follicle begin to rise. Low levels enhance the LH surge, as described above, but as concentrations increase, progesterone exerts a negative feedback effect that may serve to terminate the surge. In addition, progesterone appears to act locally to increase the distensibility of the follicle wall. Some change in the elastic properties of the follicle wall seems necessary to explain the rapid increase in follicular fluid volume just prior to ovulation, which is unaccompanied by any significant change in intrafollicular pressure. The preovulatory follicle reaches a diameter of 18–25 mm as it burgeons forth from the surface of the ovary. Acting through cyclic AMP, progesterone, or both, LH stimulates granulosa cell production of plasminogen activators that activate plasminogen in the follicular fluid to produce plasmin, which, in turn, generates collagenase and other proteolytic enzymes, ultimately causing the digestion of collagen in the follicular wall and increasing its distensibility. Until this time, plasminogen activator synthesis is suppressed by a system of inhibitors that evidence suggests may be influenced by epidermal growth factor.

The LH surge also appears to stimulate local synthesis of prostaglandins and other eicosanoids; concentrations increase markedly in the preovulatory follicle and are highest at ovulation, observations that suggest they play a role in the ovulatory process. Indeed, inhibition of prostaglandin synthesis can block follicle rupture and result in a luteinized unruptured follicle, thus providing the rationale for the clinical recommendation that treatment with nonsteroidal antiinflammatory drugs (NSAIDs) (prostaglandin synthetase inhibitors) is best avoided in the periovulatory interval. Prostaglandins act to free lysosomal enzymes to digest the follicular wall and may promote angiogenesis. In addition, they may stimulate contractions of smooth muscle fibers located in the theca externa that appear to be necessary for extrusion of the oocyte–cumulus cell mass.

As LH reaches its peak, circulating levels of estradiol plunge, possibly the result of LH down-regulation of its own receptors. The midcycle LH surge is accompanied by a simultaneous release of FSH, probably in response to a common hypothalamic releasing factor, GnRH. However, midcycle FSH release is far more than coincidental; evidence suggests several important functions: FSH may be responsible for the increased activity of intrafollicular proteolytic enzymes involved in follicle rupture. Moreover, FSH, not LH, stimulates expansion of the cumulus cell mass which supports the oocyte within the follicle; cumulus expansion allows the oocyte–cumulus cell mass to sever its follicular attachments and become free-floating just before follicle rupture. Perhaps most importantly, the induction of LH receptors on granulosa cells is a specific FSH-mediated process and a necessary prerequisite for the normal progress of luteinization and subsequent synthesis of progesterone. Clinically, a shortened or otherwise inadequate luteal phase is frequently observed in cycles in which FSH levels are low.

THE CORPUS LUTEUM

After ovulation, the selected follicle remains the dominant ovarian structure. In response to the ovulatory surge of LH, the follicle luteinizes, and in so doing, undergoes both a morphologic and a functional conversion to become the corpus luteum. The wall of the follicle becomes convoluted, and the antrum fills with blood and lymph. The now-luteinized granulosa cells enlarge and accumulate lipid and lutein pigment. Theca–lutein cells differentiate from the surrounding theca and stroma. The corpus luteum becomes richly vascular as a fine network of capillaries branches out from thecal vessels to penetrate the granulosa.

Before ovulation, the selected follicle expressed its dominance largely through its production of estrogen, thereby priming the endometrium and directing events leading to its own ovulation. After ovulation and luteinization, the follicle survives as the corpus luteum. It continues to secrete estrogen, but is also the principal source of luteal phase progesterone production. The combined influence of estrogen and progesterone mediates the maturation of the secretory endometrium and also serves to inhibit any meaningful new follicular development. Thus, the corpus luteum, itself derived from the single dominant preovulatory follicle, remains in control, directing the progress of events during the luteal phase. Indeed, removal or destruction of the corpus luteum reliably causes a prompt fall in circulating progesterone concentrations and brings about the premature onset of menses.

Requirements of Normal Luteal Function

Corpus luteum progesterone production is dependent on several factors, the first being optimal development of the preovulatory follicle. The so-called inadequate corpus luteum may often be only a reflection of similarly inadequate preovulatory follicular development. Recall that normal growth and development of the preovulatory follicle require the continued presence of FSH, estrogen, and IGF-I, which together act to induce LH receptor development on those same granulosa cells that become granulosa–lutein cells in the corpus luteum. Experimental selective suppression of FSH during the follicular phase is associated with lower preovulatory estradiol levels, a decrease in luteal phase progesterone production, and a reduction in the total number of luteal cells. This suggests that the extent to which LH receptors accumulate on granulosa cells during the follicular phase may affect the extent of luteinization and thus the functional capacity of the corpus luteum.

Because clomiphene citrate stimulates FSH release, promotes follicular development, and increases preovulatory estradiol levels, many consider such treatment a logical approach to treatment of luteal phase deficiency. According to this rationale, if one builds a better follicle one might expect it to become a better, more functionally adequate, corpus luteum. Normal luteal function also requires continued LH stimulation; administration of an LH antiserum, luteal phase hypophysectomy, or treatment with a GnRH antagonist will cause a prompt and premature luteolysis.

Further evidence that the corpus luteum is functionally dependent on LH comes from observations that progesterone is secreted in well-defined pulses that are temporally related to pituitary LH pulses during the latter half of the luteal phase. This forms the basis for another common approach to the treatment of luteal phase defects. Taking advantage of the structural and functional similarity of LH and hCG, exogenous hCG is often used to stimulate greater steroid hormone production by the corpus luteum. Another therapeutic alternative involves the use of exogenous progesterone to supplement presumably inadequate progesterone production by the defective corpus luteum.

In addition to an adequate number of LH receptors and continued LH secretion, the corpus luteum requires LDL as a source of cholesterol. The rate of de novo cholesterol synthesis is insufficient to meet the demand for this obligate precursor; the mature corpus luteum produces up to 40 mg of progesterone per day. Because of its relatively high molecular weight and poor diffusion, LDL cannot reach the luteinized granulosa until developing vessels reach the luteinized granulosa after ovulation. One way in which LH serves to support the corpus luteum is to promote LDL receptor binding, internalization, and processing.

The theca cell layer of the preovulatory follicle also luteinizes and contributes to corpus luteum steroid hormone production. Like the follicle from which it comes, the corpus luteum produces significant quantities of steroid and peptide hormones. There is growing evidence that the granulosa–lutein and theca–lutein cells of the corpus luteum are functionally, as well as morphologically, distinct. Large (granulosa–lutein) luteal cells produce peptides (relaxin, oxytocin, and possibly inhibin), as well as large quantities of estradiol and progesterone; small ("paraluteal," theca–lutein) cells make only steroid hormones. Recent immunochemical studies suggest that the functional compartmentalization of steroid synthesis that exists in the follicle may be preserved in the corpus luteum. However, precisely which cells make which steroids in response to what specific stimuli and whether these cell populations truly do functionally interact remain to be clarified.

Luteal Suppression of Folliculogenesis

Progesterone levels rise steadily after ovulation to reach a peak approximately 8 days after the LH surge. While mediating the progressive maturation of the secretory endometrium, progesterone also effectively suppresses new follicular growth, acting at the level of the ovary as well as on higher centers. In the nonhuman primate, the ovary destined to yield the next dominant follicle and ovulation can be predicted from the levels of progesterone found in the ovarian veins; the ovary with the lowest level of progesterone in its venous effluent, and presumably therefore the lowest intraovarian concentration, will most likely give rise to the next dominant follicle. This clearly suggests that intraovarian progesterone may regulate the extent of new follicular growth.

There is some evidence that progesterone may inhibit aromatization and thus limit the extent of estrogen-dependent folliculogenesis. The negative feedback effects of estrogen and progesterone on pituitary FSH release further inhibit new follicular development. In primates, evidence suggests that the corpus luteum is also a rich source of inhibin; whereas inhibin secretion is FSH dependent in the follicle, LH stimulates its release from granulosa–lutein cells in the corpus luteum. Inhibin levels rise and fall in parallel with progesterone during the luteal phase. Follicle-stimulating hormone follows a reciprocal pattern; levels fall to a nadir at midluteal phase, then increase again just before menses.

Suppression of gonadotropin secretion does appear to be important, since exogenous gonadotropins can overcome any intraovarian inhibition and stimulate follicle development and ovulation if administered during the luteal phase. The intercycle rise in FSH, which serves to recruit the next cohort of follicles and signals the beginning of a new cycle, is thus postponed until luteal regression is all but complete. Until then, reduced levels of gonadotropin secretion and local, intraovarian inhibitory mechanisms combine to effectively suppress any significant new follicular development.

Luteolysis

In the latter half of the luteal phase, progesterone levels decline gradually, again returning to basal concentrations with the onset of menses. In the nonfertile cycle, the life span of the corpus luteum, and thus luteal phase duration, is limited to 10–16 days in 95% of cycles. Unless pregnancy intervenes, the corpus luteum's demise is inevitable and cannot be prevented for long, even if one provides continuous exogenous LH/hCG support. The mechanisms responsible for corpus luteum regression remain unknown despite much investigation.

Because progesterone concentrations gradually fall as estradiol levels peak again at the midluteal phase, many investigators have speculated that estrogen might be the putative luteolytic stimulus. Several lines of experimental evidence are consistent with this view. It's also clear that exogenous estrogen, if administered in adequate amounts, can induce functional luteolysis and destroy the corpus luteum. However, the absence of estrogen receptors in luteal tissue argues against a role in luteolysis, and most investigators now agree that estrogen-induced luteolysis is a pharmacologic and not a physiologic phenomenon.

Other proposed mechanisms of spontaneous luteolysis include increased local production of luteolytic prostaglandins (most notably, prostaglandin $F_{2\alpha}$ [$PGF_{2\alpha}$]) and various processes through which the corpus luteum would be deprived of LH stimulation (eg, declining levels of LH secretion due to the negative feedback of estradiol, progesterone, and inhibin; a locally induced decrease in LH receptor concentrations; or interference with LH binding). Unfortunately, experimental alterations in LH pulse frequency and amplitude cannot provoke luteolysis, progesterone levels begin to fall before any detectable decline in LH receptor content, and LH binding affinity is unchanged throughout the luteal phase. On the other hand, as evidence from studies in nonhuman primates suggests, luteolysis might involve a functional uncoupling of LH binding and postreceptor events; the corpus luteum might thus be rendered insensitive to further LH stimulation. The true cause of spontaneous luteal regression remains one of the greatest mysteries of the menstrual cycle.

After its demise, the corpus luteum deteriorates but persists in the ovary for several subsequent cycles, then known as a corpus albicans. This disorganized mass of collagen and connective tissue is the final remnant of the first selected, then dominant, and ultimately, luteinized ovulatory follicle that became the corpus luteum, and eventually regressed, and all the while directed the events known as the normal menstrual cycle.

BIBLIOGRAPHY

Adashi EY. The ovarian life cycle. In: Yen SCC, Jaffe RB, eds. Reproductive endocrinology. Philadelphia: WB Saunders, 1991:181–237

Adashi EY. Intraovarian peptides: stimulators and inhibitors of follicular growth and differentiation. Endocrinol Metab Clin North Am 1992;21:1–17

Auletta FJ, Flint APF. Mechanisms controlling corpus luteum function in sheep, cows, nonhuman primates and women especially in relation to the time of luteolysis. Endocr Rev 1988;9:88–105

Burger H. Inhibin. Reprod Med Rev 1992;1:1–20

Carr BR. The normal menstrual cycle. In: Carr BR, Blackwell RE, eds. Textbook of reproductive medicine. Norwalk, Connecticut: Appleton and Lange, 1993:209–219

Irianni F, Hodgen GD. Mechanism of ovulation. Endocrinol Metab Clin North Am 1992;21:19–38

Yen SCC. The human menstrual cycle: neuroendocrine regulation. In: Yen SCC, Jaffe RB, eds. Reproductive endocrinology. Philadelphia: WB Saunders, 1991:273–308

Prostaglandins

Present in most human cells, prostaglandins are 20-carbon atom fatty acids. Generally intracellular mediators, prostaglandins can occasionally act as local hormones. Thus, prostaglandins are synthesized from essential fatty acids and act and are catabolized in the same cell. Prostaglandins that escape from the cell into the circulation are rapidly metabolized by the lung, kidney, and liver. There are at least 14 different types of naturally occurring prostaglandins, designated by the letters *A* through *I*. Each letter indicates the location of specific combinations of hydroxyl groups, ketone groups, and unsaturated carbon atoms on the cyclopentane ring of the molecule. The numeric subscript 1, 2, or 3 located after the alphabetic designation indicates the number of double bonds in the aliphatic side chains of the compound. The two prostaglandins with well-established biologic importance are PGE_2 and $PGF_{2\alpha}$, each with two double bonds on its aliphatic side chains (Fig. 6-2).

Prostaglandins, particularly PGE_2 and $PGF_{2\alpha}$, are synthesized from arachidonic acid, derived from the hydrolysis of cell membrane phospholipids by the lysosomal enzyme phospholipase A_2. Arachidonic acid can then be converted via the cyclooxygenase or the lipoxygenase pathway (Fig. 6-3). Through the cyclooxygenase pathway, arachidonic acid is converted into cyclic endoperoxides (PGG and PGH), which are subsequently converted into PGE_2 and $PGF_{2\alpha}$ by isomerase and reductase or into prostacyclin and thromboxane A_2 by prostacyclin synthetase and thromboxane synthetase, respectively (Fig. 6-3). The human gene encoding cyclooxygenase has been cloned. While the availability of arachidonic acid is generally thought to limit the rate of prostaglandin biosynthesis, the expression of the cyclooxygenase gene is equally important, or even more so. The lipoxygenase pathway produces hydroxyperoxide derivatives of arachidonic acid, hydroperoxyeicosatetraenoic acid and hydroxyeicosatetraenoic acid, with hydroxyperoxide functional groups being present at the 5, 12, or 15 position of the molecule. The 5- and 15-hydroxyperoxide derivatives can be further transformed into leukotrienes, which mediate the hypersensitivity response.

Nonsteroidal antiinflammatory drugs such as aspirin, indomethacin, ibuprofen, and sodium naproxen inhibit cyclooxygenase and, therefore, prostaglandin production. Glucocorticoids inhibit prostaglandin biosynthesis by rendering the cell membrane phospholipid resistant to hydrolysis by phospholipase A_2. Progesterone can exert a local antiinflammatory action when given locally by stabilizing lysosomes and therefore prevent the release of the lysosomal enzyme phospholipase A_2. Both PGE_2 and $PGF_{2\alpha}$ are metabolized in all tissues, especially the placenta, by the enzyme 15-hydroxyprostaglandin dehydrogenase to 13,14-dihydro-14-keto-PGE_2 and 13,14-dihydro-14-keto-$PGF_{2\alpha}$ and are finally reduced to 13,14-dihydro derivatives of both compounds. Thromboxane A_2 is converted to the stable metabolite thromboxane B_2, followed by transformation into 15-keto and 13,14-dihydro derivatives, as well as 11-keto derivatives, with subsequent oxidation.

MECHANISM OF ACTION

Prostaglandin exerts its action through its specific receptors found in cell membranes. The postreceptor intracellular mechanism is unclear. In the myometrium, prostaglandin brings about contractions through mobilization of calcium; $PGF_{2\alpha}$ inhibits adenylate cyclase activity and, therefore, conversion of ATP to cyclic AMP, as well as inhibition of calcium binding to cytoplasmic membrane protein, thus giving rise to increased free calcium that can mediate muscle contractions.

Prostaglandins induce contraction or relaxation of smooth muscle, including those of the gastrointestinal tract, the res-

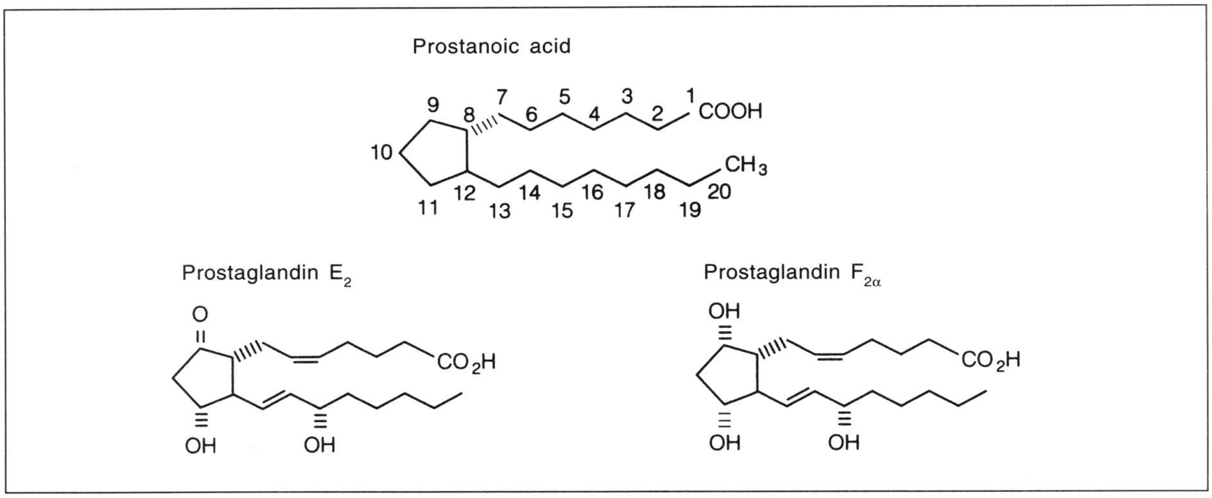

FIG. 6-2. Structure of prostanoic acid, prostaglandin E_2, and prostaglandin $F_{2\alpha}$.

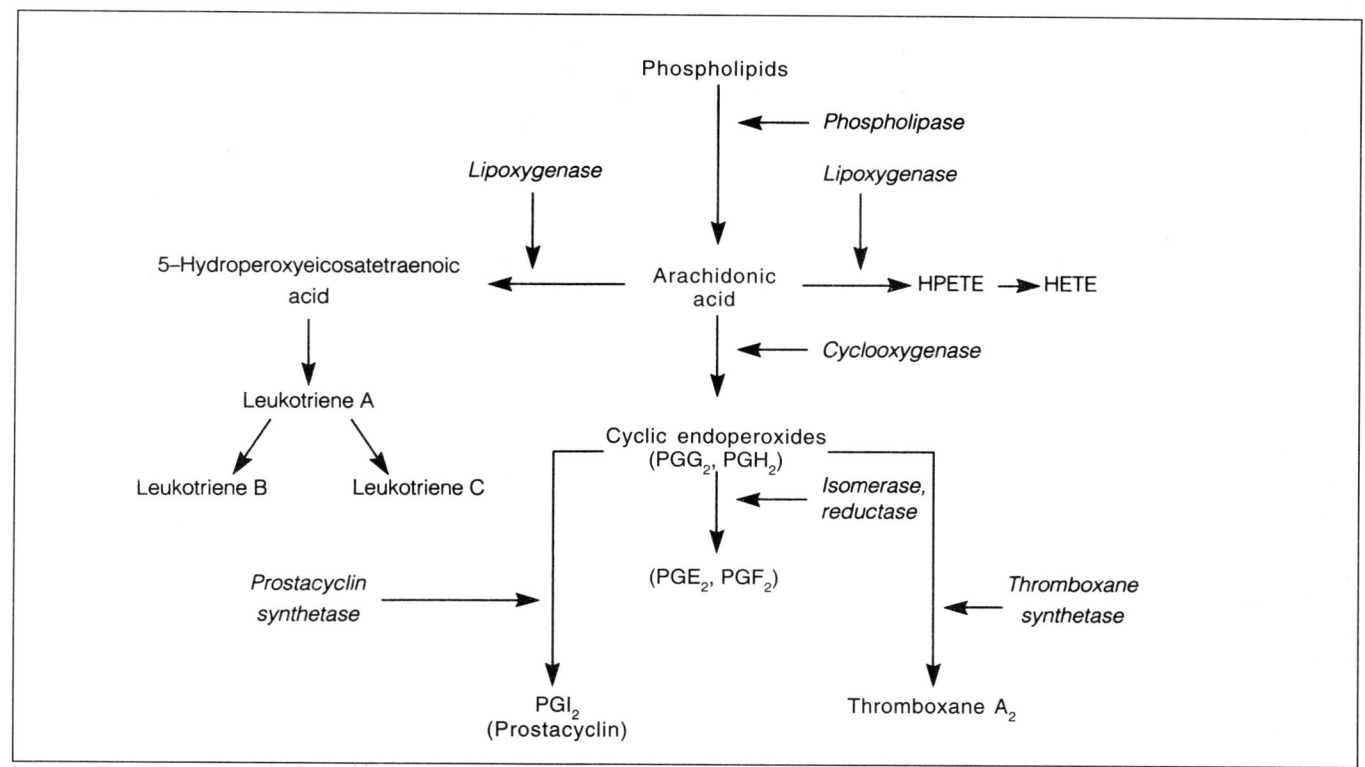

FIG. 6-3. Biosynthesis of prostaglandins through the cyclooxygenase pathway and of leukotrienes through the lipoxygenase pathway. HPETE indicates hydroperoxyeicosatetraenoic acid; HETE, hydroxyeicosatetraenoic acid.

piratory tract, the cardiovascular system, and the reproductive tract, thus explaining some of the side effects (uterine contractions, nausea, vomiting, and diarrhea) associated with prostaglandin use. Given intravenously (IV) or intrauterine, PGE_2 and $PGF_{2\alpha}$ induce human uterine contractions during all phases of the menstrual cycle. However, during menstruation intrauterine administration of PGE_2 relaxes the uterus. Prostaglandin E_2, $PGF_{2\alpha}$, and thromboxane A_2 stimulate contractions of the pregnant human uterus, PGE_2 being about 10 times more potent than $PGF_{2\alpha}$. Prostacyclin relaxes the uterus. Thromboxane is a potent vasoconstrictor and induces platelet aggregation, thus promoting clotting. A powerful vasodilator and antiaggregatory to platelets, prostacyclin slows down clotting. To prolong the half-life, biologic potency, and clinical usefulness of prostaglandins, analogues that protect the 15-hydroxyl group (eg, 15-methyl-$PGF_{2\alpha}$ and 16,16-dimethyl-PGE_2) have been developed. They are 10–100 times more potent than the parent compound.

Prostaglandins play important roles in all aspects of normal human reproduction. These include 1) the prostaglandin-mediated release of gonadotropin at the hypothalamic level for the midcycle preovulatory LH surge; 2) a local effect of prostaglandin on ovarian muscle for contractions and on the follicle for the rupture and release of the oocyte; 3) prostaglandin-mediated luteolysis in subprimate species; 4) local prostaglandin-induced relaxation and contraction of the fallopian tube to promote synchronized tubal transport of the ovum to the uterus; 5) the exertion of implantation-related effects of prostaglandin at multiple sites in both the embryo (hatching of blastocysts and fluid accumulation) and the endometrium (increase in capillary permeability and inflammatory changes); 6) fetal lung development; 7) PGE_2-mediated maintenance of ductus arteriosus patency in utero and subsequent postnatal changes; and 8) the production and release of $PGF_{2\alpha}$ and PGE_2 by fetal membranes, the decidua, and the placenta to stimulate uterine contractions at the time of spontaneous labor and parturition. Expression of the cyclooxygenase (prostaglandin synthetase) gene is undetectable in trophoblast during the first and second trimesters but is increased in amnion and trophoblast by 3.5- and 2.5-fold in association with labor.

Prostaglandins are involved with the pathophysiology of several gynecologic and obstetric disorders. Endometrial production and release of prostaglandins ($PGF_{2\alpha}$, PGE_2) are elevated in patients with primary dysmenorrhea. Similarly, elevated endometrial prostaglandins caused by an intrauterine device (IUD) are responsible for IUD-related dysmenorrhea and menorrhagia. In the absence of intrauterine pathologic lesions, some cases of menorrhagia are also due to elevated prostacyclin, other prostaglandins, or both. Prostaglandins mediate the inflammatory response that occurs in the healing process. This can give rise to postsurgical adhesion formation.

All of these prostaglandin-mediated disorders can be corrected with the use of NSAIDs to inhibit prostaglandin biosynthesis, and there is impressive clinical relief and outcome. Preterm labor is prostaglandin mediated, even when it is initiated by infection, since many bacteria possess the phospholipase enzyme that is essential for generating arachidonic acid and prostaglandins. Alternatively or additionally, the cytokines produced by the inflammatory cells and macrophages induced by chorioamnionitis can stimulate the arachidonic cascade or pathway (Fig. 6-3) and generate prostaglandins. Preterm labor can be successfully inhibited with selected NSAIDs.

A suggested etiology of preeclampsia is an imbalance in PGE_2, prostacyclin, and thromboxane. A decrease in placental production of PGE_2, a vasodilator, results in relative dominance of $PGF_{2\alpha}$ vasoconstrictor effects with ensuing hypertension. A balance between the vasodilatory, platelet antiaggregatory prostacyclin and the vasoconstrictory, platelet proaggregatory thromboxane of the placenta regulates blood pressure. The umbilical arteries and placental veins synthesize more prostacyclin than do other vessels, thus maintaining low peripheral vascular resistance in fetal circulation, which has high renin levels and high cardiac output. Women with preeclampsia have reduced prostaglandin production by umbilical arteries, placental veins, and fetal tissues, thus changing the balance in favor of thromboxane, which is vasoconstrictory.

CLINICAL APPLICATIONS

Prostaglandins E_2 and $F_{2\alpha}$ are used for the induction of labor in many countries, but not in the United States, and are as effective as oxytocin for the induction of labor at term. In early and midpregnancy, the uterus is readily stimulated by prostaglandins to contract, but it is less sensitive to oxytocin than it is at term. Besides the intravenous route, PGE_2 can be given orally, intravaginally as suppositories or a gel, and intraamniotically. Side effects are few and include nausea, vomiting, and diarrhea. Infrequently, posterior uterine tears into the cul-de-sac may occur.

Cervical softening at term is brought about by the local cervical action of prostaglandins, but the precise mechanism of action is not known. It is possible that the reduction of collagen levels, the disruption of the collagen network, or loosening of the collagen fibers, as well as the increased production of ground substance with enhanced water uptake, lead to a decrease in the structural integrity of the cervix and, therefore, softening. However, cervical softening with prostaglandin may be brought about or contributed by the uterine muscle contractions induced by prostaglandin. Rather than mechanically dilating a firm, unfavorable cervix, it can be readily and easily softened in 6–12 hours with PGE_2 or its newer analogues, given as a gel or suppository vaginally or endocervically, before the induction of labor or abortion. This can also increase the success rates of induction of labor with oxytocin. The cellulose-based PGE_2 gel has problems with long-term stability, homogeneity, and clinical handling, but the special cross-linked starch polymer gel has overcome these disadvantages. Prostaglandin E_2 chips have also been tried. Large-scale clinical trials have demonstrated the efficacy of PGE_2 gel for cervical ripening prior to induction of labor, with reduced cesarean delivery rates. Prostaglandin E_2 gel is now approved in the United States for cervical ripening prior to labor induction.

Prostaglandins play an important role in the nonsurgical treatment of postpartum hemorrhage caused by uterine atony due to a variety of obstetric conditions (see the section on Obstetrics). In neonates, PGE_2 can be given to maintain the patency of the ductus arteriosus in the presence of heart malformations that are dependent on ductus arteriosus pulmonary blood flow.

Suppression of prostaglandin production is used for the treatment of reproductive conditions caused by an excess or an imbalance of prostaglandin production and release. Primary dysmenorrhea, IUD-related dysmenorrhea, and menorrhagia are effectively corrected with NSAID therapy. For patients with primary dysmenorrhea, a prostaglandin synthetase inhibitor such as ibuprofen or naproxen is given for the first 2–3 days of menstrual flow to reduce endometrial prostaglandin production and release, with 80–90% of patients relieved of pain. For IUD-related dysmenorrhea and menorrhagia, the NSAIDs should be given throughout menstruation. Patients with menorrhagia that is not caused by a uterine anatomic pathologic lesion can also be successfully treated with NSAIDs to suppress their uterine prostaglandins throughout menstruation. Given perioperatively and postoperatively for tubal reconstructive surgery in animals, NSAIDs inhibit and reduce postoperative adhesion formation by suppressing prostaglandin release and, therefore, the postoperative surgical inflammatory response.

Based on increased placental and platelet production of thromboxane in women with preeclampsia, low-dose aspirin (60 mg/d) significantly reduced the development of preeclampsia in women at risk for developing this pregnancy complication. Low doses of aspirin (60–100 mg/d) have a remarkable ability to inhibit thromboxane production selectively without significantly suppressing PGI production, probably because the platelets that pass through the gut capillaries are exposed to higher concentrations of aspirin than they are in the peripheral circulation. The ratio of serum thromboxane A_2 to prostacyclin metabolites decreased by 35% with aspirin treatment but increased by 51% with placebo treatment. To be effective, low-dose aspirin has to be given as essentially a preventive therapy for pregnancy-induced hypertension and not as a curative therapy. In a meta-analysis of six trials of low-dose aspirin, the relative risk of pregnancy-induced hypertension was reduced to 0.35, with risks of low birth weight reduced by 44% and of cesarean delivery by 66%.

Nonsteroidal antiinflammatory drugs can inhibit renal prostaglandin biosynthesis and therefore fetal urine output leading to oligohydramnios. The degree of oligohydramnios is dependent on the dose of indomethacin, with 200 mg more likely to produce oligohydramnios. It is reversible upon stopping treatment. Indomethacin can therefore be used to reduce severe polyhydramnios by reducing amniotic fluid volumes through inhibition of fetal renal prostaglandin production and therefore urine output, but more definitive studies are needed.

Nonsteroidal antiinflammatory drugs can successfully arrest preterm labor through inhibition of prostaglandin production and are currently the only tocolytics that might be effective in stopping labor. The potential risks, however, include premature closure of the ductus arteriosus in utero, pulmonary hypertension, and oligohydramnios. Nevertheless, short-term indomethacin therapy for preterm labor has not been found to increase neonatal hypertensive complications (see the section on Obstetrics).

Indomethacin in small doses is used to obtain successful nonsurgical closure of patent ductus arteriosus in preterm infants and other newborns. The dose of indomethacin should be kept low because of the risk of renal insufficiency.

BIBLIOGRAPHY

Bennett PR, Henderson DJ, Moore GE. Changes in expression of the cyclooxygenase gene in human fetal membranes and placenta with labor. Am J Obstet Gynecol 1992;167:212–216

Bernstein P. Prostaglandin E_2 gel for cervical ripening and labour induction: a multicenter placebo-controlled trial. Can Med Assoc J 1991;145:1249–1254

Dawood MY. Dysmenorrhea. Clin Obstet Gynecol 1990;33:168–178

Dawood MY. Nonsteroidal antiinflammatory drugs and reproduction. Am J Obstet Gynecol 1993;169:1255–1265

Dekker GA, Sibai BM. Low-dose aspirin in the prevention of preeclampsia and fetal growth retardation: rationale, mechanisms and clinical trials. Am J Obstet Gynecol 1993;168:214–227

Higby K, Xenakis EM, Pauerstein CJ. Do tocolytic agents stop preterm labor? A critical and comprehensive review of efficacy and safety. Am J Obstet Gynecol 1993;168:1247–1256; discussion, 1256–1259

Imperiale TF, Petrulis AS. A meta-analysis of low-dose aspirin for the prevention of pregnancy-induced hypertensive disease. JAMA 1991;266:260–264

Schiff E, Peleg E, Goldenberg M, Rosenthal T, Ruppin E, Tamarkin M, et al. The use of aspirin to prevent pregnancy-induced hypertension and lower the ratio of thromboxane A2 to prostacyclin in relatively high risk pregnancies. N Engl J Med 1989;312:351–356

Genetics

CHROMOSOMAL DISORDERS

The normal diploid human chromosome number is 46, occurring as 23 homologous pairs. Twenty-two pairs, called autosomes, are alike in males and females. The two sex chromosomes, the remaining pair, differ in males and females. The normal male chromosomal complement is designated 46,XY; the normal female chromosomal complement is designated 46,XX.

A chromosomal error may be either a numeric change (a deviation from the normal number) or a structural change (an abnormality in chromosome morphology). Chromosome aberrations occur in approximately 1/200 live births and are associated with 50–70% of first-trimester spontaneous abortions.

Whether associated with duplication or deficiency of genetic information, chromosomal syndromes are usually characterized by multiple anomalies. Among the deleterious effects consistently associated with chromosomal abnormalities are mental retardation; intrauterine and postnatal growth retardation; and anomalies of many organ systems, especially the craniofacial, skeletal, cardiac, and genitourinary systems. The most frequently seen chromosomal disorders are trisomies (a complement in which there is one additional whole chromosome) and monosomies (a complement in which one entire chromosome is lacking).

Trisomy 21 (Down syndrome) is the most common autosomal abnormality, occurring in 1/800 liveborn infants; other autosomal trisomies, such as trisomy 18 and trisomy 13, are well recognized, though less common. Each of these trisomies shows an increased incidence with advancing maternal age.

Monosomy almost always causes early intrauterine death. Although monosomy for the X chromosomes causes early abortion in most cases, it may result in a viable fetus with Turner syndrome.

The most common chromosomal abnormalities in the general population are the balanced structural rearrangements (translocations). The translocations are reciprocal in that two chromosomes are involved in a mutual exchange of broken fragments. When the total amount of material is unchanged, it is called a balanced translocation. Of significance to the obstetrician–gynecologist is the fact that approximately 2% of couples with recurrent spontaneous abortions are found to be carriers of balanced chromosomal abnormalities that could be related to the pregnancy loss.

MENDELIAN DISORDERS

A mutation at a single genetic locus, on either an autosome or a sex chromosome, results in a mendelian disorder. Such a disorder may be manifested in a dominant or recessive manner. More than 3,000 traits are believed to be inherited in a mendelian fashion.

An autosomal recessive disorder is one that is expressed only when each parent possesses one copy of the gene in question (the heterozygous state) and the affected child has inherited a pair of the genes (the homozygous state). There is a 25%

chance that each offspring of the heterozygous parents will be affected with the disease. There is rarely a family history of the disease outside the affected siblings, and males and females are equally likely to be affected. Autosomal recessive diseases include cystic fibrosis, sickle cell disease, phenylketonuria, and Tay–Sachs disease.

An autosomal dominant trait is one that is manifest in the individual who has only a single copy of the gene (the heterozygous state). It is transmitted from generation to generation, and the probability that a person carrying the gene will pass it to his or her offspring is 50%. Examples of autosomal dominant disorders include neurofibromatosis, Marfan syndrome, achondroplasia, and adult-type polycystic kidney disease.

Because males (XY) and females (XX) differ in the number of X chromosomes they possess, the inheritance pattern of mutations carried on the X chromosome differs from that carried on autosomes. A trait controlled by a gene on the X chromosome is expressed in all males with the allele. Affected males are said to be hemizygous. Females are affected if they are homozygous or if they inactivate most of the X chromosomes with the normal allele. In X-linked inheritance, there is no male-to-male transmission; all daughters of an affected male receive the mutant gene and are carriers, however. One-half of the sons and daughters of a heterozygous female receive the mutant gene. In general, X-linked recessive traits are not clinically expressed in the heterozygous female, while X-linked dominant traits are expressed. Important X-linked disorders include hemophilia A and B, Duchenne-type muscular dystrophy, and glucose-6-phosphate dehydrogenase deficiency.

UNIPARENTAL DISOMY

Uniparental disomy is a newly identified mode of inheritance in which contributions of genetic material from each parent are unequal. Errors in cell division cause two copies of a chromosome to be inherited from one parent, whereas no copy of that chromosome is inherited from the other parent. Therefore, one chromosome pair in the individual does not conform to the normal pattern of one maternally derived and one paternally derived copy. The genetic material within gametes of each sex is differentially modified, leading to different patterns of gene expression during development, depending on parent of origin (so-called imprinting). Uniparental disomy has been associated with various genetic disorders (eg, Prader–Willi syndrome, Angelman syndrome), some cases of intrauterine growth retardation, and certain genetic cancer-predisposing syndromes (eg, Beckwith–Wiedemann syndrome).

MULTIFACTORIAL DISORDERS

It is thought that multifactorial disorders result from a combination of the effects of two or more deleterious genes and environmental influences, which are often unidentified. Certain characteristics suggest that a trait is inherited in a multifactorial fashion:

- The trait has an incidence of approximately 1/1,000 or 2/1,000 births and usually involves a single organ system.
- After one affected child, the risk of recurrence in subsequent siblings is usually 2–5%.
- If the trait is more common among members of one sex, the risk for relatives is higher if the proband belongs to the less frequently affected sex.
- The more serious the anomaly, the higher the recurrence risk.
- As the degree of relation decreases, the recurrence risk to relatives decreases more rapidly than it does for autosomal dominant traits.

The multifactorial disorders include many fairly common disorders, such as neural tube defects, congenital heart disease, cleft lip with or without cleft palate, and pyloric stenosis.

TRIPLE REPEAT MUTATIONS

Recently, a newly identified class of human mutation, consisting of an amplification of unstable contiguous trinucleotide repeat sequences, has been shown to be the genetic cause of several common diseases, including fragile X syndrome, spinal and bulbar muscular atrophy (Kennedy disease), myotonic dystrophy, and Huntington disease. This novel mutation provides a specific molecular mechanism behind the phenomenon of anticipation, which is the clinical observation that some genetic diseases manifest at either an earlier age or more severely in successive generations.

Fragile X Syndrome

The fragile X syndrome, an X-linked disorder, is the most common inherited form of mental retardation, with a prevalence of about 1/1,250 males and 1/2,000 females. In addition to moderate to severe mental retardation, affected males have facial dysmorphic features, macroorchidism, and a folate-sensitive fragile site on the X chromosome, at band Xq27.3. The responsible gene *(FMR-1)* has been cloned, and it includes the repeated CGG sequence that causes the fragile X mutation. Normal individuals have 6–54 CGG repeats at this locus, with an average of about 30 repeats. Alleles with greater than 52 repeats, including those identified in a normal family, are meiotically unstable. Individuals with no significant phenotypic abnormalities, but who are at high risk for having an affected offspring, have triple repeats ranging between 52–200. Such individuals are said to have a premutation, because it has a high probability of expanding to a full mutation in the next generation. Finally, individuals with more than 200 CGG repeats are affected with the fragile X syndrome. The passage from premutation to full mutation status occurs only with transmission from the mother. Expanded CGG repeats appear to cause abnormal methylation of the *FMR-1* gene, which in turn causes a reduction in gene transcription, resulting in disease.

Spinal and Bulbar Muscular Atrophy (Kennedy Disease)

Kennedy disease is an X-linked recessive disorder characterized by motor neuron degeneration that starts in adulthood and leads to progressive muscular weakness of the upper and lower extremities. Affected males have reduced fertility and gynecomastia; female carriers have few or no symptoms. A mutation in the N-terminus of the androgen receptor gene involving CAG repeats has been shown to be the cause of this disease. Unaffected individuals have 13–30 GAG repeats in the first exon (ie, transcribed region) of this gene; individuals with Kennedy disease have 40–62 repeats.

Myotonic Dystrophy

Myotonic dystrophy is the most common form of adult muscular dystrophy, with a prevalence of 2–14/100,000 individuals. This autosomal dominant condition is manifest by myotonia, cardiac arrhythmias, cataracts, male baldness, male infertility (hypogonadism), and other associated endocrinopathies. The age of onset and severity of the disease show extreme variation, both within and between families. The rare congenital form of myotonic dystrophy is associated with profound newborn hypotonia and mental retardation. Such children are invariably the offspring of affected mothers, never affected fathers. The mothers frequently have mild to subclinical features of myotonic dystrophy. The myotonic dystrophy gene has been cloned, and an unstable DNA sequence specific for the disease has been characterized. Detection of an enlarged DNA fragment due to the expansion of CTG repeat within the myotonic dystrophy gene can be used for direct DNA diagnosis in affected individuals and persons at risk. Furthermore, there is a strong correlation between the length of fragment expansion and the degree of disease severity in gene carriers. The gene containing the repeat has been designated myotonin protein kinase.

Huntington Disease

Huntington disease is an autosomal dominant disorder that affects about 1/100,000 individuals. This progressive neurodegenerative disorder is characterized by motor disturbances, cognitive loss, and psychiatric manifestations. Affected individuals develop a distinctive choreic movement disorder that has an insidious onset in the fourth to fifth decade of life and gradually worsens over a period of 10–20 years until death. A juvenile form of Huntington disease exists with a preponderance of paternal transmission of the disease. The gene (designated *IT15*) contains a polymorphic CAG repeat sequence. Unaffected individuals usually have about 11–24 CAG repeats, whereas patients with Huntington disease have 42–86 CAG repeats. The length of the repeat appears to correlate with the age of onset and severity of the disease.

GONADAL DYSGENESIS

The term *gonadal dysgenesis* applies to persons who have streak gonads rather than ovaries. Gonadal dysgenesis is usually associated with monosomy for the X chromosome (45,X) or structural abnormalities of the sex chromosomes. Rarely, those with apparently normal female (46,XX) or male (46,XY) chromosomal complements have gonadal dysgenesis. Affected individuals lack germ cells and show hypogonadism at puberty.

The most common chromosomal abnormality associated with gonadal dysgenesis is 45,X; however, the proportion of 45,X persons in a given sample depends on the method by which they have been identified. About 80% of cases recognized by pediatricians show this complement. In contrast, only 40% of patients in whom gonadal dysgenesis has been diagnosed as a result of primary amenorrhea have a 45,X complement; 20% show an X-chromosome structural abnormality or mosaicism, and 40% show 46,XY or 46,XX complements.

Almost all 45,X individuals have short stature (mean adult height, 141 ± 0.6 cm) and certain features of Turner syndrome. None of these features is pathognomonic, but in aggregate they form a characteristic spectrum that is more likely to occur in individuals with a 45,X complement than in individuals with most other sex chromosome abnormalities. These may include the following: epicanthal folds, high-arched palate, low nuchal hairline, webbed neck, shield chest, coarctation of the aorta, ventricular septal defect, renal anomalies, pigmented nevi, nail hypoplasia, and cubitus valgus. Hypertension is relatively frequent among adult patients. The normal gonad is usually replaced by a white fibrous streak, 2–3 cm long and approximately 0.5 cm wide. This streak gonad is characterized histologically by an interlacing dense fibrous stroma that is indistinguishable from a normal ovarian stroma. There are usually no oocytes, not because no oocytes are formed, but because oocyte atresia is increased. Inasmuch as there are germ cells in 45,X embryos, it is not surprising that a small percentage (3–5%) of 45,X individuals menstruate spontaneously. There have even been reports of a few fertile patients.

The above comments notwithstanding, menstruation and fertility occur so rarely that 45,X patients should be counseled to anticipate primary amenorrhea and sterility. However, hormone therapy (estrogen and cyclic progestogens) can lead to normal uterine size, and 45,X women can carry pregnancies achieved through donor oocytes (IVF or gamete intrafallopian transfer [GIFT]). Pregnancies with donor embryos obtained by uterine lavage is also feasible.

Lack of normal ovarian development leads to deficient secretion of sex steroids. Estrogen and androgen levels are decreased; FSH and LH levels are increased. At puberty, therefore, pubic and axillary hair fail to develop in normal quantities, breasts contain little parenchymal tissue, and the areolar tissue is only slightly darker than the surrounding skin. In addition, the well-differentiated external genitalia, vagina, and müllerian derivatives remain small. Accordingly, estrogen and cyclic progestogen replacement therapy is required.

Various treatments for short stature in 45,X patients have

been proposed: GH, anabolic steroids, and low-dose estrogens. Most pediatric endocrinologists now appear to favor use of human recombinant DNA–derived methionyl human GH.

Recombinant GH has virtually replaced human pituitary GH and does not carry with it the risk of Creutzfeldt-Jakob disease. No longer is the supply of GH limited, so treatment may be expanded to include patients with gonadal dysgenesis and even children with short stature of unknown etiology. Short-term increases in growth have been demonstrated with GH alone or in combination with steroids (estrogen or oxandrolone) in children with Turner syndrome. Likewise, GH replacement has resulted in short-term increases in height in those with idiopathic short stature.

The efficacy of GH or other therapy may be limited. Observations that epiphyses in patients with a 45,X complement are structurally abnormal suggest that Turner syndrome can be considered as a malformation syndrome. Not only are long bones abnormal but so are the teeth and skull. Persons with a 45,X karyotype might be said to have a skeletal dysplasia.

Most 45,X patients have normal intelligence, but any given 45,X patient is slightly more likely to be retarded than are 46,XX persons. Their performance IQ is lower than their verbal IQ, the latter being similar to that of 46,XX matched controls. In particular, 45,X patients have an unusual cognitive defect in which they are unable to appreciate the shapes and relationships of objects to each other (space-form blindness).

Monosomy for the X chromosome (45,X) may originate during oogenesis, during spermatogenesis, or after fertilization. In humans, 70% of liveborn 45,X individuals have lost a paternal sex chromosome. The frequency of 45,X is not correlated with advancing maternal age, consistent with the paternal origin for monosomy X.

Individuals with a 45,X/46,XX mosaic have fewer anomalies than do those with a 45,X complement. Of 45,X/46,XX individuals, 12% menstruate, compared with only 3% of 45,X individuals, and 18% undergo breast development, compared with 5% of 45,X individuals. Furthermore, the mean adult height is greater in 45,X/46,XX individuals (146 cm) than in 45,X individuals (142 cm). Detected far less often, 45,X/47,XXX individuals are phenotypically similar to 45,X/46,XX individuals.

Other chromosome abnormalities associated with gonadal dysgenesis include deletions of the short or long arms of the X chromosome, and isochromosome for the X long arm. (Division of the centromere in the transverse rather than in the longitudinal plane results in an isochromosome, a metacentric chromosome consisting of isologous arms.) An isochromosome for the X long arm is the most common X chromosome structural abnormality, but coexisting 45,X lines (mosaicism) are common.

Some individuals who have gonadal dysgenesis have an apparently normal female (46,XX) chromosomal complement. Their external genitalia and streak gonads are indistinguishable from those of individuals who have gonadal dysgenesis and an abnormal chromosomal complement. Likewise, their secondary sexual development and endocrine profiles are the same as those of other individuals with streak gonads. The somatic features of the Turner syndrome are usually absent, however, and the stature is generally normal (mean height, 165 cm). This condition is inherited in an autosomal recessive fashion. In some families, affected individuals also have neurosensory deafness (Perrault syndrome).

Gonadal dysgenesis may occur in individuals with apparently normal male (46,XY) chromosomal complements. Individuals with 46,XY gonadal dysgenesis show female external genitalia, a uterus, and fallopian tubes. At puberty secondary sexual development fails to occur. Height is normal and somatic anomalies are usually absent. However, a relationship between 46,XY gonadal dysgenesis and renal failure of uncertain pathogenesis exists. Approximately 20–30% of 46,XY gonadal dysgenesis patients develop a dysgerminoma or gonadoblastoma. Often the neoplasia arises in the first or second decade. Because of the relatively high probability of undergoing neoplastic transformation, gonads should be extirpated from all individuals with 46,XY gonadal dysgenesis. The uterus and fallopian tubes should not be removed, even though it is technically easier to remove these organs rather than to extirpate only the streaks. Retention of the uterus allows pregnancy through donor oocytes or donor embryos, as mentioned for 45,X gonadal dysgenesis. Genetic heterogeneity exists with respect to 46,XY gonadal dysgenesis. At least one form segregates in the fashion expected of X-linked kindreds. An autosomal recessive form of 46,XY gonadal dysgenesis may or may not also exist.

ANDROGEN INSENSITIVITY SYNDROMES

In complete androgen insensitivity (complete testicular feminization), 46,XY individuals show bilateral testes, female external genitalia, a blindly ending vagina, and no müllerian derivatives (ie, neither a uterus nor fallopian tubes are ordinarily present). The underlying pathogenesis is inability to respond to testosterone. In 60–70% of cases, androgen receptors are not present (receptor negative). In 30–40%, receptors are present (receptor positive). In the latter, a defect at a more distal step in androgen action must be postulated. Receptor-positive and receptor-negative cases are clinically indistinguishable. However, antimüllerian hormone is synthesized as in the normal testis; the body responds normally to antimüllerian hormone for which reason no uterus is present. Affected individuals undergo breast development, but areolae are often pale and underdeveloped. Pubertal feminization occurs; however, pubic hair and axillary hair are usually sparse, but scalp hair is normal.

Testes are usually normal in size. They may be located in the abdomen, inguinal canal, or labia (ie, anywhere along the path of embryonic testicular descent). If located in the inguinal canal, testes may produce inguinal hernias. Frequency of gonadal neoplasia is increased, but the exact magnitude is uncertain. Once stated to be relatively high, the actual risk is probably no greater than 5%. Risk of malignancy is clearly low before ages 25–30 years, albeit thereafter increasing. Benign tubular adenomas (Pick adenomas) are especially common in postpubertal patients, probably as result of increased secretion of LH. Although orchiectomy is eventually necessary, it is acceptable to leave the testes in situ until after pubertal feminization.

Despite pubertal feminization, some individuals with androgen insensitivity show clitoral enlargement and labioscrotal fusion; the term *incomplete (partial) androgen insensitivity* (incomplete testicular feminization) is applied to these patients. Both complete and incomplete (partial) androgen insensitivities are distinct, but heterogeneity exists for each. Both complete androgen insensitivity and its incomplete counterpart result from mutations in the same gene, localized to the long arm of the X chromosome.

DNA DIAGNOSTIC TECHNOLOGY

Exciting new developments have occurred in DNA-based diagnostic technologies. Techniques such as Southern blotting, restriction fragment length polymorphisms, and polymerase chain reactions (PCR) are becoming increasingly important in the diagnosis of endocrine disorders.

Southern blotting is a method by which DNA is fractionated by electrophoresis, transferred to a membrane (blotted), and detected by a complementary labeled probe that hybridizes to the DNA, revealing information about its identity, size and abundance (Fig. 6-4). Southern blotting and subsequent hybridization with DNA probes enable one to follow mutant genes in families by the use of restriction fragment length polymorphisms. When the molecular basis of a disease is known, precise tests can be designed to detect directly the underlying mutation, be it a deletion, insertion, or single base change.

Restriction enzymes are bacteria-derived enzymes that recognize specific, short nucleotide sequences and cut DNA at those sites. Restriction fragment length polymorphisms are genetic variations resulting from a difference in DNA sequence that affects the recognition sequence for restriction enzymes. When DNA is digested by a particular enzyme, the fragments will differ, depending on the presence or absence of the proper recognition sequence for the enzyme. A good example of the role of restriction fragment length polymorphisms is in evaluation of congenital adrenal hyperplasia. Most of these patients have point mutations that may not be detectable by Southern blot analysis. The restriction fragment length polymorphisms are especially helpful with this disease because the gene for 21-hydroxylase is closely linked to *HLA-DR* and *HLA-B* regions. Thus, restriction fragment length polymorphisms would be indicated for prenatal diagnosis with use of appropriate probes to identify either 21-hydroxylase per se or the *HLA-B* or *HLA-DR* regions.

Today most of the direct tests rely on the ability to amplify quickly and efficiently a specific region of DNA using the PCR. This technique allows a target sequence of up to 2 kilobases of DNA to be amplified 10^5–10^6-fold from template segments present in amounts as small as a single molecule. The method depends on the use of two flanking oligonucleotide DNA primers (usually 20–35 nucleotides long) and repeated cycles of primer extension using DNA polymerase. Thus, PCR analysis can be performed rapidly on DNA from even a single cell. The number of common mendelian diseases in which molecular genetics is sufficiently understood to allow this sort of diagnosis is now large and still rapidly expanding under the impetus of the Human Genome Project designed ultimately to determine the sequence of the entire human genome. Polymerase chain reaction is currently used for diagnosis of genetic diseases such as Duchenne muscular dystrophy and cystic fibrosis, for diagnosis of Lyme disease, and for evaluation of human papillomavirus.

Fluorescence in situ hybridization (Fig. 6-5) is a new approach that merges molecular genetics and cytogenetics. It is a physical mapping technique in which fluorescein-tagged DNA probes are hybridized to chromosome. The ability to detect and characterize chromosomal abnormalities using fluorescence in situ hybridization has been greatly enhanced by the availability of numerous chromosome-specific probes (eg, chromosomes 13, 21, 18, X, and Y) that can be used in interphase nuclei and directly on metaphase chromosomes.

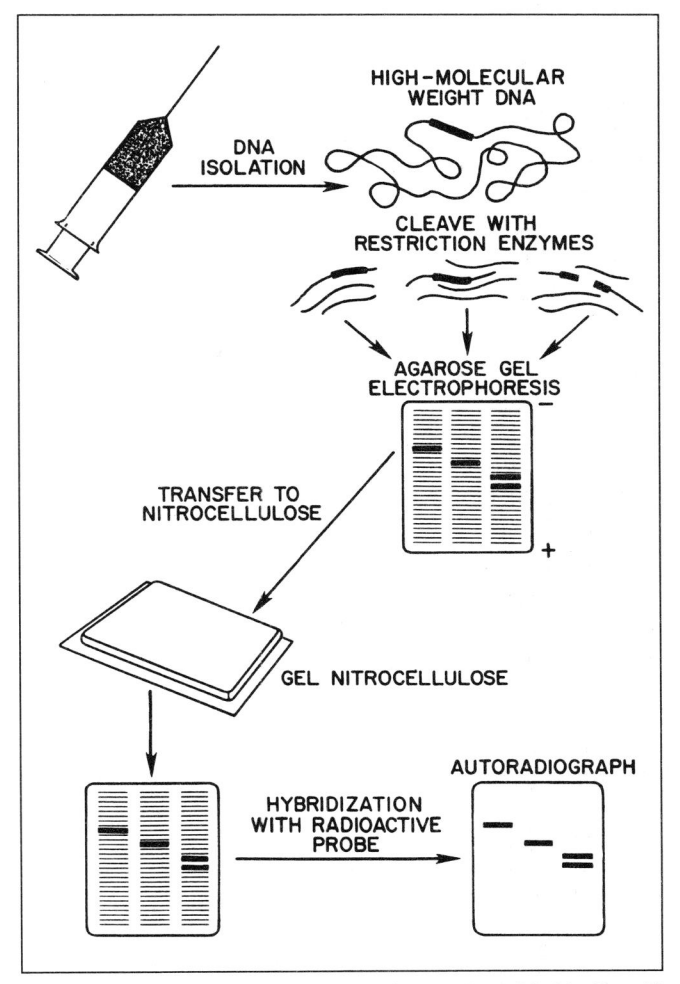

FIG. 6-4. Southern blotting analysis. (Cunningham FG, MacDonald PC, Gant NF, Leveno KJ, Gilstrap LC III. Genetics. In: Williams obstetrics. 19th ed. Norwalk, Connecticut: Appleton & Lange, 1993:935)

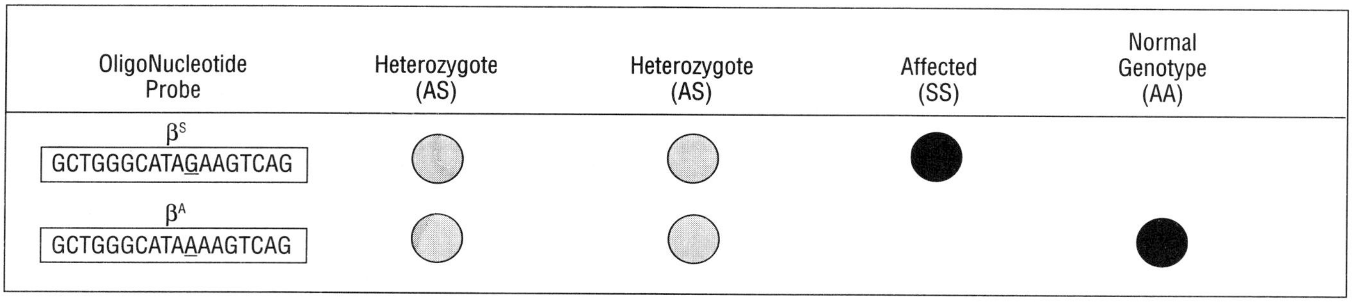

OligoNucleotide Probe	Heterozygote (AS)	Heterozygote (AS)	Affected (SS)	Normal Genotype (AA)
β^S GCTGGGCATAGAAGTCAG	◐	◐	●	
β^A GCTGGGCATAAAAGTCAG	◐	◐		●

FIG. 6-5. Dot-blot analysis. Oligonucleotides are constructed for sequences unique to normal DNA (β^A) and mutant DNA (β^S) at the sequence responsible for sickle cell anemia. The DNA challenged by the oligonucleotide probe will be hybridized if and only if the DNA contains all nucleotides connoted by the probe. Thus, AS individuals will respond to both β^A and β^S probes, whereas AA or SS individuals will respond only to one of the two probes (β^A and β^S, respectively). Homozygous individuals respond with a stronger (darker) signal than do heterozygous individuals. (Simpson JL. Genetic counseling and prenatal diagnosis. In: Gabbe SG, Niebyl JR, Simpson JL, eds. Obstetrics: normal and problem pregnancies. 2nd ed. New York: Churchill Livingstone, 1991:290; modified from Simpson JL. Genetic factors in obstetrics and gynecology. In: Scott JR, DiSaia PJ, Hammond CB, Spellacy WN, eds. Danforth's obstetrics and gynecology. 6th ed. Philadelphia: JB Lippincott, 1990:253)

BIBLIOGRAPHY

Caskey CT, Pizzuti A, Fu YH, Fenwick RG Jr, Nelson DL. Triplet repeat mutations in human disease. Science 1992;256:784–789

Hall JG. Genomic imprinting: review and relevance to human diseases. Am J Hum Genet 1990;46:857–873

The Huntington's Disease Collaborative Research Group. A novel gene containing a trinucleotide repeat that is expanded and unstable on Huntington's disease chromosomes. Cell 1993;72:971–983

Simpson JL. Genetics of sexual differentiation. In: Rock JA, Carpenter SE, eds. Pediatric and adolescent gynecology. New York: Raven Press, 1992:1–37

Simpson JL, Elias S, eds. Essentials of prenatal diagnosis. New York, Churchill Livingstone, 1993

Simpson JL, Golbus MS. Genetics in obstetrics and gynecology. 2nd ed. Philadelphia: WB Saunders, 1992

Pediatric and Adolescent Gynecology

PEDIATRIC PROBLEMS

History and Physical Examination

Neonates

The clinician's knowledge of evaluation and management of pediatric gynecologic problems begins with the neonate. The initial assessment, in the delivery room, conveys to the parents that evaluation of the genitalia is a normal and integral part of the general physical examination. Thus, in addition to the general physical examination, attention should be focused on the breast examination. At that point, not uncommonly as a reflection of maternal endogenous estrogen production, breast tissue is palpable in the neonate. Evaluation should include an attempt to elicit any nipple discharge. The abdomen is gently palpated for evidence of organomegaly, and the external genitalia are assessed for any ambiguity. The labia are gently grasped and separated to allow inspection of the introitus–hymenal area. Upon completion of the inspection segment of the genital examination, a rectal examination is performed. A midline structure indicative of a uterus is usually palpable and is often slightly enlarged as a result of exposure to the maternal estrogens. The adnexa should not be palpable at this time. A normal protuberant hymen with an associated thin, white, mucoid discharge from the vagina is frequently apparent. In the first few weeks of life, a small amount of vaginal bleeding may occur, indicative of withdrawal of estrogen of maternal origin.

Pediatric Patients

The history for pediatric patients is obtained primarily from the parents, who ideally should be integrally involved in the physical examination process. The physician must win the confidence of the pediatric patient, and this can often be accomplished with a "show and tell" approach. The child must feel a sense of control over the examination and experience no discomfort, as well as be prepared before the actual gynecologic examination.

The gynecologic examination is usually accomplished by placing the patient in a froglike position. If this proves unsatisfactory, then a knee–chest position accompanied with a Valsalva maneuver will allow adequate assessment of the introital (lower third of the vagina) area. Low-power magnification, as with a colposcope or a hand-held magnifying glass, facilitates assessment of the genitalia. The vestibule should be evaluated for any discharge. It has been advocated that an aseptic technique with use of intravenous tubing (butterfly) can be passed into a soft no. 12 bladder catheter, all of which is attached to a 1-ml tuberculin syringe, thus allowing aspiration of any fluid from the vagina as well as accomplishing lavage. A cotton-tipped swab can be used for obtaining cultures if necessary.

Other useful instrumentation includes an otoscope or a Cameron–Myers vaginoscope. Gentle traction on the labia upward and outward further exposes the vaginal introitus and permits assessment. Calcium calginate swabs are especially useful in obtaining cultures from the vagina. Familiarity with normal variance of hymenal configurations is essential. Evidence for a microperforate, imperforate, or septated hymen should be noted at this time. If an adequate examination cannot be accomplished in this manner, then sedation or examination under anesthesia becomes necessary, depending on the circumstance.

Diagnostic imaging techniques used for assessment include ultrasonography, computed tomography, and magnetic resonance imaging. An adequately distended urinary bladder is almost always required for the study. Most examinations in infants and young children can be performed abdominally with a 5.0- or a 7.5-MHz transducer. A 5.0-MHz or lower-frequency transducer is used for older children and teenaged patients.

Pediatric Gynecologic Problems

Vulvar Disorders

Vulvovaginitis is the most common childhood gynecologic problem that a clinician is likely to encounter. In part, vulvovaginal irritation is due to the lack of labial fat pads and pubic hair for protection of the external genitalia. Transfer of fecal bacteria can occur in light of the proximity of the anal orifice to the vagina. Masturbation may also be a contributing factor. In part because of the relatively low estrogenic milieu, the thin atrophic epithelium is more susceptible to bacterial invasion than the epithelium in the postpubertal child.

A number of entities can be associated with vulvovaginitis. These include nonspecific vulvovaginitis, which is a reflection of poor perineal hygiene in that primarily coliform bacteria secondary to fecal contamination result in vaginitis. Other organisms that have been associated with vulvovaginitis include beta-hemolytic streptococci and coagulase-positive staphylococci. In part, these organisms are transmitted manually from the nasopharynx. Other irritants, such as soap, detergents, and bubble bath, should be considered in the differential diagnosis. Specific organisms that cause vulvovaginitis include *Gardnerella vaginalis* as well as *Candida* species. The presence of organisms such as enterococci, anaerobic bacteria such as *Peptococcus, Peptostreptococcus,* *Veillonella parvula,* and *Bacteroides* species have been reported. Treatment, in large part, depends on the specific causative agent.

Adhesions of the labia primarily involve the labia minora and are characterized by a central line of adherence from an area immediately inferior to the clitoris to the fourchette. These are more commonly seen in the patient under age 6 years. The condition is due to local inflammation in association with the hypoestrogenic state of the preadolescent girl. Pooling of urine in the vagina and recurrent urinary tract infections can be associated with labial adhesions. Treatment includes topical estrogen cream or polymyxin B sulfate ointment applied each evening for 7–10 days. Either treatment should be accompanied by sitz baths and appropriate cleansing of the area. Mechanical separation should be gentle and certainly not traumatic.

Molluscum contagiosum is characterized by an umbilicated, dome-shaped papule. The central umbilication is usually associated with a pulpy core. Viral inclusion bodies (molluscum bodies) are noted in the central core. Treatment requires elimination of the lesions, usually by application of silver nitrate–curettage.

Lichen sclerosus et atrophicus is a chronic atrophic skin disease characterized by small, pink to ivory, flat-topped papules that are several millimeters in diameter. The papules tend to coalesce into plaques that become wrinkled and atrophic. Often, an hourglass or a figure-of-eight appearance is noted. It usually occurs in children less than age 7 years. While the cause is unknown, it is believed to be an autoimmune disorder. Treatment is symptomatic, including application of emollients and topical corticosteroids.

Lichen planus is often associated with oral mucosal and subcutaneous lesions. The vulvar lesions are characterized by angular, violaceous, flat-topped papules that may simulate leukoplakia. Treatment consists of topical intralesional corticosteroids and antihistamines to control pruritus.

Seborrheic dermatitis presents with erythematous, oily, circumscribed patches that can be found on the face, scalp, and chest, as well as on the intertriginous areas of the body. Secondary bacterial or candidal infection is quite common, causing pain, pruritus, dysuria, and vaginal bleeding. Treatment includes sitz baths and topical aluminum acetate solution (Burow solution).

Atopic dermatitis is often associated with a patient who has hay fever or asthma, as well as a family history positive for such allergies. The vulvar lesion is characterized by a chronic condition accompanied by intense pruritus, erythema, papules, and vesicles with oozing and crusting of the involved areas. Antihistamines are used to control the pruritus, and topical corticosteroids such as 1% hydrocortisone appear to be effective.

Contact dermatitis is characterized by sharp, serpiginous borders and usually is associated with soaps, powders, bubble baths, feminine hygiene sprays, topical medications, toilet paper, and rubber, as well as certain types of clothing. Treatment revolves around avoidance of the offending agent(s) and use of sitz baths or compresses with Burow solution during acute episodes.

Vulvar psoriasis is frequently associated with lesions on other parts of the body and is characterized by violaceous papules or plaques with a thick, adherent silvery scale. Use of corticosteroid cream (1% hydrocortisone) in conjunction with control of any secondary infection and pruritus is advocated.

Enterobiasis includes pinworms and helminths that may carry colonic bacteria to the perineum, causing recurrent vulvovaginitis. Diagnosis often requires use of the cellulose adhesive tape test, especially when the patient presents with intense pruritus over the anal area at bedtime as well as in the early morning hours. Treatment consists primarily of administering pyrantel pamoate.

Other lesions involving the vulva in the pediatric patient include shigellosis caused by *Shigella flexneri* and *S. sonnei*, which are associated with various gastrointestinal symptoms as well as vaginitis. Systemic antibiotics appear to be the treatment of choice.

Herpetic vulvar lesions have also been identified in the pediatric patient and are characterized by clusters of vesicles with an erythematous base. Sexual abuse should be ruled out, and suspected abuse should be reported to child protective services. The duration of primary lesions may be decreased with the use of topical acyclovir ointment. This therapy should be complemented with use of sitz baths and application of antiinflammatory agents.

Vaginal Bleeding and Discharge

A profuse, foul-smelling discharge should alert the clinician to the possibility of a foreign body. Wadded toilet paper is the most common foreign body identified in the pediatric patient's vagina.

The clinician should also consider a prolapsed urethra, which is more common in African–American children and oftentimes follows physical exertion or trauma. The patient typically presents with vulvar pain and dysuria accompanying the vaginal bleeding. Examination reveals a protruding granular-appearing mass at the urethral meatus. Treatment revolves around use of estrogen cream applied daily for 7–10 days to the affected area. It is rare that surgical intervention is necessary.

Bleeding can also be associated with condylomata acuminata and sexual abuse. Suspected cases of sexual abuse must be reported to child protective services.

A number of endocrinologic causes are associated with vaginal bleeding in this age group, including premature menarche as well as precocious puberty. Malignant neoplasms such as sarcoma botryoides, should be included in the differential diagnosis when vaginal bleeding is noted.

Sexual Abuse

A national study has estimated a rise of epidemic proportions (322%) in the incidence of child sexual abuse. Children may be sexually abused in either an intrafamilial or an extrafamilial setting. Most perpetrators are known to the child; only 10–15% are strangers. In most cases of child sexual abuse, the perpetrator is a relative of the child.

At least 0.2–0.3% of children have been involved in persistent incestuous relationships. Unfortunately, such abuse usually is not discovered before a period of approximately 5 years. Brief sexual encounters occur more frequently. The victims of incest are 90% female and 10% male. Incest is often repeated with successive daughters of the family.

Child molestation includes touching or fondling a child's genitals or asking a child to fondle the adult's genitals, or forced exposure to sexual acts or pornography. Sexual intercourse includes vaginal, oral, or rectal penetration (or attempted penetration) on a nonassaultive basis. Without detection and intervention, molestation not uncommonly progresses ultimately to full sexual intercourse. Less than 10% of sexual abuse is assaultive, forced intercourse (family-related rape).

Children are subject to more sexual abuse by family members or caretakers, whereas adolescents are at higher risk for abuse from strangers. Those children living in single-parent homes, with stepparents, or in homes of substance abusers may be at higher risk for abuse.

Most incest involves fathers and daughters. Sexual relationships usually begin gradually and without any violence. The father brings to the relationship a need for sexual gratification, and the daughter brings a need for tender affection and

---

Collecting Forensic Specimens in Sexual Abuse

Obtain 2–3 swabbed specimens from each body area assaulted (for sperm, acid phosphatase, P30, mouse antihuman semen -5[mhs-5] antigen, blood group antigen determinates). Need to be air dried.

Mouth: swab under tongue and at buccal pouch next to upper and over molars.

Vagina: Dry or moistened swab or 2cc saline wash. Overdilution of secretions may give rise to false (-) results for acid phosphatase.

Rectum: Insert swab at least 0.5–1 inch beyond anus.

Specimens should be taken from any other suspicious site in the body or clothing. Saline or sterile water-moistened swab may be used to lift any stains suspected to be dried seminal fluid.

Some forensic labs request that a dry smear be made from the vaginal sample.

Collect a saliva specimen to determine the victims antigen secretor status. Saliva may be collected using 3 or 4 sterile swabs on a 2 × 2" gauze pad placed in mouth.

Obtain a venous blood sample from victim for antigen secretor status.

Save torn, bloody or any clothing suspected to be semen stained (including tampons, pads or diapers). These items should not be packaged in plastic bags. Sealed plastic bags will promote growth of Candida and other organisms which might destroy some evidence.

Samples of combed pubic hair or scalp hair and finger nails are sometimes taken and may be used to help identify the perpetrator.

DeJong AR, Finkel MA. Sexual abuse of children. Curr Probl Pediatr 1990;20:534–535

nurturance. The father is usually rigid, patriarchal, and emotionally immature. He is unlikely to engage in extramarital relationships, but he may have a tendency toward alcoholism. Mothers of these families are often chronically depressed, unavailable to their husbands because of work or illness, and often themselves the childhood victims of sexual abuse. The families are often closely knit and socially isolated.

The diagnosis of child sexual abuse is established on the history obtained from the child. The physical examination is infrequently diagnostic in the absence of a history or specific laboratory findings. Information from the child in cases of sexual abuse takes on a sense of legal importance as the child's out-of-court statements are sometimes the only evidence in the case. The statements are an exception to the hearsay rule, in many states, that statements made by physicians providing diagnostic or treatment services are admissible in court.

The initial history should be obtained from the parent or accompanying adult, separate from the child, during which time the physician will need to inquire about name(s) the child has for her genitals. The child's history should then be taken separate from and not in the presence of accompanying adult(s). This interview should be unhurried, and the interviewer should remain calm and, in particular, nonjudgmental. It is important not to presuppose guilt, since in many cases the child is unaware of any wrongdoing.

The physical examination is normal in up to 50% of sexual abuse cases. Low-power magnification (colposcopy) may be of assistance in evaluating the child's genitalia. Ideally, assessment is accomplished within 72 hours of the assault. Careful evaluation and documentation of the introitus and hymenal orifice, despite its potential variable configuration, should be documented. The box outlines how to collect forensic specimens.

Various abnormalities of the genitalia may be confused with sexual abuse. Conditions including lichen sclerosus et atrophicus, vaginal or vulvar hemangiomas, urethral caruncle, labial agglutination, perianal cellulitis, and vulvar trauma may be present. Not all genital trauma is abuse related. Suggestive patterns of abuse include bruising, presence of pinch marks, grip marks, scratches, or burn marks on the lower trunk, genitalia, thighs, or buttocks.

Antibiotic treatment prophylaxis is not necessary in chronic or asymptomatic cases. Culture results can dictate the treatment regimen. In acute cases, ceftriaxone (125 mg IM for patients weighing < 45 kg; 250 mg for patients weighing > 45 kg) and erythromycin (50 mg/kg per day for 7 days) should be offered. Tetanus toxoid also should be administered, as with any other penetrating injury.

The presence of semen, sperm, acid phosphatase, positive gonorrhea or chlamydia culture, or a positive serologic test for syphilis establishes the diagnosis of sexual abuse as a medical certainty, even in the absence of a positive history. It is imperative that child protective services be contacted with respect to any and all alleged sexual abuse.

Sexually Transmitted Diseases

Sexually transmitted infections may be present in the pediatric patient. The atrophic vagina in this age group is a good culture medium for both gonococcal vaginitis and chlamydial infection. With respect to the latter, enzyme immunoassays such as the enzyme-linked immunosorbent assay (ELISA) and the fluorescent antibody smear technique are currently useful for establishing the diagnosis. Treatment consists of 7 days of erythromycin (50 mg/kg per day in four divided doses) or sulfisoxazole for 10 days (150 mg/kg per day in four divided doses). The presence of trichomoniasis in the pediatric patient is also suggestive of child sexual abuse, and appropriate reporting to child protective services is mandatory. The risk of acquisition of human immunodeficiency virus (HIV) from sexual abuse in this age group is likely to be the largest concern of patient and family. There has been at least one case of acquired immunodeficiency syndrome (AIDS) or HIV infection closely associated with sexual abuse. Currently, screening for HIV is considered reasonable if a child gives a history of repeated abuse by multiple perpetrators or is symptomatic or if the perpetrator is known to have AIDS or is a known bisexual, homosexual, or intravenous drug abuser. If the screening test is initially negative, a repeat screen is recommended in 3–6 months after initial assessment.

ADOLESCENT GYNECOLOGY

Normal Puberty

Puberty is a transition period between childhood and the sexually mature adult. It is marked by rapid changes in somatic growth and sexual development. Profound psychologic changes accompany these developmental events. The exact mechanism responsible for the initiation and timing of pubertal events remains unclear. It probably results from a reactivation of an intact hypothalamic–pituitary–ovarian axis, rather than immaturity of the system. Genetic and environmental influences other than those affecting body weight contribute to the differential timing of these pubertal events.

Hormonal Events

There is substantial evidence that the hypothalamic–pituitary–ovarian axis is operative as early as fetal life. Gonadotropin-releasing hormone production from the arcuate nucleus (pulse generator) stimulates gonadotropin secretion beginning around 10–13 weeks, and production of FSH and LH is maximal at midgestation, the time at which the hypothalamic nuclei and hypophysial–portal system are complete. During the remainder of pregnancy gonadotropin levels decrease due to negative feedback of ovarian sex steroid production. After delivery, with the loss of negative feedback of sex steroids, gonadotropin levels rise again, and fall to low levels by age 1–2 years. Gonadotropin levels remain low throughout childhood but rise again around the time of puberty. Gonadotropin-releasing hormone pulses manifest initially as nocturnal LH pulses, which eventually occur throughout the daytime as well. With the establishment of pulsatile gonadotropin secretion, gonadal production of estrogen occurs, resulting in somatic growth and the development of secondary sexual characteristics.

If exogenous GnRH is administered to the prepubertal female, plasma levels of FSH are greater than LH, but during puberty, LH levels exceed FSH. Agonadal females have the same temporal specific qualitative pattern of gonadotropins as eugonadal individuals. This suggests that the negative feedback of estrogen must not be required to shut down the hypothalamic–pituitary–gonadal axis, since agonadal individuals are unable to produce ovarian estrogen.

The pituitary secretion of an adrenal androgen-releasing hormone is associated with a significant rise in the adrenal androgen dehydroepiandrosterone sulfate (DHEAS), beginning about age 6–8 years. Levels of DHEAS continue to rise through the teenaged years, then gradually decrease with age. It is unlikely that the adrenal gland is necessary for the initiation of puberty, since patients with primary adrenal insufficiency have no adrenarche, but they do undergo gonadarche.

Onset

Children have been maturing earlier in North America, Europe, and Japan over the past century. Improved living standards and antenatal and postnatal nutrition have resulted in taller, heavier children who mature earlier. This trend of decreasing menarche has slowed over the past 20 years and now has plateaued. High altitude, strenuous exercise, poor nutrition, chronic disease, and severe obesity may delay the onset of puberty, while moderate obesity may be associated with earlier puberty. A relationship of the critical body mass to the onset of menarche has been postulated but remains controversial.

When environmental factors are optimal, puberty is chiefly controlled by genetic factors. The average interval between the times of menarche in identical twins is 2.2 months, whereas in dizygotic twins it is 8.2 months.

Normal Timing and Pattern

The typical sequence of events of puberty includes thelarche, adrenarche, growth spurt, and finally menarche.

Thelarche. The first sign of puberty is usually the development of the breasts. Breast budding usually occurs between 9 and 11 years of age. This sign indicates the competency of the hypothalamic–pituitary–ovarian axis. Shortly thereafter, estrogen induces vaginal changes. The pH becomes acidic and more suitable for Döderlein bacilli, which increase in number just before menarche. Breast development progresses through Tanner stage 5 (adult contour) usually within 3–3.5 years after the onset of thelarche.

Adrenarche. The second event is represented by adrenarche, the development of pubic hair. It usually occurs shortly after thelarche, between 11 and 12 years of age. It is accompanied by increasing serum levels of DHEAS. Adrenarche shows that the hypothalamic–pituitary–adrenal androgen axis is intact. Axillary hair usually does not appear until the growth of pubic hair is complete. Absence of axillary hair can be familial.

Growth Spurt. At about physiologic age 12 years, a growth spurt, expressed as growth velocity in centimeters per year, occurs. In normal puberty, GH continues to be secreted at the childhood rate and is responsible for continuing the preadolescent velocity of 4 cm/y. Steroids superimpose on this an additional increment of 5 cm/y at the peak of the curve. This maximum value of 9 cm/y, usually referred to as peak height velocity, constitutes a very helpful landmark in evaluating somatic growth. Current evidence suggests that estrogen stimulates the secretion of GH, which in turn increases the production of IGF-I or somatomedin C. Insulinlike growth factor I appears to be an important mediator of the pubertal growth process.

Menarche. Menarche occurs at an average of 2.5 years after thelarche, at an average age of 12.8 years for U.S. girls, when growth deceleration is advanced and breast development is almost complete. The relationship between growth spurt and menarche is constant, and the average increment in linear growth after menarche is about 5 cm. Initial menstrual cycles are usually anovulatory. This period of adolescent sterility can last 12–18 months after menarche and is a normal physiologic variation. Ovulation signals the maturation of estrogen's positive feedback upon gonadotropin secretion.

Relationship Between Skeletal Maturation and Sexual Maturation. Attempts have been made to correlate the ossification and subsequent fusion of certain epiphyses with landmarks in developmental growth. In the absence of sex steroids, the skeletal age of the hand and wrist remains about 12–13 years. In the presence of sex hormones, skeletal maturation progresses beyond 13 years, leading to complete fusion of all epiphyses of the hand and wrist. The iliac epiphysis ossifies over the crest of ilium in a lateral-to-medial direction. An iliac epiphysis usually indicates that ovarian steroids have been released. Complete fusion of the iliac epiphysis to the crest of the ilium occurs only at age 21–23 years.

Normal Variations in Pubertal Development

Breast development may normally occur as early as 8 years of age. Consequently, the borderline between physiologic premature thelarche and pathologic prematurity is arbitrarily set at 8 years. The interval from the appearance of the breast buds to full breast maturation is usually about 3–3.5 years, but it varies from 1.5 years to more than 6 years. Asymmetric thelarche as a physiologic variant is not uncommon and should not be interpreted as a potential unilateral breast tumor.

Adrenarche may precede thelarche in 10–15% of females. Pubic hair development to full maturity usually occurs over 3–4 years.

The peak growth velocity of 41 girls in one study averaged 9 cm/y. The average age at which the peak is reached occurs at about 12.0 years in girls, with a standard deviation of about 0.9 years. The height spurt is more an acceleration in length of the trunk.

The normal range of menarche in young girls in the United States is 5 years, from 10.5 to 15.5 years, with a mean of 12.8 years.

Delayed Puberty and Primary Amenorrhea

Etiologies for delayed puberty and primary amenorrhea may be divided into hypogonadal and eugonadal categories. Patients with hypogonadism may have hypergonadotropism secondary to ovarian failure or hypogonadotropism with abnormalities affecting hypothalamic and pituitary pubertal maturation. The eugonadal category is composed of patients with clinical evidence of steroidogenesis but delayed menarche. This latter group frequently has obstruction or developmental failure of the female müllerian system. Less common eugonadal etiologies include pituitary prolactinoma, androgen insensitivity syndrome, and failure of the development of a mature positive feedback system with cyclic LH.

Hypogonadism

Hypergonadotropic hypogonadism represents the single largest cause of delayed puberty (40%). The etiology of the ovarian failure is usually some privation or deletion of X chromosome material (eg, 45,X; 46,X; del X). However, other patients with ovarian failure and sexual infantilism may have normal 46,XX and rarely 46,XY karyotypes (Swyer syndrome).

Abnormal Sex Chromosome Group (Chromosomally Incompetent Ovarian Failure). When ascertained at puberty, mosaic forms containing a 45,X cell line in association with either a 46,XX cell line (structurally normal or abnormal X) or a 46,XY cell line are the most common genotypes. The use of high-resolution chromosome-banding techniques in conjunction with DNA probes (molecular cytogenetics) has helped to better characterize the morphologically abnormal X and Y chromosomes identified in these hypergonadotropic individuals. The latter is the principal clinical concern, since the presence of Y chromosomal material is associated with a relatively high incidence (20%) of dysgenetic gonadal tumors in such individuals (dysgerminoma, gonadoblastoma).

Southern blotting with Y chromosome–specific DNA probes or the amplification of target sequences that are Y chromosome–specific using the PCR technique allows the identification of covert Y chromosome DNA in 45,X subjects or when a putative Y chromosomal fragment is suspected. The presence of Y chromosomal material in this situation mandates removal of the dysgenetic gonads. Use of DNA probes for the X chromosome combined with PCR or PCR alone may be important in the characterization of small deletions or point mutations of the X chromosome that are not detectable by chromosome-banding techniques. Use of DNA technology may also better define sex-determining genes and statural determinants on the sex chromosomes.

Normal Sex Chromosome Group (Chromosomally Competent Ovarian Failure). This group represents normal 46,XX ovarian failure, but occasionally chromosomally competent 46,XY (Swyer syndrome) may be diagnosed.

The etiologies of the 46,XX hypergonadotropic group are as follows:

- Single gene, autosomal recessive (familial gonadal dysgenesis)
- Environmental factors in utero or during childhood (eg, viral)
- Neoplastic therapy (radiation therapy/chemotherapy)
- Autoimmune disorders with or without a polyglandular immunopathy
- Galactosemia
- Associated genetic disorders such as ataxia telangiectasia and myotonia dystrophica
- 17α-Hydroxylase deficiency

In Savage syndrome, some ovarian follicles are present, but they are resistant to gonadotropin stimulation. The etiology is not clear, but it is thought to be a gonadotropin receptor defect. A clear clinical phenotype and specific inactivating mutations in the gonadotropin receptors (FSH, LH) need to be identified before Savage syndrome can be established as a defined clinical entity.

It is possible that abnormal gonadotropins or abnormal gonadotropin receptors may be responsible for some forms of 46,XX ovarian failure. A mutation in the beta subunit of LH leading to testicular failure has recently been described. The etiology of sporadic 46,XY Swyer syndrome appears to be mutations in the sex-related gene (*SRY*) on Yp that interfere with gene activation and testicular development. Familial Swyer syndrome is problematic, but it is probably due to a second gene in the cascade of testicular development that is located on the X chromosomes. Mutations in this gene, which may be the target of the *SRY* protein, interrupts testicular development and leads to a Swyer phenotype.

Hypogonadotropic hypogonadism is due to the temporary or permanent inability to secrete GnRH. Such patients have low or low-normal pituitary gonadotropins. Multiple diverse etiologies are present within this group and may be responsible for delaying or interrupting the normal pattern of pubertal maturation within the hypothalamus and pituitary:

- Physiologic delay (reversible)
- Systemic disease processes (sustained malnutrition)
  — Gastrointestinal malabsorption
  — Anorexia nervosa
  — Exercise
- Endocrine disease processes
  — Primary hypothyroidism
  — Cushing disease or syndrome
- Irreversible hypothalamic–pituitary etiologies
  — Isolated GnRH deficiency with or without anosmia (Kallmann syndrome)
  — Pituitary insufficiency
  — Pituitary tumors (eg, craniopharyngioma, prolactinoma)

Computed axial tomographic scanning or magnetic resonance imaging with and without contrast media, coupled with serum prolactin determinations, can help diagnose early pituitary tumors in this age group.

A new ultrasensitive immunoradiometric assay for TSH allows better discrimination between low and normal values, which is useful in the diagnosis of pituitary and hypothalamic hypothyroidism. Thyrotropin-releasing hormone stimulation tests are useful in the detection of subclinical primary hypothyroidism.

Anorexia nervosa and milder variants are becoming more frequent. The psychiatric aspects remain a special challenge.

The differential diagnosis of irreversible gonadotropin failure and physiologic delay remains difficult. Pooled urine gonadotropin measurements may distinguish the two, but sequential measurements are necessary to identify the gradual gonadotropin rise in patients with physiologic delay. Identifying a normal pubertal pattern of gonadotropin release in response to GnRH may aid in the diagnosis of physiologic delay. Deletions in the GnRH gene have been identified in the mouse, but none have been identified to date in humans. However, deletions of the Kallmann gene (*KALIG-I*) on Xp have been identified in some subjects with X-linked forms of Kallmann syndrome. This gene appears to encode a cell adhesion protein that facilitates the migration of the GnRH neurons from the medial olfactory placode to the hypothalamus.

Eugonadism

The most common anatomic genital abnormality associated with delayed menarche is congenital absence of the uterus and vagina (Mayer–Rokitansky–Küster–Hauser syndrome). Less frequently, patients have functional but obstructed genital tracts, including transverse vaginal septum and imperforate hymen.

The eugonadal patient with complete androgen insensitivity syndrome has evidence of steroid production. The lack of pubic hair and normal breast development identifies these individuals who have 46,XY karyotypes, testes, and receptor defects for androgens. Their hairlessness and male levels of testosterone differentiate them from those with the Mayer–Rokitansky–Küster–Hauser syndrome. Associated urinary tract abnormalities in the latter group should be excluded by ultrasonography or intravenous pyelography. Deletions and point mutations have now been identified in the androgen receptor gene on Xq in some patients with complete androgen insensitivity syndrome.

The last patients in the eugonadal group are individuals who exhibit pubertal maturation but who never develop a mature positive feedback system for establishing LH surges and ovulation. These patients with chronic anovulation (recycling failure) are at risk for endometrial hyperplasia if tonic LH and unopposed estrogen production continue. Their workup should always include a serum prolactin measurement.

Diagnosis

Age 13 is 2.5 standard deviations from the mean for thelarche. Total absence of breast development and estrogen effects at age 13 requires some preliminary investigation. In addition to a careful general physical examination, the following should be obtained:

- Serum FSH and LH measurements
- Posteroanterior and lateral skull X-ray films
- Thyroxine (T_4), triiodothyronine (T_3) resin uptake; TSH measurement
- Prolactin measurement

An elevation in serum FSH level should be followed up by cytogenetic evaluation. Undetectable or low serum gonadotropin levels necessitate finer scrutiny for pituitary tumors with computed tomography or magnetic resonance imaging. Determination of bone age may be helpful in selected cases, since it correlates better with sexual development than does chronologic age.

Menarcheal delay accompanied by normal sexual and somatic growth requires a careful pelvic examination to exclude anatomic etiologies. This examination should be assisted by pelvic ultrasonography and intravenous pyelography. Cytogenetic studies are indicated if complete androgen insensitivity syndrome is a diagnostic consideration.

BIBLIOGRAPHY

Pediatric Problems

Bacon JL. Pediatric vulvovaginitis. Adolesc Pediatr Gynecol 1989; 2:86–93

Clark JA, Muller SA. Lichen sclerosus et atrophicus in children: a report of 24 cases. Arch Dermatol 1967;95:476–482

Muram D. Child sexual abuse—genital tract findings in prepubertal girls, I: the unaided medical examination. Am J Obstet Gynecol 1989; 160:328–333.

Muram D. Child sexual abuse: relationship between sexual acts and genital findings. Child Abuse Negl 1989;13:211–216

Paradise JE, Willis ED. Probability of vaginal body in girls with genital complaints. Am J Dis Child 1985;139:472–476

Rimsza ME, Niggeman MS. Medical evaluation of sexually abused children: a review of 311 cases. Pediatrics 1982;69:8–14

Simmons PS. Office pediatric gynecology. Prim Care 1988;15:617–628

Tilelli JA, Turek D, Jaffe AC. Sexual abuse of children: clinical findings and implications for management. N Engl J Med 1980;302:319–323

Williams TS, Callen JP, Owen LG. Vulvar disorders in the prepubertal female. Pediatr Ann 1986;15:588–589; 592–601; 604–605

Adolescent Gynecology

Bick D, Franco B, Sherins RJ, Heye B, Pike L, Crawford J, et al. Brief report: intragenic deletion of the KALIG-1 gene in Kallmann's syndrome. N Engl J Med 1992;326:1752–1755

Hardelin JP, Levilliers J, del Castillo I, Cohen-Salmon M, Legouis R, Blanchard S, et al. X chromosome-linked Kallmann syndrome: stop mutations validate the candidate gene. Proc Natl Acad Sci U S A 1992;89:8190–8194

Lee PA. Neuroendocrinology of puberty. Semin Reprod Endocrinol 1988;6:13–20

McDonough PG, Tho SP, Trill JJ, Byrd JR, Reindollar RH, Tischfield JA. Use of two different deoxyribonucleic acid probes to detect Y chromosome deoxyribonucleic acid in subjects with normal and altered Y chromosomes. Am J Obstet Gynecol 1986;154:737–748

Reindollar RH, Byrd JR, McDonough PG. Delayed sexual development: a study of 252 patients. Am J Obstet Gynecol 1981;140:371–380

Reindollar RH, Su BCJ, Tho SPT. Molecular biology: applications for pediatric and adolescent gynecology. Semin Reprod Endocrinol 1988;6:1–11

Tho SP, Behzadian A, Byrd JR, McDonough PG. Use of human alpha-satellite deoxyribonucleic acid to detect Y-specific centromeric sequences. Am J Obstet Gynecol 1988;159:1553–1557

Wilson DM, Rosenfeld RG. Treatment of short stature and delayed adolescence. Pediatr Clin North Am 1987;34:865–880

Disorders of Menstruation

SECONDARY AMENORRHEA

Secondary amenorrhea can result from dysfunction of the central nervous system, pituitary gland, thyroid or adrenal gland, ovary, or uterus or from a disorder of peripheral metabolism (see box). The most common cause of secondary amenorrhea is the development of chronic hypothalamic anovulation. This can be induced by stress, increased exercise level, a precipitous decrease in body weight, or the development of an inappropriate lean body mass–fat ratio. Once pregnancy is ruled out, patients are found to have normal gonadotropin levels with an appropriate LH:FSH ratio and show withdrawal bleeding after progestogen challenge. Any of these states carried to the extreme form, however, will result in hypothalamic amenorrhea with a fall in LH and FSH levels, an inversion of the LH:FSH ratio, and failure to respond to progestogen challenge. Other conditions may mimic these findings, including systemic illness, which generally presents as hypogonadotropism; head trauma; space-occupying lesions of the central nervous system of all types; and the intake of numerous pharmaceutical agents, most notably minor tranquilizers, monoamine oxidase inhibitors, and drugs that alter serotonin metabolism. Unusual space-occupying lesions such as fibromas from neurofibromatosis, infiltrative disorders such as histiocytosis X, and disorders such as syphilis and tuberculosis, which can form granulomas, also result in amenorrhea. Rare causes of amenorrhea include its association with temporal arteritis or cavernous sinus thrombosis.

Pituitary dysfunction can likewise result in secondary amenorrhea. Perhaps the most common cause is functional hypoprolactinemia, which is thought by many investigators to represent a disorder of central dopamine metabolism, or the presence of prolactinomas. Likewise, secondary amenorrhea can occur after resection of prolactinomas or other tumors or in association with infarction of the pituitary gland (Sheehan syndrome). In the former state, hyperprolactinemia is diagnosed by elevated prolactin levels on multiple occasions and hypopituitarism by the findings of low gonadotropin levels. Hypothalamic dysfunction can be differentiated from pituitary disorder by the use of GnRH injection following priming.

Hypothyroidism can at times result in menstrual dysfunction and may or may not be associated with hyperprolactinemia. The patient with hypothyroidism may present with dry skin, lethargy, and constipation. Frequently, the T_4 level will be normal, whereas the TSH level will be markedly elevated. At times, secondary hypothyroidism will be detected with a low T_4 level and a low TSH level. All of these conditions are treated with replacement thyroid hormones.

Disorders of adrenal metabolism likewise can result in the development of secondary amenorrhea. Dehydroepiandrosterone sulfate levels may be mildly elevated in patients with polycystic ovary syndrome (PCO) or variance of congenital adrenal hyperplasia; they may be markedly elevated and associated with virilism in patients with adrenal adenomas and other tumors. One will find hyperadrenalism in the form of Cushing syndrome. This may be ACTH dependent or independent and is best evaluated with a 24-hour urinary free cortisol associated with the creatinine.

Obesity is associated with the development of menstrual dysfunction; however, it may not be associated with PCO. The

---

Causes of Secondary Amenorrhea

Central Nervous System
Trauma
Tumors
Infiltrative disease
Granulomas
Neurofibrosis
Stress
Weight loss
Exercise
Systemic illness

Pituitary
Prolactinomas
Functional hyperprolactinemia
Other tumors
Infarction (Sheehan syndrome)
Surgery
Stalk transection

Thyroid
Hypothyroidism
Hyperthyroidism

Adrenal
Tumor
Cushing syndrome
Late-onset adrenal hyperplasia

Ovary
Premature ovarian failure (immune)
Surgical removal of ovaries
Polycystic ovary syndrome
Hyperthecosis
Other tumors

Uterus
Asherman syndrome
Endometrial ablation

relationship between excess body fat and ovulatory dysfunction appears to be stronger for early-onset obesity. Correction of ovulatory function can be achieved approximately 68% of the time with normalization of body weight.

The ovary is one of the most common sites of the development of ovulatory dysfunction. This may result from elevated androgen secretion in patients with PCO, hyperthecosis, or tumors. Patients with PCO will present with an elevated LH:FSH ratio 40% of the time, elevated DHEAS level 50% of the time, elevated prolactin level 20% of the time, an upper limit of normal total testosterone, elevated level of free testosterone, and decreased level of sex hormone–binding globulin. These patients respond to progestogen challenge and can be managed with oral contraceptive agents or clomiphene citrate if pregnancy is desired.

Premature ovarian failure (ie, cessation of menses before age 35) may be of hereditary, autoimmune, or unknown etiology. The diagnosis is usually made by finding FSH levels greater than 40 mIU/ml in association with amenorrhea or oligoovulation. These patients are best treated with replacement estrogen/progestogen therapy.

Although not frequently recognized as an ovarian cause of secondary amenorrhea, surgery, either wedge resection or resection of endometriomas, can result in ovulatory dysfunction and premature menopause. Like patients with premature ovarian failure, these individuals will have an FSH level in the range of 25–40 mIU/ml.

Finally, disorders of the endometrium are an uncommon cause of secondary amenorrhea. Uterine synechiae may be of the unintentional or intentional (endometrial ablation) type. Asherman syndrome is associated with uterine trauma, either secondary to the presence of an infected IUD, infected spontaneous abortion, or dilation and curettage (D&C). Diagnostic findings include normal gonadotropin and estrogen levels and deformity of the uterine cavity when evaluated by hysterosalpingography. The condition is treated surgically, followed by estrogen priming of the endometrium.

Although not commonly thought of as a cause of amenorrhea, numerous drugs can produce atrophy of the endometrium either primarily or secondarily. Oral contraceptive agents, with their predominance of progestogens, will frequently result in amenorrhea. Administration of depot medroxyprogesterone acetate suppresses endometrial growth directly and indirectly through the central axis, as does danazol. Finally, GnRH analogues that block estrogen production through central mechanisms will result in amenorrhea.

The workup of the patient with secondary amenorrhea consists of a careful history and physical examination with attention being paid to head trauma, intake of medication, headaches, energy level, hirsutism, body weight, and history of previous surgery. Laboratory investigation should include LH, FSH, prolactin and TSH levels. If there are signs of androgen excess, 17-hydroxyprogesterone, DHEAS, and testosterone levels should be determined. If signs or symptoms of central nervous system, adrenal, or ovarian tumors are detected, computed tomography or magnetic resonance imaging scan or ultrasonography should be carried out. Therapy is directed at correcting the specific abnormality, and often the choice of therapy will depend on whether or not the patient wishes to become pregnant. Frequent forms of therapy instituted include oral contraceptive agents or replacement hormonal therapy with estrogen/progestogens or induction of ovulation with clomiphene citrate, gonadotropins, or dopamine agonists in the case of patients with hyperprolactinemia.

Hyperprolactinemia

Patients with hyperprolactinemia will generally present with ovulatory dysfunction, galactorrhea, delayed pubescence, or signs of a polyendocrinopathy. The four primary causes of hyperprolactinemia are pituitary hyperplasia, which is the result of dopamine dysfunction; prolactinomas, which are categorized as microadenomas (less than 10 mm in size) or macroadenomas (greater than 10 mm in size); hypothyroidism; and drug intake (see box). There are numerous other causes of hyperprolactinemia, as indicated in the box.

The workup of the patient with hyperprolactinemia should consist of the measurement of prolactin levels on multiple occasions. Since prolactin is a dynamic hormone affected by stress, breast examination, exercise, and sleep, it is suggested the samples be drawn in the late morning, at least 1 hour away from meals, or in the early afternoon. Repeated determinations are strongly recommended, because not only is prolactin a dynamic hormone, the accurate measurement of prolactin is very difficult. In addition to the measurement of prolactin, it is suggested that the T_4 level, TSH level, or high-sensitivity

---

Causes of Hyperprolactinemia

Central Nervous System
Trauma
Tumors and cysts (all types)
Infections
Neurofibromas
Granulomas (tuberculosis and syphilis)
Infiltrative disease (histiocytosis X)
Cavernous sinus thrombosis
Temporal arteritis

Pituitary
Trauma
Tumor
Prolactinomas
Functional disease

Thyroid
Hypothyroidism

Body
Chest trauma, surgery, or burn
Herpes zoster
Breast manipulation
Renal failure
Hysterectomy/oophorectomy
Breast reduction or augmentation
Pregnancy

Drugs (Examples)
Tranquilizers, major and minor
Antidepressants
Steroid hormones
Oral contraceptives
Antihypertensives
H_2 receptor antagonists
Antituberculins

TSH level be determined to rule out compensated hypothyroidism. If signs of polyendocrinopathy are present, the GH or ACTH level should be measured. The use of dynamic pituitary challenge test is of historic interest only; it is used only to evaluate patients who have undergone hypophysectomy.

The use of visual field examinations is to be discouraged except in patients with macroadenomas. Microadenomas do not produce chiasmatic suppression, and patients who have macroadenomas will present with superior bitemporal hemianopsia only 68% of the time. Radiographic imaging is generally restricted to either computed tomography scanning or magnetic resonance image scanning. Each of these techniques is capable of detecting tumors approximately 2 mm in size, and there is a considerable discrepancy in cost of the two techniques. While it is true that magnetic resonance imaging technology will yield the clearest image, computed tomography scanning is perfectly adequate to differentiate a microadenoma from a macroadenoma.

The treatment of the patient with hyperprolactinemia hinges on several factors: 1) symptoms, 2) the desire for pregnancy, 3) whether the patient has a microadenoma or a macroadenoma, and 4) whether the patient is hypoestrogenic. Hypothyroidism, when treated with replacement therapy, will resolve the hyperprolactinemia. Those patients taking medication that induces hyperprolactinemia could have the medication discontinued if symptoms warrant such a move. Those individuals with functional hyperprolactinemia who have slightly elevated prolactin levels and withdrawal bleeding after progestogen challenge could be treated with progestogens, an oral contraceptive agent, or with a dopamine agonist. Patients often have side effects such as nausea with dopamine agonist intake, and it is suggested that the medication be begun at a 1.25-mg dose level at bedtime and increased slowly over the next few weeks. In addition, the vaginal administration of dopamine agonists will at times produce sustained levels of the drug and minimize side effects.

Patients with a microadenoma may be treated with oral contraceptive agents, replacement estrogen/progestogen therapy, dopamine agonists, or transsphenoidal hypophysectomy. Unfortunately, surgery results in a failure to cure the underlying endocrine disorder 50–75% of the time, although tumor recurrence is uncommon. It is strongly suggested that patients who are hypoestrogenic secondary to hyperprolactinemia be given replacement estrogen therapy or have their prolactin levels normalized, as at least four studies in the literature demonstrate that this is associated with increased bone loss. Bone loss is shown to be reversible by the administration of dopamine agonists.

Finally, patients with a macroadenoma deserve special comment. These patients in general are managed with a dopamine agonist throughout their lifetimes. Lesions that do not respond to dopamine agonist are best treated with either surgical or radiation therapy. Unfortunately, transsphenoidal hypophysectomy results in a 70% failure rate to cure either the tumor or the underlying endocrine disorder. Dopamine agonists, while not being directly tumorcidal, will oftentimes result in the long-term remission of hyperprolactinemia.

The patient who desires pregnancy and is hyperprolactinemic is best treated with a dopamine agonist in increasing doses until prolactin levels become normal. The vast majority of these patients will have a normalization of their menstrual function and achieve pregnancy in a rather short time. Once pregnancy is achieved, medication should be discontinued in those patients with functional hyperprolactinemia or microadenomas. Those individuals with macroadenomas may be either treated with dopamine agonist throughout pregnancy or followed expectantly with visual field examinations every 2 months. The use of empirical dopamine agonist therapy in the patient with euprolactinemia is to be discouraged, as well-controlled studies have not shown a beneficial effect.

Finally, the natural history of prolactinomas is unclear. At this juncture it is recommended that women entering menopause who have functional hyperprolactinemia or microadenomas be treated with conventional estrogen/progestogen replacement therapy. Those women with macroadenomas may be candidates for replacement therapy either with or without concomitant dopamine agonist administration and should be monitored by a reproductive endocrinologist or a neurosurgeon with a special interest in hyperprolactinemia.

Anorexia Nervosa

Anorexia nervosa is generally seen in white females under age 25 and is a syndrome that includes a history of weight loss, amenorrhea, and behavioral changes. This classic triad usually occurs together, although any one symptom may precede another. While the incidence of this problem has been reported as being 1/200–1/100 in white girls 12–18 years of age, there appears to be an at-risk population.

One study has shown that two thirds of a sample of adolescent girls showed at least one symptom of disturbed eating behavior during adolescence, prior to entering college, and that early physical maturation presents a definite risk factor. Professional ballet dancers, for example, have an incidence ranging from 1/20–1/5, depending on the competitive level of the company from which the survey originated. Many consider weight loss-related amenorrhea an early form of the disorder; the reasons for the progression of the illness to the syndrome of anorexia nervosa, a condition accompanied by severe psychologic changes, are unknown at present. This disorder may also progress to bulimia, a condition in which the patient may gorge and attempt to rid herself of calories by artificial means, such as vomiting or using laxatives or diuretics.

The psychologic and behavioral changes include a distorted body image so that the patient believes she is too fat, even though she may be emaciated. There is also a severe preoccupation with food, with aversions to food that is high in caloric content, and large intakes of diet soda and raw vegetables. The patient may become hyperactive and indulge in strenuous running, biking, or exercise classes. Fear of gaining weight becomes an all-consuming obsession.

A variety of physical changes occurs, and it is generally thought that the signs and symptoms of anorexia nervosa result from a physical and metabolic adaptation to semistarvation. Laboratory findings may include severe leukopenia, with relative lymphocytosis and hypercarotenemia. With the last sign, the skin may take on a yellowish hue. Analysis of electrolytes may reveal metabolic alkalosis, hypokalemia, and mild azotemia if the patient has developed bulimia.

Endocrine changes include deficient secretion of both LH and FSH. There is a particularly striking deficiency of LH secretion from the anterior pituitary. Investigation of the 24-hour secretion of LH reveals a lack of the normal episodic variation and, in some cases, a reversion to a prepubertal low pattern of secretion over a 24-hour period. Nocturnal spurting of LH, a pattern usually observed only in early puberty, also occurs. Gonadotropin secretion can be restored to a normal, adultlike pattern by the pulsatile administration of GnRH. These findings suggest that the amenorrhea seen in association with anorexia nervosa is probably due to faulty signals to the medial central hypothalamus from the arcuate nucleus, the center most likely responsible for the important episodic stimulation of GnRH.

Recent studies suggest activation of the hypothalamic–pituitary–adrenal pathways in patients with anorexia nervosa. The cortisol level is elevated, the response to ACTH-releasing hormone is abnormal, and the ACTH-releasing hormone level is increased in the cerebrospinal fluid. Corticotropin-releasing hormone is known to suppress LH pulses both in humans and animals and may augment dopaminergic and opiodergic inhibition of GnRH.

A number of other abnormalities observed in patients with anorexia nervosa suggest hypothalamic dysfunction. For example, the deficiency in the handling of a water load, which is thought to result from a mild diabetes insipidus; abnormal thermoregulatory responses on exposure to temperature extremes; and a lack of shivering are all controlled by mechanisms that probably involve hypothalamic pathways. All of these alterations seem to represent a syndrome that is too diffuse to be anything but metabolic and are primarily due to starvation. The lowered T_3 levels and, in some cases, the low T_4 levels that have been reported are probably also related to the starvation syndrome and represent a metabolic adaptation.

The management of anorexia nervosa is still a subject of wide debate. All therapeutic modalities are geared toward the attainment of normal weight. Treatment includes various combinations of psychotherapy (including family therapy), psychoanalysis, and, occasionally, drug therapy. Tricyclic antidepressants, cyproheptadine levodopa, and metoclopramide have all been used with variable success. Behavior modification has been used with some success, although opinions on its efficacy vary. Despite impressive studies on the cause and psychogenesis of anorexia nervosa, however, few specific or new therapeutic modalities are available.

Emphasis has been placed on early diagnosis and recognition of anorectic behavior so that the patient may be treated before the full-blown syndrome is established. Since amenorrhea is an early part of the disease process, it is usually the first symptom for which the patient seeks help. Gynecologists, therefore, should be particularly attentive to a history of dieting and weight loss in their young patients. Treatment of anorexia nervosa will depend on the amount of weight loss. Generally, patients weighing less than 75% of ideal weight need aggressive intervention. The extent of the electrolyte abnormalities and the presence of other problems such as diuretic, laxative, or substance abuse and the presence of immediate life-threatening medical complications should also be considered.

This evaluation is usually best done in a hospital by a team with expertise in anorexia, consisting of psychiatrists or psychologists, internists or pediatricians, and a nutritionist. The resumption of normal menses is dependent on a return to normal weight. Follow-up over a 10-year period shows that amenorrhea persists in 49% of patients but only in 11% (2 of 19) who have a normalization of weight. The LH response to GnRH may be a good predictor of outcome. Preoccupation with food and persistent dieting are not uncommon in weight-recovered patients. Recent evidence indicates that a large exercise load may compound the effects of the low body weight, and patients with recovered anorexia may need to weigh even more if they continue to be highly active.

A leading complication of amenorrhea seen with anorexia and weight loss is the loss of bone mineral content and bone density present in spinal, radial, and femoral sites and fractures. Longitudinal studies of bone density show little or no reversal with resolution of the amenorrhea. Increased cortisol levels, as well as hypoestrogenism, seen in anorexia has been suggested as a mechanism for the osteopenia.

For those patients who recover from anorexia nervosa but never menstruate again, estrogen replacement is definitely indicated to circumvent the specter of premature osteoporosis, which may result in stress fractures and collapse of the femoral neck. The effectiveness of long-term estrogen replacement is still unknown. Unfortunately, many patients who remain underweight refuse estrogen therapy because of their continuing anxiety about gaining weight. Thus, the treatment of anorexia nervosa remains a major therapeutic challenge that has yet to be met.

Exercise-Induced Amenorrhea

Psychoneuroendocrinology is a rapidly developing field that encompasses many disorders frequently seen by the practicing gynecologist. These disorders include chronic hypothalamic anovulation; stress-related amenorrhea; amenorrhea associated with weight loss and change in the lean body mass–fat ratio; athletic amenorrhea; and menstrual problems associated with eating disorders such as anorexia nervosa, bulimia, or bulimia and anorexia. These conditions blend in the modern gynecologic patient in that the practitioner is frequently faced with the young professional woman in a high-stress position who participates in a significant exercise program each week and maintains a body weight near the threshold at which menstrual dysfunction can develop. These individuals will frequently have low-normal gonadotropin levels and are hypoestrogenic. This can result in osteopenia, perhaps an increased incidence of stress fractures, change in status of lipoproteins, and specific forms of malnutrition.

A variety of activities can result in exercise-related amenorrhea. This can range from ballet dancing, which may delay puberty in young women; to long-distance running; to certain field events. The intensity and length of training has a direct correlation with amenorrhea, and in fact, amenorrhea has been found to vary with the type of exercise. For example, runners are much more prone to amenorrhea than swimmers, which is attributed to a difference in body composition among swimmers, who frequently have a higher fat ratio. Likewise, body bulk seems to be lower in runners than in swimmers.

It is virtually impossible to separate body weight and composition from exercise. It has been suggested that one of the events that triggers the onset of puberty is the acquisition of a body weight of 48 kg and an appropriate fat to lean mass ratio. It is known that undernutrition delays puberty. Fat to lean body weight changes from 1:5 to 1:3 and 22% fat are required for the maintenance of menstrual function. A loss of 10–15% body weight causes the cessation of menstruation. Athletic amenorrhea can occur prior to weight loss. This is reminiscent of the patient with anorexia nervosa, who often develops menstrual dysfunction prior to loss of body weight. In addition, once the anorectic woman regains body weight, she does not necessarily have the restoration of normal menstrual function. Acute interruption of exercise, namely through injury, can also result in the restoration of menstrual function without an appreciable change in body weight.

All of these alterations result in psychic stress, which inhibits GnRH release by altering the activity of the GnRH pulse regulator in the arcuate nucleus. This results in a sequence of events ranging from dysfolliculogenesis disorders, luteal phase defect, oligoovulation and anovulation to hypothalamic amenorrhea, and the attainment of a pubertallike state. Likewise, the process goes back through this series of events, as weight is gained or exercise is ceased. Furthermore, individuals who are subject to great exercise stress are influenced by the conditions set forth in the general adaption syndrome by Selye. These individuals show signs of hypercortisolism, and athletes in extreme training obliterate the 24-hour circadian rhythm of cortisol. Corticotropin-releasing factor release brings about the breakdown of proopiomelanocortin, which releases ACTH, endorphins, and other byproducts. Likewise, there are alterations in thyroid function, with significant reductions in serum T_3 and T_4 and elevations in GH, prolactin, melatonin, epinephrine, and norepinephrine.

The management of the patient with exercise-related amenorrhea is often difficult. Frequently, these women are addicted to the physical and psychic euphoria that they achieve through exercise and are determined to maintain a trim body habitus and a competitive life style. It is suggested that these women be given accurate information regarding the risks of maintaining a hypoestrogenic state and offered replacement hormonal therapy. Likewise, the use of calcium supplements and multivitamins may prove beneficial.

POLYCYSTIC OVARY SYNDROME

Polycystic ovary syndrome is clinically characterized by the pubertal onset of oligomenorrhea, oligoovulation, infertility, and usually mild hyperandrogenism. Hyperandrogenism may result from disorders of the pituitary–hypothalamus or ovaries or, possibly, from increased peripheral production of androgens. Hyperandrogenism and ovulatory dysfunction associated with PCO may be associated with peripheral insulin resistance and resulting hyperinsulinemia. Several recent studies have demonstrated insulin resistance in most, if not all, women with a clinical diagnosis of PCO, and women with hyperthecosis have high prevalence of clinical diabetes. One attractive hypothesis suggests that blood insulin may interact with ovarian receptors for IGF-I and may cause increased synthesis and release of both androstenedione and testosterone. Increased sex steroid levels may then feed back on the pituitary–hypothalamus to cause chronic anovulation and elevated blood levels of serum LH.

Some older data supported the concept of a primary disorder of ovarian estrogen synthesis, but more recent studies have shown the biosynthetic capability of ovarian tissues to be normal in patients with PCO. Infertility occurs because of anovulation or oligoovulation, and pregnancy rarely occurs unless ovulation is induced. The chronic anovulation, which permits uninterrupted estrogen stimulation, is associated with an increased incidence of endometrial hyperplasia and carcinoma.

The diagnosis of PCO is based on characteristic symptoms of menstrual disturbances, hyperandrogenism, and infertility. The serum LH level is usually above normal, while the serum FSH level is reduced or in the low-normal range. Increased LH secretion is a result of greater frequency of LH pulses, increased magnitude of LH pulses, or both. Measurement of serum DHEAS should replace measurement of urinary 17-ketosteroid as a diagnostic test. The level of DHEAS is usually normal or only slightly elevated. Levels more than 7 µg/ml suggest an adrenal disorder.

Serum testosterone levels are usually at the upper limits of normal or mildly elevated, rarely more than 200 ng/dl. Levels greater than 200 ng/dl suggest a tumor. The excess androgen results from increased direct secretion by the ovaries. There may be significant hirsutism without elevated serum testosterone levels, because there are decreased levels of sex hormone–binding globulin and, thus, an increase in unbound testosterone in women with PCO. The unbound fraction (in normal women, less than 1% of the total testosterone level) is thought to be the biologically active fraction.

There is an increasing body of evidence that women with PCO have an increased incidence of lipid abnormalities and vascular disease. A series of studies has shown that women with PCO commonly have increased levels of triglycerides and LDL cholesterol and reduced levels of high-density lipoprotein (HDL) cholesterol, a pattern consistent with atherogenesis and atherosclerosis. In a cross-sectional study, these patients were shown to have increased systolic and diastolic blood pressure and a high incidence of insulin resistance. The lipid abnormalities correlated with insulin resistance more closely than with blood androgens. Interestingly, this group of patients consistently had upper-body (male pattern) obesity with an increased hip–waist ratio. Both upper-body obesity and insulin resistance correlate strongly with cardiovascular disease.

One attractive hypothesis to explain the androgen–insulin–lipid relationship has been proposed. Hyperinsulinism, regardless of the cause, in the presence of gonadotropins, stimulates the thecal–stromal compartment of the ovary to produce androgens. These androgens not only directly affect insulin action but also increase the number and size of abdominal adipocytes, causing an increase in upper-body obesity and a further state of insulin resistance. Upper-body obesity and the associated lipid abnormalities are correlated with an increased incidence of arterial vascular disease. One case–control study clearly showed a higher prevalence of abnormal coronary arteriograms in hyperandrogenic women.

A small percentage of patients who have clinical characteristics and laboratory values consistent with PCO is found, on further evaluation, to have mild adrenal hyperplasia resulting from 21-hydroxylase deficiency. In members of some ethnic groups, there is a surprisingly high prevalence of this genetically transmitted disorder. Mild (or adult form) 21-hydroxylase deficiency is linked to the human leukocyte antigen (HLA) on chromosome 6. In one study, the prevalence of the disease in Ashkenazi Jews was 3.78%; in Hispanics, 1.9%; in Yugoslavs, 1.6%; and in a diverse Caucasian population, only 0.1%.

The disorder is identified by means of an ACTH stimulation test. Synthetic ACTH (cosyntropin, 0.25 mg) is administered as an intravenous bolus. Serum 17α-hydroxyprogesterone is measured before and 30 minutes after injection. Patients with normal adrenal function rarely have 17α-hydroxyprogesterone levels of greater than 200 ng/dl at 30 minutes, whereas those with 21-hydroxylase deficiency usually have levels that exceed 2,000 ng/dl. A more convenient screening procedure is measurement of serum 17α-hydroxyprogesterone at 8 AM. A morning serum 17α-hydroxyprogesterone level of greater than 2–3 ng/ml necessitates a stimulation test. It is clinically worthwhile to make this distinction, because patients with mild congenital adrenal hyperplasia who desire pregnancy may respond better to adrenal suppression than to clomiphene citrate.

Treatment of PCO is designed to alleviate symptoms and reduce the probability of uterine malignancy and vascular disease. For women who do not desire pregnancy and do not have excess hair growth, the cyclic administration of a progestational agent should be used to induce withdrawal bleeding. Medroxyprogesterone acetate, 10 mg/d for 10 days each month, usually prevents the development of endometrial hyperplasia.

Mild hirsutism is adequately controlled in most young women by the administration of a low-dose oral contraceptive. Patients who have more severe hirsutism or an absolute or relative contraindication for oral contraceptives may be treated with spironolactone, which inhibits the biologic effect of androgens at the cellular level. At the usual dosage, 150–200 mg twice daily, spironolactone is a remarkably safe and effective drug.

If pregnancy is desired, most patients respond to clomiphene citrate, although gonadotropins and hCG are occasionally required. Wedge resection is rarely necessary and has a high incidence of postoperative adhesive disease.

Women with PCO who do not respond to clomiphene citrate often are difficult management problems when ovulation induction with gonadotropins is attempted. When viewed with vaginal ultrasonography, the ovaries, even without stimulation, often contain numerous small follicles. When such large numbers of follicles are stimulated with gonadotropins, the risk of severe hyperstimulation syndrome is greatly increased. One is often confronted with a patient with numerous follicles of 10 mm or less in diameter and a serum estradiol level sufficiently high to make the administration of hCG inadvisable. Patients, therefore, are usually started on only one or two ampules of gonadotropins daily, and some investigators have suggested that the use of pure FSH may be desirable. Close monitoring with serum estradiol and vaginal ultrasonography is mandatory, and hCG is withheld if the serum estradiol is greater that 2,000 pg/ml.

More recently, several investigators have suggested placing 8–10 unipolar cautery burns in the ovarian capsule and cortex as therapy for anovulation not responsive to clomiphene citrate and have reported a high probability of ovulation and pregnancy. Laser drilling of the capsule appears to give the same success rate. In patients who are difficult to manage on human gonadotropins, either method seems to be a viable alternative.

Perhaps most importantly, hyperandrogenism in women can no longer be regarded only as a problem of cosmetics and infertility. The increased prevalence of arterial vascular disease requires that all possible risk factors be eliminated. Intervention should at a minimum include weight control, avoidance of smoking, limited intake of saturated fats and cholesterol, and a regular exercise program. Some women's lipid abnormalities may require drug therapy.

HIRSUTISM AND VIRILIZATION

While many women may complain of an increase in body hair, the term *hirsutism* should only be used for excessive hair involving areas that follow a male pattern of hair distribution. This generally is central or midline in distribution (eg, chin, intermammary area, and midline lower abdomen). Virilization, on the other hand, is extremely rare and should not be used interchangeably with hirsutism. Virilization includes defeminizing signs (decrease in breast size and change in female body contour) and masculinizing signs (temporal balding, increase in muscle mass, clitorimegaly, and deepening of the voice). The diameter of the clitoris should be less than 7 mm, or the cross-sectional area of its width and height should be less than 35 mm^2.

The evaluation of a woman who presents with hirsutism or virilization should be directed at pinpointing the sources of abnormal androgen production and specifically suppressing this increased production. It is also important to formulate a working diagnosis. A differential diagnosis of patients who present with hirsutism and occasionally virilization is presented in the box. The first two disorders (drug exposure and intersex) may be easily ruled out by history, physical examination, or both. This listing has been divided into the three potential sources of abnormal androgen production: ovary, adrenal, and peripheral. Mixed sources of abnormal production may occur in patients diagnosed as having the most common conditions: PCO and idiopathic hirsutism. These two disorders are found in more than 90% of all patients who present with hirsutism. In these patients, virilization does not occur.

As clinical markers of androgen excess, testosterone serves as an ovarian marker, DHEAS serves as an adrenal marker, and 3α-androstanediol glucuronide serves as a peripheral marker. Testosterone is not a specific marker for the ovary but best serves as a guide to abnormal ovarian androgen production. Free testosterone does not usually add more information in determining an abnormal source of androgen production, but it may be found to be elevated more frequently than the measurement of total testosterone. In patients with idiopathic disease, testosterone and DHEAS levels are usually normal but may be slightly elevated, showing an ovarian, adrenal, or mixed androgen production. The primary abnormality here, however, is that of increased androgen production by skin due to increased 5α-reductase activity. This may be reflected by elevated levels of 3α-androstanediol glucuronide, but it may be assumed, and not measured, if the assay is not available and testosterone and DHEAS levels are near normal.

Tumors of the ovary or adrenal gland are first suspected by the history of rapid progression of defeminizing and virilizing signs. These tumors are typically unilateral and may be suggested by levels of testosterone that are more than 2.5 times the upper range of the clinical laboratory or by DHEAS levels above 8 μg/ml. Currently, sophisticated scanning techniques are available to localize tumors. Vaginal ultrasonography without or with color-flow Doppler is the best technique for the ovary. Computed tomography, magnetic resonance imaging, and iodomethylnorcholesterol scans are most useful for the adrenal gland but may help with ovarian localization as well. Therefore, selective venous catheterization should be used only if these techniques fail to make a diagnosis and the patient has a suggestive history and clinical examination.

An adrenal adenoma may secrete testosterone rather than DHEAS. In such a patient, normal ovaries are seen on scan. Also, any woman with a history of virilization of recent onset needs to be evaluated further, even if testosterone and DHEAS levels are less than those noted above. This is particularly relevant in postmenopausal women in whom androgen levels in the presence of a tumor may be lower. Women with ovarian hyperthecosis may be virilized. The diagnosis is usually made and the presence of a tumor ruled out because of a long history of androgen excess and, typically, the finding of bilaterally enlarged ovaries.

Cushing syndrome is extremely rare but should be considered in the differential diagnosis. Adult-onset congenital adrenal hyperplasia (usually due to 21-hydroxylase deficiency) may occur in 5% of hirsute patients and closely mimics PCO. The prevalence of congenital adrenal hyperplasia varies in patients of different ethnic groups and is highest in Eskimos, Ashkenazi Jews, and patients of Mediterranean ancestry. Screening for this disorder is carried out with measurements of early morning serum 17-hydroxyprogesterone with care taken to avoid measurements in the luteal phase of some patients who have occasional ovulation. If it is greater than 2–3 ng/ml, but less than 6 ng/ml, an ACTH test needs to be carried out to confirm or rule out the diagnosis. If it is less than 2 ng/ml in hirsute patients, the diagnosis has been essentially ruled out. Rarely, an 11-hydroxylase deficiency may present in the same way and is diagnosed by elevated 17-hydroxyprogesterone levels. Some of these patients are also hypertensive.

Suppressive therapy should be chosen to decrease the abnormal sources of androgen production. Oral contraceptives containing 1 mg of norethindrone or ethynodiol diacetate or the newer oral contraceptives containing 250 μg of norgestimate or 150 μg of desogestrel may be used in combination with 30–35 μg of ethinyl estradiol. Dehydroepiandrosterone sulfate levels may be suppressed by approximately 30%. Ovarian wedge resection for treatment of hirsutism is ineffective and contraindicated in young women. Severe ovarian androgen excess and hyperthecosis may also be treated effectively with a GnRH agonist.

If DHEAS levels are elevated above 5 μg/ml or if the diagnosis is congenital adrenal hyperplasia, glucocorticoids may be prescribed. For patients with uncomplicated adrenal androgen excess, low doses of dexamethasone at night (0.25–0.5 mg) or prednisone (2.5–7.5 mg) may be prescribed. However, recent clinical data have suggested that dexamethasone is not particularly effective for the treatment of hirsutism even if adrenal androgen excess exists and androgen levels become suppressed. Better results may be achieved with antiandrogens.

Differential Diagnosis of Androgen Excess

Drug Induced
Examples include exogenous testosterone, danazol

Intersex Conditions
Usually with ambiguous genitalia (eg, 46,XY with incomplete androgen resistance)

Ovary
Polycystic ovary syndrome
Stromal hyperthecosis
Ovarian tumors

Adrenal
Adrenal tumors
Cushing syndrome
Congenital adrenal hyperplasia

Peripheral
Idiopathic

For patients with idiopathic disease and those patients with a strong peripheral component, the antiandrogen spironolactone (100–200 mg/d) should be prescribed. With this drug, some suppression of testosterone also occurs. Various therapeutic combinations are appropriate if a mixed source of androgen production is documented or if there is a poor clinical response in 3–6 months.

Once androgen levels are suppressed, the existing hair should be removed. This is best carried out by electrolysis. Any effective treatment for hirsutism requires at least 3–6 months to accomplish. Overall, the therapeutic success rate for hirsutism is approximately 70%. After a tumor is removed, the anabolic effects of androgen decrease and clitoromegaly recedes somewhat. This occurs more rapidly than changes in body hair, which eventually undergoes reductions in both growth and thickness.

DYSFUNCTIONAL UTERINE BLEEDING

Dysfunctional uterine bleeding (DUB) is abnormal bleeding that cannot be attributed to organic disease in the pelvis or to pregnancy. It occurs most often in association with anovulation. However, in a small percentage of patients of childbearing age complaining of DUB bleeding is in association with ovulatory cycles. In ovulatory cycles, the endometrium undergoes proliferation due to stimulation by ovarian estrogen in the follicular phase of the menstrual cycle. Estrogen also brings about the synthesis of progesterone receptors on the endometrial epithelial cells. After ovulation, the endometrium is exposed to progesterone produced by the corpus luteum and is converted to secretory endometrium. Approximately 10–14 days after ovulation, the blood levels of estrogen and progesterone decline, resulting in endometrial desquamation and withdrawal bleeding.

Pathophysiology

Ninety percent of cases of DUB are thought to be anovulatory, occurring most frequently in those in adolescent and perimenopausal age groups. This type of bleeding is commonly associated with chronic anovulation, a state in which gonadotropin release is sufficient to initiate ovarian steroidogenesis but is insufficient to stimulate normal follicular maturation and ovulation. Under the constant influence of estrogen, the endometrium continues to proliferate until endometrial breakthrough ensues, unless estrogen is increased. It is thought that, because of an absence of endometrial growth limiting progesterone and normal withdrawal bleeding, the endometrium eventually becomes excessively vascular and hyperplastic without sufficient stromal support. Frequent acyclic bleeding ensues, with the potential to end in a vicious cycle of prolonged heavy flow. This hypermenorrhea can be preceded by irregular intervals of amenorrhea and even regular cycles.

The remaining 10% of cases of DUB are ovulatory, occurring mostly in women 20–40 years of age. Some are manifested by midcycle bleeding because of a reduction in estrogen at the time of ovulation; others occur as polymenorrhea because of a short proliferative or secretory phase or subtle anomalies of the ovulatory process. This type of DUB often occurs in women at the extremes of the reproductive years and is related to a decreased follicular response to gonadotropins.

Studies also indicate that fibrinolytic activity in utero is greatly increased in patients with DUB. There is an increase in levels of $PGF_{2\alpha}$, PGE_2, and prostacyclin, with a higher $PGE_2:PGF_{2\alpha}$ ratio, which would be expected to produce vasodilation, myometrial relaxation, reduced platelet aggregation, and increased menstrual blood loss.

Initial attempts to diagnose DUB should be directed toward eliminating organic lesions of the reproductive tract, iatrogenic causes, pregnancy complications, and coagulation disorders as possible etiologic factors, as well as detecting the factors that are responsible for anovulation. Conditions that may resemble or may be confused with DUB include the following:

- Intrauterine benign neoplasia (polyp, myoma)
- Reproductive tract malignancy
- Endometriosis or adenomyosis
- Bleeding associated with pregnancy (threatened or incomplete abortion, ectopic pregnancy, trophoblastic disease) or puerperium (subinvolution of the uterus, placental polyp, retained products of conception)
- Blood dyscrasias (thrombocytopenic purpura, platelet abnormalities, von Willebrand disease)
- Pelvic inflammatory disease and chronic endometritis

Abnormal bleeding occurring in the presence of such lesions, however, does not exclude the possibility of coincidental or coexisting anovulatory flow. After a reasonable attempt has been made to exclude these entities as possible causes for abnormal uterine bleeding, conditions known to disturb ovarian function and to result in anovulatory bleeding should be considered.

Anovulation results from disturbances in the neuroendocrine regulation of ovarian function (eg, polycystic ovaries) and may be related to diverse environmental and systemic influences that affect the hypothalamus. Both amenorrhea and anovulatory cycles have been associated with vigorous exercise with or without significant weight loss. Adrenal hyperfunction (eg, congenital or acquired adrenal hyperplasia) and hyperprolactinemia may result in amenorrhea or anovulatory cycles. Both hypothyroidism and hyperthyroidism may lead to anovulatory bleeding. Primary hyperthyroidism can provoke extremely heavy bleeding. Although the pathophysiology is not entirely understood, derangement of the metabolic clearance rate of estrogens may be responsible. Many drugs, including gonadal steroids, psychopharmacologic agents, and autonomic drugs, also have well-established inhibitory effects on the ovulatory process. The latter include morphine, reserpine, phenothiazines, monoamine oxidase inhibitors, and anticholinergic drugs.

Diagnostic procedures and laboratory studies should be considered when appropriate. These include complete blood count, endometrial biopsy, hysteroscopy, and selective laboratory tests such as thyroid function tests and serum prolactin and serum androgen levels (testosterone and DHEAS) when thyroid disorders, hyperprolactinemia, and hyperandrogenism are suspected.

Management

Patients Under Age 35

Given normal pelvic and cytologic findings, bleeding in women under age 35 is rarely due to an organic abnormality. Because an occasional adolescent girl with a bleeding disorder, notably von Willebrand disease or a platelet abnormality, has her first serious bleeding at the time of menarche, the clotting mechanism should be investigated in adolescent girls with acute uterine hemorrhage.

Most adolescent girls with acute uterine hemorrhage can be managed by hormonal therapy; curettage is rarely indicated. Estrogen stimulation will produce endometrial proliferation, but progesterone alone, without preliminary exposure to estrogen (to synthesize progesterone receptors), has no effect on the endometrium. The administration of a combination oral contraceptive, with a formulation containing 35 μg of estrogen, usually controls bleeding within 24 hours. The dose may be increased in a stepwise fashion if the original dose has been ineffective in controlling the bleeding. In patients with severe bleeding, the intravenous use of conjugated estrogens in conjunction with an oral contraceptive compound may shorten the duration of bleeding. The usual dosage is 25 mg, infused slowly every 4–6 hours for 24 hours. After the acute bleeding has been controlled, the oral contraceptive compound may be continued at a reduced dosage for 2–3 weeks, at which time a withdrawal period is allowed.

For young patients with less acute bleeding, the administration of cyclic progestins usually establishes a normal bleeding pattern. Therapy may be prescribed around the calendar month; for example, 10 mg of medroxyprogesterone acetate may be administered daily for the first 10 days of each month. An occasional patient requires cyclic therapy with one of the combination oral contraceptives over prolonged time periods, especially a patient with chronic anovulation.

Most forms of estrogen–progestogen replacement therapy in women of reproductive age result in cyclic bleeding but should not be relied on to correct the anovulatory pattern. Correction of clear-cut deficiencies in specific hormones, such as thyroid or adrenal substances, is of greater value than the simple creation of artificial cycles by substitution therapy. Likewise, correction of hyperthyroidism and appropriate therapy for adrenal hyperplasia should result in the reestablishment of normal ovulatory cycles. When pregnancy, in addition to establishment of ovulatory cycles, is desirable and no specific endocrine disorder can be identified, an ovulation-inducing agent such as clomiphene citrate may be administered.

Patients Over Age 35

Women over age 35, and especially those over age 40, who have significant abnormal bleeding require endometrial sampling to rule out a malignant or premalignant lesion. After organic diseases, including an endometrial malignancy or a premalignant lesion, have been ruled out, the management of DUB is similar to that described for younger women.

Progestin therapy, such as the administration of medroxyprogesterone acetate, 10 mg, or norethindrone or its acetate, 2.5–5 mg, for 10 days each month is recommended. A low-dose estrogen–progestogen preparation may also be used in women over age 35 who do not have any other risk factors, such as smoking, hypertension, or diabetes. Progestin therapy reverses the hyperplastic process in virtually all women with benign adenomatous hyperplasia. The endometrial sample obtained after 6 months of therapy determines the course of further management.

Hysterectomy may be considered an acceptable alternative for older patients with recurrent bleeding who are unresponsive to the usual therapeutic modalities. Another potential surgical approach is ablation of the endometrium with a hysteroscopically directed laser beam or electrocautery, but the long-term effects of these procedures are unknown.

Prostaglandin synthesis inhibitors, including mefenamic acid, naproxen, and ibuprofen, reduce excessive menstrual blood loss in women with menorrhagia or idiopathic hypermenorrhea but not in women with uterine leiomyomata. When administered, these drugs would have to be taken before or at the onset of blood flow to prevent the synthesis of prostaglandins that are thought to be responsible for excessive bleeding. Gonadotropin-releasing hormone analogues have also been suggested as therapy for DUB. This therapy may be considered for patients who have a major contraindication to sex hormone therapy. Continuous administration of GnRH analogues for up to 6 months will result in amenorrhea and may be considered in highly selected cases. Gonadotropin-releasing hormone agonists may also be used along with a low-dose combination of estrogen–progestogen. The suggested regimen consists of administering a long-acting GnRH agonist continuously and a combined estrogen–progestogen formulation in cyclic fashion to effect monthly withdrawal bleeding. A major advantage of this approach is the prevention of bone loss, vasomotor symptoms, and other hypoestrogenic manifestations.

BIBLIOGRAPHY

Secondary Amenorrhea

Baker ER, Mathur RS, Kirk RF, Williamson HO. Female runners and secondary amenorrhea: correlation with age, parity, mileage, and plasma hormonal and sex-hormone-binding globulin concentrations. Fertil Steril 1981;36:183–187

Bates GW, Bates SR, Whitworth NS. Reproductive failure in women who practice weight control. Fertil Steril 1982;37:373–378

Blackwell RE. Diagnosis and management of prolactinomas. In: Wallach EE, Kempers RD, eds. Modern trends in infertility and conception control, vol 4. Chicago: Year Book Medical Publishers, 1988: 197–208

Blackwell RE, Chang RJ, Cragum JR. Prolactin disorders in infertility. In: Seibel MM, ed. Infertility: a comprehensive text. Norwalk, Connecticut: Appleton and Lange, 1990:97–109

Blackwell RE, Younger JB. Hormonal regulation of breast physiology. In: Carr BR, Blackwell RE, eds. Textbook of reproductive medicine. Norwalk, Connecticut: Appleton and Lange, 1993:171–182

Boyar RM, Katz J, Finkelstein JW, Kapen S, Weiner H, Weitzman ED, et al. Anorexia nervosa. Immaturity of the 24-hour luteinizing hormone secretory pattern. N Engl J Med 1974;291:861–865

Carr DB, Bullen BA, Skrinar GS, Arnold MA, Rosenblatt M, Beitins IZ, et al. Physical conditioning facilitates the exercise-induced secretion of beta-endorphin and beta-lipotropin in women. N Engl J Med 1981;305:560–563

Chang RJ. Anovulation of CNS origin. In: Carr BR, Blackwell RE, eds. Textbook of reproductive medicine. Norwalk, Connecticut: Appleton and Lange, 1993:265–280

Eisenberg E. Toward an understanding of reproductive function in anorexia nervosa. In: Wallach EE, Kempers RD, eds. Modern trends in infertility and conception control. Vol 2. Philadelphia: Harper and Row, 1982:99–106

Katz E, Adashi EY. Treatment of infertility using bromocriptine mesylate. In: Seibel MM, ed. Infertility: a comprehensive text. Norwalk, Connecticut: Appleton and Lange, 1990:351–362

Liu JH. Anovulation of CNS origin: functional and miscellaneous causes. In: Carr BR, Blackwell RE, eds. Textbook of reproductive medicine. Norwalk, Connecticut: Appleton and Lange, 1993:281–295

McArthur JW, Oloughlin KM, Beitins IZ, Johnson L, Hourihan J, Alonso C. Endocrine studies during the refeeding of young women with nutritional amenorrhea and infertility. Mayo Clin Proc 1976;51:607–616

Pugliese MT, Lifshitz F, Grad G, Fort P, Marks-Katz M. Fear of obesity: a cause of short stature and delayed puberty. N Engl J Med 1983;309:513–518

Stradtman EW. Thyroid dysfunction and ovulatory disorders. In: Carr BR, Blackwell RE, eds. Textbook of reproductive medicine. Norwalk, Connecticut: Appleton and Lange, 1993:297–321

Vaitukaitis JL. Anovulation and amenorrhea. In: Seibel MM, ed. Infertility: a comprehensive text. Norwalk, Connecticut: Appleton and Lange, 1990:51–59

Valk TW, Corley KP, Kelch RP, Marshall JC. Hypogonadotropic hypogonadism: hormonal responses to low dose pulsatile administration of gonadotropin-releasing hormone. J Clin Endocrinol Metab 1980;51:730–738

Warren MP, Jewelewicz R, Dyrenfurth I, Ans R, Khalaf S, Vande Wiele RL. The significance of weight loss in the evaluation of pituitary response to LH-RH in women with secondary amenorrhea. J Clin Endocrinol Metab 1975;40:601–611

Wentz AC. Body weight and amenorrhea. Obstet Gynecol 1980;56:482–487

Yen SSC. Chronic anovulation caused by peripheral endocrine disorders. In: Yen SSC, Jaffe RB, eds. Reproductive endocrinology: physiology, pathology, and clinical management. 3rd ed. Philadelphia: WB Saunders, 1991:576–630

Yen SSC. Chronic anovulation due to CNS-hypothalamic-pituitary dysfunction. In: Yen SSC, Jaffe RB, eds. Reproductive endocrinology: physiology, pathology, and clinical management. 3rd ed. Philadelphia: WB Saunders, 1991:631–688

Polycystic Ovary Syndrome

Adashi EY. Insulin and related peptides in hyperandrogenism. Clin Obstet Gynecol 1991;34:872–881

Barnes R, Rosenfield RL. The polycystic ovary syndrome: pathogenesis and treatment. Ann Intern Med 1989;110:386–399

Daniell JF, Miller W. Polycystic ovaries treated by laparoscopic laser vaporization. Fertil Steril 1989;51:232–236

Greenblatt E, Casper RF. Endocrine changes after laparoscopic ovarian cautery in polycystic ovarian syndrome. Am J Obstet Gynecol 1987;156:279–285

Nader S. Polycystic ovary syndrome and the androgen-insulin connection. Am J Obstet Gynecol 1991;165:346

Wild RA. Lipid metabolism and hyperandrogenism. Clin Obstet Gynecol 1991;34:864–871

Wild RA, Alaupovic P, Parker IJ. Lipid and apolipoprotein abnormalities in hirsute women. I. The association with insulin resistance. Am J Obstet Gynecol 1992;167:1191–1196

Wild RA, Grubb BB, Hartz A, Van Nort JJ, Bachman W, Bartholomew M. Clinical signs of androgen excess as risk factors for coronary artery disease. Fertil Steril 1990;54:255–259

Hirsutism and Virilization

Barbieri RL. Clinical aspects of the hyperandrogenism-insulin resistance acanthosis nigricans syndrome. Semin Reprod Endocrinol 1994;12:26–31

Carmina E, Lobo RA. Peripheral androgen blockade versus glandular androgen suppression in the treatment of hirsutism. Obstet Gynecol 1991;78:845–849

Lobo RA. Androgen excess. In: Mishell DR Jr, Davajan V, Lobo RA, eds. Infertility, contraception and reproductive endocrinology. 3rd ed. Boston: Blackwell Scientific Publications, 1991:422–446

Lobo RA, Goebelsmann U. Adult manifestation of congenital adrenal hyperplasia due to incomplete 21-hydroxylase deficiency mimicking polycystic ovarian disease. Am J Obstet Gynecol 1980;138:720–726

Lobo RA, Goebelsmann U, Horton R. Evidence for the importance of peripheral tissue events in the development of hirsutism in polycystic ovary syndrome. J Clin Endocrinol Metab 1983;57:393–397

Serafini P, Lobo RA. Increased 5 alpha-reductase activity in idiopathic hirsutism. Fertil Steril 1985;43:74–78

Surrey ES, de Ziegler D, Gambone JC, Judd HL. Preoperative localization of androgen-secreting tumors: clinical, endocrinologic, and radiologic evaluation of ten patients. Am J Obstet Gynecol 1988;158:1313–1322

Taylor L, Ayers JW, Gross MD, Peterson EP, Menon KM. Diagnostic considerations in virilization: iodomethyl-norcholesterol scanning in the localization of androgen secreting tumors. Fertil Steril 1986;46:1005–1010

Menopause

Menopause is the permanent cessation of menstruation that occurs after the loss of ovarian activity. The perimenopause is the period immediately before and after menopause. The climacteric is a more encompassing word, indicating the period of time when a woman passes through a transition from the reproductive stage of life to the postmenopausal years, a period marked by waning ovarian function.

In longitudinal studies the median age for menopause is approximately 51.5 years. Most patients go through a period of irregular menstrual function prior to menopause, a perimenopausal transition that lasts on the average 4 years. Because a median age of menopause means that only half the women have reached menopause at that age, it is more useful clinically to remember the range for the age of menopause, approximately ages 48–55.

Current smokers and undernourished women experience an earlier menopause. There is no correlation between age of menarche and age of menopause. Because of the contribution of body fat to estrogen production, thinner women experience a slightly earlier menopause. Race, parity, the use of oral contraception, and socioeconomic status have little influence. There is reason to believe that premature ovarian failure can occur in women who have previously had abdominal hysterectomy, presumably because ovarian vasculature has been compromised. About 1% of women will experience menopause before age 40.

SYMPTOMS

Exogenous estrogen can enhance the quality of postmenopausal life and provide additional protection against osteoporosis and cardiovascular disease. Vasomotor, psychogenic, and urogenital-related problems occur early in the menopausal transition and, because they are readily apparent to the patient, are the most frequent reasons patients consult with their physician. The two main indications for long-term therapy—cardiovascular disease and osteoporosis prevention—are asymptomatic and usually require various tests to quantify the presence and degree of risk. However, the cost-effectiveness of the various screening tests has not been established. Although menopause is a universal event, there is no generic presentation and treatment, and patients need to be evaluated individually.

Vasomotor Flushes

The hot flush is the most common menopausal symptom for which patients seek treatment: approximately 60% of women note hot flushes within 3 months of a natural or surgical menopause. Of these women, 85% have them for more than 1 year.

A hot flush is a sudden sensation of intense warmth of the upper body that typically lasts 4 minutes. This is accompanied by a visible ascending flush of the thorax, neck, and face and is followed by profuse sweating. Hot flushes frequently awaken patients from sleep, causing insomnia and fatigue. This may then lead to symptoms such as irritability, impaired memory, and poor concentration.

Hot flushes result from the acute withdrawal of estrogens, either by menopause or by discontinuation of exogenous estrogen. For example, women with Turner syndrome, who are hypoestrogenic, do not have hot flushes unless they receive and are withdrawn from exogenous estrogen. An intact pituitary is not required, since a total hypophysectomy does not prevent the occurrence of hot flushes. Thus, estrogen appears to act via central neurotransmitters that regulate the thermoregulatory center in the hypothalamus.

Estrogens are more than 95% effective in relieving hot flushes. Since the effect on hot flushes is mediated via hypothalamic neurotransmitters, a minimum of 3–4 weeks of treatment is usually necessary to achieve a therapeutic effect. The dose should not be increased before that time. If estrogens are to be discontinued, they should be tapered to avoid the return of hot flushes.

Progestins have been shown to be more than 70% effective in relieving hot flushes. Progestins also may act via central neurotransmitters, as progesterone is known to raise the hypothalamic thermoregulatory set point during the luteal phase in ovulatory women. Progestins are particularly useful in patients for whom estrogen is contraindicated.

Recent studies have suggested that women with hot flushes have a lowered thermoregulatory center set point. Biofeedback and other nondrug methods such as exercise may achieve their ameliorating effect by raising this level, thus making the increased surge in peripheral skin blood flow and temperature less noticeable.

Genital Atrophy

Estrogen and progesterone receptors are present in the vagina, and estrogen receptors have been identified in the urethra and to a lesser extent the trigone of the bladder. Estrogen receptors have not been found in the vascular network of the vaginal connective tissue. Three common problems result from an estrogen deficiency: atrophic vaginitis, urethral syndrome, and urinary incontinence.

Normal vaginal health is maintained by moisturization and a protective ecologic milieu. Both are influenced by estrogen. The normal microbial flora of the vagina is dependent on the glycogen content of the vaginal epithelial cells and the resulting pH. Estrogen increases vaginal blood flow and hence the vaginal transudate and vaginal moisturization.

Patients with atrophic vaginitis present with a variety of symptoms, often described as irritation, dryness, dyspareunia, pruritus, malodor, a grayish vaginal discharge, and sometimes bleeding. The vaginal epithelium is typically pale and may have a "strawberry" appearance. The most objective sign is an increase in the lateral wall vaginal pH. Values in excess of 4.5 are abnormal. A maturation index with more than 20% parabasal cells is also indicative of an atrophic epithelium.

Although estrogen deficiency is the most common cause of vaginitis, infections may also be present. This requires accurate identification and specific treatment of the causative agent, for example, *Gardnerella* in bacterial vaginosis or *Candida*.

Postmenopausal women frequently complain of urinary frequency, nocturia, urgency and urgency incontinence. There are three main types of incontinence: genuine stress incontinence, detrusor instability, and overflow incontinence. The cure of incontinence is dependent on making an accurate diagnosis. Apart from a surgical approach, conservative measures such as circumvaginal muscle-strengthening exercises are most helpful. Estrogen may play a complementary role in patients with stress incontinence by raising the urethral closure pressure. Although the data are conflicting, some studies report a 60–70% improvement in symptoms associated with genuine stress incontinence. Estrogen therapy is ineffective in women with detrusor instability and overflow incontinence. However, most patients have a combination of incontinence; in one series 71% of women with genuine stress incontinence had urge incontinence and 40% of women with detrusor instability had genuine stress incontinence.

Urogenital atrophy may have secondary consequences that are remote from the pelvis. For example, cardiorespiratory fitness may be compromised in women who are reluctant to exercise because of incontinence; prolonged interrupted sleep due to nocturia may lead to irritation, depression, and inability to work effectively; and vaginal dryness can lead to dyspareunia.

Psychologic and Psychiatric Disorders

Certain emotional changes commonly occur at the time of menopause and estrogen deprivation, but it is not certain whether there is a cause-and-effect relationship between the symptoms and the decrease in estrogen. There is no uniform pattern: symptoms include being out of control, mood swings, irritability, impaired short-term memory, fatigue, headaches, insomnia, and depression. The last may be due to an endogenous abnormality, and it is important to emphasize to patients that the climacteric does not induce major psychiatric illnesses.

Menopause-related psychologic symptoms can respond well to traditionally prescribed estrogens, perhaps because sleep is improved. Some patients react to progestins, especially medroxyprogesterone acetate, with an increase in mood problems. Alternatives include low-dose norethindrone-based progestins or micronized oral progesterone. Psychologic symptoms may be due to environmental stressors at the time of menopause. Resolving the situation, counseling, stress management, and regular aerobic exercise is the preferred approach to treating these patients. Androgen administration has also been proposed to bring about a sense of well-being and improve headache and psychologic problems.

Osteoporosis

Osteoporosis is a complex multifactorial condition that is characterized by reduced bone mass and a tendency to have spontaneous fractures or those caused by minimal trauma. The fractures typically occur in the vertebrae (middle to lower thoracic and lumbar spine), the femoral neck, and the distal radius. Because 70% of the strength of the bone is attributable to its mass, it is possible to identify a precondition to osteoporosis—osteopenia. Osteopenia refers to bone mass (or density) that is 20% (± two standard deviations) or greater below that of a woman aged 35 years, for a given region of the skeleton. There are no discernible fractures, but damage to the microarchitecture of the horizontal and vertical plates, which constitute the scaffolding of the trabecular bone, may indeed be present.

There are two types of bone: trabecular bone present primarily in the axial skeleton (vertebrae) and cortical bone found in the appendicular skeleton (long bones in the arms and legs). In most regions, there is a mixture of both types of bone, which varies according to the anatomic site. For example, the midradius is 95% cortical bone; the far distal radius is 75% cortical and 25% trabecular bone.

Bone is living tissue and is governed by the bone-remodeling cycle. Two cell types are involved. Osteoclasts remove "old" bone by activating their ruffle borders with an acidlike substance; when the resorption cavity has reached a predetermined depth, osteoblasts are attracted into the cavity and are responsible for new bone formation. This takes place in two stages: the secretion of a collagen-rich ground substance called osteoid and subsequent mineralization with hydroxyapatite crystals. The latter are composed primarily of calcium. The resorption cavity is normally filled with new, freshly synthesized, bone. Deficits and hence osteopenia will arise when osteoclasts are overactive or osteoblasts are unable to refill normal resorptive cavities. Estrogen and progesterone receptors have been identified in osteoblasts even though estrogen therapy's main effect has been attributed to a reduction in bone resorption.

The most rapid phase of bone mass accrual occurs from puberty (after closure of the epiphyseal plates) to the mid-20s. Bone mineral still accrues thereafter at a slower rate until the mid-30s to reach peak bone mass, after which the bone is slowly lost at the rate of 0.3–0.5% until menopause. The rate then increases to approximately 2.3% per year for the next 6 years. Osteopenia/osteoporosis results if menopause is reached with reduced peak bone mass or if the rate of bone loss after menopause is excessive.

Risk factors will identify only 30% of women with osteopenia. High-risk factors include family history, white and Asian races, body build, diet deficient in calcium, life style (excessive alcohol use, smoking, decreased exercise), and previous menstrual history. Recent studies have shown that a late menarche, infrequent or anovulatory menstrual cycles, activities that induce premenopausal amenorrhea such as excessive exercise, and eating disorders are all linked to significant reductions in bone mass.

Bone mass measurement can identify and quantify the presence and degree of osteopenia, although the routine use of this test is not recommended. Of the methods available, dual-energy X-ray absorptiometry is the most accurate. Measurements can be made of the lumbar spine (L-2 through L-4), the hip (femoral neck, trochanter, and Ward triangle), and the distal radius and ulna. Patients may have osteopenia in only one site or in all three. The far distal radius is usually reflective of bone density in the spine or hip. Radiographic absorptiometry correlates well with dual-energy X-ray absorptiometry and other related technologies. An X-ray film of the hand is made and compared with a standardized aluminum step wedge (of varying densities) placed adjacent to the hand at the time of radiography.

Women suspected of having osteoporosis secondary to a medical condition (eg, hyperthyroidism and hyperparathyroidism) may be tested. These tests include urinary calcium, alkaline phosphate, and creatinine, blood sedimentation rate, blood urea nitrogen, collagen cross-link, TSH, and, selectively, parathyroid hormone assessment. All patients require a full physical examination. Low back pain, for example, may be due to muscle spasm associated with scoliosis or a herniated disk.

The prevention and management of osteopenia (low bone mass without fracture) and osteoporosis are predicated on the same principles: exercise to stimulate new bone formation, calcium to mineralize the newly formed osteoid, and hormone therapy to control the rate of bone loss. Recent studies have shown that increased activity and calcium consumption during adolescence and young adulthood increases bone mass. The same is also true—but to a lesser extent—in menopausal and older women. Best results are obtained by prescribing all three modalities.

Exercise needs to be gravitational and should involve all relevant muscle groups with repetitive muscle-strengthening exercise. To avoid injury, the patient's repetition maximum (maximum weight that can be lifted through one movement) must be established and exercise started at about 60% of this value. Forty-five minutes of aerobic exercise three times per week (at 70% of the maximum heart rate) has been found to slow down the rate of postmenopausal bone loss. Results are better if the patient is calcium replete. Since most menopausal women have approximately 450 mg of elemental calcium in their diet, a supplement of 1,000 mg of elemental calcium per day is needed in women not taking estrogen. Because of limits in intestinal calcium absorption, 500 mg of calcium in the morning and a similar dose at night will ensure a maximal absorptive response. Older women and women with achlorhydria should take their calcium with meals.

Estrogens prevent bone loss by decreasing bone resorption, increasing calcium absorption, and reducing renal calcium clearance. Estrogen also improves the bone mass response to exercise. Most estrogen therapy is effective in reducing osteoporosis-related fractures, as long as blood estradiol levels equivalent to 40–60 pg/ml are obtained. This is especially important in women with marked degrees of osteopenia (less than 70% or more than three standard deviations below peak bone mass). Combination estrogen and progestin therapy has an additive effect on bone mass. For this reason, women with marked bone loss who have had a hysterectomy should be considered for combination hormone therapy. Early hormone therapy will secure the best results, but it is never too late to start treatment. Women over age 65 years and women with established osteoporosis also improve their bone mass on estrogen therapy. Women on estrogen therapy require calcium supplementation of only 500 mg/d. Bone loss recurs once hormone therapy is stopped. Consequently, hormone therapy for osteoporosis involves continuous and prolonged treatment.

Women with secondary osteoporosis and those who are nonresponsive to hormonal therapy or are unable to take hormones (eg, women with breast cancer) should be referred to specialists in bone metabolism.

Atherosclerosis

Cardiovascular disease—specifically coronary artery disease—is responsible for the deaths of more postmenopausal women than all other causes of death combined. Since the prevalence of this disease increases after menopause and is reduced by about 50% in postmenopausal women treated with estrogens (compared with matched, untreated women), it is believed that estrogen protects against atherosclerosis. The increase in coronary heart disease in Caucasian women lags behind that of men by about 10 years; after menopause the mortality rises to become half that of men. This gender difference is less true for African–American women (whose main cardiovascular problem is hypertension) and other races, for example, the Japanese.

The lipid hypothesis is based on the association between increased plasma cholesterol, especially LDL cholesterol, and atherogenic disease. The risk is reduced by increased HDL cholesterol. As women become menopausal, the LDL cholesterol levels, which are lower than those in men, increase to exceed those of men. The oxidized form of LDL cholesterol damages the vascular endothelium and is now believed to be the primary initiator of atherogenic disease. High-density lipoprotein levels in women remain constant throughout life and are generally higher than those of men.

Since only 25% of the cardiovascular disease protective effect of estrogen can be explained by its LDL-lowering action, other factors such as direct effect of estrogen on coronary arteries may be involved. A subfraction of LDL cholesterol, Lp(a), has been identified as a lipid risk factor independent of cholesterol and LDL cholesterol. Part of the Lp(a) molecule, apolipoprotein(a), is homologous with the profibrinolytic protein plasminogen. Recent research has incriminated platelet deposition and thrombin formation in the earlier stages of atherogenesis.

Other factors involved in atherogenesis and influenced by hormonal therapy include hyperinsulinemia, elevated triglyceride levels in the presence of low HDL cholesterol, and various endogenous vasoactive substances. These include the vasodilators endothelium-derived relaxing factor; prostacyclin; and, in normal coronary arteries, serotonin and acetylcholine. Vasoconstriction occurs in response to platelet-derived thromboxane and endothelin, synthesized by the vascular endothelium.

Most of the current literature is based on the effect of oral estrogens on HDL cholesterol (increased by 8–15%) and LDL cholesterol (decreased by 4–15%). Parenteral administration of estrogen decreases LDL cholesterol but has a lesser effect on increasing HDL cholesterol. Progestins—depending on the type and dose—can reduce the lipid effect of oral estrogen. Oral, but not parenteral, estrogen increases triglycerides by about 20%. Oral androgens decrease triglycerides and HDL cholesterol. Preliminary studies suggest that oral estrogens reduce Lp(a). Estrogen enhances the effect of insulin by preventing its breakdown and improves carbohydrate metabolism. Oral estrogen increases some procoagulant factors, but progestins enhance fibrinolysis.

Most epidemiologic studies have shown a dramatic cardioprotective effect of exogenous estrogens. As a consequence, "routine" hormone therapy is advocated by many experts. However, although these studies control for a number of other cardiovascular disease risk factors, it is still possible that healthier populations were chosen for hormonal therapy. Definitive information will need to be based on randomized, long-term, prospective studies.

HORMONE THERAPY

Prior to the initiation of hormonal therapy, the patient should be evaluated with a careful history and a physical examination, including blood pressure, breast and pelvic examination, and a Pap test. Mammography should be considered prior to therapy. The test should be repeated yearly after age 50 in all women. The endometrium should be sampled if a patient bleeds at unpredictable times or if bleeding is heavy. This is usually accomplished by office aspiration. If an adequate sample cannot be obtained and if vaginal ultrasonography suggests an intrauterine pathologic lesion, fractional D&C, with hysteroscopy if deemed necessary, may be needed. A biopsy specimen must be obtained from patients who receive unopposed estrogens prior to instituting therapy and yearly thereafter, regardless of bleeding, as the annual incidence of hyperplasia is 30%. An alternative—especially in older women—is to monitor the endometrium with annual vaginal ultrasound examinations. Endometrial biopsies are restricted to those individuals whose endometrial thickness exceeds 4 mm. Blood pressure should be monitored 3–6 months after initiation of treatment and then yearly.

The most commonly used schedule of hormone therapy in the United States is cyclic, with conjugated equine estrogens, 0.625 mg given on days 1–25, and medroxyprogesterone acetate, 5–10 mg given on days 13–25 (Tables 6-2 and 6-3). No hormones are given during the remainder of the month. On this regimen, most patients demonstrate withdrawal bleeding. This schedule may be modified by substituting other oral estrogen for conjugated equine estrogens, such as micronized estradiol, 1 mg, piperazine estrone sulfate, 0.625 mg; or esterified estrogens, 1.25 mg. Estrogen may also be administered parenterally as transdermal estradiol, 0.05 mg twice weekly. To avoid recurrence of symptoms in the hormone-free week, the estrogen is often prescribed continuously. Vaginal estrogen creams are best reserved for urogenital-related problems and are used in a dose of 1–2 g of cream by applicator three times per week. An alternative is to digitally massage small amounts of cream into the vagina each evening.

Other progestins may be substituted for medroxyprogesterone acetate. These include norethindrone, 1.25–2.5 mg, and oral micronized progesterone, 200 mg/d. For patient convenience, progestins may be used for the first 10–12 days of the calendar month.

To avoid withdrawal bleeding, continuous (rather than cyclic) treatment has been proposed. Micronized estradiol, 1 mg (or equivalent), as needed to control symptoms or for a given indication, is given continuously with norethindrone, 0.35–0.70 mg, or medroxyprogesterone acetate, 2.5 mg. Most patients initially have irregular vaginal bleeding, but within 1 year 95% of women still on treatment become amenorrheic. Higher doses of norethindrone are required with higher doses of estrogen. Higher doses of progestins are associated with abdominal bloating and mastalgia and may cause the patient to discontinue therapy. The lowest effective dose should therefore be used.

Risk Factors

The benefits and risks of hormone therapy, as they pertain to each patient, should be reviewed with her in detail. Patients should also be informed that estrogens may cause nausea, mastalgia, headaches, and mood changes, as well as pose more serious risks. Ultimately, it is the patient who must decide and give her informed consent.

Endometrial Neoplasia

Unopposed estrogen use (ie, without the addition of progestin) may induce endometrial hyperplasia and, ultimately, adenocarcinoma. Carcinomas associated with estrogen use are generally of an early stage and low grade and are less likely to have invaded the myometrium. The adjusted 5-year survival rate is 94%, possibly because of earlier diagnoses in these closely monitored patients. Unopposed estrogen use appears to increase the risk of endometrial cancer fourfold to eightfold (from 1/1,000 women per year in nonestrogen users) and is related to both the dose and duration (minimum, 1–2 years) of estrogen use. A reduction of the dose or cyclic treatment does not provide adequate protection; progestins are highly recommended in patients with an intact uterus. Progestins can both prevent and reverse hyperplasia; their use has been found to reduce the incidence of endometrial cancer to a level below that in women who do not receive hormones. The duration of progestin use is important; although 7 days of treatment per month lowers the annual incidence of hyperplasia to 3%, 13 days of treatment per month essentially reduces this to zero.

TABLE 6-2. AVAILABLE ESTROGENS

Generic Name	Brand Name	Doses Available (mg)
Oral		
Conjugated equine estrogens	Premarin	0.3, 0.625, 0.9, 1.25, 2.5
Piperazine estrone sulfate, estropipate	Ogen, Hormonin	0.3, 0.625, 1.25, 2.5, 5
Esterified estrogens	Estratab, Evex, Menest, Amnestrogen	0.3, 0.625, 1.25, 2.5
Estradiol valerate	Progynova	1, 2
Estriol hemisuccinate	Hormonion	1, 2
Micronized estradiol	Estrace	1, 2
Estriol		1, 2
Synthetic		
Diethylstilbestrol	Generic	0.1, 0.25, 0.5, 1, 5
Ethinyl estradiol	Estinyl, Feminone	0.02, 0.05, 0.5
Quinestrol	Estrovis	0.1
Mestranol		
Injectable		
Estradiol benzoate	Generic	0.5 mg/ml
Polyestradiol phosphate	Estradurin	40 mg/2 ml
Conjugated equine estrogen	Intravenous Premarin	25 mg/ml
Estrone	Generic	1, 1, 5 mg/ml
Estradiol valerate	Generic	10, 20, 40 mg/ml
	Delestrogen, Estate, Gynogen, Menaval	10, 20, 40 mg/ml
Estradiol cypionate	Generic	5 mg/ml
	Depo-Estradiol	1, 5 mg/ml
	E-Ionate, E-Cypionate	5 mg/ml
Ethinyl estradiol	Generic	1 g powder
Topical–vaginal		
Estropipate	Ogen	1.5 mg/g
Conjugated equine estrogen	Premarin	0.625 mg/g
Dinestrol	DV 0.01% in 90 g	
Diethylstilbestrol	Generic	0.1, 0.5 mg (suppositories)
Topical–transdermal		
17β-Estradiol	Oestrogel	3 mg
	Estraderm (skin patch)	0.05 mg/d, 0.1 mg/d (release rate)

Modified from Shoupe D, Mishell DR Jr. Therapeutic regimens. In: Mishell DR Jr, ed. Menopause: physiology and pharmacology. Chicago: Year Book Medical Publishers, 1987

TABLE 6-3. AVAILABLE PROGESTINS

Generic Name	Brand Name	Doses Available (mg)
Oral		
Medroxyprogesterone acetate	Provera, Curretab, Amen	2.5, 5, 10
Megestrol acetate	Megace, Pallace	20, 40
Norethindrone (norethisterone)	Norlutin, Nor-Q D, Micronor	0.35, 5
Micronized progesterone	Utrogestin	100
Northindrone acetate	Norlutate, Aygestin	5
Norgestrel	Ovrette	0.075
Injectable		
Medroxyprogesterone acetate	Depo-Provera	100, 400 mg/ml
	Prodrox	250 mg/ml
Hydroxyprogesterone caproate	Delalutin	125 mg/ml
	Generic	125 mg/ml
Progesterone	Generic	25, 50, 100 mg/ml

Shoupe D, Mishell DR Jr. Therapeutic regimens. In: Mishell DR Jr, ed. Menopause: physiology and pharmacology. Chicago: Year Book Medical Publishers, 1987

Ovarian Neoplasia

While estrogen replacement may possibly increase the risk of endometrioid cancer of the ovary (which accounts for up to 10–20% of all ovarian malignancies), this has not been established conclusively. It is not known whether progestin use reduces this risk, if it indeed exists.

Breast Neoplasia

The possibility that estrogen use may increase the risk of breast cancer was raised because 1) breast cancer can be an estrogen-sensitive tumor; 2) estrogens can induce mammary tumors in rodents; and 3) women with prolonged endogenous estrogen exposure (eg, early menarche, late menopause, nulliparity) are at increased risk for this neoplasm. Epidemiologic studies that have been reanalyzed using meta-analysis have not found an overall increased risk of breast cancer for all postmenopausal estrogen users. The data did suggest a minimally increased risk of breast cancer for those women who used estrogen for more than 10–20 years. The possibility that the addition of a progestin may protect the breast (as it does the endometrium) has been suggested, but it remains unproven. Since progestins adversely affect lipoproteins and, thus, could potentially increase mortality from cardiovascular disease, the use of progestins in women without a uterus is unnecessary. An exception may be the selective use of progestins in patients with marked osteopenia.

Gallbladder Disease

Several studies have shown a twofold increase in the incidence of gallbladder disease in women receiving estrogen replacement therapy, presumably by increasing the cholesterol saturation of bile, which leads to precipitation and stone formation. However, other case–control studies have failed to demonstrate such an increase.

Thromboembolic Disease

First-generation oral contraceptives, with a high estrogen content, have been associated with thromboembolic disease, usually in women who also smoke. There appears to be a dose–response relationship, since controlled epidemiologic studies of physiologic postmenopausal estrogen therapy have found no increase in thrombosis. A consistent and clinically relevant biochemical effect of estrogen replacement on the coagulation and fibrinolytic systems has not been universally found.

Hypertension

In general, estrogen therapy modestly lowers blood pressure in most women; on occasion, however, it may induce or exacerbate hypertension in others. This idiosyncratic elevation in blood pressure is usually reversible on discontinuation of estrogen, and it is not associated with an increased risk of stroke.

Glucose Tolerance

Although oral contraceptives are associated with a tendency toward impaired carbohydrate metabolism, the lower doses used for estrogen replacement have not been linked to impaired glucose tolerance. With estrogen use, postmenopausal women with diabetes either showed no change or exhibited improved diabetic control, as evidenced by lower fasting blood glucose levels or reduced insulin requirements.

Contraindications

Absolute contraindications to postmenopausal estrogen replacement are 1) undiagnosed genital bleeding, 2) active liver disease, 3) recent myocardial infarction, and 4) active thromboembolic disease or a history of estrogen-related thromboembolic disease.

Relative contraindications are 1) chronic liver dysfunction (the liver's ability to metabolize estrogen is impaired, leading to excessive levels of estrogen); 2) poorly controlled hypertension; 3) a history of thromboembolic disease; and 4) acute intermittent porphyria (estrogens are known to precipitate attacks). The contraindications to the use of estrogen in women known to have or suspected of having endometrial or breast cancer are presently undergoing evaluation, and specific recommendations must await the availability of further data. The sense of well-being afforded by amelioration of menopausal symptoms should be weighed against the risk of stimulating tumor growth within the context of informed decision making between the patient and her physician.

Progestins

Progestins are used primarily to reduce the risk of endometrial hyperstimulation caused by estrogen replacement. Lower doses of progestins can be used since recent studies have shown that it is not necessary to simulate a secretory endometrium. Progestins may also be used to relieve hot flushes in patients who are not candidates for estrogen replacement.

Progesterone and its derivatives are well absorbed by the vaginal, rectal, and intramuscular routes. The oral route, although convenient and commonly used, provides a highly variable degree of absorption, with as much as a threefold difference among some patients. For this reason, variable clinical effects may be seen among patients given the same oral dose. Following absorption, oral progestins are presented to the liver in high concentration, where they may affect the hepatic metabolism of serum lipoproteins.

Medroxyprogesterone acetate, 10 mg, is the most commonly used progestin in the United States; it is effective against hyperplasia, with minor effects on serum lipids. Many patients are unable to tolerate this dose, and 5 mg may be used in its place; this dose offers similar protection against hyperplasia, except for some individuals who poorly absorb oral medroxyprogesterone acetate. Given IM in its depot form, medroxyprogesterone acetate is well absorbed. However, it has a highly variable duration of effectiveness and when used alone is commonly associated with irregular vaginal bleeding in premenopausal women. It is not recommended for routine hormone replacement.

The progestins used in oral contraceptives are 19-nortestosterone derivatives; these have partial androgenic properties, with potential adverse actions on lipids. Norethindrone was initially used in a dose of 2.5–5 mg, but doses of 1 mg and less (as used in low-dose oral contraceptives) have been shown to be equally effective against hyperplasia and have a much lower impact on lipids. DL-Norgestrel, known for its more potent androgenic properties, was similarly used in 0.5-mg doses, but it appears that a 0.15-mg dose is equally effective. The newer progestins—gestodene, norgestimate, and desogestrel—are reputed to have less of a lipogenic effect and are being evaluated as substitutes for the norethindrone derivatives in combination hormone replacement.

Progestins may produce abdominal bloating, mastalgia, headaches, mood changes, and acne. Progestins, particularly the 19-nortestosterone derivatives, also have been found to adversely affect serum lipids, decreasing HDL and increasing LDL levels in a dose-dependent fashion. Since the protective activity of progestins on the endometrium appears to be related more to the duration of use (ie, 13 days) than to the dose, the minimum effective dose is best. In sequential programs it is 5 mg for medroxyprogesterone acetate and 1 mg for norethindrone; in continuous regimens it is 2.5 mg and 0.35–0.7 mg, respectively.

Clonidine, a centrally acting adrenergic agonist/antagonist, at a dose of 0.1–0.2 mg twice daily, has been found to be effective for the treatment of hot flushes. Some patients respond better to the transdermal route of clonidine administration.

BIBLIOGRAPHY

Bachmann GA, Leiblum SR, Gill J. Brief sexual inquiry in gynecologic practice. Obstet Gynecol 1989;73:425–427

Barrett-Connor E, Bush TL. Estrogen and coronary heart disease in women. JAMA 1991;265:1861–1867

Crook D, Stevenson JC. Progestogens, lipid metabolism and hormone replacement therapy. Br J Obstet Gynaecol 1991;98:749–750

Dupont WD, Page DL. Menopausal estrogen replacement therapy and breast cancer. Arch Intern Med 1991;151:67–72

Falkerborn M, Persson I, Adami HO, Bergstrom R, Eaker E, Lithell H, et al. The risk of acute myocardial infarction after oestrogen and oestrogen-progestogen therapy. Br J Obstet Gynaecol 1992;99:821–828

Fuster V, Badimon L, Badimon JJ, Chesebro JH. The pathogenesis of coronary artery disease and the acute coronary syndromes (1). N Engl J Med 1992;326:242–250

Kronenberg F. Hot flashes: epidemiology and physiology. Ann N Y Acad Sci 1990;592:52–86; discussion 123–133

Lobo RA. Treatment of the postmenopausal woman: where we are today. In: Lobo RA, ed. Treatment of the postmenopausal woman: basic and clinical aspects. New York: Raven Press, 1994;427–432

Moyer DL, De Lignieres B, Driguez P, Pez JP. Prevention of endometrial hyperplasia by progesterone during long-term estradiol replacement: influence of bleeding pattern and secretory changes. Fertil Steril 1993;59:992–997

Notelovitz M. Estrogen replacement therapy: indications, contraindications, and agent selection. Am J Obstet Gynecol 1989;161:1832–1841

Notelovitz M. Osteoporosis: screening, prevention, and management. Fertil Steril 1993;59:707–725

Padwick ML, Pryse-Davies J, Whitehead MI. A simple method for determining the optimal dosage of progestin in postmenopausal women receiving estrogens. N Engl J Med 1986;315:930–934

Sherwin BB. The impact of different doses of estrogen and progestin on mood and sexual behavior in postmenopausal women. J Clin Endocrinol Metab 1991;72:336–343

Voigt LF, Weiss NS, Chu J, Daling JF, McKnight B, van Belle G. Progestogen supplementation of exogenous oestrogens and risk of endometrial cancer. Lancet 1991;338:274–277

Walsh RW, Schiff I, Rosner B, Greenberg L, Ravnikar V, Sacks FM. Effects of postmenopausal estrogen replacement on the concentrations and metabolism of plasma lipoproteins. N Engl J Med 1991;325:1196–1204

The Thyroid Gland

Thyroid homeostasis is modulated by a complex set of interrelated mechanisms that involve TRH, a peptide hormone that is synthesized by the anterior hypothalamus and transported to the anterior pituitary by the way of the hypothalamic–pituitary portal system; TSH, a glycopeptide that is secreted by the anterior pituitary; and autoregulatory mechanisms within the thyroid gland itself.

The biologically active thyroid hormones are T_4 and T_3. Measurement of these hormones is commonly used to test thyroid function. Feedback of thyroid hormones on TSH secretion appears to affect the pituitary gland. The set point for feedback control of the pituitary–thyroid axis, however, is regulated by alterations in TRH secretion. Intrathyroidal stores of thyroid hormones are maintained by autoregulatory mechanisms within the gland itself. Various environmental stimuli, including temperature alterations, starvation, and excessive iodine ingestion, may influence synthesis and release of thyroid hormones.

Abnormalities of thyroid function, including thyrotoxicosis and hypothyroidism, may have profound effects on gonadal function and fertility. Either hypothyroidism or hyperthyroidism may lead to anovulation or other abnormalities of reproductive function and thus must be considered part of the differential diagnosis in reproductive disorders.

TESTS OF THYROID FUNCTION

Both T_4 and T_3 circulate in plasma bound to a specific protein, thyroid-binding globulin (TBG). Thyroxine is bound more firmly than T_3. The free, or non–protein-bound, fractions of T_4 and T_3 may be measured and are in equilibrium with the bound hormones. The level of free T_4 correlates well with the clinical appraisal of thyroid function, while total T_4 and T_3, as a result of changes in TBG, may show considerable variation in euthyroid individuals.

Serum Thyroxine Concentration

In the older methods used to determine the level of thyroid hormone, protein-bound iodine or butanol-extractable iodine was measured. While some nonhormonal iodine was eliminated, a variable proportion of the measured iodine was not hormonal. Even the more recently developed measurement of T_4 by column chromatography failed to separate these contaminants completely. Therefore, most laboratories have now adopted very specific radioimmunoassay techniques that measure only T_4. The direct measurement of T_3 by radioimmunoassay is a useful assay in some patients for the diagnosis of T_3 thyrotoxicosis. Under some circumstances, most notably in pregnant women whose TBG levels are markedly elevated, free T_4 measurement by radioimmunoassay is useful when either hypofunction or hyperfunction of the thyroid is suspected.

Measurements Reflecting Hormone Binding

The most common method used to determine thyroid hormone binding is the in vitro T_3 uptake assay. In this test, radioactive T_3 is added to the patient's serum, which is treated with an insoluble particulate material (resin or cross-linked dextran beads) that competes with TBG for available hormone. The percentage of radioactive hormone in the particulate phase is determined. It is inversely related to the unoccupied binding sites on TBG and is directly related to the non–protein-bound hormone. The product of the serum T_4 and T_3 uptake results in the free T_4 index, a measurement that correlates closely with the level of free circulating T_4.

Measurements Reflecting Iodine Accumulation

Radioiodine uptake measures the uptake of radioactive iodine by the thyroid and, as such, is a direct test of thyroid function. While generally useful as a diagnostic tool in patients with hyperthyroidism, its use in the diagnosis of hypothyroidism has been compromised in recent years by iodine additives to food products.

Measurement of Serum Thyroid-Stimulating Hormone

Serum TSH is determined by radioimmunoassay. The serum TSH level is elevated in patients with primary hypothyroidism and is decreased or absent in patients with thyrotoxicosis. The serum concentration of TSH is a sensitive indicator of thyroid function and a useful guide in following thyroid replacement therapy. When combined with the TRH stimulation tests, it allows the accurate diagnosis of subtle degrees of thyroid dysfunction that are not detectable by standard methods.

Thyrotropin-Releasing Hormone Stimulation Test

Thyrotropin-releasing hormone has been made commercially available and is a useful diagnostic tool in patients with suspected thyroid disease. The negative feedback of the T_4 and T_3 on TSH release operates at the pituitary level. Therefore, in patients with thyrotoxicosis resulting from autonomous overproduction of thyroid hormones, there is no increase in TSH level when TRH is administered; in patients with primary hypothyroidism, the response is exaggerated.

The test is also useful in differentiating between primary (thyroprival), secondary (pituitary), and tertiary (hypothalamic) hypothyroidism. The TRH test is performed as follows:

1. Obtain a baseline serum TSH level.
2. Rapidly administer TRH, 500 µg IV (transient hypertension, flushing, and nausea may occur).
3. Determine the serum TSH concentration 30 minutes after injection.

THYROID THERAPY IN GYNECOLOGY

Thyroid therapy has been used extensively in patients with infertility and menstrual disorders. In the absence of demonstrable hypothyroidism, there is no clear evidence of any benefit from such therapy, and it probably represents nothing more than a placebo. Thyroid function should be evaluated in all patients with hyperprolactinemia. Prolactin levels may be grossly elevated in patients with primarily hypothyroidism and enlargement of the pituitary suggesting a tumor. The serum prolactin concentration promptly returns to normal with adequate replacement therapy with T_4. The adequacy of replacement therapy should be monitored by determinations of the serum levels of T_4 and TSH.

BIBLIOGRAPHY

Burrow GN. Management of thyrotoxicosis in pregnancy. N Engl J Med 1985;313:562–565

Davis LE, Leveno KJ, Cunningham FG. Hypothyroidism complicating pregnancy. Obstet Gynecol 1988;72:108–112

Larsen PR, Ingbar SH. The thyroid gland. In: Wilson JD, Foster DW, eds. Williams textbook of endocrinology. 8th ed. Philadelphia: WB Saunders, 1992:357–487

Momotani N, Noh J, Oyanagi H, Ishikawa N, Ito K. Antithyroid drug therapy for Graves' disease during pregnancy. N Engl J Med 1986;315:24–28

The Adrenal Gland

ADRENAL ANATOMY AND STEROID BIOCHEMICAL PATHWAYS

The anatomy of the adrenal gland in the fetus differs from that in both pregnant and nonpregnant women. After 8 weeks of gestation, the fetal adrenal cortex has two distinct zones. The inner fetal zone makes up 80% of the newborn adrenal gland weight (6.5 g). This fetal zone produces dehydroepiandrosterone (DHEA), a precursor of placental estrogen, and rapidly involutes in the weeks after birth. The definitive zone, the outer zone of the fetal adrenal cortex, gives rise to the three adrenal cortex zones in the adult.

The adult adrenal gland weighs approximately 5 g. The gland is divided into an outer (cortex) and an inner (medulla) portion. Eighty percent of the gland's weight is in the cortex, which is divided into three zones: 1) the outer zone, the zona glomerulosa; 2) the middle zone, the zona fasciculata; and 3) the inner zone, the zona reticularis. During pregnancy, the zona fasciculata increases in width. The total weight of the adrenal gland may or may not increase slightly during pregnancy.

Low-density lipoprotein cholesterol is the precursor of the active adrenal steroids that are enzymatically synthesized in specific adrenal zones. Corticotropin from the anterior pituitary gland interacts with adrenocortical cellular receptors, increasing the level of intracellular cyclic AMP. Through activation of the enzyme protein kinase, cyclic AMP subsequently initiates steroidogenesis by converting cholesterol to pregnenolone. Several of the steroidogenic enzymes are members of the cytochrome P-450 group of oxygenases.

The outer zone of the adult adrenal cortex, the zona glomerulosa, synthesizes and secretes aldosterone. The absence of 17α-hydroxylase (P-450c17) and the presence of 18-hydroxysteroid dehydrogenase (P-450c11) result in the conversion of cholesterol to aldosterone. The biosynthesis of aldosterone is regulated by the renin–angiotensin system and is stimulated by the octapeptide angiotensin II and by the increased level of serum potassium.

Corticotropin stimulates the middle adrenocortical zone, the zona fasciculata, to synthesize cortisol. This classic pathway sequentially converts cholesterol to pregnenolone, progesterone, and 17α-hydroxyprogesterone. In this Δ^4 pathway, the enzyme 17α-hydroxylase (P-450c17) converts progesterone to 17α-hydroxyprogesterone. The 21-hydroxylase enzyme, a microsomal cytochrome (P-450c21) enzyme, is encoded in two genes (A and B) on chromosome 6. The enzyme 21-hydroxylase converts 17α-hydroxyprogesterone to 11-deoxycortisol, which, in turn, is converted to the final product, cortisol, by the enzyme 11β-hydroxylase (P-450c11) (Fig. 6-6).

LABORATORY EVALUATION OF ADRENAL FUNCTION

Plasma cortisol levels undergo a diurnal variation in nonpregnant women, with normal 8-AM plasma levels ranging from 8 to 25 µg/dl (220–660 nmol/L). The 4-PM plasma cortisol levels range from 2 to 15 µg/dl (50–410 nmol/L). During pregnancy, the diurnal cortisol variation is decreased in amplitude, and plasma cortisol levels increase progressively, reaching maximal morning levels of approximately 35 µg/dl in the third trimester. The glycoprotein transcortin (ie, corticosteroid-binding globulin) is the main binding protein for cortisol, and its mean concentration range increases from 17 to 25 µg/dl in nonpregnant women to 45–55 µg/dl in pregnant women in the third trimester. The fetus is protected from the high maternal cortisol levels because 1) maternal corticosteroid-binding globulin levels are approximately twice as high as fetal corticosteroid-binding levels, thereby facilitating fetal-to-maternal transplacental passage of glucocorticoids; and 2) the placenta converts 80% of the cortisol to cortisone as it passes from the maternal to the fetal compartment.

The urinary free cortisol level is an accurate indication of adrenocortical function, although care must be taken in the 24-hour urine collection, and both cortisol and creatinine levels must be determined. Urinary free cortisol values in excess of 100–150 µg/24 h are associated with Cushing syndrome in nonpregnant women. In a normal pregnancy, however, urinary free cortisol values range from 200 to 500 µg/24 h. During a pregnancy complicated by Cushing syndrome, levels of 600 µg/24 h and higher have been recorded.

Urinary 17-hydroxycorticosteroids measure 1) cortisol and its metabolite cortisone, 2) 11-deoxycortisol, and 3) the tetrahydro metabolites of these three steroids. In nonpregnant women, the level of 17-hydroxycorticosteroids ranges from 2 to 10 mg/24 h; this level does not change during normal pregnancies. Similarly, the level of 17-ketosteroids has a range of 4–15 mg/24 h (14–52 µmol/d) in nonpregnant women, and these levels are relatively constant until late in the pregnancy, when they increase.

In nonpregnant women, total and free serum testosterone levels are 0.2–0.8 ng/ml (0.7–2.8 nmol/L) and 1.5–9.5 pg/ml, respectively. Total serum testosterone values greater than 2 ng/ml (eg, or two and one-half times the upper normal limit for the individual laboratory's testosterone range) in nonpregnant patients may be associated with an ovarian tumor. Polycystic ovary syndrome, ovarian stromal hyperthecosis, and, to some degree, congenital adrenal hyperplasia may mimic an ovarian neoplasm. During pregnancy, the total testosterone value rises, but the percentage of free testosterone is reduced because of the increased plasma concentration of the sex hormone–binding globulin.

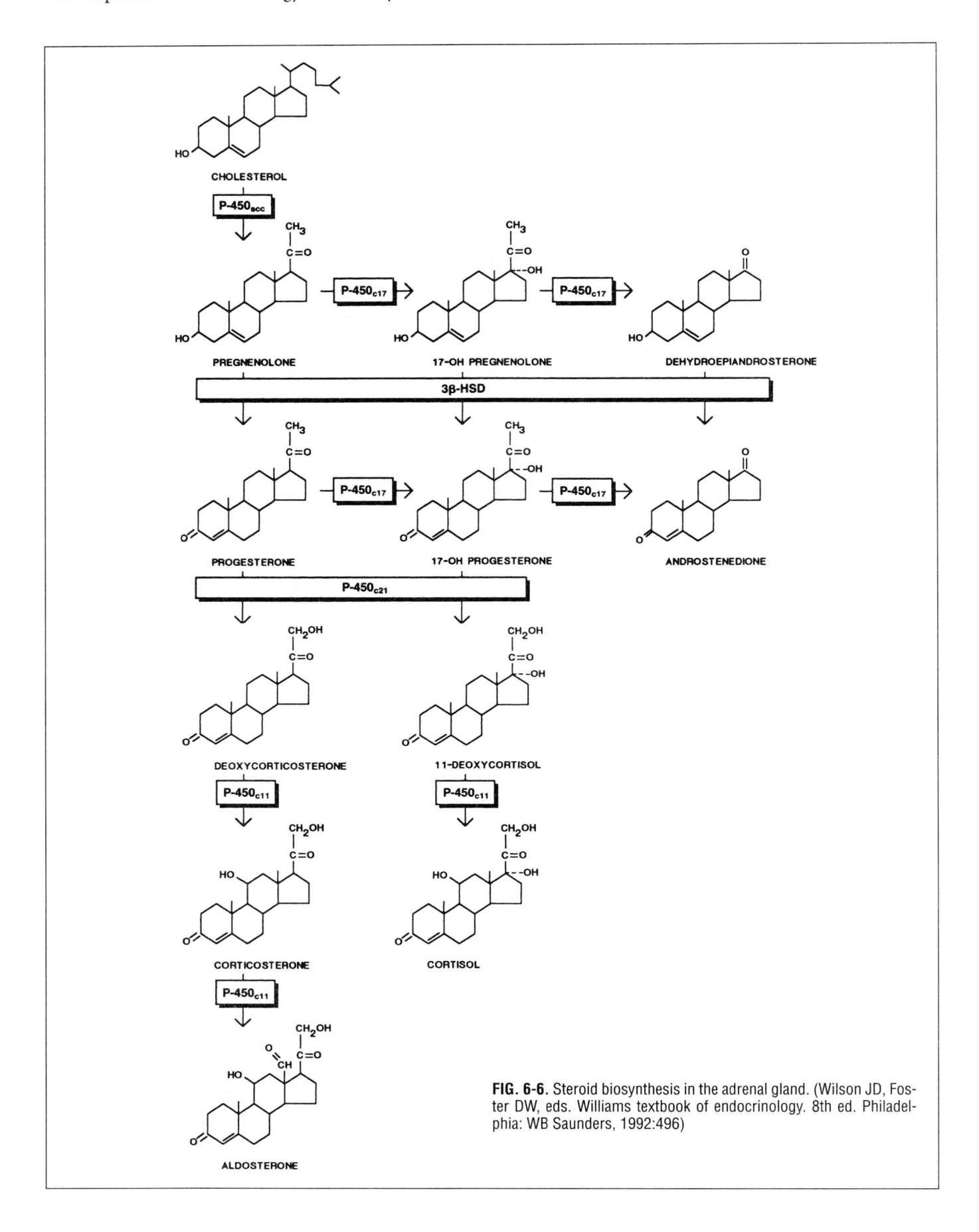

FIG. 6-6. Steroid biosynthesis in the adrenal gland. (Wilson JD, Foster DW, eds. Williams textbook of endocrinology. 8th ed. Philadelphia: WB Saunders, 1992:496)

All virilized patients require evaluation regardless of the testosterone level. Postmenopausal women with testosterone levels greater than 1 ng/ml and androstenedione levels greater than 2 ng/ml require investigation.

The ACTH value has a diurnal variation, with maximum levels reached in the morning. The adult range is 20–100 pg/ml (4–22 pmol/L). The plasma ACTH concentration can be useful in differentiating the cause of Cushing syndrome. Patients with adrenal adenomas or carcinomas usually have undetectable (<20 pg/ml) ACTH levels, whereas patients with pituitary ACTH-secreting adenomas and one third of patients with ectopic ACTH syndrome have normal to mildly elevated ACTH levels. Corticotropin levels in excess of 200–250 pg/ml suggest an ectopic source. Computed tomography scanning of the abdomen and bronchoscopy are useful in localizing adrenal and ectopic tumors. Data concerning ACTH levels in pregnancy are conflicting.

Dehydroepiandrosterone sulfate is primarily of adrenal origin and ranges from 0.6 to 3.4 μg/ml (5.4–9.2 μmol/L) in nonpregnant women; these levels are markedly and progressively decreased during pregnancy. Adrenal DHEAS levels greater than 8 μg/ml in nonpregnant, premenopausal women and greater than 4 μg/ml in postmenopausal women suggest the presence of a neoplasm and require further evaluation and dexamethasone suppression testing.

The metyrapone test evaluates pituitary ACTH reserve by blocking 11α-hydroxylase, thus preventing cortisol and corticosterone production and increasing 11-deoxycortisol secretion. A twofold or 10-mg increase in the 24-hour urinary 17-hydroxycorticosteroid level suggests normal pituitary ACTH reserve, whereas less than 3 mg in 24 hours suggests "frank insufficiency." In principle, patients with Cushing disease show an exaggerated response, while those with adrenal adenomas or carcinomas show an impaired or absent response. The test takes 2–3 days and may also include an ACTH stimulation test. Data on the use of these tests during pregnancy are limited.

The single-dose overnight dexamethasone test is the first screening test to be performed in patients with symptoms that suggest Cushing syndrome. The patient is given 1 mg of dexamethasone at 11 PM, and the plasma cortisol level is determined from a sample drawn at 8 AM the following morning. An 8-AM plasma cortisol level of less than 5 μg/dl excludes Cushing syndrome. If the result of the overnight dexamethasone suppression test is abnormal, the patient may be hospitalized for the low-dose and high-dose dexamethasone suppression tests. These tests are used to monitor urinary 17-hydroxycorticosteroid and plasma cortisol levels. After 2 days of baseline data have been obtained, the low-dose test is conducted with the administration of 0.5 mg of dexamethasone every 6 hours for 2 days. The low-dose test is followed immediately by the 2-day high-dose test, in which the dexamethasone dose is increased to 2 mg and is also administered every 6 hours for an additional 2 days.

Comparison of hormonal levels (ie, 24-hour urinary 17-hydroxycorticosteroids, free cortisol, and creatinine; and blood for cortisol, ACTH, and dexamethasone) on the second day of both low-dose and high-dose dexamethasone treatment with the basal levels dictates whether the patient's glucocorticoid secretion is suppressible. Normal individuals have hormone levels on the second day of the low-dose dexamethasone administration as follows: urinary 17-hydroxycorticosteroids < 2.5 mg/24 h, urinary free cortisol < 20 μg/24 h, plasma cortisol < 5 μg/dl, ACTH <20 pg/ml, and a dexamethasone value of 3–4 ng/ml. Failure to suppress urinary 17-hydroxycorticosteroids and plasma cortisol on the low-dose test suggests Cushing syndrome. Corticotropin will 1) remain elevated or high normal in the ectopic ACTH syndrome, 2) be within the normal range in Cushing disease, and 3) be undetectable in adrenal tumor. Failure to suppress these hormones, or suppression of less than 40%, on the high-dose regimen suggests an adrenal neoplasm or an ectopic ACTH-secreting tumor. Patients with pituitary-dependent hypercortisolism (ie, Cushing disease) should have at least a 50% suppression of urinary hormone and plasma cortisol and ACTH.

In patients with suspected adrenocortical insufficiency (eg, primary adrenocortical deficiency and Addison disease), the adrenal reserve must be evaluated. The rapid ACTH test measures plasma cortisol at 60 and 120 minutes after a single cosyntropin injection and has been shown to cause an increase in plasma cortisol of 20 μg/dl in the nonpregnant patient. Although a normal response to the rapid test excludes the diagnosis of primary adrenal insufficiency, it does not exclude the possibility of secondary adrenal insufficiency, and the in-hospital 48-hour ACTH infusion test may be necessary. The metyrapone test also evaluates pituitary ACTH reserve.

The rapid intravenous ACTH stimulation test is used to identify patients with congenital adrenal hyperplasia. Cosyntropin is given as a 250-μg intravenous bolus. Baseline, 30-minute, and 60-minute blood samples are collected. A 17α-hydroxyprogesterone level less than 4 ng/ml at 30 minutes excludes 21-hydroxylase enzyme deficiency, whereas levels of about 15 ng/ml suggest nonclassic deficiency or heterozygotes with 21-hydroxylase deficiency. Levels above 30 ng/ml suggest classic 21-hydroxylase deficiency.

ADULT ADRENAL ANDROGEN EXCESS

Clinically, androgen excess manifests itself not only with hirsutism but also with anovulation; irregular menstrual periods; infertility; increased libido; defeminization; and, in extreme cases, virilization with temporal balding, clitoromegaly, deepening voice, increased muscle mass, and male body habitus. The androgen excess may arise from any one of several distinct clinical syndromes. It may be either of ovarian or adrenal origin. Ovarian syndromes characterized by androgen overproduction include 1) simple hirsutism, 2) PCO, 3) hyperthecosis, or 4) an ovarian androgen-secreting tumor (eg, hilus cell tumors, benign cystic teratomas, arrhenoblastomas, luteinized thecoma, and adrenal rest tumor). The adrenal syndromes that may lead to androgen excess include 1) congenital adrenal hyperplasia as a result of partial deficiencies in 21-hydroxylase, 11-hydroxylase, or rarely, 3β-hydroxysteroid dehydrogenase; 2) Cushing syndrome; 3) an adrenal androgen-secreting tumor; 4) hypothyroidism; or 5) acromegaly. Nonclassic congenital adrenal hyperplasia (eg, late onset, partial, acquired, or attenuated) is believed to arise in patients with either one severe 21-hydroxylase deficiency allele (ie, "compound heterozygotic") or two mild alleles (ie, "homozygous mild").

The ovaries produce only small percentages of total DHEAS (0–5%), DHEA (1–10%), and testosterone (5–20%) but 50% of androstenedione (Fig. 6-7). The adrenal glands produce 95% of DHEAS, 90% of DHEA, 0–30% of testosterone, and 50% of androstenedione. The largest androgen pool is the circulating mild androgen DHEAS (2,000 ng/ml), which has a serum concentration that is 200 times that of DHEA.

The laboratory tests needed for the woman with suspected androgen excess depend on the physician's preliminary clinical diagnosis. The androgen excess in a hirsute woman may be evaluated by determining serum levels of free and total testosterone, DHEAS, and 17α-hydroxyprogesterone. In some instances, especially if the results of these tests are normal, serum androstenedione, DHEA, and dihydrotestosterone are measured. The condition of hirsute women with minimal menstrual irregularity and only an elevation in serum free testosterone may be diagnosed as simple hirsutism; the condition of those with no hormonal abnormality, as idiopathic hirsutism. Mild elevations of DHEAS may indicate a 3β-hydroxysteroid dehydrogenase deficiency. A serum 17α-hydroxyprogesterone level greater than 3 ng/ml is evidence of a 21-hydroxylase–deficient or 11β-hydroxylase–deficient form of congenital adrenal hyperplasia. Serum testosterone or DHEAS levels greater than 2 ng/ml (free testosterone greater than 40 pg/ml) or 7 μg/ml, respectively, suggest an androgen-secreting ovarian or adrenal tumor.

Treatment depends on the source and type of androgen excess and the patient's desire for pregnancy. The abnormal androgen level associated with the simple hirsutism of PCO may be treated with a low-dose oral contraceptive if the patient does not want to become pregnant. Androgen levels should be remeasured after 1 month of therapy and continued if adequate androgen suppression is obtained. Treatment with spironolactone may be necessary. If the patient's goal is pregnancy, suppression therapy is withheld and ovulation induction is begun with clomiphene citrate.

Patients with adult-onset congenital adrenal hyperplasia are treated with a corticosteroid (eg, prednisone or dexamethasone); the androgen level should be remeasured 30 days into the treatment to confirm suppression. If the patient plans pregnancy but does not ovulate, clomiphene citrate therapy is begun.

CONGENITAL ADRENAL HYPERPLASIA

The term *congenital adrenal hyperplasia* describes a group of enzyme disorders of adrenal steroid biosynthesis that are inherited as autosomal recessive traits. Unaffected carriers of such a trait have a one-in-four risk of having an affected child.

A patient with this condition has a partial or complete blockage of one of the enzymes in the steroid biosynthetic pathway.

The specific enzymatic block is identified by determining which steroids have an elevated level just before the blockage and demonstrating a deficiency in those steroids after the enzymatic block. Ratios of steroid levels before and after the enzyme block, with and without ACTH adrenal stimulation, can be helpful in the diagnosis of specific forms of incomplete congenital adrenal hyperplasia. In the most common form of congenital adrenal hyperplasia, the 21α-hydroxylase deficiency, the steroids that are elevated preceding the blockage are progesterone and 17α-hydroxyprogesterone. The urinary metabolite of 17α-hydroxyprogesterone classically used to diagnose this condition is urinary pregnanetriol. Prenatal diagnosis of congenital adrenal hyperplasia is possible through the determination of abnormal steroid levels in the amniotic fluid (second trimester) and of amniotic cells or by HLA typing and DNA analysis of 21-hydroxylase genes, C4 genes, or HLA genotyping genes from first-trimester chorionic villus cells or second-trimester amniotic fluid cells. The goal is accurate early first-trimester diagnosis and treatment (ie, dexamethasone) attempting to prevent the virilization of the genitalia in female fetuses with congenital adrenal hyperplasia.

21-Hydroxylase Deficiency

21-Hydroxylase deficiency is the most common cause (95%) of congenital adrenal hyperplasia and is estimated to occur in 1/14,000 births, although a much higher incidence is reported in Ashkenazi Jews and Eskimos. It causes increased levels of urinary 17-ketosteroids and plasma DHEA. Serum levels of 17α-hydroxyprogesterone and its urinary excretion product pregnanetriol are also elevated. The serum 17α-hydroxyprogesterone level normally ranges from 0.3 to 4.2 ng/ml. It is usually much greater than 8 ng/ml in patients with congenital adrenal hyperplasia; however, intermediate levels (3–8 ng/ml) do occur, and patients with nonclassic 21-hydroxylase deficiency and heterozygotes may present with nondiagnostic levels and require the rapid ACTH test for diagnosis. Intermediate levels that result from congenital adrenal hyperplasia must be differentiated from those that result from ovarian production in patients with PCO.

The 21α-hydroxylase deficiency may take 1) a simple virilizing form; 2) a less common, but more severe, salt-wasting form; or 3) the nonclassic, or late-onset, form with virilization during childhood or adolescence and in females subsequent hirsutism, acne, and infertility. In the newborn female the extent of virilization causing ambiguous genitalia varies as a function of the severity of the 21-hydroxylase deficiency (ie, the classic simple virilizing form versus the salt-losing form). Rapid diagnosis and gender assignment based on chromosomal and gonadal sex is required. In its severe form, the 21-hydroxylase deficiency causes a deficiency in aldosterone, resulting in dehydration, sodium depletion, and hyperkalemia (ie, adrenal crisis). The salt-wasting crisis can be fatal in the first weeks of life unless it is diagnosed and treated promptly

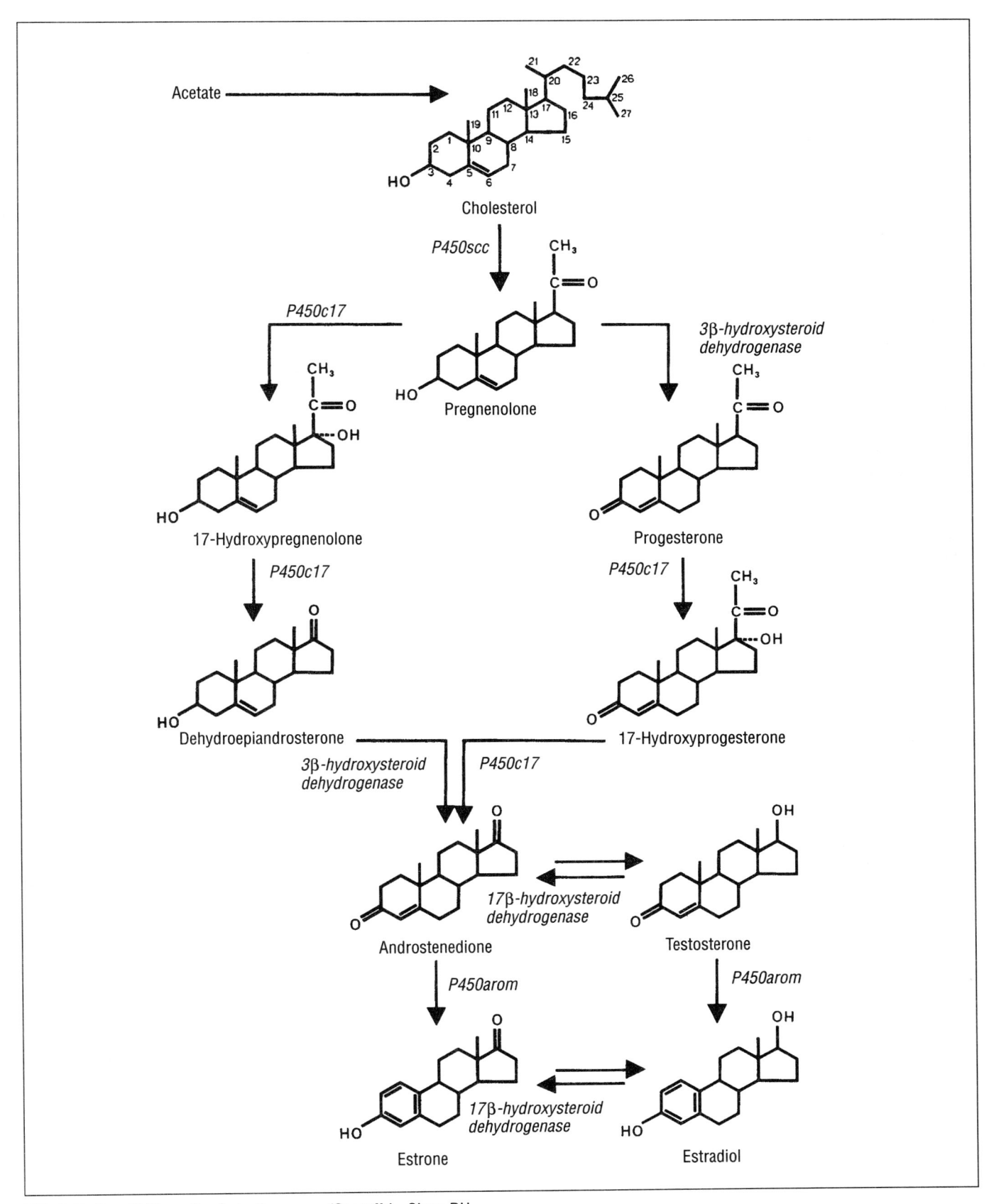

FIG. 6-7. Steroid biosynthesis in the ovary. (Speroff L, Glass RH, Kase NG. Clinical gynecologic endocrinology and infertility. 5th ed. Baltimore: Williams and Wilkins, 1994:40)

(eg, with corticosteroids, mineralocorticoids, and sodium chloride). The neonate should be observed for signs of adrenal insufficiency and abnormalities of serum sodium and potassium levels that require appropriate replacement therapy.

During childhood, milder forms of congenital adrenal hyperplasia cause accelerated growth and skeletal maturation that can result in early closure of the epiphyses and, therefore, short stature in untreated patients. The late-onset form of congenital adrenal hyperplasia is characterized by the onset of virilization during or within a few years of puberty. Androgen excess caused by adult-onset congenital adrenal hyperplasia may be differentiated from that caused by PCO by the rapid ACTH stimulation test. A stimulated level of 17α-hydroxyprogesterone less than 4 ng/ml usually indicates normal adrenal function, whereas intermediate levels are indicative of nonclassic or heterozygote 21-hydroxylase deficiency. Levels above 30 ng/ml indicate classic 21-hydroxylase deficiency.

Treatment depends on the severity of the 21-hydroxylase deficiency. Glucocorticoid replacement therapy (eg, dexamethasone, 0.25–0.5 mg at bedtime; prednisone, 5 mg at bedtime and 2.5 mg in the morning) is the primary treatment. Glucocorticoid therapy restores fertility in young girls and women with 21-hydroxylase deficiency and should be continued during pregnancy, although at the lowest effective dosage to minimize the possibility of adverse effects. Early first-trimester prenatal diagnosis by chorionic villus sampling is available. If the fetus is female and has the 21-hydroxylase deficiency, the mother may be treated with dexamethasone in an attempt to prevent fetal virilization. All patients undergoing treatment for congenital adrenal hyperplasia should be monitored periodically by determination of serum or urinary steroid values to guide therapeutic dosages.

Poor growth in children and Cushing syndrome in children and adults are side effects of excessive treatment while inadequate glucocorticoid replacement can result in accelerated skeletal maturation, premature epiphyseal fusion, short stature, hirsutism, amenorrhea, infertility, and adrenal rest tumors. Patients with the salt-wasting form of congenital adrenal hyperplasia require mineralocorticoid replacement (ie, Flurocortisone, Fluorinef).

11β-Hydroxylase Deficiency

Congenital adrenal hyperplasia is associated with 11β-hydroxylase deficiency in less than 5% of cases. The incidence is 1/100,000 live births. 11β-Hydroxylase arises from a single gene (P-450c11), which also gives rise to the 18-hydroxysteroid dehydrogenase activity, converting corticosterone to aldosterone. 11β-Hydroxylase deficiency blocks the conversion of 11-deoxycortisol to cortisol, resulting in excessive pituitary ACTH secretion and adrenal hyperplasia. The 11β-hydroxylase deficiency also blocks the conversion of 11-deoxycorticosterone to corticosterone in the aldosterone pathway. Thus, at least two types of 11β-hydroxylase deficiency exist, depending on the pathway affected and the severity of the deficiency. Levels of 11-deoxycorticosterone, 11-deoxycortisol, androgens, and total urinary 17-ketosteroids are all elevated in patients with 11β-hydroxylase deficiency.

The virilization manifestations of this form of congenital adrenal hyperplasia can result in female pseudohermaphroditism. The excessive adrenal production of 11-deoxycorticosterone, a mild mineralocorticoid, can cause hypertension, sodium and water retention, volume expansion, and, possibly, hypokalemia. The absence of hypertension, however, does not rule out the diagnosis. This condition is diagnosed by elevated baseline and ACTH-stimulated preblock steroids (eg, 11-deoxycorticosterone and 11-deoxycortisol) and their urinary metabolites. It is distinguished from Cushing syndrome by a normal result on the low-dose dexamethasone suppression test. Treatment requires glucocorticoid replacement to suppress ACTH secretion. Prenatal diagnosis is possible, but prenatal treatment has not yet been established.

3β-Hydroxysteroid Dehydrogenase Deficiency

The enzymatic block caused by 3β-hydroxysteroid dehydrogenase deficiency occurs early in the steroid biochemical pathways and blocks conversion of Δ^5 (ie, double bond in the B ring between positions 5 and 6, with a 3-hydroxy configuration such as in pregnenolone, 17α-hydroxypregnenolone, and DHEA) to Δ^4 steroids (ie, double bond in the A ring between positions 4 and 5 such as in progesterone, 17α-hydroxyprogesterone, and androstenedione).

In the neonate, if the deficiency is partial, adrenal insufficiency and—in females—mild virilization of the external genitalia are present. Males have abnormal external genital development, varying from hypospadias to nearly normal-appearing female genitalia. In the adult the late-onset form may cause hirsutism and menstrual irregularities. The variability of clinical features and the salt-wasting component may be caused not only by deficiencies of the presumed single 3β-hydroxysteroid dehydrogenase enzyme but also by abnormalities of one or more isozymes of the Δ^5–Δ^4 isomerase that occur in a specific pathway (eg, the glucocorticoid, the mineralocorticoid, or the sex steroid pathway). The resultant overactivity of the Δ^5 steroid pathway leads to abnormally elevated levels of pregnenolone, 17α-hydroxypregnenolone, and DHEA. In addition, some individuals have also demonstrated elevations in 17α-hydroxyprogesterone levels. Diagnosis is based on increased ratios of the Δ^5:Δ^4 steroids, although ACTH stimulation testing may be required. Treatment involves replacing the deficient cortisol, aldosterone, and gonadal hormones (Fig. 6-6).

17α-Hydroxylase Deficiency

A deficiency of 17α-hydroxylase blocks the conversion of progesterone to 17α-hydroxyprogesterone in the Δ^4 pathway and the conversion of pregnenolone to 17α-hydroxypregnenolone in the Δ^5 pathway, resulting in cortisol and sex steroid deficiencies. Serum levels of 11-deoxycorticosterone are elevated, but plasma levels of cortisol and urinary levels of 17-hydroxycorticosteroids and 17-ketosteroids are subnormal. Clinical manifestations of this rare disorder include hypertension, sexual infantilism (in females), and male pseudohermaphroditism (in males). Treatment comprises the replacement of glucocorticoid and appropriate sex steroids.

CUSHING SYNDROME

Cushing syndrome results from chronic excessive circulating levels of cortisol and is either ACTH dependent or ACTH independent. The ACTH-dependent causes of Cushing syndrome are 1) primary pituitary ACTH hypersecretion (ie, Cushing disease), 2) the ectopic ACTH syndrome (ie, ACTH secretion by nonpituitary tumors), and 3) the ectopic ACTH-releasing hormone syndrome (ie, a nonhypothalamic tumor secreting ACTH-releasing hormone and causing pituitary hypersecretion of ACTH). The excessive ACTH production causes bilateral adrenal hyperplasia resulting in the hypersecretion of cortisol. The ACTH-independent causes of Cushing syndrome are 1) autonomous primary adrenocortical adenoma or carcinoma, 2) rare adrenal bilateral micronodular dysplasia or rare bilateral ACTH-independent macronodular hyperplasia, and 3) iatrogenic administration of glucocorticoids.

Cushing syndrome, which is three to four times more common in women than in men, is associated with pituitary ACTH-dependent hyperplasia (Cushing disease) in 70% of cases; adrenal adenoma, adrenal carcinoma, and ectopic ACTH syndrome are each seen in 10% of cases.

The clinical manifestations of Cushing syndrome are central obesity, moon face, "buffalo hump," atrophic skin with striae, moderate hypertension (diastolic blood pressure > 100 mm Hg), polydipsia and polyuria, true diabetes mellitus (10–15%), osteoporosis, weakness, hirsutism, menstrual disorders, psychiatric complications (eg, emotional lability, depression, anxiety), weight gain, and other symptoms. As result of protein wasting, the skin becomes thin and fragile, develops purple striae, and is easily bruised. Because the clinical manifestations of Cushing syndrome are somewhat similar to the changes that occur in a normal pregnancy, it can be difficult to diagnose this disorder during pregnancy. Markedly increased acne and hirsutism during pregnancy suggest hyperandrogenism and require evaluation. Although hypertension during pregnancy is more commonly associated with toxemia or chronic hypertension, the possibility of Cushing syndrome should not be overlooked.

In nonpregnant patients, the plasma cortisol level in the morning is 8–25 µg/dl; in the late evening it is 1–8 µg/dl. Patients with Cushing syndrome frequently have plasma cortisol levels of 15–35 µg/dl, regardless of the time of day. The initial screening tests for Cushing syndrome are the 24-hour urinary free cortisol determination, followed by the overnight 1-mg dexamethasone suppression test. If Cushing syndrome has not yet been excluded, low-dose and, possibly, high-dose, dexamethasone suppression tests are performed. High-resolution, thin-section computed tomography or magnetic resonance imaging scans are useful in tumor localization.

Treatment for an adrenal tumor is primarily surgical, and adrenal exploration is recommended. Adrenal tumors are usually unilateral. Patients undergoing unilateral adrenalectomy must be given operative and postoperative glucocorticoid replacement therapy, generally hydrocortisone, 100 mg every 6 hours, beginning with the operation. On each of the subsequent 3 days, the dosage is reduced by one half, until a maintenance dosage of approximately 25 mg of hydrocortisone two times per day is reached. This dose is continued for several months until normal pituitary–adrenal function is demonstrated. The surgical cure rate for benign adrenal adenomas approaches 100% but is very poor for malignant adrenocortical tumors.

The main ACTH-dependent cause of Cushing syndrome is ACTH-secreting anterior pituitary corticotrope microadenoma, and treatment by transsphenoidal hypophysectomy yields a success rate of 70–90%. Success rates with macroadenomas are approximately 50%. Possible complications include transient diabetes insipidus, cortisol deficiency, and rarely, cerebrospinal fluid rhinorrhea and meningitis. Pituitary irradiation has also been used successfully. In the past, bilateral adrenalectomy was used as a treatment; however, this treatment caused adrenal insufficiency necessitating lifelong hormone replacement and also resulted in Nelson syndrome, a rapidly growing pituitary adenoma.

Maternal Cushing syndrome is very detrimental to a fetus, and therefore early diagnosis and treatment are important to avoid the high rate of stillbirths and premature labor associated with this disorder. Postpartum, the neonate of a mother with Cushing syndrome must be evaluated for adrenal insufficiency. If Cushing syndrome in a pregnant woman is corrected by adrenal or pituitary surgery, replacement hormonal therapy may be required. Successful treatment should allow normal continuation of the pregnancy.

PRIMARY ADRENOCORTICAL DEFICIENCY

Destruction of the adrenal cortex results in primary adrenocortical deficiency (Addison disease). In the past, the primary cause of adrenocortical destruction was tuberculosis. Today, the most common cause (75%) is idiopathic atrophy of the adrenal glands secondary to an autoimmune process. One half of patients with autoimmune adrenal insufficiency will have other associated endocrine or autoimmune disorders, termed polyglandular autoimmune syndromes. These other associated diseases, listed in order of decreasing incidence, include ovarian failure (20%), diabetes mellitus (11%), hypoparathyroidism, hypothyroidism, thyrotoxicosis, nontoxic goiter, pernicious anemia, and testicular failure. Rare causes of Addison disease include histoplasmosis, amyloidosis, adrenal apoplexy, metastatic carcinoma to the adrenal glands, mitotane treatment, use of heparinlike drugs, and congenital aplasia.

Nonpregnant women with Addison disease may have no menstrual irregularities, although severe debilitating disease results in amenorrhea. Twenty-five percent of women with idiopathic Addison disease are amenorrheic. Adrenal insufficiency should be suspected when a tetralogy of symptoms occurs: 1) hypotension, 2) weight loss, 3) anorexia, and 4) weakness. Patients with severe adrenal insufficiency show signs of cortisol deficiency (eg, gastrointestinal symptoms, anorexia, nausea, vomiting, hypochlorhydria, abdominal pain, and weight loss), as well as signs of aldosterone deficiency (eg, hyponatremia, hypovolemia, weight loss, hypotension, and shock). Hyperpigmentation occurs secondary to pituitary hypersecretion of ACTH and other peptides. Hyperkalemia and acidosis also occur.

Addison disease is rarely associated with pregnancy. Primary adrenal insufficiency may be difficult to diagnose in pregnant patients because of the similarity of its symptoms to those of pregnancy (eg, nausea, weakness, fatigue, and hyperpigmentation). When adrenal insufficiency is suspected in pregnant patients, early laboratory confirmation and simultaneous treatment are required. Adrenal insufficiency is evaluated by measuring adrenal reserve (ie, by determining basal and ACTH-stimulated plasma cortisol and urinary 24-hour 17-hydroxycorticosteroid levels).

All patients with adrenal insufficiency must be observed for the development of an adrenal crisis. Characterized by hypotension, shock, anorexia, nausea, abdominal pain, weakness, fatigue, lethargy, confusion, and coma in a patient who has been subjected to a major physiologic stress, an adrenal crisis is a life-threatening medical emergency. Treatment is primarily directed at rapid elevation of circulating glucocorticoid and replacement of sodium and water deficits. Therefore, rapid administration of 5% glucose in normal saline and dexamethasone or hydrocortisone IV is recommended.

Although Addison disease does not appear to affect the spontaneous abortion rate or prematurity, maternal antibodies in the adrenal cortex have been demonstrated in neonatal serum. In addition, maternal Addison disease, even if treated, has been associated with low neonatal birth weight. Secondary adrenal cortical insufficiency occurs when ACTH secretion has been chronically suppressed by 1) long-term glucocorticoid treatment and then its withdrawal, 2) postsurgical removal of an adrenal tumor or a pituitary ACTH-producing tumor, and 3) by pituitary (ie, Sheehan syndrome) or hypothalamic destruction. Adrenal crisis can occur with secondary adrenal cortical insufficiency and requires immediate treatment.

PHEOCHROMOCYTOMA

Pheochromocytoma is a rare adrenal medullary tumor that can be inherited as an autosomal dominant trait, producing excessive catecholamines (ie, norepinephrine, epinephrine, and dopamine from some tumors). Although 90% of these tumors are benign, their local infiltrating tendency often makes it impossible to rule out a malignancy until subsequent years bring no recurrence of metastases. The tumors are in the abdominal cavity 95% of the time, most frequently near the adrenal gland. Reports of the tumor's incidence in hypertensive patients have ranged from 0.05% to as high as 2%. Of 139 reported cases of pheochromocytoma associated with pregnancy, two thirds occurred in multigravidas and one third occurred in primigravidas. Remissions may occur between pregnancies, but subsequent pregnancies may lead to a recurrence with more severe symptoms. A malignant pheochromocytoma with thyroid carcinoma, called Sipple syndrome, may arise in association with pregnancy.

The signs and symptoms of a pheochromocytoma are variable, but they often include headache, labile or sustained hypertension that is resistant to conventional treatment, profuse sweating, paroxysmal attacks of blanching or flushing, palpitations, tachycardia, headache, anxiety during episodes, and increased fasting blood glucose levels. The classic manifestation of a pheochromocytoma is the paroxysm or crisis caused by sudden catecholamine release from the tumor and resulting in symptoms of headache, hypertension, and tachycardia. The paroxysm may last minutes or several hours.

During pregnancy, pheochromocytoma should be suspected in cases of paroxysmal hypertension or severe preeclampsia. Paroxysmal attacks can be initiated by postural changes, uterine contractions, or fetal movement. Shock may follow the induction of anesthesia for vaginal delivery in patients with or without previous symptoms, or it may occur in the postpartum period. The possibility of a pheochromocytoma should be considered when any patient experiences unexpected hypertension, hypotension, or shock after delivery.

The presence of a pheochromocytoma can be confirmed by 24-hour urine examination revealing elevated levels of vanillylmandelic acid, total metanephrines (normetanephrine–metanephrine), and total urinary catecholamines. Plasma catecholamines are of limited usefulness. Tumor locations have been pinpointed by computed tomography scans, magnetic resonance imaging, and scintiphotography using metaiodobenzylguanidine. A tumor should be localized by roentgenography during pregnancy only after the fetal risks have been carefully considered. Although surgical removal of the tumor is the primary treatment, interim medical management uses alpha-adrenergic blocking agents. Exploratory laparotomy or abdominal exploration at the time of cesarean delivery has been necessary to localize some tumors.

Maternal pheochromocytoma is associated with a very high proportion of fetal loss. A review of 162 pregnancies complicated by this disease showed fetal survival in only 47%, with intrauterine death in 23%, intrapartum or postpartum death in 17%, and spontaneous abortion in 12%. Medical maternal intervention with appropriate blocking agents may decrease fetal wastage.

Pregnancy complicated by a pheochromocytoma is associated with maternal mortality in 40–50% of cases. The mortality rate is much higher in the postpartum period than in the antenatal period. Once the condition has been diagnosed during pregnancy, surgical or temporizing medical management depends on the stage of gestation and the severity of the maternal condition. The question of vaginal versus cesarean delivery is controversial, because both are associated with a high maternal death rate (31% and 19%, respectively). It may be prudent to consider medical management of the pregnancy, followed by cesarean delivery with abdominal exploration for the tumor.

BIBLIOGRAPHY

Barbieri RL. Hyperandrogenism: new insights into etiology, diagnosis, and therapy. Curr Opin Obstet Gynecol 1992;4:372–379

Buescher MA, McClamrock HD, Adashi EY. Cushing syndrome in pregnancy. Obstet Gynecol 1992;79:130–137

Harrison TR, Stone RM. Principles of internal medicine. 12th ed. New York: McGraw-Hill, 1991

Holt JP Jr. Disorders of the adrenal glands in pregnancy. In: Gleicher N, ed. Principles and practice of medical therapy in obstetrics. 2nd ed. New York: Plenum Publishing, 1992:211–238

Lobo RA. Ovarian hyperandrogenism and androgen-producing tumors. Endocrinol Metab Clin North Am 1991;20:773–805

Pang S, Pollack MS, Marshall RN, Immken L. Prenatal treatment of congenital adrenal hyperplasia due to 21-hydroxylase deficiency. N Engl J Med 1990;322:111–115

Schenker JG, Granat M. Phaeochromocytoma and pregnancy—an updated appraisal. Aust N Z J Obstet Gynaecol 1982;22:1–10

Shapiro B, Gross MD. Endocrine crises. Pheochromocytoma. Crit Care Clin 1991;7:1–21

Speroff L, Glass RH, Kase NC. Clinical gynecologic endocrinology and infertility. 4th ed. Baltimore: Williams and Wilkins, 1989

Tulchinsky D, Ryan KJ. Maternal-fetal endocrinology. Philadelphia: WB Saunders, 1980:137–145

Wilson JD, Foster DW, eds. Williams textbook of endocrinology. 8th ed. Philadelphia: WB Saunders, 1992

Yen SSC, Jaffe RB. Reproductive endocrinology: physiology, pathophysiology, and clinical management. 3rd ed. Philadelphia: WB Saunders, 1991

Infertility

Infertility may be defined as failure to conceive after 12 months of unprotected intercourse. Couples who are unable to establish a pregnancy may be infertile or sterile. Infertility is an involuntary reduction in reproductive ability; sterility is a total inability to reproduce. In either case, the situation may or may not be reversible. If there has never been a pregnancy, the infertility is termed primary. If there is a documented history of pregnancy, including spontaneous abortion or ectopic pregnancy, the infertility is termed secondary.

Normal couples have approximately a 20% chance that conception will occur after 1 month of unprotected intercourse (fecundity rate). The chance of conception increases to 60–70% after 6 months and reaches 85–90% after 1 year. Thus, it has been estimated that 10–15% of couples in the United States who are attempting to conceive will be infertile. However, a recent survey of a specific population suggests that 20–35% of couples may try for more than one year to conceive at some stage in their reproductive cycle.

At least four factors have been instrumental in increasing the absolute number of infertile couples at the beginning of the 1980s. First, the largest number of births in the United States actually occurred between 1956 and 1961. Thus, the median age of this group in 1983 was 25 years. Because persons in the middle of their reproductive years are most likely to be trying to conceive, a larger number of women are discovering their infertility. Second, the age-specific rates of infertility have increased, primarily because sexually transmitted disease that leads to pelvic inflammatory disease has become more prevalent. Furthermore, increasing numbers of women are entering the work force and are thus being exposed to potential occupational hazards that affect reproduction, and more couples are being exposed to environmental toxins that decrease fertility. Third, the current tendency to delay childbearing into the later reproductive years allows more time for the infectious, occupational, and environmental factors to exert their cumulative effect on fertility. Inherent, age-related biologic factors further reduce the ability to conceive. Finally, couples who have delayed their childbearing until their later reproductive years have condensed the interval of desired fertility into a shorter time span and thus may feel a greater pressure to conceive within a shorter period of time. These couples tend to seek infertility services earlier if they are unsuccessful.

Infertility as experienced by most couples is a life crisis. Feelings of frustration and anger are common. The infertile couple may feel powerless and isolated. A careful history may often reveal feelings of guilt and depression. Physician acceptance of the responsibility for the care of the infertile couple includes a commitment to provide for the educational and emotional needs of the patient. A careful explanation of the reproductive process, examinations, and testing are necessary. The anxiety associated with infertility may often be relieved by empathetic counseling and a prompt and orderly evaluation.

INITIAL EVALUATION

Both members of the infertile couple should undergo a rational and orderly examination. The evaluation, which includes a history, physical examination, and laboratory studies, is designed to identify all significant causes of infertility. Potential etiologies and their generally accepted incidence include:

- Male factors (30–40%)
- Ovulation factors (15–20%)

- Tubal and peritoneal factors (25–30%)
- Cervical and uterine factors (10%)
- Immunologic incompatibility (5%)
- Miscellaneous factors (5%)

Because several factors may contribute to failure to conceive, all major factors should be evaluated initially. Although the history or physical examination may delineate a potential etiology, it is still important to perform a thorough evaluation, as infertility is often due to multiple factors. This is especially likely if a relative cause rather than absolute cause of infertility is noted. Thus, even if azoospermia is noted, an evaluation of female factors is still desirable. In the initial evaluation it is essential to establish whether ovulation occurs, whether adequate sperm numbers are present, and whether the fallopian tubes are patent. Once these factors are assessed, other potential causes of subfertility can be studied as indicated.

The goal of the evaluation is to identify the etiology of reduced fertility in the couple and, if possible, to provide a prognosis for future fertility based on the condition or conditions identified. The extent of the evaluation will be determined by factors such as age, length of infertility, historic factors, and study findings. The initial evaluation, including laparoscopy if indicated, can be completed in 3 months or longer. For the young couple who have failed to conceive in 6 months reassurance and delay may be indicated; for the couple with infertility of greater than 3 years, however, spontaneous conception is unlikely, and aggressive evaluation is indicated.

The interval of the infertility investigation presents an excellent opportunity for preconceptional counseling. Family and medical history can be assessed and medical factors affecting the pregnancy treated. Diabetes can be brought under control, genetic studies obtained, and rubella inoculations given. Further medical consultations can be sought, and prescriptions can be adjusted. Life style factors such as smoking, alcohol consumption, and exercise can be addressed as well.

INVESTIGATION AND TREATMENT OF THE INFERTILE MALE

Nearly half of all infertility is at least partially, if not totally, attributable to the male. Since obstetrician–gynecologists are the health care providers most frequently consulted for diagnosis and treatment of infertility problems, it is incumbent on them to obtain a working knowledge of male infertility diagnosis and treatment.

History and Physical Examination

As in other medical encounters, the first step in evaluation includes a careful and complete history and physical examination. The history should attempt to discover conditions such as cryptorchidism, hypospadias, abnormal puberty, impotence, hypogonadism (decreased need for shaving, diminished libido, erectile or ejaculatory dysfunction), diabetes, or thyroid abnormality, which suggest possible endocrine dysfunction that could impinge on sperm production and sexual function. Prior genital trauma, infection (especially adult mumps orchitis), or surgery suggests possible anatomic or immunologic causes of male infertility. History of recent febrile illness and environmental, medication, or drug exposure should also be elicited; febrile illness may depress spermatogenesis for up to 3 months. The general physical examination should search for evidence of an endocrine abnormality such as inadequate virilization, in addition to evidence of other systemic illness. Careful genital examination includes evaluation of the penis and position of the meatus; palpation of the spermatic cords, searching for varicocele, nodularity, or epididymal enlargement; and assessment of the position, size, and consistency of the testis. Since the seminiferous tubules comprise 85% of the adult testicular volume, a decrease in testicular volume implies loss of germinal epithelium.

Laboratory Tests

The differential diagnosis of male infertility includes pretesticular, testicular, or posttesticular causes of abnormal semen production, and decreased fertilizing ability of spermatozoa despite apparently normal semen. The pretesticular causes are:

- Hypopituitarism
- Hyperprolactinemia
- Hypothalamic dysfunction or failure

The testicular causes are:

- Testicular dysgenesis (Klinefelter syndrome, Noonan syndrome)
- Androgen resistance syndromes
- Anorchidism
- Cryptorchidism
- Orchitis
- Selective germinal cell dysfunction
- Germinal cell aplasia
- Sertoli-cell-only syndrome
- Chemotherapy or radiotherapy
- Environmental exposure and drugs

The posttesticular causes are:

- Varicocele
- Obstruction of the vas deferens (congenital aplasia, vasectomy, gonococcal infection, tuberculosis)
- Obstruction of the epididymis (congenital aplasia, gonococcal infection, tuberculosis)
- Retrograde ejaculation (autonomic dysfunction from diabetes or surgery, ganglionic blockade)
- Seminal vesicle or prostate dysfunction (infection, drugs)
- Coital dysfunction
- Impaired sperm function with normal semen
- Immunologic (antisperm antibodies [ASAs])
- Idiopathic

Following several screening semen analyses, recognition of these potential abnormalities directs the remainder of the diagnostic evaluation. Normal semen analyses do not exclude male causes of the couple's infertility; if the complete evaluation of both partners still fails to disclose a cause of their infertility, sperm fertility testing is indicated even when the semen analysis results are normal.

At least two, and preferably three, semen analyses obtained over a 75–90-day interval are adequate to screen for male infertility. Each should be obtained after a period of abstinence equal to the male's usual ejaculatory interval. If the semen analyses show a sperm count greater than 20 million/ml with at least 2 ml of seminal plasma; at least 50% motility, with a significant proportion moving with rapid, progressive motility; and normal morphology greater than 50%, further initial laboratory evaluation of the male is not necessary. Most cases of oligospermia are idiopathic or are associated with endocrine dysfunction, varicocele, or germinal epithelium dysfunction or failure. Low semen volume suggests inadequate collection, ductal obstruction, atresia, destruction or dysfunction of the seminal vesicles or prostate, or retrograde ejaculation. Abnormalities of motility (asthenospermia) may be due to varicocele, infection, ASAs, epididymal dysfunction, cigarette or marijuana smoking, environmental toxins, androgen deficiency, infrequent ejaculation, ultrastructural tail or ciliary defects (Kartagener syndrome).

Computer programs have been developed for objective classification of sperm morphology, although such systems are neither standardized nor widely available. Hence, the percentage of morphologically normal sperm and classification of morphologic defects is subjectively determined. Many sperm head defects are associated with abnormal chromatin, and recent evidence suggests that viable spermatozoa with abnormal chromatin have reduced fertilizing capacity and are more likely to result in an abnormal embryo if fertilization does occur. New, strict (Kruger) criteria for morphologic classification have recently been introduced that appear to be better predictors of fertilization in vitro. Whether these criteria reliably predict fertilization in vivo and pregnancy from coitus remains to be demonstrated.

Other tests of male reproductive function include biochemical evaluation of semen, which allows assay of markers from the accessory glands that could suggest sites of ductal or glandular obstruction, atresia, or dysfunction (eg, fructose and prostaglandins from the seminal vesicles, acid phosphatase and zinc from the prostate). Determination of a normal hypothalamic–pituitary–testicular axis by radioimmunoassay of serum levels of gonadotropins, prolactin, and sex steroids eliminates various hypogonadal syndromes such as hypothalamic failure (Kallmann syndrome), pituitary failure, or testicular failure (Klinefelter syndrome). Karyotypic evaluation is used to further evaluate apparent testicular (hypergonadotropic) failure. Scrotal Doppler ultrasonography is the preferred method for detection and confirmation of varicocele, and its use is indicated even in patients with palpable varicocele to evaluate the contralateral spermatic vein prior to surgical ligation. Seminal cultures for microorganisms, including *Mycoplasma*, *Ureaplasma*, and *Chlamydia* species are indicated in select cases.

Retrograde vasography may be used to define obstructive conditions. Finally, testicular biopsy may be indicated in selected cases of testicular dysfunction to differentiate patients who are candidates for endocrine or surgical therapy from those who are irreversibly sterile.

Sperm antibody testing is indicated when an immunologic cause of male infertility is suspected from other studies (ie, significant agglutination on semen analysis, abnormal in vivo or in vitro tests of sperm–cervical mucus interaction, evidence of decreased sperm fertilization potential by laboratory test or failed fertilization in vitro) or in cases of unexplained infertility. Antisperm antibodies may be present in the semen attached to sperm, free in seminal plasma, or in serum. Although the correlation between the presence of antibody and infertility is not perfect, sperm from men with significant levels of ASA may have diminished cervical mucus penetration, altered migration through the upper female reproductive tract, or inhibition of sperm binding to the zona pellucida and oolemma. Antisperm antibodies can be demonstrated by using various biologic end points, such as agglutination (Kibrick) or immobilization (Isojima), the mixed antiglobulin reaction, or the immunobead test.

Videomicrographic computed systems for the analysis of sperm motion and morphology are available and are appearing in more and more laboratories over the past few years. Such instruments can replace the corresponding subjective portions of the routine semen analysis, allowing precise computation of various movement (percentage of motile sperm, average velocity, path straightness, head and flagellar beat amplitude, and frequency) and morphology (sperm head size, area, shape, and staining density) parameters with accuracy, reproducibility, and speed. At present, the normal ranges for these motion parameters are under investigation. Important correlation between these movement measurements and the in vitro fertilizing capacity of spermatozoa has been reported, and additional prospective studies are under way attempting to relate them with male fertility potential outside the laboratory. However, at this time computed sperm motility analysis offers no particular advantage over conventional semen analysis, and its use cannot be recommended except in the research setting.

Functional Evaluation of Spermatozoa

Functional evaluation of the fertilization potential of spermatozoa includes determination of sperm transport, sperm–oocyte recognition, the acrosome reaction and sperm–egg fusion. Sperm transport is assessed by the Sims–Huhner postcoital test, performed during the periovulatory phase of the menstrual cycle. Abnormalities of sperm–cervical mucus interaction can be investigated further by using antibody testing or one of the various in vitro tests. These include slide tests for evaluating sperm penetration through the mucus interface or shaking sperm; the crossed hostility test that uses donor mucus and sperm; and quantitative assessment of the speed and depth of sperm penetration into a mucus column. The postcoital and slide tests require only a microscope and can easily be performed in the office. Other tests of sperm transport, such as cervical insemination followed either by culdocentesis or laparoscopy, have been described but are not used clinically.

Although fertilization in vitro demonstrates that capacitation, the acrosome reaction and sperm–egg fusion have been successful (the so-called diagnostic IVF), the normality of these steps in the fertilization process is evaluated most easily by the zona-free hamster oocyte sperm penetration assay. Removal of the zona pellucida from hamster oocytes prepared for the sperm penetration assay allows cross-species sperm penetration and head decondensation. These oocytes are then inseminated with a prepared, capacitated sperm sample from the patient and a fertile control, and the percentage of ova showing sperm binding and penetration is recorded. Greater than 20% oocytes penetrated is considered normal, while less than 10% is an abnormal result. The value of the sperm penetration assay lies in its 80–90% concordance with IVF, although its ability to predict fertility in other situations is considerably lower. Repetitive abnormal sperm penetration assay results suggest an abnormality in sperm function that may be amenable to gamete micromanipulation.

The first contact between sperm and egg involving specific receptors is at the zona pellucida, an important site not assessed in the sperm penetration assay. The hemizona assay was described in an attempt to evaluate this important interaction. In the hemizona assay, human oocytes are microbisected to obtain two matched half (hemi) zona surfaces, which are then separately exposed to capacitated sperm from the patient and a fertile control. The ratio of tightly bound patient and control sperm to these hemizonae determines the hemizona index. Preliminary results suggest that the hemizona index may predict fertilization, although its routine use for predicting IVF results requires further study and validation. Failed sperm–zona interaction may be amenable to assisted fertilization with micromanipulation. In the future, recombinant human DNA-derived zona receptors may take the place of these hemizonae in assessing sperm–zona interaction.

Another assay of sperm function is the hypoosmotic swelling test, which evaluates sperm membrane integrity in a hypotonic medium. Several studies have suggested that the results of this test may be an independent predictor of sperm fertilizing ability, although the data at present are not sufficient to recommend its routine use. Similarly, measurement of acrosin—a sperm acrosomal proteinase—levels and other aspects of the acrosome, including determination of the proportion of acrosome-reacted sperm after capacitation, may offer additional probes of the functional competence of spermatozoa.

Treatment of Male Infertility

The treatment of male infertility (Table 6-4) ultimately depends on an accurate determination of the underlying pathophysiologic process leading to disordered sperm production, delivery, or function. In addition, the reproductive potential of the female partner must be fully evaluated. When the specific pathophysiology is not known—or when specific therapy is not available—empirical endocrine treatment and homologous insemination have been suggested, although their value in many situations is unconfirmed by prospective, controlled trials. Others may be candidates for assisted reproduction alone or with micromanipulation procedures such as partial zona dissection, subzona sperm insertion, or microinjection of sperm into the oocyte. When the male infertility problem is refractory to all therapy, insemination with donor semen remains a treatment option that provides an excellent prognosis.

If varicocele is thought to be the cause of subfertility, surgical ligation of the spermatic vein improves semen quality in about 80% of patients, and half of those can be expected to impregnate their partners. Men with ASAs have been treated with corticosteroids or sperm washing and intrauterine insemination. Seminal fluid volume and liquefaction distur-

TABLE 6-4. AVAILABLE TREATMENT OPTIONS FOR MALE INFERTILITY

Treatment Option*	Indication
Agent	
Gonadotropins	Hypogonadotropic testicular failure, empirical
GnRH	Hypothalamic failure (Kallmann syndrome)
Alpha-sympathomimetics	Ejaculation or emission failure
Anticholinergics	Ejaculation or emission failure
Antibiotics	Genital tract infection, antisperm antibodies, empirical
Clomiphene	Hypogonadotropic testicular failure, idiopathic oligospermia, empirical
Immunosuppressive agents (eg, steroids)	Antisperm antibodies, empirical
Androgens	Empirical
Zinc, vitamins	Empirical
Procedures	
Vasovasostomy and related reanastomoses	Acquired vas deferens obstruction, congenital vas deferens obstruction, or vasectomy reversal
Varicocelectomy	Varicocele
Sperm washing and separation	Empirical, impaired sperm function with normal semen
Intrauterine insemination	Cervical factor infertility, impaired sperm function with normal semen or oligospermia, unexplained infertility
IVF, GIFT	Empirical, impaired sperm function with normal semen or oligospermia
Assisted fertilization (micromanipulation)	Empirical, impaired sperm function with normal semen or severe oligospermia

* GnRH indicates gonadotropin-releasing hormone; IVF, in vitro fertilization; GIFT, gamete intrafallopian tube transfer.

bances can be treated by either obtaining a split ejaculate or administering sympathomimetic or anticholinergic medications. These medications may also facilitate normal ejaculation when autonomic dysfunction results in failed emission, ejaculation, or retrograde ejaculation. Alternatively, motile sperm can often be recovered from the alkalinized urine of men with retrograde ejaculation. Intracervical or washed intrauterine insemination is then performed with these recovered sperm samples. Vasovasostomy or vasoepididymostomy can be contemplated for correction of congenital or acquired obstruction of the vas deferens.

Hypogonadotropic hypogonadism is amenable to endocrine therapy using gonadotropins, which have been successful in restoring normal spermatogenesis and fertility in carefully selected and adequately evaluated patients. However, when hormonal therapy (including clomiphene citrate) is used empirically, improvement in semen quality may be delayed and transitory. Pregnancy rates are often disappointing in these situations. Empirical intrauterine insemination of washed spermatozoa, combined with controlled superovulation of the female partner, has been shown to be efficacious in a few studies for treatment of male infertility in which sperm function appears normal. Many different procedures for preparation of sperm have been described, including washing in a variety of different media followed by separation (swim-up, centrifugation, migration through gradients of a colloidal suspension of silica or columns of glass wool), although no procedure has been shown to be clearly superior to others. Prospective, controlled trials are attempting to confirm these results in large series of patients.

Modifications of assisted reproductive procedures have improved success in male factor infertility; as the efficiency of IVF and related procedures has improved, fewer and fewer competent, motile sperm are required to obtain embryos for transfer back to the uterus. Microfertilization is the newest and most promising development for treatment of these patients. A specialized laboratory and trained personnel are required for handling gametes, using micromanipulators under high-power magnification. Both partial zona dissection (creation of a small slit in the zona pellucida to facilitate sperm entry into the perivitelline space) and subzona insertion of several spermatozoa directly into the perivitelline space frequently result in fertilization and have approximately equal pregnancy rates of 20–30% per embryo transfer in experienced programs. Direct injection of sperm heads into the oocyte cytoplasm has resulted in fertilization and early embryo cleavage, but no pregnancies have yet been reported from this technique.

INVESTIGATION AND TREATMENT OF THE FEMALE

Ovulation Failure and Ovulation Disorders

Patients with ovulatory disorders may report amenorrhea, oligomenorrhea, menorrhagia, or infertility. Persistent anovulation should be evaluated prior to ovulation induction to aid in selection of the appropriate treatment method and to rule out significant disease (Table 6-5).

Evaluation

The hypothalamic–pituitary–ovarian axis is sensitive to stimuli at many sites. It can be disrupted by hypothalamic dysfunction, cranial tumors, obesity, anorexia, systemic disease, or abnormalities in the ovaries, thyroid, or adrenal gland that affect circulating steroid levels.

Anovulation is presumed in women with amenorrhea or cycles of 42 days or longer. Anovulation can be present even in women with regular menstrual cycles and can be documented by a monophasic basal body temperature (BBT) graph or serum progesterone levels (5–10 days prior to anticipated menses) of 4 ng/ml or lower. Proliferative endometrial biopsies are consistent with anovulation, but they should be reserved for evaluation of the luteal phase in ovulatory women or to assess endometrial histology associated with long-standing anovulation.

Evaluation of the etiology of anovulation should include assay of serum levels of FSH, LH, and prolactin, and thyroid function tests. In cases of hirsutism and hyperandrogenism with signs of Cushing disease, measurement of serum testosterone levels, DHEAS, and 17α-hydroxyprogesterone, or overnight dexamethasone suppression may be helpful. Com-

TABLE 6-5. TREATMENT OF OVULATION DISORDERS*

Disorder and Treatment	Treatment Regimen
Hyperprolactinemia	
Dopamine agonist	2.5–7.5 mg/d
Hypothalamic amenorrhea	
Pulsatile GnRH	Initially at 5 μg/pulse every 90 min
Gonadotropins–hCG	Initially 75–150 IU/d, beginning cycle day 3; thereafter individualized by response
Hypothalamic pituitary dysfunction	
Clomiphene citrate	50–150 mg/d, beginning cycle day 2–5
Pure FSH–hCG	Initially 75 IU/d, beginning cycle day 3; thereafter individualized by response
Gonadotropins–hCG	As for pure FSH
GnRH (with/without pretreatment with GnRH analogue)	Initially at 5 μg/pulse every 90 min
Hyperandrogen states	
Prednisone	5–7.5 mg/d in divided doses
Dexamethasone	0.5 mg/d at bedtime
Clomiphene citrate	50–150 mg/d in addition to glucocorticoid therapy (if continued anovulation)

* GnRH indicates gonadotropin-releasing hormone; hCG, human chorionic gonadotropin; FSH, follicle-stimulating hormone.

puted tomography scans may be required in women with hypoestrogenic amenorrhea or hyperprolactinemia, to rule out cranial tumors. Elevated levels of FSH (>40 mIU) are diagnostic of ovarian failure. Tests to evaluate autoimmune causes of ovarian failure (antinuclear antibody, rheumatoid factor, sedimentation rate, thyroid and ovarian antibodies) are suggested, since some women with autoimmune diseases and apparent ovarian failure will ovulate and become pregnant after immunosuppression with prednisone. In general, however, increased FSH levels indicate an absence of ovarian follicles, and ovulation induction rarely succeeds.

Most anovulatory patients have low or normal LH, FSH, and prolactin levels. These patients are often combined under a diagnosis of hypothalamic dysfunction or chronic anovulation and are excellent candidates for ovulation induction. It is important that other causes of infertility be excluded. Evaluation of male factors and hysterosalpingography should be performed as a minimal evaluation prior to ovulation induction. When tubal or peritoneal diseases are suspected, laparoscopy is indicated.

Ovulation Induction Regimens

Clomiphene Citrate. The primary indication for the use of clomiphene citrate is normogonadotropic (or inappropriate) euprolactinemic anovulation. Amenorrheic women who respond to a progesterone challenge test are good candidates for treatment with clomiphene. Clomiphene citrate is an antiestrogen with some agonistic activity that binds to estrogen receptors in the hypothalamus to stimulate increased GnRH pulsatility, thereby stimulating pituitary FSH and LH secretion.

Therapy is initiated at a starting dose of 50 mg daily for 5 days, starting on day 2–5 after spontaneous or progestin-induced withdrawal bleeding. Dosage should be increased at 50-mg increments until normal ovulatory cycles are obtained. Failure to ovulate with 150–200 mg daily for 5 days usually necessitates use of other induction agents. Once an ovulatory dose is reached, further increases will not result in increased rates of conception. Clinical experience has demonstrated that about 75% of women will conceive while taking ≤100 mg of clomiphene citrate daily for 5 days.

Ovulation can be monitored by BBT, serum progesterone levels, or urinary LH tests or some combination of these. Adequate corpus luteum function should be confirmed by an in-phase timed endometrial biopsy. Pregnancy will usually occur within four to six ovulatory cycles, and other regimens should be considered if clomiphene fails after this interval. Failure to ovulate with 100–150 mg of clomiphene citrate may be associated with an abnormal LH surge, and addition of hCG (10,000 IU) may facilitate ovulation. Administration of hCG should be timed by follicular ultrasonography, as premature administration can produce premature luteinization. Dominant follicles should approach a mean diameter of 18–20 mm prior to hCG administration during clomiphene-induced cycles.

Cervical mucus should be evaluated during clomiphene citrate therapy, as dysmucorrhea results in about 15% of patients and may respond to supplemental estrogen therapy. Alternatively, intrauterine inseminations of partner's sperm will bypass viscous cervical mucus. Endometrial biopsy should also be evaluated, as up to 25% of cycles induced by clomiphene citrate may demonstrate luteal phase defect. Patients should be monitored periodically by pelvic examination to rule out ovarian enlargement.

Although wide variations in results have been reported, approximately 80% of patients will ovulate with clomiphene citrate. In contrast, the reported pregnancy rate is only about 40%. The discrepancy may result from the effect of clomiphene citrate on cervical mucus and endometrium, as well as other causes of infertility. In the absence of other infertility factors, conception rates of 80–90% have been reported. Although clomiphene is generally well tolerated, side effects can include ovarian enlargement (13%), hot flushes (10%), abdominal discomfort (5%), breast tenderness (2%), visual symptoms (1–2%), and headaches (1–2%). Multiple gestations, primarily twins, have been reported in 6–12% of pregnancies. Congenital anomalies and spontaneous abortion rates are not increased.

Gonadotropins. Although first indicated only for treatment of hypogonadotropic hypogonadism, in which a pregnancy rate of 80–90% has been reported, gonadotropins are also indicated for women who fail to ovulate or to conceive within six cycles of clomiphene citrate. Gonadotropins are also used to treat unexplained infertility and for assisted reproductive techniques. Contraindications to gonadotropin therapy include ovarian failure and untreated hyperprolactinemia, because alternative treatment methods are more appropriate. Inability to monitor follicular response adequately as well as lack of expertise in administration are other contraindications. Patients should be carefully counseled regarding realistic expectations and the extent of monitoring involved. Risks of therapy, including multiple gestation, hyperstimulation, and spontaneous abortion must be discussed before gonadotropin therapy is started. All patients should be thoroughly evaluated for additional causes of infertility prior to its use, and these factors should be corrected.

Treatment cycles with gonadotropins must be carefully monitored with serum estrogen determination and ultrasonographic evaluation of follicular growth. Transvaginal ultrasonography adds information on follicle number and size. Gonadotropins are started on cycle day 3 after baseline ultrasonography and an estradiol level, using an initial dosage of 75–150 units daily for 3 days. The subsequent regimen is determined by the patient's response. Transvaginal ultrasonography is begun when the serum estradiol level approaches 300 pg/ml and is performed every 1 to 3 days until ovulation is imminent. Human chorionic gonadotropin (5,000–10,000 U) is administered to simulate the LH surge when the lead follicle achieves a mean diameter of 18 mm in association with an estradiol level of 250–300 pg/ml per mature follicle. Most centers withhold hCG if the estradiol level is >2,000 pg/ml or there are four or more dominant follicles, thus reducing the risk of hyperstimulation and multiple gestation.

Most pregnancies occur within four to six cycles of therapy. Ovulation rates of 90% are usually observed. Success of gonadotropin ovulation induction varies with the etiology of anovulation. Women with hypothalamic amenorrhea have a cumulative pregnancy rate of 91%, while women with hypothalamic–pituitary dysfunction (PCO, normoestrogenic anovulation) who fail to conceive with clomiphene citrate have pregnancy rates ranging from 40% to 60%. Abortion rates are reported to be 25–30%. Complications include multiple gestation (20%) and ovarian hyperstimulation.

Regimens combining clomiphene citrate and gonadotropins–hCG have been used, resulting in decreased amounts of gonadotropins required. Clomiphene citrate, 100 mg, is begun on day 3 and gonadotropins are given in a serial or overlapping manner. Monitoring is the same as for gonadotropins alone.

Follicle-Stimulating Hormone. Although pure FSH has been suggested to improve pregnancy rates and decrease the risk of hyperstimulation in patients with PCO by providing a physiologic equalization of the LH:FSH ratio, pregnancy rate and ovarian hyperstimulation have not been significantly improved by use of pure FSH. High endogenous LH levels have been associated with abnormal ovulation and increased risk of spontaneous abortion.

Gonadotropin-Releasing Hormone. Although hypothalamic amenorrhea is the only approved indication for pulsatile GnRH, this agent has also been used successfully to induce ovulation and pregnancy in women with other forms of anovulation. For ovulation induction GnRH is given in a pulsatile fashion IV or subcutaneously by a computed pump. Ovulation rates of 55–60% have been reported. Ovulation has been induced with pulsatile GnRH in the presence of high prolactin levels and in patients with luteal phase defect refractory to other therapy. Patients with PCO typically respond poorly. However, new approaches using pretreatment with GnRH analogues may normalize the pituitary response to pulsatile GnRH and improve response. In a variety of intermittent injection protocols, GnRH is administered at 90–120-minute intervals through subcutaneous or intravenous routes. Hyperstimulation is uncommon, and multiple gestations, mostly twins, occur in about 7% of pregnancies.

Dopamine Agonists. In patients with elevated prolactin levels, treatment with a dopamine agonist, 2.5 mg two or three times daily, leads to the return of cyclic menses and ovulation in 2–3 months. Studies suggest low complication rates in pregnancies induced with the drug if the patients have normal computed tomography scans or microadenomas. Ovulation is restored in approximately 90% of patients, with an 80% pregnancy rate and a low incidence of spontaneous abortion. The incidence of multiple births is not increased. Dopamine agonists are usually discontinued as soon as pregnancy is established. Teratogenic effects have not been described. Nausea, headache, and faintness are common initial problems; however, tolerance is usually developed within several weeks.

Glucocorticoids. Glucocorticoids are a form of treatment for patients with excess adrenal androgen production resulting in ovulatory disorders. These agents suppress ACTH secretion and subsequently adrenal androgens. In addition to its adrenal effects, glucocorticoid treatment has been found to inhibit ovarian androgen secretion. To maximize suppression, prednisone, 5.0–7.5 mg, or dexamethasone, 0.5 mg, should be given as a single or split dose in such a way that most of the drug is given at night. Combined clomiphene–glucocorticoid therapy may improve ovulation rates when glucocorticoid therapy or clomiphene alone is unsuccessful.

Gonadotropin-Releasing Hormone Analogues. Use of GnRH analogues has been proposed prior to ovulation induction regimens using gonadotropins, pure FSH, or pulsatile GnRH. A regimen of at least 2–3 weeks of daily administration of GnRH analogues is necessary to suppress pituitary gonadotropins, resulting in suppression of tonic LH, premature LH surges, and improved follicular development. The major application has been in patients with PCO and in IVF.

Confirmation of Ovulation and Evaluation of Corpus Luteum Function

Assessment of ovulation is an important step in the infertility investigation. Until recently, methods based on progesterone secretion by the corpus luteum have been the primary methods to confirm ovulation. The three primary methods to document progesterone production and corpus luteum formation are BBT, serum progesterone levels, and endometrial biopsy. Basal body temperature, the daily record of oral, rectal, or vaginal temperature recorded by the patient on awakening, is biphasic in ovulatory cycles because of progesterone secretion, which produces a 0.5–1.0°F increase in basal temperature. Basal body temperature is most useful in evaluating the approximate day of ovulation and in assessing the length of the luteal phase. It does not confirm adequate luteal function. A temperature elevation of less than 11 days is abnormal.

Midluteal serum progesterone levels are helpful in confirming ovulation. Physician visits are not required, and numeric values that are reproducible from laboratory to laboratory are obtained. Pulsatility in progesterone secretion may make interpretation difficult; however, by the midluteal phase the frequency of progesterone pulses is reduced and a pattern similar to the diurnal pattern of cortisol production is noted. Serial sampling gives a more representative picture of corpus luteum function throughout the cycle. While progesterone levels >4 ng/ml confirm an ovulatory cycle, conception cycles usually are associated with levels >10 ng/ml. Although progesterone levels are an easy way to document ovulation, they are inadequate to exclude luteal phase defect.

Endometrial biopsy confirms ovulation but should be reserved for assessing endometrial maturity in the presence of an ovulatory BBT chart or elevated midluteal progesterone level. Biopsy should be obtained approximately 10–12 days after the LH surge and assessed by strict criteria. If abnormal, the biopsy should be repeated in a subsequent cycle. Biopsies are abnormal if they are desynchronous by more than 2 days from the cycle day, calculated prospectively from ovulation (based on LH surge). Evaluation and treatment of luteal phase defect is an extremely controversial issue. Optimal luteal phase assessment may require BBT, serum progesterone level, and an endometrial biopsy.

Tests such as BBT, progesterone levels, and endometrial biopsy are retrospective tests that confirm luteinization of the follicle but do not predict impending ovum release. Recently, in-home test kits to detect the LH surge and serial ultrasound examinations to detect follicle rupture have gained popularity. The LH surge kits predict ovulation 12–24 hours before follicle collapse in approximately 90% of women. Serial ultrasonography detects follicle rupture on the day of ovulation and excludes the diagnosis of luteinized unruptured follicle syndrome. Both tests are useful to time intercourse or procedures such as insemination but not to assess the quality of the corpus luteum function. Tests to predict ovulation and to evaluate corpus luteum function are summarized below:

- Tests to evaluate/predict ovulation
  —Serial transvaginal ultrasonography
  —LH surge kits
- Tests to evaluate corpus luteum function
  —BBT
  —Midluteal serum progesterone
  —Endometrial biopsy

Tubal and Peritoneal Factors

There are four basic types of tubal obstruction: 1) obstruction at the cornu, 2) obstruction in the isthmus, 3) fimbrial obstruction (see box), and 4) peritubal adhesions. The site of the obstruction can usually be determined by hysterosalpingography (cornual and isthmic obstructions) or by laparoscopy (fimbrial obstruction and peritubal adhesions).

Persistent pelvic adhesions may occur as a consequence of previous inflammatory conditions such as pelvic inflammatory disease, endometriosis, appendicitis with rupture, ruptured ovarian cysts such as dermoids, previous surgery, and foreign body reaction. Adhesive disease may result in infertility or may be associated with pelvic pain. Infertility may be the result of extrinsic adhesions involving the fallopian tubes or ovaries that prevent the development of a normal tuboovarian interface for oocyte retrieval, or infertility may be the result of intrinsic damage to the endosalpinx, creating intratubal synechiae and loss of the normal luminal surface. The latter cause is not amenable to surgical repair.

Resections of functional ovarian cysts, uterine suspensions, removal of small subserous fibroids, wedge resection of the ovaries before trial with clomiphene citrate, and unnecessary appendectomies may result in pelvic adhesions and impaired reproductive capacity. An aggressive approach to therapy early in the course of gonorrhea and chlamydial infection is always in order. If reparative tubal surgery is performed, avoidance of glove powder and foreign bodies (eg, suture fragments) in

---

Classification of the Extent of Tubal Disease with Distal Fimbrial Obstruction

Mild
Absent or small hydrosalpinx <15 mm diameter
Inverted fimbria easily recognized when patency achieved
No significant peritubal or periovarian adhesions
Preoperative hysterogram reveals a rugal pattern

Moderate
Hydrosalpinx 15–30 mm diameter
Fragments of fimbria not readily identified
Periovarian and/or peritubular adhesions without fixation, minimal cul-de-sac adhesions
Absence of a rugal pattern on preoperative hysterogram

Severe
Large hydrosalpinx >30 mm diameter
No fimbria
Dense pelvic or adnexal adhesions with fixation of the ovary and tube to either the broad ligament, pelvic sidewall, omentum, and/or bowel
Obliteration of the cul-de-sac
Frozen pelvis (adhesion formation so dense that limits of organs are difficult to define)

Rock JA, Katayama KP, Martin EJ, Woodruff JD, Jones HW Jr. Factors influencing the success of salpingostomy techniques for distal fimbrial obstruction. Reprinted with permission from The American College of Obstetricians and Gynecologists (Obstetrics and Gynecology, 1978, 52, 591)

---

the abdominal cavity; meticulous care in handling of tissues; use of delicate instruments, fine suture material, and magnification; and complete hemostasis are necessary.

Distal tubal occlusion is the most common site of tubal obstruction. Several options exist for reestablishing tubal patency, including fimbrioplasty, which is used when the adhesive disease is minimal and nearly normal fimbrial architecture is preserved, and neosalpingostomy, which is performed when a new opening is created in the oviduct.

Both procedures may be performed through the laparoscope or at the time of laparotomy. Comparable success rates have been reported, but laparoscopic surgery requires additional equipment and expertise. Successful term pregnancies have been reported in 5–30% of women who undergo treatment for moderate or severe distal tubal disease and 50–70% of women with mild disease. Patients with severe disease have a low rate of success and should be encouraged to consider IVF.

Proximal tubal disease is encountered less frequently, but it may be the consequence of previous tubal ligation, cornual polyps, salpingitis isthmica nodosa, endometriosis, or pelvic inflammatory disease. Surgical options include tubal reimplantation, tubocornual anastomosis, isthmic–isthmic anastomosis, or a cannulation of the proximal fallopian tube through the uterus. Tubocornual anastomosis is well suited for cornual or proximal tubal occlusion, and the results are considerably better than those with uterine implantation. Uterine cannulation of the proximal fallopian tube has been performed successfully by directing a cannula through the hysteroscope or under fluoroscopic visualization and dilating a balloon or advancing a catheter through the site of obstruction. Successful term pregnancies have been reported in 20–40% of women who undergo treatment.

Patients with combined proximal and distal tubal disease have a poor prognosis for fertility following surgical correction, probably reflecting extensive disease of the entire fallopian tube. These individuals are best treated by IVF, as are patients who have undergone previously unsuccessful tubal surgery or who are unwilling to proceed with tubal surgery.

Tubal Anastomosis

Approximately 1% of women who undergo tubal ligation regret their decisions and subsequently have a microsurgical tubal anastomosis procedure, usually after remarriage and the desire for additional children. Incorporation of the surgical microscope and fine nonreactive suture material into this procedure have dramatically improved the outcome. The success rate following tubal anastomosis depends on the type of anastomosis performed; isthmic–isthmic anastomosis yields the highest success rate, and ampullary–cornual anastomosis is associated with the poorest outcome. The type of sterilization procedure selected and the length of the remaining viable tube have been reported to affect the outcome. Procedures that result in the least amount of tissue destruction or removal, such as the Pomeroy procedure, and clip and ring applications are preferred. Unipolar tubal cautery and fimbriectomy are associated with the poorest results. Patients with tubal lengths of less than 4 cm following anastomosis generally have an unfavorable prognosis. Two to four percent of patients experience an ectopic pregnancy after tubal anastomosis.

Endometriosis

Endometriosis is associated with infertility in a significant number of women who are thoroughly evaluated. Severe or extensive endometriosis may cause tubal and ovarian adhesions and distortions. The etiology of infertility associated with mild to moderate endometriosis (stages I and II, American Fertility Society classification; see Fig. 4-3 in the Gynecology section) is not clearly understood, however. In infertile patients who are otherwise normal, laparoscopy should be carried out to determine whether endometriosis is present. It is found in approximately one third of infertile women.

Individual treatment of endometriosis should be based on the extent of the disease, the patient's desire for childbearing, the patient's age, and other coexisting medical and surgical factors. Three modalities of treatment are available: expectant, hormonal, and surgical.

Ovarian suppression or surgical excision has not been shown to improve pregnancy rates for mild to moderate endometriosis-associated infertility. However, medical therapy has been shown to relieve pain and reduce the amount of endometriosis visible at laparoscopy. Thus, medical therapy may be indicated for women with pain but not infertility.

Pseudopregnancy. Pseudopregnancy consists of a regimen with a continuous (acyclic) combined estrogen–progestogen preparation such as oral contraceptives containing no more than 35 μg of estrogen. The treatment may begin with one pill per day and should be increased to two pills per day if breakthrough bleeding occurs. Alternatively, a progestin such as medroxyprogesterone acetate may be prescribed at a dose of 10 mg three times daily (30 mg/d) orally. Other progestational agents have also been used, but their effectiveness has not been documented.

Pseudomenopause. Danazol, an isoxazol derivative of the synthetic steroid 17α- ethinyltestosterone, is given orally at a dose of 400–800 mg/d to induce pseudomenopause.

Gonadotropin-Releasing Hormone Agonists. Nafarelin acetate at a dose of 200 μg twice daily is administered intranasally. Leuprolide, 3.75 mg, is given IM each month. Goserelin, 3.6 mg, is given subcutaneously each month.

Women with minimal endometriosis have an approximate 30–70% chance of conceiving within 6 months of discontinuation of therapy if other infertility factors are corrected. Thus, in an asymptomatic woman in her 20s with minimal disease, a 6-month period of observation is in order. However, if pregnancy does not occur within a reasonable time period and the patient becomes symptomatic, a medical treatment plan with one of the several medical approaches listed above is recommended, either before or after conservative surgery.

Laparoscopy with electrocoagulation or laser vaporization of endometriomas and lysis of adhesions may be performed for patients with mild to moderate disease. For extensive endometriosis, a conservative surgical procedure is performed. Endometriomas should be resected, while superficial disease may be vaporized or fulgurated. Tubal adhesions are freed, and the uterus may be suspended. If midline pain has been severe, a presacral neurectomy may ameliorate dysmenorrhea. Pregnancy rates range approximately from 60% for moderate disease to 35% for severe disease.

Cervical Factors

The role of cervical factors in infertility remains a controversial one; however, the majority of practitioners believe that cervical mucus abnormalities in combination with other factors may contribute to subfertility and should be evaluated. There are two types of cervical problems: structural abnormalities of the cervix and inadequate or abnormal mucus production. Structural problems are often iatrogenic and result from surgical procedures such as conization. In these cases destruction of the endocervical epithelium or stenosis leads to inadequate mucus production and cervical crypts for sperm storage. Extensive cauterization or laser ablation may impair cervical function. However, there is no evidence that cryosurgery affects cervical factors in normal women. A decrease in mucus amount and cervical canal size is often noted in women with in utero exposure to diethylstilbestrol (DES). The significance of this observation is unclear.

Abnormalities of cervical mucus may involve both quantity and quality. This may include scant, qualitatively normal mucus; thick or cloudy mucus; or normal-appearing mucus that appears to immobilize or kill spermatozoa. Cervical factors are commonly evaluated by the postcoital test. This study is noninvasive, relatively inexpensive, and usually performed early in the workup. This test assesses both mucus quality and sperm–mucus interaction. It is scheduled for the preovulatory phase of the menstrual cycle, and timing is crucial. Mucus production occurs in response to estrogen stimulation, and even a small amount of progesterone produced early in the ovulatory period can adversely affect the quality of cervical mucus and the test. The study is usually done 1–2 days prior to ovulation, but if timing proves difficult, home LH monitoring can be performed and the test completed on the morning of the LH surge.

There are a variety of opinions regarding the timing of the assessment in relation to intercourse. Early testing (2–8 hours postcoitus) assesses mucus penetration, whereas a delay to 12–18 hours also permits the study of sperm storage and survival or screening for sperm antibodies.

At the time of the postcoital examination, the cervix is visualized and the size of the os and the quantity of mucus are assessed qualitatively. If a tightly closed os or scant mucus is seen, the practitioner should be alert to a high probability of either incorrect timing or an abnormal test. The cervix is swabbed, if necessary, and a sample of mucus removed from the external and midcanal. The samples are evaluated for quantity, spinnbarkeit, fluidity, ferning, and cell numbers. Vaginal epithelial cells are of no significance and represent vaginal contamination. The observation of white blood cells suggests infection requiring culture and appropriate antibiotic therapy. A numeric scoring system is recommended for scoring mucus samples.

Only after the mucus is evaluated is attention turned to sperm numbers and mobility. If mucus quality is poor and no sperm are seen, the test must be repeated either with better timing (ie, use of LH kit) or after mucus quality is corrected. Good-quality mucus with immotile or absent sperm in a couple with normal semen analysis suggests the presence of ASAs in the male or female partner, and sperm antibody testing is recommended. Further information about these couples can be obtained by studying sperm penetration into donor human or bovine mucus.

If visualization of the cervix reveals a tight os or no mucus, sounding should be performed and timing checked. If conization has been performed, one should have a high index of suspicion that endocervical epithelia have been destroyed.

Treatment of cervical factor varies with the cause. Stenosis and scarring may be treated with dilatation either surgically or with laminaria. In the past, estrogen was administered during the follicular phase of the cycle to treat abnormal cervical mucus. Currently, intrauterine insemination with washed sperm suspended in a buffer is used either to bypass the hostile cervical mucus or because of stenosis. Timing of the procedure is important, as no cervical reservoir exists to store sperm until oocyte release. Patients with cervical factor have a high pregnancy rate when treated with intrauterine insemination and may conceive promptly, even in unstimulated cycles.

Uterine Factors

A variety of uterine conditions have been implicated in infertility. These include endometritis, leiomyomata, intrauterine synechiae, congenital malformations, and polyps. Foreign bodies can also affect implantation. Most of these abnormalities can also cause recurrent abortion. However, tuberculous endometritis is clearly associated with infertility.

Several factors are postulated to cause infertility by distorting the cavity or preventing implantation either mechanically or by their effect on endometrial development. Most are detected by hysterosalpingography and confirmed by hysteroscopy. There is also increasing interest in the use of ultrasonography in combination with fluid distention of the uterus to evaluate uterine anomalies. Endometritis is identified by endometrial biopsy and culture.

Acute endometritis, which is associated with instrumentation of the uterus, foreign bodies, or gonorrhea, may cause transient infertility but is usually self-limiting. Occasionally a retained IUD or fetal tissue is noted.

Chronic endometritis is more likely to be a cause in long-standing infertility. Cultures for *Mycoplasma* species have been recommended in the past, but at present bacterial infections and tuberculosis are more significant, as *Mycoplasma* is a ubiquitous organism. If endometritis is noted on endometrial biopsy, bacterial culture, careful evaluation of histology for granulomas, and specific tuberculosis culture (if indicated) are recommended. Bacterial endometritis is managed by D&C supplemented by the administration of a broad-spectrum antibiotic, which is then continued for 10–14 days after the procedure.

Tuberculous endometritis is treated with a combination drug therapy for 18–21 months, with follow-up D&C and cultures. Because of associated tubal damage, pregnancy is infrequent.

Other endometrial abnormalities such as hyperplasia or carcinoma may cause infertility. Diagnosis is by endometrial biopsy or D&C. Treatment of hyperplasia is hormonal, either with progestins or ovulation induction. An occasional young, infertile patient with carcinoma in situ may be a candidate for hormonal therapy with careful follow-up.

Intrauterine adhesions following postabortal or postpartum curettage are associated with infertility if amenorrhea results or an extensive amount of endometrium is destroyed. Diagnosis is made by hysterosalpingography with confirmation and therapy by hysteroscopy. Uterine perforation is a common complication with severe adhesions, and special expertise is required. After resection, continuous estrogen therapy is given for 1–3 months, followed by progestin withdrawal. Restoration of menses and fertility in at least 50% of patients is common.

Support for the concept that infertility results from polyps, leiomyomata, or minor synechiae is minimal. A few reports detail pregnancies in previously infertile women after resection; however, no controlled series exists. In patients in whom no other factors are detected or who have failed to conceive with treatment of other factors, it is recommended that the physician evaluate any abnormalities noted on hysterosalpingography by hysteroscopy and resect lesions that are readily removable. This includes incising synechiae, resecting septa, shaving off small submucous leiomyomata, or removing intracavitary pedunculated leiomyomata. Abdominal myomectomy is recommended only when the uterus is judged to be sufficiently large to cause symptoms during pregnancy or when all other causes of infertility have been excluded and infertility is believed to be due to a large submucous or intramural leiomyoma.

There is little evidence to support a role for uterine anomalies in failure to conceive unless they involve obstruction of the vagina or cervix or significant atresia of the müllerian structures. The septate uterus is associated with fetal wastage, and many surgeons discuss resection of the septa at hysteroscopy prior to expensive ovulation therapy or assisted reproductive technologies.

Evaluation of the uterus is essential to a thorough evaluation of infertility. Several factors may have an impact on conception and should be treated if other fertility factors have been addressed or no other etiology is identified.

Clinical Applications of Gonadotropin-Releasing Hormone and Its Analogues

Gonadotropin-releasing hormone is produced and released in a pulsatile fashion from the arcuate nucleus and preoptic anterior hypothalamic area. It reaches the anterior pituitary through the portal system and is believed to bind to specific receptors in the anterior pituitary, where it stimulates the synthesis, storage, and secretion of LH and FSH in both males and females. Follicle-stimulating hormone and LH, in turn, are essential for gonadal function. Gonadotropin-releasing hormone is a decapeptide with an identical structure in all mammals, including humans. Like several other brain peptides, GnRH is synthesized as part of a much larger precursor peptide. When administered to females or males, GnRH stimulates a prompt and large release of LH and a smaller secretion of FSH.

Gonadotropin-releasing hormone is rapidly degraded by a peptidase and is cleared by glomerular filtration. Its half-life in peripheral circulation is short (2–4 minutes). To increase the potency and duration of action of GnRH, analogues with agonistic or antagonistic properties have been synthesized.

Substitution of an amino acid at position 6 or 10 results in analogues with agonistic activities, whereas modifications at positions 1, 2, 3, 5, 6, and 10 result in analogues with antagonistic properties. Administration of GnRH agonists produces an initial stimulation of pituitary gonadotropes, resulting in secretion of FSH and LH and the expected gonadal response. However, continuous or repeated administration of an agonist in an inappropriate (nonpulsatile) fashion or at nonphysiologic doses ultimately produces an inhibition of the pituitary–gonadal axis. Functional changes resulting from this inhibition include pituitary GnRH receptor down-regulation, gonadal gonadotropin receptor down-regulation, attenuated gonadotropin secretion, and decreased steroidogenesis and gametogenesis.

In normal men and women, GnRH agonists also suppress GH release stimulated by GH-releasing hormone; in persons with hyperprolactinemia, prolactin levels are suppressed. The hypothalamic pituitary–adrenal axis is not altered by GnRH agonists. The inhibitory effects of analogues are fully reversible. Agonists may also act directly on extrapituitary reproductive and nonreproductive target sites such as the gonads, uterus, placenta, and prostate.

Gonadotropin-releasing hormone antagonists have a direct inhibitory effect on reproductive processes. They compete for and occupy pituitary GnRH receptors, thus blocking the access of endogenous GnRH or exogenously administered agonists to their required recognition sites.

Gonadotropin-releasing hormone agonists are potent therapeutic agents with considerable advantages for clinical use. They cannot be administered orally but may be given parenterally, by nasal spray, or in vaginal pessaries. Implants that contain GnRH analogues and that are capable of slow drug release have been developed, and some are currently in use while others are undergoing clinical trials. The biologic tolerance of agonists is excellent. Their side effects are minimal.

Gonadotropin-releasing hormone and its analogues have been used or are being tried in patients with a large number of clinical conditions (see box). These are briefly reviewed.

Diagnostic Use

Acute injection of native GnRH to males or females elicits an immediate response that may be used to evaluate the status of hypothalamic–pituitary–gonadal function in a variety of neuroendocrine conditions in which amenorrhea, infertility, or both, are presenting symptoms. These provocative tests may differentiate hypothalamic disorders from primary pituitary deficiencies. Repeated daily infusions of GnRH rather than single-bolus administration have been recommended to overcome pituitary resistance and to activate a quiescent pituitary gland.

Clinical Applications

Ovulation Induction. Intravenous or subcutaneous pulsatile administration of GnRH by means of portable computerized infusion pumps in an appropriate amount and at a frequency that mimics endogenous release stimulates ovarian function and induces the menstrual cycle, ovulation, and pregnancy in women with hypothalamic amenorrhea.

For intravenous use, GnRH in doses of 20–100 ng/kg is commonly used, whereas larger doses of 5–20 mg given every 90 minutes are required for subcutaneous administration. Higher

> **Actual and Potential Indications for the Use of GnRH and Its Analogues***
>
> **GnRH**
> Diagnostic tests
> Ovulation induction (pulsatile)
> Delayed puberty
> Male hypogonadotropic hypogonadism
> Cryptorchidism
>
> **GnRH Analogues**
> Female application
> - Ovulation
>   — Induction (polycystic ovary syndrome, in vitro fertilization)
>   — Suppression (? contraception)
>   — Dysfunctional uterine bleeding
> - Hirsutism and virilization
> - Premenstrual syndrome
> - Endometriosis and ? adenomyosis
> - Leiomyomata
> - Hormone-dependent cancers
>   — Breast
>   — ? Endometrial and ovarian
> - Precocious puberty
>
> Male application
> - Precocious puberty
> - Contraception
> - Prostate cancer
>
> * GnRH indicates gonadotropin-releasing hormone; ?, suspected or possible indication.

doses are more effective for induction of ovulation but are also more likely to cause ovarian hyperstimulation. Gonadotropin-releasing hormone analogues have also been used for induction of ovulation in patients with PCO and in those who are undergoing ovarian stimulation for IVF or GIFT. For these indications, the pituitary function is initially suppressed with a preparation of a GnRH analogue to inhibit the endogenous source of gonadotropin, and then the ovary is stimulated with human gonadotropins and hCG to initiate follicular development and ovulation.

Endometriosis. The ability of GnRH to produce amenorrhea and anovulation has provided the basis for the use of GnRH agonists in the management of endometriosis. A relationship between endometriosis and infertility has been documented repeatedly. Approximately 30–60% of women with unexplained infertility are found to have pelvic endometriosis. Mild and moderate stages of endometriosis are usually treated with medication, whereas the more severe cases are managed surgically. Several GnRH analogues have been evaluated clinically for the management of endometriosis (Table 6-6). Three of these preparations, namely, nafarelin acetate, leuprolide acetate, and goserelin, are available for the management of endometriosis. Their suppressive effect on endometriosis is comparable to that of danazol. Preliminary studies indicate that GnRH analogues may also be of benefit for adenomyosis.

Uterine Leiomyomata. The hypoestrogenic condition induced by GnRH analogues may bring about a marked decrease (40–50%) in the size of leiomyomata within 3 months of treatment. After discontinuation of the treatment, however, the leiomyomata regrow to their original size within a few months. Thus, this treatment may become a valuable adjunct for preoperative management of larger leiomyomata or for arrest of bleeding and correction of anemia. The drug may also be used for small symptomatic leiomyomata, particularly in perimenopausal women.

Hormone-Dependent Tumors. Suppression of gonadotropin secretion by high doses of GnRH agonists is beneficial in some hormone-dependent and malignant tumors of the breast and the prostate. The mechanism of action of these drugs involves a decrease in the secretion of pituitary gonadotropin and gonadal steroids, resulting in medical castration. Agonists may also have a direct effect on steroidogenesis. Specific binding sites of GnRH and analogues have been demonstrated in both ovarian and endometrial cancers. These GnRH-binding sites could mediate a direct inhibitory effect of its analogues on the proliferation of these malignancies. Clinical studies in progress should elucidate the usefulness of the analogues in managing these neoplasms.

Other Indications

Suppression of ovarian function by GnRH analogues is accompanied by a reduction of both estrogen and androgen production. In hirsute or virilized females, this property of GnRH agonists can be used to reduce hair growth and alleviate the clinical manifestation of hyperandrogenism. For long-term use, a combination of a GnRH analogue and an oral contraceptive has been shown to successfully reduce hirsutism and prevent undesirable side effects of GnRH analogues.

Maturation of the pituitary–gonadal system in both males and females requires pulsatile GnRH stimulation. Idiopathic

TABLE 6-6. GONADOTROPIN-RELEASING HORMONE AGONISTS STUDIED FOR GYNECOLOGIC CONDITIONS

Generic Name	Route of Administration	Dosage
Buserelin	Subcutaneous	200 µg/d
	Intranasal	300–344 µg × 4 d
Decapeptyl	Intramuscular depot	3 mg/mo
Goserelin	Subcutaneous implant	3.6 mg/mo
Histerelin	Subcutaneous injection	100 µg/d
Leuprolide	Subcutaneous injection	500–1,000 µg/d
	Intranasal	400 µg × 4 d
	Intramuscular depot	3.75–7.5 mg/mo
Nafarelin	Intranasal	200 µg × 2 d
	Intramuscular depot	3 mg/mo
Tryptorelin	Intramuscular depot	2–4 mg/mo

precocious puberty may be viewed as a disease characterized by premature hypothalamic GnRH activity. Suppression of pituitary gonadal function in patients with this condition has been the aim of various therapeutic modalities. Chronic administration of GnRH agonists has proven to be a remarkably safe and effective therapy for children of both sexes with precocious puberty. Within 6–18 months after beginning daily treatment, pubertal levels and patterns of secretion of gonadotropins and sex steroids revert to prepubertal levels and patterns. A more striking aspect of this therapy is the regression of secondary sexual characteristics and the cessation of menstrual bleeding.

Since administration of GnRH superagonists results in the down-regulation of pituitary activity and suppression of gonads, they also have been evaluated for their potential as a contraceptive in both females and males. Their usefulness for this purpose, however, awaits further study regarding their safety and effectiveness.

Side effects of GnRH analogue therapy include symptoms of hypoestrogenism, such as dryness of the vagina and hot flushes. A modest decrease in bone density has been observed in patients treated with GnRH analogues for a period of 3 months or longer. In most cases there is recovery from osteopenia following the cessation of treatment. Occasionally, however, there may be a delay in the restoration of bone density. For this reason, caution should be exercised in prolonged or repetitive use of these agents. To prevent bone loss and symptoms of hypoestrogenism when prolonged use of GnRH analogues is desirable, addition of a small dose of a progestogen alone or with estrogen has been advocated. Preliminary studies indicate that the add-back regimen may be useful in conditions such as endometriosis, leiomyomata, DUB, and hirsutism when chronic administration of GnRH analogues is contemplated. The rationale behind add-back therapy is that sufficient steroids are added to GnRH analogue treatment to diminish the symptoms and sequelae of hypoestrogenism without compromising their efficacy.

Gonadotropin-Releasing Hormone Antagonists

Gonadotropin-releasing hormone antagonists have a half-life of more than 24 hours and have the advantage of inducing an immediate inhibition of LH and FSH release and, hence, suppression of gonadal activity.

The administration of a GnRH antagonist is associated with histamine release, which may be related to a basic amino acid in position 6. Clinical evaluation of GnRH antagonists is limited. Primate studies and preliminary human experience indicate that these compounds may be useful for suppression of ovulation, for contraception in males or females, and for IVF. Further clinical application of these antagonists awaits the development of safer and better tolerated formulations.

IMMUNOLOGIC ASPECTS OF INFERTILITY

The ability of spermatozoa coated with antibody to penetrate and survive within cervical mucus is often impaired. The extent of this impairment depends on 1) the proportion of spermatozoa in the ejaculate coated with immunoglobulin, 2) the amount of antibody coating the sperm surface, and 3) the immunoglobulin class (immunoglobulin G [IgG] versus IgA). Hence, postcoital testing timed to detection of the preovulatory urinary LH surge and BBT charts remains the best initial method available to screen for ASAs. The presence of fewer than five motile sperm per high-power field, in association with normal preovulatory cervical mucus and normal semen parameters, is highly suggestive of the presence of an immunologic problem. Suspicion should be aroused when complete immobilization of sperm is detected or when spermatozoa are observed shaking in place within cervical mucus.

The behavior of sperm in the cervical mucus depends on the types of antibodies present and their specificity for the sperm surface. In men with autoimmunity to the sperm, when 100% of spermatozoa in the ejaculate are coated with antibody, it is rare to find even one or two motile sperm per high-power field in a well-timed postcoital test despite millions of motile spermatozoa in the ejaculate. These men should then be considered functionally oligospermic; that is, their spermatozoa cannot enter the female reproductive tract, although they may be present in high numbers in semen. In contrast, antibody binding to limited regions of the sperm surface, such as the tail tip, results in no loss in sperm penetrating ability, and these ASAs should not impair the likelihood of fertilization.

In women, high concentrations of non–complement-fixing IgA antibodies present in cervical mucus may result in sperm entrapment, leading to their shaking in place. Conversely, complement-fixing antibodies of the IgG and IgM class, which promote sperm plasma membrane damage, will lead to their immobilization. This process may take as long as 6–7 hours, and for this reason, overnight postcoital testing (8–10 hours) provides a clearer indication of antibody-mediated sperm damage than does a short interval (2 hours) of observation after coitus.

Antibody Testing

Antibody studies done in humans have generally focused on circulating ASAs in serum that show immobilizing or agglutinating activities against the spermatozoa. However, the presence of sperm antibodies in the reproductive tract in semen or cervical mucus appears to be of greater clinical importance.

In men, the amount of immunoglobulin bound to the sperm surface at the time of ejaculation depends on 1) the transudation of ASAs from serum into epididymal, prostatic, and seminal vesicle secretions and their mixing with sperm at ejaculation; 2) the local production of IgA antibodies within the genital tract; and 3) the elapsed time since the last ejaculation. Hence, those ASAs coating the sperm surface reflect the additive effects of several mechanisms of immunoglobulin secretion within the male reproductive tract. Thus, tests capable of detecting immunoglobulin on living sperm recovered from the ejaculate provide an important means to determine when autoimmunity to sperm exists, and if so, to determine its clinical significance. As a corollary, the presence of humoral ASA in serum is not relevant to an individual's fertility unless these antibodies are also present within the reproductive tract.

The diagnosis of clinically relevant immunity to sperm in women is difficult, given the current inability to adequately sample secretions of the uterus and fallopian tubes. In addition, immunoglobulin secretion within each of the reproductive compartments (cervix, uterus, fallopian tubes) is under hormonal control and exhibits different mechanisms in the regulation of antibody transport. As an example, estradiol lowers the content of immunoglobulins within cervical mucus while stimulating the active transport of IgA and transudation of IgG into the uterine lumen.

In a study of serum samples from known fertile women, supplied by the World Health Organization reference bank, 40% contained immunoglobulins that reacted with spermatozoa, usually directed against the tail tip. These results suggest that there is a continuum in the extent of the immunity to sperm and that those mechanisms in women that prevent immunization to paternally derived antigens on sperm are imperfect. Hence, care must be exercised in distinguishing between a "positive" result and a clinically significant result, whether based on immunobead binding or any ASA assay. It is clear that results of these tests should not be interpreted in the absence of clinical correlates. This is true despite the development of better ASA assays and increasing laboratory evidence that these phenomena may lead to infertility.

Specific Laboratory Tests

Spontaneously occurring antibodies that react with intracellular antigens within permeable sperm have been detected by indirect immunofluorescence in 90% of sera of children and 60% of adults. Conversely, ASAs directed against antigens located on the sperm surface (which have the potential to cause infertility) are uncommon and occur in only 5–10% of unselected infertile men and women. These clinically significant ASAs must be distinguished from the high incidence of "immunologic background noise."

Agglutinating Antibody
Sperm agglutination tests are sensitive and specific means of detecting ASAs directed against the sperm surface. Both macroscopic (gel agglutination) and microscopic tests are available. However, failure to give careful attention to controls may lead to false-positive results.

Immobilizing Antibody
The percentage of motile sperm observed after incubation of spermatozoa, heat-inactivated patient serum, and complement is determined and compared with sperm motility after an incubation in which heat-inactivated normal human serum replaces that of the patient. While it correlates well with infertility and is associated with a low incidence of false-positive results, this test will not detect ASAs of the IgA class that do not interact with complement.

Immunobead Binding
Immunobead binding allows the direct detection of immunoglobulins on the surface of living spermatozoa. The region of the spermatozoon surface to which spermatozoa antibodies have bound, the proportion of spermatozoa in the ejaculate that is coated with antibody, and the isotypes of these antibodies can be determined. The test can be used directly to assess antibody binding to sperm in a semen specimen or, indirectly, to study seminal plasma, serum, follicular fluid, or solubilized cervical mucus.

Treatment

The impact of immunity to spermatozoa on sperm function is complex. The immunologic response to spermatozoa in men and women is polyclonal; that is, several different antibodies to different sperm-associated antigens are produced. These may be of different immunoglobulin classes (IgG, IgA, and IgM), which are structurally different molecules that interact with complement in different ways. The additive effects of four loci of action (sperm transport, the kinetics of the acrosome reaction, the interaction of sperm with the zona pellucida, and the oolemma) must all be placed within a complex equation. Several studies have shown that ASAs present in serum of men and serum of women reduce but do not inhibit the ability of spermatozoa to bind to and fertilize the egg.

Once the specificities of the various ASAs for their antigenic determinants on spermatozoa are known, these varying and perhaps opposing effects should be more clinically predictable for each individual. Currently, however, given the inability to predict the effects of these antibodies on sperm function and the fact that the etiology of immunities to sperm remains unknown, the most practical clinical treatment approach is an empirical one, directed not against the cause but rather against an abnormal response.

While initially reported to be promising in the treatment of women with immunity to spermatozoa, condom therapy has been found to be ineffective and has been abandoned.

The use of high-dose corticosteroids has been advocated because they have an immunosuppressive effect, acting at the level of antigen processing by macrophages and impairing complement-mediated cytotoxicity. Several uncontrolled reports have noted success with various regimens, but only a few studies have documented a reduction in antibody titer. Given the possibility of peptic ulcers, abnormalities in glucose tolerance, and the rare but serious complication of aseptic hip joint necrosis during treatment, one must currently remain conservative about their use pending further, more controlled, studies.

Controlled ovarian hyperstimulation and intrauterine insemination with washed sperm has also been used for the management of immunologic infertility, with modest success.

In men with autoimmunity to sperm, although ASAs remain bound to the sperm surface after their recovery from semen and cannot be removed by washing or during capacitation of sperm, it is good laboratory practice to produce the semen specimen directly on hospital premises into the sperm-processing solution, rather than transport it from home, during which time ASAs continue to accumulate on spermatozoa, increasing the likelihood of their agglutination and immobilization. The technique of ejaculating directly into the collection buffer, with immediate centrifugation through a colloidal suspension of silica, appears to maximize the sperm recovery while minimizing the proportion of antibody-coated spermatozoa obtained.

If this approach does not succeed within a reasonable clinical trial period (four to six intrauterine insemination treatment cycles), IVF should be performed to document whether sperm attachment to the zona pellucida, its penetration, and fertilization are normal or impaired. In vitro fertilization, although technically intense and expensive, offers the couple a significant chance of achieving pregnancy whether in the presence of autoantibodies to sperm in men or ASAs in women. If the normalcy of fertilization is documented, three to four additional attempts at IVF would be reasonable. Conversely, a severely impaired fertilization rate might be an indication for micromanipulation of the gametes with subzonal injection of spermatozoa into the perivitelline space in subsequent cycles. However, this procedure must be regarded as investigational. The effectiveness of these procedures as applied to immunologic infertility needs to be clearly documented through future studies.

GENERAL STRATEGY OF TREATMENT

All factors should be carefully investigated to determine whether the infertility has multiple causes. All factors should be treated concurrently to maximize the chance for a subsequent pregnancy. Alternative therapies should be clearly presented to the patient. Decisions are not always clear, especially when multiple factors are involved or when the factors that have been identified are associated with relative infertility. Couples who are well informed about the disease process and the options available can often assess their chances for success realistically. To facilitate this, patient education materials should be made available to them. A referral base of other professionals should be developed and made available, such as a urologist with expertise in male infertility, a mental health professional, and a reproductive endocrinologist for consultation and referral as necessary. In addition, a trained office nurse can be a valuable resource for monitoring therapy and providing patient education.

If the results of the infertility evaluation are normal, the prognosis for a pregnancy is good. In one study, patients with unexplained infertility had a cumulative pregnancy rate of 65%, with 81% of these couples achieving a full-term pregnancy. Because the potential for a spontaneous cure is high, it is important to be cautious in the application of untried empirical treatments that may actually delay conception.

Patients who have specific disorders should be treated by standard means first. For example, anovulatory women should be treated with the lowest effective dose of the cheapest medication (ie, clomiphene citrate) and should use timed intercourse. The fact that use of gonadotropins and intrauterine insemination may yield a higher per-cycle pregnancy rate does not justify using this expensive and time-consuming modality as the initial therapy.

Patients with tubal disease have high pregnancy rates with assisted reproductive technologies, but women with findings amenable to surgical correction, especially by laparoscopic means, should be offered surgery as the first-line therapy unless there is extensive damage to the reproductive organs.

Couples with unexplained infertility or those who fail to conceive with conventional therapy for identified causes should be reevaluated periodically to determine whether a particular factor has become inadequate since the last evaluation. Infertility is a dynamic process, and reevaluation may well reveal a new factor that is affecting the couple's ability to conceive. Patients who do not conceive after 1 year of interventional therapy or 3 years of observation, after thorough evaluation, and women approaching age 40 have a low probability of conception and more aggressive means are indicated. Assisted reproductive technologies are an appropriate recommendation.

Whether infertility results from identifiable factors or the cause is unknown, these couples face intense and often overwhelming emotional turmoil. Often, they have been frustrated by previous therapeutic interventions. The anxiety may lead to interpersonal and sexual problems for the couple, and the physician should address these issues early in therapy.

The practitioner should remain alert to patient preferences, should always recommend the least invasive and expensive therapy first, and should ensure the availability of the physician or staff for counseling as needed.

BIBLIOGRAPHY

Investigation and Treatment of the Male

Aitken RJ. Evaluation of human sperm function. Br Med Bull 1990;46:654–674

Cohen J, Edwards R, Fehilly C, Fishel S, Hewitt J, Purdy J, et al. In vitro fertilization: a treatment for male infertility. Fertil Steril 1985; 43:422–432

Colpi GM, Pozza D, eds. Diagnosing male infertility: new possibilities and limits. Basel: S Karger AG, 1992

Laufer N, Simon A. Treatment of male infertility by gamete micromanipulation. Hum Reprod 1992;7(1 suppl):73–80

Liu DY, Baker HW. Tests of human sperm function and fertilization in vitro. Fertil Steril 1992;58:465–483

Oehninger S, Franken D, Alexander N, Hodgen GD. Hemizona assay and its impact on the identification and treatment of human sperm dysfunctions. Andrologia 1992;24:307–321

Santen RJ, Swerdloff RS, eds. Male reproductive dysfunction: diagnosis and management of hypogonadism, infertility and impotence. New York: Marcel Dekker, 1986

Siegal MS. The male fertility investigation and the role of the andrology laboratory. J Reprod Med 1993;38:317–334

Tanagho EA, Lue TF, McClure RD, eds. Contemporary management of impotence and infertility. Baltimore: Williams and Wilkins, 1988

Investigation and Treatment of the Female

Aiman J. Infertility, diagnosis and management. New York: Springer-Verlag, 1984

American College of Obstetricians and Gynecologists. Infertility. ACOG Technical Bulletin 125. Washington, DC: ACOG, 1989

Blacker CM. Ovulation stimulation and induction. Endocrinol Metab Clin North Am 1992;21:57–84

Collins JA, Wrixon W, Janes LB, Wilson EH. Treatment-independent pregnancy among infertile couples. N Engl J Med 1983;309:1201–1206

Crowley WF Jr, Filicori M, Spratt DI, Santoro NF. The physiology of gonadotropin-releasing hormone (GnRH) secretion in men and women. Recent Prog Horm Res 1985;41:473–531

Dmowski WP. Danazol-induced pseudomenopause in the management of endometriosis. Clin Obstet Gynecol 1988;31:829–839

Dodson WC, Hughes CL, Whitesides DB, Haney AF. The effect of leuprolide acetate on ovulation induction with human menopausal gonadotropins in polycystic ovary syndrome. J Clin Endocrinol Metab 1987;65:95–100

Dodson WC, Whitesides DB, Hughes CL Jr, Easley HA 3d, Haney AF. Superovulation with intrauterine insemination in the treatment of infertility: a possible alternative to gamete intrafallopian transfer and in vitro fertilization. Fertil Steril 1987;48:441–445

Filicori M, Flamigni C, Meriggiola M, Cognigni G, Valdiserri A, Ferrari P, et al. Ovulation induction with pulsatile gonadotropin-releasing hormone: technical modalities and clinical perspectives. Fertil Steril 1991;56:1–13

Friedman AJ, Harrison-Atlas D, Barbieri RL, Benacerraf B, Gleason R, Schiff I. A randomized, placebo-controlled, double-blind study evaluating the efficacy of leuprolide acetate depot in the treatment of uterine leiomyomata. Fertil Steril 1989;51:251–256

Friedman AJ, Hornstein MD. Gonadotropin-releasing hormone agonist plus estrogen-progestin "add-back" therapy for endometriosis-related pelvic pain. Fertil Steril 1993;60:236–241

Friedman AJ, Reim MS, Harrison-Atlas D, Garfield JM, Doubilet PM. A randomized, placebo-controlled, double-blind study evaluating leuprolide acetate depot treatment before myomectomy. Fertil Steril 1989;52:728–733; errata 54:749

Griffith CS, Grimes DA. The validity of the postcoital test. Am J Obstet Gynecol 1990;162:615–620

Gysler M, March CM, Mishell DR Jr, Bailey EJ. A decade's experience with an individualized clomiphene treatment regimen including its effect on the postcoital test. Fertil Steril 1982;37:161–167

Halman LJ, Abbey A, Andrews FM. Why are couples satisfied with infertility treatment? Fertil Steril 1993;59:1046–1054

Hammond MG, Talbert LM, eds. Infertility: A practical guide for the physician. 3rd ed. Boston: Blackwell Scientific Publications, 1992

Henzl MR, Corson SL, Moghissi K, Buttram VC, Berquist C, Jacobson J. Administration of nasal nafarelin as compared with oral danazol for endometriosis: a multicenter double-blind comparative clinical trial. N Engl J Med 1988;318:485–489

Hughes EG, Fedorkow DM, Collins JA. A quantitative overview of controlled trials in endometriosis-associated infertility. Fertil Steril 1993;59:963–970

Hughes EG, Fedorkow DM, Daya S, Sagle MA, Van de Koppel P, Collins JA. The routine use of gonadotropin-releasing hormone agonists prior to in vitro fertilization and gamete intrafallopian transfer: a meta-analysis of randomized controlled trials. Fertil Steril 1992;58:888–896

Kelly AC, Jewelewicz R. Alternate regimens for ovulation induction in polycystic ovarian disease. Fertil Steril 1990;54:195–202

Luborsky JL, Visintin I, Boyers S, Asari T, Caldwell B, DeCherney A. Ovarian antibodies detected by immobilized antigen immunoassay in patients with premature ovarian failure. J Clin Endocrinol Metab 1990;70:69–75

Moghissi KS. Cervical and uterine factors in infertility. Obstet Gynecol Clin North Am 1987;14:887–904

Moghissi KS. Treatment of endometriosis with estrogen-progestin combination and progestogens alone. Clin Obstet Gynecol 1988;31:823–828

Moghissi KS. Gonadotropin releasing hormones: clinical applications in gynecology. J Reprod Med 1990;35:1097–1107

Page H. Estimation of the prevalence and incidence of infertility in a population: a pilot study. Fertil Steril 1989;51:571–577

Reichel RP, Schweppe KW. Goserelin (Zoladex) depot in the treatment of endometriosis. Zoladex Endometriosis Study Group. Fertil Steril 1992;57:1197–1202

Rock JA. Uterine reconstructive surgery. In: Rock JA, Murphy AA, Jones HW Jr, eds. Female reproductive surgery. Baltimore: Williams and Wilkins, 1992:113–145

Rock JA, Katayama KP, Martin EJ, Woodruff JD, Jones HW Jr. Factors influencing the success of salpingostomy techniques for distal fimbrial obstruction. Obstet Gynecol 1978;52:591–596

Rock JA, Markham SM. Endometriosis. In: Rakel R, ed. Conn's current therapy. Philadelphia: WB Saunders, 1989:942–943

Schlaff WD, Rock JA, eds. Decision making in reproductive endocrinology. Boston: Blackwell Scientific Publications, 1993

Schlaff WD, Hassiokos DK, Damewood MD, Rock JA. Neosalpingostomy for distal tubal obstruction: prognostic factors and impact of surgical technique. Fertil Steril 1990;54:984–990

Shoham Z, Balen A, Patel A, Jacobs HS. Results of ovulation induction using human menopausal gonadotropin or purified follicle-stimulating hormone in hypogonadotropic hypogonadism patients. Fertil Steril 1991;56:1048–1053

Shoham Z, Homburg R, Jacobs HS. Induction of ovulation with pulsatile GnRH. Baillieres Clin Obstet Gynaecol 1990;4:589–608

Siegler AM, Valle RF. Therapeutic hysteroscopic procedures. Fertil Steril 1988;50:685–701

Singh KB, Dunnihoo DR, Mahajan DK, Bairnsfather LE. Clomiphene-dexamethasone treatment of clomiphene-resistant women with and without the polycystic ovary syndrome. J Reprod Med 1992;37:215–218

Immunologic Aspects of Infertility

Ayvaliotis B, Bronson RA, Rosenfeld D, Cooper GW. Conception rates in couples where autoimmunity to sperm is detected. Fertil Steril 1985;43:739–742

Bronson RA, Cooper GW, Phillips DM. Effects of anti-sperm antibodies on human sperm ultrastructure and function. Hum Reprod 1989;4:653–657

Bronson RA, Cooper GW, Rosenfeld DL. Correlation between regional specificity of antisperm antibodies to the spermatozoan surface and complement-mediated sperm immobilization. Am J Reprod Immunol 1982;2:222–224

DeAlmeida M, Gazagne I, Jeulin C, Herry M, Belaisch-Allart J, Frydman R, et al. In vitro processing of sperm with autoantibodies and in-vitro fertilization results. Hum Reprod 1989;4:49–53

Hellstrom WJ, Overstreet JW, Samuels SJ, Lewis EL. The relationship of circulating antisperm antibodies to sperm surface antibodies in infertile men. J Urol 1988;140:1039–1044

Hendry WF, Hughes L, Scammell G, Pryor JP, Hargreave TB. Comparison of prednisolone and placebo in subfertile men with antibodies to spermatozoa. Lancet 1990;335:84–88

Jager S, Kremer J, Kuiken J, Mulder I. The significance of the Fc part of antispermatozoal antibodies for the shaking phenomenon in the sperm-cervical mucus contact test. Fertil Steril 1981;36:792–797

Meinertz H, Linnet L, Fogh-Andersen P, Hjort T. Antisperm antibodies and fertility after vasovasostomy; a follow-up study of 216 men. Fertil Steril 1990;54:315–321

Moghissi KS, Sacco AG, Borin K. Immunolgic infertility. I. Cervical mucus antibodies and postcoital test. Am J Obstet Gynecol 1980;136:941–950

Vazquez-Levin M, Kaplan P, Guzman I, Grunfeld L, Garrisi GJ, Navot D. The effect of female antisperm antibodies on in vitro fertilization, early embryonic development, and pregnancy outcome. Fertil Steril 1991;56:84–88

Recurrent Spontaneous Abortion

Clinically recognized spontaneous abortion occurs in 15% of married women aged 15–44 in the United States, and 3–4% experience recurrent spontaneous abortions. Dealing with spontaneous abortion in office practice takes patience, understanding, and time. Therapy begins with education.

RECURRENT RISK

For decades, it was believed that with each pregnancy loss, the risk of subsequent losses escalated to the point that after three spontaneous abortions a patient was thought to have an 80–90% chance of a pregnancy loss. This belief was refuted in 1964 when studies by Warburton reassessed the risks of women experiencing pregnancy losses (Table 6-7). The true risk of pregnancy loss is approximately 15–20% in the first pregnancy and rises to 35% after one spontaneous abortion, but does not increase thereafter. If the woman has at least one liveborn, the risk of her first spontaneous abortion is 15%, and after one spontaneous abortion rises to 25% with no further increase.

The prevalence of spontaneous abortion increases with maternal age. The risk of spontaneous abortion begins to increase rapidly at age 35 and at age 40 is approximately twice that at age 20. Although one might suspect that the reason for the increase is the known increase in aneuploid conception with increasing maternal age, this does not wholly account for the rapid rise in spontaneous abortion. Indeed, larger numbers of euploid pregnancies are lost with increasing maternal age. This suggests that some unknown uterine factor, perhaps decreased uterine blood supply, chronic infections, or diminished luteal response, changes with age. However, there is no increased risk with gravidity.

Most spontaneous abortions occur because of karyotypic abnormalities in the fetus. Approximately 50–70% of first-trimester abortuses are karyotypically abnormal; 30% of second-trimester abortuses and 3% of stillbirths are karyotypically abnormal. The remaining nongenetic causes include anatomic, infectious, hormonal, immune, and environmental factors. Patients should be evaluated for causes of repeated spontaneous abortion and treated for all those identified. In addition, avoidance of smoking, drinking alcohol, and exposure to environmental chemicals known to increase the risk of spontaneous abortion is recommended.

GENETICS

The most common single cause of first trimester spontaneous abortion is genetic abnormalities. Of the 50–70% of first-trimester abortuses that are karyotypically abnormal, approximately 50% have autosomal trisomy. All chromosomal trisomies except trisomy 1 have been found in spontaneous abortuses, the most common being trisomy 16. In about 25% of chromosomally abnormal abortuses, monosomy X (45,X) is found. Polyploidy accounts for another 20%. Patients having a karyotypically abnormal abortus are more likely to have another abortus that is abnormal. Conversely, if the first abortus has a normal karyotype, subsequent abortuses are likely to be normal. Although no therapy can be offered a patient with recurrent karyotype abnormalities, at least she can be advised of the reason for her pregnancy failures. Most

TABLE 6-7. RECURRENCE RISK FIGURES USEFUL FOR COUNSELING WOMEN WITH REPEATED SPONTANEOUS ABORTIONS

	Prior Abortions	% Risk
Women with liveborn infants	0	12
	1	24
	2	26
	3	32
	4	26
Women without liveborn infants	2 or more	40–45

Data from Warburton D, Fraser FC. Spontaneous abortion risks in man: data from reproductive histories collected in a medical genetics unit. Am J Human Genet 1964;16:1–25; Poland BJ, Miller JR, Jones DC, Trimble BK. Reproductive counseling in patients who have had a spontaneous abortion. Am J Obstet Gynecol 1977;127:685–691

abnormalities result from the disorders of meiosis in gamete formation or in mitosis after fertilization, but in 5% of couples a chromosomal abnormality may be found in the parents.

About 5% of couples experiencing recurrent abortions and having an anomalous child or a stillbirth will carry a translocation. This risk rises to 10% if the couples themselves have a sibling who is the parent of an anomalous child or a stillborn infant. Artificial insemination with donor sperm or IVF with donor oocytes may be offered to patients whose chromosome abnormality would prohibit a normal liveborn (for example, a 21–21 translocation).

CONGENITAL UTERINE ANOMALIES

Uterine anomalies occur in 0.04–0.13% of women; hysterosalpingography demonstrates uterine anomalies in 1–3% of women with any reproductive problem and in 10–15% of women with repeated abortion. These anomalies result from derangement of müllerian ducts fusion. In addition to embryologic errors that typically occur between 6 and 12 embryologic weeks (ie, 8–14 weeks after the last menstrual period), first-trimester exposure to DES is associated with uterine anomalies that are included in classification systems of these problems.

Nomenclature and Classification

The American Fertility Society's revised classification is a helpful guide in discussing the various clinical presentations and treatment of uterine anomalies.

Class I: Hypoplasia/agenesis—Hypoplasia/agenesis anomalies include congenital absence of the vagina, cervix, fallopian tubes, or uterus, or various combinations thereof.

Class II: Unicornuate uterus—Unicornuate uterus may be truly unicornuate with total agenesis of one side of the müllerian duct or a dominant uterus with an attached rudimentary horn. The rudimentary horn may or may not have a cavity of its own; if a cavity is present, it may or may not communicate with the dominant uterine cavity. The importance of these anatomic combinations lies in the various clinical presentations, depending on the variant that is present.

Class III: Uterus didelphys—Resulting from failed fusion of the müllerian ducts, uterus didelphys is often associated with two cervices, two vaginas, and a longitudinal vaginal septum.

Class IV: Bicornuate uterus—A bicornuate uterus is a less severe failure of fusion than uterus didelphys and is not associated with a double cervix or vagina.

Class V: Septate uterus—Failure of resorption of the midline uterine septum of varying degrees produces a septum of varying lengths; clinical severity tends to be related to the amount of the cavity that is bisected by the septum.

Class VI: Arcuate uterus—Considered by most to be either a normal variant or the least involvement possible in a class V uterus, an arcuate uterus is classically described as a saddle-shaped uterus with fundal depression, with very little effect on the overall size or shape of the endometrial cavity.

Class VII: DES related—Women exposed in utero to DES may experience reproductive difficulties because of uteri with very small T-shaped cavities or other disturbances in the genital tract.

Clinical Presentations and Management

Somatic growth and sexual development are otherwise normal in women with congenital absence or anomaly of the müllerian ducts. The clinical presentations may be best discussed within the context of the classification (Revised American Fertility Society) system described here.

Class I: Hypoplasia/agenesis—Patients with müllerian agenesis present with amenorrhea or, less commonly, with cyclic pain caused by isolated atresia of the uterine cervix. These patients can have endometriosis if outflow of the endometrium is prevented by an atretic cervix or vagina.

Young women with a functioning endometrium and cervical atresia are usually best treated by hysterectomy. A few successful attempts at uterovaginal fistula formation have allowed cyclic flows; others report severe infections, sepsis, and even death.

Class II: Unicornuate uterus—Unicornuate uterus represents a small proportion of anomalies, about 2% overall. Women with unicornuate uteri are at greater risk of first-trimester losses (about 50% abort) and preterm labor and delivery (about 15%). Older series report some risk of a second-trimester loss and stillbirth. The unicornuate uterus is rarely responsible for primary infertility.

The rudiment without a cavity rarely produces symptoms and may be confused with a leiomyoma at surgery; it is distinguished as a uterine horn by its attachment to the tube and uteroovarian ligament. Patients with a cavity with egress possible through a patent tube present with symptoms that are attributable to endometriosis; patients with a cavity without uterine or tubal egress present with cyclic cramping pain. Evaluation in any patient with a unicornuate anomaly must include evaluation of the urinary tract; up to 70% of these women have ipsilateral renal agenesis.

Treatment options include prophylactic cerclage, which, at present, must be considered empirical treatment. Symptomatic rudimentary horns should be excised, with care taken to maintain the integrity of the dominant uterine horn.

Class III: Uterus didelphys—Preterm labor and delivery is the most common presenting fertility-related symptom, occurring in up to 40% of cases. Didelphys uteri are associated with a vaginal septum in 75% of cases. Up to 9% of these patients have renal agenesis, and 20% have duplicative ureteric systems; intravenous pyelography is thus warranted.

Diagnosis is suspected from physical examination findings of the vaginal septum or double cervices, with possible palpation of two fundi. Hysterosalpingography further identifies two patent uterine cavities; laparoscopy distinguishes the didelphys from the rarer bicollis unicornuate uterus. The distinction between anomalies has been reported from the use of transabdominal and transvaginal ultrasonography, computed tomography, and magnetic resonance imaging.

Prophylactic cerclage is recommended by some investigators, but proof of its efficacy is lacking. Metroplasty is rarely, if ever, indicated in women with uterus didelphys and is possible only by the Strassman unification procedure. Hysteroscopic metroplasty of bicollis septate uteri has been successful, with the cervices left intact.

Class IV: Bicornuate uterus—Patients with a bicornuate uterus present with repeated abortion most frequently. They present less commonly with preterm labor. Diagnosis may be suspected by hysterosalpingography, but laparoscopy is required to distinguish this anomaly from didelphys or septate uteri.

Hysteroscopic metroplasty is not advised because of the increased risk of perforation between the horns; the Strassman unification may be the procedure of choice, but others perform Tompkins or Jones metroplasty. Metroplasty is indicated in habitual aborters only after all other causes have been eliminated. Prophylactic cerclage is recommended by some investigators.

Class V: Septate uterus—Septate uterus is the anomaly most often associated with first-trimester loss (up to 20% of cases), but it is also the anomaly found most frequently by careful examination of the uterus at the time of cesarean delivery or hysteroscopy. Other symptoms are rare. This anomaly is due to failure of resorption of the septum that is present in all female fetuses at 18 weeks of gestation. As such, one would expect rare concomitant urinary tract anomalies. An intravenous pyelogram is usually normal and is considered elective by most investigators in the evaluation of women with septate uteri.

Hysteroscopic incision of the septum with scissors, a resectoscope, or a fiber laser is the treatment of choice. Particularly wide septa may be removed in a two-stage hysteroscopic procedure. If another indication warrants laparotomy and transfundal metroplasty is elected, the techniques of Strassman, Tompkins, and Jones have all been associated with excellent results—up to 80% fetal salvage rates. Postoperative estrogen therapy (eg, conjugated equine estrogens, 2.5 mg twice daily) is prescribed for 1 month after therapy to encourage endometrial repair.

Class VI: Arcuate uterus—Probably a normal variant, arcuate uterus is typically identified at hysterosalpingography in women who are being evaluated for infertility or habitual abortion. No specific treatment is indicated.

Class VII: DES related—Women with the classic T-shaped, small uterus have a high rate of first-trimester losses (up to 50%) and preterm delivery (13–40%). The hysterosalpingographic picture of a T-shaped uterus is occasionally found in the woman with infertility but with no history of fetal exposure to DES. Metroplastic approaches have been largely unsuccessful. More than any other approach, prophylactic cerclage has been suggested as being efficacious in patients with this anomaly.

Anomalies associated with fetal loss are often treated, despite the lack of controlled studies demonstrating improved efficacy over expectant management or bed rest. This is particularly noteworthy in the case of repeated abortion, as women who have experienced three or more first-trimester losses successfully deliver a viable infant without specific treatment in most cases. Thus, fetal salvage rates of 70–80% may not be too different than what would be expected without intervention.

It is of extreme importance, however, to be certain that the uterine anomaly is the sole factor that is responsible for the pregnancy loss. The most common anomaly is the septum, which is best treated hysteroscopically in most cases, with similar success reported for transabdominal approaches as well. Following transabdominal metroplasty, women should subsequently undergo cesarean delivery, whereas those treated hysteroscopically may safely undergo vaginal delivery.

Cervical Incompetence: Congenital and Acquired

Cervical incompetence is usually due to cervical trauma from overvigorous D&C, cervical conization, or laceration from a previous delivery, but it may be congenital. Diagnosis is confirmed by history, a cervix that admits a no. 8 Hegar dilator, balloon hysterography, or vacuum cap hysterography during the luteal phase of the cycle. A careful prenatal observation of the cervix is also useful in confirming the diagnosis. Depending on the extent of the defect and the procedure that is performed (Shirodkar, McDonald, interval Lash procedure), successful pregnancy rates range from 50% to 85%.

ENDOCRINE FACTORS

Corpus luteum deficiencies are suspected in approximately 30–40% of women who have habitual abortions. A recent study demonstrated an incidence of 23% in patients in whom an endocrine etiology could be identified. An inadequate luteal phase is a specific entity that reflects abnormal folliculogenesis with inadequate progesterone production and with a subsequent insufficient progestational effect on the glands and stroma of the endometrium. This effect does not allow for proper implantation or normal placentation.

Stimulation by FSH early in the cycle must be adequate to induce follicular growth and to ensure granulosa cell proliferation. Furthermore, the LH surge must be adequate to induce ovulation and steroidogenesis, and a sufficient tonic LH level is necessary in the luteal phase to maintain luteal function. Finally, normal levels of prolactin are required for normal luteal function. Alternatively, certain luteolytic agents, such as synthetic progestins or prostaglandins, may also be responsible for an inadequate luteal phase. It has been shown that inadequate endometrial progesterone receptors may also prevent the normal maturation of the endometrium.

ABNORMALITIES IN PLACENTATION

Abnormalities in placentation are responsible for approximately 6% of recurrent abortions. These are represented chiefly by a circumvallate placenta.

Intrauterine Synechiae

Intrauterine synechiae (Asherman syndrome), once thought to be a cause of recurrent spontaneous abortion, are commonly a result of multiple uterine curettages. Adhesions may follow overzealous curettage of the uterus during the postpartum or postabortal period, intrauterine surgery (eg, myomectomy), or endometritis. Dense, avascular adhesions may interfere with placentation, and patients often benefit by hysteroscopic lysis. In one series, 89.6% of patients conceived after lysis with the spontaneous abortion rate ranging from 5.9% to 21.4%. However, no randomized, controlled data exist to confirm efficacy of hysteroscopic lysis of adhesions in preventing subsequent spontaneous abortion.

Leiomyomata

Uterine leiomyomata are usually multiple and may contribute to pregnancy wastage, but the pathophysiology is unknown. Location rather than size is probably most important. Submucous leiomyomas may result in fetal loss through several theoretic mechanisms: 1) endometrial thinning over the surface of the myomas may impair decidualization and implantation; 2) necrosis within the myomas (red degeneration) from hormonally stimulated growth exceeding the blood supply may lead to uterine contractions and fetal expulsion; and 3) the myomas may encroach upon the space required by the developing fetus and lead to fetal expulsion in the second trimester.

Controlled clinical trials to document therapeutic efficacy of myomectomy have not been performed. However, several reports indicate that after myomectomy 50% of patients with repeated pregnancy loss achieve a viable pregnancy.

ENDOCRINE ABNORMALITIES

Thyroid Disease

Overt hypothyroidism and hyperthyroidism are uncommon but real causes of spontaneous abortion. Serum tests to diagnose these disorders are commonly available and thwart the need to treat "subclinical" disease empirically.

Diabetes Mellitus

Uncontrolled insulin-dependent diabetes mellitus may increase the risk of spontaneous abortion. However, euglycemic patients with diabetes mellitus do not have an increased risk of pregnancy loss. Therefore, unless a patient has symptoms of the disease, there is no reason to screen for diabetes mellitus in those patients presenting only with recurrent spontaneous abortion.

Luteal Phase Defect

The luteal phase defect presumably results when the endometrium fails to develop appropriately for implantation and cannot support placentation, either secondary to deficient progesterone or a poor endometrial response to adequate progesterone. Endometrial histologic dating lagging at least 2 days or more behind the actual postovulatory date in two menstrual cycles is diagnostic of the luteal phase defect. Because of the pulsatile nature of progesterone secretion, random serum progesterone levels are inadequate for diagnosis.

Early pregnancy losses secondary to disordered placentation in an unsupportive endometrial environment is a plausible explanation for spontaneous abortion. Unfortunately, no study exists comparing the prevalence of luteal phase defect in a normal fertile population with a population of women experiencing recurrent spontaneous abortions. There is also variation in interpretation among pathologists, leading to altered management. The prevalence of luteal phase defect in fertile women is unclear. Some studies indicate a prevalence of 27%. Less-well-controlled studies in women experiencing recurrent spontaneous abortions suggest that the prevalence of abnormal biopsy results is 35%. Even if the populations were comparable, the prevalences in the two groups may not be different. Thus, the association is not firm, and one can only presume that the prevalence of luteal phase defect is higher in the latter cohort.

Randomized studies have not been performed to document efficacy of preferred therapeutic regimes for luteal phase defect. In one study involving a small group of infertile women, a higher abortion rate was observed in women with untreated luteal phase defect.

Patients with luteal phase defect may be treated with progesterone vaginal suppositories, 25 mg twice daily beginning 2 days after the LH surge or on day 3 after the temperature shift as determined by BBT and continuing until 8 weeks of gestation. Alternatively, clomiphene citrate, 50–100 mg, may be administered for 5 days beginning day 3–5 of the menstrual cycle. Since not all patients will correct the histologic dating of their endometrial biopsy with these therapies, an endometrial biopsy should be performed during the treatment cycle before another pregnancy is contemplated.

INFECTIONS

Many infections have been implicated in causing recurrent spontaneous abortion. The mechanism whereby infections may result in spontaneous abortion is unclear. Perhaps maternal fever, bacterial toxins, destruction of a fetal cell vital to embryogenesis, or even maternal treatment itself may cause spontaneous abortion.

Very few prospective studies exist comparing a cohort of patients with spontaneous abortions compared with a fertile population in terms of the prevalence of any suggested organism. Women who have *Mycoplasma* infection of the endometrium seem to have a higher prevalence of spontaneous abortion. Furthermore, doxycycline treatment has been shown to increase resultant term pregnancy. Women who have endometrial cultures positive for ureaplasma should be treated, along with their partners, with 100 mg of doxycycline twice daily for 2 weeks. Other infections implicated in early fetal wastage include *Toxoplasma gondii*, herpes virus, and cytomegalovirus.

IMMUNOLOGIC DISORDERS

The nature of the immunologic process responsible for tolerating a fetus containing 50% foreign antigens is complex. Both autoimmune and alloimmune factors have been identified as causes of pregnancy losses.

Antifetal Antibodies

Fetal wastage occurs when an otherwise normal mother produces antibodies against her fetus on the basis of genetic dissimilarities at a given locus. The most obvious example is D (Rh) incompatibility.

Autoimmune Disease

Patients with an autoimmune disease such as systemic lupus erythematosus have an increased risk of spontaneous abortion. These patients seem to form antibodies not only against their own tissue but against placental tissue, which ultimately leads to thrombi in the placental bed and rejection of early pregnancy.

Antiphospholipid Antibodies

A relationship between the antiphospholipid antibodies including lupus anticoagulant and anticardiolipin antibodies and recurrent spontaneous abortion has been established (Table 6-8). Therefore, tests for lupus anticoagulant and anticardiolipin should be performed in these patients.

Shared Parental Histocompatibility Antigens

The fetal allograft containing foreign paternal antigens logically should be rejected by the mother; however, an unknown gestational mechanism invokes immune tolerance. It is thought that the paternal antigens that are foreign to the mother invoke a protecting blocking antibody that prevents the normal maternal immune cells of rejection from recognizing the fetus as foreign. These protective antibodies form only when maternal and paternal histocompatibility antigens are dissimilar, and they account for the widely recognized maternal antipaternal–leukocyte antibodies. If similarity exists, the protective antibodies are thought not to form and therefore the fetus is rejected by the mother's immune cells.

TABLE 6-8. THE RISK OF SPONTANEOUS ABORTION IN PATIENTS WITH ANTIPHOSPHOLIPID ANTIBODIES

Patient Category	Patients (%) with Titer (IgG Phospholipid Units) of 16–80	≥ 80
Primipara	6	38
Previous spontaneous abortion	30	85

Adapted from information appearing in *The New England Journal of Medicine*; Lockshin MD, Sammaritano LR. Antiphospholipid antibodies and fetal loss. N Engl J Med 1992;326:951–952

The major histocompatibility antigens were the first antigens suggested to be involved in this recognition. However, multiple studies have now shown that parental sharing of HLAs does not increase the risk of spontaneous abortion. Others have suggested that trophoblast lymphocyte cross-reacting antigens may be the antigen system involved.

In addition to parental antigen sharing, other circumstantial evidence exists to support that parental histoincompatibility is beneficial. Only 16.6% of women with repetitive abortions have antipaternal antileukocytoxic antibodies, in contrast to 64% of multiparous women and 20% of primiparous women. Similarly, 50% of women with three or more recurrent abortions show no blocking factors, as evidenced by failure to demonstrate a mixed lymphocyte reaction when their lymphocytes are exposed to their partner's lymphocytes.

Immunization of women lacking blocking antibodies but sharing HLAs with various paternal cells to invoke a blocking antibody that would protect the fetus has been suggested as a treatment modality. If fetal rejection occurs as a result of diminished fetal–maternal immunologic interaction, it seems logical that immunotherapy to enhance interaction at few differing loci is plausible. Such therapy is experimental, however, and its efficacy remains to be established.

ENVIRONMENTAL FACTORS

A variety of teratogenic agents and environmental factors may result in spontaneous abortion. These include drugs and chemicals, occupational and environmental agents, cigarette smoking and alcohol ingestion, illicit drugs, ionizing radiation, and trauma (see "Teratogenic Agents" in the Obstetrics section).

Psychologic Factors

That impaired psychologic well-being predisposes to early fetal losses has been claimed but not proved. Neurotic or mentally ill women abort, but whether the frequency of losses is higher than in normal women is unknown. Confounding factors have not been excluded in studies claiming a relationship.

Generalized Effects of Severe Maternal Illness

Maternal diseases not previously mentioned that may be associated with fetal wastage include Wilson disease, maternal phenylketonuria, cardiac insufficiency (eg, cyanotic heart disease), and hematologic disorders (eg, hemoglobinopathies or aplastic anemia). In fact, any life-threatening disease would be expected to be associated with increased abortion rates. Seriously ill women rarely become pregnant, but in some cases the disease process may deteriorate after onset of pregnancy. Overall, only a small fraction of all fetal losses can be attributable to severe maternal disease. Thus, general probes for maternal health should be sought; however, detailed disease-by-disease assessment is probably unnecessary.

EVALUATION AND FOLLOW-UP

Patients experiencing recurrent pregnancy loss would benefit from undergoing evaluation of the following:

- Karyotype of woman and partner
- Karyotype of any subsequent abortus
- TSH level
- Prolactin level
- Timed endometrial biopsy and histologic dating
- *Ureaplasma urealyticum* culture
- Hysterosalpingography or hysteroscopy or both
- Antiphospholipid antibodies
  —Lupus anticoagulant
  —Anticardiolipin antibodies

These tests are usually performed after three spontaneous abortions or in the woman older than age 35 years after two spontaneous abortions. These tests should be repeated after appropriate treatments have been completed and before another pregnancy is attempted.

Perhaps more important than evaluation and treatment in the patient experiencing spontaneous pregnancy loss is the care for the patient during her next pregnancy. The emotional turmoil experienced during a pregnancy by the patient with a history of spontaneous abortions cannot be overstated. These patients will benefit emotionally by seeing their physicians frequently during the first trimester. Early ultrasound examinations will establish viability, as well as allow the patient to be reassured weekly that the pregnancy is continuing. Patients who have fetal cardiac activity demonstrated on ultrasonography at 8 weeks of gestation have a 3–5% risk of spontaneously aborting. The demonstration of fetal cardiac activity at 8 weeks of gestation enables patients to have a shorter period of anxiety. Another reason to follow the patient frequently in early pregnancy is to rule out the risk of ectopic pregnancy. Patients who are experiencing repetitive spontaneous abortions have a fourfold increased risk of subsequent ectopic pregnancy. After reaching 8 weeks of gestation, patients may then undergo routine obstetric care.

BIBLIOGRAPHY

American Fertility Society. Myomas and reproductive dysfunction: guideline for practice. Birmingham, Alabama: AFS, 1992

Barlow SM, Sullivan FM. Reproductive hazards of industrial chemicals: an evaluation of animal and human data. London: Academic Press, 1982

Beer AE, Quebbeman JF, Semprini AE. Immunopathological factors contributing to recurrent and spontaneous abortion in humans. In: Bennet MJ, Edmonds DK, eds. Spontaneous and recurrent abortions. Oxford: Blackwell, 1987:90–108

Daly DC, Walters CA, Soto-Albors CE, Riddick DH. Endometrial biopsy during treatment of luteal phase defects is predictive of therapeutic outcome. Fertil Steril 1983;40:305–310

Davis OK, Berkley AS, Nause GJ, Cholst IN, Freedman KS. The incidence of luteal phase defect in normal, fertile women, determined by serial endometrial biopsies. Fertil Steril 1989;51:582–586

Fija-Talamanaca I, Settimi L. Occupational factors and reproductive outcome. In: Hafez ESE, ed. Spontaneous abortion. Lancaster [Lancashire]: MTP Press, 1984:61–80

Fizet D, Bousquet J. Absence of a factor blocking cellular cytotoxicity reaction in the serum of women with recurrent abortion. Br J Obstet Gynaecol 1983;90:453–456

Heidam LZ. Spontaneous abortions among laboratory workers: a follow-up study. J Epidemiol Community Health 1984;38:36–41

Malpas P. A study of abortion sequence. J Obstet Gynaecol Br Emp 1938;45:932–949

Mowbray JF, Gibbings C, Liddell H, Reginald PW, Underwood JL, Beard RW. Controlled trial of treatment of recurrent spontaneous abortion by immunisation with paternal cells. Lancet 1985;1:941–943

Ohno M, Maeda T, Matsunobu A. A cytogenetic study of spontaneous abortions with direct analysis of chorionic villi. Obstet Gynecol 1991;77:394–398

Poland BJ, Miller JR, Jones DC, Trimble BK. Reproductive counseling in patients who have had a spontaneous abortion. Am J Obstet Gynecol 1977;127:685–691

Rocklin RE, Kitzmiller JL, Carpenter CB, Garovoy MR, David JR. Maternal-fetal relation. Absence of an immunologic blocking factor from the serum of women with chronic abortions. N Engl J Med 1976;295:1209–1213

Scott RT, Synder RR, Strickland DM, Tyburski CC, Bagnall JA, Reed KR. The effect of interobserver variation in dating endometrial histology on the diagnosis of luteal phase defects. Fertil Steril 1988;50:888–892

Stimson WH, Strachnan AF, Shepard A. Studies on the maternal immune response to placental antigens: absence of a blocking factor from the blood of abortion-prone women. Br J Obstet Gynaecol 1979;86:41–45

Taskinen H, Lindbohm ML, Hemminki K. Spontaneous abortions among women working in the pharmaceutical industry. Br J Ind Med 1986;43:199–205

The American Fertility Society classifications of adnexal adhesions, distal tubal occlusion, tubal occlusion secondary to tubal ligation, tubal pregnancies, müllerian anomalies, and intrauterine adhesions. Fertil Steril 1988;49:944–955

Thomas ML, Harger JH, Wagener DK, Rabin BS, Gill TJ 3d. HLA sharing and spontaneous abortion in humans. Am J Obstet Gynecol 1985;151:1053–1058

Warburton D, Fraser, FC. Spontaneous abortion risks in man: data from reproductive histories collected in a medical genetics unit. Am J Human Genet 1964;16:1–25

Wentz AC. Physiologic and clinical considerations in luteal phase defects. Clin Obstet Gynecol 1979;22:169–185

Assisted Reproductive Technologies

Assisted reproductive technology refers to a group of procedures that have in common the handling of oocytes/embryos outside of the body, with gametes or concepti replaced into the body to establish pregnancy to cure infertility. The initial and still most commonly used procedure, IVF, involves extraction of oocytes, fertilization in the laboratory, and transfer of embryos across the cervix into the uterine cavity. Since the first successful birth in 1978, numerous variations have been brought into practice. This section describes each procedure and offers perspective to understand the choice among them.

Assisted reproductive technology is a complex discipline requiring a team of individuals with training and expertise in reproductive surgery, pelvic ultrasonography, reproductive endocrinology, embryology, and andrology. For this reason, discrete programs are usually organized to provide this service, a director having overall responsibility, and each function being provided by various members of the team.

Because of the complexity of these procedures and because relatively few aspects of techniques have been defined and universally accepted, each program varies in a multitude of aspects throughout each part of the process. It is not surprising, therefore, that success rates have also varied widely. It is the responsibility of the referring physician to be aware of the various programs' results, which are available in a yearly publication through the American Fertility Society, as well as the inherent difficulties in assessing quality of care discussed at the end of the section.

IN VITRO FERTILIZATION—EMBRYO TRANSFER

Patient Selection and Preparation

Women with abnormal fallopian tubes or endometriosis, idiopathic infertility, male infertility, and immunologic infertility all respond well to IVF. Women who have failed to conceive with donor insemination or ovulation induction are also excellent candidates. Rough guidelines as to when assisted reproductive technology may be considered are 2 years of unexplained infertility or 2 years following treatment of a particular defect or at least 1 year of donor insemination or ovulation induction. These may be modified, depending on factors such as age, presence of severe defects, or multiple infertility factors.

Levels of FSH and estradiol can be used to identify women with abnormal ovarian function and a reduced prognosis. When the FSH level exceeds 25 mIU/ml on day 3 of menses, successful birth is rarely achieved with IVF. Age alone predicts prognosis, with successful births occurring in less than half as many women over age 40 as in women under age 40. *Chlamydia* should be tested for or empirically treated, since serologic evidence of infection has been associated with a reduced birth rate and increased fetal loss.

Many programs test the fertilizing capacity of sperm using zona-free hamster eggs, since some males may fail to fertilize with routine methods of sperm preparation, and alternative methods may enhance sperm penetration. Testing for ASAs is essential if the patient's own serum is to be used in the culture medium; it is also helpful to identify very high levels in one or both partners, allowing the use of a higher than usual number of sperm for insemination.

The uterine cavity should be assessed with hysterography, transvaginal ultrasonography, and hysteroscopy if necessary to ensure the absence of any significant uterine defects. A thorough semen analysis should be done close to the time of the cycle of treatment, and all attempts should be made to resolve pyospermia, which can reduce sperm function. Finally, a rehearsal of the transfer has been shown to increase the rate of pregnancy.

Ovarian Stimulation and Monitoring

Most IVF cycles are conducted with ovarian stimulation, since the pregnancy rate increases with the number of embryos transferred. A metaanalysis of randomized trials has shown a twofold odds ratio for pregnancy with the combination of an agonist of GnRH and gonadotropins, compared with other stimulation regimens. This method is used by almost all IVF programs and also reduces cancellations for poor responses and premature LH surges, yields more extra embryos for cryopreservation, and gives patients and the program more flexibility in scheduling by varying the duration of ovarian suppression prior to stimulation. It is also possible to retrieve the single mature oocyte from the natural menstrual cycle, although approximately three such cycles are needed to achieve a cumulative pregnancy rate comparable to one stimulated cycle. It avoids any risk of stimulation and multiple pregnancy.

Both transvaginal ultrasonography and serum estradiol levels are used to determine when hCG should be injected to initiate resumption of meiosis. With the natural cycle, serum or urinary LH levels must be monitored to ensure that the LH surge has not begun or to time retrieval according to the onset of the LH surge. The ultrasonographic appearance and thickness of the endometrium have been found to be prognostic for successful pregnancy, with a sonolucent superficial layer and a thickness more than 8–9 mm being ideal.

Oocyte Retrieval

The follicle aspiration is scheduled for 34–36 hours after hCG injection. With GnRH agonist/gonadotropins, this can be extended to as late as 38 hours with minimal risk of ovulation. Prophylactic antibiotics are commonly given. Retrieval is almost always done by ultrasound-guided transvaginal aspiration, even if it is necessary to transverse the uterus when an ovary is adherent to the uterine fundus. In most cases intravenous sedation is sufficient for analgesia, making it an outpatient or even office-based procedure. A povidone–iodine vaginal preparation is a wise precaution to prevent pelvic infection, but the agent must be thoroughly removed before the procedure.

Insemination

Usually 50,000–5,000,000 sperm are added to each oocyte, depending on sperm parameters, after a period of 2–8 hours of preincubation to allow further oocyte maturation. The oocytes are stripped of their surrounding cells and examined 12–20 hours after insemination. Visualization of two pronuclei confirms normal fertilization. Concepti with three or more pronuclei are discarded. Extra embryos are most commonly cryopreserved at the two-pronucleus stage.

Embryo Culture and Quality Control

A variety of media have been used with success. Electrolyte concentrations are often adjusted to simulate the levels measured in the human fallopian tube. Serum from the patient, umbilical cord blood, or designated donors has been most often added to media to provide protein and growth factors. Some preparations of serum albumin have also been used successfully. Various bioassays have been also been used for quality control of the media (eg, mouse embryos or human or hamster sperm) to detect toxicity. Various methods are used to control the environment, such as heating blocks, a layer of oil over the medium, or carbon dioxide- and temperature-controlled mobile chambers, so that temperature, pH, and osmolarity are kept within narrow limits.

Embryo Transfer

Embryos are most often replaced 2 days after oocyte retrieval. Embryos are graded, and those chosen for transfer are loaded in a minute volume into a transfer catheter. The catheter tip is advanced into the uterine fundus and the embryos are expelled. The catheter is checked for retained embryos, and the patient rests for a period of time before returning home.

Luteal Phase Supplementation

With GnRH agonist/gonadotropin cycles, the luteal phase must be supported with hCG or progesterone. The latter is probably as effective and carries less risk of ovarian hyperstimulation. Progesterone supplementation is generally continued until 10–12 weeks of gestation.

Early Pregnancy

Pregnancy is diagnosed by rising levels of hCG. Clinical pregnancy is confirmed by the presence of a gestational sac. It is inappropriate for a program to count biochemical pregnancies (rising hCG only) in its "pregnancy" rate. Viable deliveries are births at more than 20 weeks of pregnancy productive of at least one living infant. Since about 5% of clinical pregnancies are ectopic, a careful transvaginal ultrasound scan should be done at 4 and 6 weeks after transfer. Cornual pregnancies are not rare and are easily visualized. Cervical pregnancies have also occurred. A tubal pregnancy can usually be detected, but the patient with an intrauterine pregnancy should be cautioned not to ignore significant pain. If a heterotopic (ectopic and intrauterine) pregnancy is found, the ectopic pregnancy can usually be excised laparoscopically without disturbing the intrauterine gestation.

Elevated hCG levels with no sign of an intrauterine sac by 4 weeks from transfer should raise suspicion of a tubal pregnancy. Tubal pregnancy can occur in an adherent tube that normally would not pick up an egg. If the tube is found to be inaccessible laparoscopically, methotrexate can be used instead of laparotomy. Methotrexate can also be used primarily without laparoscopy if the ultrasonography is diagnostic or if a D&C fails to reveal chorionic villi.

Complications

There has been a very low incidence of pelvic infection after follicle aspiration. This can be minimized by using prophylactic antibiotics and a povidone–iodine vaginal preparation. Ovarian hyperstimulation occurs in about 0.2% of stimulated cycles but is more common in anovulatory women. Multiple pregnancy occurred in 30% of pregnancies in 1991, but it is more common in programs with higher success rates, in younger women, when more embryos are transferred, and when the embryos are of superior quality. Tubal pregnancy occurs almost exclusively in women with tubal disease and has the highest incidence in those who have had tubal surgery. Cornual pregnancy primarily occurs when the tube had been removed previously.

Cryopreserved Embryos

There is no known limit on duration of embryo storage. Women who were successful with fresh embryos are more likely to be successful with frozen embryos from the same cycle than women who were not successful. About two thirds of embryos survive the process, but each woman is highly individual, just as there are some men with high-quality sperm whose germ cells do not freeze well. The embryos can be transferred during a natural cycle or a hormonally controlled cycle. It has not yet been confirmed whether the latter yields superior pregnancy rates.

Pregnancy Outcome

There is a minor trend toward premature labor in singleton pregnancies. The rate of spontaneous abortion is mildly increased (about 20%). The rate of congenital anomalies has not been increased.

Micromanipulation of Oocytes and Embryos

In cases of previous failed fertilization or very poor semen quality, fertilization can be aided by mechanically creating a slit in the zona pellucida with a micropipette (partial zona dissection) or by inserting a small number of sperm under the zona (subzonal insertion). There is no lower limit of semen parameters with subzonal insertion as long as viable sperm are present. Success is possible even with sperm that are completely immotile due to flagellar defects. Approximately 20% of oocytes have monospermic fertilization, but since the women of male factor partners generally stimulate well, the rate of pregnancy can still be reasonable, although reduced. Very recently a successful technique has been reported with injection of a single sperm directly into the cytoplasm of the egg.

Embryos can be micromanipulated to assist them in hatching from the zona pellucida (assisted hatching) by making an artificial opening in the zona pellucida. Assisted hatching increases implantation per embryo about twofold in women aged 39 or older and also increases the pregnancy rate in women with an elevated level of FSH (15–25 mIU/ml). Assisted hatching also increases implantation for embryos of lesser quality or with a thick zona and for cryopreserved embryos.

Use of Donor Gametes

The fertilization rate is entirely normal with frozen donor sperm. The pregnancy rate with donated oocytes is generally 1½–2-fold higher than with routine IVF, because donors are generally young or fertile or both. Both known and anonymous oocyte donors are used. This has allowed women who have failed multiple IVF attempts, who have abnormal ovarian function (elevated FSH, poor response to stimulation), or who are advanced in age to have an excellent chance of pregnancy. Other advantages of egg donation are that amniocentesis is not required, provided that the donor is young and the rate of spontaneous abortion is low.

Choosing an In Vitro Fertilization Program for Referral

Success rates are generally reported as clinical pregnancies and deliveries per retrieval. These rates are available for individual programs through the American Fertility Society on an annual basis. For 1991, the average delivery rate per retrieval was 15%. Rates are separated for women more than 39 years of age and for couples with abnormal sperm count or motility (Table 6-9). Women less than 40 years of age and without any male factor represent a group that can be compared across programs. Individual rates vary dramatically, but many programs are consistently achieving rates of more than 20% deliveries per retrieval. Since the average of 15% is pulled down by many inferior and inexperienced centers, a good rule of thumb is that a center should achieve an above-average rate, preferably over 20%, to warrant the confidence of a referral. At the same time, many factors can influence these rates. With many programs reporting relatively small numbers of cases, rates will vary widely based on chance alone (for example with $n = 50$, the 95% confidence limits of 15% extends from 5% to 25%). Ideally, rates should be based on at least 100–200 re-

TABLE 6-9. IN VITRO FERTILIZATION RESULTS BY AGE AND PRESENCE OF MALE FACTOR*

Age, Male Factor (MF)	Canceled Stimulations (%)	Retrievals (No.)	Deliveries/ Retrieval (%)
<40, no MF	14.1	13,564	18.0
>40, no MF	25.1	2,257	8.0
<40, MF	9.1	4,013	13.0
>40, MF	18.8	739	5.5
Total	14.7	20,573	15.5

* Data were reported to the American Fertility Society by 215 U.S. and Canadian assisted reproductive technology programs.

trievals, which may require accumulation of more than 1 year's results.

Programs that are well known will accumulate referrals of more difficult cases. As a rule of thumb, one could adjust by adding 5% for such programs. Programs that transfer more embryos or hold more embryos until cleavage before a choice is made for transfer will bias upward their fresh embryo transfer results while compromising their frozen embryo results. Programs at the other extreme, which freeze all extra embryos at the two-pronucleus stage without picking the best for fresh transfer, will compromise their fresh results and will have more pregnancies from cryopreservation. The former extreme, given similar quality of all other aspects of the program, will have a higher overall delivery rate, but at the expense of more multiple pregnancy.

The proper balance of the risks of multiple pregnancy versus the likelihood of achieving pregnancy between these extremes is controversial. In some countries these decisions have been taken out of the programs' hands because of the risks and high costs of multiple pregnancies, with laws or strict guidelines limiting transfer to no more than three embryos.

Another factor that is very difficult to assess is the selection of patients for IVF. The longer the duration of infertility and the more extensive and effective are the routine infertility treatments, the more hard-core will be the remaining patients going through IVF. In all, the best one can do is to limit referrals to a well-known program with conscientious, well-trained individuals and at least a 15–20% delivery rate per retrieval and good results with embryo freezing.

GAMETE INTRAFALLOPIAN TRANSFER

Gamete intrafallopian transfer refers to the placement of sperm and eggs into the fallopian tube. This has generally been done by laparoscopy or minilaparotomy. The average delivery rate for GIFT in 1991 was 27%, compared with 15% for IVF. For programs whose IVF success rate is substantially below the national average for GIFT, their patients with normal tubes will probably fare better with GIFT. Since IVF is less invasive, programs with IVF rates close to or exceeding the national average for GIFT are likely to do relatively little GIFT, both by their recommendation and by patient choice. As more uniformly high success rates are achieved with IVF, GIFT may play a progressively smaller role in the future. Results of GIFT for 1991 are shown in Table 6-10.

Women with significantly abnormal tubes should not have GIFT, because in such women the success rate is no higher than that for IVF, and their rate of tubal pregnancy is also increased. Women with significant male factors also do less well with GIFT, and fertilization is better documented with IVF. The rate of tubal pregnancy may be higher with GIFT, although it appears to have decreased as fewer women with tubal disease have undergone GIFT (5% ectopic in 1988, 2.9% in 1991). This rate still exceeds the rate in women with normal tubes having IVF.

Gamete intrafallopian transfer has been done in combination with IVF, placing fewer oocytes into the tubes, leaving more for IVF, and also performing a transcervical transfer of embryos. This allows better documentation of fertilization but somewhat compromises the objective of the GIFT procedure.

Gamete intrafallopian transfer is also sometimes done at the time of diagnostic laparoscopy. The disadvantages of this approach are that pregnancy might occur with further time and further treatments specific to the laparoscopic diagnosis, the additional expense (including multiple pregnancies) with GIFT, and any compromise of the laparoscopic treatment due to the coexisting GIFT procedure. However, in cases with an adequate duration of infertility and no indication of pelvic disease, the procedure seems reasonable, particularly since the additional cost and pregnancy rate are roughly equivalent to the pregnancy rate and cost of a limited series of gonadotropin/intrauterine insemination cycles.

ZYGOTE OR TUBAL EMBRYO TRANSFER

The placement of fertilized oocytes (zygote intrafallopian transfer) or cleaving embryos (tubal embryo transfer) into the fallopian tubes allows fertilization to be maximized and confirmed, while still taking advantage of the tubal environment for part of the early development of the embryo. While the success rate theoretically should be higher, the rate of success with these procedures was only modestly increased over that of IVF in 1991 (20% versus 15%, respectively) and two randomized studies in programs with good IVF success rates failed to find a difference in outcome with the tubal procedures. Transfer efficiency may be a factor with zygote intrafallopian transfer and tubal embryo transfer, and probably a small transfer volume and accurate placement are critical. Whether the increased cost and the need for a second surgical procedure are worthwhile must depend on each program's individual experience with these procedures.

OTHER PROCEDURES

Attempts have been made over the last few years to cannulate the tubes transcervically to avoid the need for laparoscopy and anesthesia to deposit gametes or embryos into the fallopian tubes. This procedure has met with very irregular and generally inferior results, compared with standard GIFT or tubal embryo transfer.

Peritoneal oocyte and sperm transfer is a procedure in which the oocytes are retrieved, and the oocytes and sperm are placed into the pelvic cavity under ultrasound guidance. A randomized trial must be done to prove that this method is superior to superovulation/intrauterine insemination before the procedure can be shown to be worthwhile. Even sperm injection directly into the follicle has been reported to be successful. Again, this must be directly compared with superovulation/intrauterine insemination.

FUTURE DEVELOPMENTS

Using gene amplification by PCR it is possible to obtain a diagnosis of sex genotype and cystic fibrosis genotype from a single cell of an eight-cell embryo. Results are then available so that later that day, only embryos of one sex (as with sex-linked genetic disorders) or those having a normal genotype can be replaced. This avoids the need for testing by amniocentesis and subsequent abortion but is much more invasive and expensive, thus limiting its application. In the future, tests for many other genetic disorders should be available. Insertion of genetic material to cure genetic diseases may also be possible, although this methodology is currently limited by the inefficiency of methods by which to incorporate genetic material into cells.

Various attempts are being made to improve embryo growth by culturing embryos on a layer of other cells (cocultures) from both reproductive and nonreproductive tissues. As more knowledge accumulates regarding optimal in vitro conditions, it can be expected that IVF and transcervical transfer will become the procedure of choice for almost all patients and programs.

BIBLIOGRAPHY

American Fertility Society. Revised minimum standards for in vitro fertilization, gamete intrafallopian transfer, and related procedures. Fertil Steril 1990;53:225–226

Assisted reproductive technology in the United States and Canada: 1991 results from the Society for Assisted Reproductive Technology generated from the American Fertility Society Registry. Fertil Steril 1993;59:956–962

TABLE 6-10. GAMETE INTRAFALLOPIAN TRANSFER RESULTS BY AGE AND PRESENCE OF MALE FACTOR*

Age, Male Factor (MF)	Canceled Stimulations (%)	Retrievals (No.)	Deliveries/Retrieval (%)
<40, no MF	17.0	2,798	30.4
>40, no MF	30.0	620	10.8
<40, MF	12.7	720	26.9
>40, MF	29.2	156	13.5
Total	19.2	4,474	26.5

* Data were reported to the American Fertility Society for 215 U.S. and Canadian assisted reproductive technology programs.

Cohen J, Alikani M, Trowbridge J, Rosenwaks Z. Implantation enhancement by selective assisted hatching using zona drilling of human embryos with poor prognosis. Hum Reprod 1992;7:685–691

Hughes EG, Fedorkow DM, Daya S, Sagle MA, Van de Koppel P, Collins JA. The routine use of gonadotropin-releasing hormone agonists prior to in vitro fertilization and gamete intrafallopian transfer: a meta-analysis of randomized controlled trials. Fertil Steril 1992;58:888–896

Meldrum DR. In vitro fertilization and embryo transfer. In: Sciarra JJ, ed. Gynecology and obstetrics. Vol 5. Philadelphia: JB Lippincott, 1992:1–15

Endocrine Assays

The number of endocrine assays available to the physician or researcher has increased rapidly in recent years. Assays that are becoming obsolete or that are only rarely of use are not discussed. The normal ranges for most of these assays are somewhat laboratory specific, since antibodies are used and they have variable cross-reactions with other compounds present in the specimen unless chromatographic steps are performed. The individual laboratory's normal ranges should be used for interpreting results, making sure that normal ranges appropriate to age, sex, and medical condition of the patient being evaluated are obtained.

UNITS

The units used for reporting results are not constant between laboratories. Values currently may be expressed in milligrams (10^{-3} g), micrograms (10^{-6} g), nanograms (10^{-9} g), or picograms (10^{-12} g) per milliliter or deciliter (100 ml). There is growing pressure to change to yet another unit system called Système International (SI) units which express the concentration in moles per liter. It is not clear at present if and when the SI units will be used at the level of the clinical laboratory in the United States, but if they do, they will inevitably produce the potential for dangerous errors during the transition.

ESTROGENIC STEROIDS

Estradiol

Estradiol immunoassay is useful for monitoring treatment with FSH and LH for infertility, as well as for use as a diagnostic test in cases of amenorrhea. Because there is considerable variation in the concentration of estradiol during the normal menstrual cycle, individual determinations must be interpreted with correction for the timing of onset of the menses preceding and following the date of the blood sample. Very low values (< 50 pg/ml) tend to suggest lack of estrogen secretion by the ovary. Some estrogen is produced in the body by peripheral conversion of adrenal or ovarian androgens, and exogenously administered estrogens can be picked up by the assay as well. When used for monitoring treatment with FSH and LH, the estradiol secretion usually increases exponentially, requiring semilog plots (log of estradiol on the vertical axis and day of treatment on the horizontal axis) to predict future estradiol concentrations accurately.

Estrone

Specific measurements of estrone are possible but require column chromatography. Such determinations are used only for research at the present time.

Estriol

Estriol immunoassay is being used in the midtrimester in combination with determinations of hCG and alpha-fetoprotein to detect patients with an increased probability of carrying a fetus with Down syndrome.

PROGESTATIONAL STEROIDS

Progesterone

Immunoassay for progesterone is useful for detecting progesterone production by the corpus luteum or the placenta. Other sources of small amounts of progesterone include the adrenal gland and the ovarian stroma. These may contribute to basal concentrations of progesterone in congenital adrenal hyperplasia or PCO, respectively. The peak of progesterone secretion in a normal menstrual cycle is 1 week before onset of menses with a slow rise to the peak over the 7 days after ovulation and a slow drop from the peak over the last 7 days before menses. Pulsatile secretion of progesterone is linked to the pulsatile secretion of LH, so there is considerable variability in the progesterone concentration seen during the luteal phase depending on the timing of the blood sample with respect to ovulation or the LH peak. Values of more than 5 ng/ml are generally accepted as confirmatory of ovulation, making progesterone determinations useful in assessing ovulatory function. However, because of the large swings produced during the luteal phase, the interpretation of an isolated progesterone concentration must be correlated with BBT charts and the dates of the preceding and subsequent menses.

An isolated serum progesterone determination should not be used to diagnose a luteal phase defect, since the biologic variability in individual serum progesterone concentrations is too great. During pregnancy, the progesterone level rises progressively to term, reaching far higher values than during the luteal phase. A value of progesterone below 4.5 ng/ml at 5–7 weeks after the last menstrual period in conjunction with an abnormal hCG doubling time, suggests an ectopic pregnancy or a blighted ovum.

17α-Hydroxyprogesterone

Immunoassay for 17α-hydroxyprogesterone is particularly useful in monitoring and diagnosing congenital adrenal hyperplasia due to 21-hydroxylase deficiency. 17α-Hydroxyprogesterone is secreted in large amounts by the corpus luteum, leading to potential confusion in women if the timing of the menstrual cycle is not taken into account during interpretation of results. Since 17α-hydroxyprogesterone is not secreted by the placenta, determination of 17α-progesterone has been used to demonstrate corpus luteum function during pregnancy when the progesterone production due to the corpus luteum cannot be distinguished from that of the placenta. In normal women who do not have a functioning corpus luteum the concentration of 17α-hydroxyprogesterone is generally less than 2 ng/ml. Values near this upper limit can originate from the thecal compartment of the ovary in PCO. Very high values may be secreted by the adrenal gland in congenital adrenal hyperplasia and during the luteal phase in normal women. In congenital adrenal hyperplasia, the cortisol dosage can usually be adjusted to maintain values at or below 2 ng/ml.

ANDROGENIC STEROIDS

Dehydroepiandrosterone Sulfate

The serum concentration of DHEAS is approximately 1,000 times higher than that of DHEA. More than 90% of DHEAS originates from the adrenal gland, making it the best marker of adrenal androgen secretion available. Because of its long half life and stable secretion pattern, DHEAS undergoes essentially no diurnal variation. Dehydroepiandrosterone sulfate is secreted in large quantities in utero by the fetal adrenal gland. Following birth of the infant, DHEAS concentrations fall rapidly. Low plasma concentrations are found in both males and females until shortly prior to puberty, when the increasing concentrations are the first sign of impending puberty. Following puberty the plasma DHEAS concentration remains high in both sexes, reaching a peak in the 20s and then slowly tailing off. The DHEAS concentration eventually drops to very low levels in both sexes late in life.

Testosterone

Testosterone immunoassay is useful in women to evaluate the cause of hirsutism and amenorrhea. In normal women, approximately equal quantities are secreted from the ovary and the adrenal gland. Much of the testosterone in normal women is produced indirectly in the bloodstream from prehormones such as androstenedione and androstenediol. Concentrations of 2 ng/ml or greater are frequently associated with ovarian or adrenal tumors, and, as a rule of thumb, such tumors should be ruled out when concentrations of testosterone exceed 2 ng/ml or greater. The testosterone in blood is bound to a binding globulin (testosterone-binding globulin) very much as T_4 is bound to its own binding globulin. Only free or unbound testosterone is biologically active. Interpretation of testosterone concentrations is made more accurate by use of either a testosterone free index or a determination of dialyzable free testosterone.

Androstenedione

Immunoassay of androstenedione is of less clinical utility than that of either DHEAS or testosterone. Androstenedione is produced in approximately equal amounts by the ovary and adrenal gland in normal women. An increase in the serum androstenedione concentration can be produced by either ovarian or adrenal hypersecretion. Thus, interpretation of elevated values is difficult, since the source of the elevation is not obvious. Androstenedione can serve as a prehormone for production of both testosterone and estrogens.

Dehydroepiandrosterone

Immunoassay of DHEA is one of the least useful of all the assays discussed here. Dehydroepiandrosterone is secreted episodically primarily by the adrenal gland, with approximately 10% by the ovary. It is subject to large diurnal variations in secretion by the adrenal gland (it follows cortisol) and by swings in its secretion, depending on the activity of the ovary. It is potentially useful as a research tool, but for clinical purposes the serum DHEAS concentration is much more informative.

5α-Androstane-3α, 17β-diol Glucuronide

An extensive literature has established that 5α-androstane-3α, 17β-diol glucuronide is a marker of the activity of peripheral 5α-reductase enzyme. This steroid is presumed to reflect paracrine activity of the hormone dihydrotestosterone formed from testosterone and inactivated at its site of action. Serum 5α-androstane-3α, 17β-diol glucuronide correlates highly with genital skin 5α-reductase activity responsible for conversion of testosterone to dihydrotestosterone. Approximately 83% of the steroid is conjugated at position 17 in women. A major fraction of 5α-androstane-3α, 17β-diol glucuronide is derived from other unstudied sources, potentially including DHEAS, DHEA, and androstenedione of adrenal origin. It can be used to obtain a measure of the relative activity of 5α-reductase in hirsute patients.

GLUCOCORTICOID STEROIDS (CORTISOL)

Cortisol is the natural glucocorticoid secreted by the adrenal gland. It is under the control of ACTH and is normally suppressed when exogenous glucocorticoids such as dexamethasone or prednisone are administered. Cortisol is secreted episodically by the adrenal gland, with a marked diurnal variation, producing high morning values and low evening values. In order to interpret cortisol concentrations, careful attention must be paid to the timing of blood sampling and the stress to which the individual has been placed at the time of blood sampling. Cortisol is principally of concern if undersecreted (Addison disease) or oversecreted (Cushing disease or syndrome). A simple test for ruling out Cushing disease is to give 1 mg of dexamethasone orally at 11 PM and to draw an 8-AM blood sample for cortisol determination, which should be less than 5 µg/dl.

PROTEIN HORMONES OF THE REPRODUCTIVE SYSTEM

Prolactin

Prolactin is a protein hormone whose only established function is in milk secretion. Breast-feeding stimulates short-term elevations in serum prolactin levels. The serum concentration of prolactin is frequently increased in patients with pituitary tumors and brain tumors that impinge on the hypothalamic region. Serum prolactin is increased throughout pregnancy. In normal women, serum prolactin concentrations may increase transiently following many stimuli, including painful procedures, anesthesia, pelvic and breast examinations or stimulation, sexual relations, and meals. Many medications produce increases in serum prolactin concentrations, including rauwolfia derivatives, phenothiazine derivatives, substituted butyrophenones, tricyclic antidepressants, opiates, methydopa, TRH, and estrogens.

Gonadotropins

Follicle-stimulating hormone and LH are glycoprotein hormones comprising an alpha subunit and a beta subunit. They share the same alpha subunit as hCG. Determination of serum FSH is useful in diagnosing cases of amenorrhea, since it rises to very high levels in cases of ovarian failure (or menopause). Tests yielding values in the menopausal range should be repeated in younger women on another sample, since sample mixup is possible. Use of the LH:FSH ratio in the diagnosis of PCO is fashionable but unreliable, since some cases of PCO have normal LH:FSH ratios. Abnormal samples should be correlated with the onset of the subsequent menses to rule out sampling during the preovulatory LH surge, which occurs approximately 2 weeks prior to onset of menses in a normal cycle. Values obtained during the LH surge show elevations of both FSH and LH and an elevated LH:FSH ratio in normal women. Due to extensive sharing of peptide sequences between hCG and LH, most LH determinations will cross-react with hCG, and pregnant women appear to have marked elevation in their serum LH concentration (as well as prolactin) but a normal value for FSH.

Human Chorionic Gonadotropin

Human chorionic gonadotropin is a glycoprotein hormone that shares identical alpha subunits with FSH, LH, and TSH. To measure low concentrations of hCG reliably, the use of an antiserum specific for segments of the beta subunit of hCG that are not shared with the beta subunit of LH is required. Zero values for hCG are not seen in most assay systems. Thus, a lower limit of sensitivity must be established for each system below which hCG cannot be reliably detected. This value is in the range of 2–5 mIU/ml in most good systems. In a normal pregnancy, hCG levels rise exponentially for the first 8 weeks after the missed period. They peak at about 10 weeks and slowly tail off to reach a lower plateau that persists throughout the remainder of pregnancy. Ectopic pregnancies and abnormal pregnancies frequently produce lower serum concentrations of hCG, which rise more slowly than normal or fall.

Because of the lack of a universally used hCG standard, there may be significant differences in the value assigned to a single sample by different laboratories. Computing a doubling time from two hCG determinations on blood samples obtained several days apart allows detection of many ectopic and other abnormal pregnancies, due to the abnormal rate of rise found in using the doubling time. The doubling time is independent of the standard used, since it involves computing the ratio of the two samples, and all units cancel out except for time. The doubling time can be calculated by using the formula: Doubling time = $Ln(2) \cdot t / Ln(X2/X1)$, where Ln is the natural log function, t is the time elapsed between the two blood samplings in days (eg, 3 days and 13 hours would be entered in the formula as 3.54 days), and $X1$ and $X2$ are the values for the first and second hCG concentrations, respectively. The mean doubling time of hCG in normal pregnancies is 2.31 days. Confidence limits of 95% include doubling times up to 6 days and as short as 0.9 days. Decreasing values for hCG indicate that a pregnancy is nonviable. Such values inserted into the equation above produce negative results. Values from the equation with a negative sign are called half-life values. The half-life value is also useful to determine whether residual tissue is present. The normal half-life of hCG in women is 24–36 hours (1–1.5 days). Longer half-lives suggest that some viable trophoblast is still present in the body, and this can, of course, include an ectopic pregnancy.

BIBLIOGRAPHY

Jaffe SB, Jewelewicz R. The basic infertility investigation. Fertil Steril 1991;56:599–613

McClamrock HD, Adashi EY. Gestational hyperandrogenism. Fertil Steril 1992;57:257–274

Navot D, Bergh PA, Laufer N. Ovarian hyperstimulation syndrome in novel reproductive technologies: prevention and treatment. Fertil Steril 1992;58:249–261

Rittmaster RS. Androgen conjugates: physiology and clinical significance. Endocr Rev 1993;14:121–132

Schenker JG. Prevention and treatment of ovarian hyperstimulation. Hum Reprod 1993;8:653–659

Shoham Z, Jacobs HS, Insler V. Luteinizing hormone: its role, mechanism of action, and detrimental effects when hypersecreted during the follicular phase. Fertil Steril 1993;59:1153–1161

Speroff L, Glass RH, Kase NG. Clinical gynecologic endocrinology and infertility. 4th ed. Baltimore: Williams and Wilkins, 1989

Wilson JD, Foster DW, eds. Williams textbook of endocrinology. 8th ed. Philadelphia: WB Saunders, 1992

Yen SSC, Jaffe RB, eds. Reproductive endocrinology. 3rd ed. Philadelphia: WB Saunders, 1991

APPENDIX A
REFERENCE VALUES

Measure	SI	Conventional (C)	Conversion Factor (CF) C × CF = SI
Acetoacetate, plasma	<100 µmol/L	<1.0 mg/dl	97.95
Adrenal steroids, plasma			
Aldosterone, supine, saline suppression	<220 pmol/L	<8 ng/dl	27.74
Cortisol			
8 AM	220–660 nmol/L	8–24 µg/dl	27.59
4 PM	50–410 nmol/L	2–15 µg/dl	27.59
Overnight dexamethasone suppression	<140 nmol/L	<5 µg/dl	27.59
Dehydroepiandrosterone (DHEA)	0.6–70 nmol/L	0.2–20 µg/L	3.467
Dehydroepiandrosterone sulfate (DHEAS)	5.4–9.2 µmol/L	820–3380 ng/ml	0.002714
11-Deoxycortisol (compound S)	<60 nmol/L	<2 µg/dl	28.86
17α-Hydroxyprogesterone, women	1–13 nmol/L	0.3–4.2 µg/L	3.026
Adrenal steroids, urinary excretion			
Aldosterone	15–70 nmol/d	5–26 µg/d	2.774
Cortisol, free	30–300 nmol/d	10–100 µg/d	2.759
17-Hydroxycorticosteroids	5.5–28 µmol/d	2–10 mg/d	2.759
17-Ketosteroids, women	14–52 µmol/d	4–15 mg/d	3.467
Ammonia (as NH_3), venous whole blood	6–45 µmol/L	10–80 µg/dl	0.5872
Angiotensin II, plasma, 8 AM	10–30 ng/L	10–30 pg/ml	1.0
Arginine vasopressin (AVP), plasma, random fluid intake	2.3–7.4 pmol/L	2.5–8 ng/L	0.92
Bicarbonate, serum	18–23 mmol/L	18–23 meq/L	1.0
Calciferols (see vitamin D)			
Calcitonin, serum	<50 ng/L	<50 pg/ml	1.0
Calcium			
Ionized serum	1–1.5 mmol/L	4–4.6 mg/dl	0.2495
Total serum	2.2–2.6 mmol/L	9–10.5 mg/dl	0.2495
β-Carotene, serum	0.9–4.6 µmol/L	50–250 µg/dl	0.01863
Catecholamines, plasma			
Epinephrine, basal supine	170–520 pmol/L	30–95 pg/ml	5.458
Norepinephrine, basal supine	0.3–2.8 nmol/L	15–475 pg/ml	0.005911
Catecholamines, urinary			
Epinephrine	<275 nmol/d	<50 µg/d	5.458
Normetanephrine	0–11 µmol/d	0–2.0 mg/d	5.458
Total catecholamines (as norepinephrine)	<675 nmol/d	<120 µg/d	5.911
Vanillylmandelic acid (VMA)	<35 µmol/d	<68 mg/d	5.046
Chloride, serum	98–106 mmol/L	98–106 meq/L	1.0
Cholesterol, plasma			
Total cholesterol			
Desirable	<5.20 mmol/L	<200 mg/dl	0.02586
Borderline high	5.2–6.18 mmol/L	200–239 mg/dl	0.02586
High	≥6.21 mmol/L	≥240 mg/dl	0.02586
High-density lipoprotein (HDL) cholesterol			
Desirable	≥1.29 mmol/L	≥50 mg/dl	0.02586
Borderline high	0.9–1.27 mmol/L	36–49 mg/dl	0.02586
High	≤0.91 mmol/L	≤35 mg/dl	0.02586
Low-density lipoprotein (LDL) cholesterol			
Desirable	<3.36 mmol/L	<130 mg/dl	0.02586
Borderline high	3.39–4.11 mmol/L	131–159 mg/dl	0.02586
High	≥4.14 mmol/L	≥160 mg/dl	0.02586

Measure	SI	Conventional (C)	Conversion Factor (CF) C × CF = SI
Corticotropin (ACTH), plasma	4–22 pmol/L	20–100 pg/ml	0.2202
C peptide, plasma	0.5–2 µg/L	0.5–2 ng/ml	1.0
Creatinine, serum	<133 µmol/L	<1.5 mg/dl	88.40
Fatty acids, nonesterified or free (FFA), plasma	<0.7 mmol/L	<18 mg/dl	0.03906
Gastrin, serum	<120 ng/L	<120 pg/ml	1.0
Glucagon, plasma	50–100 ng/L	50–100 pg/ml	1.0
Glucose, plasma			
Overnight fast, normal	4.2–6.4 mmol/L	75–115 mg/dl	0.05551
Overnight fast, diabetes mellitus	7.8 mmol/L	>140 mg/dl	0.05551
72-h fast, normal women	>2.2 mmol/L	>40 mg/dl	0.05551
Glucose tolerance test, 2-h postprandial plasma glucose			
Normal	<7.8 mmol/L	<140 mg/dl	0.05551
Impaired glucose tolerance	7.8–11.1 mmol/L	140–200 mg/dl	0.05551
Diabetes mellitus	>11.1 mmol/L	>200 mg/dl	0.05551
Gonadal steroids, plasma			
Androstenedione, women	3.5–7.0 nmol/L	1–2 ng/ml	3.492
Estradiol, women			
Basal	70–220 pmol/L	20–60 pg/ml	3.671
Ovulatory surge	>740 pmol/L	>200 pg/ml	3.671
Dihydrotestosterone, women	0.17–1.0 nmol/L	0.05–3 ng/ml	3.467
Progesterone, women			
Luteal phase	6–64 nmol/L	2–20 ng/ml	3.180
Follicular phase	<6 nmol/L	<2 ng/ml	3.180
Testosterone			
Women	<3.5 nmol/L	<1 ng/ml	3.467
Prepubertal boys and girls	0.2–0.7 nmol/L	0.05–0.2 ng/ml	3.467
Gonadotropins, plasma			
Women, basal			
Follicle-stimulating hormone	5–20 IU/L	5–20 mIU/ml	1.0
Luteinizing hormone	5–25 IU/L	5–25 mIU/ml	1.0
Women, ovulatory peak			
Follicle-stimulating hormone	12–30 IU/L	12–30 mIU/ml	1.0
Luteinizing hormone	25–100 IU/L	25–100 mIU/ml	1.0
Prepubertal boys and girls			
Follicle-stimulating hormone	<5 IU/L	<5 mIU/ml	1.0
Luteinizing hormone	<5 IU/L	<5 mIU/ml	1.0
Growth hormone, plasma			
After 100 g glucose orally	<5 µg/L	<5 ng/ml	1.0
After insulin-induced hypoglycemia	>9 µg/L	>9 ng/ml	1.0
Human chorionic gonadotropin, beta subunit, plasma; nonpregnant women	<3 IU/L	<3 mIU/ml	1.0
β-Hydroxybutyrate, plasma	<300 nmol/L	<3.0 mg/dl	96.05
Insulin, plasma			
Fasting	35–145 pmol/L	5–20 µU/ml	7.175
During hypoglycemia (plasma glucose <2.8 nmol/L [<50 mg/dl])	<35 pmol/L	<5 µU/ml	7.175
Insulin-like growth factor I (IGF I, somatomedin-C), women	0.45–2.2 kU/L	0.45–2.2 U/ml	1.0
Lactate, plasma	0.56–2.2 mmol/L	5–20 mg/dl	0.111
Magnesium, serum	0.8–1.20 mmol/L	1.8–3.0 mg/dl	0.4114
Osmolality, plasma	285–295 mmol/kg	285–295 mosm/kg	1.0

Measure	SI	Conventional (C)	Conversion Factor (CF) C × CF = SI
Oxytocin, plasma			
Random	1–4 pmol/L	1.25–5 ng/L	0.80
Ovulatory peak in women	408 pmol/L	5–10 ng/L	0.80
Parathyroid hormone, serum (intact PTH using immunoradiometric assay [IRMA])	10–65 ng/L	10–65 pg/ml	1.0
Phosphorus, inorganic, serum	1–1.5 mmol/L	3.0–4.5 mg/dl	0.3229
Potassium, serum	3.5–5.0 mmol/L	3.5–5.0 meq/L	1.0
Prolactin, serum	2–15 µg/L	2–15 ng/ml	1.0
Pyruvate, blood	39–102 µmol/L	0.3–0.9 mg/dl	0.01129
Renin activity, plasma, normal-sodium diet			
Supine	3.2 ± 1 µg/L/h	3.2 ± 1.1 ng/ml/h	1.0
Standing	9.3 ± 4.3 µg/L/h	9.3 ± 4.3 ng/ml/h	1.0
Sodium, serum	136–145 mmol/L	136–145 meq/L	1.0
Thyroid function tests			
Radioactive iodine uptake, 24 h	0.05–0.30	5–30%	—
Reverse triiodothyronine (rT_3), serum	0.15–0.61 nmol/L	10–4 ng/dl	0.01536
Thyrotropin (TSH), highly sensitive assay, serum	0.6–4.6 mU/L	0.6–4.6 µU/ml	1.0
Thyroxine (T_4), serum	51–42 nmol/L	4–11 µg/dl	12.87
Thyroxine-binding globulin, serum (as thyroxine)	150–360 nmol/L	12–28 µg/ml	12.87
Triiodothyronine (T_3), serum	1.2–3.4 nmol/L	75–220 ng/dl	0.01536
Triiodothyronine resin uptake, serum	0.25–0.35	25–35%	—
Triglycerides, plasma (as Triolein)	<1.80 mmol/L	<160 mg/dl	0.01129
Uric acid, serum	120–420 µmol/L	2–7 mg/dl	59.48
Vitamin D (as vitamin D, cholecalciferol), plasma			
1, 25-Dihydroxycholecalciferol (1,25(OH)$_2$D)	36–144 pmol/L	15–60 pg/ml	2.400
25-Hydroxycholecalciferol (25-OHD)	20–100 nmol/L	8–40 ng/ml	2.496

Modified from Wilson JD, Foster DW. Williams textbook of endocrinology. 8th ed. Philadelphia: WB Saunders, 1991

APPENDIX B
ACOG RESOURCES

The ACOG Technical Bulletin series of the American College of Obstetricians and Gynecologists is designed to provide practicing physicians with the latest proven techniques of clinical practice. ACOG Committee Opinions are intended to provide timely information on controversial issues, ethical concerns, and emerging approaches to clinical management. Subscriptions and complete sets of all Technical Bulletins or Committee Opinions in print, with or without a three-ring binder, are available for sale. Contact the ACOG Resource Center for a current list and order forms for both series. (Because individual Technical Bulletins and Committee Opinions are withdrawn from and added to the series, some of the titles listed here may no longer be current.)

ACOG Technical Bulletins

Number	Title	Publication Date
68	Dysmenorrhea	March 1983
75	Septic Shock	March 1984
78	Blood Component Therapy	July 1984
82	Hemorrhagic Shock	December 1984
83	Genitourinary Fistulas	January 1985
84	Teratology	February 1985
86	Grief Related to Perinatal Death	April 1985
91	Management of Preeclampsia	March 1986
92	Management of Diabetes Mellitus in Pregnancy	May 1986
95	Management of the Breech Presentation	August 1986
100	Urinary Incontinence	January 1987
103	Evaluation and Treatment of Hirsute Women	April 1987
106	Oral Contraception	July 1987
108	Antenatal Diagnosis of Genetic Disorders	September 1987
109	Methods of Midtrimester Abortion	October 1987
111	Prophylactic Oophorectomy	December 1987
112	Obstetric Anesthesia and Analgesia	January 1988
113	Sterilization	February 1988
115	Premature Rupture of Membranes	April 1988
117	Antimicrobial Therapy for Obstetric Patients	June 1988
119	Gynecologic Herpes Simplex Virus Infections	August 1988
120	Medical Induction of Ovulation	September 1988
122	Perinatal Herpes Simplex Virus Infections	November 1988
124	The Battered Woman	January 1989
125	Infertility	February 1989
127	Assessment of Fetal and Newborn Acid–Base Status	April 1989
128	Amenorrhea	May 1989
129	Chronic Pelvic Pain	June 1989
130	Diagnosis and Management of Postterm Pregnancy	July 1989
131	Multiple Gestation	August 1989
132	Intrapartum Fetal Heart Rate Monitoring	September 1989
133	Preterm Labor	October 1989
134	Dysfunctional Uterine Bleeding	October 1989
135	Vulvovaginitis	November 1989
136	Ethical Decision-Making in Obstetrics and Gynecology	November 1989
137	Dystocia	December 1989
138	Diagnosis and Management of Invasive Cervical Carcinomas	December 1989
139	Vulvar Dystrophies	January 1990
140	New Reproductive Technologies	March 1990
141	Cancer of the Ovary	May 1990
142	Male Infertility	June 1990

ACOG Technical Bulletins (continued)

Number	Title	Publication Date
143	Diagnosis and Management of Postpartum Hemorrhage	July 1990
145	The Adolescent Obstetric–Gynecologic Patient	September 1990
146	Laser Technology	September 1990
147	Prevention of D Isoimmunization	October 1990
148	Management of Isoimmunization in Pregnancy	October 1990
149	Stress in the Practice of Obstetrics and Gynecology	November 1990
150	Ectopic Pregnancy	December 1990
151	Automobile Passenger Restraints for Children and Pregnant Women	January 1991
152	Operative Vaginal Delivery	February 1991
153	Antimicrobial Therapy for Gynecologic Infections	March 1991
154	Alpha-Fetoprotein	April 1991
155	Classification and Staging of Gynecologic Malignancies	May 1991
156	Nonmalignant Conditions of the Breast	June 1991
157	Induction and Augmentation of Labor	July 1991
158	Carcinoma of the Breast	August 1991
159	Fetal Macrosomia	September 1991
160	Immunization During Pregnancy	October 1991
161	Trauma During Pregnancy	November 1991
162	Carcinoma of the Endometrium	December 1991
163	Fetal and Neonatal Neurologic Injury	January 1992
164	The Intrauterine Device	February 1992
166	Hormone Replacement Therapy	April 1992
167	Osteoporosis	May 1992
168	Cardiac Disease in Pregnancy	June 1992
169	Human Immunodeficiency Virus Infections	June 1992
170	Group B Streptococcal Infections in Pregnancy	July 1992
171	Rubella and Pregnancy	August 1992
172	Sexual Assault	September 1992
173	Women and Exercise	October 1992
174	Hepatitis in Pregnancy	November 1992
175	Invasive Hemodynamic Monitoring in Obstetrics and Gynecology	December 1992
176	Diagnosis and Management of Fetal Death	January 1993
177	Perinatal Viral and Parasitic Infections	February 1993
178	Management of Gestational Trophoblastic Disease	March 1993
179	Nutrition During Pregnancy	April 1993
180	Smoking and Reproductive Health	May 1993
181	Thyroid Disease in Pregnancy	June 1993
182	Depression in Women	July 1993
183	Cervical Cytology: Evaluation and Management of Abnormalities	August 1993
184	Endometriosis	September 1993
185	Hemoglobinopathies in Pregnancy	October 1993
186	Vulvar Cancer	November 1993
187	Ultrasonography in Pregnancy	December 1993
188	Antepartum Fetal Surveillance	January 1994
189	Exercise During Pregnancy and the Postpartum Period	February 1994
190	Gonorrhea and Chlamydial Infections	March 1994
191	Hysteroscopy	April 1994
192	Uterine Leiomyomata	May 1994
193	Genital Human Papillomavirus Infections	June 1994
194	Substance Abuse	July 1994
195	Substance Abuse in Pregnancy	July 1994

ACOG Committee Opinions

Number	Title	Publication Date
16	Effectiveness of Tubal Sterilization *Committee on Gynecologic Practice*	December 1981 (Reaffirmed 1992)
38	Withholding or Withdrawing Life-Sustaining Medical Therapy *Committee on Ethics*	June 1985
41	Contraception for Women in Their Later Reproductive Years *Committee on Gynecologic Practice*	December 1985 (Reaffirmed 1988)
45	Guidelines for Relationships Between Industry and the American College of Obstetricians and Gynecologists and Its Fellows *Committee on Ethics*	October 1985
46	Endorsement of Institutional Ethics Committees *Committee on Ethics*	October 1985
47	Ethical Issues in Human In Vitro Fertilization and Embryo Placement *Committee on Ethics*	July 1986
49	Use and Misuse of the Apgar Score *Committee on Obstetric Practice* *(Joint with AAP Committee on Fetus and Newborn)*	November 1986 (Reaffirmed 1991)
55	Patient Choice: Maternal–Fetal Conflict *Committee on Ethics*	October 1987
56	Ethical Issues Relating to Expert Testimony by Obstetricians and Gynecologists *Committee on Ethics*	October 1987
60	Estrogen Dose in Oral Contraceptives *Committee on Gynecologic Practice*	March 1988 (Reaffirmed 1991)
61	Ethical Issues in Pregnancy Counseling *Committee on Ethics*	March 1988
63	Sterilization of Women Who Are Mentally Handicapped *Committee on Ethics*	September 1988
64	Guidelines for Vaginal Delivery After a Previous Cesarean Birth *Committee on Obstetric Practice*	October 1988 (Reaffirmed 1991)
66	Premenstrual Syndrome *Committee on Gynecologic Practice*	January 1989 (Reaffirmed 1990)
69	Chorionic Villus Sampling *Committee on Obstetric Practice*	November 1989 (Reaffirmed 1991)
73	Ethical Considerations in Sterilization *Committee on Ethics*	September 1989
75	Qualifications and Privileges for Performing Gynecologic Intraabdominal Laser Therapy *Committee on Gynecologic Practice*	November 1989 (Reaffirmed 1992)
76	Maternal Serum Alpha-Fetoprotein *Committee on Obstetric Practice*	December 1989 (Reaffirmed 1991)
79	Scope of Services for Uncomplicated Obstetric Care *Committee on Obstetric Practice*	January 1990 (Reaffirmed 1993)
86	CPT Coding: Unbundled Services *Committee on Health Economics Analysis*	October 1990 (Reaffirmed 1992)
87	Deception *Committee on Ethics*	November 1990
88	Ethical Issues in Surrogate Motherhood *Committee on Ethics*	November 1990

ACOG Committee Opinions (continued)

Number	Title	Publication Date
89	Qualifications and Privileges for Performing Gynecologic Laser Therapy in the Lower Genital Tract *Committee on Gynecologic Practice*	December 1990 (Reaffirmed 1992)
90	Safety of Oral Contraceptives for Teenagers *Committee on Adolescent Health Care*	February 1991
92	Statement on Surgical Assistants *Committee on Obstetric Practice* *(Joint with Committee on Gynecologic Practice)*	March 1991 (Reaffirmed 1993)
93	Screening for Tay–Sachs Disease *Committee on Obstetric Practice*	March 1991 (Reaffirmed 1992)
94	Multifetal Pregnancy Reduction and Selective Fetal Termination *Committee on Ethics*	April 1991
98	Fetal Maturity Assessment Prior to Elective Repeat Cesarean Delivery *Committee on Obstetric Practice*	September 1991 (Reaffirmed 1993)
100	Second-Look Surgery for Ovarian Carcinoma *Committee on Gynecologic Practice*	November 1991 (Reaffirmed 1993)
101	Current Status of Cystic Fibrosis Carrier Screening *Committee on Obstetric Practice*	November 1991 (Reaffirmed 1993)
104	Anesthesia for Emergency Deliveries *Committee on Obstetric Practice*	March 1992 (Reaffirmed 1993)
105	Postpartum Tubal Sterilization *Committee on Obstetric Practice*	March 1992 (Reaffirmed 1993)
106	Credentialing Guidelines for Operative Laparoscopy *Committee on Gynecologic Practice*	April 1992
107	Credentialing Guidelines for Operative Hysteroscopy *Committee on Gynecologic Practice*	April 1992
108	Ethical Dimensions of Informed Consent *Committee on Ethics*	May 1992
110	Recertification *ABOG/ACOG Liaison Committee*	May 1992
112	Vitamin A Supplementation During Pregnancy *Committee on Obstetric Practice*	August 1992
114	Cocaine in Pregnancy *Committee on Obstetric Practice*	September 1992
115	Home Uterine Activity Monitoring *Committee on Obstetric Practice*	September 1992
116	Utility of Antepartum Doppler for Estimating Umbilical and Uterine Artery Flow *Committee on Obstetric Practice*	November 1992
117	Genetic Risk and Screening Techniques for Epithelial Ovarian Cancer *Committee on Gynecologic Practice*	December 1992
118	Pain Relief During Labor *Committee on Obstetric Practice*	January 1993
119	Zygote Intrafallopian Transfer *Committee on Gynecologic Practice*	February 1993
120	Folic Acid for the Prevention of Recurrent Neural Tube Defects *Committee on Obstetric Practice*	March 1993

ACOG Committee Opinions (continued)

Number	Title	Publication Date
121	Obstetric Management of Patients with Spinal Cord Injury *Committee on Obstetric Practice*	April 1993
122	Adolescent Acquaintance Rape *Committee on Adolescent Health Care*	May 1993
123	Prostaglandin E$_2$ Gel for Cervical Ripening *Committee on Obstetric Practice*	June 1993
124	Contraceptives and Congenital Anomalies *Committee on Gynecologic Practice*	July 1993
125	Placental Pathology *Committee on Obstetric Practice*	July 1993
126	Estrogen Replacement Therapy and Endometrial Cancer *Committee on Gynecologic Practice*	August 1993
127	Office Mammography *Committee on Gynecologic Practice*	August 1993
128	Routine Cancer Screening *Committee on Gynecologic Practice*	October 1993
129	Commercial Ventures in Medicine: Concerns About the Patenting of Procedures *Committee on Ethics*	November 1993
130	Human Immunodeficiency Virus Infection: Physicians' Responsibilities *Committee on Ethics*	November 1993
131	Diethylstilbestrol *Committee on Gynecologic Practice*	December 1993
132	Maximizing Pregnancy Rates Resulting from Donor Insemination with Frozen Semen *Committee on Gynecologic Practice*	January 1994
133	Colposcopy Training and Practice *Committee on Gynecologic Practice*	March 1994
134	Length of Hospital Stay for Gynecologic Procedures *Committee on Gynecologic Practice*	March 1994
135	Estrogen Replacement Therapy in Women with Previously Treated Breast Cancer *Committee on Gynecologic Practice*	April 1994
136	Preembryo Research: History, Scientific Background, and Ethical Considerations *Committee on Ethics*	April 1994
137	Fetal Distress and Birth Asphyxia *Committee on Obstetric Practice*	April 1994
138	Utility of Umbilical Cord Blood Acid–Base Assessment *Committee on Obstetric Practice*	April 1994
139	Adolescents' Right to Refuse Long-Term Contraceptives *Committee on Adolescent Health Care*	June 1994
140	The Role of the Obstetrician–Gynecologist in the Diagnosis and Treatment of Breast Disease *Committee on Gynecologic Practice*	June 1994

INDEX

A

Abdominal pain
  low, 66–71
    history-taking with, 66
    physical examination with, 67
    with pelvic inflammatory disease, 94–95
    with peptic ulcer disease, 30
Abdominal wall, ultrasound evaluation of, 221
Abdominal wound, failure, 285–286
ABO incompatibility, 156
Abortifacients, steroidal, 295
Abortion
  failed, 292–293
  hysterectomy for, 294–295
  hysterotomy for, 294–295
  incomplete, 292–293
  induced. *See also* Pregnancy, termination
    ethical issues related to, 113–114
    first-trimester, 291–293
    oral contraceptive use after, 58
    second-trimester, 293–294
    subsequent reproduction after, 295
  septic, pelvic pain with, 68
  spontaneous
    and chromosomal abnormalities, 135, 433–434
    congenital uterine anomalies and, 434–435
    in diabetes mellitus, 436
    endocrine factors in, 435
    environmental factors and, 437
    evaluation and follow-up with, 438
    with immunologic disorders, 437
    with infection, 436
    leiomyomata and, 436
    with luteal phase defect, 436
    pelvic pain with, 68
    placentation abnormalities and, 435–436
    psychologic factors and, 437
    recurrent, 433–438
      genetics of, 135, 433–434
      risk, 433, 433t
    with severe maternal illness, 437
    in thyroid disease, 436
Abruptio placentae, 155
Abscess
  Bartholin duct, 227–228
  brain, sinusitis-related, 16
  breast, 76
  dural, sinusitis-related, 16
  pelvic, postoperative, 281
  tuboovarian, pelvic pain with, 67–68
Abstinence, periodic, 56–57
Acetaminophen
  for headache, 45
  for osteoarthritis, 34

Acetic acid, vulvar washing with, 227
Acid aspiration, 271–272
Acid–base analysis, umbilical cord blood, 143–144
Acid–base balance, fetal, 143–144
Acidemia, fetal or newborn, 143
Acidosis, fetal or newborn, 143
Acne, 51
  and oral contraceptive use, 58
  in pregnant patient, 177
ACOGNET, 120
Acquired immunodeficiency syndrome, 91–93
  clinical features of, 92
  diagnosis of, 92–93
  epidemiology of, 91
  management of, 93
  in pregnant patient, 182
Acrochordon, vulvar, 227
Actinomycin D, for gestational trophoblastic tumors, 340–341
Activins, 371
Acute fatty liver of pregnancy, 166
Acute intermittent porphyria, abdominal pain with, 68
Addison disease, 415–416
  in pregnant patient, 176
Adenocarcinoma
  endometrial, 321
    prognosis for, 322
  vaginal, diethylstilbestrol and, 315–316
  vulvar, 307, 312
Adenofibroma(s), 250
  endometrioid, 257
  ovarian, 257
    mucinous, 257
    serous, 257
Adenoma(s)
  adrenal, 397
  ovarian, 257
  pituitary. *See also* Prolactinoma(s)
    hyperthyroidism with, 48–49
Adenomatoid tumor(s), of uterus, 250
Adenomyosis
  chronic pelvic pain with, 70
  diagnosis of, 249
  histogenesis of, 248–249
  incidence of, 248
  pathogenesis of, 248
  pathology of, 248–249
  signs and symptoms, 249
  treatment of, 249
Adenosis, with intrauterine diethylstilbestrol exposure, 316
Adhesion barrier materials, and wound healing, 264
Adhesions
  intestinal, surgical management, complications of, 274–275

Adhesions *(continued)*
  intrauterine, 426–427
    hysteroscopy for, 212
  labial, in pediatric patient, 385
Admission, for surgery, 225
Adnexa
  removal, uterine conservation with, 250
  ultrasound evaluation of, 220
Adnexal mass(es)
  diagnosis of, 258–259
  management of, 330, 330t
Adnexal problems, pelvic pain with, 68
Adolescent gynecology, 387–390
Adolescents, oral contraceptives for, 58
Adrenal crisis, in pregnant patient, 176
Adrenal gland(s), 409–417
  anatomy of, 409
  disorders, amenorrhea secondary to, 391
  fetal, 149
  function, laboratory evaluation of, 409–411
  maternal, in pregnancy, 150, 176
  tumors of, 397
Adrenal steroid(s), synthesis and secretion, 409, 410f
Adrenarche, 388
Adrenocortical deficiency, primary, 415–416
Adult respiratory distress syndrome, 271
  pregnant patient with, 165
Aerobic capacity, and exercise, 10
AFAFP. *See* Alpha-fetoprotein, amniotic fluid
Affect, definition of, 40
Affective disorders, 40
Alanine phosphatase, in gallbladder disease, 31
Albuterol, 17
Alcohol
  abuse, 12–13
    detection of, CAGE technique for, 13
  injection, for vulvar pruritus, 229
  teratogenicity, 140
Aldosterone, synthesis and secretion, 409
Alkaline phosphatase
  in gallbladder disease, 31
  in Paget disease of bone, 37
Alkylating agents, teratogenicity, 346–347, 347t
Allergy, dermatitis in, 50
Alloimmune thrombocytopenia, neonatal, fetal therapy for, 131–132
Allopurinol, for gout, 35
Alpha and beta blockers, mixed, for hypertension, 22
Alpha blockers, for hypertension, 22–23
Alpha-fetoprotein
  amniotic fluid, 137

Alpha-fetoprotein *(continued)*
  maternal serum, 136–137
Alprazolam, in management of premenstrual syndrome, 75
Amaurosis fugax, in giant cell arteritis, 35
Ambulation, early, postoperative, 268
Amenorrhea
  in anorexia nervosa, 393–394
  exercise-induced, 394–395
  with hyperprolactinemia, 392–393
  post-pill, 58
  primary, 389–390
  secondary, 391–395
    causes of, 391
American College of Obstetricians and Gynecologists, Resource Center, 120–121
American Fertility Society, classification of endometriosis, 253, 254f
Aminopterin, teratogenicity, 346, 347t
Amitriptyline, 42
  for migraine prevention, 46
  side effects of, 43
Amniocentesis, 137–138
Amniotic fluid
  dynamics, 144–145
  production, 144–145
  volume, 144–145
    assessment of, 128, 130
Amniotic fluid index, 128, 130–131, 162
Amoxapine, 42
  side effects of, 43
Amoxicillin
  for cystitis, 20
  for gonorrhea, 84
  for *Helicobacter pylori* infection, 30
  for syphilis, 85
Ampicillin, for cystitis, 20
Amsacrine, teratogenicity, 347t
Analgesia
  obstetric, 196–198
  postoperative, 269–270
Analgesics
  for back pain, 39
  for headache, 45
  overuse of, 46–47
Anal wink reflex, 236
Anatomic support defects and dysfunction. *See also* Genital prolapse
  classification of, 230
  nonsurgical management of, 232
  physical examination with, 231–232
  surgical management of, 231–237
  treatment of, 232–237
Androgen(s), in follicular development, 369
Androgen excess, 395–398, 411–412
  differential diagnosis of, 397
  laboratory evaluation for, 412
  treatment of, 428
Androgen insensitivity syndromes, 382–383

5α-Androstane-3α,17β-diol glucuronide, assays, 444
Androstenedione
  assays, 444
  synthesis and secretion of, 412, 413f
Anemia
  fetal, 157
  perioperative management of, 268
  postoperative, 268
  in pregnant patient, 172
Anesthesia
  complications of, 270–273
  for laparoscopy, 213
  obstetric, 196–198
  during pregnancy, 344
Aneuploidy
  detection of, in uncultured amniocytes, 138
  and multiple spontaneous abortions, 135
  parental, 135
Anger, as defense mechanism, for dying patient, 355
Angioma(s), uterine, 250
Angiotensin converting enzyme inhibitors
  for hypertension, 22–23
  for incipient diabetic nephropathy, 26
Anorexia nervosa
  amenorrhea secondary to, 393–394
  incidence of, 393
  management of, 393
  pathophysiology of, 393–394
Anoscopy, 222–223
Anovulation
  chronic hypothalamic, 391
  investigation and treatment of, 421–422
Antacids, for gastroesophageal reflux, 30
Antepartum care, 124–143
  follow-up visits in, 126
  initial history-taking in, 124
  laboratory tests in, 124–125
  patient education in, 124
  physical examination in, 124
  routine, 124–126
  ultrasonography in, 126–129
Antepartum testing, 129–131
  indications for, 129
  techniques, 129–131
Antibiotic therapy
  for acne, 51
  for bronchitis, 16
  for cystitis, 20
  for *Helicobacter pylori* infection, 30
  for necrotizing infections, 282
  for pneumonia, 17–18
  prophylactic
    for rape victim, 106
    for surgery patient, 225–226
  for sinusitis, 15
  for surgical pelvic infection, 281
  for tuberculosis, 18
  for urethritis, 19

Antibiotic therapy *(continued)*
  and wound healing, 264–265
Anticardiolipin antibodies, and spontaneous abortion, 437
Anticipation, 380
Anticoagulants, teratogenicity, 139
Anticoagulation, for deep vein thrombosis, 284–285
Anticonvulsants
  for migraine prevention, 46
  teratogenicity, 139
Antidepressants, 41–43
  in management of premenstrual syndrome, 75
  for migraine prevention, 46
Antidiuretic hormone, secretion, 364
Antifetal antibodies, and spontaneous abortion, 437
Antihypertensive therapy, in management of pregnancy-induced hypertension, 153–154
Antimetabolites, teratogenicity, 346–347, 347t
Antimuscarinic drugs, for peptic ulcer disease, 30
Antiphospholipid antibodies, and spontaneous abortion, 437
Antiphospholipid antibody syndrome, in pregnant patient, 179
Antirheumatoid drugs, for rheumatoid arthritis, 33–34
Antiseptics, topical, and wound healing, 264
Antithyroid drugs
  for hyperthyroidism, 49
  teratogenicity, 139
Apnea of prematurity, 201
Arachidonic acid metabolism, 376, 377f
ARDS. *See* Adult respiratory distress syndrome
Arterial blood gases, in asthma, 16–17
Arthritis
  epidemiology of, 32
  gouty, 35–36
  psoriatic, differential diagnosis of, 33
  in viral infection, differential diagnosis of, 33
Asherman syndrome, spontaneous abortion and, 435–436
Aspiration, of gastric contents, 271–272
Aspirin
  for headache, 45
  low-dose, to prevent pregnancy-induced hypertension/preeclampsia, 154
  for osteoarthritis, 34
  for rheumatoid arthritis, 33
Assessment
  initial, of patient, 2
  routine periodic, 8
Assisted reproductive technology, 421, 439–443
  future developments in, 442

Assisted reproductive technology
        (*continued*)
    laparoscopy in, 214
    procedures, 439–442
Asthma
    clinical features of, 16
    epidemiology of, 16
    management of, 16–17
    pathophysiology of, 16
    pregnant patient with, 165
Atenolol
    for hypertension, 22
    for migraine prevention, 46
Atherosclerosis
    and diabetes, 26
    postmenopausal, 403–404
Atopic dermatitis, 50
    in pediatric patient, 385
Atrophic vaginitis, 81
Atropine sulfate, for cardiac arrest, 272
Atypical squamous cells of undetermined
        significance, 216
Autoimmune disorder(s), 145
    and spontaneous abortion, 437
Autoimmune thyroiditis, 47–48
Autonomy, 112–113
    ethical principle of, 356–357
Autosomal chromosomal alterations, and
        malignancy, 298–299
Autosomal dominant traits, 380
Autosomal recessive disorders, 379–380
Autosomes, 379
Azithromycin
    for *Chlamydia* infection, 83
    for gonorrhea, 84

B

Back pain
    diagnosis of, 38–39
    management of, 39–40
    physical examination with, 39
    spectrum of, 37
    tests with, 39
Bacteria, commensal, of genital tract, 280
Bacterial infection(s)
    sexually transmitted, 82–85
    sinusitis caused by, 15
    of skin, 51
Bacterial vaginosis, diagnosis and
        management of, 78–79
Bacteriuria
    asymptomatic, 20
        in pregnant patient, 184
    management of, 20
    and urinary incontinence, 236
Bacteroides, pelvic inflammatory disease
        caused by, 94
Balanced anesthesia, obstetric, 198
Balanced translocation(s), parental, 133–134
Bargaining, as defense mechanism, for
        dying patient, 355

Barium enema, in diagnosis of colorectal
        cancer, 32
Bartholin duct
    abscess, 227–228
    cyst, 227–228
Bartholin gland
    cancer of, 312
    tumors, 227
Basal body temperature
    in confirmation of ovulation and
        assessment of luteal function,
        423–424
    in fertile interval prediction, 57
Basal cell carcinoma, vulvar, 313
Base deficit, 143
Base excess, 143
Battered child syndrome, 103–104
Battered wife syndrome, 107–109
Battered woman, 107–109
Beneficence, 112, 114
    ethical principle of, 356
Benzathine penicillin, for syphilis, 85
Benzoyl peroxide, for acne, 51
Bereavement, 354–355
Beta blockers
    for hypertension, 22
    for hyperthyroidism, 49
    for migraine prevention, 46
    for tocolysis, 159–160
Betamethasone, with preterm labor and
        delivery, 160
Bethesda system, for reporting cervical
        cytology, 216
Bias, statistical, 118
Biliary colic, 31
Biliary tract cancer, 352
Bilirubin, serum, 31
Bioethics, 111
Biofeedback, for detrusor instability, 241
Biophysical profile, 129–130
Biopsy. *See also* Fine-needle aspiration
        biopsy; Cervical biopsy
    of thyroid nodule, 49
Biostatistics, 118–120
Biparietal diameter, 162
Birth defects, and oral contraceptive use,
        59
Birth injury, 195
Birth weight, and maternal smoking, 140
Bismuth emulsion, for *Helicobacter pylori*
        infection, 30–31
Bladder
    infections, management of, 19–20
    intraoperative injury and fistulas, 279–280
    irritative problems of, 242–244
    postoperative care, 269
    retraining, for detrusor instability, 241
    ultrasound evaluation of, 221
Blastomere biopsy, 138
Bleeding. *See also* Dysfunctional uterine
        bleeding; Hemorrhage

Bleeding (*continued*)
    menstrual, with oral contraceptives, 59
    postoperative
        ovarian vessel, management, 274
        retroperitoneal venous, management, 274
        uterine vessel, management, 274
        vaginal, management, 274
    in second half of pregnancy, 154–155
    uterine
        abnormal, hysteroscopic diagnosis
            of, 211
        with intrauterine devices, 60
    vaginal
        with endometrial carcinoma, 322
        in pediatric patient, 386
Bleomycin, effect on ovarian function, 343t
Blood, occult, in stool, 32
Blood glucose. *See also* Hyperglycemia;
        Hypoglycemia
    in diagnosis of diabetes, 24–25
Blood group incompatibility, fetal–
        maternal, 156–158
Blood pressure. *See also* Hypertension
    classification of, 21
    measurement of, 21
Blood transfusion
    autologous, 268
    risks of, 268
Body mass index, 11
Bone density, measurement of, 36, 402–403
Bone disease, 32–37
Bone loss, age-associated, 36, 402–403
Bone mass, 36
    accrual, 402–403
    measurement of, 36, 402–403
Bowel care, postoperative, 268–269
Bowel preparation, preoperative, 268
Bowen disease, and human papillomavirus
        infection, 88
Brain disorders, in neonates and infants,
        intrapartum-related, 195–196
Breast(s)
    abscess, 76
    benign neoplasms of, 76–77
    cancer of, 76, 301–306
        adjuvant treatment, 305–306
        and diethylstilbestrol exposure in
            utero, 316
        diagnosis of, 28–29
        ductal, 302–303
        epidemiology of, 28, 301–302
        histology of, 302–303
        and hormone therapy, 406
        incidence of, 301
        lifetime risk of, 301
        lobular, 302–303
        management of, 27–29
        medical–legal considerations, 306
        metastatic, 306
        mortality with, 301

Breast(s), cancer of *(continued)*
    and oral contraceptive use, 58–59
    pathology of, 302–303
    in pregnancy, 350
    prognosis for, 306
    protective factors for, 301–302
    recurrence, predictors of, 305
    risk factors for, 301–302
    screening for, 28
    staging, 303
    treatment options, 303–305
  clinical examination of, 28
  congenital absence of, 75
  cystic mass in, management of, 29
  developmental anomalies, 75
  development of, 388
    asymmetric, 75
    premature, 75
  disorders of, 75–77
  fibroadenoma of, 76
  fibrocystic changes of, 75
  hypertrophy, 75
  intraductal papilloma, 76
  lipoma of, 76
  mass(es) or lump in, management of, 28–29
  overdevelopment, 75
  physical examination of, 28–29
  reconstruction, after breast cancer surgery, 305
  self-examination of, 28–29
  squamous metaplasia, 76
  superficial angiitis of, 76
  tenderness, 76–77
  trauma, 76
Breast-feeding, 204
  oral contraceptive use during, 58
Breast implant(s), silicone, 305
Breech delivery, vaginal, 194
Brenner tumors, 257–258
Bretylium, in cardiopulmonary resuscitation, 272–273
Bromocriptine, in management of premenstrual syndrome, 75
Bronchitis
  chronic, 16
  management of, 16
BSE. *See* Breast(s), self-examination of
Bullae, 50
Bupropion, 42
  side effects of, 43
Buserelin, dosage and administration, 428t
Busulfan
  effect on ovarian function, 343t
  teratogenicity, 347t
Butalbital, for headache, 45

C

CA 125, 258–259
  as marker for ovarian cancer, 327, 330, 333–334
  serum elevations, causes of, 330

Caffeine, for headache, 45
CAGE technique, for detection of alcohol abuse, 13
Calcitonin, therapy
  for osteoporosis, 37
  in Paget disease of bone, 37
Calcium
  dietary, intake, 36–37
  supplementation, in management of premenstrual syndrome, 74
Calcium channel blockers
  for hypertension, 22–23
  for migraine prevention, 46
  for tocolysis, 160
Calcium homeostasis, fetal, 149
Calendar rhythm method, in fertile interval prediction, 57
Calorie requirement, postoperative, 267
Cancer
  biliary tract, 352
  breast. *See* Breast(s), cancer of
  cervical. *See* Cervical cancer
  and chromosomal abnormalities, 298
  colon. *See* Colorectal cancer
  colorectal. *See* Colorectal cancer
  endometrial. *See* Endometrial carcinoma
  of fallopian tube. *See* Fallopian tube(s), cancer of
  fetal–placental metastasis, 347
  genetics and, 298–301
  hematologic, in pregnancy, 351–352
  hereditary factors in, 298
  liver, in pregnancy, 352–353
  lung. *See* Lung cancer
  ovarian. *See* Ovarian cancer
  pain control for, 356–357
  pancreatic, 352
  and pregnancy, 342–353
  during pregnancy, 343–353
    diagnosis of, 343
    embryology of, 343–344
    immunology of, 343
    incidence of, 343
    non–reproductive tract, 350–353
    radiation therapy for, 345–346
    reproductive tract, 347–350
    signs and symptoms of, 343
    surgery for, 344–345
    treatment of, 343–347
  previously treated, and pregnancy, 342–343
  and sexual dysfunction, 98
  and smoking, 8
  of stomach, 352
  terminal, management of, 354–357
  thyroid. *See* Thyroid cancer
  vaginal. *See* Vagina, cancer of
Candidiasis, 50
  recurrent, 81
  vulvovaginal, diagnosis and management of, 80–81

Captopril, for hypertension, 22
Carbamazepine, teratogenicity, 139
Carbon dioxide, in respiratory acidosis, 143
Cardiac arrest
  anesthesia-related, 272–273
  in sterilization, 289
Cardiac disease, pregnant patient with, 163–164
Cardiac output, in pregnancy, 164
Cardiopulmonary resuscitation, 272
Cardiovascular disease
  management of, 21–24
  postmenopausal, 403–404
  risk, effects of oral contraceptives on, 57–58
Cardiovascular fitness, 10
Carminatives, 30
Case–control studies, 116–118
Catheter(s), and wound healing, 264
CBE. *See* Breast(s), clinical examination of
Cefazolin, preoperative prophylaxis with, 226, 264
Cefixime, for gonorrhea, 84
Cefoperazone, side effects and adverse reactions to, 226
Cefotetan
  for pelvic inflammatory disease, 94
  side effects and adverse reactions to, 226
Cefoxitin
  for pelvic inflammatory disease, 94
  preoperative prophylaxis with, 226
Ceftriaxone
  for gonorrhea, 84
  for pelvic inflammatory disease, 94
  for syphilis, 85
  for urethritis, 19
Cellular immunity (cell-mediated immunity), 145
Cellulitis, 51
Central nervous system, malignancy, 353
Central venous pressure, monitoring, in hemorrhaging patient, 273
Cephalosporins
  first-generation, for cystitis, 20
  preoperative prophylaxis with, 226
Cephalothin, preoperative prophylaxis with, 226
Cerebral palsy, 195–196
Cerebrovascular disease, in pregnant patient, 168
Cervical biopsy, with cervical lesion, 318
Cervical cancer
  bulky, with positive pelvic nodes, treatment of, 320–321
  epidemiology of, 317
  FIGO staging for, 318–319
  microinvasive
    definition of, 319–320
    treatment of, 320
  persistent, treatment of, 321
  in pregnancy, 347–348

Cervical cancer (continued)
    prognosis for, 320, 320t
    recurrent, treatment of, 321
    risk factors for, 317
    screening, 317–318
    stage at diagnosis, and survival, 326, 327t
    stages IB and IIA, treatment of, 320
    staging, 318
    treatment of, 318–321
Cervical cap, 56
Cervical conization, with cervical lesion, 318
Cervical incompetence, clinical features and management of, 435
Cervical intraepithelial neoplasia, 317
    and human papillomavirus infection, 88
    treatment of, 217–218, 318
Cervical mucus
    abnormalities, 425–426
    examination of, 78
Cervical neoplasia, 317–321
    diagnosis of, 318
    etiology of, 318
    screening, 317–318
Cervical shock, 292
Cervicitis, 77
    differential diagnosis of, 19
Cervix
    condylomata acuminata, diagnosis of, 89–90
    histopathology of, 216
    structural problems, 425–426
    ultrasound evaluation of, 220
Cesarean delivery, 193
    infection after, 205
    and puerperal hysterectomy, 193
    vaginal birth after, 193–194
Chemical(s), teratogenic, 138–140
Chemonucleolysis, 39
Chemotherapy
    for breast cancer, 303–305
    for endometrial cancer, 324
    for epithelial ovarian cancer, 333
    fertility subsequent to, 342–343
    for gestational trophoblastic tumors, 340–341
    for invasive squamous cell carcinoma of vulva, 311
    ovarian dysfunction related to, 342, 343t
    during pregnancy, 346–347
    teratogenicity, 346–347, 347t
Chenodeoxycholic acid, for gallstones, 31
Child abuse
    physical, 103–104
    sexual, 104–105, 386–387
Chlamydia trachomatis
    acute urethral syndrome, 82, 243
    cervicitis caused by, 82
    culture, 82

Chlamydia trachomatis (continued)
    infection
        diagnosis of, 82–83
        epidemiology of, 82
        in pregnancy, 83–84
        spectrum of, 82
        treatment of, 83
    infertility caused by, 82
    in pediatric patient, 387
    pelvic inflammatory disease caused by, 94–95
    pneumonia caused by, 17
    postpartum endometritis caused by, 82
    salpingitis caused by, 68, 82
    urethritis caused by, 19
Chloasma, and oral contraceptive use, 58
Chlorambucil
    effect on ovarian function, 343t
    teratogenicity, 347t
Cholangitis, 31
Cholecystectomy, in gallbladder disease, 31
Cholecystitis, acute, 31
Cholelithiasis
    management of, 31
    and oral contraceptive use, 58
Cholestasis of pregnancy, 165–166
Cholesterol
    gallstones, 31
    serum
        classification of, 23
        and diet, 11
        management of, 23–24
Chondrocalcinosis, 36
Chorioamnionitis, subclinical, and preterm birth, 158
Choriocarcinoma, 338–341
    hyperthyroidism with, 48–49
Chorionic villus sampling, 137–138
Chromosomal abnormalities
    and cancer, 298
    and maternal age, 133–134
    and multiple spontaneous abortions, 135
    prenatal diagnosis of, 133–135
    and spontaneous abortion, 433–434
Chromosomal disorder(s), 379
Chromosomal inversion(s), parental, 134–135
Chromosomal translocations, 379
    parental, 133–134
    and spontaneous abortion, 434
Chronic pain syndrome, 70–71
Cigarette smoking. See also Smoking cessation
    and cervical cancer, 317
    cessation, 8–9
        strategies, 8–9
        weight gain with, 9
    effects on childbearing, 8
    health risks of, 8
    and lower esophageal sphincter pressure, 30

Cigarette smoking (continued)
    and oral contraceptive use, 58–59
    and peptic ulcer disease, 30
    and postoperative pulmonary care, 268
    in pregnancy, 8–9
    teratogenicity, 140
Cimetidine
    for gastroesophageal reflux, 30
    for peptic ulcer disease, 30
Ciprofloxacin
    for cystitis, 20
    for gonorrhea, 84
    for urethritis, 19
Cisplatin
    effect on ovarian function, 343t
    teratogenicity, 347t
Clavicular fracture, intrapartum-related, 195
Clear cell adenocarcinoma, vaginal, diethylstilbestrol and, 315–316
Clear cell tumor(s), ovarian, 257
Climacteric, 401
Clindamycin
    for bacterial vaginosis, 79
    for pelvic inflammatory disease, 94–95
Clinical trials, randomized, 116
Clobetasol propionate, for lichen sclerosus et atrophicus, 229
Clomiphene citrate
    mechanism of action, 374
    for ovulation induction, 422
    therapy, in polycystic ovary syndrome, 396
Clomipramine, 42
    in management of premenstrual syndrome, 75
Clonidine
    for hot flushes, 407
    for hypertension, 22
Clostridium sordellii, toxic shock syndrome caused by, 95–96
Cluster headache. See Headache, cluster
c-myc proto-oncogene, in gynecologic cancer, 299–300
Cocaine
    abuse, 13
    teratogenicity, 141
Codeine, for headache, 45
Codeine phosphate, for headache, 45
Cohort studies, 116–117
Colchicine, for gout, 35–36
Colon, injuries, intraoperative or obstetric, management of, 276–277
Colon cancer. See Colorectal cancer
Colonoscopy, 32
Colorectal cancer
    diagnosis of, 32
    epidemiology of, 32
    management of, 32
    in pregnancy, 352–353
    screening for, 32

Color-flow Doppler imaging, 126
Colpectomy, indications for, 233
Colpocleisis, indications for, 233
Colpopexy, 233
Colporrhaphy, 233
    anterior, for stress urinary incontinence, 240
Colposcopy, 215–218
    with cervical neoplasia, 318
    of diethylstilbestrol-exposed daughters, 316
    findings with, 217
    technique, 215–216
    of vagina, 218
    of vulva, 218, 307
Complete blood count, preoperative, 225
Compression stockings, in prevention of deep vein thrombosis, 284
Computed tomography, of adnexal masses, 258
Conditioning, 10
Condoms
    female, 56–57
    male, 56–57
Condylomata acuminata, 87–88
    anatomical distribution, 88
    diagnosis of, 88–90
    management of, 90–91
    in pediatric patient, 386
    in pregnant patient, 177
Confidence interval, 119–120
Confounding, 118, 120
Congenital adrenal hyperplasia, 397, 412–415
    fetal therapy for, 131
Congenital anomalies/malformations, 200
    incidence of, 65
    in infants of diabetic mothers, 170
    polygenic/multifactorial, 135, 380
    teratogen-related, 138
Congenital heart disease, pregnant patient with, 163–164
Connective tissue disease, abdominal pain with, 68
Contact dermatitis, 50
    in pediatric patient, 385
Contraception, for rape victim, 106
Contraceptives
    effectiveness of, 56
    failure, factors affecting, 56
    use, in United States, 56
Contraction stress test, 129–131
Contrast venography, for diagnosis of deep vein thrombosis, 283
Coping behaviors, 12
Coronary artery disease, 21
    prevention of, 23–24
    risk factors for, 23
Corpus albicans, 375
Corpus luteum
    deficiency, and spontaneous abortion, 435

Corpus luteum (continued)
    function
        evaluation of, 423–424
        normal, requirements for, 374
    of pregnancy, 146–147
    suppression of folliculogenesis, 374–375
Corticosteroids
    for asthma, 17
    for gout, 35
    for lichen sclerosus et atrophicus, 229
    with preterm labor and delivery, 160
    for vulvar squamous cell hyperplasia, 229
Corticotropin
    deficiency, 365
    for gout, 35
    laboratory evaluation of, 411
    synthesis and secretion, 365, 365t, 409
Corticotropin stimulation test, 396, 411
Cortisol
    assays, 444–445
    plasma, laboratory evaluation of, 409
    synthesis and secretion, 409
    urinary free, laboratory evaluation of, 409
Cosyntropin stimulation test, 396, 411
Cough, in bronchitis, 16
Coumarin
    teratogenicity, 139
    therapy, for deep vein thrombosis, 285
Counseling
    about nutrition and weight control, 11
    by age group, 2–6
Countershock, in cardiopulmonary resuscitation, 272
Crisis intervention, 103–111
Crohn disease, in pregnant patient, 166
Cross-sectional studies, 116–117
Crown–rump length, 128, 162
Cryocautery, for prolapsed urethral mucosa, 228
Cryotherapy, for human papillomavirus infection, 90
Culdeplasty, indications for, 233
Culdocentesis, indications for, 67–68
Curettage, vacuum, first-trimester, 291–293
    anesthesia for, 292
    complications of, 292–293
    technique, 291–292
Cushing disease, 365, 415
Cushing syndrome, 397
    clinical features of, 415
    etiology of, 415
    laboratory diagnosis of, 415
    maternal, fetal effects of, 415
    pathophysiology of, 415
    treatment of, 415
Cyclooxygenase pathway, 376, 377f
Cyclophosphamide
    effect on ovarian function, 343t
    teratogenicity, 347t

Cystadenofibroma(s), 250
    ovarian, 257
Cystadenoma(s)
    mucinous, ovarian, 257
    serous, ovarian, 256–257
Cystic fibrosis, genetics of, 135–136
Cystic structures, in fetus, draining of, 132–133
Cystitis
    acute, in pregnant patient, 184
    interstitial, 243–244
    management of, 19–20
    pain with, 68
Cystocele
    causes of, 230
    displacement type, 230
    distention type, 230
    severity gradings, 230
    types of, 230
Cystometry, 237–238, 238f
Cystoscopy, for genitourinary fistulas, 277
Cystourethroscopy, 237
Cytarabine, teratogenicity, 347t
Cytogenetic diagnosis, prenatal, 137–138
Cytokines, intraovarian regulatory role, 372
Cytomegalovirus, in pregnant patient, 182
Cytosine arabinoside, effect on ovarian function, 343t
Cytotoxic chemotherapy
    secondary malignancy after, 347
    teratogenicity, 346–347, 347t

D

Danazol
    for endometriosis, 253
    for leiomyomata uteri, 246–247
    in management of premenstrual syndrome, 75
    teratogenicity, 139
Date rape, 105
Daunorubicin, teratogenicity, 347t
Death, leading causes of, by age group, 2–6
Decapeptyl, dosage and administration, 428t
Deep vein thrombophlebitis, pregnant patient with, 164–165
Deep vein thrombosis
    postoperative, 282–285
        diagnosis of, 282–283
        epidemiology of, 282
        prevention of, 283–284
        risk factors for, 283–284
        surgical management, 285
        treatment of, 284–285
Defenses, 12
Defibrillation, 272
Dehiscence, 285–286
Dehydroepiandrosterone, 409
    assays, 444
    synthesis and secretion of, 412, 413f

Dehydroepiandrosterone sulfate
  assays, 411, 444
  in menstrual disorders, 397–398
  in pregnancy, 147–148
  synthesis and secretion of, 412, 413f
Delivery, preterm, 158–160
Denial, as defense mechanism, for dying patient, 355
Depot-medroxyprogesterone acetate, 62–63
  in management of premenstrual syndrome, 75
Depression
  definition of, 40
  diagnosis of, 41
  diagnostic criteria for, 40
  in dying patient, 355–356
  epidemiology of, 40–41
  etiology of, 40–41
  and oral contraceptive use, 58
  postpartum, 41, 204
  premenstrual, 41
  and reproductive events, 41
  risk factors for, 40–41
  treatment of, 41–43
  types of, 40
Dermatitis, 50
Dermatofibrosarcoma protuberans, vulvar, 313
Dermatologic conditions
  management of, 50–51
  in pregnant patient, 176–178
Dermatophytoses, 50
Dermatoses, vulvar, 229
  in pediatric patient, 385
Dermoids, ovarian, 258
Descending perineal syndrome, 233–234
Desipramine, 42
  side effects of, 43
Detrusor hyperreflexia, 235
Detrusor instability, 235, 244
  pharmacotherapy for, 241, 241t
  treatment of, 241
Dexamethasone
  for androgen excess, 397
  with preterm labor and delivery, 160
Dexamethasone suppression test, 411
Dextran, prophylaxis, 284
Diabetes mellitus
  classification of, 24
  complications of, 24
  diagnosis of, 24–25
  management of, 25
  preconceptional care with, 64–65
  in pregnant patient, 149–150
    gestational, 170–171
    preexisting, 169–170
  risk factors for, 24
  screening for, 24–25
  skin disorders in, 51
  and spontaneous abortion, 436
  type II (non–insulin-dependent), 24, 26–27

Diabetes mellitus (continued)
  type I (insulin-dependent), 24–26
Diabetic nephropathy, 26–27
  in pregnant patient, 176
Diagnostic test(s), 116
Diaphragm, 56
  for stress urinary incontinence, 240
Diazepam, for bladder and urethral disorders, 243, 245
Dichloralphenazone, for headache, 45
Diclofenac sodium, for headache, 45
Dicyclomine hydrochloride, for detrusor instability, 241t
Diet
  for diabetic patient, 25, 27
  evaluation of, 11
  health problems influenced by, 11
  in management of premenstrual syndrome, 74
  in prevention of coronary artery disease, 23
  recommendations for, 11
Diethylstilbestrol
  exposure in utero
    and adenocarcinoma of vagina, 315–316
    benign anomalies related to, 316
  teratogenicity, 139
Dihydroergotamine mesylate, for headache, 45
Dilation and evacuation, for second-trimester abortion, 293–294
Diltiazem
  for hypertension, 22
  for migraine prevention, 46
Dimethyl sulfoxide
  for interstitial cystitis, 243–244
  side effects and adverse reactions to, 243–244
D immune globulin, 156–158
Diphenylhydantoin, teratogenicity, 139
Disease processes
  and infectious morbidity, 280–281
  and wound healing, 265
D isoimmunization, 156–158
Disseminated intravascular coagulation, 152
Diuretics, for hypertension, 22
Divalproex sodium, for migraine prevention, 46
DMPA. See Depot-medroxyprogesterone acetate
DNA analysis, in prenatal diagnosis, 136
DNA diagnostic technology, 383
Domestic violence, 107–109
Do not resuscitate orders, 357
Dopamine agonists, in ovulation induction, 423
Doppler ultrasonography, 126
Dot-blot analysis, 383, 384f
Down syndrome. See also Trisomy 21
  prenatal diagnosis of, 136

Doxepin, 42
  for migraine prevention, 46
  side effects of, 43
Doxorubicin, effect on ovarian function, 343t
Doxycycline
  for Chlamydia infection, 83
  for gonorrhea, 84
  for pelvic inflammatory disease, 94–95
  for urethritis, 19
Drain(s), surgical
  in postoperative patient with pelvic infection, 281–282
  and wound healing, 264
Drug(s)
  amenorrhea secondary to, 392
  illicit, teratogenicity, 140–141
  teratogenic, 138–140
Durable power of attorney for health care, 357
Dying patient
  advance directives by, 357
  management of, 354–357
Dysfunctional uterine bleeding, 398–399
  management of, 399
  pathophysiology of, 398–399
Dysgerminoma, ovarian, 327–328
Dysmenorrhea, 69
  prostaglandins in, 377–378
Dyspareunia, 69
  management, 101
Dyspepsia
  with gallbladder disease, 31
  with peptic ulcer disease, 30
Dysuria, 19

E
Early embryonic size, 128
Ectopic pregnancy, 250–253
  combined with intrauterine pregnancy, 251
  diagnosis of, 67–68, 251–252
  and first-trimester abortion, 292–293
  incidence of, 250
  laparoscopy for, 214
  mortality with, 250
  and pelvic inflammatory disease, 95
  pelvic pain with, 68
  persistent, 252
  risk factors for, 250–251
  sites of, 251
  subsequent fertility after, 251
  treatment of, 252–253
Eisenmenger syndrome, pregnant patient with, 163–164
Elderly. See also Geriatric patient
  bacteriuria in, 20
  hyperthyroidism in, 48
  joint and bone disease in, 32–33
  pneumonia in, 17–18
Electrocautery, 214–215
  for endometriosis, 253

Electrocautery (continued)
    for human papillomavirus infection, 90
Electrolytes, in postoperative care, 266–267
Electromyography, in diagnosis of urinary incontinence, 239
Embryo(s)
    cryopreservation, 440
    micromanipulation of, 440–441
    transfer
        after in vitro fertilization, 440
        tubal, 442
Embryo biopsy, 138
Enalapril, for hypertension, 22
Endocervical canal, hysteroscopic evaluation of, 210–211
Endocrine assays, 443–446
    for estrogenic steroids, 443
    for progestational steroids, 443–445
    units for, 443
Endocrine system, maternal, in pregnancy, 149–150
Endometrial ablation, hysteroscopy for, 212
Endometrial biopsy, to confirm ovulation, 423–424
Endometrial carcinoma
    diagnosis of, 322
    epidemiology of, 321–322
    estrogen replacement therapy after, 324
    FIGO staging for, 322–323
    hereditary factors in, 298
    in pregnancy, 350
    prognosis for, 322
    risk, and oral contraceptive use, 58
    risk factors for, 322
    stage at diagnosis, and survival, 326, 327t
    and tamoxifen therapy, 306
    treatment of, 323–324, 324t
    ultrasound evaluation of, 219
Endometrial hyperplasia, 324–325, 426
    atypical, 325
    ultrasound evaluation of, 219
Endometrial neoplasia, with hormone therapy, 404
Endometrioma(s)
    ovarian, 257
    treatment of, 425
Endometriosis
    American Fertility Society classification of, 253, 254f
    chronic pelvic pain with, 70
    clinical features of, 253
    diagnosis of, 253
    etiology of, 253
    infertility with, 425
    laparoscopy for, 214
    ovarian involvement in, 257
    prevalence of, 253
    treatment of, 253–254, 425, 428
Endometritis, 426
    postpartum, 205–206

Endometritis (continued)
    ultrasound evaluation of, 219
Endometrium, disorders, amenorrhea secondary to, 392
Endothelin-1, intraovarian regulatory role, 372
Endotoxic shock, 282
Enterobacter, cellulitis caused by, 51
Enterobiasis, in pediatric patient, 386
Enterocele
    causes of, 230, 231t
    surgical approach for, 231t
Enterococcus, cystitis caused by, 19
Environmental agents, teratogenicity, 140
Epidemiologic studies
    analytic, 116–118
    methodologic limitations of, 118
Epidemiology, 116–120
Epidermal growth factor, intraovarian regulatory role, 372
Epidural analgesia, obstetric, 197
Epilepsy, in pregnant patient, 167
Epinephrine, for cardiac arrest, 272
Episiotomy, infection of, 206
Epithelioid sarcoma, vulvar, 313
Erectile dysfunction, management, 101–103
Ergotamine tartrate
    for headache, 45
    overuse of, 46–47
Error(s), types I and II, 118–119
Erysipelas, 51
Erythroblastosis fetalis, 156
Erythromycin
    for *Chlamydia* infection, 83
    for gonorrhea, 84
    for pneumonia, 18
    for urethritis, 19
Escherichia coli
    cellulitis caused by, 51
    cystitis caused by, 19
    pelvic inflammatory disease caused by, 94
Estradiol
    assays, 443
    in ovulation, 373
Estriol, assays, 443
Estrogen
    and breast cancer risk, 301–302
    in corpus luteum function, 374–375
    effects on bone mass, 36
    and endometrial cancer, 322
    in leiomyomata uteri, 245–246
    in ovulation, 373
    in pregnancy, 147–148
    protective effects
        against atherosclerosis, 23–24, 403–404
        against cardiovascular disease, 23–24, 403–404
        against coronary artery disease, 23–24, 403–404

Estrogen, protective effects (continued)
    against hypertension, 23
    against osteoporosis, 403
    regulation of menstrual cycle by, 368
    replacement therapy, after endometrial cancer, 324
    therapy
        for anatomic support defects and dysfunction, 232
        for dysfunctional uterine bleeding, 399
        for hot flushes, 401
        for osteoporosis, 36–37
        in Paget disease of bone, 37
        postmenopausal, 404–406, 405t
    topical
        for prolapsed urethral mucosa, 228
        for stress urinary incontinence, 239
        for vaginal atrophy, 232
Estrone, assays, 443
Ethambutol, for tuberculosis, 18
Ethical issues, in obstetrics and gynecology, 111–115
Ethical principles, 112–113, 356–357
Ethics
    analysis in, 111–112
    contextual issue in, 113
    issues in, 111–115
Etidronate
    for osteoporosis, 37
    in Paget disease of bone, 37
Etoposide, effect on ovarian function, 343t
Etretinate, teratogenicity, 139
Eugonadism, 390
Evaluation, by age group, 2–6
Evisceration, 285–286
Exercise
    benefits of, 9
        with rheumatoid arthritis, 33
    counseling about, 9–10
    in management of premenstrual syndrome, 75
    in prevention of coronary artery disease, 23
    target heart rate in, 10
    and weight control, 9–10
Exercise-induced amenorrhea, 394–395
Exercise program, development of, 10
External cephalic version, 194

F

Facial nerve palsy, intrapartum-related, 195
Fallopian tube(s)
    anastomosis, 425
    cancer of, 335–336
        operative staging of, 335–336
        in pregnancy, 348–349
        spread of, 336
        treatment of, 336
    ligation, abdominal, 288

Fallopian tube(s) *(continued)*
    obstruction, proximal, hysteroscopy for, 212
    occlusion, laparoscopic, 288–289
Family planning. *See also* Fertility control
    natural, 57
Famotidine
    for gastroesophageal reflux, 30
    for peptic ulcer disease, 30
Fatty food intolerance, with gallstones, 31
Fecal incontinence, 222–223
Fecundity rate, 417
Femur length, and gestational age, 162
Fertility
    after oral contraceptive use, 58–59
    after previously treated cancer, 342–343
    after radiation therapy, 346, 346*t*
    potential, after ectopic pregnancy, 251
Fertility control, 56–63
Fetal anomalies
    and chorionic villus sampling, 138
    monogenic, 135–136
    polygenic/multifactorial, 135, 380
Fetal heart rate
    intrapartum monitoring, 190*t*, 190–191
    nonreassuring, response to, 191, 192*f*
    testing, 129–130
Fetal movement, assessment of, 131
Fetal surgery, open, 133
Fetal therapy, 131–133
    intravenous, 132
    invasive, 132–133
    medical, 131–132
Fetal umbilical artery velocimetry, 131
Fetoscopic tissue sampling, 138
Fetus
    acid–base balance in, 143–144
    anatomy survey, ultrasound, 128–129
    endocrinology of, 148–149
    ethical issues related to, 114
    growth retardation, 158
    immunocompetence of, 146
    tachyarrhythmia, fetal therapy for, 131
    ultrasound assessment of, 127–129
Fibrinogen I 125 scanning, for diagnosis of deep vein thrombosis, 283
Fibroadenoma, of breast, 76
Fibroma(s)
    ovarian, 258
    vulvar, 227
FIGO staging
    for cervical cancer, 318–319
    for endometrial cancer, 322–323
    of gestational trophoblastic tumors, 339
    of ovarian cancer, 329
    of vaginal carcinoma, 315
    of vulvar carcinoma, 309–310
Fine-needle aspiration biopsy
    of breast mass, 29
    of thyroid nodule, 49
Fitness, 9
Fitz–Hugh–Curtis syndrome, 82

Flavoxate hydrochloride, for detrusor instability, 241*t*
Flexible sigmoidoscopy, in diagnosis of colorectal cancer, 32
Fluid(s), in postoperative care, 266–267
Fluorouracil
    effect on ovarian function, 343*t*
    for human papillomavirus infection, 90
    teratogenicity, 347*t*
    topical
        for vaginal intraepithelial neoplasia, 314
        for vulvar intraepithelial neoplasia, 308
Fluoxetine, 42
    in management of premenstrual syndrome, 75
    for migraine prevention, 46
    side effects of, 43
Folic acid
    deficiency, in pregnant patient, 172
    recommended intake, for reproductive-age women, 66
Folic acid antagonists, teratogenicity, 346–347, 347*t*
Follicle(s)
    antral, 369–370
    dominant, selection of, 370–371
    preantral, 368–369
    preovulatory, 372–373
    primordial, 368
Follicle-stimulating hormone
    fetal, 148–149
    in folliculogenesis, 369–371
    in ovulation induction, 423
    in puberty, 367
    synthesis and secretion of, 364–366, 365*t*
Folliculitis, 51
Folliculogenesis, 368–372
    feedback regulators, 372
    intraovarian regulators, 371–372
    luteal suppression of, 374–375
Follow-up studies, 117
Foot, passive dorsiflexion, with back pain, 38–39
Forceps delivery, 191*t*, 191–192
Fractures, in osteoporosis, 36
Fragile X syndrome, 380
Fungal infections
    sinusitis caused by, 15
    of skin, 50
Furosemide, for hypertension, 22

G

Galactocele, 76
Gallbladder disease
    and hormone therapy, 406
    management of, 31
Gallstones, management of, 31
Gamete intrafallopian transfer, 441–442

Gardnerella
    pelvic inflammatory disease caused by, 94
    vaginitis caused by, 78–79
Gastroesophageal reflux, management of, 29–30
Gastrointestinal bypass, pregnancy after, 166–167
Gastrointestinal disorders
    acute versus chronic, 29
    management of, 29–32
Gastrointestinal malignancy, in pregnancy, 352–353
General anesthesia, obstetric, 197–198
Gene therapy, in gynecologic cancer, 300–301
Genetic assessment, preconceptional, 65–66
Genetic disorder(s)
    prenatal diagnosis of, 133–138
    screening for, 135–136
Genetics, 379–384
    and gynecologic cancer, 298–301
Genital atrophy, menopausal, 401–402
Genital prolapse. *See also* Anatomic support defects and dysfunction
    acquired, 230
    with aging, 230
    causes of, 230
    congenital, 230
    recurrent, 233
Genitourinary fistula(s)
    diagnosis of, 277
    management of, 277–280
Gentamicin, for pelvic inflammatory disease, 94
Geriatric patient. *See also* Elderly
    genital prolapse in, 230
    physical examination of, 231
    preoperative antibiotic prophylaxis for, 225–226
Germinal epithelial cysts, 256
Gestational age, determination of, 162
Gestational trophoblastic disease, 337–341. *See also* Hydatidiform mole
    treatment of
        follow-up after, 341
        reproductive performance after, 341
        secondary malignancy after, 341
        surveillance after, 341
Gestational trophoblastic tumor(s), 338–341
    after molar pregnancy, 338
    classification of, 339
    diagnosis of, 339
    follow-up after successful treatment, 341
    metastatic, treatment of, 340–341
    nonmetastatic, treatment of, 339–340
    signs and symptoms of, 339
    staging, 339
    treatment of, 339–341

Gestational trophoblastic tumor(s) (continued)
  types of, 338–339
  World Health Organization prognostic scoring system for, 339, 340t
Ghon complex, 18
Giant cell arteritis, management of, 34–35
Glomerulonephritis, in pregnant patient, 175
Glucocorticoids
  assays, 444–445
  in ovulation induction, 423
  for rheumatoid arthritis, 34
Glucose tolerance, and hormone therapy, 406
Glucose tolerance test, in pregnant patient, 170, 170t
Goiter, toxic multinodular, 48–49
Gold therapy, for rheumatoid arthritis, 34
Gonadal dysgenesis, 381–382
  and malignancy, 298
Gonadotropin-releasing hormone
  clinical applications, 427–429
  hypothalamic secretion of, 362–364, 363f
  in ovulation induction, 364, 423, 427–428
  in puberty, 367
Gonadotropin-releasing hormone agonists
  for adenomyosis, 249
  clinical applications, 427–429
  for dysfunctional uterine bleeding, 399
  for endometriosis, 253, 425
  for leiomyomata uteri, 246–247
  mechanism of action, 364
Gonadotropin-releasing hormone analogues
  clinical applications, 427–429
  in ovulation induction, 423, 427–428
  side effects and adverse reactions to, 429
Gonadotropin-releasing hormone antagonists, 429
Gonadotropins
  assays, 445
  for ovulation induction, 422–423
Gonads, fetal, 149
Gonorrhea
  diagnosis of, 83–84
  follow-up, 84
  in pregnancy, 84–85
  spectrum of, 83
  symptoms of, 83
  treatment of, 83–84
Goserelin
  dosage and administration, 428t
  for treatment of endometriosis, 425
Gout
  clinical features of, 35
  treatment of, 35–36
Gouty nephropathy, 35
Granulosa–stromal cell tumors, ovarian, 258

Graves disease, 48–49
Grief, 103, 109–110, 354–355
  stages of, 355–356
Group B streptococcal infection, in pregnant patient, 185
Growth factors
  intraovarian regulatory role, 371
  and wound healing, 265
Growth hormone
  in leiomyomata uteri, 246
  synthesis and secretion of, 365t, 366
  therapy, for short stature, 382
Growth retardation, fetal, 158
Growth spurt, pubertal, 388
Guaiac test, in diagnosis of colorectal cancer, 32
Gynecology, ethical issues in, 114–115

H

Haemophilus influenzae
  pelvic inflammatory disease caused by, 94
  pneumonia caused by, 17
  sinusitis caused by, 15
Hair, changes, in pregnancy, 177
Hashimoto thyroiditis, 47–48
HBeAg. See Hepatitis B envelope antigen
HBsAg. See Hepatitis B surface antigen
Headache, 43–47
  acute, 45
  acute recurrent, 45
  chronic daily, 45
  classification of, 43–44
  cluster, clinical features of, 44
  diagnosis of, 44–46
  drug therapy for, 45–47
  epidemiology of, 43
  in giant cell arteritis, 35
  migraine
    clinical features of, 43–44
    and oral contraceptive use, 58
    in pregnant patient, 168–169
    prophylactic medication for, 46
  prophylactic medication for, 46
  sinusitis-related, 15–16
  subacute, 45
  tension-type, clinical features of, 43–44
Head flexion, in nerve root irritation, 38
Health care resources, allocation of, 113, 115
Health maintenance, 8–14
Health promotion, preconceptional, 64
Heart rate, target, in exercise, 10
Helicobacter pylori, and peptic ulcer disease, 30–31
Hematologic cancer, in pregnancy, 351–352
Hematologic disorders, in pregnant patient, 172–174
Hematometra, with first-trimester abortion, 292
Hemizygous state, 380

Hemoglobin S, 173
Hemoglobin SC, 173–174
Hemolytic disease of newborn, 156
Hemorrhage. See also Bleeding
  control of bleeding in, 274
  in first-trimester abortion, 292
  perioperative, 273–274
  postpartum
    early, 204–205
    late, 205
Heparin
  prophylaxis, 284
  therapy, for deep vein thrombosis, 284–285
Hepatitis A, in pregnant patient, 179
Hepatitis B, 20
  neonatal immunoprophylaxis, 180, 181t
  in pregnant patient, 179–180
  vaccine, 20–21, 180, 180t
Hepatitis B envelope antigen, 21
Hepatitis B immune globulin, 21
Hepatitis B surface antigen, 21
Hepatitis D, 180
Hepatocellular carcinoma, in pregnancy, 352–353
HER-2/neu gene, in gynecologic cancer, 299–300
Hernia(s), incisional, 285–286
Heroin
  abuse, 13
  teratogenicity, 141
Herpes gestationis, 176–177
Herpes simplex virus
  and genital cancer, 86
  infection, 51, 85–87
    clinical features of, 86–87
    complications of, 86–87
    diagnosis of, 87
    epidemiology of, 85–86
    reactivation, 87
    treatment of, 87
  in pregnant patient, 183–184
  types of, 85–86
Herpes zoster, 51
  pain with, 68
Herpetic lesions, vulvar, in pediatric patient, 386
Heterozygous state, 379
Hidradenocarcinoma, clear-cell, vulvar, 312
Hidradenoma, vulvar, 227
High-density lipoproteins, 23
High-risk factors
  descriptions of, 7
  identification of, 2
Hilar cell hyperplasia, 256
Hirsutism, 396–398, 411–412
Histamine H_2-receptor antagonists
  for gastroesophageal reflux, 30
  for peptic ulcer disease, 30
Histerelin, dosage and administration, 428t

History-taking
  preoperative, 224–225
  in urogynecology, 235–236
Hodgkin disease, in pregnancy, 351–352
Homeostasis, 12
Homozygous state, 379
Honesty, ethical issues related to, 114
Hormonal agents, teratogenicity, 139
Hormone(s). See also specific hormone(s)
  anterior pituitary, 364–366
  posterior pituitary, 364
  protein
    assays, 445
    mechanism of action, 360–361
  receptor physiology, 360–361
  steroid. See Steroid(s)
Hormone-dependent tumors, treatment of, 428
Human chorionic gonadotropin
  assays, 445
  discriminatory zone, in diagnosis of ectopic pregnancy, 251–252
  monitoring, after molar pregnancy, 338
  in ovulation induction, 364, 422–423
  in pregnancy, 148
  serial measurements, in diagnosis of normal versus abnormal pregnancy, 68
  β-subunit, radioimmunoassay, in diagnosis of ectopic pregnancy, 251
Human chorionic somatomammotropin, 366
Human immunodeficiency virus
  and cervical cancer, 317
  ethical issues related to, 114
  infection, 91–93
    clinical features of, 92
    diagnosis of, 92–93
    epidemiology of, 91
    management of, 93
    pathogenesis of, 91–92
  in pediatric patient, 387
  in pregnant patient, 185–186
  transmission, 91
  and substance abuse, 13
Human leukocyte antigen, shared parental, and spontaneous abortion, 437
Human papillomavirus
  acetowhite change with, 227, 307
  and cervical cancer, 317–318
  and genital cancer, 88
  infection, 87–91
    clinical features of, 88
    diagnosis of, 88–90
    epidemiology of, 87
    management of, 90–91
    subclinical
      diagnosis of, 89
      types of, 89

Human papillomavirus (continued)
  and invasive squamous cell carcinoma of vulva, 309
  and vulvar cancer, 307
  and vulvar vestibulitis syndrome, 228
Humoral immunity, 145
Huntington disease, 380–381
Hyaline membrane disease, 201
Hydatidiform mole, 337–338. See also Invasive mole; Molar pregnancy
  complete (classic), 337
  diagnosis of, 337–338
  follow-up care with, 338
  incidence of, 337
  and malignancy, 298
  partial, 337
  treatment of, 338
Hydramnios, 145
Hydrocephalus, fetal therapy for, 132
Hydrochlorothiazide, for hypertension, 22
Hydroxychloroquine, for rheumatoid arthritis, 34
17-Hydroxycorticosteroids, urinary, laboratory evaluation of, 409
11-Hydroxylase deficiency, 397, 411, 414
  incidence of, 414
  pathophysiology of, 414
  treatment of, 414
17α-Hydroxylase deficiency
  clinical features of, 415
  pathophysiology of, 414–415
  treatment of, 415
21-Hydroxylase deficiency, 396–397, 411–414
  treatment of, 414
17α-Hydroxyprogesterone, assays, 444
3β-Hydroxysteroid dehydrogenase deficiency, 411–412
  clinical features of, 414
  diagnosis of, 414
  pathophysiology of, 414
  treatment of, 414
Hyperandrogenism, 395–398. See also Androgen excess
Hyperglycemia, in diabetes, 24
Hyperpigmentation, in pregnant patient, 177
Hyperprolactinemia
  amenorrhea secondary to, 392–393
  causes of, 392–393
Hyperreactio luteinalis, 256
Hypertension, 21–23
  in diabetic patient, 24
    management of, 26
  diagnosis of, 21–22
  drug therapy for, 22
    monitoring during, 23
  epidemiology of, 21
  and hormone therapy, 406
  laboratory evaluation with, 21–22
  in pregnancy, 152–154

Hypertension (continued)
  secondary, causes of, 22
  treatment of, 22–23
Hyperthermia, maternal, teratogenicity, 139
Hyperthyroidism, 407–408
  causes of, 48
  clinical features of, 48
  diagnosis of, 48–49
  epidemiology of, 48
  medication-induced, 48
  in pregnant patient, 171
  and spontaneous abortion, 436
  treatment of, 49
Hyperuricemia, 35
Hypoadrenalism, in pregnant patient, 176
Hypoglycemia, with insulin therapy, 26
Hypogonadism, 389
  hypogonadotropic, treatment of, 421
Hypothalamic–pituitary axis
  fetal, 148
  hormone secretion and, 364–366, 365t
  maturation of, 366–367
Hypothalamus
  dysfunction, amenorrhea secondary to, 391
  maternal, in pregnancy, 150
Hypothyroidism, 407–408
  amenorrhea secondary to, 391
  causes of, 47
  clinical features of, 47
  diagnosis of, 47–48
  in pregnant patient, 171–172
  and spontaneous abortion, 436
Hysterectomy
  for abortion, 294–295
  for adenomyosis, 249
  bladder injury in, 279
  for dysfunctional uterine bleeding, 399
  for endometrial cancer, 323
  for endometriosis, 254
  for leiomyomata uteri, 248
  puerperal, and cesarean delivery, 193
  vaginal, indications for, 233
  for vaginal carcinoma, 315
Hysterosalpingography, 426–427
Hysteroscopy, 210–212
  complications of, 212
  contact, 210
  contraindications to, 212
  equipment, 210
  indications for, 210–212
  panoramic, 210
  therapeutic, with endometrial polyps, 250
Hysterotomy, for abortion, 294–295

I

Ibuprofen
  for headache, 45
  for osteoarthritis, 34
  for rheumatoid arthritis, 33

IDDM. See Diabetes mellitus, type I (insulin-dependent)
Ileus, postoperative, 269
Illicit drugs, teratogenicity, 140–141
Imipramine hydrochloride, 42
 for detrusor instability, 241t
 side effects of, 43
 for stress urinary incontinence, 239–240
Immune system
 fetal, 146
 functions of, 145
 maternal, in pregnancy, 145–146
Immune thrombocytopenic purpura, in pregnant patient, 174
Immunization(s), 3–6
 during pregnancy, 187
Immunobiology, 145
Immunoglobulin M, fetal, 146
Immunologic disorders
 in pregnant patient, 178–179
 and spontaneous abortion, 437
Immunotherapy, for human papillomavirus infection, 90–91
Impedance plethysmography, for diagnosis of deep vein thrombosis, 283
Impetigo, 51
Impetigo herpetiformis, 177
Implantation, 146
Implants, contraceptive, 61–62
Impotence, management, 101–103
Inborn errors of metabolism, neonatal screening for, 135
Incest, 104–105, 386–387
Incision(s), and wound healing, 261, 285–286
Incisional hernia(s), 285–286
Indium-111-labeled platelet imaging, for diagnosis of deep vein thrombosis, 283
Indomethacin
 for closure of patent ductus arteriosus, 379
 for headache, 45
 for rheumatoid arthritis, 33
Infection(s). See also Pelvic infection(s); Sexually transmitted disease
 necrotizing, 282
 pelvic, pelvic pain with, 67–68
 postoperative
  antibiotic therapy for, 281
  failure of, 281
  prevention of, 225–226
 postpartum, 205–206
 in pregnant patient, 179–187
 and spontaneous abortion, 436
 vulvovaginal, 77
Infectious problems, management of, 18–21
Infertility, 417–433
 definition of, 417
 female

Infertility, female (continued)
 after previously treated cancer, 342, 343t
 after radiation therapy, 346, 346t
 cervical factors in, 425–426
 evaluation, laparoscopy for, 213–214
 investigation of, 421–431
 and intrauterine device use, 61
 with leiomyomata uteri, 246–247
 treatment of, 421–431
 uterine factors in, 426–427
 immunologic aspects of, 429–431
 initial evaluation for, 417–418
 male
  investigation of, 418–420
  treatment of, 420t, 420–421
 rate, factors affecting, 417
 risk factors for, 417–418
 treatment of
  advances in, 359
  general strategy for, 431
Inflammatory bowel disease, 68
 in pregnant patient, 166
Influenza
 management of, 18–19
 vaccine, 19–20
Information retrieval, 120–121
Informed consent, for surgery, 225
Inhalation anesthesia, obstetric, 198
Inhibin, 371
In situ hybridization, 383, 384f
Insulin, in diabetes, 24
Insulinlike growth factor(s), intraovarian regulatory role, 371–372
Insulinlike growth factor-1, 366
Insulin therapy, for diabetes, 25–27
Interferon
 for human papillomavirus infection, 90–91
 intralesional, for vulvar vestibulitis syndrome with human papillomavirus infection, 227
International Federation of Gynecology and Obstetrics. See FIGO
Interstitial cystitis, 243–244
Intervertebral disc, degeneration, 37
Interviewing, for detection of substance abuse, 13–14
Intestine(s), intraoperative injuries and fistulas, 274–277
 in sterilization, 289
Intraamniotic injections, 132
Intrapartum management, 189–199
Intrauterine device, 60–61
 adverse effects of, 60–61
 dysmenorrhea with, prostaglandins in, 377–378
 expulsion, 60
 infection-related complications with, 61
 and infertility, 61
 localization, ultrasonography for, 220
 missing strings with, 60

Intrauterine device (continued)
 and pelvic inflammatory disease, 61
 perforation with, 60
 pregnancy-related complications with, 60–61
 retrieval, hysteroscopic, 211
 types of, 60
 uterine bleeding with, 60
Intrauterine growth retardation, 158
 and chromosomal abnormalities, 135
 diagnosis of, ultrasonography for, 128
Intravenous anesthesia, obstetric, 198
Intravenous urography, for genitourinary fistulas, 277
Intraventricular hemorrhage, in premature infant, 201
Invasive mole, 338–341
In vitro fertilization, 421
 complications of, 440
 with donor gametes, 441
 early pregnancy monitoring after, 440
 embryo culture and quality control, 440
 embryo transfer after, 440
 indications for, 431
 insemination for, 440
 luteal phase supplementation with, 440
 oocyte retrieval for, 439–440
 oocytes for, 370–371
 ovarian stimulation and monitoring for, 439
 patient selection and preparation, 439
 pregnancy diagnosis after, 440
 pregnancy outcome with, 440
 program, selection for referral, 441
Involutional changes, 202
Iodide, teratogenicity, 139
Iodine. See also Radioactive iodine uptake
 radioactive
  contraindications to, in pregnancy, 353
  for hyperthyroidism, 49
Iodine 131
 for hyperthyroidism, 49
 teratogenicity, 140
Ionizing radiation, teratogenicity, 140
Ipratropium bromide, 17
Iron, supplementation, in pregnancy, 172
Iron-deficiency anemia, in pregnant patient, 172
Irritable bowel syndrome, management of, 31–32
Isocarboxazid, 42
Isoimmunization, 156–158
Isometheptene, for headache, 45
Isoniazid, for tuberculosis, 18
Isotretinoin, teratogenicity, 139
Itching, 50–51. See also Pruritus

J

Jaundice, with gallbladder disease, 31
Jaw claudication, in giant cell arteritis, 35
Joint disease, 32–37

Justice, principle of, 113, 356–357

K
Kallmann syndrome, 390
Karyotype abnormalities, and malignancy, 298–299
Kegel exercises
    for genital prolapse, 232
    for stress urinary incontinence, 240
Kennedy disease, 380–381
Ketoprofen, for headache, 45
Ketorolac tromethamine, for postoperative pain control, 269
Keyes punch biopsy, of vulva, 227
Kidney(s), ultrasound evaluation of, 221
Klebsiella, pneumonia caused by, 17
Knot(s), and wound healing, 263

L
Labetalol, for hypertension, 22
Labia, adhesions of, in pediatric patient, 385
Labor
    active management of, 189
    initiation of, 150
    physiology of, 150–151
    preterm, 158–160
        physiology of, 151
        prostaglandins in, 377–379
    stimulation, 189–190
Laboratory assessment, preoperative, 225
Lactase deficiency, 32
Lactation
    inappropriate, 75
    neuroendocrine regulation of, 203
    nutrition in, 125
Lactobacilli, in normal flora, 280
Lactogenesis, 202–203
Laparoscopy, 212–215
    complications of, 215
    diagnostic, 213–214
        with low abdominal or pelvic pain, 67–69
        of ovarian lesions, 259
        in pelvic inflammatory disease, 94
    in ectopic pregnancy, 252
    in gallbladder disease, 31
    indications for, 213–215
    operative, 214–215
    in postoperative patient with pelvic infection, 281
    small intestinal injury in, 275
    technique, 213
    therapeutic, for endometriosis, 253, 425
    tubal occlusion procedure, 288–289
        bipolar, 288–289
        clip technique, 289
        complications of, 289–290
        Silastic band technique, 289
        single versus double puncture, 288
        unipolar, 288
        Waters cautery technique, 289

Large bowel, intraoperative injuries and fistulas, 276–277
Laser therapy, 214–215
    for endometriosis, 253
    for human papillomavirus infection, 90
    for vaginal intraepithelial neoplasia, 314
    for vulvar intraepithelial neoplasia, 308
Late luteal phase dysphoric disorder, 71
LeFort colpocleisis, indications for, 233
Legionella pneumophila, pneumonia caused by, 17–18
Leiomyomata uteri, 245–248
    anatomic classification of, 246
    degeneration of, 246
    diagnosis of, 247
    etiology of, 245–246
    and fertility, 246–247
    malignant degeneration, incidence of, 246
    prevalence of, 245
    recurrence, after myomectomy, 248
    risk, and oral contraceptive use, 58
    signs and symptoms, 246–247
    spontaneous abortion and, 436
    submucous, excision or resection, hysteroscopy for, 211
    treatment of, 247–248, 428
    ultrasound evaluation of, 219
Leiomyosarcoma(s)
    vaginal, 316
    vulvar, 312–313
Leukemia(s), in pregnancy, 351–352
Leukoplakia, 217
Leuprolide
    dosage and administration, 428t
    for treatment of endometriosis, 425
Leydig cell hyperplasia, 256
Lice, 51
Lichen planus
    desquamative vaginitis with, 81
    erosive, of vulva and vagina, 229
    in pediatric patient, 385
Lichen sclerosus et atrophicus
    in pediatric patient, 385
    vulvar, 228–229
Lichen simplex chronicus, vulvar, 229
Lidocaine, in cardiopulmonary resuscitation, 272–273
Life-sustaining treatment, 357
Ligating clips, and wound healing, 263–264
Lipoma(s)
    of breast, 76
    uterine, 250
    vulvar, 227
Lipomyoma(s), uterine, 250
Lipoproteins, and coronary artery disease, 23
Lipoxygenase pathway, 376, 377f
Literature, interpretation of, 120
Lithium, teratogenicity, 139
Lithotripsy, for gallstones, 31

Liver
    cancer of
        and oral contraceptive use, 58
        in pregnancy, 352–353
    and oral contraceptive use, 58–59
Liver disease, in pregnant patient, 165–166
Local block, obstetric, 196–197
Logistic regression, 120
Longitudinal studies, 117
Loop electrosurgery, with cervical lesion, 318
Loss, 109–110
Low back pain, 37
    causes of, 37–38
Low-density lipoproteins, 23–24
Lower esophageal sphincter, pressure, decreased, 29–30
L-PAM, effect on ovarian function, 343t
Lung cancer, 8
Lung disease, chronic, in premature infant, 201
Lupus anticoagulant, and spontaneous abortion, 437
Lupus nephritis, in pregnant patient, 175–176
Luteal phase defect, and spontaneous abortion, 436
Luteinizing hormone
    fetal, 148–149
    in puberty, 367
    surge, and ovulation, 372–373
    synthesis and secretion of, 364–366, 365t
Luteolysis, 375
Luteoma of pregnancy, 256
Lymphedema, superficial, 51
Lysergic acid diethylamide, teratogenicity, 141

M
Macules, 50
Magnesium, supplementation, in management of premenstrual syndrome, 74
Magnesium sulfate
    in management of pregnancy-induced hypertension, 153–154
    for tocolysis, 159
Magnetic resonance imaging
    of adnexal masses, 258
    for diagnosis of deep vein thrombosis, 283
Malignant hyperthermia, 270
Malignant melanoma, risk, and oral contraceptive use, 58
Malnutrition, diagnosis of, 11
Mammography
    in breast cancer patient, 303
    of breast lesions, 29
    screening, 28
M-AMSA, effect on ovarian function, 343t
Manchester operation, indications for, 233

Manipulative therapy, for back pain, 39
Maprotiline, 42
    side effects of, 43
Marfan syndrome, pregnant patient with, 163–164
Marijuana
    abuse, 13
    teratogenicity, 140–141
Mastalgia, 75
Mastectomy, for breast cancer, 303–305
Mastitis, 76, 206
Mastodynia, 75
Maternal serum testing, in prenatal diagnosis, 136–137
Mathematical modeling, 120
Mayer–Rokitansky–Küster–Hauser syndrome, 390
Mechlorethamine hydrochloride, teratogenicity, 347t
Meclofenate sodium, for headache, 45
Meconium aspiration, 162, 200
Medical ethics. See Ethics
Medical history, in preconceptional care, 64–65
MEDLINE, 120–121
Medroxyprogesterone acetate
    depot, 62–63
    for endometriosis, 253
    for leiomyomata uteri, 246
    in management of premenstrual syndrome, 75
    postmenopausal therapy, 404, 405t, 406–407
Melanoma
    in pregnancy, 350–351
    vaginal, 316–317
    vulvar, 307, 312
Menarche, 388
    delayed, 389–390
    premature, 386
Mendelian disorder(s), 379–380
Meningitis, sinusitis-related, 16
Menopause, 401–407
    age of, 401
    genital atrophy with, 401–402
    hormone therapy in, 404–407
        contraindications to, 406
        risk factors in, 404–406
    osteoporosis and, 402–403
    psychological and psychiatric disorders with, 402
    and sexual dysfunction, 98
    symptoms of, 401–404
    vasomotor flushes in, 401
Menorrhagia, prostaglandins in, 377–378
Menstrual cycle, 363f, 368–375
    changes, ultrasound evaluation of, 219
    length of, 368
Menstrual extraction, 291
Menstruation
    disorders of, 391–400
    postpartum, 202

Mercaptopurine
    effect on ovarian function, 343t
    teratogenicity, 347t
MeSH, 121
Mesonephroid tumor(s), ovarian, 257
Metabolic acidosis, fetal, 143
Metaproterenol, 17
Methadone, teratogenicity, 141
Methimazole
    for hyperthyroidism, 49
    teratogenicity, 139
Methotrexate
    effect on ovarian function, 343t
    for gestational trophoblastic tumors, 340–341
    for rheumatoid arthritis, 34
    teratogenicity, 347t
    therapy, for ectopic pregnancy, 252
Methyldopa, for hypertension, 22
Methylergonovine, for postpartum hemorrhage, 205t
Methylergonovine maleate, for migraine prevention, 46
Methysergide maleate, for migraine prevention, 46
Metronidazole
    for bacterial vaginosis, 79
    for *Helicobacter pylori* infection, 30
    for pelvic inflammatory disease, 94
    for trichomoniasis, 80
Metyrapone test, 411
Microfertilization, 421
Mifepristone, as abortifacient, 295
Migraine. See Headache, migraine
Misoprostol
    as abortifacient, 295
    for peptic ulcer disease, 30
Mitral valve prolapse, pregnant patient with, 163–164
Mixed acidosis, fetal or newborn, 143
Molar pregnancy. See also Hydatidiform mole
    and malignancy, 298, 338
Molecular genetics, clinical applications of, 299–301
Molluscum contagiosum, 50–51
    in pediatric patient, 385
Mondor disease, 76
Monitoring, central, in hemorrhaging patient, 273
Monoamine oxidase inhibitors, 42
    for migraine prevention, 46
    side effects of, 43
Monosomy, 379
Monosomy X, 135. See also 45,X karyotype
Mood, definition of, 40
Morbidity, leading causes of, by age group, 3–6
Mosaicism
    confined placental, 137–138
    fetal, 137–138
Mourning, 355

Moxalactam, side effects and adverse reactions to, 226
MSAFP. See Alpha-fetoprotein, maternal serum
Müllerian tumors, mixed, uterine, 321
Multichannel urodynamics, 238–239
Multifactorial disorders, 135, 380
Multiple gestation, 155–156
Multiple sclerosis, in pregnant patient, 168
Mutation(s)
    proto-oncogene and tumor suppressor gene, and malignancy, 299, 300t
    triple repeat, 380–381
Myasthenia gravis, in pregnant patient, 167–168
Mycobacterium tuberculosis, 18
Mycoplasma pneumoniae
    bronchitis caused by, 16
    pneumonia caused by, 17–18
    urethritis caused by, 19
Myomata uteri. See Leiomyomata uteri
Myomectomy, 247–248
Myotonic dystrophy, 380–381

N

Nabumetone, for osteoarthritis, 34
Nadolol, for migraine prevention, 46
Nafarelin
    dosage and administration, 428t
    for treatment of endometriosis, 425
Naproxen sodium, for headache, 45
Narcotics
    for headache, 45
    for postoperative pain control, 269–270
National Library of Medicine subject headings, 121
Nausea and vomiting, and oral contraceptive use, 58
Necrotizing enterocolitis, in premature infant, 202
Necrotizing fasciitis, 282
Neisseria gonorrhoeae
    antibiotic-resistant, 82–83
    infection, epidemiology of, 82
    pelvic inflammatory disease caused by, 94–95
    penicillinase-producing versus penicillinase-negative, 82–83
    urethritis caused by, 19
Neonatal alloimmune thrombocytopenia, in pregnant patient, 174
Neonatal loss, contributing factors, 65
Neonatal resuscitation, 200
Neonate(s)
    history and physical examination of, 384
    umbilical cord blood pH and blood gas values, 144
Nephrotic syndrome, in pregnant patient, 175

Nerve root
  decompression, 40
  irritation
    diagnosis of, 38–39
    management of, 39
Neural tube defects, 135
  prenatal diagnosis of, 136–137
  prevention of, maternal folic acid intake for, 65
  risk of, in children of diabetics, 65
Neuroendocrinology, 361–367
Neurofibroma, vulvar, 227
Neurohormones, 361–362
Neurologic disease, in pregnant patient, 167–168
Neuroma(s), uterine, 250
Neurosecretion, 361–362
Neurotransmitters, 361–362
Nevi, pigmented, in pregnant patient, 177
Nicotine replacement therapy, 9
Nifedipine
  for hypertension, 22
  for migraine prevention, 46
Nipple discharge, 75–76
Nitrofurantoin, for cystitis, 20
Nitrogen mustard, effect on ovarian function, 343t
Nocturia, 235
Nocturnal penile tumescence, 101–102
Nodules
  skin, 50
  thyroid, management of, 49–50
Non-A, non-B hepatitis, in pregnant patient, 180–181
Non-Hodgkin lymphoma, in pregnancy, 351–352
Non–insulin-dependent diabetes. *See* Diabetes mellitus, type II (non–insulin-dependent)
Nonmaleficence, 112, 356
Nonsteroidal antiinflammatory drugs
  adverse effects of, 33
  antiprostaglandin activity, 378–379
  for gout, 35
  for headache, 45
  in management of premenstrual syndrome, 75
  and peptic ulcer disease, 30, 33
  for rheumatoid arthritis, 33
Nonstress test, 129–130
Norfloxacin
  for cystitis, 20
  for urethritis, 19
Normal flora, 280
Nortriptyline, 42
  for migraine prevention, 46
  side effects of, 43
Nutrition, 11–12
  counseling about, 11
  in lactating woman, 125
  management of, 12
  in pregnancy, 124–125

Nutrition *(continued)*
  recommendations for, 11
Nutritional care, preconceptional, 66
Nutritional status, evaluation of, 11

O

Obesity
  and gallbladder disease, 31
  and infectious morbidity, 280–281
  management, in diabetic patient, 27
  menstrual dysfunction with, 391–392
  postoperative pulmonary care with, 268
Obstetrics, ethical issues in, 113–114
Obstructive uropathy, fetal therapy for, 132
Occupational agents, teratogenicity, 140
Odds ratio, 118–119
Ofloxacin
  for *Chlamydia* infection, 83
  for cystitis, 20
  for gonorrhea, 84
  for pelvic inflammatory disease, 94
  for urethritis, 19
Oligohydramnios, 145
Omeprazole, for peptic ulcer disease, 30
Oncogene(s)
  expression, abnormalities, and malignancy, 299
  structural abnormalities, and malignancy, 299
Oncology, recent advances in, 297
Oocyte(s), 368
  micromanipulation of, 440–441
  retrieval, for in vitro fertilization, 439
Oocyte harvest, ultrasonography in, 221
Oogonia, 368
Oophorectomy
  for endometriosis, 254
  prophylactic, 260
Operative obstetrics, 191–196
Oral contraceptives
  for adenomyosis, 249
  for adolescents, 58
  for androgen excess, 397
  androgenic side effects of, 58
  and breast cancer risk, 302
  and *Candida* vulvovaginitis, 80
  and *Chlamydia trachomatis* infection, 82
  combination, 57
  contraindications to, 59
  for dysfunctional uterine bleeding, 399
  effects of, 57–59
    on breasts, 58
    on cardiovascular disease risk, 57–58
    on central nervous system, 58
    on liver and bile ducts, 58
    on reproductive tract, 58
    on skin, 58
    on subsequent fertility, 58–59
  for endometriosis, 253
  formulations, 57

Oral contraceptives *(continued)*
  multiphasic, 57
  noncontraceptive health benefits of, 59
  prescribing guidelines, 58
  protective effects, against ovarian cancer, 326
  and smoking, 58–59
  use
    after abortion, 58
    during breast-feeding, 58
    in United States, 56
Orbital inflammation, with hyperthyroidism, 48
Orgasm, lack of, management, 100–101
Osteoarthritis
  clinical features of, 34
  differential diagnosis of, 33
  epidemiology of, 32, 34
  treatment of, 34
Osteopenia, 402–403
Osteoporosis
  fractures in, 36
  hyperthyroidism and, 48
  management of, 36–37
  postmenopausal, 402–403
Ovarian cancer, 259, 326–336
  autosomal chromosome abnormalities and, 298–299
  CA 125 as marker for, 327, 330, 333–334
  diagnosis of, 329–330
  epidemiology of, 326, 326f
  epithelial, 327–328, 330–334
    chemotherapy for, 333
    follow-up care with, 333–334
    palliative surgery for, 332–333
    radiation therapy for, 333
    recurrence, 333–334
    second-look laparotomy for, 332
    surgery for, 330–333
    treatment of, 330–333, 331t
  FIGO staging of, 329
  germ cell, 327–328
    diagnosis of, 334
    prognosis for, 334
    serum markers for, 334, 334t
    treatment of, 334
  granulosa cell, 328, 335
  hereditary factors in, 298
  histology, 327–329
  metastasis, 326–327, 329
  in pregnancy, 348–349
  prevalence of, 260
  prophylactic oophorectomy and, 260
  relationship to other gynecologic cancers, 326, 327f
  risk, and oral contraceptive use, 58
  risk factors for, 326
  screening for, 327
  Sertoli–Leydig cell, 328–329, 335
  sex cord–mesenchymal, 334–335
  sex cord–stromal, 327–329, 334–335

Ovarian cancer *(continued)*
 stage at diagnosis, and survival, 326, 327*t*
 survival, 326–327
 World Health Organization classification of, 327–328
Ovarian cycle, 363*f*
Ovarian cyst(s)
 follicular, 255–256
 germinal epithelial, 256
 luteinized, 255–256
 nonneoplastic, 255–256
 and oral contraceptive use, 58
 rupture, pelvic pain with, 68
 surgical therapy, 259
Ovarian failure
 chromosomally competent, 389
 chromosomally incompetent, 389
 primary, 389
Ovarian hemorrhage, extracapsular, pelvic pain with, 68
Ovarian hyperstimulation syndrome, 255
Ovarian neoplasia, with hormone therapy, 406
Ovarian neoplasms, benign, 256–258
Ovarian preservation, for benign ovarian disease, 259–260
Ovarian stromal hyperplasia, 256
Ovarian stromal hyperthecosis, 256
Ovarian stromal proliferative disorders, 256
Ovarian torsion, pelvic pain with, 68
Ovarian vessel bleeding, postoperative, management, 274
Ovaries
 cystadenofibromas, 257
 disorders of, 255–260
  amenorrhea secondary to, 392
  surgical therapy, 259
 intraovarian signaling systems, 371–372
 mucinous cystadenomas, 257
 serous cystadenomas, 256–257
 steroid biosynthesis in, 412, 413*f*
 tumors, 397
  Brenner, 257–258
  clear cell, 257
  endometrioid, 257
  germ cell, 258
  mesonephroid, 257
  stromal, 258
Ovulation
 confirmation of, 423–424
 disorders, investigation and treatment of, 421*t*, 421–424
 failure, investigation and treatment of, 421–424
 hormonal regulation of, 373
 induction, 372–373, 427–428
  hormones for, 364
  regimens for, 422–423
 Luteinizing hormone surge and, 372–373
 postpartum, 202

Ovulation *(continued)*
 steroid hormone actions in, 366
Oxybutynin hydrochloride, for detrusor instability, 241*t*
Oxytocin
 high-dose, for second-trimester abortion, 294
 inhibitors, 160
 in labor, 151
 for labor induction, 189*t*, 189–190
 in lactation, 203
 for postpartum hemorrhage, 205*t*
 secretion, 364

P

Paget disease
 of bone, management of, 37
 of vulva, 308–309
Pain control
 for cancer patient, 356–357
 ethical issues related to, 115
 postoperative, 269–270
Pamidronate, in Paget disease of bone, 37
Pancreas
 endocrine
  fetal, 149
  maternal, in pregnancy, 150
 transplantation, 26
Pancreatic cancer, 352
Pancreatitis, with gallstones, 31
Pap test
 abnormal, management of, 216–217
 and cervical cancer, 317
 with cervical neoplasia, 318
 diagnosis of trichomoniasis, 79–80
 recommended schedule for, 317–318
Papular dermatitis of pregnancy, 177
Papules, 50
Paracervical block, obstetric, 196–197
Paramethadione, teratogenicity, 139
Paraplegia, and pregnancy, 168
Parathyroid gland, fetal, 149
Paroxetine, 42
 side effects of, 43
Parturition, physiology of, 150–151
Patent ductus arteriosus, symptomatic, 201
Patient-controlled analgesia, 269
Patient Self-Determination Act, 115, 357
Pediatric gynecology, 384–387
Pediatric patient(s), history and physical examination of, 384–385
Pelvic congestion syndrome, chronic pelvic pain with, 70
Pelvic examination
 preoperative, 224–225
 in urogynecology, 236
Pelvic floor rehabilitation, for stress urinary incontinence, 240
Pelvic infection, 94–96. *See also* Pelvic inflammatory disease; Toxic shock syndrome; Tuberculosis, pelvic
 pelvic pain with, 67–68

Pelvic infection *(continued)*
 surgical, 280–282
  antibiotic therapy for, 281
   failure of, 281
  microbiology of, 280
  necrotizing, 282
  risk factors for, 280–281
Pelvic inflammatory disease, 94–95
 abdominal pain with, 94
 atypical, 95
 diagnosis of, 94
 and ectopic pregnancy risk, 95
 and infertility, 95
 prevention of, 95
 risk, with intrauterine device, 61
 sequelae, 95
 treatment of, 94–95
 ultrasound evaluation of, 221
Pelvic masses
 biopsy, ultrasonography in, 221
 laparoscopy for, 214
 ultrasound evaluation of, 220
Pelvic pain, 66–71
 acute, 67–68
  nongynecologic causes, 68
 with adenomyosis, 70
 with adnexal problems, 68
 chronic, 67–71
  continuous, 67, 69–71
  episodic, 67, 69
  nongynecologic causes, 71
 with chronic salpingitis, 70
 with early pregnancy complications, 68
 with endometriosis, 70, 253–254
 gynecologic causes of, 67
 history-taking with, 66
 in irritable bowel syndrome, 32
 laparoscopy for, 214
 with leiomyomata uteri, 246
 midcycle, 69
 with pelvic congestion syndrome, 70
 with pelvic infection, 67–68
 physical examination with, 67
Penicillin
 allergy, and preoperative antibiotic prophylaxis, 226
 for gonorrhea, 84
 for pneumonia, 17–18
Penicillin G, for syphilis, 85
Penile implant, 102–103
Peptic ulcer disease
 management of, 30–31
 and nonsteroidal antiinflammatory drugs, 30, 33
Peptostreptococcus, pelvic inflammatory disease caused by, 94
Percutaneous umbilical cord blood sampling, 138
Perforation, in first-trimester abortion, 292
Perihepatitis, pelvic pain with, 67–68
Perimenopause, 401
Perineal defect, causes of, 230
Perineal prolapse, 233–234

Perineum
    injuries, intraoperative or obstetric, management of, 276–277
    lacerations of, severity grading of, 234
Peripheral artery cannulation, in hemorrhaging patient, 273
Peritoneum, wound healing in, 264
Periventricular hemorrhage, in premature infant, 201
Periventricular leukomalacia, in premature infant, 201
Pessary
    for genital prolapse, 232
    for stress urinary incontinence, 240
Petechiae, 50
pH, of blood or tissue, 143
Phencyclidine, teratogenicity, 141
Phenelzine, 42
    for migraine prevention, 46
Phenobarbital, teratogenicity, 167
Phenoxybenzamine, for bladder and urethral disorders, 243, 245
Phenylpropanolamine, for stress urinary incontinence, 239
Phenytoin, teratogenicity, 167
Pheochromocytoma, 416–417
    in pregnant patient, 176
Physical examination
    with anatomic support defects and dysfunction, 231–232
    preoperative, 224–225
    in urogynecology, 236
Physical therapy, for back pain, 39
Pituitary adenoma, hyperthyroidism with, 48–49
Pituitary cycle, 363f
Pituitary gland
    anterior, hormones, 364–366
    dysfunction, amenorrhea secondary to, 391
    hyperplasia, hyperprolactinemia due to, 392–393
    maternal, in pregnancy, 150
    posterior, hormones, 364
Pituitary hormone(s), 364–366
    fetal, 149
Placenta
    endocrinology of, 146–148
    management, with abdominal pregnancy, 251
Placental calcium pump, 149
Placental lactogen, 150, 366
    in pregnancy, 148
Placental site trophoblastic tumor, 338–341
Placenta previa, 154–155
Placentation, abnormalities, and spontaneous abortion, 435–436
Ploidy abnormalities, and malignancy, 298
PMS. See Premenstrual syndrome
Pneumococcal vaccine, 20
Pneumonia
    etiology of, 17
    management of, 17–18

Pneumonia (continued)
    mortality with, 17
    signs and symptoms of, 17
Pneumoperitoneum, for laparoscopy, 213
Podophyllin, for human papillomavirus infection, 90
Polycystic kidney disease, in pregnant patient, 175
Polycystic ovaries, ultrasound evaluation of, 220–221
Polycystic ovary disease, 255
Polycystic ovary syndrome, 391–392, 395–396
    clinical features of, 395
    diagnosis of, 395
    pathophysiology of, 395–396
Polymerase chain reaction, 383
Polymyalgia rheumatica, management of, 34
Polyploidy, and spontaneous abortion, 433
Polyps, endometrial
    epidemiology of, 249
    etiology of, 249
    histopathology of, 249–250
    hysteroscopy for, 211
    incidence of, 249
    pathogenesis of, 249
    signs and symptoms, 250
    treatment of, 250
Popliteal nerve compression, 38
Postabortal syndrome, 292
Postcoital test, 426
Postoperative care, 266–269
Postpartum blues, 41
Postpartum care, 203–204
Postpartum depression. See Depression, postpartum
Postpartum psychosis, 41
Postterm gestation, 161–162
Prazosin
    for bladder and urethral disorders, 243, 245
    for hypertension, 22
Precision, of epidemiologic studies, 118
Precocious puberty, 386, 428–429
Preconceptional care, 64–66
    for diabetic, 64–65
    genetic assessment in, 65–66
    medical history in, 64–65
    nutritional care in, 66
    reproductive history in, 65
Predictive value, of test results, 116
Prednisone
    for androgen excess, 397
    for asthma, 17
    for giant cell arteritis, 35
    for polymyalgia rheumatica, 34
Preeclampsia
    definition of, 152
    management of, 153–154
    pathophysiology of, 152–153
    severity of, indicators of, 152

Pregnancy. See also Antepartum care
    abdominal, 251
    after sterilization, 289–290
    anesthesia during, 344
    asymptomatic bacteriuria in, 20
    bleeding in, in second half, 154–155
    cancer and, 342–353
    cervical, 251
    chemotherapy during, 346–347
    Chlamydia infection in, 83–84
    cigarette smoking in, 8–9
    complications of, 152–163
        early, pelvic pain with, 68
    cystitis in, treatment of, 20
    diagnosis of, 124
    endocrinology of, 146–150
    extrauterine. See also Ectopic pregnancy
        sites of, 251
    gonorrhea in, 84–85
    hematologic cancer in, 351–352
    heterotopic, 251
    hypertension in, 152–154
    immunology of, 145–146
    with intrauterine device in place, 60–61
    medical complications of, 163–188
    nutrition in, 124–125
    and pheochromocytoma, 416–417
    physiology of, 143–151
    prevention, for rape victim, 106
    sarcoma in, 353
    selective reduction, 295
    and sexual dysfunction, 98
    spouse abuse in, 107
    syphilis in, 85
    termination, 290–295
        mortality in, 290t, 290–291, 291t
    thyroid cancer management in, 49
    thyroid nodule management in, 49
    trichomoniasis in, 80
    ultrasonography in, 126–129
    weight gain in, 124–125
    work during, 125–126
Pregnancy-induced hypertension
    definition of, 152
    management of, 153–154
    pathophysiology of, 152–153
    and premature fetus, management, 154
Pregnancy loss, contributing factors, 65
Premature infant, umbilical cord blood pH and blood gas values, 144
Premature ovarian failure, 392
Premature rupture of membranes, 160–161
Premenstrual dysphoric disorder, 71
Premenstrual symptoms, epidemiology of, 71
Premenstrual syndrome, 71–74
    diagnosis of, 72–73
    differential diagnosis of, 72–73
    epidemiology of, 71
    etiology of, 73
    history-taking with, 71–72
    management of, 73–74
    symptoms of, 72

Premstrual syndrome *(continued)*
　　treatment of
　　　medical, 74
　　　nonmedical, 73–74
Prenatal diagnosis, techniques, 136–138
Preoperative care, 224–226
Preoperative orders, 225
Preterm birth, 158–160
　　complications of, 201–202
Prevention, 2. *See also* Preconceptional care
Primidone, teratogenicity, 167
Probenecid
　　for gout, 35
　　for pelvic inflammatory disease, 94
Procarbazine
　　effect on ovarian function, 343*t*
　　teratogenicity, 347*t*
Progesterone
　　assays, 433–444
　　in assessment of luteal function, 423–424
　　in corpus luteum function, 374–375
　　in management of premenstrual syndrome, 75
　　in ovulation, 373
　　in petrolatum, for lichen sclerosus et atrophicus, 229
　　in pregnancy, 146–147
　　serum, in viable versus unsuccessful pregnancy, 251
Progestins
　　for dysfunctional uterine bleeding, 399
　　for endometriosis, 253
　　for hot flushes, 401
　　for leiomyomata uteri, 247
　　long-acting, 61–63
　　　implants, 61–62
　　postmenopausal therapy, 404–407, 405*t*
Prolactin
　　assays, 445
　　in lactation, 203
　　and nipple discharge, 75
　　synthesis and secretion of, 365, 365*t*
Prolactinoma(s), 392–393
Proopiomelanocortin, 365
Propantheline bromide, for detrusor instability, 241*t*
Propranolol
　　for hypertension, 22
　　for migraine prevention, 46
Propylthiouracil, teratogenicity, 139
Prostaglandin(s), 376–379
　　actions of, 376
　　clinical applications, 378–379
　　disorders mediated by, 377–378
　　intrauterine, for second-trimester abortion, 294
　　mechanism of action, 376–378
　　nomenclature for, 376
　　for peptic ulcer disease, 30
　　for postpartum hemorrhage, 205*t*
　　structure of, 376, 376*f*

Prostaglandin(s) *(continued)*
　　synthesis of, 376, 377*f*
　　systemic, for second-trimester abortion, 294
　　types of, 376
Prostaglandin synthetase inhibitors
　　for dysfunctional uterine bleeding, 399
　　for tocolysis, 160
Prosthetic heart valve(s), pregnant patient with, 164
Proteus
　　cellulitis caused by, 51
　　cystitis caused by, 19
Proto-oncogene(s)
　　mutations, and malignancy, 299, 300*t*
　　prognostic significance, in gynecologic cancer, 300
Protriptyline, 42
　　side effects of, 43
Prurigo gestationis, 177
Pruritus
　　in pregnancy, 165–166
　　vulvar, 229
Pseudogout, management of, 36
Pseudohermaphroditism, female, 414
Pseudomenopause, for treatment of endometriosis, 425
Pseudomonas, cellulitis caused by, 51
Pseudomosaicism, fetal, 138
Pseudomyxoma ovarii, 257
Pseudomyxoma peritonei, 257
Pseudopregnancy, for treatment of endometriosis, 425
Psoriasis, 51
　　in pregnant patient, 177–178
　　vulvar, in pediatric patient, 386
Psychotherapy, for depression, 41
Puberty. *See also* Precocious puberty
　　delayed, 389
　　hormonal events in, 387–388
　　neuroendocrinology of, 366–367
　　normal, 387–388
　　　timing and pattern of, 388
　　　variations in, 388
　　onset of, 388
Pudendal block, obstetric, 196–197
Puerperium, 202–206
　　complications in, 204–206
　　physiology of, 202–203
Pulmonary care, postoperative, 268
Pulmonary disorders
　　management of, 15–18
　　pregnant patient with, 164–165
Pulmonary edema
　　cardiogenic (high-pressure), 271
　　noncardiogenic, 271
Pulmonary embolism
　　postoperative, 282–285
　　　diagnosis of, 282–283
　　　epidemiology of, 282
　　　pregnant patient with, 164–165
　　　risk factors for, 283–284

Pulmonary embolism *(continued)*
　　surgical management, 285
Purified protein derivative, 18
Purpura, 50
Pustules, 50
P value, 119
Pyelonephritis, 19–20
　　acute, in pregnant patient, 184–185
Pyosalpingitis, pelvic pain with, 67–68
Pyrazinamide, for tuberculosis, 18

Q

Quadriplegia, and pregnancy, 168
Quality of life, 113, 354–357

R

Radiation
　　effects on fetus, 345–346
　　risk of sterility or amenorrhea after, by dose, 346*t*
Radiation therapy
　　for breast cancer, 303–305
　　for cervical cancer, 318–319
　　for endometrial cancer, 323–324
　　for epithelial ovarian cancer, 333
　　fertility subsequent to, 342–343
　　for gestational trophoblastic tumors, 341
　　for invasive squamous cell carcinoma of vulva, 311
　　during pregnancy, 345–346
　　for vaginal carcinoma, 315
Radioactive iodine uptake, 48, 408
Ranitidine
　　for gastroesophageal reflux, 30
　　for peptic ulcer disease, 30
Rape, 105–107
Rash, 50–51
Receptor(s), hormone
　　cell surface, 360
　　intercellular, 361
　　physiology, 360–361
Reciprocal translocation(s), parental, 133–134
Rectal prolapse, 222
Rectocele, causes of, 230
Rectovaginal fistula, 276
Rectum, intraoperative or obstetric injuries, management of, 276–277
Reflex, deep tendon, testing, 38
Regional analgesia, obstetric, 196–197
Regional anesthesia, complications of, 270
Relationship factors, and sexual dysfunction, 97–98
Relative risk, 118–119
Renal colic, pain with, 68
Renal disease, in pregnant patient, 174–176
Renal failure, acute, in pregnant patient, 175
Renal transplantation, pregnancy after, 176

Reproductive endocrinology, advances in, 359
Reproductive history, in preconceptional care, 65
Reproductive tract, effects of oral contraceptives on, 58
Resistant ovary syndrome, 368
Respiratory acidosis, fetal, 143
Respiratory depression, with postoperative analgesia, 270
Respiratory disorders, management of, 15–18
Respiratory distress syndrome, 201
Respiratory insufficiency, acute, anesthesia-related, 271
Restriction fragment length polymorphism, 299–300, 383
Retained products of conception, ultrasound evaluation of, 219
Retinoic acid, for acne, 51
Retinopathy of prematurity, 202
Retroperitoneal venous bleeding, postoperative, management, 274
Rhabdomyosarcoma, vulvar, 312
Rheumatism, epidemiology of, 32
Rheumatoid arthritis
  clinical features of, 33
  differential diagnosis of, 33
  epidemiology of, 33
  in pregnant patient, 178
  risk, and oral contraceptive use, 58
  treatment of, 33–34
Rifampin
  for pneumonia, 18
  for tuberculosis, 18
Risk factors, identification of, 2
Robertsonian translocation(s), parental, 133–134
RU 486, as abortifacient, 295
Rubella, in pregnant patient, 181–182

S

Saline, hypertonic, instillation, for second-trimester abortion, 294
Salpingectomy, in ectopic pregnancy, 252
Salpingitis
  chronic, chronic pelvic pain with, 70
  pelvic pain with, 67–68
  risk, and oral contraceptive use, 58
  silent, 95
Salpingocentesis, for ectopic pregnancy, 253
Salpingo-oophorectomy
  for endometrial cancer, 323
  for endometriosis, 254
Salpingostomy, in ectopic pregnancy, 252
Salpingotomy, in ectopic pregnancy, 252
Salsalate, for osteoarthritis, 34
Sarcoma(s)
  in pregnancy, 353
  uterine, 321, 325
    classification of, 325

Sarcoma(s) (continued)
  vaginal, 316
  vulvar, 307, 312–313
Scabies, 51
Scalpel(s), and wound healing, 261
Sciatica, 37
  management of, 39
Scleroderma, in pregnant patient, 179
Screening, 2–8
  breast cancer, 28
  for colorectal cancer, 32
  for diabetes, 24–25
  for dietary/nutrition problems, 11
Screening test(s), 116
  sensitivity of, 2
  specificity of, 2
Seborrheic dermatitis, 51
  in pediatric patient, 385
Seizure disorders, in pregnant patient, 167
Semen analysis, 418–419
Sensitivity
  of screening tests, 2
  of tests, 116
Septic shock, 282
Serotonin antagonists
  for headache, 45
  for migraine prevention, 46
Sertoli–stromal cell tumors, ovarian, 258
Sertraline, 42
  side effects of, 43
Sex chromosome(s), 379
  abnormalities, ovarian failure due to, 389
  normal, ovarian failure with, 389
Sexual abuse, of child, 104–105, 386–387
  forensic specimen collection in, 386
Sexual arousal, lack of, management, 99–100
Sexual assault, 105–107
Sexual counseling, 99–103
Sexual desire, lack of, management, 99
Sexual dysfunction, 97–103
  management, 99–103
  sources of, 97–99
Sexuality, 97
Sexually transmitted disease, 82–93
  bacterial, 82–85
  in pediatric patient, 387
  and substance abuse, 13
  transmission
    and condom use, 56–57
    and diaphragm use, 56
    and spermicide use, 56
  viral, 85–93
Sexual response cycle, 97
Sheehan syndrome, 365
Shigellosis, in pediatric patient, 386
Shock
  cervical, 292
  endotoxic, 282
  hemorrhagic, 273
  septic, 282

Short stature, growth hormone therapy for, 382
Shoulder dystocia, 195
Sickle cell crisis, abdominal pain with, 68
Sickle hemoglobinopathy, in pregnant patient, 173
Sigmoidoscopy, 32, 222–223
Silicone breast implants, 305
Sinobronchial syndrome, 15
Sinusitis
  acute, 15
  causes of, 15
  chronic, 15–16
  management of, 15–16
Skeletal maturation, and sexual maturation, 388
Skin disorders, 50–51. See also Dermatoses
Small bowel, intraoperative injuries and fistulas, 274–276
Smoking. See Cigarette smoking
Sodium bicarbonate, in cardiopulmonary resuscitation, 273
Somatization, 40
Somatomedins. See Insulinlike growth factor(s)
Southern blotting, 383, 383f
Specificity
  of screening tests, 2
  of tests, 116
Sperm
  functional evaluation of, 419–420
  hypoosmotic swelling test, 420
  immobilizing antibody test, 430
  immunobead binding test, 430
Sperm agglutination tests, 430
Sperm antibody testing, 419, 429–430
Spermicide, vaginal, 56
Sperm penetration assay, 419–420
Spinal analgesia, obstetric, 197
Spinal and bulbar muscular atrophy, 380–381
Spine, physical examination of, 38–39
Spirometry, in asthma, 16
Spironolactone
  for androgen excess, 398
  in management of premenstrual syndrome, 75
Spondylolisthesis, 37, 39–40
Spondylolysis, 37, 39–40
Sponge, vaginal, 56
Spontaneous abortion. See Abortion, spontaneous
Spouse abuse, 107–109
Sputum, Gram stain, 17
Squamous cell carcinoma
  vaginal, 314
    diagnosis of, 314–315
    FIGO staging of, 315
    invasive, 314–315
    survival, 315
    treatment of, 315
  vulvar, 307

Squamous cell carcinoma, vulvar (continued)
  invasive, 309–311
  versus verrucous carcinoma, 311–312
Squamous cell hyperplasia, vulvar, 228–229
Squamous intraepithelial lesions
  high-grade, 216–217
  low-grade, 216–217
Staphylococcus, cystitis caused by, 19
Staphylococcus aureus
  sinusitis caused by, 15
  skin infection, 51
  toxic shock syndrome caused by, 95–96
Staphylococcus saprophyticus, cystitis caused by, 19
Staples, and wound healing, 263–264
Status asthmaticus, 17
Status migrainosus, 43
Statutory rape, 105
Stem cell transplantation, to fetus, 132
Sterility, definition of, 417
Sterilization, 287–290
  complications of, 289–290
  failure rate of, 288
  female, laparoscopy for, 213
  frequency of, 287
  involuntary, 288
  medicolegal considerations, 288
  patient selection and counseling for, 287–288
  pregnancy after, 289–290
  rates, in United States, 56
  reversal of, 288, 290
  techniques, 288–289
Steroid(s). *See also* Adrenal steroid(s); *specific hormone(s)*
  androgenic, assays, 444
  estrogenic, assays, 433
  feedback, 366
  glucocorticoid, assays, 444–445
  mechanism of action, 361
  progestational, assays, 433–434
Stomach, cancer of, 352
Stool guaiac test, in diagnosis of colorectal cancer, 32
Straight leg raising, 38–39
Strawberry cervix, 79
Streptococci
  alpha, sinusitis caused by, 15
  group A beta-hemolytic, skin infection, 51
Streptococcus agalactiae
  cystitis caused by, 19
  pelvic inflammatory disease caused by, 94
Streptococcus pneumoniae
  pelvic inflammatory disease caused by, 94
  pneumonia caused by, 17–18

Streptococcus pneumoniae (continued)
  sinusitis caused by, 15
Streptococcus pyogenes
  pelvic inflammatory disease caused by, 94
  sinusitis caused by, 15
  toxic shock syndrome caused by, 95
Streptokinase, therapy, 285
Streptomycin, for tuberculosis, 18
Stress management, 12
Stress reduction, in management of premenstrual syndrome, 75
Striae, abdominal, clinical significance of, 231
Stroke, in pregnant patient, 168
Struma ovarii, 258
  hyperthyroidism with, 48–49
Subarachnoid hemorrhage, in pregnant patient, 168
Substance abuse, 12–14
  barriers to care and, 13
  detection of, interviewing techniques for, 13–14
Sucralfate, for peptic ulcer disease, 30
Sulfasalazine, for rheumatoid arthritis, 34
Sulfisoxazole
  for *Chlamydia* infection, 83
  for cystitis, 20
Sulfonylurea drugs, for diabetes, 27
Sumatriptan, for headache, 45
Superficial angiitis, of breast, 76
Surgery
  complications of, 270–286
  postoperative care for. *See* Postoperative care
  preoperative care for. *See* Preoperative care
Surgical instruments, and wound healing, 261
Surrogate decision makers, 112–113
Suture material(s)
  currently available, 262, 262t
  inflammatory response to, 262–263
  selection of, 262–263
Suturing
  tight, and wound healing, 262, 263f
  and wound healing, 261–264
Swan–Ganz catheter
  applications of, 273–274
  indications for, 273
Swyer syndrome, 389
Sympathomimetics, for headache, 45
Synechiae, uterine
  hysteroscopic diagnosis of, 211
  spontaneous abortion and, 435–436
Syphilis
  congenital, 85
  course of, 85
  diagnosis of, 85
  epidemiology of, 82
  in pregnancy, 85

Syphilis *(continued)*
  testing, for gonorrhea patient, 84
  treatment of, 85
Systemic lupus erythematosus
  differential diagnosis of, 33
  in pregnant patient, 178–179

T

T_3. *See* Triiodothyronine
T_4. *See* Thyroxine
Tachyarrhythmia, fetal therapy for, 131
Tamoxifen
  for breast cancer treatment, 305–306
  and endometrial cancer, 322
Tampon, for stress urinary incontinence, 240
Telogen effluvium, postpartum, 177
Tension headache. *See* Headache, tension-type
Teratogenic agents, 138–141
Teratoma(s)
  cystic, 258
    ovarian, 327–328
    ovarian, hyperthyroidism with, 48–49
Terazosin, for hypertension, 22
Terminal care, ethical issues related to, 114–115
Testicular feminization, 382–383
Testosterone
  assays, 444
  in petrolatum, for lichen sclerosus et atrophicus, 229
  synthesis and secretion of, 412, 413f
  total and free serum, laboratory evaluation of, 409
Tetracycline
  for cystitis, 20
  for gonorrhea, 84
  for *Helicobacter pylori* infection, 30
  for urethritis, 19
Thalassemia, in pregnant patient, 172–173
Thecomas, 258
Thelarche, 388
Theophylline, 17
Thermal knives, and wound healing, 261
Third spacing, 267
Thrombocytopenia, in pregnancy-induced hypertension, 152
Thromboembolism. *See also* Deep vein thrombosis; Pulmonary embolism
  and hormone therapy, 406
  risk, effects of oral contraceptives on, 57–58
Thrombolytic therapy, indications for, 285
Thromboxane, 376
Thyroid adenoma, 48
Thyroid cancer
  management of, 49–50
  in pregnancy, 353

Index

Thyroid disease
  postpartum, 172
  in pregnant patient, 171–172
  and spontaneous abortion, 436
Thyroid disorders. *See also* Hyperthyroidism; Hypothyroidism; Thyroid cancer; Thyroid nodules
  clinical physiology of, 47
  fetal and neonatal, 47
Thyroid function tests, 47, 408
  in pregnant patient, 171
Thyroid gland, 407–408
  fetal, 148
  maternal, in pregnancy, 150
Thyroid hormone(s), 407–408
Thyroiditis
  autoimmune, 47–48
  postpartum (painless, silent, lymphocytic), 48
  subacute (painful), 48–49
Thyroid nodules, management of, 49–50
Thyroid-stimulating hormone, 47
  serum, measurement of, 408
  synthesis and secretion of, 364–366, 365t
Thyroid therapy, in gynecology, 408
Thyrotoxicosis, 48–49, 407–408
Thyrotropin-releasing hormone, 47
Thyrotropin-releasing hormone stimulation test, 408
Thyroxine, 47, 407–408
  serum, measurement of, 408
  therapy, for hypothyroidism, 48
Thyroxine-binding globulin, 47
Timolol maleate, for migraine prevention, 46
Tineas, 50
TNM staging system, 303–304
Tocolysis, 159–160
Toluidine blue, vulvar staining with, 227
Toxic shock syndrome, 95–96
  Clostridium sordellii-associated, 95–96
  management, 96
  risk, with vaginal sponge, 56
  staphylococcal, 95–96
  streptococcal, 95–96
Toxoplasmosis
  congenital, 183
  in pregnant patient, 182–183
Transformation zone, abnormal, 216–218
Transforming growth factor, intraovarian regulatory role, 372
Transfusion, fetal, 132
Tranylcypromine, 42
Trazodone, 42
  side effects of, 43
Tretinoin, teratogenicity, 139
Triamterene, for hypertension, 22
Trichloroacetic acid, for human papillomavirus infection, 90

Trichomonas vaginalis, urethritis caused by, 19
Trichomoniasis
  diagnosis and management of, 79–80
  in pediatric patient, 387
Tricyclic drugs (tricyclic antidepressants), 42
  in management of premenstrual syndrome, 75
Triethylenemelamine, teratogenicity, 347t
Triiodothyronine, 47, 407–408
Triiodothyronine uptake assay, 408
Trimethadione, teratogenicity, 139
Trimethoprim, for cystitis, 20
Trimethoprim–sulfamethoxazole, for cystitis, 20
Trimipramine, 42
  side effects of, 43
Triple screen, for prenatal diagnosis of Down syndrome, 136
Trisomy, 379
  prenatal diagnosis of, 133, 136
  and spontaneous abortion, 433
Trisomy 13, 379
Trisomy 18, 379
Trisomy 21, 379
Tryptorelin, dosage and administration, 428t
Tubal embryo transfer, 442
Tuberculosis
  management of, 18
  pelvic, 96
  in pregnant patient, 186–187
  treatment of, 96
Tuboovarian abscess, pelvic pain with, 67–68
Tumor(s). *See also* Ovaries, tumors; Vulva, tumors
Tumor markers, 297
Tumor suppressor gene(s), 299
  mutations, and malignancy, 299, 300t
  prognostic significance, in gynecologic cancer, 300
Turner syndrome, 379, 381–382
  and malignancy, 298
Twin gestation, 194–195

U

Ulcerative colitis, in pregnant patient, 166
Ultrasonography
  in antepartum care, 126–129
    basic examinations, 127–129
    comprehensive examinations, 129
    indications for, 127
    routine, 127
    types of examinations, 127–129
  of breast lesions, 29
  diagnostic, 219–221
    of adnexal masses, 258
    for deep vein thrombosis, 283
    in ectopic pregnancy, 251–252

Ultrasonography *(continued)*
  in evaluation of low abdominal or pelvic pain, 67–68
  in gynecology, 218–221
  operative procedures with, 221
  technical advances in, 126
Umbilical cord blood. *See also* Percutaneous umbilical cord blood sampling
  acid–base determinations, 143–144
  pH and blood gas values
    normal, 144
    in premature infant, 144
  sample collection, 143–144
Uniparental disomy, 380
Ureaplasma, urethritis caused by, 19
Urea–prostaglandin, for second-trimester abortion, 294
Ureter(s)
  anatomy of, 277
  ectopic, 235
  intraoperative injury and fistulas, 277–279
  ultrasound evaluation of, 221
Urethra
  prolapsed, in pediatric patient, 386
  ultrasound evaluation of, 221
Urethral diverticula, treatment of, 241–242
Urethral diverticulum, 235
Urethral mucosa, prolapse of, 228
Urethral pressure profilometry, 239, 239f
Urethral spasm, treatment of, 243
Urethral syndrome, 242–243
Urethritis
  chronic. *See* Urethral syndrome
  management of, 19
Urethrocystometry, 239
Urethropexy, needle, for stress urinary incontinence, 240
Urethrovaginal fistulas, 280
Urethrovesical junction mobility, 236–237
Urinalysis
  in cystitis, 19
  preoperative, 225
  in urethritis, 19
Urinary catheterization, clean, intermittent self-catheterization, 244
Urinary diverticulum, 235
Urinary fistula, 235
Urinary frequency, 235
Urinary incontinence, 234–242
  bacteriuria and, 236
  causes of, 235
  definition of, 234
  diagnosis of, 234–239
    stress test for, 237
  with genital prolapse, 232
  genuine stress, 235
    diagnosis of, 235–237
    history-taking with, 235–236
  overflow, 235, 244

Urinary incontinence (continued)
　physical examination with, 236
　in postmenopausal patient, 402
　prevalence of, 234
　stress
　　mechanical devices for, 240
　　pelvic floor rehabilitation for, 240
　　pharmacotherapy, 239–240
　　surgical intervention for, 240–241
　　treatment of, 239–241
　treatment of, 239–242
　urge, 235
Urinary leakage, clinical significance of, 235
Urinary retention
　causes of, 244
　diagnosis of, 244
　treatment of, 244–245
Urinary tract
　intraoperative injury and fistulas, management of, 277–280
　lower
　　physical examination of, 236
　　symptoms. See also Urinary incontinence
　　　workup for, 235–236
Urinary tract infection
　management of, 19–20
　postpartum, 206
　in pregnant patient, 184–185
Urinary tract malignancy, in pregnancy, 352
Urine output
　normal, 267
　postoperative, 267
Urodynamics, multichannel, 238–239
Uroflowmetry, 237
　and pressure voiding studies, 239
Urogynecology, 234–245
Urolog, 236
Ursodeoxycholic acid, for gallstones, 31
Uterine bleeding. See also Dysfunctional uterine bleeding
　with intrauterine devices, 60
Uterine corpus, cancer of, 321–326. See also Endometrial carcinoma
Uterine evacuation, ultrasonography in, 221
Uterine infection, postpartum, 205–206
Uterine prolapse
　causes of, 230
　severity gradings, 230
Uterine vessel bleeding, postoperative, management, 274
Uterus
　arcuate, clinical features and management of, 435
　bicornuate, clinical features and management of, 435
　congenital anomalies
　　classification of, 434
　　clinical features of, 434–435

Uterus, congenital anomalies (continued)
　　management of, 434–435
　　nomenclature for, 434
　　and spontaneous abortion, 434–435
　　ultrasound evaluation of, 219
　congenital malformations of, hysteroscopic evaluation of, 211
　conservation, with adnexal removal, 250
　diethylstilbestrol-related anomalies, clinical features and management of, 435
　didelphys, clinical features and management of, 434–435
　disorders of, 245–250
　evaluation of, in infertility work-up, 426–427
　hypoplasia/agenesis, clinical features and management of, 434
　involutional changes, postpartum, 202
　postoperative, ultrasound evaluation in, 219–220
　postpartum, ultrasound evaluation in, 219–220
　sarcomas of, 321, 325
　septa, incision of, hysteroscopy for, 211–212
　septate, clinical features and management of, 435
　ultrasound evaluation of, 219
　unicornuate, clinical features and management of, 434

V

Vaccine
　hepatitis B virus, 20–21
　influenza, 19–20
　pneumococcal, 20
Vacuum extraction, 192–193
Vagina
　cancer of, 314–317. See also specific malignancy
　　epidemiology of, 314
　　in pregnancy, 349
　　risk factors for, 314
　colposcopy of, 218
　condylomata acuminata, diagnosis of, 89
　epithelial changes, with intrauterine diethylstilbestrol exposure, 316
　normal flora of, 77
　pH of, 77
　　determination of, 78
　postmenopausal, 81
Vaginal atrophy, 81, 401–402
　estrogen therapy for, 232
Vaginal birth after cesarean delivery, 193–194
Vaginal bleeding
　in pediatric patient, 386
　postoperative, management, 274

Vaginal delivery, breech, 194
Vaginal discharge
　amine test, 78
　examination of, 78
　excessive, 78
　normal, 77
　in pediatric patient, 386
　wet preparation, 78
Vaginal foam, cream, suppositories jelly, and sponges, 56
Vaginal intraepithelial neoplasia, 314
　diagnosis of, 314
　and human papillomavirus infection, 88
　treatment of, 314
Vaginectomy, for vaginal carcinoma, 315
Vaginismus, 69
　management, 101
Vaginitis, 77–82
　atrophic, 81, 401–402
　desquamative, 81. See Lichen planus, erosive
　diagnosis of, 78
　differential diagnosis of, 19
　evaluation of, 77–78
　foreign-body, 81
　gonococcal, in pediatric patient, 387
　history-taking with, 77
　management of, 78
　physical examination with, 77–78
Validity, of epidemiologic studies, 118
Valproic acid, teratogenicity, 139
Varicocele, 418, 420
Vascular injury, in sterilization, 289
Vasomotor flushes, in menopause, 401
Ventricular fibrillation, 272
Verapamil
　for hypertension, 22
　for migraine prevention, 46
Verrucous carcinoma, of vulva, 311–312
Vesicles, 50
Vesicocervical fistulas, 280
Vesicovaginal fistulas, 279–280
Vestibular gland, tumors, 227
Vinblastine
　effect on ovarian function, 343t
　teratogenicity, 347t
Vincristine, effect on ovarian function, 343t
Viral infections
　bronchitis caused by, 16
　sexually transmitted, 85–93
　sinusitis caused by, 15
　of skin, 50–51
Virilization, 396–398, 411–412
　laboratory evaluation with, 411
　with luteoma of pregnancy, 256
Vitamin A, teratogenicity, 139–140
Vitamin B$_{12}$, deficiency, 172
Vitamin D, therapy, for osteoporosis, 36
Voiding
　abnormalities, 244–245

Voiding (continued)
    normal, 244
Vulva
    cancer of, 307–313. *See also specific malignancy*
        FIGO staging system for, 309–310
        in pregnancy, 349
        verrucous, 311–312
    carcinoma in situ, 307–308
    colposcopy of, 218, 227, 307
    condylomata acuminata, diagnosis of, 88–89
    examination of, 227
    hidradenoma, 227
    nonmalignant disorders of, 227–229
    Paget disease of, 308–309
    staining, with toluidine blue, 227
    tumors
        benign, 227–228
        cystic, 227
        solid, 227
    washing, with acetic acid, 227, 307
Vulvar biopsy, office, 227
Vulvar disorder(s), in pediatric patient, 385–386
Vulvar dystrophies, 228–229
Vulvar intraepithelial neoplasia, 229, 307–308
    and human papillomavirus infection, 88
Vulvar vestibulitis syndrome, 228
Vulvectomy
    for invasive squamous cell carcinoma of vulva, 309–311

Vulvectomy (continued)
    for vaginal carcinoma, 315
Vulvovaginal infection, 77
Vulvovaginitis, in pediatric patient, 385

W

Walthard rests, 257
Warfarin
    prophylaxis, 284
    teratogenicity, 139
Wart(s), genital, 88
Weight, evaluation of, 11
Weight control, 11–12
    and exercise, 9–10
    management of, 12
Weight gain
    in pregnancy, 124–125
    with smoking cessation, 9
Weight reduction
    in obese diabetic patient, 27
    in prevention of coronary artery disease, 23
Wheals, 50
Word catheter, for Bartholin duct abscess treatment, 228
Wound(s)
    blood supply to, 265
    disruptions, 285–286
    drainage, and wound healing, 264
    infection
        closure technique and, 263, 263f
        risk factors for, 265
    irrigation, 264
    management, principles of, 260

Wound healing, 260–265
    absorbable ligating clips and, 263–264
    adhesion barrier materials and, 264
    advances in, 265
    antibiotics and, 264–265
    catheters and, 264
    disease processes and, 265
    drainage and, 264
    factors affecting, 264–265, 285–286
    incision and, 261, 285–286
    knots and, 263
    in peritoneum, 264
    stages of, 260–261
    staples and, 263–264
    surgical instruments and, 261
    suturing and, 261–264
    topical agents and, 264

X

45,X karyotype, 381–382
    ovarian failure with, 389
    and spontaneous abortion, 433
X-linked inheritance, 380
46,XX karyotype, 381–382
    ovarian failure with, 389
45,X/46,XX mosaicism, 382
46,XY karyotype, 381–382
    ovarian failure with, 389

Z

Zygote intrafallopian transfer, 442